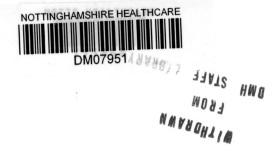

KAUFMAN'S CLINICAL NEUROLOGY FOR PSYCHIATRISTS

KAUFMAN'S CLINICAL NEUROLOGY FOR PSYCHIATRISTS

Eighth Edition

David Myland Kaufman, MD

Departments of Neurology and Psychiatry
Montefiore Medical Center
Albert Einstein College of Medicine
Bronx, New York

Howard L. Geyer, MD, PhD

Department of Neurology
Montefiore Medical Center
Albert Einstein College of Medicine
Bronx, New York

Mark J. Milstein, MD

Department of Neurology
Montefiore Medical Center
Albert Einstein College of Medicine
Bronx, New York

ELSEVIER

ELSEVIER

First edition 1981
Second edition 1985
Third edition 1990
Fourth edition 1995
Fifth edition 2001
Sixth edition 2007
Seventh edition 2013

Notices

Knowledge and best practice in this field are constantly changing. As new research and experience broaden our understanding, changes in research methods, professional practices, or medical treatment may become necessary.

Practitioners and researchers must always rely on their own experience and knowledge in evaluating and using any information, methods, compounds, or experiments described herein. In using such information or methods they should be mindful of their own safety and the safety of others, including parties for whom they have a professional responsibility.

With respect to any drug or pharmaceutical products identified, readers are advised to check the most current information provided (i) on procedures featured or (ii) by the manufacturer of each product to be administered, to verify the recommended dose or formula, the method and duration of administration, and contraindications. It is the responsibility of practitioners, relying on their own experience and knowledge of their patients, to make diagnoses, to determine dosages and the best treatment for each individual patient, and to take all appropriate safety precautions.

To the fullest extent of the law, neither the Publisher nor the authors, contributors, or editors, assume any liability for any injury and/or damage to persons or property as a matter of products liability, negligence or otherwise, or from any use or operation of any methods, products, instructions, or ideas contained in the material herein.

ISBN: 978-0-323-41559-0;
E-ISBN: 978-0-323-46131-3

Senior Content Strategist: Charlotta Kryhl
Senior Content Development Specialist: Ailsa Laing/Sharon Nash
Senior Content Coordinator: John Leonard
Senior Project Manager: Beula Christopher
Senior Designer: Christian Bilbow
Illustration Manager: Amy Faith Heyden
Illustrator: Marie Dean
Marketing Manager: Michele Milano

Printed in the United States of America

Last digit is the print number: 9 8 7 6 5 4 3

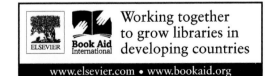

CONTENTS

DEDICATION

I dedicate Kaufman's Clinical Neurology for Psychiatrists *to Rita, my wife of more than 45 years, whose love has made everything possible, and our grandchildren – Lila, Owen, Aaron, Penelope, Eliana, and Benjamin.*
David Myland Kaufman

To my parents, my wife, and my daughters, with gratitude, admiration, and love.
Howard L. Geyer

I dedicate this book to my husband, Chris, who always makes me laugh, and my parents, David and Nancy, who will always inspire me to make the most of my life and career.
Mark J. Milstein

ACKNOWLEDGMENTS

My wife and best friend, Rita, acted as my muse by originally suggesting writing this book by expanding the syllabus for my course, "Clinical Neurology for Psychiatrists," and then giving me numerous ideas for each future edition.

David Myland Kaufman, MD

I am privileged to have worked with and learned from many wonderful mentors, colleagues, and patients over the years, and am thankful for all they have taught me. I am especially grateful to my wife Laurence for her love, encouragement, and patience, during my work on this project and always.

Howard L. Geyer, MD, PhD

I would like to thank Dr. David Kaufman who not only taught me invaluable lessons during my residency training but *also* brought me into this project and Dr. Steven Herskovitz (Director of the Neuromuscular Division) who always pushes me to examine all angles of a problem and answer medical questions as precisely as possible. Additionally, I owe tremendous gratitude to Dr. Sheryl Haut, whose mentorship and support has helped me achieve success in student and resident teaching and personal academic endeavors.

Mark J. Milstein, MD

Drs. Steven M. Safyer (President of the Medical Center), Allen M. Spiegel (Dean of the Albert Einstein College of Medicine), Byram Karasu (Chair of Psychiatry), Herbert Schaumburg (Chair Emeritus of Neurology), Mark Mehler (Chair of Neurology), and Michael Swerdlow (partner at Neurologic Associates) have provided the framework and encouragement to pursue the writing of this book and undertake other academic work in the midst of our clinical responsibilities. At the same time, they have grown Montefiore into a vibrant, world-renowned, patient-centered, urban medical center that is the teaching hospital of the Albert Einstein College of Medicine.

Our housestaff and faculty-colleagues at Montefiore Medical Center/Albert Einstein College of Medicine and other academic medical centers have reviewed chapters and in other ways offered invaluable help with this edition: Susan Duberstein, Jelena Pavlović, Gail Solomon, Renee Monderer, Jack Farinhas, Jacqueline Bello, Judah Burns, Lisa Ferber, and Michael Kaufman. Ms. Meryl Ranzer, Mr. Barry Morden, and Ms. Ann Mannato captured the sense of neurology in wonderful illustrations.

The library staffs of Montefiore Medical Center Cherkasky Library and the D. Samuel Gottesman Library of the Albert Einstein College of Medicine have graciously provided us with modern-day technology information. Our attorneys, Mr. Jeffrey A. Lowin, of Morris Cohen LLP, and Mr. H. Joseph Mello, of Winston & Strawn LLP, provided excellent council.

We also thank our editors at Elsevier, Charlotta Kryhl, Ailsa Laing, John Leonard, and Sharon Nash, who have opened their doors and provided many improvements for this edition. Finally, our thanks go to the Elsevier production team for their hard work and dedication including Beula Christopher, Christian Bilbow, and Amy Faith Heyden.

David Myland Kaufman, MD
Howard L. Geyer, MD, PhD
Mark J. Milstein, MD

Notes About References

Most chapters provide specific references from the neurologic and general medical literature. In addition, several standard, well-written textbooks contain relevant information about many topics:

Aminoff, M. J., & Faulkner, L. P. (Eds.), (2012). *The American Board of Psychiatry and Neurology: Looking Back and Moving Ahead*. Washington: American Psychiatric Press.

Biller, J. (2013). *Practical Neurology DVD Review* (2nd ed.). Philadelphia: Wolters Kluwer.

Blumenfeld, H. (2010). *Neuroanatomy Through Clinical Cases* (2nd ed.). Sunderland, MA: Sinauer.

Ellison, D., Love, S., Chimelli, L., et al. (2013). *Neuropathology: A Reference Text of CNS Pathology* (3rd ed.). Philadelphia: Elsevier.

Goetz, C. G. (2011). *Textbook of Clinical Neurology* (3rd ed.). Philadelphia: WB Saunders.

Heilman, K. M., & Valenstein, E. (2003). *Clinical Neuropsychology* (5th ed.). New York: Oxford University Press.

Howard, J. (2013). *Neurology Video Textbook*. New York: DemosMedical.

Jones, K. L., Jones, M. C., & del Campo, M. (2013). *Recognizable Patterns of Human Malformations* (7th ed.). Philadelphia: Elsevier.

Kanner, A. M. (2012). *Depression in Neurologic Disorders*. Oxford, UK: Wiley-Blackwell.

Lyketos, C. G., Rabins, P. V., Lipsey, J. R., et al. (Eds.), (2008). *Psychiatric Aspects of Neurologic Diseases: Practical Approaches to Patient Care*. New York: Oxford University Press.

Posner, J. B., Saper, C. B., Schiff, N., et al. (2007). *Plum and Posner's Diagnosis of Stupor and Coma (Contemporary Neurology Series)* (4th ed.). New York: Oxford University Press.

Ropper, A. H., & Samuels, M. A. (Eds.), (2009). *Adams and Victor's Principles of Neurology* (9th ed.). New York: McGraw Hill, Waltham Mass., Academic Press, 2014.

Rosenberg, R. N., & Pascual, J. M. (2015). *Rosenberg's Molecular and Genetic Basis of Neurological and Psychiatric Disease* (5th ed.). New York: Elsevier.

Schapira, A. H. V. (Ed.), (2007). *Neurology and Clinical Neuroscience*. Philadelphia: Mosby Elsevier.

Scheiber, S. C., Kramer, T. A. M., & Adamowski, S. E. (Eds.), (2003). *Core Competencies for Psychiatric Practice: What Clinicians Need to Know. A Report of the American Board of Psychiatry and Neurology, Inc*. Washington, D.C.: American Psychiatric Publishing, Inc.

Walker, A., Kaufman, D. M., Pfeffer, C., et al. (2008). *Child and Adolescent Neurology for Psychiatrists*. Philadelphia: Lippincott Williams & Wilkins.

Web Sites That Offer Information About Several Areas

(Sites relevant to single areas are listed in each chapter's references and in Appendix 1.)

American Academy of Neurology's Practice Guidelines: http://www.aan.com/professionals/practice/guideline

Gene Clinics: http://geneclinics.org/

Medlink Neurology (a commercial neurology textbook): http://www.medlink.com

National Institute of Health: http://health.nih.gov/category/BrainandNervousSystem

Online Mendelian Inheritance in Man: http://www.ncbi.nlm.nih.gov/omim

Pubmed: http://www.ncbi.nlm.nih.gov/pubmed

Registry and results database of publicly and privately supported clinical studies of human participants conducted around the world: http://ClinicalTrials.gov

PHYSICIAN-READERS, PLEASE NOTE

Kaufman's Clinical Neurology for Psychiatrists discusses medications, testing, procedures, and other aspects of medical care. Despite their purported effectiveness, many are fraught with side effects and other adverse outcomes. Discussions in this book neither recommend nor offer medical advice, and they do not apply to individual patients. The physician, who should consult the package insert and the medical literature, remains responsible for medications' indications, dosage, contraindications, precautions, side effects, adverse reactions, and alternatives, including doing nothing. Some aspects of medical care that this book discusses are widely and successfully used for particular purposes not approved by the Food and Drug Administration (FDA). Regarding these "off-label" treatments, as well as conventional ones, this book is reporting – not endorsing – their use by neurologists or other physicians. Finally, because medical practices rapidly evolve, readers should expect that sooner or later new diagnostic criteria and treatments will replace those discussed in this edition.

PURPOSE

We have written *Kaufman's Clinical Neurology for Psychiatrists* – a collegial straightforward guide – from our perspective as neurologists at a major, urban academic medical center. In a format combining traditional neuroanatomic correlations with symptom-oriented discussions, the book will assist psychiatrists in learning modern neurology. It emphasizes neurologic conditions that are frequently occurring, common to psychiatry and neurology, illustrative of a scientific principle, or have prominent psychiatric manifestations. It also includes descriptions of numerous neurologic conditions that may underlie aberrant behavior, disturbances in mood, or cognitive impairment – symptoms that prompt patients or medical colleagues to solicit psychiatry consultations. *Kaufman's Clinical Neurology for Psychiatrists* does not intend to replace comprehensive neurology textbooks or convert psychiatrists into semiprofessional neurologists; however, this book contains essential information required of psychiatrists.

ORGANIZATION AND CONTENT

The organization and content of *Kaufman's Clinical Neurology for Psychiatrists* arose from our experience as faculty at the Albert Einstein College of Medicine, attending physicians at Montefiore Medical Center, and supervisors of numerous neurology and psychiatry residents; consultation with our colleagues, many of whom are world-renowned physicians; and feedback from many of the 20,000 psychiatrists who have attended the course, "Clinical Neurology for Psychiatrists," and the more than 50,000 individuals who have purchased previous editions of this book. Learning the material in this book should help readers prepare for examinations, perform effective consultations, and improve their practice and teaching.

Section 1 reviews classic anatomic neurology and describes how to approach patients with a suspected neurologic disorder, identify central or peripheral nervous system disease, and correlate physical signs. Section 2 discusses common and otherwise important clinical areas, emphasizing aspects a psychiatrist may encounter. Topics include neurologic illnesses, such as multiple sclerosis, brain tumors, strokes, and traumatic brain injury; and common symptoms, such as headaches, chronic pain, epilepsy, and involuntary movement disorders. For each topic, chapters describe the relevant symptoms including psychiatric comorbidity, easily performed office and bedside examinations, appropriate laboratory tests, differential diagnoses, and some management options.

Many chapters contain outlines for a bedside examination; reproductions of standard bedside tests, such as the Montreal Cognitive Assessment (MoCA) and Abnormal Involuntary Movement Scale (AIMS), references to recent medical literature, and pertinent web sites. One chapter provides a compilation of computed tomography (CT), magnetic resonance imaging (MRI), and positron emission tomography (PET) images that other chapters reference. Appendices contain information pertaining to most chapters: Patient and Family Support Groups (Appendix 1); Costs of Various Tests and Treatments (Appendix 2); Diseases Transmitted by Chromosome or Mitochondria Abnormalities (Appendix 3); and Chemical and Biological Neurotoxins (Appendix 4).

In addition, the book reviews neurologic conditions that have entered the public arena because, willingly or unwillingly, psychiatrists are liable to be drawn into debates involving their own patients or the medical community. Psychiatrists should be well versed in the intricacies of the following conditions that this book describes:

- Amyotrophic lateral sclerosis and multiple sclerosis as battlegrounds of assisted suicide
- Meningomyelocele with Arnold–Chiari malformation as an indication for abortion and the value of spending limited resources on this fatal or severely debilitating condition
- Chronic pain as the fulcrum for legalizing marijuana and heroin
- Parkinson disease, spinal cord injury, and other disorders amenable to research and treatment with stem cells
- Persistent vegetative state and continuing life-support technology
- Cost of medical testing and treatment.

ADDITIONS AND OTHER CHANGES FOR THE EIGHTH EDITION

The first seven editions of *Kaufman's Clinical Neurology for Psychiatrists* have enjoyed considerable success in the United States, Canada, and abroad. The book has been translated into Japanese, Italian, Korean, and Spanish. In the eighth edition, written 3 years after the seventh, we have clarified the presentations, discussed recent developments in many areas, and added many clinical, anatomic, and radiologic illustrations. To give the question-and-answer sections greater power, we have increased the number of questions, refined them, expanded the discussions, and provided more illustrations. We have increased the usage of questions based on clinical vignettes because they mimic the clinical experience and the trend of national specialty examinations.

In a major new feature of this edition, *Kaufman's Clinical Neurology for Psychiatrists* refers to the diagnostic criteria for various neurologic disorders in the *Diagnostic and Statistical Manual of Mental Disorder, 5th Edition (DSM-5)*. It compares and contrasts DSM-5 diagnostic criteria to neurologists' diagnostic criteria, which admittedly remain for the most part uncodified and variable. With a few exceptions, DSM-5 criteria rely entirely on the nature and duration of symptoms, but neurologists, depending on the illness, rely on genetic testing, biopsy results, blood tests, various laboratory testing, or physical findings, but only sometimes exclusively on the patient's symptoms, to make a diagnosis in their field.

This edition updates and expands most topics and adds new ones:

- New nomenclature for seizures and epilepsy
- Revised diagnostic criteria for multiple sclerosis
- New treatments for epilepsy, Alzheimer disease, Parkinson disease, multiple sclerosis, and headaches
- New diagnostic modalities and treatments for several movement disorders
- New imaging techniques
- New organization of sleep–wake disorders
- Current guidelines for the diagnosis of concussions and their management
- Psychiatric comorbidity of neurologic illnesses
- New paraneoplastic disorders.

DIDACTIC DEVICES: THE VISUAL APPROACH AND QUESTION-AND-ANSWER SECTIONS

Kaufman's Clinical Neurology for Psychiatrists – like much of the practice of neurology – relies on a visual approach. It provides abundant illustrations, including numerous sketches of "patients" that personify or reinforce clinical descriptions, correlate the basic science with clinical findings, and serve as the basis for question-and-answer learning. The visual approach conforms to neurologists' predilection to "diagnose by inspection." For example, they rely on their observations for the diagnoses of gait abnormalities, psychogenic neurologic deficits, neurocutaneous disorders, strokes, and involuntary movements.

In addition, the book reproduces neurologic test results, which are also visual records, such as CT, MRI, and electroencephalography (EEG).

Kaufman's Clinical Neurology for Psychiatrists complements the text with question-and-answer sections at the end of most chapters and at the conclusion of the book. Sections at the end of chapters generally refer to material discussed within that chapter, whereas those questions at the book's conclusion tend to require comparison of neurologic disorders that have appeared under different headings. In Chapter 4, before the question-and-answer review of the preceding chapters' material, the book offers a guide to preparing for standardized tests.

The Albert Einstein College of Medicine and many other medical schools rely on similar "problem-based interactive studying" – case-based question-and-answer problems – as the optimum meaningful and efficient learning strategy. Not merely quizzing the reader, the book's questions-and-answers form an integral part of the learning experience. In fact, many readers find that these sections are the single most informative portion of the book and term them "high yield." In keeping with the visual emphasis of the book, many of the questions are based on visual material, including sketches of patients and reproductions of MRIs, CTs, and EEGs.

ONE CAVEAT

Kaufman's Clinical Neurology For Psychiatrists expects well-educated and thoughtful readers. It demands attention and work, and asks them to follow a rigorous course. Readers should find the book, like the practice of medicine, complex and challenging, but at the same time rich and fulfilling.

Even with the additions of text, illustrations, and questions, the eighth edition of *Kaufman's Clinical Neurology for Psychiatrists* remains manageable in size, depth, and scope, but still succinct enough for psychiatrists to read and enjoy from cover to cover.

David Myland Kaufman, MD
Howard L. Geyer, MD, PhD
Mark J. Milstein, MD

CLASSIC ANATOMIC NEUROLOGY

FIRST ENCOUNTER WITH A PATIENT: EXAMINATION AND FORMULATION

Despite the ready availability of sophisticated tests, the "hands on" examination remains the fundamental aspect of neurology. Beloved by neurologists, the neurologic examination provides a vivid portrayal of both function and illness. When neurologists say they have seen a case of a particular illness, they mean that they have really *seen* a patient with it.

When a patient's history suggests a neurologic illness, the neurologic examination may unequivocally demonstrate it. Even if psychiatrists themselves do not perform the examination, they should be able to appreciate neurologic signs and assess a neurologist's conclusion.

Neurologists systematically examine the nervous system's major components, paying particular attention to areas of interest in an individual patient in light of his or her symptoms. Neurologists try to adhere to the routine while avoiding omissions and duplications. Despite obvious dysfunction of one part of the nervous system, they evaluate all major areas. A neurologist can usually complete an initial or screening examination in 20 minutes or less and return to perform detailed or otherwise special testing of particular areas, such as the mental status.

EXAMINATION

Neurologists usually begin by noting a patient's age, sex, and handedness, and then review the primary symptom, present illness, medical history, family history, and social history. They explore the primary symptom, associated symptoms, and possible etiologic factors. If a patient cannot relate the history, the neurologist might interrupt the process to look for language, memory, or other cognitive deficits. Many chapters in Section 2 contain outlines of the standard questions that relate to common symptoms.

After obtaining the history, the neurologist should be able to anticipate the patient's deficits and prepare to look for disease primarily of the central nervous system (CNS) or the peripheral nervous system (PNS). At this point, without yielding to rigid preconceptions, the physician should have developed some sense of the problem at hand.

Then neurologists should look for the site of involvement (i.e., "localize the lesion"). "Localization," one of the initial goals of most neurologic examinations, is valuable in the majority of cases. However, it is often able in the majority of cases. However, it is often somewhat of an art and inapplicable in several important neurologic illnesses, such as Alzheimer disease.

The examination is not only of historical interest, but also remains irreplaceable in diagnosis. It consists of a functional neuroanatomy demonstration: mental status, cranial nerves, motor system, reflexes, sensation, cerebellar system, and gait (Box 1.1). This format should be followed during most examinations. Trainees still mastering this structure may bring a printed copy to the patient's bedside to serve both as a reminder and as a place to record neurologic findings.

The examination usually starts with an assessment of the mental status, because cognition is the most fundamental neurologic function and cognitive impairments may preclude an accurate assessment of other neurologic functions. The examiner should consider specific intellectual deficits, such as language impairment (see Aphasia, Chapter 8), as well as general cognitive impairment (see Dementia, Chapter 7). Tests of cranial nerves may reveal malfunction of nerves either individually or in groups, such as the *ocular motility nerves* (III, IV, and VI) or the *cerebellopontine angle nerves* (V, VII, and VIII) (see Chapter 4).

The examination of the motor system is usually performed more to detect the pattern than the severity of weakness. Whether weakness is mild to moderate (*paresis*) or complete (*plegia*), the pattern rather than severity offers more clues to localization. On a practical level, of course, the severity of the paresis determines the patient's functional capacity, e.g., whether a patient walks, requires a wheelchair, or stays bedridden.

When neurologists detect paresis they attempt to classify its pattern. They frequently speak of three patterns. If the lower face, arm, and leg on one side of the body are paretic, they call the pattern *hemiparesis*. They usually attribute hemiparesis to damage in the contralateral cerebral hemisphere or brainstem. They call weakness of both legs *paraparesis* and usually attribute it to spinal cord damage. If the paresis predominantly involves the distal portion of all four limbs, *distal quadriparesis*, they usually ascribe it to PNS rather than CNS damage.

Eliciting two categories of reflexes assists in determining whether paresis – or other neurologic abnormality – originates in CNS or PNS injury. *Deep tendon reflexes* (*DTRs*) are normally present with uniform reactivity (speed and forcefulness) in all limbs, but neurologic injury often alters their activity or symmetry. In general,

BOX 1.1	**Neurologic Examination**

Mental status
  Attention
  Cooperation
  Orientation (to month, year, place, and any physical or mental deficits)
  Language
  Memory for immediate, recent, and past events
  Higher intellectual functions: arithmetic, similarities/differences
Cranial nerves
  I Smell
  II Visual acuity, visual fields, optic fundi, pupil size and reactivity (afferent limb)
  III, IV, VI Pupil size and reactivity (efferent limb), extra-ocular movements
  V Corneal reflex and facial sensation
  VII Strength of upper and lower facial muscles, taste
  VIII Hearing
  IX–XI Articulation, palate movement, gag reflex
  XII Tongue movement
Motor system
  Limb strength
  Tone (e.g., spasticity, flaccidity)
  Abnormal movements (e.g., tremor, chorea, fasciculations)
Reflexes
  Deep tendon reflexes
    Biceps, triceps, brachioradialis, quadriceps/patellar, Achilles
  Pathologic reflexes
    Extensor plantar response (Babinski sign), frontal release
Sensation
  Position, vibration, stereognosis, light touch
  Pain
Cerebellar system
  Finger-to-nose and heel-to-shin tests
  Rapid alternating movements
Gait

with CNS injury that includes corticospinal tract damage DTRs are hyperactive, whereas with PNS injury DTRs are hypoactive.

In contrast to DTRs, *pathologic reflexes* are not normally elicitable beyond infancy. If these are found, they are a sign of CNS damage. The most widely recognized pathologic reflex is the famous *Babinski sign*. After plantar stimulation, the great toe normally moves downward (i.e., it has a flexor response). With brain or spinal cord damage, plantar stimulation typically causes the great toe to move upward (i.e., to have an extensor response). This reflex extensor movement, which is a manifestation of CNS damage, is the Babinski sign (see Fig. 19.3). Neurologists say that the Babinski sign and other pathologic reflexes are "present," "found," or "elicited," but not "positive" or "negative." The terminology is similar to a traffic stop sign: It may be present or absent, but not positive or negative.

Frontal release signs, which are also pathologic reflexes, reflect frontal lobe injury. When present they point to an "organic" basis for a change in personality and, to some degree, correlate with cognitive impairment (see Chapter 7).

Unlike abnormal DTRs and Babinski signs, which are reproducible, objective, and difficult to mimic, the sensory examination relies almost entirely on the patient's report. Its subjective nature has led to the practice of disregarding reports of disturbances inconsistent with the rest of the examination. Under most circumstances, the best approach is to test the major sensory modalities in a clear anatomic order and tentatively accept the patient's report.

Depending on the nature of the suspected disorder, physicians may first test light touch sensation with their finger-tips or a wood stick cotton swab, and then three sensations carried by the posterior columns of the spinal cord: position, vibration, and stereognosis (appreciation of an object's form by touching it). Neurologists might test pain (pinprick) sensation, which is carried in the lateral columns, but only in a careful manner with a non-penetrating, disposable instrument, such as with a broken wood shaft of the cotton swab.

Neurologists evaluate cerebellar function by observing several standard maneuvers that include the *finger-to-nose test* and *rapid alternating movement test* (see Chapter 2). These tests may demonstrate intention tremor or incoordination.

If at all possible, neurologists watch the patient walk, because a normal gait requires intact CNS and PNS motor pathways, coordination, proprioception, and balance. Moreover, all these systems must be well-integrated. Examining the gait is probably the single most valuable assessment of noncognitive functions of the nervous system. Neurologists watch for gait abnormalities that characterize many neurologic illnesses (see Table 2.1). In addition, they should expect certain gait abnormalities to be comorbid with cognitive impairment. Whatever the abnormality, gait impairment is not merely a neurologic sign, but a condition that routinely leads to fatal falls and permanent incapacity for numerous people each year.

FORMULATION

Although somewhat ritualistic, a succinct and cogent *formulation* remains the basis of neurologic problem solving. A neurologist's classic formulation consists of an appraisal of the four aspects of the examination: symptoms, signs, localization, and differential diagnosis. A neurologist might also have to support a conclusion that neurologic disease explains the patient's symptoms and signs or, equally important, does not. For this step, neurologists at least tentatively separate psychogenic signs from neurologic ("organic") ones.

Localization of neurologic disease requires the clinician not only to determine whether the illness affects the CNS, PNS, or muscles (see Chapters 2–6), but precise localization of lesions within these regions of the nervous system is also generally expected. The physician must also establish whether the illness affects the nervous system diffusely or in a focal, discrete area. The site and extent of neurologic damage generally indicates certain diseases. A readily apparent example is that strokes and tumors usually involve a discrete area of the brain, but

Alzheimer disease usually causes widespread, symmetrical changes.

Finally, neurologists create a differential diagnosis that lists the disease or diseases most consistent with the patient's symptoms and signs. They should include unlikely but potentially life-threatening conditions. In addition, many neurologists, in a flourish of intellectualism, conclude with unlikely but fascinating explanations. However, even at tertiary care institutions, common conditions arise commonly. Just as "hoof beats are usually from horses, not zebras," patients are more likely to have hemiparesis from a stroke than a mitochondrial disorder.

A typical formulation might be as follows: "Mr. Jones, a 56-year-old right-handed bartender, has had left-sided headaches for 2 months and, on the day before admission, had a generalized seizure. He is lethargic. He has papilledema, a right hemiparesis with hyperactive DTRs, and a Babinski sign. The lesion is probably situated in the left cerebral hemisphere. It is most likely a tumor or stroke, but possibly a bacterial abscess." This formulation briefly recapitulates the salient elements of the history and physical findings. In this case, neurologists would tacitly assume that neurologic disease is present because of the obvious, objective physical findings. The history of seizures, the right-sided hemiparesis, and abnormal reflexes localize the lesion. Neurologists would base their differential diagnosis on the high probability that a discrete cerebral lesion is causing these abnormalities.

A house officer presenting a case to a superior is well advised to separate the wheat from the chaff and complete the presentation within 2 minutes, which is the limit of most listeners' attention spans. The clinician should also practice the presentation before rounds, bearing in mind Benjamin Franklin's proverb, "By failing to prepare, you are preparing to fail."

In summary, the neurologist should present a succinct, well-rehearsed formulation that answers *The Four Questions of Neurology*:
- What are the *symptoms* of neurologic disease?
- What are the *signs* of neurologic disease?
- *Where* is the lesion?
- *What* is the lesion?

RESPONDING AS A NEUROLOGIST TO CONSULTATIONS

During their training, psychiatry residents often rotate through a neurology service where they are required to answer requests for neurology consultations. Consultants at all levels must work with a variation of the traditional summary-and-formulation format. While the patient's interests remain paramount, the consultant's "client" is the referring physician. Both the referring physician and consultant should be clear about the reason for the consultation. Reasons for consultations typically concern a neurologic symptom, the significance of a neuroimaging report, or a treatment recommendation. Sometimes physicians request a broad review, such as when they ask the consultant to provide a second opinion or offer a prognosis. On the other hand, the referring physicians may not want to know the diagnosis or treatment options, but simply want the neurology service to assume the primary care of the patient.

Without belaboring the obvious, the consultation note must be organized, succinct, and practical. The primary physician in an acute care hospital should be able to digest it in 2 minutes. Long notes are usually boring and inadvertently hide useful information. Cutting and pasting information and conclusions in computerized medical records by a consultant is redundant, liable to repeat errors, and, if a previous physician made an astute diagnosis, appears to take credit for someone else's idea. Notes that are bad, for whatever reason, reflect poorly on the consultant and the consultant's service, and they hamper the patient's care. At least in an academic setting, the consultant should offer at least one teaching point about the case and provide general guidelines for handling similar inquires.

Finally, consultants should show an awareness of the entire situation, which often contains incomplete and conflicting elements. They should also be mindful of the situation of the referring physician and patient. Consultants in emergency situations might help by ordering – not merely suggesting – routine tests, such as blood studies, and important but innocuous treatments, such as thiamine injections. Except in unusual circumstances, consulting residents should not suggest hazardous tests or treatments without first presenting the case to their supervisor. Consultants should not divert the primary physicians' efforts from the patient's most important medical problems. They should not suggest embarking on elaborate, time-consuming testing for obscure, unlikely diagnoses when the patient's illness is obvious and requires the primary medical team's full attention. The consultant should ask, "How can I help?"

NEUROLOGIC DIAGNOSIS

Neurologists confirm a clinical diagnosis using different frames of reference. For some diseases, such as migraine and chronic pain, neurologists rely almost entirely on a patient's symptoms. For others, such as Parkinson disease, they base their diagnosis on physical abnormalities or constellations of findings. For many other diseases, regardless of the patient's symptoms and signs, their diagnosis rests on an abnormal test result. For example, the diagnosis of stroke or a brain tumor requires imaging studies, and confirmation of seizures often necessitates an EEG. Neurologists diagnose many asymptomatic individuals as having a neurologic disease on the basis of a single test, such as genetic analysis or MRI (see Chapter 20).

The clinical formulation remains the mainstay of neurologic diagnosis, but abnormal findings on MRI or other studies routinely trump clinical impressions. For example, the clinical examination may indicate the presence, location, and etiology of a cerebral lesion, but if an MRI indicates a different process, neurologists generally forsake their clinical formulation and accept the MRI findings as the diagnosis.

Overall, neurologists' and psychiatrists' diagnoses routinely differ in several respects. Neurologists shift the basis of their diagnosis from clinical constellation, to image, to pathologic specimen, or to another test – whichever is the most specific. In contrast, psychiatrists base diagnoses, with the exception of sleep disorders and perhaps a few others, entirely on their patient's history and observable clinical presentation without performing a physical examination. Neurologists routinely diagnose illnesses in asymptomatic individuals, such as those with genetic mutations for Huntington disease or a spinocerebellar ataxia, but psychiatrists almost always require symptoms. Finally, neurologists do not have a *Diagnostic and Statistical Manual (DSM) of Neurologic Disorders*. While the lack of a DSM prevents uniformity, neurologists remain flexible in their diagnostic criteria and freed from pigeonholing patients' symptoms and signs, which may considerably vary with the same illness from patient to patient, into diagnostic boxes.

CHAPTER 2

SIGNS OF CENTRAL NERVOUS SYSTEM DISORDERS

Disorders of the brain and the spinal cord – the two major components of the central nervous system (CNS) – typically cause readily recognizable combinations of paresis, sensory loss, visual deficits, and neuropsychologic disorders (Box 2.1). Such signs of CNS disorders differ from those of the peripheral nervous system (PNS) and both differ from the signs of psychogenic disorders. Neurologists formulate their preliminary diagnosis and often initiate treatment on the basis of the patient's history and the examination, but if results of investigations – such as laboratory testing or magnetic resonance imaging (MRI) – contradict the initial clinical impression, they will usually revise or at least reconsider it.

SIGNS OF CEREBRAL HEMISPHERE LESIONS

Hemiparesis, usually accompanied by changes in reflexes and muscle tone, is one of neurology's most prominent and reliable signs. Damage to the *corticospinal tract*, also called the *pyramidal tract* (Fig. 2.1), in the cerebrum or brainstem above (rostral to) the decussation of the pyramids, causes contralateral hemiparesis (Box 2.2) with weakness of the arm and leg – and, if the lesion is high enough, the lower face – opposite the side of the lesion. Damage to this tract within the spinal cord causes *ipsilateral* arm and leg or only leg paresis, but no face paresis.

The division of the motor system into upper and lower motor neurons is a basic construct of clinical neurology. During the corticospinal tract's entire path from the cerebral cortex to the motor cranial nerve nuclei and the anterior horn cells of the spinal cord, this tract consists of *upper motor neurons (UMNs)* (Fig. 2.2). The anterior horn cells, which are part of the PNS, begin the *lower motor neuron (LMN)*. Cerebral lesions that damage the corticospinal tract cause *signs of UMN injury* (Figs. 2.2–2.5):
- Paresis with muscle spasticity
- Hyperactive deep tendon reflexes (DTRs)
- Babinski signs.

In contrast, PNS lesions, including motor neuron diseases (diseases of the anterior horn cells) and disorders of nerves (neuropathy), cause *signs of LMN injury*:
- Paresis with muscle flaccidity and atrophy
- Hypoactive DTRs
- No Babinski signs.

Another indication of a cerebral lesion is loss of certain sensory modalities over one half of the body, i.e., *hemisensory loss* (Fig. 2.6). A patient with a cerebral lesion characteristically loses contralateral position sensation, two-point discrimination, and the ability to identify objects by touch (stereognosis). Neurologists often describe loss of those modalities as "cortical" sensory loss.

Pain sensation, a "primary" sense, is initially received by the thalamus, from which it is relayed to the cortex, limbic system, and elsewhere. Because the thalamus is situated above the brainstem but below the cerebral cortex, most patients with cerebral lesions still perceive painful stimuli. For example, patients with cerebral infarctions may be unable to specify a painful area of their body, but they will still feel the pain's intensity and discomfort (see Chapter 14).

Visual loss of the same half-field in each eye, *homonymous hemianopia* (Fig. 2.7), is a characteristic sign of a contralateral cerebral lesion. Other equally characteristic visual losses are associated with lesions involving the eye, optic nerve, or optic tract (see Chapters 4 and 12). Because they are situated far from the visual pathway, lesions in the brainstem, cerebellum, or spinal cord do not cause visual field loss.

Another conspicuous sign of a cerebral hemisphere lesion is *focal (partial)* or *focal-onset seizures* (see Chapter 10). In fact, the majority of focal seizures that alter awareness or induce psychomotor phenomena originate in the temporal lobe.

Signs of Damage of the Dominant, Nondominant, or Both Cerebral Hemispheres

Although hemiparesis, hemisensory loss, homonymous hemianopia, and focal seizures may result from lesions of either cerebral hemisphere, several neuropsychologic deficits are referable to either the dominant or nondominant hemisphere. Neurologists usually ask a patient's handedness when taking a history, but if this information is unavailable, because approximately 85% of people are right-handed, they assume with reasonable confidence that the left hemisphere serves as the dominant hemisphere.

Lesions of the dominant hemisphere may cause language impairment, *aphasia*, a prominent and frequently occurring neuropsychologic deficit (see Chapter 8). Because the corticospinal tract sits adjacent to the language centers, right hemiparesis often accompanies aphasia (see Fig. 8.1).

Lesions of the nondominant parietal lobe tend to produce one or more striking neuropsychologic disturbances (see Chapter 8). For example, patients may neglect or ignore left-sided visual and tactile stimuli (*hemiinattention*). They may fail to use their left arm and leg because they neglect their limbs rather than because of

BOX 2.1	Signs of Common CNS Lesions

Cerebral hemisphere*
  Hemiparesis with hyperactive deep tendon reflexes, spasticity, and Babinski sign
  Hemisensory loss
  Homonymous hemianopia
  Focal (partial) seizures
  Aphasia, hemi-inattention, and dementia
  Pseudobulbar palsy
Basal ganglia*
  Movement disorders: parkinsonism, athetosis, chorea, and hemiballismus
  Postural instability
  Rigidity
Brainstem
  Cranial nerve palsy with contralateral hemiparesis
  Internuclear ophthalmoplegia (MLF# syndrome)
  Nystagmus
  Bulbar palsy
Cerebellum
  Tremor on intention^
  Impaired rapid alternating movements (dysdiadochokinesia)^
  Ataxic gait
  Scanning speech
Spinal cord
  Paraparesis or quadriparesis
  Spasticity
  Sensory loss up to a "level"
  Bladder, bowel, and sexual dysfunction

*Signs contralateral to lesions
#MLF, Medial longitudinal fasciculus
^Signs ipsilateral to lesions

BOX 2.2	Signs of Common Cerebral Lesions

Either hemisphere*
  Hemiparesis with hyperactive deep tendon reflexes and a Babinski sign
  Hemisensory loss
  Homonymous hemianopia
  Focal seizure
Dominant hemisphere
  Aphasia: fluent, nonfluent, conduction, or isolation
  Gerstmann syndrome: acalculia, agraphia, finger agnosia, and left–right confusion
  Alexia without agraphia
Nondominant hemisphere
  Hemi-inattention
  Anosognosia
  Constructional apraxia
Both hemispheres
  Dementia
  Pseudobulbar palsy

*Signs contralateral to lesions

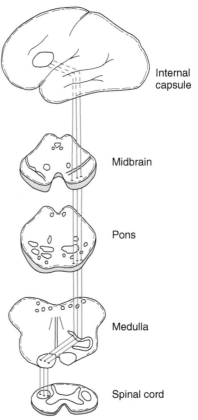

FIGURE 2.1 ■ Each corticospinal tract originates in the cerebral cortex, passes through the internal capsule, and descends into the brainstem. The tracts cross in the pyramids, which are protuberances on the inferior portion of the medulla, to descend in the spinal cord mostly as the *lateral corticospinal tract*. The corticospinal tracts synapse with the *anterior horn cells* of the spinal cord, which give rise to peripheral nerves. Neurologists often call the corticospinal tract the *pyramidal* tract because it crosses in the pyramids. The *extrapyramidal* system, which modulates the corticospinal tract, originates in the basal ganglia and cerebellum, and remains within the brain.

Labels in figure: Internal capsule, Midbrain, Pons, Medulla, Spinal cord

paresis. When they have left hemiparesis, patients may not appreciate it (*anosognosia*). Many patients lose their ability to arrange matchsticks into certain patterns or copy simple forms (*constructional apraxia*, Fig. 2.8).

As opposed to signs resulting from unilateral cerebral hemisphere damage, bilateral cerebral hemisphere damage produces several important disturbances that psychiatrists are likely to encounter in their patients. One of them, *pseudobulbar palsy*, best known for producing emotional lability, results from bilateral *corticobulbar tract* damage (see Chapter 4). The corticobulbar tract, like its counterpart the corticospinal tract, originates in the motor cortex of the posterior portion of the frontal lobe. It innervates the brainstem motor nuclei, which in turn innervate the head and neck muscles. Traumatic brain injury (TBI), multiple cerebral infarctions (strokes), and frontotemporal dementia (see Chapter 7), are apt to strike the corticobulbar tract, as well as the surrounding frontal lobes, and thereby cause pseudobulbar palsy.

Damage to both cerebral hemispheres – from large or multiple discrete lesions, degenerative diseases, or metabolic abnormalities – also causes dementia (see Chapter 7). In addition, because CNS damage that causes dementia must be extensive and severe, it usually also produces at least subtle physical neurologic findings, such as hyperactive DTRs, Babinski signs, mild gait impairment, and frontal lobe release reflexes. However, many neurodegenerative illnesses that cause dementia, particularly

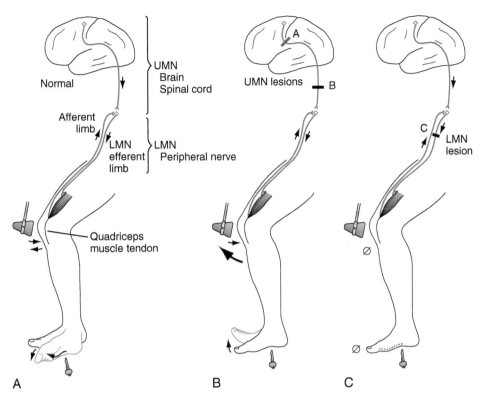

FIGURE 2.2 ■ A, Normally, when neurologists strike a patient's quadriceps tendon with a percussion hammer, the maneuver elicits a DTR. In addition, when they stroke the sole of the foot to elicit a plantar reflex, the big toe bends downward (flexes). B, When brain or spinal cord lesions injure the corticospinal tract, producing upper motor neuron (UMN) damage, DTRs react briskly and forcefully, i.e., DTRs are hyperactive. As another sign of UMN damage, the plantar reflex is extensor (a Babinski sign). C, In contrast, peripheral nerve injury causes lower motor neuron (LMN) damage, the DTR is hypoactive and the plantar reflex is absent.

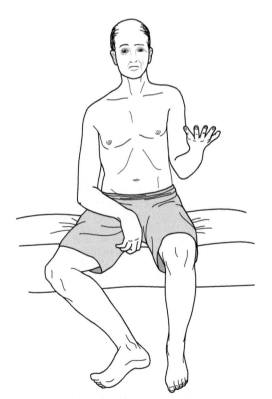

FIGURE 2.3 ■ This patient shows right hemiparesis with weakness of the right arm, leg, and lower face. The right-sided facial weakness causes the flat nasolabial fold; however, the forehead muscles remain normal (see Chapter 4 regarding this discrepancy). The right arm moves little, and the elbow, wrist, and fingers take on a flexed position; the right leg is externally rotated; and the hip and knee are flexed.

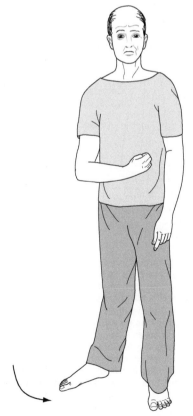

FIGURE 2.4 ■ When the patient stands up, his weakened arm retains its flexed posture. His right leg remains externally rotated, but he can walk by swinging it in a circular path. This maneuver is effective but results in *circumduction* or a *hemiparetic gait*.

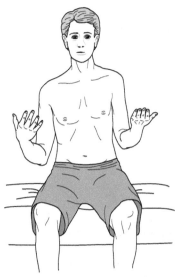

FIGURE 2.5 ■ Mild hemiparesis may not be obvious. To exaggerate it, the physician has asked this patient to extend both arms with his palms held upright, as though his outstretched hand were supporting a pizza box. His weakened arm sinks (drifts) and his palm turns inward (pronates). The imaginary pizza box would slide to his right. His arm drift and pronation represent a *forme fruste* of the posture seen with severe paresis (Fig. 2.3).

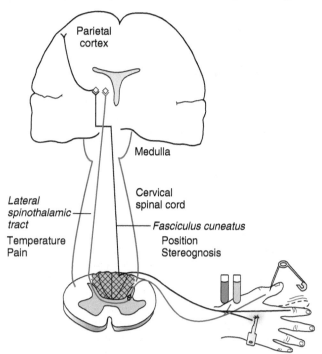

FIGURE 2.6 ■ Peripheral nerves carry pain and temperature sensations to the spinal cord. After a synapse, these sensations cross and ascend in the *contralateral lateral spinothalamic tract* (*pink*) to terminate in the thalamus. From there, tracts relay the sensations to the limbic system, reticular activating system, and other brainstem regions as well as the cerebral cortex. In parallel, the peripheral nerves also carry position and vibration sense and stereognosis to the *ipsilateral fasciculus cuneatus* and *fasciculus gracilis*, which together constitute the spinal cord's *posterior columns* (*cross-hatched*) (Fig. 2.15). Unlike pain and temperature sensation, these sensations ascend in the spinal cord via ipsilateral tracts (*black*). They cross in the decussation of the medial lemniscus, which is in the medulla, synapse in the thalamus, and terminate in the parietal cortex. (To avoid spreading blood-borne illnesses, examiners should use a disposable instrument when testing pain.)

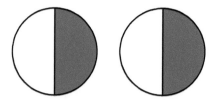

FIGURE 2.7 ■ In homonymous hemianopia, the same half of the visual field is lost in each eye. In this case, damage to the left cerebral hemisphere has caused a right homonymous hemianopia. This sketch portrays visual field loss, as is customary, from the patient's perspective; the colored area represents the defect (see Figs. 4.1 and 12.7).

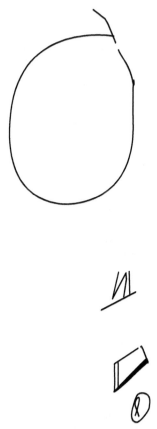

FIGURE 2.8 ■ A patient showing constructional apraxia from a right parietal lobe infarction was unable to complete a circle (*top figure*), draw a square on request (*second figure*), or even copy one (*third figure*). She spontaneously tried to draw a circle and began to retrace it (*bottom figure*). Her constructional apraxia consists of rotation of the forms, perseveration of certain lines, and the incompleteness of the second and lowest figures. In addition, the figures tend toward the right-hand side of the page, which indicates that she has neglect of the left-hand side of the page, i.e., left hemi-inattention (see Chapter 8).

Alzheimer disease, do not cause overt findings such as hemiparesis.

While certainly not peculiar to cerebral lesions and even typically absent in early Alzheimer disease, gait impairment is a crucial neurologic finding. Because walking requires intact and well-integrated strength, sensation, and coordination, testing the patient's gait is the single most reliable assessment of a patient's noncognitive neurologic function. Gait impairment constitutes the primary physical component of the subcortical dementias, such as vascular dementia, dementia with Lewy

TABLE 2.1 **Gait Abnormalities Associated With Neurologic Disorders**

Gait	Associated Illness	Figure
Apraxic	Normal pressure hydrocephalus	7.10
Astasia-abasia	Psychogenic disorders	3.4
Ataxic	Cerebellar damage	2.13
Festinating (*marche à petits pas*)	Parkinson disease	18.9
Hemiparetic/ hemiplegic	Strokes, congenital injury (cerebral palsy)	
• Circumduction		2.4
• Spastic hemiparesis		13.4
Diplegic	Congenital injury	13.3
Steppage	Tabes dorsalis (CNS syphilis)	2.20
Waddling	Duchenne dystrophy and other myopathies	6.4

bodies disease, and Parkinson disease dementia (see Chapter 7). Several distinct gait abnormalities are clues to specific neurologic disorders, such as normal pressure hydrocephalus (Table 2.1). As a general rule, slow gait speed, e.g., 0.7 m/sec or less, is associated with an increased risk of dementia, stroke, falls, disability, hospitalization, and death.

SIGNS OF BASAL GANGLIA LESIONS

The basal ganglia, located subcortically in the cerebrum, consist of the caudate and putamen (together constituting the *striatum*), globus pallidus, substantia nigra; and subthalamic nucleus (corpus of Luysii) (see Fig. 18.1). They give rise to the extrapyramidal motor system, which modulates the corticospinal (pyramidal) tract. It controls muscle tone, regulates motor activity, and generates postural reflexes. Its efferent fibers play on the cerebral cortex, thalamus, and other CNS structures. Because its efferent fibers are confined to the brain, the extrapyramidal tract does not act directly on the spinal cord or LMNs.

Signs of basal ganglia disorders include a group of fascinating, often dramatic, *involuntary movement disorders* (see Chapter 18):

- *Parkinsonism* is the combination of resting tremor, rigidity, bradykinesia (slowness of movement) or akinesia (absence of movement), and postural abnormalities. It usually results from Parkinson disease and related neurodegenerative illnesses, exposure to dopamine receptor-blocking antipsychotic medications, or toxins.
- *Athetosis* is the slow, continuous, writhing movement of the fingers, hands, face, and throat. Kernicterus or other perinatal basal ganglia injury usually causes it.

- *Chorea* is intermittent, randomly located, jerking of limbs and the trunk. The best-known example occurs in *Huntington* disease (previously called "Huntington chorea"), in which the caudate nuclei characteristically atrophy.
- *Hemiballismus* is the intermittent flinging of the arm and leg of one side of the body. It is classically associated with small infarctions of the contralateral subthalamic nucleus, but similar lesions in other basal ganglia may be responsible.

In general, when damage is restricted to the extrapyramidal system, patients have no paresis, DTR abnormalities, or Babinski signs – hallmarks of corticospinal (pyramidal) tract damage. More important, in many of these conditions, such as hemiballismus and athetosis, patients have no cognitive impairment or other neuropsychologic disorder. On the other hand, several conditions – such as Huntington disease, Wilson disease, and advanced Parkinson disease – affect the cerebrum as well as the basal ganglia. In them, dementia, depression, and psychosis frequently accompany involuntary movements (see Box 18.4).

With unilateral basal ganglia damage, signs develop in the contralateral limbs. For example, an infarction of the subthalamic nucleus causes contralateral hemiballismus, and degeneration of the substantia nigra causes contralateral parkinsonism ("hemiparkinsonism").

SIGNS OF BRAINSTEM LESIONS

The brainstem contains, among a multitude of structures, the cranial nerve nuclei, the corticospinal tracts, other "long tracts" that travel between the cerebral hemispheres and the limbs, and cerebellar afferent (inflow) and efferent (outflow) tracts. Combinations of cranial nerve and long tract signs, and the *absence* of signs of cerebral injury, such as visual field cuts and neuropsychologic deficits, indicate the presence and location of a brainstem lesion. For example, brainstem injuries cause *diplopia* (double vision) because of cranial nerve impairment, but visual acuity and visual fields remain normal because the visual pathway, which passes from the optic chiasm to the cerebral hemispheres, does not travel within the brainstem (see Fig. 4.1). Similarly, a right hemiparesis associated with a left third cranial nerve palsy localizes the lesion to the brainstem (particularly the left midbrain). Moreover, that pair of findings indicates that further examination will reveal neither aphasia nor dementia.

Several brainstem syndromes illustrate critical anatomic relationships, such as the location of the cranial nerve nuclei or the course of the corticospinal tract; however, none of them involves neuropsychologic abnormalities. Although each syndrome has an eponym, for practical purposes it is only necessary to identify the clinical findings and, if appropriate, attribute them to a lesion in one of the *three major divisions of the brainstem: midbrain, pons, or medulla* (Fig. 2.9). Whatever the localization, most brainstem lesions result from occlusion of a small branch of the basilar or vertebral arteries.

In the midbrain, where the oculomotor (third cranial) nerve fibers pass through the descending corticospinal

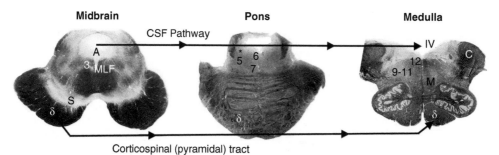

FIGURE 2.9 ■ Myelin stains of the three main divisions of the brainstem – midbrain, pons, and medulla – show several clinically important tracts, the cerebrospinal fluid (CSF) pathway, and motor nuclei of the cranial nerves. (*Midbrain*) The midbrain is identifiable by its distinctive silhouette and gently curved (pale, unstained in this preparation) substantia nigra (S). The aqueduct of Sylvius (A) is surrounded by the periaqueductal gray matter. Ventral to the aqueduct, near the midline, lie the oculomotor (3) and trochlear (not pictured) cranial nerve nuclei. The nearby MLF, which ascends from the pons, terminates in the oculomotor nuclei. The large, deeply stained cerebral peduncles, ventral to the substantia nigra, contain the corticospinal (pyramidal [Δ]) tract. Originating in the cerebral cortex, the corticospinal tract (Δ) descends ipsilaterally through the midbrain, pons, and medulla until it crosses in the medulla's pyramids to continue within the contralateral spinal cord. CSF flows downward from the lateral ventricles through the aqueduct of Sylvius into the fourth ventricle (IV), which overlies the lower pons and medulla. CSF exits from the fourth ventricle into the subarachnoid space. (Also see a functional drawing [Fig. 4.5], computer-generated rendition [Fig. 18.2], and sketch [Fig. 21.1].) (*Pons*) The pons (Latin, bridge) houses the trigeminal motor division (5), abducens (6), facial (7), and acoustic/vestibular (not shown) cranial nerve nuclei and, inferior and lateral to the fourth ventricle, the locus ceruleus (*). In addition to containing the descending corticospinal tract (Δ), the basilar portion of the pons (*basis pontis*) contains large crisscrossing cerebellar tracts. (Also see a functional drawing [Fig. 4.7] and an idealized sketch [Fig. 21.2].) (*Medulla*) The medulla (Latin, marrow), readily identifiable by the pair of unstained scallop-shaped inferior olivary nuclei, includes the cerebellar peduncles (C), which contain afferent and efferent cerebellar tracts; the corticospinal tract (Δ); and the floor of the fourth ventricle (IV). It also contains the decussation of the medial lemniscus (M), the nuclei for cranial nerves 9–11 grouped laterally and 12 situated medially, and the trigeminal sensory nucleus (not pictured) that descends from the pons to the cervical–medullary junction. (Also see a functional drawing [Fig. 2.10].)

tract, a single small infarction can damage both pathways. Patients with oculomotor nerve paralysis and contralateral hemiparesis typically have a lesion in their midbrain ipsilateral to the paretic eye (see Fig. 4.9). In an analogous situation, patients with an abducens (sixth cranial) nerve paralysis and contralateral hemiparesis have a lesion in the pons ipsilateral to the paretic eye (see Fig. 4.11).

Lateral medullary infarctions create a classic but complex picture, *the lateral medullary syndrome*. Patients have dysarthria because of paralysis of the ipsilateral palate from damage to cranial nerves IX through XI; ipsilateral facial numbness (*hypalgesia*) (Greek, decreased sensitivity to pain) because of damage to cranial nerve V, with contralateral anesthesia of the body (*alternating or crossed hypalgesia*) because of ascending spinothalamic tract damage; and ipsilateral ataxia because of inferior cerebellar peduncle dysfunction. They also have nystagmus and vertigo from damage to the vestibulocochlear nerve and ipsilateral Horner syndrome (ptosis, miosis, anhydrosis) due to interruption of sympathetic fibers. In other words, the most important elements of this syndrome consist of damage to three groups of nuclei (V, VIII, and IX–XI) and three white matter tracts (spinothalamic, sympathetic, and inferior cerebellar peduncle). Although the lateral medullary syndrome commonly occurs and provides an excellent example of clinical-pathologic correlation, physicians need not recall all of its pathology or clinical features; however, they should know that lower cranial nerve palsies accompanied by alternating hypalgesia, without cognitive impairment or limb paresis, result from a lesion in the lower brainstem (Fig. 2.10). They should also know that the lateral medullary syndrome causes bulbar palsy (see Chapter 4).

Nystagmus, repetitive jerk-like eye movements that are usually conjugate (i.e., affecting both eyes equally and simultaneously), is not peculiar to the lateral medullary syndrome, but rather may result from any type of injury to the brainstem's large vestibular nuclei. Nystagmus can be a manifestation of various disorders, including intoxication with alcohol, phenytoin (Dilantin), phencyclidine (PCP), or barbiturates; ischemia of the vertebrobasilar artery system; multiple sclerosis (MS); Wernicke–Korsakoff syndrome; or viral labyrinthitis. Among individuals who have ingested PCP, coarse vertical and horizontal (three directional or multidirectional) nystagmus characteristically accompanies an agitated delirium and markedly reduced sensitivity to pain and cold temperature. Unilateral nystagmus may be a component of *internuclear ophthalmoplegia*, which is usually a manifestation of MS or a small brainstem infarction (see Chapters 4 and 15).

SIGNS OF CEREBELLAR LESIONS

The cerebellum (*Latin*, diminutive of cerebrum) consists of two hemispheres and a central portion, the *vermis*. Each hemisphere controls coordination of the ipsilateral limbs, and the vermis controls coordination of "axial" or "midline structures": the head, neck, and trunk. Because the cerebellum controls coordination of the limbs on the same side of the body, it differs from the cerebrum wherein each hemisphere governs the contralateral body.

Another unique feature of the cerebellum is that when one hemisphere is damaged, the other will eventually assume the functions for both. In other words, although loss of one cerebellar hemisphere will temporarily cause

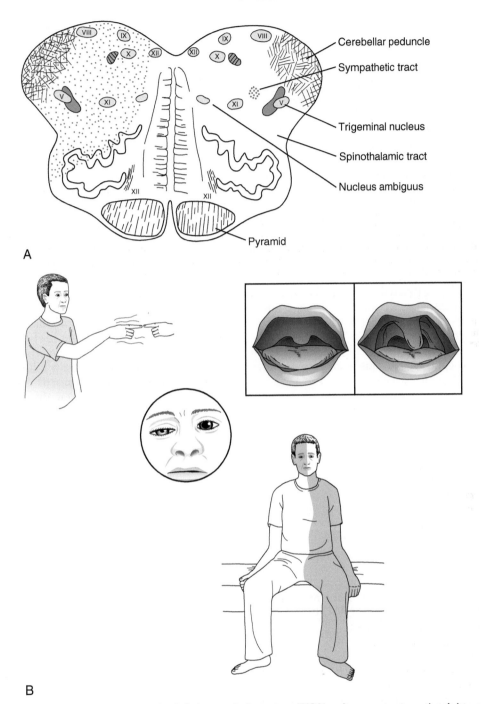

FIGURE 2.10 ■ A, An occlusion of the right posterior inferior cerebellar artery (PICA) or its parent artery, the right vertebral artery, has caused an infarction of the lateral portion of the right medulla (stippled). This infarction damages important structures: the inferior cerebellar peduncle, the spinal trigeminal nerve (V) sensory nucleus, the spinothalamic tract (which arose from the contralateral side of the body), the nucleus ambiguus (cranial nerves IX and X motor nuclei), and poorly delineated sympathetic fibers. However, this infarction spares medial structures: the corticospinal tract, medial longitudinal fasciculus (MLF), and hypoglossal nerve (XII) nucleus. B, Because he has sustained an infarction of his right lateral medulla, this patient has a right-sided Wallenberg syndrome. He has a right-sided Horner syndrome (ptosis and miosis) because of damage to the sympathetic fibers (also see Chapter 12). He has right-sided ataxia because of damage to the ipsilateral cerebellar tracts. He has an alternating or crossed hypalgesia: diminished pain sensation on the *right* side of his face, accompanied by loss of pain sensation on the *left* trunk and extremities (shaded). Finally, he has hoarseness and paresis of the right soft palate because of damage to the right nucleus ambiguus. Because of the right-sided palate weakness, the palate deviates upward toward his left on voluntary phonation (saying "ah") or in response to the gag reflex.

incapacitating ipsilateral incoordination, the patient's deficit lessens as the remaining hemisphere compensates almost entirely. For example, patients who lose one cerebellar hemisphere to a stroke or TBI typically regain their ability to walk, although they may never dance.

Children who sustain such an injury are more resilient and often can learn to ride a bicycle and participate in athletic activities.

In addition to causing incoordination, cerebellar lesions cause subtle motor changes, such as muscle hypotonia and pendular DTRs. However, cerebellar lesions do not cause paresis, hyperactive DTRs, or Babinski signs.

Although several technically sophisticated studies have shown that the cerebellum contributes to cognition and emotion, it does not play a discernible role in these functions in everyday endeavors. For example, lesions restricted to the cerebellum do not lead to dementia, language impairment, or other cognitive impairment. A good example is the normal intellect of children and young adults despite having undergone resection of a cerebellar hemisphere for removal of an astrocytoma (see Chapter 19).

On the other hand, several conditions damage the cerebrum as well as the cerebellum. For example, alcohol, phenytoin (Dilantin), lithium, and toluene may cause prominent ataxia and cognitive impairment.

For practical purposes, neurologists assess cerebellar function in tests of coordinated motor function. Thus, *intention tremor*, demonstrable in the finger-to-nose (Fig. 2.11) and heel-to-shin tests (Fig. 2.12), characterizes cerebellar dysfunction. This tremor is evident when the patient moves to a target but is absent when the patient rests. In a classic contrast, Parkinson disease causes a *resting tremor* that is present when the patient sits quietly and reduced or even abolished when the patient moves (see Chapter 18). Physicians should not confuse the neurologic term "intention tremor" with "intentional tremor," which would be a self-induced or psychogenic tremor.

Another sign of incoordination due to a cerebellar lesion is *dysdiadochokinesia*, impaired rapid alternating movements of the limbs. When asked to slap the palm and then the back of the hand rapidly and alternately on his or her own knee, for example, a patient with dysdiadochokinesia will do so with uneven force and irregular rhythm, and lose the alternating pattern.

Damage to either the entire cerebellum or the vermis alone causes incoordination of the trunk (*truncal ataxia*). This manifestation of cerebellar damage forces patients to place their feet widely apart when standing and leads to a lurching, unsteady, and wide-based pattern of walking (*gait ataxia*) (Table 2.1 and Fig. 2.13). A common example is the staggering and reeling of people intoxicated by alcohol. In addition, such cerebellar damage prevents people from walking heel-to-toe, i.e., performing "tandem gait." Another common example of ataxia occurs in individuals who have inherited genetic mutations that cause combinations of cerebellar and spinal cord degeneration. In several disorders, patients have abnormalities beyond the nervous system (Fig. 2.14). Extensive damage of the cerebellum causes *scanning speech*, a variety of dysarthria. Scanning speech, which reflects incoordination of speech production, is characterized by poor modulation, irregular cadence, and

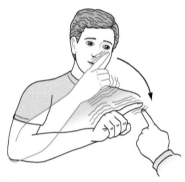

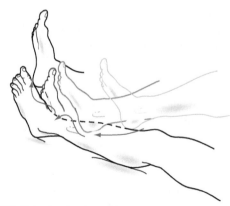

FIGURE 2.11 ■ This young man has a multiple sclerosis plaque in the right cerebellar hemisphere. During the *finger-to-nose* test, his right index finger touches his nose and then the examiner's finger by following a coarse, irregular path. The oscillation in his arm's movement is an *intention tremor*, and the irregularity in the rhythm is *dysmetria*.

FIGURE 2.12 ■ In the *heel-to-shin test*, the patient with the right-sided cerebellar lesion in the previous sketch displays limb *ataxia* as his right heel wobbles when he pushes it along the crest of his left shin.

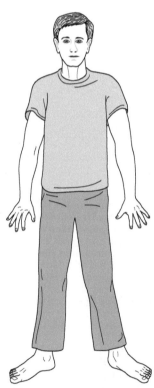

FIGURE 2.13 ■ Because this man has developed cerebellar degeneration from alcoholism, he has a typical *ataxic gait*. His stance is broad-based. His gait is unsteady, and he is uncoordinated.

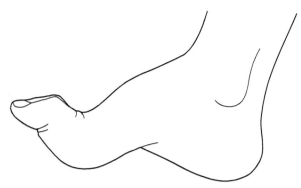

FIGURE 2.14 ■ The *pes cavus* foot deformity consists of a high arch, elevation of the dorsum, and retraction of the first metatarsal. When pes cavus occurs in families with childhood-onset ataxia and posterior column sensory deficits, it is a reliable sign of Friedreich ataxia, which is the most common hereditary ataxia in the United States and Europe.

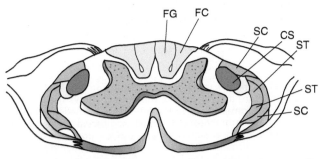

FIGURE 2.15 ■ In this sketch of the spinal cord, the centrally located gray matter is stippled. The surrounding white matter contains myelin-coated ascending and descending tracts. Clinically important ascending tracts are the spinocerebellar tracts (SC), the lateral spinothalamic tract (ST), and the posterior columns [fasciculus cuneatus (FC), from the upper limbs, and fasciculus gracilis (FG), from the lower limbs]. The most important descending tract is the lateral corticospinal (CS) tract.

inability to separate adjacent sounds. Physicians should be able to distinguish dysarthria – whether caused by cerebellar injury, bulbar or pseudobulbar palsy, or other neurologic disorder – from aphasia (see Chapter 8).

Before considering the illnesses that damage the cerebellum (see Section 2), physicians must appreciate that the cerebellum normally undergoes age-related changes that appear between ages 50 and 65 years in the form of mildly impaired functional ability and abnormal neurologic test results. For example, as people age beyond 50 years, they walk less rapidly and less sure-footedly. They begin to lose their ability to ride a bicycle and to stand on one foot while putting on socks. During a neurologic examination they routinely topple during tandem walking.

SIGNS OF SPINAL CORD LESIONS

The spinal cord's gray matter, which when viewed in the axial plane appears as a broad H-shaped structure in the center of the spinal cord, consists largely of neurons that transmit nerve impulses at one horizontal level. The spinal cord's white matter, composed of myelinated tracts that convey information in a vertical direction, surrounds the central gray matter (Fig. 2.15). This pattern – gray

matter on the inside with white outside – is opposite that of the cerebrum. Interruption of the myelinated tracts causes most of the signs of spinal cord injury, which neurologists call "myelopathy."

The major *descending* pathway, entirely motor, is the *lateral corticospinal tract*.

The major *ascending* pathways, entirely sensory, include the following:

- *Posterior columns* (or *dorsal columns*), comprised of the *fasciculi cuneatus* and *gracilis*, carry position and vibration sensations to the thalamus.
- *Lateral spinothalamic tracts* carry temperature and pain sensations to the thalamus.
- *Anterior spinothalamic tracts* carry light touch sensation to the thalamus.
- *Spinocerebellar tracts* carry joint position and movement sensations to the cerebellum.

Spinal Cord Transection

If an injury severs the spinal cord, the *transection's* location – cervical, thoracic, or lumbosacral – determines the pattern of the ensuing motor and sensory deficits. Cervical spinal cord transection, for example, blocks all motor impulses from descending and sensory information from arising through the neck. This lesion causes paralysis of the arms and legs (*quadriparesis*) and, after 1–2 weeks, hyperactive DTRs, and Babinski signs. In addition, it prevents the perception of all limb, trunk, and bladder and bowel sensation. Similarly, a midthoracic spinal cord transection causes paralysis of the legs (*paraparesis*) with similar reflex changes, and sensory loss in the trunk and below (Fig. 2.16). In general, all spinal cord injuries disrupt bladder control and sexual function, which rely on delicate, intricate systems (see Chapter 16).

Another motor impairment attributable to spinal cord damage, whether from a specific lesion or a neurodegenerative illness, is pathologically increased muscle tone, which neurologists label *hypertonicity* or *spasticity*. It often creates more disability than the accompanying paresis. For example, because spasticity causes the legs to be straight, extended, and unyielding, patients tend to walk on their toes (see Fig. 13.3). Similarly, spasticity greatly limits the usefulness of patients' hands and fingers.

In a variation of the complete spinal cord lesion, when a penetrating injury severs only the lateral half of the spinal cord, neurologists refer to the injury as a spinal cord hemitransection. The lesion causes the classic *Brown–Séquard syndrome*, which consists of ipsilateral paralysis of limb(s) from corticospinal tract damage and loss of vibration and proprioception from dorsal column damage combined with loss of temperature and pain (hypalgesia) sensation in the opposite limb(s) from lateral spinothalamic tract damage (Fig. 2.17). In the vernacular of neurology, one leg is weak and the other is numb.

Even with devastating spinal cord injury, cerebral function is preserved. In a frequently occurring and tragic example, soldiers surviving a penetrating gunshot wound of the cervical spinal cord, although quadriplegic, retain intellectual, visual, and verbal facilities. Nevertheless, veterans and other individuals with spinal cord injuries

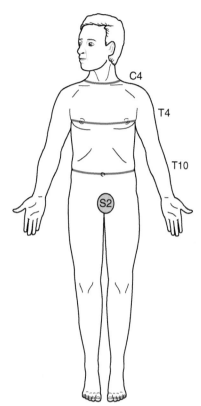

FIGURE 2.16 ■ In a patient with a spinal cord injury, the "level" of hypalgesia indicates the site of the damage. The clinical landmarks are C4, T4, and T10. C4 injuries cause hypalgesia below the neck; T4 injuries, hypalgesia below the nipples; T10 injuries, hypalgesia below the umbilicus.

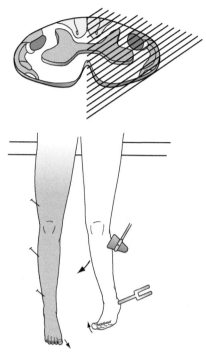

FIGURE 2.17 ■ In this case of hemitransection of the thoracic spinal cord from a knife wound, the patient shows the Brown–Séquard syndrome. Injury to the left lateral corticospinal tract results in the combination of left-sided leg paresis, hyperactive DTRs, and a Babinski sign; injury to the left posterior column results in impairment of left leg vibration and position sense. Most striking, injury to the left spinothalamic tract causes loss of temperature and pain sensation in the right leg. Loss of pain sensation contralateral to paresis is the signature of the Brown–Séquard syndrome.

often despair from isolation, lack of social support, and loss of their physical abilities.

Syringomyelia

A lesion that often affects only the cervical spinal cord consists of an elongated cavity, *syringomyelia* or simply a *syrinx* (Greek, *syrinx*, pipe or tube + *myelos* marrow). The syrinx occurs in the substance of the spinal cord, adjacent to its *central canal*, which is the thin tube running vertically within the gray matter. It usually develops, for unclear reasons, during adolescence. Traumatic intraspinal bleeding may cause a variety of syrinx, a *hematomyelia*. These conditions produce clinical findings that reflect their neuroanatomy (Fig. 2.18). In both cases, as the cavity expands, its pressure rips apart the lateral spinothalamic tract fibers as they cross from one to the other side of the spinal cord. It also presses on the anterior horn cells of the anterior gray matter. The expansion not only causes neck pain, but a striking loss in the arms and hands of pain and temperature sensation, muscle bulk, and DTRs. Because the sensory loss is restricted to patients' shoulders and arms, neurologists frequently describe it as *cape-* or *shawl-like*. Moreover, the sensory loss is characteristically restricted to loss of pain and temperature sensation because the posterior columns, merely displaced, remain functional.

NEUROLOGIC ILLNESSES

Several illnesses damage only specific ascending and descending spinal cord tracts (Fig. 2.19). The posterior columns – *fasciculus gracilis* and *fasciculus cuneatus* – seem particularly vulnerable. For example, tabes dorsalis (syphilis), combined system degeneration (vitamin B_{12} deficiency, see Chapter 5), and the spinocerebellar ataxias (SCAs) each damages the posterior columns alone or in combination with other tracts (also see Box 15.1). In these conditions, impairment of the posterior columns leads to a loss of position sense that prevents patients from being able to stand with their eyes closed (*Romberg's sign*). When they walk, this position sense loss produces an ataxic gait or possibly a *steppage gait* (Fig. 2.20).

In another example, the human T-lymphotropic virus type 1 (HTLV-1) infects the spinal cord's lateral columns. The infection, which is endemic in Caribbean islands, causes *HTLV-1 associated myelopathy* (or simply *HTLV-1 myelopathy*) in which patients develop spastic paraparesis that resembles MS. Perhaps more than in any other common myelopathy, the spasticity is disproportionately greater than the paresis.

Several toxic-metabolic disorders – some associated with substance abuse – damage the spinal cord. For example, nitrous oxide (N_2O), a gaseous anesthetic that may be inhaled as a drug of abuse by thrill-seeking

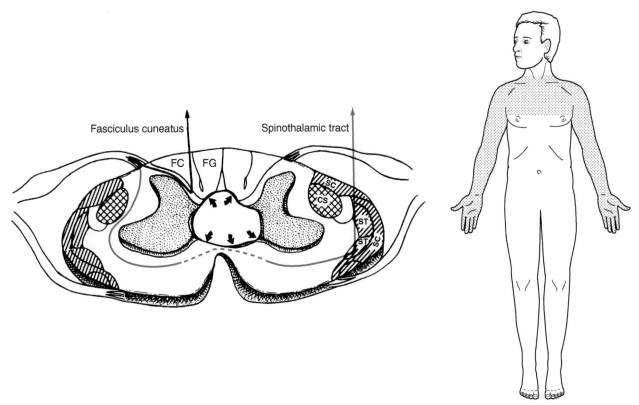

FIGURE 2.18 ■ *Left,* A syringomyelia (syrinx) is an elongated cavity in the spinal cord. Its expansion disrupts the lateral spinothalamic tract as it crosses, and compresses the anterior horn cells of the gray matter. It does not impair the function of the posterior columns and corticospinal tracts. *Right,* The classic finding is a shawl-like pattern of loss of pain and temperature sensation in the arms and upper chest (in this case, C4–T4) that is accompanied by weakness, atrophy, and areflexia in the arms.

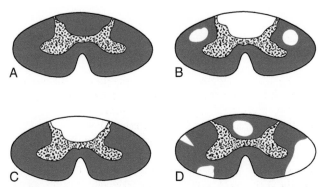

FIGURE 2.19 ■ A, A standard spinal cord histologic preparation stains normal myelin (white matter) black and leaves the central H-shaped column gray. B, In combined system degeneration (vitamin B$_{12}$ deficiency), posterior column and corticospinal tract demyelination causes their lack of stain. C, In tabes dorsalis (tertiary syphilis), damage to the posterior column leaves them unstained. D, MS leads to asymmetric, irregular, demyelinated unstained plaques.

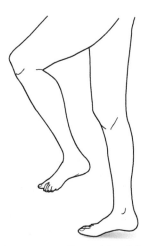

FIGURE 2.20 ■ The steppage gait consists of the patient's raising each knee excessively, as if perpetually climbing a staircase. This maneuver compensates for a loss of position sense by elevating the feet to ensure that they will clear the ground. Although the steppage gait is a classic sign of posterior column spinal cord damage from tabes dorsalis, peripheral neuropathies that impair position sense are a more frequent cause of this gait abnormality.

dentists, causes a pronounced myelopathy by inactivating vitamin B$_{12}$ (see Chapter 5). Copper deficiency, often from excess consumption of zinc by food faddists or inadvertently ingested from excess denture cream, leads to myelopathy. Also, unless physicians closely monitor and replace vitamins and nutrients following gastric bypass surgery, patients remain at risk of developing myelopathy for up to several years after the surgery.

Most important, dementia accompanies myelopathy in several illnesses because of concomitant cerebral damage. Examples of this association include tabes dorsalis, vitamin B$_{12}$ deficiency, AIDS, and, when disseminated throughout the cerebrum, MS.

CHAPTER 3

PSYCHOGENIC NEUROLOGIC DEFICITS

Classic studies of hysteria, conversion disorders, and related conditions included patients who underwent only rudimentary physical examinations and minimal, if any, laboratory testing. Studies that re-evaluated the same patients after many years reported that in as many as 15% of them, specific neurologic conditions, such as movement disorders, multiple sclerosis (MS), or seizures, emerged. Another interesting aspect of these studies is that physicians in the first two-thirds of the 20th century assumed that many illnesses were entirely "psychogenic," but today's physicians consider these same illnesses to be neurologic disorders, such as *Tourette disorder*, writer's cramp and other focal dystonias, erectile dysfunction, migraines, and trigeminal neuralgia.

Neurologists currently have an arsenal of high-tech tests, including computed tomography (CT), magnetic resonance imaging (MRI), functional MRI (fMRI), positron emission tomography (PET), electroencephalography (EEG), EEG-video monitoring, genetic analyses, and a full array of subspecialty consultants. Nevertheless, they still fail to reach 100% accuracy in their diagnoses. They also may hesitate before diagnosing a deficit as psychogenic, which is unfortunate, because delay in diagnosis adversely affects outcome. In some cases they may be forced to "undiagnose" a neurologic illness, such as MS, when further testing, observation, or consultation shows that the deficits actually constitute manifestations of a conversion disorder.

NEUROLOGIST'S ROLE

Even in the face of flagrant psychogenic signs, neurologists generally test for neurologic illness that could explain the patient's symptoms, particularly those illnesses that would be serious or life-threatening. Although frequently observing, the course of the illness proves most informative, at the initial consultation neurologists tend to request extensive evaluations to obtain objective evidence of disease or its absence. They typically do not specify whether a patient's symptoms and signs are of conscious or unconscious origin, subsuming both under the category of psychogenic disorders. Moreover, they consider malingering and exaggerations of a known neurologic deficit, *embellishment*, as psychogenic disorders. For example, they do not differentiate one person with "blindness" as a manifestation of an unconscious conflict from another one deliberately pretending to be blind to gain insurance money.

Within the framework of this potential oversimplification, neurologists reliably separate psychogenic disorders from ones that have a physiologic, organic basis. They also seek to recognize when patients have mixtures of neurologic and psychogenic deficits, disproportionately severe posttraumatic disabilities, and minor neurologic problems that preoccupy them.

When concluding that patients actually have a psychogenic disturbance, neurologists usually offer reassurances, suggest that the deficits will resolve by a certain date, and refer them for psychiatric consultation. Sometimes neurologists provide patients acceptable, face-saving exits by prescribing placebos or nonspecific treatment, such as physical therapy. They avoid ordering invasive diagnostic procedures, surgery, and medications, especially habit-forming or otherwise potentially dangerous ones. Occasionally, they hospitalize patients with conversion disorders to repeat an evaluation, provide treatment, and offer a refuge.

Neurologists working with psychiatrists will probably attribute most psychogenic symptoms or deficits to a *conversion disorder* (*functional neurological symptom disorder*), which constitutes a category under the new class of Somatic Symptom and Related Disorders in the *Diagnostic and Statistical Manual of Mental Disorders, 5th edition* (DSM-5). The diagnostic criteria for conversion disorder include one or more symptoms of altered voluntary motor or sensory function, incompatibility of the symptoms with neurologic and medical conditions, and distress or impairment in an important area of functioning. A defining characteristic of the class is that the symptoms provoke abnormal thoughts, feelings, and behaviors; however, the diagnosis rests on the neurologic examination. This chapter discusses several well-known, general psychogenic voluntary motor or sensory deficits. Other chapters describing neurologic illnesses discuss specific psychogenic deficits, such as psychogenic nonepileptic seizures (PNES) (see Chapter 10), psychogenic diplopia and blindness (see Chapter 12), and psychogenic tremors (see Chapter 18).

PSYCHOGENIC DEFICITS

What general clues prompt a neurologist to suspect a psychogenic deficit? When a deficit violates the *laws of neuroanatomy*, neurologists almost always deduce that it has a psychogenic origin. For example, if temperature sensation is preserved but pain perception is "lost," the deficit is *nonanatomic* and therefore likely to be psychogenic. Likewise, tunnel vision, which clearly violates these laws, is a classic psychogenic disturbance (see Fig. 12.7). One caveat is that migraine sufferers sometimes experience tunnel vision as an aura (see Chapter 9).

Other clues include a sudden onset and variable presence. For example, if someone who appears to have suddenly developed hemiparesis either walks when unaware of being observed or walks despite seeming to have paraparesis while in bed, neurologists conclude that the paresis has a psychogenic basis. A clear example occurs when someone with a "seizure" momentarily "awakens" and stops convulsive activity, but resumes it when assured of being observed. The psychogenic nature of a deficit can be confirmed if it is reversed during an interview while under the influence of hypnosis or hypnotic infusion.

Motor Signs

In general, signs of psychogenic weakness and gait impairment compared to signs of sensory loss are more sensitive and specific and carry greater predictive value. One indication of psychogenic weakness is a nonanatomic distribution of deficits, such as loss of strength in the arm and leg accompanied by blindness in one eye and deafness in one ear – all on the same side of the body. Another indication is the absence of functional impairment despite the appearance of profound weakness, such as ability to walk on heels and then toes even though manual testing seems to show marked ankle weakness.

Deficits that are intermittent also suggest a psychogenic origin. For example, a "give-way" effort, in which the patient offers a brief (several seconds) exertion before returning to an apparent paretic position, indicates a fluctuating condition that is probably psychogenic. Similarly, the *face–hand test*, in which the patient momentarily exerts

sufficient strength to deflect their falling hand from hitting their own face (Fig. 3.1), also indicates a psychogenic paresis.

An indication of psychogenic unilateral leg weakness is *Hoover sign* (Fig. 3.2). Normally, when someone attempts to raise a genuinely paretic leg, the other leg presses down. The examiner can feel the downward force at the patient's normal heel and can use the straightened leg, as a lever, to raise the entire leg and lower body. In contrast, Hoover sign consists of the patient unconsciously pressing down with a "paretic" leg when attempting to raise the unaffected leg and failing to press down with the unaffected leg when attempting to raise the "paretic" leg.

A similar test involves abduction (separating) the legs. Normally, when asked to abduct one leg, a person reflexively and forcefully abducts both of them. Someone with genuine hemiparesis will abduct the normal leg, but will be unable to abduct the paretic one. In contrast, someone with psychogenic weakness will reflexively abduct the "paretic" leg when abducting the normal leg (*abductor sign*) (Fig. 3.3).

Gait Impairment

Many psychogenic gait impairments closely mimic neurologic disturbances, such as tremors in the legs, ataxia, or weakness of one or both legs. The most readily identifiable psychogenic gait impairment is *astasia-abasia* (Greek, inability to stand, inability to walk). In this disturbance, patients stagger, balance momentarily, and appear to be in great danger of falling; however, catching themselves at "the last moment" by grabbing hold of railings, furniture, and even the examiner, they never actually injure themselves (Fig. 3.4).

Another blatant psychogenic gait impairment occurs when patients drag a "weak" leg as though it were a

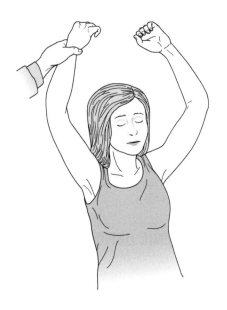 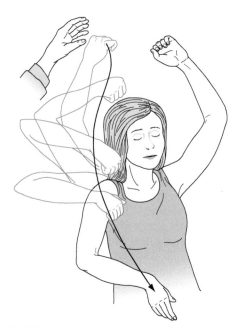

FIGURE 3.1 ■ In the face–hand test, a young woman with psychogenic right hemiparesis inadvertently demonstrates her preserved strength by deflecting her falling "paretic" arm from striking her face as the examiner drops it.

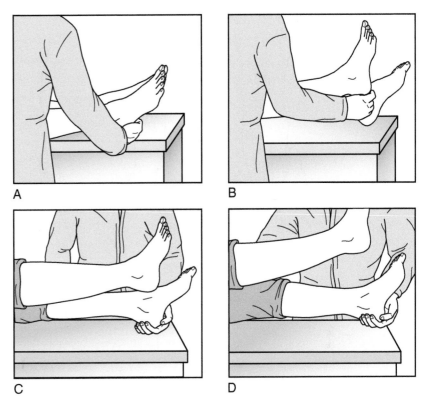

FIGURE 3.2 ■ A neurologist demonstrates Hoover sign in a 23-year-old man who has a psychogenic left hemiparesis. *A,* She asks him to raise his left leg as she holds her hand under his right heel. *B,* Revealing his lack of effort, the patient exerts so little downward force with his right leg that the neurologist easily raises it. *C,* When the neurologist asks him to raise his right leg while cupping his left heel, the patient reveals his intact strength as he unconsciously forces his left, "paretic" leg downward. *D,* As if to carry the example to the extreme, the patient forces his left leg downward with enough force to allow the neurologist to use his left leg as a lever to raise his lower torso.

completely lifeless object. In contrast, patients with a true hemiparetic gait swing their paretic leg outward with a circular motion, i.e., "circumduct" their leg (see Fig. 2.4). Still other characteristics that signify a psychogenic gait include a robotic pattern to walking and intermittent buckling at the knees.

Sensory Deficits

Although the sensory examination is the least reliable portion of the neurologic examination, several sensory abnormalities indicate a psychogenic deficit. For example, loss of sensation to pinprick* with a sharply demarcated boundary in the middle of the face and body constitutes the classic *splitting the midline*. This finding suggests a psychogenic loss because the sensory nerve fibers of the skin normally extend across the midline (Fig. 3.5). In a variation of this test, because vibrations naturally spread across bony structures, loss of vibration sensation over only half of the forehead, jaw, or sternum strongly suggests a psychogenic disturbance.

A similar abnormality is loss of sensation throughout the entire face but not past the hairline. This pattern is inconsistent with the anatomic distribution of the trigeminal nerve, which innervates the face and scalp anterior to the vertex but not the angle of the jaw (see Fig. 4.12).

As already mentioned, a discrepancy between pain and temperature sensations, which are normally carried together

by the peripheral nerves and then the lateral spinothalamic tracts, suggests psychogenic sensory loss. By contrast, discrepancy between pain and *position* sensations in the fingers is indicative of syringomyelia (Fig. 2.18). In a syringomyelia, the expanding central canal disrupts the central fibers of the spinal cord, which carry pain sensation.

Testing for sensory loss when the arms are twisted, placed out of sight behind the patient's back, or viewed in a mirror may also expose psychogenic sensory deficits.

Finally, because sensory loss impairs function, patients with genuine sensory loss in their feet or hands cannot perform many tasks if their eyes are closed. Also, those with true sensory loss in both feet – from severe peripheral neuropathy or injury of the spinal cord posterior columns, usually from vitamin B_{12} deficiency, tabes dorsalis, or MS – tend to fall when standing erect with their eyes shut: the *Romberg sign* (see Chapter 2). By contrast, patients with psychogenic sensory loss can still generally button their shirts, walk short distances, and stand with their feet together and their eyes closed.

Special Senses

When patients' blindness, tunnel vision, diplopia, or other disorders of vision violate the laws of neuroanatomy, which are firmly based on the laws of optics, neurologists diagnose those symptoms as psychogenic. Neurologists and ophthalmologists can readily separate psychogenic and neurologic visual disorders (see Chapter 12).

A patient with psychogenic deafness usually responds to unexpected noises or words. Unilateral hearing loss in the ear ipsilateral to a hemiparesis is highly suggestive of a psychogenic etiology because extensive auditory tract

---

*Neurologists avoid using actual pins to avoid blood-borne infections. Rather, they usually test for pain with nonpenetrating, disposable single-use instruments, such as broken cotton-tipped applicators.

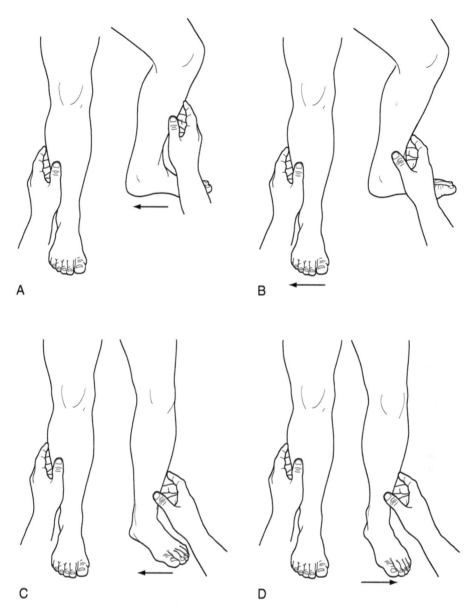

FIGURE 3.3 ■ Upper series: Left hemiparesis from a stroke: The examiner's hands are pushing the legs together, i.e., adducting them. *A,* When asked to abduct the left leg, that leg's weakness cannot resist a physician's pressure, which moves the leg toward the midline (adducts it). At the same time, the normal right leg reflexively abducts. *B,* When asked to abduct the normal right leg, the patient forcefully abducts it. The paretic left leg cannot resist the examiner's pressure, and the examiner pushes the leg inward. Lower series: Psychogenic left hemiparesis: *C,* When asked to abduct both legs, the patient fails to resist the examiner's hand pushing the left leg inward (adducting it). In addition, because of the patient's failure to abduct the right leg, the examiner's hand also presses it inward. *D,* When asked to abduct the normal right leg, the patient complies and forcefully abducts it; however, the left leg, which has psychogenic weakness, reflexively resists the physician's inward pressure and abducts – *the abductor sign.*

synapses in the pons ensure that some tracts reach the upper brainstem and cerebrum despite central nervous system (CNS) lesions (see Fig. 4.16). If doubts about hearing loss remain, neurologists often request audiometry, brainstem auditory evoked responses, and other objective tests.

Patients can genuinely lose the sense of smell (anosmia) from head injury (see Chapter 22), neurodegenerative disorders, or advanced age; however, these patients can usually still perceive noxious volatile chemicals, such as ammonia or alcohol, which irritate the nasal mucosa endings of the trigeminal nerve rather than the olfactory nerve. This distinction is usually unknown to individuals with psychogenic anosmia, who typically claim inability to smell any substance.

Other Conditions

A distinct but common psychogenic disturbance, the *hyperventilation syndrome,* occurs in people with an underlying anxiety disorder, including panic disorder. It leads to lightheadedness and paresthesias around the mouth, fingers, and toes, and, in severe cases, to *carpopedal spasm* (Fig. 3.6). Although the disorder seems distinctive,

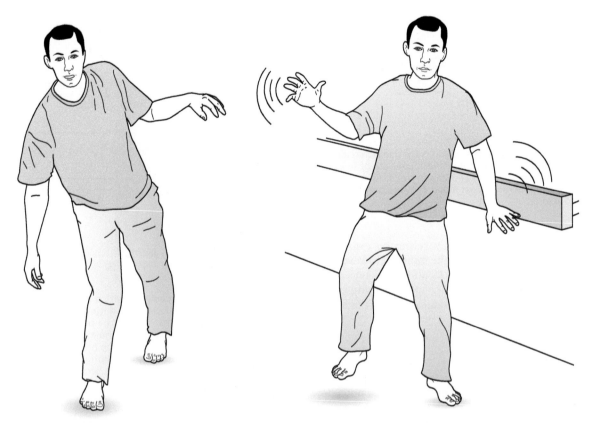

FIGURE 3.4 ■ A young man demonstrates astasia-abasia by seeming to begin to fall when walking, but then catching himself by balancing carefully. He even staggers the width of the room to grasp the rail. He sometimes clutches physicians and pulls them toward himself and then drags them toward the ground. While dramatizing his purported impairment, he actually displays good strength, balance, and coordination.

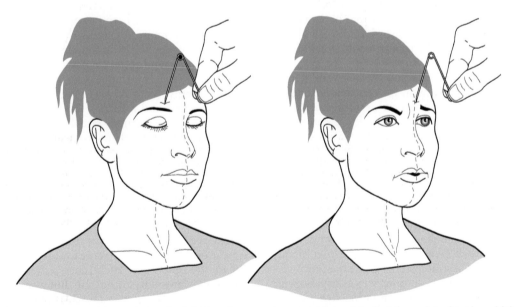

FIGURE 3.5 ■ A young woman with psychogenic right hemisensory loss appears not to feel the point of a pin, which is used only for illustrative purposes, on her right forehead, but when it crosses to the left of center, she immediately appears to feel it, i.e., she splits the midline.

physicians should be cautious before diagnosing it because focal seizures and transient ischemic attacks (TIAs) may produce similar symptoms.

In this condition, hyperventilation first causes a fall in carbon dioxide tension that leads to respiratory alkalosis. The alkalosis produces hypocalcemia, which induces the tetany of muscles and paresthesias. To demonstrate the cause of the spasms, physicians may recreate them by having a patient hyperventilate. This procedure may also induce giddiness, anxiety, or confusion. The conventional wisdom dictates that if hyperventilation produces those symptoms, the physician should abort the demonstration

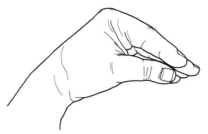

FIGURE 3.6 ■ Carpopedal spasm, which is the characteristic neurologic manifestation of hyperventilation, consists of flexion of the wrist and proximal thumb and finger joints. Also, although the thumb and fingers remain extended, they are drawn together and tend to overlap.

by having the patient continually rebreathe expired air from a paper bag cupped around the mouth. However, that remedy does not stop such attacks and physicians might mistakenly put a bag to the face of people breathing rapidly because of an asthma attack or congestive heart failure.

POTENTIAL PITFALLS

The examination of a patient suspected of having a psychogenic deficit requires particular sensitivity. It need not follow the conventional format and can be completed in two or more sessions. A threatening, embarrassing, or otherwise inept evaluation may obscure the diagnosis, harden the patient's resolve, or precipitate a catastrophic reaction.

An unreliable indication of a psychogenic deficit is a patient's absence of concern or affect, *la belle indifférence*, concerning it. In fact, the expectation that patients with somatic symptoms and related disorders display abnormal thoughts, feelings, and behaviors would preclude the diagnosis in those with *la belle indifférence*. In any case, neurologists see this emotional posture in several neurologic disorders, particularly hemi-inattention, Anton syndrome, and frontal lobe injury. Psychiatrists should give *la belle indifférence* no diagnostic credibility in conversion disorders.

Although the neurologic examination itself seems rational and reliable, some findings are potentially misleading. For example, many anxious or "ticklish" individuals, with or without psychogenic hemiparesis, have brisk deep tendon reflexes and extensor plantar reflexes.

Neurologists may misdiagnose disorders as psychogenic when they are unique or bizarre, or when their severity is greater than expected. This error may simply reflect an individual neurologist's lack of experience.

They may also misdiagnose disorders as psychogenic when a patient has no accompanying objective physical abnormalities. This determination might be faulty in illnesses where objective signs are often transient or subtle, such as MS, myasthenia gravis, focal seizures, and small strokes. Neurologists given an incomplete history may not appreciate certain disorders, such as transient hemiparesis induced by migraines, postictal paresis, or TIAs, or transient mental status aberrations induced by alcohol, medications, or seizures (see Box 9.3).

Another potential pitfall is dismissing an entire case because a patient is grossly exaggerating a deficit. Patients

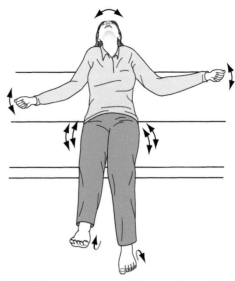

FIGURE 3.7 ■ This young woman with a psychogenic nonepileptic seizure (PNES) is screaming during an entire 30-second episode. Several features reveal its nonneurologic nature. In addition to verbalizing throughout the episode rather than only at its onset (as in an epileptic cry), she maintains her body tone, which is required to keep her sitting upright. She has alternating flailing limb movements rather than organized bilateral clonic jerks. She has subtle but suggestive pelvic thrusting.

may feel that they must overstate a genuine medical problem to gain the necessary attention. In addition, the prospect of having developed a neurologic disorder may trigger overwhelming anxiety. For example, patients with a persistent headache may so fear a brain tumor that they embellish their history with additional symptoms to obtain an MRI.

Another common error is failure to recognize a protean disorder – MS is the classic example – because its early signs tend to be evanescent, exclusively sensory, or so disparate as to appear to violate several laws of neuroanatomy. Neurologists usually arrive at the correct diagnosis early and reliably – even in ambiguous cases – with MRI and sometimes visual evoked response testing and cerebrospinal fluid analysis (see Chapter 15). On the other hand, trivial sensory or motor symptoms accompanied by normal variations in these highly sensitive tests may lead to false-positive diagnoses of MS.

Neurologists are also liable to err in diagnosing involuntary movement disorders as psychogenic. These disorders, in fact, often carry some stigmata of psychogenic illness (see Chapter 2). For example, the movements may appear bizarre, precipitated or exacerbated by anxiety, or apparently relieved by tricks, such as when walking backwards alleviates a dystonic gait. Because laboratory tests are not available for many disorders – chorea, tics, tremors, and focal dystonia – the diagnosis rests on the neurologist's clinical evaluation. As a general rule, physicians should assume, at least initially, that movement disorders are not psychogenic (see Chapter 18).

Physicians may misdiagnose epilepsy as psychogenic nonepileptic seizures (PNES) and vice versa (see Chapter 10). In general, but certainly not always, episodes of PNES are clonic and unaccompanied by incontinence, tongue biting, or loss of body tone (Fig. 3.7). Furthermore, while exceptions occur, patients tend to regain awareness and have no retrograde or anterograde amnesia immediately after the movements cease. On the other hand, both seizures originating in the frontal lobe and mixtures of epileptic and psychogenic seizures notoriously mimic purely psychogenic ones. EEG-video monitoring almost always enables neurologists to categorize seizure-like events. It is imperative to keep in mind that many patients with PNES have epileptic seizures as well, so demonstrating that a single episode is psychogenic does not refute the diagnosis of epilepsy; conversely, a patient with epileptic seizures may also have episodes that are psychogenic.

REFERENCES

Baker, G. A., Hanley, J. R., Jackson, H. F., et al. (1993). Detecting the faking of amnesia: Performance differences between simulators and patients with memory impairments. *Journal of Clinical and Experimental Neuropsychology, 15*, 668–684.

Daum, C., Hubschmid, M., & Aybek, S. (2014). The value of "positive" clinical signs for weakness, sensory and gait disorders in conversion disorder: A systematic and narrative review. *Journal of Neurology, Neurosurgery, and Psychiatry, 85*, 180–190.

Eisendrath, S. J., & McNiel, D. E. (2002). Factitious disorders in civil litigation: Twenty cases illustrating the spectrum of abnormal illness-affirming behavior. *The Journal of the American Academy of Psychiatry and the Law, 30*, 391–399.

Hayes, M. W., Graham, S., Heldorf, P., et al. (1999). A video review of the diagnosis of psychogenic gait. *Movement Disorders: Official Journal of the Movement Disorder Society, 14*, 914–921.

Jordbru, A. A., Smedstad, L. V., Klungsoyr, O., et al. (2014). Psychogenic gait disorder: A randomized controlled trial of physical rehabilitation with one-year follow-up. *Journal of Rehabilitation Medicine, 46*, 181–187.

Kanaan, R. A., & Wessely, S. C. (2010). Factitious disorders in neurology: An analysis of reported cases. *Psychosomatics, 51*, 47–51.

Letonoff, E. J., Williams, T. R., & Sidhu, K. S. (2002). Hysterical paralysis: a report of three cases and a review of the literature. *Spine, 27*, E441–E445.

Sonoo, M. (2004). Abductor sign: a reliable new sign to detect unilateral non-organic paresis of the lower limb. *Journal of Neurology, Neurosurgery, and Psychiatry, 75*, 121–125.

Stone, J., Carson, A., Duncan, R., et al. (2012). Which neurological diseases are most likely to be associated with "symptoms unexplained by organic disease." *Journal of Neurology, 259*, 33–38.

Stone, J., Smyth, R., Carson, A., et al. (2006). *La belle indifférence* in conversion symptoms and hysteria: Systematic review. *The British Journal of Psychiatry: The Journal of Mental Science, 188*, 204–209.

Stone, J., Warlow, C., & Sharpe, M. (2010). The symptom of functional weakness: A controlled study of 107 patients. *Brain: A Journal of Neurology, 133*, 1537–1551.

Voon, V., Gallea, C., Hattori, N., et al. (2010). The involuntary nature of conversion disorder. *Neurology, 74*, 223–228.

CHAPTER 4

CRANIAL NERVE IMPAIRMENTS

Various conditions may strike the cranial nerves individually, in pairs, or in groups. Moreover, when patients have symptoms of cranial nerve impairment, the underlying problem might not be damage to the cranial nerve itself, but rather a cerebral or brainstem lesion, neuromuscular junction problem, or psychogenic disturbance. Following custom, this chapter reviews the 12 cranial nerves and their disorders according to their Roman numeral designations, which readers may recall with the classic mnemonic device, "On old Olympus's towering top, a Finn and German viewed some hops" (Box 4.1).

OLFACTORY (FIRST)

Olfactory nerves transmit the sensation of smell to the brain. As the work that led to the 2004 Nobel Prize in Physiology or Medicine has shown, olfaction begins with highly complex, genetically determined specific G protein-coupled olfactory receptors. Odiferous molecules bind to one or more receptors that lead to their identification. Rats, which live by their sense of smell, have about 1400 olfactory receptor genes. Humans have about 350 olfactory receptor genes, but they comprise almost 1.5% of our total genome.

From the olfactory receptors located deep in the nasal cavity, branches of the pair of olfactory nerves pass upward through the multiple holes in the cribriform plate of the skull to several areas of the brain. Some branches terminate in entorhinal cortex and other regions on the undersurface of the frontal lobe. Others terminate deep in the hypothalamus and amygdala – cornerstones of the limbic system (see Fig. 16.5). The olfactory nerves' input into the limbic system accounts, at least in part, for the influence of smell on sexual behavior and memory. Also, unlike other sensations – touch, vision, and hearing – whose pathways synapse in the thalamus or geniculate bodies en route to the cerebral cortex, some olfactory pathways project directly to cortex without an intervening synapse in the diencephalon.

To test the olfactory nerve, neurologists compress one nostril and ask the patient to identify certain substances by smelling through the other. Neurologists use readily identifiable and aromatic but innocuous substances, such as coffee. They do not use volatile or irritative substances, such as ammonia and alcohol, because they may trigger intranasal trigeminal nerve receptors and bypass a possibly damaged olfactory nerve. Patients are unreliable when estimating their sense of smell. For qualitative and quantitative testing, especially for research, neurologists utilize a commercial, standardized set of "scratch and sniff" odors, such as the University of Pennsylvania Smell Identification Test.

When disorders impair both olfactory nerves, patients cannot perceive smells or appreciate the aroma of food. Neurologists say that these patients have *anosmia*. Anosmia carries potentially life-threatening consequences, for example when patients cannot smell escaping gas. More commonly, their food, without perceptible aroma, is left tasteless. Thus, people with anosmia, to whom food is bland, tend to have a decreased appetite and lose weight.

Lack of smell sensation in one nostril may result from head trauma or a tumor adjacent to the olfactory nerve, such as an olfactory groove meningioma. In the classic *Foster–Kennedy syndrome*, a meningioma compresses the olfactory nerve and the nearby optic nerve. Damage to those two nerves causes the combination of unilateral blindness and anosmia. If the tumor grows into the frontal lobe, it can also produce personality changes, dementia, or seizures.

Anosmia commonly afflicts anyone with nasal congestion and those who regularly smoke cigarettes. With advancing age, otherwise normal individuals begin to lose their sense of smell. More than 50% of individuals older than 65 years and 75% of those older than 80 years have some degree of anosmia. Also, individuals with genetic mutations in their G protein-coupled receptor complex have anosmia for one or more specific odors.

Although mundane problems underlie most cases of bilateral anosmia, it may reflect more serious issues. Inadvertently inhaling zinc, which had been a constituent of popular "cold remedies," has caused anosmia. Another situation where inhaled metal caused anosmia has occurred in welders who routinely inhale fumes containing vaporized iron, chromium, aluminum, and other metals. Head trauma, even from minor injuries, can shear the olfactory nerves as they pass through the cribriform plate and cause anosmia (see Traumatic Brain Injury, Chapter 22).

Loss of the sense of smell is also a manifestation of many neurodegenerative illnesses. For example, almost 90% of patients with Parkinson, dementia with Lewy bodies, Wilson, Creutzfeldt–Jakob, and Alzheimer diseases develop anosmia. In fact, among Parkinson disease patients, more have anosmia than tremor, and anosmia correlates with the most disabling manifestation of the illness – dementia. Similarly, anosmia serves as a risk factor for Alzheimer disease. Recent studies have found that the olfactory bulb manifests the same pathology as the cerebral cortex (see Chapter 7) in Alzheimer and Creutzfeldt–Jakob diseases. Schizophrenic patients also have an increased incidence of anosmia, but not to the degree brought on by neurodegenerative diseases.

In a situation opposite to anosmia, sometimes individuals have a heightened sense of smell: hyperosmia. Migraine patients before or during an attack and pregnant women frequently report hypersensitivity to smells or irritation by common, innocuous ones.

Anosmia may, of course, be psychogenic. A psychogenic origin can be revealed when a patient reports being unable to "smell" irritative substances. Such a complete sensory loss would be possible only if an illness completely obliterated both pairs of trigeminal as well as olfactory nerves.

Olfactory hallucinations may represent the first phase or *aura* (Latin, breeze) of seizures that originate in the medial-inferior surface of the temporal lobe, the uncus. These auras usually consist of a series of several-second episodes of ill-defined and unpleasant, but occasionally sweet or otherwise pleasant, smells preceding or superimposed on impaired consciousness and behavioral disturbances (see Chapter 10). Also, although most migraine auras consist of visual hallucinations, sometimes olfactory hallucinations represent an aura (see Chapter 9).

On the other hand, olfactory hallucinations as well as anosmia can be psychogenic. In contrast to smells induced by seizures, psychogenic "odors" are typically foul-smelling, continuous, and not associated with impaired consciousness. Olfactory hallucinations or delusions may constitute a manifestation of a psychiatric illness. As for identifying malingering, two tests are helpful. Malingerers may claim inability to "smell" a noxious, volatile substance, such as ammonia, that actually stimulates the trigeminal nerve. In the other test, given a forced-choice test of four smells, the malingering individual chooses a correct response less frequently than by chance, i.e., less than 25%.

OPTIC (SECOND)

The optic nerves have two main functions: vision and adjustment of the size of the pupil depending on the intensity of light. The optic nerves each begin in a common initial path that splits. The optic nerve fibers carrying visual information ultimately project to the cerebral cortex, while the others, carrying light information, project to the midbrain.

As for vision, those optic nerve fibers originate in visual receptors in the retina and project posteriorly to the otic chiasm. At the chiasm, nasal fibers of the nerves cross, but temporal fibers continue uncrossed (Fig. 4.1).

BOX 4.1		Cranial Nerves	
I	Olfactory	VII	Facial
II	Optic	VIII	Acoustic
III	Oculomotor	IX	Glossopharyngeal
IV	Trochlear	X	Vagus
V	Trigeminal	XI	Spinal accessory
VI	Abducens	XII	Hypoglossal

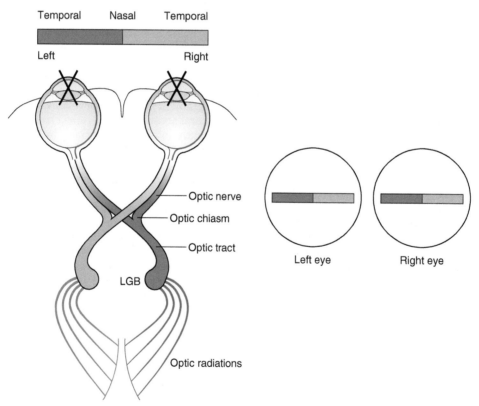

FIGURE 4.1 ■ *Left,* The optic nerves originate in the retinas. Their medial fibers cross at the optic chiasm while the temporal portions continue uncrossed. The recombinations form the optic tracts that synapse at the *lateral geniculate bodies (LGB).* The optic radiations sweep through the posterior cerebral hemispheres to terminate at the occipital ("visual") cortex. This system projects the impulses from each visual field to the contralateral occipital lobe cortex. For example, as in this sketch, impulses conveying the shaded half of the bar, which is in the patient's left visual field, project to the right occipital cortex. *Right,* As in this case, medical illustrations typically show a patient's visual fields from the patient's perspective. This illustration portrays the shaded portion of the bar in the left visual field of each eye.

Temporal fibers of one *optic nerve* join the nasal fibers of the other to form the *optic tracts*. The tracts travel to the lateral geniculate nuclei, from which the *optic radiations* emerge and pass through the temporal and parietal lobes to terminate in the calcarine cortex of the occipital lobe. Thus, each occipital lobe receives its visual information from the contralateral visual field. Further projections relay the visual information to other areas of the cerebral cortex for higher-level processing, such as tracking moving objects, reading, and interpreting.

Visual field deficits are considered among the most important findings in neurology. Many of them point to specific neurologic disorders, such as optic neuritis, pituitary adenomas, and migraine (see Chapter 12). In addition, visual field deficits are comorbid with certain neuropsychiatric conditions, such as left homonymous hemianopia with anosognosia, right homonymous hemianopia with aphasia or alexia, and tubular vision with a psychogenic disturbance.

As for their role in regulating pupil size, the optic nerves and tracts form the afferent limb of the *pupillary light reflex* by sending small branches containing impulses proportional to light intensity to the midbrain. The oculomotor nerves (the third cranial nerves) form the efferent limb. These nerves contain parasympathetic, as well as motor fibers, which innervate the pupils' constrictor muscles. Overall, the light reflex – optic nerves to midbrain and midbrain to oculomotor nerves – constricts pupil size in response to the intensity of light striking the retina. Simply put, when a neurologist shines a bright light into one or both eyes, the light reflex constricts both pupils (Fig. 4.2).

Because of the pupillary light reflex, shining light into one eye will normally result in bilateral pupillary constriction. In an example of an abnormality detectable by testing the light reflex, if neurologists shine light into the *right* eye and *neither* pupil constricts, and then into the *left* eye and *both* pupils constrict, *the right optic nerve* (afferent limb) is impaired. In a different example, if neurologists shine light into the *right* eye and it produces no constriction of the right pupil but succeeds in provoking *left* eye pupil constriction, the *right oculomotor nerve* (efferent limb) is impaired.

In contrasting the optic nerves' two functions, the visual system includes a high-level cortical system, whereas the light reflex remains a basic brainstem function. Thus, devastating occipital cortex injuries – from trauma, anoxia, or degenerative illnesses – produce blindness ("cortical blindness"). However, no matter how terrible the cerebral cortex damage – even to the point of patients being severely demented, bedridden, and blind – the pupils continue to react to light. In the absence of ocular trauma, if an unresponsive patient's pupils fail to constrict in response to light, neurologists may take the absence of that light reflex as a sign of brain death.

Routine testing of the optic nerve includes examination of (1) visual acuity, (2) visual fields (Fig. 4.3), and (3) the ocular fundi (Fig. 4.4). Because the visual system is important, complex, and subject to numerous ocular, neurologic, iatrogenic, and psychogenic disturbances, this book dedicates an entire chapter to visual disturbances particularly relevant to psychiatry (see Chapter 12).

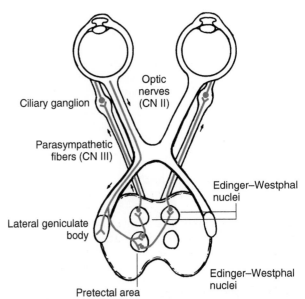

FIGURE 4.2 ■ The light reflex begins with its afferent limb in the optic nerve (cranial nerve II). The optic nerve transmits light impulses from the retinas to two important structures: (1) In conveying vision, axons synapse on the lateral geniculate body. Then the postsynaptic optic radiations convey visual information to the occipital lobe's visual cortex. (2) Optic nerve axons that participate in the light reflex travel to the *pretectal area* in the dorsal midbrain where they form a synapse. Postsynaptic neurons travel a short distance to both the ipsilateral and contralateral *Edinger–Westphal nuclei*, which are the parasympathetic divisions of the oculomotor (third cranial nerve) nuclei. Those nuclei give rise to parasympathetic oculomotor nerve fibers, which constitute the reflex's efferent limb (see Fig. 12.15 Top). Those fibers synapse in the ciliary ganglia and postsynaptic fibers terminate in the iris constrictor (sphincter) muscles. Thus, light shone into one eye constricts the pupil of that eye (the "direct" [ipsilateral] light reflex) and that of the contralateral eye (the "consensual" [indirect or contralateral] light reflex). This anatomical arrangement explains how oculomotor nerve injuries, because they usually include damage to the parasympathetic component, dilate the pupil. Similarly, it indicates how damaged sympathetic nervous innervation with unopposed parasympathetic innervation, as in the lateral medullary and Horner syndromes, produces pupil constriction (*miosis*). Finally, it shows how ciliary ganglion damage produces a dilated but extremely sensitive "Adie pupil" (see Fig. 12.15 Bottom).

The origin of the optic nerves explains their involvement in certain illnesses and not in others. Unique among the cranial nerves, the optic nerves (and a small proximal portion of the acoustic nerves) are actually projections of the brain coated by myelin derived from *oligodendrocytes*. In other words, these cranial nerves are extensions of the central nervous system (CNS). Thus, CNS illnesses, particularly childhood-onset metabolic storage diseases and multiple sclerosis (MS)-induced optic neuritis (see Chapter 15), are apt to involve the optic nerves. On the other hand, the optic nerves remain relatively immune from diseases that exclusively attack the peripheral nervous system (PNS) myelin, such as the Guillain–Barré syndrome. Whereas *oligodendrocytes* generate the myelin that covers optic nerve axons and other CNS structures, *Schwann cells* produce the myelin sheath of both the remaining cranial nerves and all myelinated nerves in the PNS.

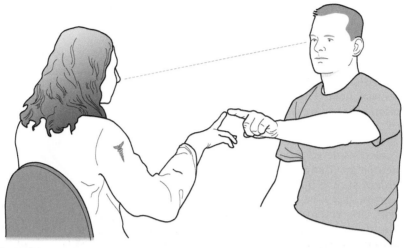

FIGURE 4.3 ■ In testing visual fields by the confrontation method, this neurologist extends her index finger as the patient points to it without diverting his eyes from her nose. She tests the four quadrants of each eye's visual field. (Only by testing each eye individually will she detect a bitemporal hemianopia, which is the visual field defect characteristic of pituitary adenomas.) Neurologists test young children and others unable to comply with this method in an abbreviated but still meaningful manner. In this case, the neurologist might assess the response to an attention-catching object introduced to each visual field. For example, a stuffed toy animal, dollar bill, or glass of water should capture a patient's attention. If the patient does not respond, the neurologist should primarily consider visual field deficit(s). In some cases, psychogenic visual loss (see later) or inattention (neglect, see Chapter 8) may explain the patient's failure to respond.

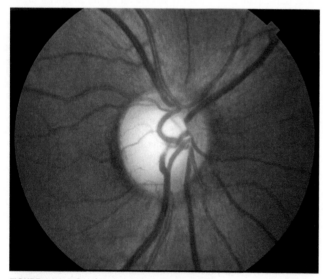

FIGURE 4.4 ■ On fundoscopy, the normal optic fundus or disk appears yellow, flat, and well-demarcated from the surrounding red retina. The retinal veins, as everywhere else in the body, are broader than their corresponding arteries. A neurologist will usually see retinal veins pulsate except when elevated intracranial pressure compresses them.

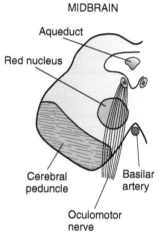

MIDBRAIN

FIGURE 4.5 ■ The oculomotor (third cranial) nerves arise from nuclei in the dorsal portion of the midbrain (see Fig. 2.9). Each travels ventrally to pass through the red nucleus, which receives fibers from the contralateral cerebellum, and then through the cerebral peduncle, which carries the corticospinal tract containing the upper motor neurons that control the contralateral limbs.

OCULOMOTOR, TROCHLEAR, AND ABDUCENS NERVES (THIRD, FOURTH, AND SIXTH)

The oculomotor, trochlear, and abducens nerves constitute the "extraocular muscle system" because, acting in unison, they move the eyes together in parallel to provide normal *conjugate gaze*. Damage to any of these nerves or the muscle or muscles they innervate causes *dysconjugate*

gaze, which results in characteristic patterns of *diplopia* (double vision). In addition, with oculomotor nerve damage, patients also lose their pupillary constriction to light as well as the elevation of their eyelid.

The oculomotor nerves (third cranial nerves) originate in the midbrain (Fig. 4.5) and supply each eye's pupil constrictor, eyelid (levator palpebrae superioris), and muscles that adduct (medial rectus), depress (inferior rectus), and elevate (superior rectus and inferior oblique) the eye. Oculomotor nerve impairment, a common condition, thus leads to a distinctive constellation: a dilated pupil, ptosis, and outward deviation (abduction) of the eye (Fig. 4.6). As discussed, oculomotor nerve injury also

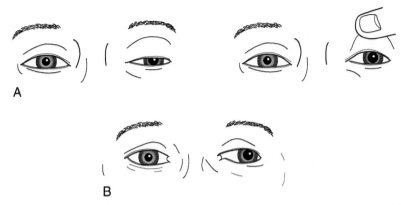

FIGURE 4.6 ■ *A*, This patient, who is looking straight ahead, has paresis of the left oculomotor nerve with typical findings: the eye is deviated laterally; the pupil is dilated and unreactive to light; and the upper eyelid covers a portion of the pupil (ptosis). *B*, In a milder case, with the patient looking ahead, close inspection reveals subtle ptosis, lateral deviation of the eye, and dilation of the pupil. In both cases, patients have diplopia that increases when looking to the right because this movement requires adducting the left eye, but the paretic left medial rectus muscle cannot participate and the patient's gaze becomes dysconjugate (also see Fig. 12.12).

impairs the efferent limb of the light reflex. In addition, it impairs the efferent limb of the *accommodation reflex*, in which the visual system adjusts the shape of the lens to focus on either near or distant objects. (Impaired focusing ability in older individuals, *presbyopia* [Greek, *presbys*, old man; *opia*, eye] results from the loss of flexibility in the aging lens, not from oculomotor nerve impairment.)

The trochlear nerves (fourth cranial nerves) also originate in the midbrain. They supply only the superior oblique muscle, which is responsible for depression of the eye when it is adducted (turned inward). To compensate for an injured trochlear nerve, patients tilt their head away from the affected side. Unless physicians observe a patient with diplopia perform this telltale maneuver, they may miss a diagnosis of a trochlear nerve injury.

Unlike the third and fourth cranial nerves, the abducens nerves (sixth cranial nerves) originate in the pons (Fig. 4.7 and see Fig. 2.9). They perform only a single function and innervate only a single muscle. Each abducens nerve innervates its ipsilateral lateral rectus muscle, which abducts the eye. Abducens nerve impairment, which is relatively common, leads to inward deviation (adduction) of the eye from the unopposed medial pull of the medial rectus, but does not cause ptosis or pupil changes (Fig. 4.8).

To review: the lateral rectus muscle is innervated by the sixth cranial (abducens) nerve and the superior oblique by the fourth (trochlear), but all the others by the third (oculomotor). A mnemonic device, "LR₆SO₄," captures this relationship.

To produce conjugate horizontal eye movements, the oculomotor nerve on one side works in tandem with the abducens nerve on the other. For example, when an individual looks to the left, the left sixth nerve and right third nerve simultaneously activate the left lateral rectus and right medial rectus muscles to produce conjugate leftward eye movement. Such complementary innervation is essential for conjugate gaze. If both third nerves were simultaneously active, the eyes would look toward the nose; if both sixth nerves were simultaneously active, the eyes would look toward opposite walls.

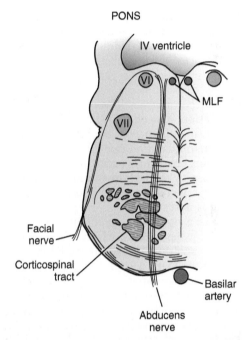

FIGURE 4.7 ■ The abducens (sixth cranial) nerves arise from nuclei located in the dorsal portion of the pons. These nuclei are adjacent to the medial longitudinal fasciculus (*MLF*; see Fig. 15.3). As the abducens nerves course ventrally, they pass medial to the facial nerves, and then between UMN neurons of the corticospinal tract.

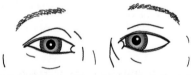

FIGURE 4.8 ■ This patient with palsy of the left abducens nerve has medial deviation of the left eye due to left lateral rectus weakness. He will have diplopia on looking ahead and toward the left, but not when looking to the right (see Fig. 12.13).

Neurologists most often attribute horizontal diplopia to a lesion affecting the oculomotor nerve on one side or the abducens nerve on the other. For example, if a patient has diplopia when looking to the left, then either the left lateral rectus or the right medial rectus is paretic. As a clue, the presence or absence of other signs of oculomotor nerve palsy (a dilated pupil and ptosis, for example) usually indicates whether that nerve is responsible.

Lesions within the brainstem, the nerves' course from the brainstem to the ocular muscles, or the neuromuscular junctions, but not in the cerebral hemispheres (the cerebrum), also weaken the extraocular muscles. Because cerebral damage does not injure the cranial nerves, patients' eyes remain conjugate despite cerebral infarctions or tumors. Even patients with advanced Alzheimer disease, ones who have sustained cerebral anoxia, and those lingering in a persistent vegetative state retain conjugate eye movement.

Similarly, in motor neuron diseases, most notably amyotrophic lateral sclerosis (ALS) and poliomyelitis, the oculomotor and abducens nerves retain normal function despite destruction of large numbers of motor neurons. Patients with motor neuron diseases may have full, conjugate eye movements despite being unable to breathe, lift their limbs, or move their head.

Because the brainstem anatomy is so compact, lesions that damage cranial nerves typically produce classic combinations of injuries of the ocular nerves and the adjacent corticospinal (pyramidal) or cerebellar outflow tracts. These lesions cause diplopia accompanied by contralateral hemiparesis or ataxia. The pattern of the diplopia localizes the lesion. The etiology in almost all cases is an occlusion of a small branch of the basilar artery causing a small brainstem infarction (see Chapter 11).

The following frequently occurring, classic brainstem syndromes, despite their pronounced physical deficits, typically do not include cognitive impairment because the cerebrum is unscathed.

Patients with a right-sided midbrain infarction have a right oculomotor nerve palsy, which causes right ptosis, a dilated pupil, and diplopia–accompanied by left hemiparesis (Fig. 4.9). With a slightly different right-sided midbrain infarction, patients have right oculomotor nerve palsy and tremor of left-sided limbs (Fig. 4.10).

A right-sided pons lesion typically translates into a right abducens nerve paresis and left hemiparesis (Fig. 4.11).

Another brainstem syndrome, which includes ocular motility impairment, results from damage to the *medial longitudinal fasciculus* (MLF). This structure is a heavily myelinated midline tract that carries fibers linking the nuclei of the abducens and oculomotor nerves (see Figs. 2.9, 4.11, 12.11, 15.3, and 15.4). Its interruption produces the *MLF syndrome*, also called *internuclear ophthalmoplegia* (INO). This classic syndrome consists of nystagmus of the abducting eye and failure of the adducting eye to cross the midline. It most often signifies MS.

The oculomotor and abducens nerves are particularly vulnerable to injury in their long paths between their brainstem nuclei and ocular muscles. Lesions in those nerves produce simple, readily identifiable clinical pictures: extraocular muscle impairment without hemiparesis, ataxia, or mental status impairment. *Diabetic infarction*, the most frequent lesion of the oculomotor nerves, produces a sharp headache and paresis of the affected muscles. Diabetic oculomotor infarctions characteristically spare the pupil. In other words, diabetic

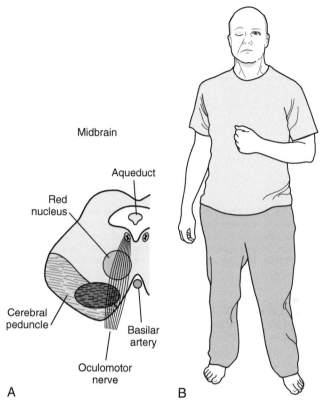

FIGURE 4.9 ■ *A,* A right midbrain infarction (red oval) damages the oculomotor nerve that supplies the ipsilateral eye and the adjacent cerebral peduncle, which contains the corticospinal tract that subsequently crosses in the medulla and ultimately controls the contralateral arm and leg. *B,* This patient has right-sided ptosis from the right oculomotor nerve palsy and left hemiparesis from the corticospinal tract injury. Also note that the ptosis elicits a compensatory unconscious elevation of the eyebrow to uncover the eye. Neurologists also see eyebrow elevation in other conditions that cause ptosis, such as the lateral medullary syndrome (Fig. 2.10), myasthenia gravis (Fig. 6.3), and cluster headache (Fig. 9.4).

infarctions cause ptosis and ocular abduction, but the pupil remains equal in size to its counterpart and normally reactive to light.

Ruptured or expanding aneurysms of the posterior communicating artery may compress the oculomotor nerve just as it exits from the midbrain. In this case, oculomotor nerve palsy – which would be the least of the patient's problems – is just one manifestation of a life-threatening subarachnoid hemorrhage. In this case, pupillary enlargement accompanies the ptosis and abduction. In a more benign condition, children occasionally have migraine headaches accompanied by temporary oculomotor nerve paresis (see Chapter 9).

Disorders of the neuromuscular junction – where the motor nerve terminal of cranial and peripheral nerves synapses with a muscle – also produce oculomotor or abducens nerve paresis. In myasthenia gravis (see Fig. 6.3) and botulism, for example, impaired acetylcholine neuromuscular transmission leads to combinations of ocular and other cranial nerve paresis. These deficits may puzzle clinicians because the muscle weakness is often subtle and variable in severity and pattern. Neurologists

MIDBRAIN

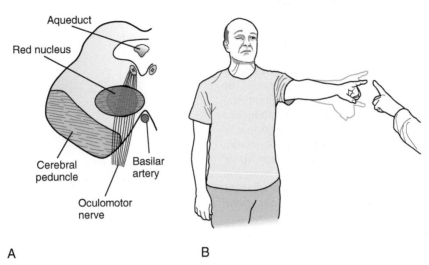

A   B

FIGURE 4.10 ■ *A*, The red nucleus is the intermediate step in conveying information from the cerebellum to the arm and leg. Each cerebellar hemisphere projects to the contralateral red nucleus which in turn, crosses back over the midline to control the contralateral arm and leg. Because this pattern involves two steps that cross the midline, neurologists often call it a "double decussation." In this case, a right midbrain infarction (red oval) damages the right oculomotor nerve and adjacent red nucleus, which governs the left arm and leg. *B*, This patient has right ptosis from the oculomotor nerve palsy and left arm ataxia from the damage to the red nucleus.

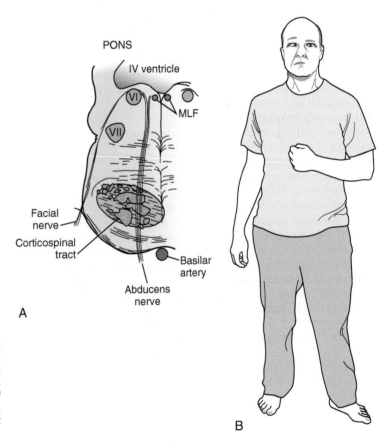

A

FIGURE 4.11 ■ *A*, A right pontine infarction (oval) damages the abducens nerve, which supplies the ipsilateral eye, and the adjacent corticospinal tract, which supplies the contralateral limbs. (The corticospinal tract involvement is analogous to that of midbrain infarctions; Fig. 4.9.) *B*, This patient has inward deviation of the right eye from paresis of the right abducens nerve, and left hemiparesis from right corticospinal tract damage.

B

may overlook mild cases or misdiagnose them as a psychogenic disorder.

A related condition, congenital dysconjugate or "crossed" eyes, *strabismus*, does not cause double vision because the brain suppresses one of the images. If uncorrected in childhood, strabismus leads to blindness of the deviated eye, *amblyopia*.

People can usually feign ocular muscle weakness only by staring inward, as if looking at the tip of their nose. Children often do this playfully; however, neurologists readily identify adults with their eyes in this position as displaying voluntary, bizarre activity. (Another disturbance, found mostly in health-care workers, comes from their surreptitiously instilling eye drops into one or both of the eyes to dilate their pupils so that they mimic ophthalmologic or neurologic disorders.)

Even though these brainstem syndromes do not impair cognitive function, others do. *Wernicke encephalopathy*, for example, consists of memory impairment (amnesia) accompanied by nystagmus and oculomotor or abducens nerve impairment (see Chapter 7). Another example is *transtentorial herniation*, in which a cerebral mass lesion, such as a subdural hematoma, forces the anterior tip or medial edge of the temporal lobe through the tentorial notch. It compresses the oculomotor nerve and adjacent brainstem to cause coma, decerebrate posturing, and a dilated pupil (see Fig. 19.3).

TRIGEMINAL (FIFTH)

In contrast to the exclusively sensory function of cranial nerves I, II, and VIII, and the exclusively motor functions of cranial nerves III, IV, VI, XI, and XII, the trigeminal nerves have both sensory and motor functions. The trigeminal (Latin, *threefold*) nerves convey sensation from the three sensory areas of the face and innervate the large, powerful muscles that protrude and close the jaw. Because these muscles' main function is to chew, neurologists often call them "muscles of mastication."

The trigeminal motor nucleus is situated in the pons, but the sensory nuclei extend from the midbrain through the medulla and into the upper spinal cord. The trigeminal nerves leave the brainstem at the side of the pons, together with the facial and acoustic nerves, to become the three cranial nerves – V, VII, and VIII – that pass through the *cerebellopontine angle*.

Examination of the trigeminal nerve begins by testing sensation in its three sensory divisions (Fig. 4.12). Neurologists touch the side of the patient's forehead, cheek, and jaw. Areas of reduced sensation, hypesthesia should conform to anatomic outlines.

Assessing the *corneal reflex* is useful, especially in examining patients whose sensory loss does not conform to neurologic expectations. The corneal reflex is a "superficial reflex" that is essentially independent of upper motor neuron (UMN) status. Its testing begins with stimulation of the cornea by a wisp of cotton or a breath of air that triggers the trigeminal nerve's V_1 division, which forms the corneal reflex's afferent limb. A brainstem synapse innervates both facial (seventh cranial) nerves, which form the efferent limb of a reflex arc. The facial nerves, which form the efferent limb, innervate both sets of orbicularis oculi muscles.

The corneal reflex – trigeminal nerves to pons to facial nerves – produces an ipsilateral direct and a contralateral consensual response, analogous to the pupillary light reflex. Stimulating one cornea will normally provoke a bilateral blink. If neurologists apply the cotton tip to the *right* cornea and *neither* eye blinks, but then applying the cotton tip to the *left* cornea prompts *both* eyes to blink, the *right trigeminal nerve* (afferent limb) is impaired. In a

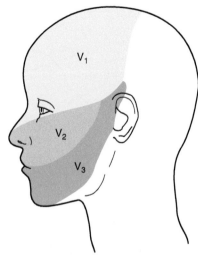

FIGURE 4.12 ■ The three divisions of the trigeminal nerve convey sensory innervation of the face. The first division (V_1) supplies the forehead, the cornea, and the scalp up to the vertex; the second (V_2) supplies the malar area; and the third (V_3) supplies the lower jaw, except for the angle. These dermatomes hold more than academic interest. Herpes zoster infections (shingles), trigeminal neuralgia (see Chapter 9), and facial angioma in the Sturge–Weber syndrome (see Fig. 13.13) each typically affect one or another dermatome. In contrast, psychogenic disturbances do not confine themselves to a single dermatome.

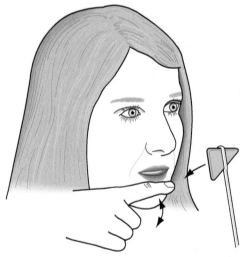

FIGURE 4.13 ■ Tapping the normal, open, relaxed jaw will move it slightly downward. The normal jaw jerk reflex is the soft rebound. Abnormalities are mostly a matter of the rebound's rapidity and strength. In a hypoactive reflex, as found in bulbar palsy and other lower motor neuron injuries, patients show little or no rebound. In a hyperactive reflex, as in pseudobulbar palsy and other upper motor neuron (corticobulbar tract) lesions, patients show a quick and forceful rebound.

different scenario, if cotton stimulation on the *right* cornea fails to provide a right eye blink, but it succeeds in provoking a *left* eye blink, the *right facial nerve* (efferent limb) is impaired.

In testing the trigeminal nerve's motor component, neurologists assess jaw muscle strength by asking the patient to clench and then protrude the jaw. The *jaw jerk reflex* consists of a prompt but not overly forceful closing after a tap (Fig. 4.13). Alterations in the response follow the rules of a deep tendon reflex. A hyperactive response indicates a UMN (corticobulbar tract) lesion, and a hypoactive response indicates a lower motor neuron (LMN) or cranial nerve lesion. The neurologist should include testing of the jaw jerk reflex in patients with dysarthria, dysphagia, and emotional lability – mostly to assess them for the likelihood of pseudobulbar palsy (see later).

Injury of a trigeminal nerve causes facial hypesthesia afferent corneal reflex impairment, jaw jerk hypoactivity, and deviation of the jaw toward the side of the lesion. A variety of conditions – nasopharyngeal tumors, gunshot wounds, and tumors of the cerebellopontine angle, such as acoustic neuromas (see Fig. 20.27) – may cause trigeminal nerve injury.

In *trigeminal neuralgia*, an aberrant vessel or other lesion in the cerebellopontine angle, MS plaques in the pons, or other disorder irritates the trigeminal nerve. Patients typically suffer lancinating jabs in the distribution of the third or less frequently the second division of the nerve (see Chapter 9). Similarly, when herpes zoster infects the trigeminal nerve, it causes a rash in the distribution of one division of the trigeminal nerve, sometimes followed by excruciating pain (*postherpetic neuralgia*) (see Chapter 14).

Finally, psychogenic sensory loss involving the face usually encompasses the entire face or the lateral half of the body, i.e., a hemisensory loss. In almost all cases, the following three nonanatomic features will be present: (1) the sensory loss will not involve the scalp (although the portion supplied by the trigeminal nerve extends to the vertex); (2) the corneal reflex will remain intact; and (3) when only one half of the face is affected, sensation will be lost sharply rather than gradually at the midline (i.e., the patient will "split the midline") rather than gradually (see Fig. 3.5).

FACIAL (SEVENTH)

The facial nerves' functions, like the trigeminal nerves' functions, are both sensory and motor: to convey taste sensation and innervate the facial muscles. Also, like the trigeminal nerves, the facial nerves' motor and sensory nuclei are situated in the pons and their nerves exit at the cerebellopontine angle.

Just as the trigeminal nerves supply the muscles of mastication, the facial nerves supply the "muscles of facial expression." In a unique and potentially confusing arrangement in their neuroanatomy, cerebral impulses innervate both the contralateral and ipsilateral facial nerve motor nuclei. Each facial nerve supplies its ipsilateral temporalis, orbicularis oculi, and orbicularis oris muscles – muscles responsible for a frown, raised eyebrows, wink, smile, and grimace. In the classic explanation, because of their crossed and uncrossed supply, the upper facial muscles are essentially innervated by both cerebral hemispheres, whereas the lower facial muscles are innervated by only the contralateral cerebral hemisphere (Fig. 4.14). A newer explanation proposes that interneurons in the brainstem link the facial nerve nuclei.

Whatever the actual underlying neuroanatomy, facial nerve injuries cause ipsilateral paresis of both upper and lower face muscles. Neurologists term this pattern a

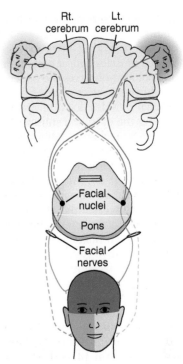

FIGURE 4.14 ■ In the classic portrayal, corticobulbar tracts originating in the ipsilateral, as well as in the contralateral, cerebral hemisphere supply each facial nerve nucleus. Each facial nerve supplies the ipsilateral muscles of facial expression. Because the upper half of the face receives cortical innervation from both hemispheres, cerebral injuries lead to paresis only of the lower half of the contralateral face. In contrast, facial nerve injuries lead to paresis of both the upper and lower half of the ipsilateral side of the face.

"peripheral facial" or "lower motor neuron weakness." In contrast, injuries of the cerebral cortex or upper brainstem, which interrupt the corticobulbar tract, cause paresis of only the lower contralateral face. Neurologists term that pattern a "central" or "upper motor neuron weakness."

Taste sensation is more straightforward. The facial nerves convey impulses from taste receptors of the anterior two-thirds of the tongue to the brainstem. The glossopharyngeal nerves (the ninth cranial nerve) convey taste information from the posterior third. A remarkable aspect of taste sensation is that, despite the extraordinary variety of foods, taste perceptions are limited. According to conventional wisdom, taste receptors detect only four fundamental sensations: bitter, sweet, sour, and salty. However, reconsideration of an idea proposed 100 years ago by a Japanese researcher confirmed that people are able to perceive a fifth taste sensation, originally labeled *umami* (Japanese, delicious flavor), that people often describe as "richness" or "savory." This taste is based on detecting L-glutamate, which is an amino acid abundant in high-protein foods and a major constituent of the flavoring monosodium glutamate (MSG). Present-day researchers have proposed that humans also taste unsaturated fats. The ions H^+, K^+, and Na^+ trigger salty and sour tastes, and G-protein receptors trigger the others.

Food actually derives most of its flavor from the aroma that the olfactory nerves detect. The olfactory nerve, not the facial nerve, conveys sensations to the frontal lobe and limbic system.

Routine facial nerve testing involves examining the strength of the facial muscles and, at certain times, assessing taste. The neurologist observes the patient's face, first at rest and then during a succession of maneuvers that employ various facial muscles: looking upward to furrow the forehead, closing the eyes, and smiling. When weakness is present, the neurologist determines whether it involves both the upper and lower, or only the lower, facial muscles. Upper and lower facial paresis suggests a lesion of the facial nerve itself. (As previously mentioned, this pattern of paresis may be termed a peripheral or LMN weakness.) In this case, the lesion also probably impairs taste sensation on the same side of the tongue.

With unilateral or even bilateral facial nerve injuries, patients have no cognitive impairment. In contrast, paresis of only the lower facial muscles suggests a lesion of the contralateral cerebral hemisphere, which may also cause hemiparesis or aphasia. As expected, weakness of the right lower face often accompanies aphasia.

To test taste, neurologists apply either a dilute salt or sugar solution to the anterior portion of each side of the tongue, which must remain protruded to prevent the solution from spreading. A patient will normally be able to identify the fundamental taste sensations, but not those "tastes" that depend on aroma, such as onion and garlic.

Facial nerve damage typically produces paresis of the ipsilateral upper and lower face muscles with or without loss of taste sensation. Sudden-onset idiopathic facial paralysis, usually with loss of taste sensation, generically labeled *Bell palsy*, has traditionally been attributed to an inflammation or infection of the nerve (Fig. 4.15). In many of these cases, herpes simplex virus has been the culprit. *Lyme disease*, due to the tick-borne spirochete *Borrelia burgdorferi*, may produce unilateral or bilateral facial weakness (see Chapters 5 and 7). Destructive injuries, including lacerations, cerebellopontine angle tumors, and carcinomatous meningitis, damage not only the facial nerve, but sometimes also its neighboring cerebellopontine angle nerves.

Lesions that stimulate the nerve have the opposite effect. For example, aberrant vessels in the cerebellopontine angle can irritate the facial nerve and produce intermittent, completely involuntary, prolonged contractions of the muscles of the ipsilateral side of the face. This disorder, *hemifacial spasm* (see Chapter 18), which casual observers might misdiagnose as a "nervous tic," represents the facial nerve counterpart of trigeminal neuralgia.

Facial nerve motor functions are essentially free of psychologic influence. People cannot mimic unilateral facial paresis. Some people, particularly children, who refuse to undergo an examination might forcefully close their eyelids and mouth. The willful nature of this strategy becomes evident when the neurologist finds resistance on opening the eyelids and jaw, and observes, when the eyelids are pried open, that the eyeballs retrovert (Bell phenomenon).

Although impairment of taste, *dysgeusia* (Greek, *geusis*, taste), usually occurs along with facial muscle weakness, as in Bell palsy and other facial nerve injuries, large brainstem lesions, such as MS plaques, may cause it. However, lesions of this size would also produce problems that would overshadow impaired taste. On the other hand, dysgeusia may develop in isolation, as when medications cause it. For example, tricyclic antidepressants, acetazolamide (for treatment of pseudotumor cerebri), and levodopa (for Parkinson disease) can diminish or distort taste. Radiotherapy directed at the head and neck causes a combination of salivary secretion loss and tongue damage.

Normal age-related changes may lead to a loss of taste sensation. Older individuals routinely lose taste sensitivity and discrimination. In addition, both age-related decrease in salivary secretions and several medications lead to "dry mouth" that markedly impairs taste function and the enjoyment of eating. Many older individuals require enhanced flavors and special preparations to make food desirable.

ACOUSTIC (EIGHTH)

Each acoustic nerve is composed of two divisions with separate courses and functions: hearing and balance. The *cochlear nerve*, one of the two divisions, transmits auditory impulses from each inner ear to the superior temporal gyri of both cerebral hemispheres (Fig. 4.16). This bilateral cortical representation of sound explains the observation that damage to an ear or only its acoustic nerve may cause deafness in that ear, but the patient will still hear sounds and speech because they pass through the other ear's acoustic nerve. The bilateral cortical representation of sound also explains why unilateral lesions of the brainstem or cerebral hemisphere do not cause deafness. For example, cerebral lesions such as tumors or strokes that involve the temporal lobes may cause aphasia and hemiparesis, but they do not impair hearing.

The neurologist simply tests hearing by whispering numbers or words into one of the patient's ears while covering the other and asking the patient to repeat them. Detailed testing requires an audiogram.

Acoustic nerve injury may result from ototoxic medications, such as aspirin or streptomycin, skull fractures' severing the nerve, or cerebellopontine angle tumors, particularly acoustic neuromas, which may be associated with neurofibromatosis (see Chapter 13). Although cognitive impairment does not generally accompany deafness, in utero rubella infections or kernicterus (see Chapter 13) commonly cause syndromes involving mental retardation and deafness. In a related situation, children with congenital hearing impairment, deprived of proper intervention, may grow-up to appear mentally retarded and have some features of autism. *Cochlear implants*, a unique, life-improving innovation, have allowed hearing-impaired infants and children to develop hearing and speaking abilities, such that most of them can enter mainstream education.

Hearing loss associated with older age, *presbycusis* (Greek, *presbys*, old man; *acusis*, hearing) affects about 25% of people older than 65 years. It typically begins with loss of high frequencies and eventually progresses to involve all frequencies. Early in its course, presbycusis impairs the

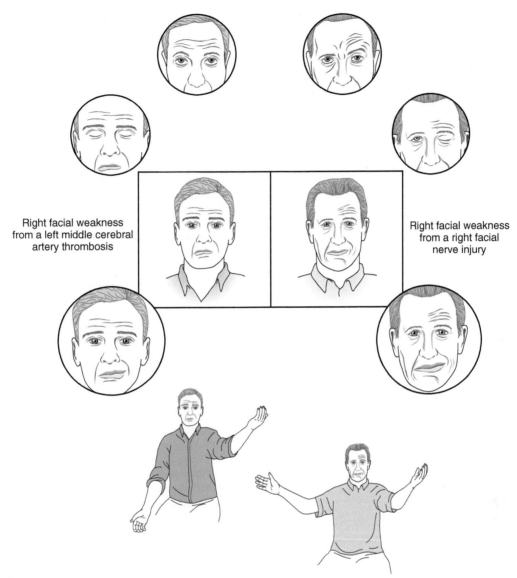

Right facial weakness from a left middle cerebral artery thrombosis

Right facial weakness from a right facial nerve injury

FIGURE 4.15 ■ The man on the left has weakness of his right lower face from thrombosis of the left middle cerebral artery: Neurologists might say that he has a "central" (CNS) facial paralysis. In contrast, the man on the right has right-sided weakness of both his upper and lower face from a right facial nerve injury (Bell palsy): Neurologists might say that he has a "peripheral" (cranial nerve) facial paralysis. In the *center boxed sketches*, the man with the central palsy (left) has flattening of the right nasolabial fold and sagging of the mouth downward to the right. This pattern of weakness indicates paresis of only the lower facial muscles. The man with the peripheral palsy (right), however, has right-sided loss of the normal forehead furrows in addition to flattening of his nasolabial fold. This pattern of weakness indicates paresis of the upper as well as the lower facial muscles. The neurologist has asked the men in the *circled sketches at the top* to look upward – a maneuver that would exaggerate upper facial weakness. The man with central weakness has normal upward movement of the eyebrows and furrowing of the forehead. The man with peripheral weakness has no eyebrow or forehead movement, and the forehead skin remains flat. The neurologist has asked the men in the *circled sketches second from the top* to close their eyes – a maneuver that also would exaggerate upper facial weakness. The man with the central weakness has very slight widening of the palpebral fissure, but he is able to close his eyelids and cover the eyeball. The man with the peripheral weakness is unable to close the affected eyelid, although his genuine effort is made apparent by the retroversion of the eyeball (Bell phenomenon). In the *lowest circled sketches* the neurologist has asked the men to smile – a maneuver that would exaggerate lower facial weakness. Both men have strength only of the left side of the mouth, and thus it deviates to the left. If tested, the man with Bell palsy would have loss of taste on the anterior two-thirds of his tongue on the affected side. The neurologist in the *bottom sketches* has asked both men to elevate their arms. The man with the central right facial weakness also has paresis of the right arm, but the man with the peripheral weakness has no arm paresis. In summary, the man on the left with the left middle cerebral artery occlusion has paresis of his right lower face and arm. The man on the right with right Bell's palsy has paresis of his right upper and lower face and loss of taste on the anterior two-thirds of his tongue.

ability to distinguish between consonants, for example, "b" and "v." One of the first and generally the most troublesome problem for individuals with presbycusis is impaired speech discrimination, especially in rooms crowded with people talking simultaneously, such as restaurants and cocktail parties. Characteristically, older individuals' inability to understand conversational speech is disproportionately greater than their hearing loss.

As with many age-related impairments, presbycusis results more from degeneration of the special sensory

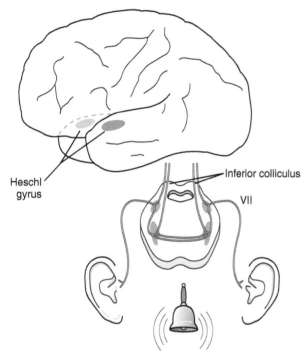

Heschl gyrus

Inferior colliculus

VII

FIGURE 4.16 ■ The cochlear division of the acoustic nerve synapses extensively in the pons. Crossed and uncrossed fibers pass upward through the brainstem to terminate in the ipsilateral and contralateral auditory (Heschl gyrus) cortex of each temporal lobe; however, Heschl gyri, which sit in the planum temporale, receive auditory stimuli predominantly from the contralateral ear. In addition, the dominant hemisphere Heschl gyrus almost abuts the Wernicke language area (see Fig. 8.1) and predictably has a major role in language function.

BOX 4.2	Age-Related Special Sense Impairments
Smell	Some degree of anosmia in 75% of individuals older than 80 years
Vision	Presbyopia: mostly inability to accommodate to see closely held or small objects; cataracts (see Chapter 12)
Taste	Loss of taste sensitivity and discrimination, as well as anosmia for aroma
Hearing	Presbyacusis: loss of speech discrimination, especially for consonants; poor high-pitched sound detection; tinnitus

organ than the cranial nerve itself (Box 4.2). In this case, the cochlear mechanism, rather than the acoustic nerve itself, deteriorates. Presbycusis potentially leads to inattention and social isolation. In addition, when hearing loss accompanies visual impairments, the resulting sensory deprivation may precipitate hallucinations. Hearing impairments no matter what their cause may also lead to misdiagnoses of apathy or dementia. For the limited problem of age-related hearing impairment in the elderly, physicians should generally dispense hearing aids readily and even on a trial basis.

Another problem for the elderly with hearing impairment consists of seeming to hear incessant ringing, buzzing, hissing, or whistling (*tinnitus*). Medications, particularly aspirin, which damage the inner ear, or ischemia,

from atherosclerotic cerebrovascular disease, may cause or exacerbate tinnitus; however, studies have not implicated psychiatric medications. If tinnitus develops unilaterally in a young or middle-aged adult, it may be a symptom of an acoustic neuroma. Otherwise, it is usually only a nuisance.

Sometimes the tinnitus is rhythmic. This variation, *pulsatile tinnitus*, while often the result of heightened sensitivity, may be a manifestation of atherosclerotic cerebrovascular disease.

When individuals feign deafness, neurologists may attempt to startle them with a loud sound or watch for an *auditory-ocular reflex* (involuntarily looking toward a noise). Neurologists wishing to confirm a diagnosis of psychogenic hearing loss may order brainstem auditory evoked response (BAER) testing (see Chapter 15). Audiometry is advisable in children with autism symptoms, cerebral palsy, intellectual disability, speech impediments, and poor school performance, as well as those suspected of having a psychogenic hearing impairment.

The other division of the acoustic nerve, the *vestibular nerve*, transmits impulses governing equilibrium, orientation, and change in position from the labyrinth to the brainstem. The signature of vestibular nerve damage is *vertigo*, a sensation of spinning within the environment or spinning of the environment itself. The most common cause of *vertigo* is vestibular injury, as from viral infections or ischemia of the inner ear (*labyrinthitis*). When vertigo is induced in an otherwise normal patient by placing the head in certain positions or merely changing positions, neurologists call the disorder *benign paroxysmal positional vertigo* (*BPPV*). One theory suggests that BPPV, which is relatively common among middle-aged and older individuals, results from free-floating stone-like debris, *otoliths*, that disturb the semicircular canals. Exercises that place the head in certain positions may alleviate the symptom, presumably by securing the offending material in innocuous places.

Ménière disease is a relatively common chronic vestibular disorder of unknown etiology that causes attacks of disabling vertigo accompanied by nystagmus – conjugate rhythmic jerking movements of the eyes – and unilateral tinnitus. More prevalent in woman than in men, it also leads to progressive hearing loss. Although most attacks of Ménière disease are obvious, they are occasionally indistinguishable from basilar artery transient ischemic attacks (TIAs), basilar artery migraines, mild hyperventilation, and BPPV.

A clinical caveat when assessing individuals who report "dizziness" is that this term encompasses lightheadedness, vertigo, anxiety, fatigue, a sense of impending doom, and a multitude of other conditions – many neither neurologic nor psychiatric. In some quarters, physicians might appropriately take "dizziness" as a *Cultural Idiom of Distress*.

GLOSSOPHARYNGEAL, VAGUS, AND SPINAL ACCESSORY NERVES (NINTH, TENTH, AND ELEVENTH)

The *bulbar* cranial nerves (IX through XII) arise from nuclei in the medulla. They innervate the muscles of the soft palate, pharynx, larynx, and tongue, and control speaking and swallowing. They also have afferent functions: the glossopharyngeal nerve brings taste sensations from the posterior third of the tongue and the vagus nerve carries autonomic nervous system impulses. The bulbar cranial nerve group is the most caudal of the three cranial nerve groups: the ocular (III, IV, and VI), cerebellopontine (V, VII, and VIII), and bulbar (IX–XII).

The medulla not only contains the nuclei and initial portions of these bulbar cranial nerves, but also several important CNS tracts, including the descending corticospinal, ascending sensory, sympathetic nervous system, and cerebellar inflow. The lateral medullary infarction, the most common brainstem stroke, illustrates the bulbar cranial nerves' relationship to these tracts (see Fig. 2.10).

Although the bulbar cranial nerves originate in the caudal end of the brainstem, located nowhere near the cerebral cortex, and execute only simple and mechanical functions, they are involved in several neurologic conditions that have psychiatric implications. For example, in *vagus nerve stimulation* for depression or epilepsy (see Chapter 10), a pacemaker-like device stimulates the vagus nerve as it ascends through the neck and terminates in the medulla's solitary nucleus. Surgeons usually attach the electrodes to the left-sided vagus nerve rather than the right-sided one to reduce the adverse cardiac effects of vagus nerve stimulation.

Bulbar Palsy

Bulbar cranial nerve injury within the brainstem or along the course of the nerves leads to *bulbar palsy*, which consists primarily of *dysarthria* (speech impairment) and *dysphagia* (swallowing impairment) (Table 4.1). An examination of bulbar palsy patients will also characteristically reveal a hypoactive jaw jerk (see Fig. 4.13) and gag reflex (Fig. 4.17). Most important, as in other conditions that strike only the brainstem or cranial nerves, neither cognitive impairment nor emotional instability is a component of bulbar palsy.

To assess bulbar nerve function, the physician should listen to the patient's spontaneous speech during casual conversation and while recounting the history. Then the patient should be asked to repeat syllables that require lingual ("la"), labial ("pa"), and guttural or pharyngeal ("ga") speech production. Most patients with bulbar palsy speak with a thick, nasal intonation. Some remain mute. Even if a patient's speech sounds normal during casual conversation, attempts at repeating a syllable with a guttural consonant, "ga…ga…ga…" will typically evoke thickened, nasal sounds, uttered "gna…gna…gna…." In addition, when saying "ah," the patient will have limited or asymmetric palate elevation because of paresis. If a brainstem lesion that causes bulbar palsy also damages the corticospinal tract, patients additionally will have limb weakness, hyperactive deep tendon reflexes (DTRs), and Babinski signs, but these signs are not part of the constellation of bulbar palsy findings.

In contrast to the dysarthria of bulbar palsy, the speech abnormality of patients with cerebellar dysfunction consists of an irregular rhythm (*scanning speech*) akin to ataxia (see Chapter 2). The speech of patients with spasmodic dysphonia has a "strained and strangled" quality, perhaps further impaired by a superimposed vocal tremor (see Chapter 18). Unlike patients with aphasia (see Chapter 8) and many of those with pseudobulbar palsy, patients with dysarthria, scanning speech, and spasmodic dysphonia have normal comprehension and can express themselves in writing or typing.

In bulbar palsy, paresis of palatal and pharyngeal muscles also causes dysphagia. Food tends to lodge in the trachea or go into the nasopharyngeal cavity. Liquids tend to regurgitate through the nose. When patients attempt to eat, they often aspirate food and saliva and remain at risk of developing aspiration pneumonia.

Finally, extensive bulbar damage will injure the medulla's respiratory center or the cranial nerves that innervate respiratory muscles. It presents a life-threatening situation. For example, the bulbar form of poliomyelitis

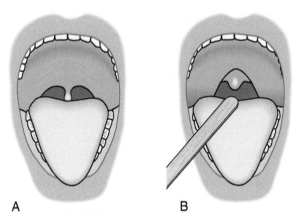

A   B

FIGURE 4.17 ■ *A,* The soft palate normally forms an arch from which the uvula seems to hang. *B,* The gag reflex consists of stimulation of the pharynx leading to pharyngeal muscle contraction. Because of the pharyngeal muscle contraction, the soft palate rises and the uvula remains in the midline. With bulbar nerve injury (bulbar palsy) – lower motor neuron injury – the palate has little, no, or asymmetric movement. With corticobulbar tract injury (pseudobulbar palsy) – upper motor neuron injury – the reaction is brisk and forceful. Unfortunately, the gag reflex often precipitates retching, coughing, or crying. (If the purpose of the examination is to assess the patient's ability to swallow, the neurologist might simply observe the patient swallow a few sips of water.)

TABLE 4.1	Comparison of Bulbar and Pseudobulbar Palsy	
	Bulbar	**Pseudobulbar**
Dysarthria	Yes	Yes
Dysphagia	Yes	Yes
Movement of palate		
Voluntary	No	No
Gag reflex	Hypoactive	Hyperactive
Jaw jerk	Hypoactive	Hyperactive
Respiratory impairment	Yes	No
Emotional lability	No	Yes
Intellectual impairment	No	Yes

(polio) forced its childhood victims into "iron lungs" to support their respiration. Even today, many patients with Guillain–Barré syndrome, myasthenia gravis, ALS, and similar conditions develop bulbar palsy that forces them to undergo tracheal intubation, tracheostomy, and mechanical ventilation.

Illnesses that commonly cause bulbar palsy by damaging the cranial nerves within the brainstem are ALS, poliomyelitis, and lateral medullary infarction. Those that damage the nerves after they have emerged from the brainstem include Guillain–Barré syndrome, chronic meningitis, and tumors that grow along the base of the skull or within the adjacent meninges. In contrast, myasthenia gravis, botulism, and several nerve agents (poison gases) cause bulbar palsy by impairing neuromuscular junction transmission (see Chapter 6).

Pseudobulbar Palsy

When cerebral damage, rather than brainstem damage, causes dysarthria and dysphagia, neurologists label the condition *pseudobulbar palsy*. Psychiatrists are more apt to encounter patients with pseudobulbar palsy than bulbar palsy because of its prominent neuropsychologic manifestation – unprovoked episodes of emotional outbursts. In addition, because the underlying lesion usually involves both frontal lobes and perhaps even more of the cerebrum, aphasia and dementia often complicate the picture.

Speech with a variable rhythm and intensity that is intermittently "explosive" characterizes the dysarthria of pseudobulbar palsy. For example, when neurologists ask pseudobulbar patients to repeat the syllable "ga," they typically blurt out "GA... GA... GA... ga... ga... GA." The dysphagia of pseudobulbar palsy often leads to aspiration and inadequate nutrition. Installing a gastrostomy tube may be required to help provide nutrition, but it does not prevent aspiration.

Similar to patients with bulbar palsy, those with pseudobulbar palsy have little or no palatal or pharyngeal movement in response to voluntary effort, as when attempting to say "ah." What separates these conditions is that in pseudobulbar palsy the gag reflex causes a brisk and forceful elevation of the palate, rapid contraction of the pharynx, and often coughing, crying, and retching (see Fig. 4.17). Hyperactivity of the jaw jerk typically accompanies hyperactivity of the gag reflex in pseudobulbar palsy (Fig. 4.18).

In pseudobulbar palsy, frontal lobe damage also leads to corticobulbar tract damage that makes the face sag and impairs expression (Fig. 4.19). Accompanying corticospinal tract damage leads to signs of bilateral corticospinal tract damage, such as hyperactive DTRs and Babinski signs.

Although the physical manifestations of pseudobulbar palsy are crucial, the most conspicuous feature of pseudobulbar palsy is the emotional lability. Pseudobulbar palsy patients tend to burst into tears or, less often, laugh, but not in response to an underlying change in their mood. Sometimes seeming to be awash with emotions, these patients appear to alternate between inexplicable euphoria and depression. Neurologists refer to their unprovoked

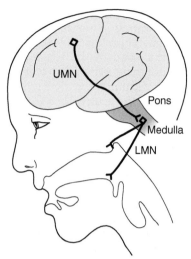

FIGURE 4.18 ■ As with damage to other lower motor neurons, damage to the bulbar cranial nerves in bulbar palsy abolishes the jaw jerk and gag reflexes. By way of contrast, in pseudobulbar palsy, upper motor neuron damage in the corticobulbar tract leads to hyperactivity of these reflexes (see Fig. 2.2).

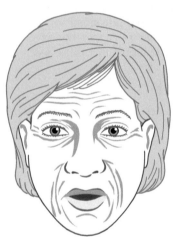

FIGURE 4.19 ■ Patients with pseudobulbar palsy, such as this woman who has sustained multiple cerebral infarctions, often remain with slack jaw, furrowed forehead, and vacant stare.

emotional expressions as *pathologic laughing and crying*, *pseudobulbar affect*, or *involuntary emotional expression disorder*. Amitriptyline, selective serotonin reuptake inhibitors, or a combination of dextromethorphan and quinidine (Nuedexta) reportedly suppresses this behavior.

Physicians should not automatically ascribe easy tearfulness, sadness, or laughter to pseudobulbar palsy. They should appreciate that neurologic illness causes a great deal of true sadness and inappropriate emotions. If carefully examined, physicians may find, for example, that their patients have both depression and pseudobulbar palsy. They may also find comorbid dementia and, if the left cerebral hemisphere is heavily damaged, aphasia, usually of the nonfluent variety (see Chapter 8).

A wide variety of structural lesions and neurodegenerative disorders that damage the frontal lobes or the entire cerebrum may cause pseudobulbar palsy. Multiple cerebral infarctions, traumatic brain injury, MS, Alzheimer disease, and frontotemporal dementia comprise the most common causes. In a special case, congenital cerebral injury (i.e., cerebral palsy) may cause pseudobulbar palsy along with bilateral spasticity and choreoathetosis. And because ALS causes both UMN and LMN damage, this illness leads to a mixture of bulbar and pseudobulbar palsy.

HYPOGLOSSAL (TWELFTH)

The hypoglossal nerves originate from paired nuclei near the midline of the medulla and descend through the base of the medulla (see Fig. 2.9). They pass through the skull and travel down to innervate the tongue muscles. Each nerve innervates the ipsilateral tongue muscles. These muscles move the tongue within the mouth, protrude it, and push it to the contralateral side. With equal muscle innervation, each side's strength is balanced and the tongue sits or protrudes in the midline.

If one hypoglossal nerve is injured that side of the tongue will become weak and, with time, atrophic. When protruded, the partly weakened tongue deviates toward the weak side (Fig. 4.20). The ipsilateral deviation illustrates the adage, "the tongue points toward the side of the lesion." If both nerves are injured, as in bulbar palsy, the tongue will become immobile. ALS patients have tongue fasciculations as well as weakness and atrophy due to loss of neurons in the hypoglossal nucleus (see Fig. 5.10).

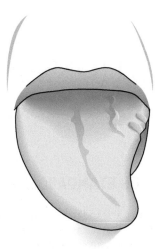

FIGURE 4.20 ■ With left hypoglossal nerve damage, the tongue deviates toward the weaker side and its affected left side demonstrates atrophy and fasciculations.

The most frequently occurring conditions that damage a hypoglossal nerve are penetrating neck wounds and nasopharyngeal tumors. Guillain–Barré syndrome, myasthenia gravis, and ALS usually impair tongue movement bilaterally. However, no matter the severity of the dysarthria and dysphagia, these conditions do not cause cognitive impairment.

QUESTIONS AND ANSWERS

PREPARING FOR STANDARDIZED TESTS

When studying for a standardized test, particularly the one offered by the American Board of Psychiatry and Neurology (APBN), many psychiatrists rely on *Clinical Neurology for Psychiatrists*. This book presents well-illustrated neurologic clinical and pathologic information for those examinations. It reinforces the material with question-and-answers sections in most chapters and at the conclusion of the book. Studies have shown that completing question-and-answer exercises remains the most efficient test preparation strategy. With that in mind, we offer several guidelines:

1. Try to extract the question's underlying idea even if it does not explicitly state one.
2. Read each question twice, reword unclear questions, and chose the simplest answer. Test-takers often answer incorrectly because they have misread the question.
3. Mentally underline key words and phrases, such as "never," "all of the following except," and "always." Because these terms often define the question, rereading the question based on them may clarify it.
4. Test-takers can usually simplify potential answers to bite-sized "yes–no" or "true–false" statements. To give an example of this and the previous point: If the question asks, "Which of the following symptoms is never a feature of disease X?" the test-taker might approach the question as, "Is *a* ever a feature of X?" "Is *b* ever a feature of X?" "Is *c* ever a feature of X?"
5. Narrow the choices as much as possible and then select the answer with the greatest likelihood of being correct. Even if the test-graders enact a penalty for incorrect answers, the odds remain in favor of the test-taker who eliminates even a single incorrect answer.
6. When approaching a lengthy question, read the question's introductory material, but concentrate on the last sentence because it typically contains the question. The test-taker might ask, "What do they want from me?" The following is an example of a typical time-consuming, misleading, and potentially frustrating question that initially hides the main idea: "Bus fare is $2, and the cost of a transfer $1. A bus begins its route with five passengers. At North Street, three additional passengers buy a ticket and board and two depart. At Mechanic Street, eight buy a ticket and board and three depart. One purchases a transfer before leaving, two buy a ticket and board, and five depart when the bus stops at Tulip Street. How many times did the bus stop?"
7. Individuals should practice sitting in isolation for stretches of 2 to 3 hours while answering series of questions. Prospective test-takers should build up their physical and mental endurance until they can spend 9 straight hours, except for a 1-hour lunch and brief breaks between test blocks, answering question after question.
8. Candidates for the ABPN and other standardized tests should form study groups that meet on a weekly basis. They can review confusing, uninteresting, or new material, as well as commiserate.

QUESTIONS AND ANSWERS: CHAPTERS 1–4

1–7: Match the description with the visual field pattern (a–f):

1. Right homonymous hemianopia
2. Bilateral superior nasal quadrantanopia
3. Right homonymous superior quadrantanopia
4. Blindness of the right eye
5. Left homonymous superior quadrantanopia
6. Bilateral inferior nasal quadrantanopia
7. Visual field deficit produced by a protuberant nose

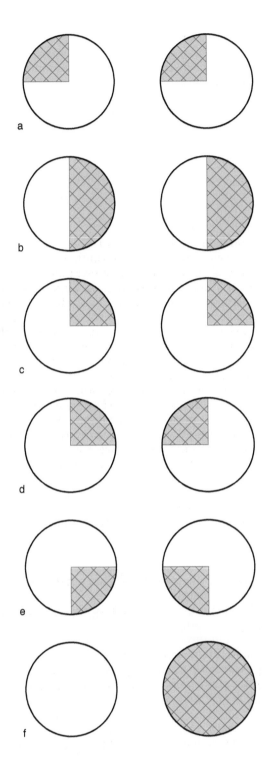

Answers: 1–b, 2–d, 3–c, 4–f, 5–a, 6–e, 7–e.

8. A 68-year-old man has sudden, painless onset of paresis of the right upper and lower face, inability to abduct the right eye, and paresis of the left arm and leg. Where is the lesion?
   a. Cerebrum (cerebral hemispheres)
   b. Cerebellum
   c. Midbrain
   d. Pons
   e. Medulla
   f. None of the above

Answer: d. The damaged structures include the right-sided abducens (VI) and facial (VII) nerves and the corticospinal tract destined to supply the left limbs, which are on the right side of the brainstem above the lower medulla. The corticospinal tract has a long course. An injury anywhere above the cervical spinal cord would produce a hemiparesis; however, cranial nerves VI and VII originate in the pons and travel a short course to leave the brainstem. A small lesion, such as a stroke, in the right side of the pons would damage all three of these structures. (If the lesion pictured in Fig. 4.11 extended slightly more laterally, it would create these deficits.)

9. An elderly man has left ptosis and a dilated and unreactive left pupil with external deviation of the left eye; right hemiparesis; right-sided hyperactive deep tendon reflexes (DTRs); and a right-sided Babinski sign. He does not have either aphasia or hemianopia. Where is the lesion?
   a. Cerebrum
   b. Cerebellum
   c. Midbrain
   d. Pons
   e. Medulla
   f. None of the above

Answer: c. Because the patient has a left oculomotor (III) nerve palsy and right hemiparesis, the lesion must be in the left midbrain. As in the previous question, the right hemiparesis may originate in corticospinal tract damage anywhere along its long course. Its presence has relatively limited localizing value. His left oculomotor nerve palsy must originate in the midbrain or the nerve's course between the brainstem and the orbit. The intersection of the corticospinal tract and oculomotor nerve is the midbrain (see Fig. 4.9.) The absence of aphasia and hemianopia exonerates the left cerebral cortex.

10. A 32-year-old waitress with multiple sclerosis (MS) developed a wide-based, lurching, unsteady gait; bilateral horizontal nystagmus; and slurred speech with variable cadence and volume. Which is the term that neurologists would use to describe her speech?
    a. Scanning
    b. Strained and strangled
    c. Aphasic
    d. Stuttering

Answer: a. Her flare-up of MS is centered in her cerebellum and adjacent structures. The cerebellar dysfunction is causing scanning speech. Strained and strangled speech is indicative of spasmodic dysphonia. Although dysarthria is sometimes comorbid, aphasia is a disturbance of language (a cognitive function) and dysarthria is a disturbance of speech (a motor function). Stuttering is usually a developmental speech disturbance characterized by impaired fluency, with blocks and repetitions of consonants.

11. A 20-year-old professional ice-skater reports having lost all vision in her right eye, right hemiparesis, and a right hemisensory loss. Her pupillary light reflexes

and DTRs are normal. During an examination, she does not press down with her left leg while attempting to lift her right leg. Where is the lesion?
a. Cerebrum
b. Cerebellum
c. Midbrain
d. Pons
e. Medulla
f. None of the above

Answer: f. No single lesion can explain all the symptoms. Her symptoms have no objective signs to confirm them. Moreover, she fails to exert maximum effort with one leg while "trying" to lift the other against resistance (Hoover sign, see Chapter 3). Neurologists would probably order various tests to exclude multiple sclerosis (MS) and other illnesses that may cause multifocal symptoms.

12. A 50-year-old woman describes having many years of gait impairment and right-sided decreased hearing. Lightly touching the right cornea elicits no response, while lightly touching the left cornea elicits a direct corneal reflex but not an indirect (consensual) one. Auditory acuity is diminished on the right. She has left-sided hyperactive DTRs with a Babinski sign, and right-sided dysdiadochokinesia. Which structures are impaired?
a. Optic nerves
b. Cerebellopontine angle structures
c. Extraocular motor nerves
d. Bulbar cranial nerves
e. None of the above

Answer: b. The right-sided corneal reflex loss, facial weakness, and hearing impairment reflect damage to the trigeminal (V), facial (VII), and acoustic (VIII) cranial nerves. These nerves emerge together from the brainstem at the cerebellopontine angle. In addition, right-sided dysdiadochokinesia reflects right-sided cerebellar damage. The left-sided hyperactive DTRs with a Babinski sign are referable to compression of the corticospinal tract in the right side of the pons. Common cerebellopontine lesions are meningiomas and acoustic neuromas, which are often manifestations of the NF2 variant of neurofibromatosis.

13. A 60-year-old man has mid-back pain, paraparesis with spasticity and hyperreflexia, loss of sensation below the umbilicus, and incontinence. Where is the spinal lesion?
a. C7
b. T4
c. T10
d. L1
e. S2

Answer: c. The lesion, which causes spastic leg weakness and other signs of upper motor neuron (UMN) injury, is located in the thoracic spinal cord at the T10 level. (The umbilicus is the landmark for T10 [see Fig. 2.16].)

14. After a minor motor vehicle crash, a young man describes having visual loss, paralysis of his legs, and loss of sensation to pin and position below the waist; however, sensation of warm versus cold remains intact. He can only see an area of 2 m² at a distance of one foot and a distance of 20 feet. He is unable to raise his legs or walk. He has brisk DTRs, but his plantar responses are flexor. Where is his lesion?
a. C7
b. T4
c. T10
d. L1
e. S2
f. None of the above

Answer: f. Many features of the examination indicate that the basis of his symptoms and signs is not from injury to his nervous system: (1) the constant area (2 m²) of visual loss at both distances – "tunnel vision" – is contrary to the optics of vision, in which vision encompasses an increasingly larger area at greater distances from the eye (see Fig. 12.7); (2) the loss of pin sensation is inconsistent with preservation of warm versus cold sensation because the spinothalamic tract transmits both pain and temperature sensory information; and (3) despite his apparent paraparesis, the normal plantar response indicates that both the UMNs and lower motor neurons (LMNs) are intact. His DTRs are brisk because of anxiety.

15. Where in the CNS do the vagus nerves' afferent fibers terminate?
a. Diencephalon
b. Midbrain
c. Pons
d. Medulla

Answer: d. The vagus nerves' afferent fibers originate in the thoracic and abdominal viscera. They travel upward through the neck to terminate in the medulla. From there, neurons project to more rostral portions of the brainstem and throughout the cerebral cortex. Surgeons must know the course of the vagus nerves' ascending fibers, particularly the left-sided vagus nerve in the neck, to implant stimulators in the nerve for the treatment of depression and epilepsy.

16. Physicians find that a 55-year-old woman, who has had increasing severe depressive symptoms for 3 years, has right-sided optic atrophy and left-sided papilledema. Where is the lesion?
a. Frontal lobe
b. Parietal lobe
c. Occipital lobe
d. Temporal lobe

Answer: a. This woman has the classic Foster–Kennedy syndrome. In her case, a right frontal lobe tumor probably compresses the underlying right optic nerve, causing optic atrophy. The tumor also increases intracranial pressure, which causes papilledema of the left optic nerve. If the physicians had tested her sense of smell, they would have found that she has anosmia on her right side.

17. After enjoying excellent health except for hypertension, a 65-year-old man becomes distraught when he develops erectile dysfunction. A neurologic examination reveals that he has orthostatic hypotension and lightheadedness, but no other abnormalities. Which neurologic system is most likely impaired?
    a. Cerebrum only
    b. The entire CNS
    c. Autonomic nervous system
    d. The cerebrum and the spinal cord's posterior columns

Answer: c. Erectile dysfunction accompanied by orthostatic hypotension is most likely to be the result of autonomic nervous system dysfunction. In this patient, the erectile dysfunction may be medication-induced. Men taking tamsulosin (Flomax), which selectively antagonizes α-1a adrenergic receptors, along with antihypertensives risk orthostatic hypotension severe enough to cause syncope. Giving sildenafil (Viagra), which inhibits phosphodiesterase, may ameliorate the erectile dysfunction but intensify the orthostatic hypotension.

18. During a 2-week period, a 60-year-old man with carcinoma of the right upper lobe of his lung develops lumbar spine pain, weak and areflexic legs, loss of sensation below the knees, and urinary and fecal incontinence. Where is the lesion?
    a. Cerebrum
    b. Brainstem
    c. Spinal cord
    d. Peripheral nervous system

Answer: d. The lumbar spine pain and absent lower-extremity DTRs indicate that the lesion is in his cauda equina. This structure is composed of lumbosacral nerve roots, which are LMNs and therefore part of the peripheral nervous system.

19. The man in Question 18 then develops a flaccid, areflexic paresis of the right arm and right-sided miosis (constricted pupil) and ptosis. Where is that lesion?
    a. Cerebrum
    b. Brainstem
    c. Spinal cord
    d. Peripheral nervous system

Answer: d. The tumor in the right upper lung has now grown to involve his right brachial plexus and adjacent sympathetic fibers. Tumor infiltration of the sympathetic fibers has caused Horner syndrome. Computed tomography (CT) of the chest will usually reveal an upper lobe lung (Pancoast) tumor.

20. Of the following, which *two* structures comprise the posterior columns of the spinal cord?
    a. Spinocerebellar tract
    b. Fasciculus cuneatus
    c. Fasciculus gracilis
    d. Posterior horn cells
    e. Lateral spinothalamic tract

Answers: b, c. The fasciculus cuneatus carries position and vibration sensations from the upper extremities and the fasciculus gracilis carries those sensations from the lower extremities.

21. Of the structures listed in Question 20, which one carries temperature sensation?

Answer: e. The lateral spinothalamic tract carries pain and temperature sensations.

22. A 40-year-old man has interscapular spine pain, paraparesis with hyperactive DTRs, bilateral Babinski signs, and complete sensory loss below his nipples. Where is the lesion?
    a. C7
    b. T4
    c. T10
    d. L1

Answer: b. The lesion clearly affects the spinal cord at the T4 level because the nipples represent the T4 landmark. Common causes include benign lesions (such as a herniated thoracic intervertebral disk), tumors (epidural metastatic tumor and meningioma), infection (abscess or tuberculoma), and inflammation (MS). Although human immunodeficiency virus (HIV) infection may involve the spinal cord, it does not produce such a discrete lesion; however, complications of HIV infection, such as lymphoma, may create a mass lesion that compresses the spinal cord. Neurologists order magnetic resonance imaging (MRI), when possible, to diagnose lesions affecting the spinal cord.

23. Which cranial nerves are covered totally or partly by CNS-generated myelin?
    a. Optic and acoustic
    b. Facial, acoustic, and trigeminal
    c. Bulbar
    d. All

Answer: a. CNS-generated myelin covers the optic and a small, proximal portion of the acoustic cranial nerves.

24. An elderly, hypertensive man develops vertigo, nausea, and vomiting. He has right-sided Horner syndrome, loss of right corneal reflex, and dysarthria because of paresis of the palate. Examination also shows that his right face, left limbs, and left side of the trunk have hypalgesia. Which way does the uvula deviate?
    a. Right
    b. Left
    c. Up
    d. Down

Answer: b. The patient has a right-sided lateral medullary (Wallenberg) syndrome (see Fig 2.10). This syndrome includes crossed hypalgesia (right face and left "body" pinprick loss, in this case), ipsilateral ataxia, and ipsilateral palate weakness. His uvula deviates to the left because of right-sided palatal muscle weakness. Because the cerebrum is spared in this condition, patients do not have cognitive impairment or physical signs of cerebral damage, such as visual field cuts or seizures.

25. In her last trimester of a normal pregnancy, a 28-year-old physician developed pain in her lower back. Immediately before delivery, the pain spread down her right antero-lateral thigh. That quadriceps muscle was slightly weak and its DTR was hypoactive. Two weeks after delivery of a healthy 10-pound baby girl, all signs and symptoms resolved. Which of the following was the most likely diagnosis?
    a. Endometriosis
    b. Compression of the lateral femoral cutaneous nerve (meralgia paresthetica)
    c. Compression of the lumbosacral plexus or femoral nerve
    d. Multiple sclerosis

Answer: c. An enlarged uterus often compresses the lumbosacral plexus or the origin of the femoral nerve. Meralgia paresthetica, which results from nerve compression in the inguinal region, is painful but not associated with weakness or DTR loss. Herniated disks occur in pregnancy because of weight gain, hyperlordosis, and laxity of ligaments; however, sciatica usually causes low back pain that radiates to the posterior portion of the leg. The presence and distribution of the pain, as well as hypoactive DTRs, exclude multiple sclerosis.

26. Where is the primary damage in Wilson disease, Huntington chorea, and choreiform cerebral palsy?
    a. Pyramidal system
    b. Extrapyramidal system
    c. Entire CNS
    d. Cerebellar outflow tracts

Answer: b. These diseases, like Parkinson disease, damage the basal ganglia – a fundamental part of the extrapyramidal motor system. Basal ganglia dysfunction may cause tremor, chorea, athetosis, rigidity, bradykinesia, and other involuntary movements. In contrast, corticospinal (pyramidal) tract dysfunction causes weakness, spasticity, DTR hyperreflexia, clonus, and Babinski signs.

27. Which one of the following is not a "frontal release" reflex?
    a. Snout reflex
    b. Rooting reflex
    c. Cremasteric reflex
    d. Palmomental reflex
    e. Grasp reflex
    f. Suck reflex

Answer: c. The frontal release reflexes involve the face (snout, suck, and rooting reflexes), jaw (jaw jerk), and palm (palmomental and grasp reflexes). Almost all frontal release signs are normally present in infants.

Depending on their context, the presence of several frontal release reflexes suggests a congenital cerebral injury, frontal lobe damage, or neurodegenerative condition. In contrast, Babinski signs and clonus are reliable signs of corticospinal tract damage. The parachute and Moro reflexes are normal responses to change in position or posture in infants. The cremasteric and anal reflexes are normally occurring superficial reflexes that depend on the integrity of the nerves of the lumbosacral plexus and the CNS.

28. A 30-year-old Marine, who already carried the diagnoses of *major neurocognitive disorder due to traumatic brain injury (TBI)* and posttraumatic epilepsy, began to laugh uncontrollably at small jokes or minor incidents, and then switch between laughter and crying. He would also cry with little or no provocation, and switch back and forth between crying and laughing. Which is the most appropriate term for his behavior?
    a. Posttraumatic stress disorder (PTSD)
    b. Emotional lability
    c. Delirium
    d. Depressive disorder

Answer: b. When minor events provoke outbursts of laughter and crying that inexplicably switch back and forth neurologists call the behavior *emotional lability*.

29. When a neurologist examined the patient in the previous question, she found that he had dysarthria, mild spastic quadriparesis, and moderately severe cognitive impairment. To which condition would the neurologist most likely ascribe his emotional lability?
    a. Bulbar palsy
    b. Pseudobulbar palsy
    c. Major neurocognitive disorder due to traumatic brain injury

Answer: b. The dysarthria, which would undoubtedly be accompanied by dysphagia, and the corticospinal tract signs (spastic quadriparesis) indicate that his emotional lability is attributable to frontal lobe damage. Some of the features – the dysarthria and the corticospinal tract signs – could have reflected a lower brainstem (bulbar) injury; however, the combination of emotional lability and cognitive impairment indicates involvement of both frontal lobes.

30. Further neurologic testing of this patient would likely reveal all of the following neurologic signs except which one?
    a. Hyperactive jaw jerk
    b. Hyperactive gag reflex
    c. Hoover sign
    d. Grasp reflex

Answer: c. Hyperactive jaw jerk and gag reflexes are hallmarks of pseudobulbar palsy and reflect corticobulbar damage, i.e., upper motor neuron damage. The presence of a grasp reflex, which is normal in infants, is a manifestation of frontal lobe damage in an adult. The presence of grasp and sucking reflexes is also normal in infants but pathologic in adults. Hoover sign indicates psychogenic weakness.

31. On his third postoperative day after cardiac surgery, a 78-year-old man was found to have no movement of his left arm or leg. Not only did he seem oblivious to the apparent left hemiparesis, the patient did not seem to care about it when his family and physicians pointed it out to him. What is the best description of the patient's response?
    a. *La belle indifférence*
    b. Apathy
    c. Anosognosia
    d. Depression

    Answer: c. This patient is unaware of his deficit. He has sustained a nondominant cerebral hemisphere stroke that caused his left hemiparesis and hemi-inattention, denial, or other neuropsychologic sequelae. Physicians may encounter patients with seeming indifference, *la belle indifférence*, to deficits; however, this is neither a sign nor criterion of conversion disorder. Physicians may find it in patients with Anton syndrome, frontal lobe injury, and, as in this case, nondominant hemisphere syndromes, but not in most cases of conversion disorder.

32. Which of the following is one of the criteria for conversion disorder?
    a. Recent psychologic stress
    b. Significant distress or impairment in an important area of functioning
    c. *La belle indifférence*
    d. Secondary gain

    Answer: b. The criteria for conversion disorder include a symptom or deficit that "causes significant distress or impairment in social, occupational, or other important area of functioning or warrants medical evaluation." However, recent psychologic stress and other precipitant are no longer criteria. Both *la belle indifférence* and secondary gain are too nonspecific and too inconsistent to be signs or criteria of conversion disorder.

33. When examining a 25-year-old waitress who presented with sudden onset of inability to move her left arm and leg, a neurologist found that she was unable to raise (flex) her left leg while lying supine, but when raising her right leg against resistance, she pushed down (extended) her left leg. Which is the name for this sign?
    a. Hoover
    b. Babinski
    c. Lasègue
    d. Romberg

    Answer: a. The physician found a Hoover sign, which relies on demonstrating the natural downward exertion (extension) of one leg while raising (flexing) the other (see Fig. 3.2). The Hoover sign is highly sensitive and specific for psychogenic weakness. A Lasègue sign (see Fig. 5.13) indicates lumbosacral nerve root irritation, usually from a herniated intervertebral disc. A Babinski sign indicates corticospinal tract injury. A Romberg sign indicates loss of position sense, usually from a peripheral neuropathy or, classically, posterior spinal cord damage.

34. Which of the following is not a taste perceived by humans?
    a. L-glutamate
    b. Umami
    c. Success
    d. Sweet
    e. Sour
    f. Salty

    Answer: c. Umami, which is perception of L-glutamate, lends food a "rich" taste. It has joined the four basic tastes: sweet, salty, sour, and bitter.

35. Dilation of the pupil is a common finding in patients in transtentorial herniation with compression of the ipsilateral oculomotor cranial nerve (see Fig. 19.3). What is the explanation for this finding?
    a. Sympathetic fibers, traveling with this cranial nerve, are damaged by compression.
    b. Parasympathetic fibers, traveling with this cranial nerve, are damaged by compression.
    c. Compression of the temporal lobe through the tentorial notch causes the pupil dilation.
    d. None of the above

    Answer: b. Compression damages the parasympathetic fibers traveling with the third cranial nerve. The unopposed sympathetic fibers dilate the pupil.

36. After campus police bring an incoherent, agitated college student to the emergency room, the physicians see that he is wearing only light, indoor clothing despite freezing outdoor temperatures. He seems oblivious to frostbite on his nose and fingertips. He is hypervigilant and possibly hallucinatory, but disoriented and completely uncooperative to examination. The physicians could determine only that he has pronounced vertical and horizontal (three-directional or multidirectional) and rotatory nystagmus. Which is the most likely intoxicant?
    a. Phenytoin (Dilantin)
    b. Vodka
    c. Heroin
    d. Phencyclidine (PCP)

    Answer: d. Nystagmus is a component of many but not all intoxication syndromes. The presence or absence of a rotatory component and accompanying physical and psychological features helps distinguish them. In the Wernicke–Korsakoff syndrome and phenytoin intoxication nystagmus is rarely rotatory. More important, amnesia and ataxia characterize the Wernicke–Korsakoff syndrome and a depressed level of consciousness characterizes phenytoin intoxication. Heroin intoxication causes stupor, respiratory depression, and small pupils, but not nystagmus. Unlike other common intoxication syndromes, those caused by PCP, because it is an anesthetic agent, produce insensitivity to pain and cold as well as an agitated delirium. Its hallmark is prominent multidirectional or rotatory nystagmus.

37. Which CNS area is most susceptible to permanent damage from a toxic serum concentration of lithium?
    a. Basal ganglia
    b. Cerebellum
    c. Spinal cord
    d. Cerebral cortex

Answer: b. Whether administered as treatment for cluster headache, bipolar disorder, or another condition, lithium at therapeutic levels causes tremor. At toxic levels, it may cause cerebellar damage and diabetes insipidus.

38. A 72-year-old edentulous man began using a denture cream containing zinc. After 1 year, he developed a stiff gait. Neither he nor any family member had any history of neurologic illness. A neurologist found that he had spastic paraparesis with hyperactive DTRs and bilateral Babinski signs. Which term would the neurologist use to describe his impediment?
    a. Myelopathy
    b. Neuropathy
    c. Ataxia
    d. Apraxia

Answer: a. Although bilateral deep cerebral or bifrontal lesions are occasionally the cause of spastic paraparesis, spinal cord injury (myelopathy) is the most common. Among older individuals and those in certain occupations, cervical spondylosis that compresses the cervical spinal cord is the most common cause of myelopathy. Among young adults, MS, trauma, and congenital injuries are the most common causes.

39. Further testing of the patient in the previous question found normal results of MRIs of the patient's head and cervical spine, vitamin B_{12}, syphilis, HTLV-1, and other routine tests, but an abnormal serum copper concentration. Which was the most likely abnormality?
    a. Elevated serum copper concentration
    b. Decreased serum copper concentration
    c. Elevated serum mercury concentration
    d. An absent serum ceruloplasmin concentration

Answer: b. Individuals who use certain zinc-containing denture creams or supplement their diet with large quantities of minerals may absorb large quantities of zinc. Excessive intake of zinc from any source results in decreased copper absorption in the gut. Low serum copper concentrations cause myelopathy. Ceruloplasmin is a copper-carrying protein. Its concentration is low or absent in Wilson disease.

40. A 65-year-old neurologist was attending a party when a colleague described a patient with "PD" (Parkinson disease); however, he thought that she had said "TD" (tardive dyskinesia) and proceeded to discuss iatrogenic illness. When speaking directly with someone in a quiet room, he could hear clearly; however, even then, he conceded that he was unable to distinguish consonants. Which of the following is most likely to be the explanation of the neurologist's problem?
    a. Aphasia
    b. Normal age-related presbycusis
    c. Mild cognitive impairment
    d. An acoustic neuroma

Answer: b. His hearing impairment is normal age-related presbycusis, which typically begins with loss of high-frequency hearing and inability to distinguish between consonants. Individuals with presbycusis characteristically describe impaired speech discrimination in rooms with many people speaking (competing conversations), but not in one-to-one talks. Elderly individuals with hearing impairment often withdraw. They may appear depressed or, because they frequently misunderstand, cognitively impaired.

41. Three months after a young man sustained a closed head injury, he has insomnia, fatigue, cognitive impairment, and personality changes. He also reports that food is tasteless. What is the most specific origin of his symptoms?
    a. PTSD
    b. Frontal lobe, head, and neck trauma
    c. Focal seizures
    d. Frontal lobe and olfactory nerve trauma

Answer: d. He probably has had a contusion of both frontal lobes that resulted in changes in behavior, sleep, cognition, and personality. In addition, he has anosmia from having sheared the thin olfactory nerve fibers in their passage through the cribriform plate. He may, of course, also suffer from PTSD. In fact, the comorbidity of PTSD and mild TBI is about 50%.

42. A middle-aged woman has increasing blindness in her right eye, where the visual acuity is 20/400 and the optic disc is white. The right pupil does not react either directly or consensually to light. The left pupil reacts directly, although not consensually. All motions of the right eye are impaired. In which area is the lesion?
    a. Neuromuscular junction
    b. Orbit
    c. Retro-orbital structures
    d. Cerebrum

Answer: c. The cause of her right-sided impaired visual acuity, optic atrophy, and loss of the direct light reflex with loss of the indirect (consensual) light reflex in the left eye is right-sided optic nerve damage. In addition, the loss of a consensual light reflex in the right eye is a sign of right oculomotor nerve injury. Her complete extraocular muscle paresis also indicates oculomotor, trochlear, and abducens nerve damage. A lesion located immediately behind the orbit, such as a sphenoid wing meningioma, would damage all these nerves. Neuromuscular junction diseases do not cause optic atrophy.

43. Which condition impairs pupils' constriction to light but allows them to constrict to accommodation?
    a. Psychogenic disturbances
    b. Oculomotor nerve injury
    c. Optic nerve injury
    d. Argyll–Robertson pupil

Answer: d. An Argyll–Robertson pupil will accommodate but not react. It is a classic sign of syphilis.

44. Which of the following conditions causes an agitated and confused state with abnormally large pupils?
    a. Heroin overdose
    b. Multiple sclerosis
    c. Atropine, scopolamine, or sympathomimetic intoxication
    d. Hyperventilation

Answer: c.

45. In which condition is a patient typically comatose with respiratory depression and pinpoint-sized pupils?
    a. Heroin overdose
    b. MS
    c. Atropine, scopolamine, or sympathomimetic intoxication
    d. Hyperventilation

Answer: a. Heroin, morphine, and other opioid overdoses typically cause the combination of coma with respiratory depression and miosis. Less commonly, infarctions and hemorrhages in the pons produce the same picture. In a classic finding, pulmonary edema complicates heroin overdose.

46. Which cranial nerve carries the afferent limb of the light reflex?
    a. Optic nerve
    b. Oculomotor nerve
    c. Facial nerve
    d. Trigeminal nerve

Answer: a.

47. Which cranial nerve carries the efferent limb of the light reflex?
    a. Optic nerve
    b. Oculomotor nerve
    c. Facial nerve
    d. Trigeminal nerve

Answer: b.

48. Which structure hangs from the soft palate?
    a. Hard palate
    b. Tonsils
    c. Vermis
    d. Uvula
    e. Inferior olivary nucleus

Answer: d.

49. Which nerve is responsible for abducting the left eye?
    a. Left III
    b. Right III
    c. Left VI
    d. Right VI

Answer: c.

50. A patient has right-sided ptosis; the right eye is abducted; and its pupil is dilated. Which nerve or region is injured?
    a. Left III
    b. Right III
    c. Left VI
    d. Right VI

Answer: b.

51. After returning home from a party, a 15-year-old girl was lethargic and disoriented. Her parents bring her to the hospital where the intern finds that she walks with an ataxic gait and has slurred speech. She also has bilateral horizontal and vertical nystagmus. What is the most likely cause of her findings?
    a. MS
    b. A cerebellar tumor
    c. A psychogenic disturbance
    d. Intoxication

Answer: d. She is most likely to be intoxicated with alcohol, barbiturates, phencyclidine (PCP), antihistamine, or other drug. A cerebellar tumor is an unlikely possibility without headache, signs of raised intracranial pressure, or corticospinal tract damage. Multiple sclerosis is unlikely because of her lethargy, disorientation, and sudden onset of symptoms. Nystagmus may be a congenital abnormality, sign of a toxic-metabolic aberration, or manifestation of a structural brainstem lesion, but it would not be present in a psychogenic sign.

52. After swimming, a young man suddenly developed vertigo, nausea, vomiting, and left-sided tinnitus. He has nystagmus to the right, but no headache, paresis, DTR abnormality, or sensory loss. What is the most likely etiology?
    a. Multiple sclerosis
    b. A cerebellar tumor
    c. A psychogenic disturbance
    d. Labyrinthine dysfunction

Answer: d. The unilateral nystagmus, hearing abnormality, nausea, and vomiting are most likely caused by left-sided inner ear disease, such as water accumulation or labyrinthitis.

53. In which neurocognitive disorder is sense of smell preserved?
    a. Parkinson disease
    b. Alzheimer disease
    c. Vascular disease
    d. Traumatic brain injury

Answer: c. Patients with neurodegenerative illness, such as Parkinson and Alzheimer diseases, lose their sense of smell before or along with a decline in cognitive function. In fact, the olfactory neurons and the cerebral cortex tend to show the same neuropathology in neurodegenerative diseases. Patients with traumatic brain injury lose their sense of smell because of direct olfactory nerve damage. In contrast, vascular disease patients usually have a preserved sense of smell.

54. What is the most caudal (lowermost) level of the CNS?
    a. Foramen magnum
    b. Slightly caudal to the thoracic vertebrae
    c. The sacrum
    d. None of the above

Answer: b. The spinal cord, which is one of the two major components of the CNS, extends to the T12–L1 vertebrae area. Neurologists who perform spinal taps in the lumbar region bear this relationship in mind to avoid injuring the spinal cord. Gunshot wounds, tumors, or other lesions below that level can still be devastating if they disrupt the cauda equina.

55. A 25-year-old man, who has been shot in his posterior thorax, has paresis of the right leg and loss of position and vibration sensation at the right ankle. Pinprick sensation is preserved in his right leg, but lost in the left leg. His upper extremities are normal. Where is the lesion?
    a. Right side of the cervical spinal cord
    b. Left side of the cervical spinal cord
    c. Right side of the thoracic spinal cord
    d. Left side of the thoracic spinal cord
    e. Right side of the lumbosacral spinal cord
    f. Left side of the lumbosacral spinal cord
    g. One or both lumbar plexuses

Answer: c. The gunshot wound has caused hemitransection of the right side of the thoracic spinal cord (the Brown–Séquard syndrome, see Fig. 2.17).

56. Which group of cranial nerves do neurologists refer to as bulbar nerves?
    a. III, IV, and VI
    b. V, VII, and VIII
    c. IX–XII
    d. None of the above

Answer: c. Neurologists refer to cranial nerves III, IV, and VI as the ocular motor nerves; V, VII, and VIII as the cerebellopontine angle nerves; and IX–XII as the bulbar nerves.

57. If the bulbar cranial nerves are damaged, which symptoms usually result?
    a. Dysarthria and dysphagia
    b. Aphasia and dementia
    c. Seizures and epilepsy
    d. Trigeminal and glossopharyngeal neuralgia

Answer: a. Damage to bulbar cranial nerves leads to bulbar palsy. Dysarthria and dysphagia are its primary manifestations, but in severe cases patients often have potentially lethal respiratory difficulty.

58. Which other clinical findings are associated with bulbar palsy?
    a. Emotional lability
    b. Dementia
    c. Hyperactive gag reflex and jaw jerk
    d. Hypoactive gag reflex and jaw jerk

Answer: d. Because the pathology in bulbar palsy afflicts the cranial nerves, which are essentially lower motor neurons, the gag reflex and jaw jerk are hypoactive or absent. Also because the pathology of bulbar palsy involves the caudal brainstem and lower cranial nerves, emotional disturbances and cognitive impairment are not components.

59. Of the following, which category of illness is the most likely cause of bulbar palsy?
    a. Dementia-producing illnesses, e.g., Alzheimer and Parkinson diseases
    b. Traumatic brain injury
    c. Motor neuron diseases
    d. Mood disorders

Answer: c. Motor neuron illnesses, particularly ALS and poliomyelitis, routinely cause bulbar palsy. Neuromuscular junction diseases, such as myasthenia and botulism, also cause bulbar palsy.

60. Which of the following illnesses is least closely associated with a slow gait (≤0.7 m/sec)?
    a. Alzheimer disease
    b. Parkinson disease
    c. Normal-pressure hydrocephalus
    d. Vascular dementia

Answer: a. Until patients enter a moderate to severe stage of Alzheimer disease, they preserve their noncognitive functions, including their ability to walk. Most illnesses that cause dementia also cause a slow and often a distinctly abnormal gait. Some neurologists group illnesses that cause dementia and gait abnormalities into the category of "subcortical dementias" (see Chapter 7). In addition to a slow gait often being comorbid with dementia, it is also a risk factor for falls, disability, hospitalizations, and death.

61. In the development of syringomyelia (syrinx), which tract is most vulnerable to injury?
    a. Lateral spinothalamic
    b. Corticospinal
    c. Spinocerebellar
    d. Fasciculus cuneatus

Answer: a. As a syrinx expands within the spinal cord, it stretches and eventually disrupts the lateral spinothalamic tract fibers as they cross anterior to the syrinx (see

Fig. 2.18). Because a syrinx typically develops in the cervical spinal cord, it usually interrupts the pain and temperature-carrying tracts of the arms but not the legs. Neurologists often describe the analgesia of the upper trunk and arms as "suspended sensory loss."

62–66. This patient is attempting to look straight head and raise both arms. Her right eye cannot abduct and she cannot lift the left arm.

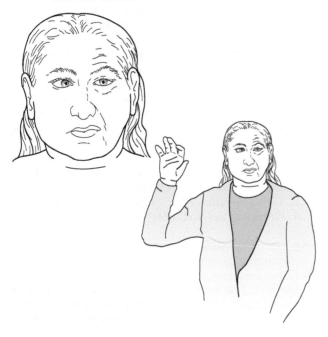

62. Paresis of which extraocular muscle prevents her right eye from abducting?
a. Right superior oblique
b. Right abducens
c. Right lateral rectus
d. Left lateral rectus

Answer: c.

63. The left side of her face is not included in the left hemiparesis. Which would be the best explanation?
a. The face, like the hand, has a small cortical representation.
b. The problem is in the right cerebral hemisphere.
c. The corticospinal tract is injured caudal to where the corticobulbar tract has innervated the facial nerve.
d. The problem is best explained by postulating two lesions.

Answer: c.

64. On which side of the body would a Babinski sign most likely be elicited?
a. Right
b. Left
c. Both
d. Neither

Answer: b.

65. What is the most likely etiology?
a. Midbrain infarction
b. Pons infarction
c. Medulla infarction
d. Bell's palsy

Answer: b.

66. With which condition is such a lesion most often associated?
a. Homonymous hemianopia
b. Diplopia
c. Impaired monocular visual acuity
d. Nystagmus

Answer: b. In summary, this patient has weakness of the right lateral rectus muscle, which prevents the right eye from abducting; weakness of the right upper and lower face; and weakness of the left arm. Because of the right eye's inability to abduct, she would have diplopia on right lateral gaze. The proper clinical assessment would be that she has injury of the right abducens and facial cranial nerves and the corticospinal tract before it crosses in the medulla. Because the lesion is not in the cerebral cortex, it would cause neither anosognosia nor a homonymous hemianopia. The lesion is undoubtedly located in the base of the right side of the pons. Its most likely etiology is an occlusion of a small branch of the basilar artery.

67. In an accident while driving his truck at work, a 30-year-old deliveryman sustained head injury. He had no loss of consciousness, seizure, or laceration. Two months later he claimed to have inability to smell or taste foods, incessant headache, insomnia, and forgetfulness. When a neurologist was asked to evaluate him for anosmia, the neurologist asked him to smell 10 samples of aromatic substances and insisted that he choose – guess if necessary – one of four possibilities for each. The truck driver correctly identified none of the 10 samples. What does his score indicate?
a. He sustained olfactory nerve injury in the accident.
b. He sustained olfactory and gustatory nerve damage in the accident.
c. He is deliberately choosing the incorrect answers.
d. He has PTSD.

Answer: c. His apparent anosmia is deliberate because he chose fewer correct responses than he would have by chance alone in this "forced choice" test of smell. The neurologist might support a diagnosis of malingering by seeing if the truck driver denied "smelling" alcohol or another irritative substance that bypasses the olfactory nerve but is detected by the trigeminal nerve.

68. Where does the corticospinal tract cross as it descends?
a. Internal capsule
b. Base of the pons
c. Pyramids
d. Anterior horn cells

Answer: c. Because the corticospinal tracts cross in the medulla's pyramids, neurologists call them the "pyramidal tract."

69. Which artery supplies Broca's area and the adjacent corticospinal tract?
    a. Anterior cerebral
    b. Middle cerebral
    c. Posterior cerebral
    d. Basilar

Answer: b. The left middle cerebral artery supplies Broca's area and the adjacent corticospinal tract.

70. Which of the following statements is *false* regarding cochlear implants in children with congenital deafness?
    a. Postoperative meningitis and other complications are rare.
    b. Cochlear implants are effective in restoring useful hearing.
    c. Cochlear implants will allow most deaf children to receive mainstream education.
    d. The benefits of cochlear implants in most children are equal to or better than their learning sign language.
    e. They are equally effective for congenital hearing loss and for presbycusis.

Answer: e. Cochlear implants have been a major advance in compensating for deafness in infants and young children. However, adults frequently cannot translate cochlear implant's electronic signals into words.

71. In which group of illnesses are muscles paretic, atrophic, and areflexic?
    a. Poliomyelitis, diabetic peripheral neuropathy, traumatic brachial plexus injury
    b. Guillain–Barré syndrome, multiple sclerosis, and muscular dystrophy
    c. Spinal cord trauma, cerebral infarction, congenital cerebral injuries
    d. Brainstem infarction, cerebellar infarction, spinal cord infarction

Answer: a. The common denominator is LMN injury.

72. Which *two* of the following would result from ciliary ganglion damage?
    a. Miosis
    b. Mydriasis
    c. Hypersensitivity to mydriatic agents (medications that dilate the pupil)
    d. Hypersensitivity to miotic agents (medications that constrict the pupil)

Answers: b, d. Damage to the ciliary ganglion will interrupt parasympathetic innervation of the pupil's sphincter muscles and leave sympathetic innervation unopposed. The unopposed sympathetic innervation will tend to dilate the pupil. Because of denervation hypersensitivity, the pupil's sphincter muscles will be unusually sensitive to miotic agents, such as pilocarpine eye drops. Thus, in an *Adie pupil*, because of ciliary ganglion damage, a dilated pupil readily constricts when examiners apply dilute solutions of pilocarpine eye drops, though the same pilocarpine drops are too dilute to constrict a normal pupil.

73. During spring break, a college student dove into the shallow end of a swimming pool. He struck his forehead firmly against the bottom. His friends noted that he was unconscious and resuscitated him. On recovery in the hospital several days later, he has severe neck pain, weakness in both hands and absent DTRs in the arms. Although pain sensation is diminished in his hands, position and vibration sensations are preserved. His legs are strong and have normal sensation; however, their DTRs are brisk and Babinski signs are present. A large, tender ecchymotic area overlies his forehead. Which of the following is the most likely cause of the hand weakness?
    a. Cerebral concussion with frontal lobe damage
    b. Intoxication
    c. Syringomyelia
    d. Herniated cervical intervertebral disk

Answer: c. Striking the forehead against the bottom of a swimming pool produces a high-impact, forceful hyperextension cervical injury as well as head trauma and possible TBI. The immediate problem in this case is that the spinal cord probably developed a hematomyelia, which is a variety of a syrinx. In this condition, the cervical spinothalamic tracts, as they cross within the spinal cord, are severed. The lesion compresses the corticospinal tracts destined for the legs, but does not interrupt them. Similar injuries occur in motor vehicle crashes where the victim's forehead strikes the dashboard or inside of the windshield, and in sports accidents where the athlete's head and neck suddenly hyperextend. In these types of accident, physicians should evaluate victims for alcohol and drug intoxication as well as for TBI and cervical spinal cord injury.

74. A 50-year-old woman, who recently came to the United States from the Dominican Republic, saw a neurologist because she had stiffness in her legs that prevented her from walking at her normal speed. The neurologist found spasticity with little or no paresis, but no sensory loss in her legs. MRIs of her head and spinal cord were normal. Tests showed normal serum concentration of vitamin B_{12} and copper. Which of the following infections is most likely the cause of her myelopathy?
    a. Human T-lymphotropic virus type 1 (HTLV-1)
    b. Human immunodeficiency virus (HIV)
    c. Syphilis
    d. Polio

Answer: a. In view of her having lived in the Dominican Republic and showing leg spasticity disproportionate greater than paresis, the neurologist correctly attributed this patient's myelopathy to HTLV-1 myelopathy. Blood tests confirmed infection with HTLV-1. HIV spinal cord infection may also cause myelopathy, but one characterized by sensory loss with little spasticity. Although syphilis may also infect the spinal cord, this infection causes tabes dorsalis. Its main findings are loss of position and vibration sensations, lightning-like pains, and Argyll–Robinson pupils. Poliovirus causes an acute febrile illness and paresis of one or more limbs, which are flaccid, areflexic, and beset with fasciculations.

75. In the neurologic examination, which maneuver reveals most about the function of a patient's motor system?
    a. Testing plantar reflexes
    b. Manual muscle testing
    c. Deep tendon reflex testing
    d. Observation of the patient's gait

Answer: d. To walk normally a person must have intact corticospinal tracts and LMNs, coordination, proprioception, and balance. Observing the patient's gait offers the most comprehensive assessment of noncognitive neurologic function.

76. A 20-year-old member of a college ski team shattered her right ankle and had to wear a cast from her foot to her knee. After the orthopedist removed the cast, he found that she had a right foot drop. Which nerve was probably injured?
    a. Tibial
    b. Fibular (previously called peroneal)
    c. Perineum
    d. Sciatic

Answer: b. Previously referred to as the *peroneal* nerve, but renamed because it sounded too similar to *perineal*, the fibular nerve lies laterally and subcutaneously at the knee. Constricting casts and lateral knee injuries may compress the fibular nerve and weaken the fibular muscles it innervates, leading to a foot drop.

77. A 29-year-old woman with a long history of depression including multiple somatic complaints reports that when she awoke she was unable to rise from bed. During the examination, she failed to move her left arm and leg either spontaneously or on request, but raised her arm to catch a ball. She denied that she was paralyzed on the left. She ignored attractive objects, such as a $1 bill brought into her left visual field. Her left nasolabial fold was flatter on her left than right side when she attempted to smile. She had a left-sided Babinski sign. Which is the most likely explanation for the left arm and leg immobility?
    a. Left hemiparesis from multiple sclerosis, stroke, or other right cerebral lesion
    b. A conscious attempt to mimic hemiparesis
    c. An unconscious process producing the appearance of hemiparesis
    d. Hemi-inattention and anosognosia from a right cerebral lesion

Answer: d. She probably has sustained a right cerebral lesion in view of the left visual field cut and flattened

(paretic) left lower face as well as her hemi-inattention (hemineglect) and anosognosia. Parietal lobe lesions that spare motor function still produce these neuropsychologic deficits.

78. Which two cranial nerves convey taste sensation from the tongue to the brain?
    a. V and VII
    b. VII and IX
    c. IX and X
    d. IX and XI

Answer: b. The facial nerve (VII) conveys taste sensation from the anterior two-thirds and the glossopharyngeal nerve (IX) conveys taste sensation from the posterior one-third of the tongue.

79. Which will be the pattern of a myelin stain of the cervical spinal cord's ascending tracts several years after a thoracic spine gunshot wound?
    a. The entire cervical spinal cord will be normal.
    b. The myelin will be unstained.
    c. The *fasciculus cuneatus* will be stained black, and the *fasciculus gracilis* will be unstained.
    d. The *fasciculus gracilis* will be stained black, and the *fasciculus cuneatus* will be unstained.

Answer: c. Because the *fasciculus cuneatus* arises from the arms and upper trunk, it remains uninjured and normally absorbs the black stain. In contrast, the *fasciculus gracilis* will be unstained because its myelin will be lost distal (downstream) from the lesion. As for the other major tracts, the corticospinal tract, which is descending, will be normally stained black because it originates proximal to the lesion. Similarly, the portion of the spinothalamic tract that originates in the legs and lower trunk will remain unstained. Overall, the loss of staining reflects *Wallerian degeneration*, in which axon injury leads to loss of their myelin and axons distal (downstream) from the injury, whether the axons are flowing toward or away from the brain.

80. A 20-year-old man has become progressively dysarthric during the previous 2 years. He has no mental impairments or cranial nerve abnormalities. His legs have mild weakness and Babinski signs, but poorly reactive DTRs. All his limbs are ataxic and his speech is scanning. He has impaired position and vibration sensation in his hands and feet. His feet have a high arch, elevated dorsum, and retracted first metatarsal. A cardiac evaluation reveals hypertrophic cardiomyopathy. His two younger brothers appear to have developed the same problem. His parents, three aunts and uncles, and two older siblings have no neurologic symptoms or physical abnormalities. Which of the following genetic abnormalities most likely cause his illness?
    a. Excessive trinucleotide repeats on both alleles of chromosome 9
    b. Excessive trinucleotide repeats on only one allele of chromosome 6
    c. Two Y chromosomes, giving him an XYY karyotype

d. Two X chromosomes, giving him an XXY karyotype

Answer: a. The patient and his two younger brothers have a spinocerebellar ataxia (SCA), which characteristically causes posterior column abnormalities (sensory loss), Babinski signs, limb ataxia, scanning speech, and *pes cavus* (see Fig. 2.14). In most cases, SCA results from a genetic defect consisting of excessive trinucleotide repeats. In his case, the illness followed an autosomal recessive pattern with both alleles carrying the mutation.

81. A man with diabetic neuropathy is unable to stand erect with feet together and eyes closed. When attempting this maneuver, he tends to topple, but he catches himself before falling. What is the name of this sign?
    a. Hoover
    b. Babinski
    c. Chvostek
    d. Romberg

Answer: d. He shows a Romberg sign. Falling over when standing erect while deprived of visual input suggests a loss of joint position sense from the lower extremities. When deprived of vision and joint position sense, people must rely on vestibular input.

Neurologists have classically attributed the Romberg sign to injury of the spinal cord's posterior columns because, when injured, these tracts cannot convey position sense up the spinal cord to the brain. The Romberg sign indicates combined system disease and tabes dorsalis – conditions in which the posterior columns are destroyed. Neurologists now attribute Romberg sign most often to diabetic or other forms of peripheral neuropathy because patients with peripheral neuropathy usually have lost position sensation emanating from their feet and ankles to the spinal cord.

82. A neurologist suspects that a 29-year-old man has psychogenic left-hemiparesis because he is unconcerned by it. On examination, when asked to abduct his legs against the examiner's hands, the patient's right leg abducts against the force of the neurologist's hand. At the same time, the examiner's hand meets considerable resistance when trying to push the left leg medially. Then, the examiner asks the patient to abduct his left leg against the examiner's hand. That leg fails to abduct and, at the same time, the right leg exerts so little force that the examiner

easily pushes it medially. The patient also reports sensory loss of all modalities in the left pelvis and trunk. Which one of the following statements concerning this case is most likely to be *false*?
    a. This patient's abductor test suggests a psychogenic basis.
    b. The patient will probably display a Hoover sign.
    c. The patient's sensory "loss" will probably stop abruptly at the midline.
    d. Recent studies have confirmed that psychogenic hemiparesis much more often affects the left than the right side.

Answer: d. A left-sided predominance of psychogenic hemiparesis had been observed in small series and attributed on the rationale that, given the choice, individuals would garner the same primary and secondary gains but endure less impairment with a left than a right hemiparesis. However, recent studies have failed to confirm earlier observations that psychogenic hemiparesis much more often affects the left than the right side. Studies have also discredited *la belle indifférence* as a sign of psychogenic deficits. This patient's examination illustrated the abductor sign, which more reliably indicates a psychogenic basis of a hemiparesis involving a leg (see Fig. 3.3). The Hoover sign, which also involves reflexive or unconscious movement of the legs, is another reliable indication of psychogenic hemiparesis (see Fig. 3.2). In general, these and other motor signs are more reliable than sensory findings in detecting psychogenic neurologic deficits.

83. A 35-year-old man who has had diabetes mellitus since childhood develops erectile dysfunction. He has absent DTRs at the wrists and ankles, loss of position and vibration sensation at the ankles, and no demonstrable anal or cremasteric reflexes. Which other disturbance is unlikely to be present?
    a. Urinary bladder hypotonicity
    b. Bilateral Babinski signs
    c. Gastroparesis
    d. Anhidrosis

Answer: b. He has a combination of peripheral and autonomic neuropathy, both presumably due to diabetes. The distal sensory and reflex loss and the absent anal and cremasteric reflexes indicate the peripheral neuropathy. Common manifestations of autonomic neuropathy are urinary bladder hypotonicity, gastroparesis, anhidrosis, retrograde ejaculation, and erectile dysfunction.

PERIPHERAL NERVE DISORDERS

By relying on clinical findings, physicians can distinguish peripheral nervous system (PNS) from central nervous system (CNS) disorders. In PNS disorders, damage to one, a group, or all peripheral nerves causes readily observable patterns of paresis, deep tendon reflex (DTR) loss, and sensory impairments. Some PNS disorders are characteristically associated with mental changes, systemic illness, or a fatal outcome.

ANATOMY

The spinal cord's *anterior horn cells* are the lower motor neurons (LMNs), whose axons constitute the peripheral nerves – the starting point of the PNS. The peripheral nerves are the final link in the pathway that transmits motor commands from the brain through the spinal cord to muscles (Fig. 5.1). Nerve roots emerging from the anterior spinal cord mingle within the brachial or lumbosacral plexus to form the major peripheral nerves, such as the radial and femoral. Although peripheral nerves are quite long, especially in the legs, they faithfully conduct electrochemical impulses over considerable distances. Because *myelin*, the lipid-based sheath generated by Schwann cells, surrounds peripheral nerves and acts as insulation, the impulses are transmitted without degradation.

When stimulated, motor nerves release packets of acetylcholine (ACh) from storage vesicles at the neuromuscular junction. The ACh packets traverse the junction and bind to specific ACh receptors on the muscle end plate. The interaction between ACh and its receptors depolarizes the muscle membrane and initiates a muscle contraction (see Chapter 6). Neuromuscular transmission culminating in muscle depolarization is a discrete, quantitative action: ACh does not merely seep out of the presynaptic terminal as loose molecules and drift across the neuromuscular junction to trigger a muscle contraction.

Peripheral nerves also transmit sensory information, but in the reverse direction: from the PNS to the CNS. For example, after receptors located in the skin, tendons, and joints detect pain, temperature, vibration, or joint position, peripheral nerves transmit this information to the spinal cord.

MONONEUROPATHIES

Disorders of single peripheral nerves, *mononeuropathies*, are characterized by flaccid paresis, DTR loss (*areflexia*),

and reduced sensation, particularly for pain (*hypalgesia* [Greek *hypo*, under + *algos*, pain] or *analgesia* [Greek, insensitivity to pain]) (Table 5.1). Paradoxically, mononeuropathies and other peripheral nerve injuries sometimes lead to spontaneously occurring sensations, *paresthesias* (Greek *para*, near + *aisthesis*, sensation) that may be painful, *dysesthesias*. Peripheral nerve injuries also convert stimuli that ordinarily do not cause pain, such as a light touch or cool air, into painful sensations, *allodynia*; exaggerate painful responses to mildly noxious stimuli, such as the point of a pin, *hyperalgesia*; or delay but then exaggerate and prolong pain from noxious stimuli, *hyperpathia*.

Several mononeuropathies are common, important, and readily identifiable. They usually result from penetrating or blunt trauma, compression, diabetic infarctions, or other damage to single nerves.

Compression, especially of nerves protected only by overlying skin and subcutaneous tissue rather than by bone, viscera, or thick layers of fat, occurs frequently. People most susceptible are diabetics; those who have rapidly lost weight, thereby depleting nerves' protective myelin covering; workers in certain occupations, such as seamstresses or watchmakers; and those who have remained in disjointed positions for long periods, often because of drug or alcohol abuse. One of the most common compressive mononeuropathies – "Saturday night palsy" – affects the radial nerve, which is vulnerable at the point where it winds around in the spiral groove of the humerus. Thus, people in alcohol-induced stupor who lean against their upper arm against a hard surface for several hours are liable to develop a *wrist drop* (Fig. 5.2). *Foot drop*, its lower-extremity counterpart, often results from common fibular nerve* damage from prolonged leg crossing compressing the nerve, lower knee injuries traumatizing the nerve, or a constrictive lower-leg cast pushing against the nerve as it winds around the head of the fibula.

Carpal tunnel syndrome (CTS), the most common mononeuropathy, results from damage of the median nerve as it travels through the carpal tunnel of the wrist (Fig. 5.3, left). Forceful and repetitive wrist movements can traumatize the nerve in that confined passage. Meat and fish processing, certain assembly-line work, and carpentry are all closely associated with CTS; however, contrary to initial claims, word processing and other keyboarding actually have a weak association with the

---

*Anatomists have renamed the *peroneal* nerves and muscles because of their similarity in sound to *perineum*. Their new name, which this book has adopted, is *fibular* nerves and muscles.

TABLE 5.1   **Major Mononeuropathies**

Nerve	Motor Paresis	DTR Lost	Pain or Sensory Loss	Examples
Median	Thumb abduction with thenar atrophy	None	Thumb, 2nd, 3rd finger and lateral 1/2 of 4th	Carpal tunnel syndrome
Ulnar	Finger and thumb adduction	None	5th and medial 1/2 of 4th fingers	Cubital tunnel syndrome Claw hand
Radial	Wrist, thumb, and finger extensors	Brachioradialis*	Dorsum of hand	Saturday night palsy Wrist drop
Femoral	Knee extensors	Quadriceps (knee)	Anterior thigh, medial calf	Femoral neuropathy from prolonged obstetric delivery
Sciatic	Ankle dorsiflexors and plantar flexors	Achilles (ankle)	Buttock, lateral calf, and most of foot	Flail foot
Fibular	Ankle dorsiflexors and evertors	None		Dorsum of foot and lateral calf

*Compression of the radial nerve: the spiral groove of the humerus spares the triceps deep tendon reflex

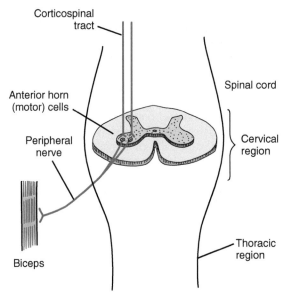

FIGURE 5.1 ■ The corticospinal tracts, as discussed in Chapter 2 and as their name indicates, consist of upper motor neurons (UMNs) that travel from the motor cortex to the spinal cord. They synapse on the spinal cord's *anterior horn cells*, which give rise to the lower motor neurons (LMNs). The LMNs join sensory fibers to form peripheral nerves.

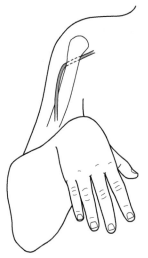

FIGURE 5.2 ■ As the radial nerve winds around the humerus, it is vulnerable to compression and other forms of trauma. Radial nerve damage leads to the readily recognizable *wrist drop*, which results from paresis of the extensor muscles of the wrist, finger, and thumb.

disorder. In another mechanism, fluid retention during pregnancy or menses entraps the median nerve in the carpal tunnel. Similarly, inflammatory tissue changes in the wrist from rheumatoid arthritis may compress the median nerve.

Whatever the mechanism, CTS causes paresthesias and pains that shoot from the wrist to the palm, thumb, and adjacent two or sometimes three fingers (Fig. 5.3, right). Symptoms worsen at night and awaken the victims, who shake their hands in an attempt to find relief. Neurologists test for the syndrome's characteristic *Tinel sign* by lightly percussing the ventral wrist: The test is positive when the percussion generates electric sensations that shoot from the wrist into the palm and fingers. *Phalen's maneuver*, holding the dorsum of the hands together with wrists flexed at 90 degrees, also may reproduce symptoms.

With chronic CTS, median nerve damage leads to thenar (thumb) muscle weakness and atrophy. Patients report impaired fine movements of the thumb and adjacent two fingers, which are instrumental in precision movements, such as writing, grasping small objects, and fastening buttons.

Most CTS patients respond to rest and, sometimes, splints. Diuretics and antiinflammatory drugs are also helpful. In refractory cases, a surgeon might inject steroids into the carpal tunnel or incise the transverse carpal ligament to decompress the tunnel.

In another example of upper-extremity nerve damage, pressure on the ulnar groove of the elbow, also known as the cubital tunnel (the "funny bone"), may damage the ulnar nerve. For instance, when individuals rest their weight on their elbows, the compression often injures the ulnar nerve. These individuals develop atrophy and weakness of their hand muscles (Fig. 5.4). The ulnar nerve damage also leads to loss of sensation of the fourth and fifth fingers and the medial surface of the hand.

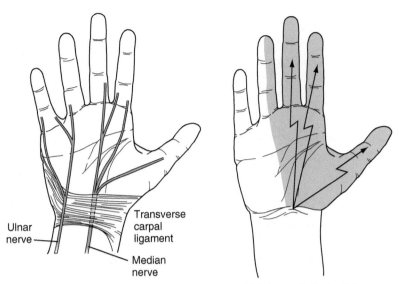

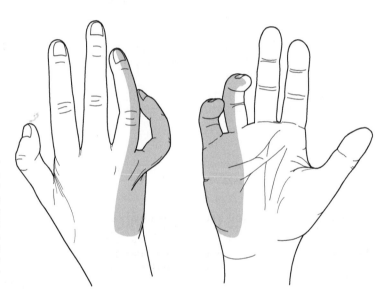

FIGURE 5.3 ■ *Left,* The median nerve passes through the carpal tunnel, which is a relatively tight compartment. In it, the median nerve is vulnerable to repetitive movement and compression from fluid accumulation. The ulnar nerve, taking a different route, passes above and medial to the roof of the tunnel, the *transverse carpal ligament,* thus escaping damage. *Right,* The usual sensory distribution of the median nerve encompasses the palm, thenar eminence (thumb base), thumb, and adjacent two fingers. In carpal tunnel syndrome, pain shoots distally from the wrist over this area. Physicians may elicit the Tinel sign, a reliable indication of the carpal tunnel syndrome, by tapping the patient's palmar wrist surface and finding that paresthesias emanate from the wrist and radiate in the median nerve distribution.

FIGURE 5.4 ■ *Left,* With ulnar nerve injuries, the palmar view shows that intrinsic muscles of the hand, particularly those of the hypothenar eminence (fifth finger base), undergo atrophy. The fourth and fifth fingers are flexed and abducted. When raised, the hand and fingers assume the *benediction sign.* In addition, the medial two fingers and palm are anesthetic (numb). *Right,* Ulnar nerve injuries also produce a *claw hand* because of atrophy of the muscles between the thumb and adjacent finger (first dorsal interosseous and adductor pollicis), as well as of those of the hypothenar eminence.

A common form of lower-extremity compressive neuropathy is *meralgia paresthetica*, entrapment of the lateral femoral cutaneous nerve by the inguinal ligament at the lateral groin. Patients report numbness and burning in a large but discrete oval patch on the lateral thigh, not extending above the hip or below the knee (Fig. 5.5). Obesity, pregnancy, tight clothing, and use of heavy utility belts are all risk factors for meralgia paresthetica. Behavior modification usually improves the symptoms. Of note, anatomists named the lateral femoral cutaneous nerve based on its sensory distribution rather than its origin. Many students mistakenly label this nerve as a branch of the femoral nerve; however, it comes directly from the L2–3 sensory roots.

Mononeuropathies can result from systemic illnesses, such as diabetes mellitus, vasculitis (e.g., lupus erythematosus,

polyarteritis nodosa), and lead intoxication (see later) – as well as from trauma. In most of the systemic conditions, pain, weakness, and other symptoms have an abrupt onset. In addition, systemic illnesses often cause stroke-like CNS insults along with the mononeuropathies.

MONONEURITIS MULTIPLEX

Mononeuritis multiplex is a serious, complex PNS condition that consists of a simultaneous or stepwise development of multiple peripheral injuries, sometimes accompanied by cranial injuries. For example, a patient might suddenly develop left radial, right sciatic, and right third cranial nerve deficits. Mononeuritis multiplex is usually a manifestation of a systemic illness, such as Lyme

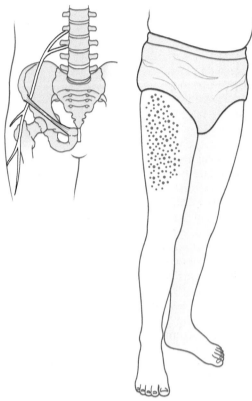

FIGURE 5.5 ■ Tight clothing, an overhanging abdominal fat pad, or an equipment belt will compress or trap the lateral femoral cutaneous nerve under the lateral edge of the inguinal ligament in the groin. The nerve damage causes simultaneous numbness and burning pain on the anterolateral aspect of the thigh (*stippled*), which neurologists call *meralgia paresthetica*.

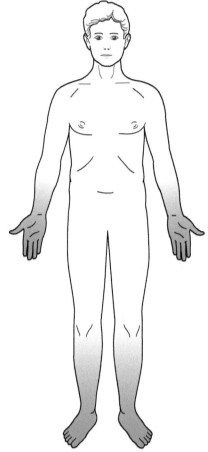

FIGURE 5.6 ■ Patients with polyneuropathy lose pain and other sensations. The loss is symmetric, more severe distally than proximally, and more severe in the legs than arms. Neurologists term this pattern of sensory loss *stocking-glove hypalgesia*.

disease or lupus erythematosus, but leprosy commonly causes it in Africa and Asia.

POLYNEUROPATHIES (NEUROPATHIES)

The most frequently occurring PNS disorder, *polyneuropathy* or simply *neuropathy*, is generalized, symmetric involvement of all peripheral nerves. Some neuropathies also attack cranial nerves. Neurologists divide neuropathies into those that predominantly damage either the myelin (demyelinating neuropathies) or axons (axonopathies). Most cases of demyelinating neuropathies fall into the category of inflammatory illness; however, cases of axonopathy include ones from porphyria, toxins, metabolic illnesses, and nutritional deficiencies. Although psychiatrists should be aware of that distinction, they must concentrate on neuropathies associated with mental status changes.

In addition, neurologists divide neuropathies into *sensory*, *motor*, or *mixed sensory-motor neuropathy*. Patients with sensory neuropathy usually suffer predominately or exclusively from numbness, paresthesias, or burning in their fingers and toes (i.e., a *stocking-glove pattern*, Fig. 5.6). The pain may reach intolerable proportions (see neuropathic pain, Chapter 14). When sensory neuropathy affects the feet, it may provoke leg movements, such

as restless legs syndrome (see Chapter 17). Patients with *motor neuropathy* usually have *distal* limb weakness. They have hand weakness that impairs fine, skilled hand and finger movements, such as buttoning a shirt; they may also present with a foot droop, which leads to difficulty raising their feet when they walk. In chronic cases their neuropathy usually also leads to muscle atrophy and flaccidity. As with other LMN injuries, it diminishes DTRs (see Fig. 2.2C); first at the Achilles, and then more proximal sites. Mixed sensory-motor neuropathy causes a combination of those symptoms and signs.

Neurologists who care for psychiatric patients may meaningfully divide neuropathies into those with and those without comorbid changes in mental status (Box 5.1).

Neuropathies Without Comorbid Mental Status Changes

Guillain–Barré Syndrome

Acute inflammatory demyelinating polyradiculoneuropathy (AIDP) or postinfectious demyelinating polyneuropathy, commonly known as Guillain–Barré syndrome, is both the quintessential PNS illness and the primary

BOX 5.1	Important Causes of Neuropathy

Endogenous toxins
  Acute intermittent and variegate porphyria*
  Diabetes mellitus
  Uremia*
Nutritional deficiencies
  Celiac disease
  Vitamin B_{12} (combined system degeneration)*
  Combined system disease*
  Starvation, malabsorption, alcoholism*
Excessive intake
  Vitamin B_6 (pyridoxine)
Medicines
  Antibiotics:
    Anti-HIV (ddI, ddC)
    Dapsone
    Isoniazid (INH)*
    Nitrofurantoin
  Antineoplastic agents
  Vitamin B_6 (pyridoxine), in high doses
  Disulfiram*
Industrial, chemical, or marine toxins
  Ciguatera fish poisoning*
  Metals: arsenic, lead, mercury, thallium
  Nitrous oxide N_2O^{+*}
  Organic solvents: n-hexane[+], toluene[+*]
Infectious/inflammatory conditions
  Guillain–Barré syndrome
  Mononucleosis, hepatitis, Lyme disease*, leprosy, syphilis*, AIDS*
  Vasculitides: systemic lupus erythematosus, polyarteritis*
Genetic diseases
  Adrenoleukodystrophy*
  Charcot–Marie–Tooth disease*
  Metachromatic leukodystrophy*
  Spinocerebellar ataxias

*Associated with mental status abnormalities
[+]May be substances of abuse

example of a demyelinating neuropathy. Although often idiopathic, this syndrome typically follows an upper respiratory or gastrointestinal illness. Cases following a week's episode of watery diarrhea are apt to be associated with a gastrointestinal *Campylobacter jejuni* infection and be more extensive and severe than idiopathic cases. Many cases seem to be a complication of other infectious illnesses, including human immunodeficiency virus (HIV) infection, Lyme disease, mononucleosis, hepatitis, cytomegalovirus (CMV), and West Nile virus. Although Guillain–Barré syndrome has followed administration of influenza vaccinations, it is a very rare complication of current ones vaccinations.

When first affected, young and middle-aged adults feel paresthesias and numbness in the fingers and toes. Then they develop flaccid paresis of their feet and legs with characteristically absent knee and ankle DTRs. Weakness, a much greater problem than numbness, ascends to involve the hands and arms. Many patients progress to respiratory insufficiency because of involvement of the phrenic and intercostal nerves, and require intubation for ventilation. If weakness ascends still further, patients develop cranial nerve involvement that may lead to dysphagia and other aspects of bulbar palsy (see Chapter 4). Additional involvement causes facial weakness and then sometimes even ocular immobility. Nevertheless, possibly because optic and acoustic nerves are protected by myelin generated by the CNS – not the PNS – patients continue to see and hear.

Even if the illness worsens to the point of total paralysis, patients usually remain conscious with a normal mental status – allowing for anxiety and depressive symptoms from enduring a life-threatening illness. Completely immobile and anarthric Guillain–Barré syndrome patients, typically with preserved consciousness and mental status, exist in a *locked-in syndrome* (see Chapter 11). Cerebrospinal fluid (CSF) exhibits an elevated protein concentration, but with few white cells (i.e., the classic *albumino-cytologic dissociation*) (see Table 20.1). *Nerve conduction studies* (see Chapter 6) show evidence of peripheral nerve demyelination.

The illness usually resolves almost completely within 3 months as the PNS myelin is regenerated. By way of treatment, plasmapheresis (plasma exchange), which extracts circulating inflammatory mediators, particularly autoantibodies, complement, and cytokines, reduces the severity and duration of the paresis. Alternatively, administration of intravenous human immunoglobulin (IVIG), which "blocks" the abnormal immune response, also restores patients' strength. Steroids will not help, which is surprising because they are helpful in other inflammatory diseases of the nervous system, such as myasthenia gravis (see Chapter 6), multiple sclerosis (MS) (see Chapter 15), and the chronic form of Guillain–Barré syndrome (chronic inflammatory demyelinating polyneuropathy [CIDP]). Of note, neurologists have additional treatments against CIDP. They use steroids as first-line therapy, a treatment that is not successful for Guillain–Barré syndrome. When they cannot be weaned from steroids, patients receive additional immunosuppressants, such as azathioprine and mycophenolate mofetil, to avoid the long-term side effects of steroid use, such as hypertension, cataracts, diabetes, osteoporosis, and myopathy. In the most treatment-resistant forms, neurologists have prescribed the monoclonal antibody, rituximab (see Chapter 6).

Not only is Guillain–Barré syndrome a life-threatening illness, but also it epitomizes the distinction between PNS and CNS diseases. Although paraparesis or quadriparesis might be a feature common to PNS and CNS illnesses, different patterns of muscle weakness, changes in reflexes, and sensory distribution characterize PNS and CNS illnesses (Table 5.2). Also, in Guillain–Barré syndrome, as in most neuropathies other than diabetic neuropathy (see later), bladder, bowel, and sexual functions are preserved. In contrast, patients with spinal cord disease usually have incontinence and impotence at the onset of the injury.

Another contrast arises from the difference between demyelinating diseases of the CNS and PNS. Despite performing a similar insulating function, CNS and PNS myelin differ in chemical composition, antigenicity, and cells of origin. Oligodendrocytes produce CNS myelin, and Schwann cells produce PNS myelin. In other words, oligodendrocytes are to Schwann cells as the CNS is to the PNS. Also, each oligodendrocyte produces myelin

TABLE 5.2　Central (CNS) and Peripheral Nervous System (PNS) Signs

		CNS	PNS
Motor system		Upper motor neuron	Lower motor neuron
Paresis		Patterns*	Distal
Tone		Spastic+	Flaccid
Bulk		Normal	Atrophic
Fasciculations		No	Sometimes
Reflexes			
	DTRs	Hyperactive++	Hypoactive
	Babinski sign	Present	Absent
Sensory loss		Patterns*	Hands and feet

*Examples: motor and sensory loss of one side or lower half of the body
+May be flaccid initially
++May be absent initially

that covers many nearby CNS axons, but each Schwann cell produces myelin that covers only one portion of a single PNS axon. From a clinical viewpoint, Schwann cells regenerate damaged PNS myelin and thus Guillain–Barré patients usually recover. In contrast, because oligodendrocytes do not regenerate damaged CNS myelin, impairments are permanent in patients who have lost CNS myelin to toxins and infections. For example, the CNS demyelination that results from toluene use represents a permanent loss.

MS appears to be a partial exception to the rule that CNS demyelinating damage is permanent. In MS, episodes of demyelination of several CNS areas, including the optic nerves, partially or even completely resolve (see Chapter 15). However, the improvement results from resolution of myelin inflammation rather than myelin regeneration. When MS-induced demyelination eventually encompasses large areas of cerebral CNS myelin, it results in permanent quadriparesis and dementia.

From another perspective, patients with uncomplicated cases of Guillain–Barré syndrome, despite profound motor impairment, generally should not have an altered mental status because it is a disease of the PNS. Thus, when Guillain–Barré syndrome patients develop mental changes, consulting physicians should look for complications involving the CNS, particularly cerebral hypoxia from respiratory insufficiency, hydrocephalus from impaired reabsorption of CSF that has an elevated protein concentration, hyponatremia from inappropriate antidiuretic hormone secretion (SIADH), or sleep deprivation. Guillain–Barré syndrome patients with the most pronounced impairments – quadriparesis, dependency on artificial ventilation, and multiple cranial nerve involvement – are the ones most apt to experience a psychotic episode.

Thus, psychiatric consultants should look first for hypoxia and other life-threatening medical complications in Guillain–Barré patients who develop mental aberrations. Also, unless the patient is already on a respirator, psychiatrists should avoid prescribing medications that depress respirations, such as benzodiazepines and opioids.

Diabetes

Although strict treatment of diabetes may delay or even prevent diabetic neuropathy, most patients who have diabetes for more than 10 years show its symptoms and signs. In addition, risk factors for vascular disease, such as obesity and cigarette smoking, exacerbate the neuropathy.

The classic finding is loss of sensation in a stocking-glove distribution. Strength remains relatively normal, but patients lose the DTRs in their ankles then knees. With long-standing diabetic neuropathy, impaired sensation in their fingertips prevents blind diabetic patients from reading Braille. In addition to the distal symmetric sensory loss, diabetic patients may suffer from suddenly occurring painful mononeuropathies and mononeuritis multiplex or continuous intense burning sensations, especially in the feet. These are especially distressing at night and prevent sleep. By a different mechanism – damaging blood vessels – diabetes can lead to cerebrovascular disease that eventually may cause vascular dementia (Vascular Neurocognitive Disorder in DSM-5 terminology, see Chapter 7).

A few groups of medicines suppress the pain of diabetic neuropathy and other neuropathies. Narcotics (opioids), but not less potent analgesics, help. Certain antiepileptic drugs (AEDs), such as gabapentin (Neurontin) and pregabalin (Lyrica), reduce pain and promote sleep. The third group, tricyclic antidepressants, in doses too low to relieve depression, reduces pain and promotes sleep. Duloxetine (Cymbalta), a selective serotonin norepinephrine (noradrenaline) reuptake inhibitor (SSNRI) helps alleviate pain caused by diabetic peripheral neuropathy. Curiously, though, selective serotonin reuptake inhibitors (SSRIs) provide little if any pain relief. In an alternative approach, a skin cream containing capsaicin, which depletes substance P, the putative neurotransmitter for pain, provides some analgesia, along with numbness, to limited areas. In contrast to their usefulness in most painful conditions, nonsteroidal antiinflammatory drugs (NSAIDs) provide little benefit in diabetic neuropathy.

Patients with diabetic neuropathy may also have autonomic nervous system involvement that causes gastrointestinal immobility, bladder muscle contraction, and sexual dysfunction. In fact, erectile dysfunction is occasionally the first or most disturbing symptom of diabetic autonomic neuropathy (see Chapter 16).

Toxic-Metabolic Disorders

Numerous metabolic derangements and toxins, including medications, frequently cause neuropathy. For example, renal insufficiency (uremia) is a common cause of neuropathy that occurs almost universally in patients undergoing maintenance hemodialysis. Also, cancer chemotherapy agents and antibiotics, including those for tuberculosis and HIV disease (see later), routinely cause neuropathy; however, antipsychotics, antidepressants, and AEDs, except for phenytoin, do not. When medications, chemicals, or other substances cause CNS or PNS damage, neurologists label them neurotoxins.

Several heavy metals cause combinations of PNS and CNS impairments. It is important to note that while heavy metal intoxication can frequently present with mental status or cognitive changes in children, this is an uncommon symptom in adult patients (see mercury poisoning, later). For example, lead poisoning causes a neuropathy in adults, but cognitive impairment and other problems in children. Pica (craving for unnatural foods), mostly from hunger, in young children prompts them to eat lead-pigment paint chips from toys or decaying tenement walls. (Lead paint on interior walls has been illegal in most cities for decades.) Even at low concentrations lead is neurotoxic in children. Lead ingestion is associated with inattention, learning disabilities, and poor school performance. High serum concentrations are associated with seizures and mental retardation. Because lead has a different deleterious effect on the mature nervous system, adults with lead poisoning develop motor mononeuropathies, such as a foot drop or wrist drop, rather than cerebral impairments. Adults most often develop lead poisoning from industrial exposure, drinking homemade alcohol distilled in equipment with lead pipes ("moonshine"), or burning car batteries for heat.

Chronic, low-level intoxication by several other heavy metals causes polyneuropathy, dermatologic abnormality, and mental changes. In recent years, neurologists have diagnosed cobalt toxicity in patients presenting with progressive sensory deficits, hearing loss, and visual problems. The culprit was found to be newer models of hip replacement prostheses, which contained cobalt. Erosion from metal-on-metal contact probably released cobalt into the patient's bloodstream, which lead to distal axonopathy and auditory and optic neuropathy. Accordingly, several models of these hip prostheses have been recalled.

In contrast, acute heavy metal poisoning typically leads to fatal gastrointestinal symptoms and cardiovascular collapse. Arsenic, which is tasteless and odorless, is a popular poison used in murder mystery cases. With chronic low-level intoxication – whether deliberate, accidental, or industrial – arsenic causes anorexia, malaise, and a distal neuropathy that might mimic Guillain–Barré syndrome. It also causes several characteristic dermatologic abnormalities: Mees' lines on the fingernails (Fig. 5.7), hyperpigmentation, and hyperkeratosis.

Mercury intoxication is more complex than arsenic poisoning. Individuals with mercury poisoning may develop a neuropathy and various CNS deficits, including cognitive impairment, tremor, ataxia, dysarthria, and visual field changes. Their gums accumulate a telltale dark line just below their teeth (Fig. 5.8).

Organic mercury compounds, such as methylmercury, typically enter the food chain at the lowest level and progress upward to saturate edible fish. Pregnant women who consume even modest quantities of mercury-containing food place their fetus at risk of mental retardation. Fish highest on the food chain carry the highest mercury concentrations. Thus, the fish group with the highest concentrations includes tuna (white meat), swordfish, and Chilean sea bass; the next highest, bluefish, halibut, and striped bass; the next highest is sole; and the lowest, herring and sardines.

Poisoning with inorganic mercury, which is widely used in industry, causes kidney damage but only mild cognitive impairment. Studies have not established definitively safe environmental or workplace levels.

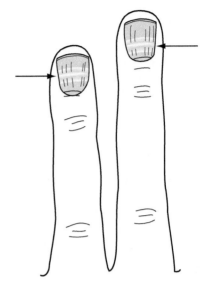

FIGURE 5.7 ■ Mees' lines, white bands (arrows) that stretch across the fingernails, characteristically indicate arsenic poisoning. In addition, poisoning by other heavy metals and trauma can cause them.

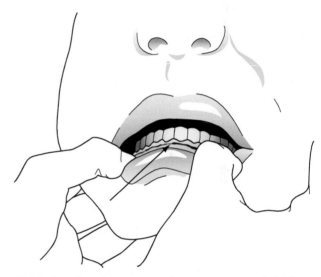

FIGURE 5.8 ■ Chronic mercury poisoning causes a dark blue or black line (arrow) along the gum. Individuals with this sign usually also have neuropathy and CNS signs, such as ataxia and dysarthria.

Investigators at one time proposed that mercury-based dental amalgams ("fillings") caused Alzheimer disease and other neurodegenerative illnesses either by dissolving in saliva and allowing mercury to enter the circulation or emitting a mercury vapor those individuals inhaled. In another inquiry, because ethyl mercury was a major component of the common vaccine preservative, *thimerosal*, investigators suspected that routine childhood immunizations caused autism (see Chapter 13). However, statistically powerful epidemiologic studies disproved both of those suspicions. In the case of vaccinations, the original "investigators" possibly engaged in fraud.

Thallium, another heavy metal, is the active ingredient in many foreign countries' rodenticides. Murderers, at least in mystery novels, lace food with it. Chronic thallium intoxication typically causes a painful neuropathy followed by hair loss (alopecia).

Aging

As people age, they develop sensory loss – akin to a sensory neuropathy – from peripheral nerve degeneration. Almost all individuals who are older than 80 years have lost some joint position and a great deal of vibratory sensation in their feet. This sensory neuropathy, which is accompanied by absent ankle DTRs, prevents older individuals from standing with their feet placed closely together, walking normally, and walking with a heel-to-toe (*tandem*) gait. It also predisposes them to falling. In addition, age- and work-related degenerative changes in the lumbar spine compress the lumbar nerve roots as they exit their neural foramina (see later, lumbar spondylosis).

Neuropathies With Comorbid Mental Status Changes

Although most neuropathies, as described in the previous section, may be painful, incapacitating, or even devastating to the PNS, they generally do not cause mental changes in adults. For example, most people who are elderly, diabetic, on hemodialysis, or receiving chemotherapy remain intelligent, thoughtful, and competent even though beset by pain, sensory loss, and weakness. In contrast, only a few diseases (Box 5.1) cause the combination of dementia and neuropathy, which would indicate both cerebral cortex and peripheral nerve damage. An analogous combination would be dementia and movement disorders, which would indicate cerebral cortex and basal ganglia damage (see Box 18.4).

Nutritional Deficiencies

Deficiencies of thiamine (vitamin B_1), niacin (nicotinic acid, B_3), or vitamin B_{12} (*cobalamin*), each produce a predominantly sensory neuropathy accompanied by dementia or other mental status abnormality (Table 5.3). From a worldwide perspective, starvation has been the most common cause of deficiencies of vitamins, their carrier-fats,

minerals, and other nutrients. For example, *beriberi* was the starvation-induced neuropathy attributable to thiamine deficiency endemic in eastern Asia. In the United States, alcoholism, bariatric surgery, and malabsorption syndromes have replaced starvation as the most common causes of nutritional neuropathies. Curiously, few patients with anorexia nervosa or self-imposed extreme diets develop a neuropathy. Their protection may lie in a selective, possibly secret, intake of food or vitamins.

Bariatric surgery remains a unique example. After its rapid introduction and widespread acceptance, postoperative "micronutrient" deficiencies caused various neurologic illnesses. Thiamine, copper, and vitamins B_{12} and E deficiencies frequently caused neuropathy, but also occasionally encephalopathy or myelopathy (see Chapter 4), i.e., CNS problems. Routine postoperative administration of these micronutrients has prevented the problem.

Alcohol-induced neuropathy has been virtually synonymous with thiamine deficiency because most cases are found in alcoholics who typically subsist on alcohol and carbohydrate-rich foods devoid of thiamine. Nevertheless, alcohol and thiamine deficiency may not be the only culprits. Studies have shown that alcohol itself did not cause a neuropathy and that thiamine deficiency is not present in all cases of this neuropathy.

Whatever the cause, thiamine deficiency generally leads to absent DTRs and loss of position sensation. Unless patients walk in the dark – a task relying on position sense generated in the legs and feet – their deficits may actually remain asymptomatic. In the well-known *Wernicke–Korsakoff syndrome*, amnesia, dementia, and cerebellar degeneration accompany the neuropathy associated with alcoholism (see Chapter 7).

In another example of vitamin deficiency-causing neuropathy, niacin deficiency is associated with or causes *pellagra* (Italian, rough skin). This starvation-induced disorder consists of dementia, dermatitis, and diarrhea – the "three D's." Despite pellagra's status as a classic illness, the role of niacin deficiency has been challenged: deficiencies of other nutrients either co-exist with or are more likely to be the actual cause.

TABLE 5.3 **Neurologic Aspects of Vitamins**

Vitamin	Diseases Associated With Deficiency	Diseases Associated With Excess	Miscellaneous Actions
A (e.g., retinol)	Night blindness	Pseudotumor cerebri	
B_1 Thiamine	Wernicke–Korsakoff syndrome* Beriberi*		
B_2 Riboflavin	Stomatitis		Migraine prophylaxis
B_3 Niacin	Pellagra*		
B_6 Pyridoxine	Seizures, psychosis	Neuropathy	
B_9 Folic acid/folate	Neural tube defects		Reduces elevated homocysteine levels
B_{12} Cobalamin	Combined system disease*		
C Ascorbic acid	Scurvy		
E Alpha-tocopherol	Ataxia, neuropathy		Scavenges free radicals

*Includes neuropathy as part of the illness

Among its many functions, vitamin B$_{12}$ sustains both CNS and PNS myelin. Thus, B$_{12}$ deficiency leads to the combination of CNS and PNS damage – *combined system degeneration*. Although its manifestations include a neuropathy, cognitive impairment and sensory loss reflecting demyelination of the posterior columns of the spinal cord (see Fig. 2.19B) predominate. Patients also develop a characteristic megaloblastic anemia. Most important, neurologists refer to combined system *degeneration* as a "correctable cause of dementia" because B$_{12}$ injections can reverse the cognitive impairment as well as the other CNS and PNS manifestations. The usual causes of B$_{12}$ deficiency include pernicious anemia, malabsorption, a pure vegetarian diet, or prolonged exposure to nitrous oxide (N$_2$O), a gaseous dental anesthetic. (N$_2$O inactivates B$_{12}$ by oxidizing its cobalt.)

The screening test for B$_{12}$ deficiency consists of determining the serum B$_{12}$ level, which is more sensitive, specific, and practical than the traditional Schilling test. In equivocal cases, especially when cognitive impairment or spinal cord abnormalities are not accompanied by anemia, determining the serum homocysteine and methylmalonic acid levels can corroborate the diagnosis: in B$_{12}$ deficiency, both homocysteine and methylmalonic acid levels rise to abnormally high levels (Fig. 5.9). Intrinsic factor antibodies, a classic finding in pernicious anemia, will be detectable in only about 60% of cases.

A variation on nutritional deficiencies causing neuropathy is celiac disease. In this condition, foods containing wheat gluten or similar protein constituents of rye and barley trigger an immune response. Affected individuals develop not only malabsorption, which is not always readily apparent, but also neuropathy and sometimes ataxia. Those severely affected develop osteoporosis, cardiac disease, and cancer.

In contrast to malnutrition causing neuropathy, excessive intake of certain vitamins causes neurologic problems. For example, although the normal adult daily requirement of vitamin B$_6$ (pyridoxine) is only 2 to 4 mg daily, several food faddists who consumed several grams daily as part of a special diet developed a profound sensory neuropathy. Similarly, high vitamin A intake may cause

pseudotumor cerebri (see Chapter 9) or induce fetal abnormalities (see Chapter 13).

Medication Adverse Effects

Several medications are well known to cause peripheral neuropathy without concomitant mental status changes (see above). One notable exception is disulfiram (Antabuse), a medication addiction psychiatrists give to alcoholics, which may have prominent neuropathy with associated encephalopathy. Because disulfiram blocks full ethanol metabolism, alcoholics develop acute severe nausea and vomiting if they consume alcohol while on the medication. However, the drug itself can be toxic, causing a prominent axonal neuropathy and even psychosis or seizures. Some patients may even have movement disorders related to bilateral basal ganglia lesions. Neurologists reassure most patients that these problems are reversible, but in severe cases residual effects may persist.

Infectious Diseases

Several common organisms have a predilection for infecting the peripheral nerves and sparing the CNS. For example, herpes zoster infects a single nerve root or a branch of the trigeminal nerve, usually in people older than 65 years or those with an impaired immune system. An infection with herpes (Greek *herpes*, spreading skin eruption) causes an ugly, red, painful, vesicular eruption ("shingles") that may remain excruciating long after the skin infection has resolved (see Postherpetic Neuralgia, Chapter 14). As another example, leprosy (Hansen disease), due to infection with *Mycobacterium leprae*, causes anesthetic, hypopigmented patches of skin, anesthetic fingers and toes, and palpable nerves. It particularly affects the cool portions of the body, such as the nose, ear lobes, and digits; however, depending on its variety, the infection may strike the ulnar or another large nerve either singly or along with others.

Some infections involve the CNS as well as the PNS. Named for the town in Connecticut where it was discovered, *Lyme disease* has risen to endemic levels in New England, Westchester, eastern Long Island, Wisconsin, Minnesota, and the Pacific Northwest. Infection by *Borrelia burgdorferi*, a spirochete whose vector is a certain tick, causes Lyme disease. The illness' peak incidence occurs in June through September, when people spend time in tick-infested wooded areas.

Acute Lyme disease typically produces multiple problems, such as arthritis, malaise, low-grade fever, cardiac arrhythmias, and a pathognomonic bull's-eye-shaped expanding rash, *erythema migrans* (Greek *erythema* flush + *migrans*, move), surrounding the tick bite. In addition, Lyme disease frequently causes facial nerve paresis, similar to Bell palsy, either unilaterally or bilaterally (see Fig. 4.15). Its PNS manifestations range from a mild neuropathy causing only paresthesias to a severe Guillain–Barré-like illness.

With CNS involvement, patients typically have headache, delirium (see Chapter 7), and other signs of meningitis or encephalitis. Their CSF may show a pleocytosis, elevated protein, decreased glucose concentrations, and

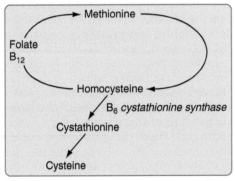

FIGURE 5.9 ■ B$_{12}$, acting as a co-enzyme, along with folate, facilitates the conversion of homocysteine to methionine. Other enzymes complete the cycle by converting methionine back to homocysteine. An absence of B$_{12}$ leads to the accumulation of both methionine and homocysteine. Whatever the cause, an elevated homocysteine level is a risk factor for neural tube defects, cerebrovascular and cardiovascular disease, and other neurologic conditions.

Lyme antibodies. Serologic tests for Lyme disease remain unreliable. Another confusing aspect of the diagnosis is that patients may have a biologic false-positive test for syphilis because *B. burgdorferi* is a spirochete (see Chapter 7).

Numerous individuals and physicians attribute years of symptoms – cognitive impairment, weakness, fatigue, and arthralgias – after an attack of adequately treated Lyme disease to a persistent Lyme infection or disordered immunologic response to it. The concept, "chronic Lyme disease," meets with skepticism in the neurologic community because it lacks consistent clinical criteria, pathology, and test results. Moreover, chronic Lyme disease symptoms do not respond to additional antibiotic treatment (see Chapters 6 and 7).

Even though Lyme disease is common, the most widespread infection of the CNS and PNS is *acquired immunodeficiency syndrome (AIDS)*. Although direct HIV infection probably causes neuropathy associated with AIDS, alternative potential etiologies include opportunistic infectious agents, such as CMV, and HIV medicines, such as nucleoside reverse transcriptase inhibitors (ddI [didanosine], Videx, and ddC [zalcitabine]). AIDS-associated peripheral neuropathy usually develops insidiously and consists of distal, symmetrical painful dysesthesias, which can be agonizing, and numbness of the soles of the feet. In contrast to the pronounced sensory symptoms, the motor symptoms consist of only relatively mild ankle and foot weakness with loss of ankle DTRs.

HIV-associated polyneuropathy generally develops late in the course of the illness when many other problems overshadow it. By then, the plasma HIV RNA titer is elevated and the CD4 count is low. In addition, depression and decreased physical function have supervened. Treatments for diabetic neuropathy often ameliorate the pain of AIDS neuropathy.

Inherited Metabolic Illnesses

Although numerous genetically determined illnesses cause neuropathy, two also cause psychosis.

Acute intermittent porphyria (AIP), the classic autosomal dominant genetic disorder of porphyrin metabolism, causes dramatic attacks of quadriparesis and colicky, often severe, abdominal pain. In about 25% to 50% of attacks AIP patients develop any of a variety of psychiatric symptoms, including agitation, delirium, depression, and psychosis. During attacks, excess porphyrins color the urine red. Quantitative tests, which replace the classic Watson–Schwartz test, readily detect urinary porphobilinogen and 5-aminolevulinic acid (ALA) in urine and serum. Although barbiturates and phenytoin may exacerbate an attack, phenothiazines are relatively safe. Notwithstanding its prominence as a standard examination question, AIP is rare in the United States.

Metachromatic leukodystrophy (MLD), an autosomal recessive illness carried on chromosome 22, derives its name from the colored granules (lipid sulfatides) that accumulate in the lysosomes of the brain, peripheral nerves, and many nonneurologic organs, such as the gallbladder, pancreas, and liver. Most important, MLD, like MS, causes a demyelination process in the CNS white matter (*leukodystrophy*) and, to a lesser extent, the PNS (see Chapter 15).

MLD symptoms usually first appear in infants and children, in whom the illness pursues a rapidly fatal course. In young adults, MLD presents with personality and behavioral changes, thought or mood disorders, and cognitive impairment. MLD-induced cognitive impairments typically progress slowly to dementia. Neurologists describe MLD-induced cognitive impairment as a "frontal dementia" because of its combination of personality, behavioral, and cognitive manifestations (see Chapter 7). Peripheral neuropathy and signs of CNS demyelination – spasticity and ataxia – follow and eventually overshadow the frontal dementia.

MLD is characterized by decreased activity of the lysosomal enzyme arylsulfatase A. Neurologists diagnose the illness by demonstrating a deficiency of this enzyme in leukocytes or cultured fibroblasts and the presence of metachromatic lipid material in biopsy specimens of peripheral nerves. In many cases, appropriate stains detect metachromatic lipid material in the urine. Autopsy specimens will show metachromatic material in cerebral tissue. As in MS, magnetic resonance imaging (MRI) shows demyelinated lesions in the brain (see Chapters 15 and 20). No treatment arrests the illness, but experimental treatments with bone marrow transplant and gene therapy hold promise.

Volatile Substance Exposure

Industrial organic solvents, which are generally lipophilic and volatile at room temperature, enter the body through inhalation, absorption through the skin, or occasionally by ingestion. Workers at risk of toxic exposures are those exposed to metal degreasing agents, paint and varnish, and shoe manufacturing chemicals; however, the danger depends more on poor ventilation and inadequate safety barriers than with particular industries.

Because of their lipophilic properties, industrial solvents, such as *n*-hexane, toluene, ethylene oxide, and carbon disulfide, penetrate the nervous system. Although these neurotoxins readily damage the CNS, PNS, or both, industrial solvents primarily cause a neuropathy. In addition, they sometimes cause various neuropsychologic symptoms – cognitive impairment, personality changes, inattention, depression, headaches, fatigue, and even psychosis – together termed *solvent-induced encephalopathy*.

Some individuals self-inflict solvent-induced encephalopathy through substance abuse. Recreational inhaling of certain volatile substances, "huffing," also damages one or both components of the nervous system. For example, in "glue sniffing," where the intoxicating component is the common hydrocarbon solvent *n*-hexane, sensation-seekers typically develop polyneuropathy and other PNS complications.

In contrast, recreationally inhaling toluene, a component of spray paint and marker pens, predominantly damages CNS rather than PNS myelin. In single exposures, inhaling toluene produces an alcohol-like euphoria, but chronic overexposure, whether deliberate or accidental, may cause personality changes, psychosis, and cognitive impairment that can reach the severity of dementia. Toluene-induced dementia falls into the category of subcortical dementia in which gait is impaired but language function is relatively preserved (see Chapter 7). Toluene may also cause ataxia, spasticity, and visual impairment. MRI can detect toluene-induced CNS demyelination (leukoencephalopathy, see Chapter 15). Thus, toluene exposure's clinical findings and MRI abnormalities mimic those of MS.

Nitrous oxide, the dental anesthetic, is also potentially toxic to the PNS and CNS, particularly the spinal cord (see previously). It is readily available in both gas cartridges, which are used in production of whipped cream, and large, safeguarded medical containers. Individuals who inhale nitrous oxide experience a few minutes of euphoria and relaxation as well as anesthesia. Frequently inhaling nitrous oxide, even intermittently for several weeks, may induce a profound neuropathy as well as spinal cord damage (see previously). Succumbing to nitrous oxide abuse and suffering the neurologic consequences remains an occupational hazard for dentists.

Pseudoneurotoxic Disease

Neurologists often diagnose occupational neurotoxicity when a group of workers has similar neurologic symptoms and signs, environmental tests detect elevated concentrations of a potential toxin in their workplace, the substance is an established cause of similar symptoms and signs in animals or humans, and laboratory testing of the workers shows abnormalities consistent with the symptoms. To be fair, symptoms of solvent-induced encephalopathy and other alleged neurotoxic states are usually nonspecific and largely subjective. Moreover, generally accepted diagnostic criteria often do not exist, relevant psychologic tests are often unreliable, and studies have not yet established safe exposure limits.

Sometimes workers' disorders have an explanation other than neurotoxin exposure. In *pseudoneurotoxic disease*, individuals attributing an illness to a neurotoxin have actually suffered the emergence or worsening of a neurologic or psychiatric disorder – alone or in combination – coincident with a neurotoxin exposure. In other words, despite their symptoms and signs, the neurotoxin has caused no ill effects. Attributing their illness to the neurotoxin constitutes a post hoc fallacy.

Sometimes the symptoms in pseudoneurotoxic cases may represent manifestations of an unequivocal neurologic illness, such as Parkinson disease or MS, which has emerged or worsened following the exposure. Similarly, patients may attribute age-related changes and variations in normal neurologic function to a neurotoxin exposure. Alternatively, the patients may have a somatic disorder, mood disorder, alcohol abuse, or other psychiatric disturbance whose manifestations mimic solvent-induced encephalopathy or other neurotoxic disorder.

The *multiple chemical sensitivity syndrome* serves as a prime example of pseudoneurotoxic disease. This disorder consists of miniscule exposures to environmental chemicals, ones usually volatile and unavoidable in day-to-day life, such as commercial cleaning agents or air fresheners, allegedly producing multiple but variable symptoms. According to affected individuals, exposure to innumerable chemicals causes attacks, which are often incapacitating, consisting of headache, alterations in level of consciousness, paresis, or various physical problems. Despite these individuals' dramatic and compelling histories and their remaining apparently free of psychiatric disturbances between episodes, scientific analysis has shown that the symptoms are unrelated to chemical exposure and have no underling physiologic basis.

Marine Toxicology

Shellfish, free-swimming fish, and other forms of sea-life produce, carry, or become contaminated by various toxins, such as organic mercury compounds (see above). *Ciguatera fish poisoning*, the best-understood and most commonly occurring example of "marine toxicology," produces gastrointestinal and unique neurologic symptoms. The toxin, *ciguatoxin*, reaches humans by moving up the food-chain from toxin-producing dinoflagellates to large, edible reef fish, particularly grouper, red snapper, and barracuda. These fish inhabit the waters off Caribbean or Indian Ocean islands, where seafood diners often fall victim.

Unlike other toxins, ciguatoxin causes a prolonged opening of voltage-gated sodium channels in nerves and muscles. Individuals who ingest ciguatoxin first have nausea and vomiting, as with most food poisonings, but then many develop the characteristic symptoms of an acute painful neuropathy with paresthesias, pain, and lack of sensation in their limbs. Victims also experience a unique symptom, *cold allodynia* or *cold reversal*, in which they misperceive cold objects as feeling hot. For example, they will sense that iced tea is hot tea served in a tall glass with ice. Although victims eventually recover, malaise, depression, and headaches may persist for months.

Puffer fish, a Japanese delicacy, and some crabs on rare occasion, contain *tetrodotoxin*. Unlike ciguatoxin, tetrodotoxin is potentially lethal. Victims first develop numbness around the mouth and face, and then flaccid quadriparesis, which leads to respiratory failure.

MOTOR NEURON DISORDERS

Amyotrophic Lateral Sclerosis

For decades, neurologists referred to amyotrophic lateral sclerosis (ALS) as "Lou Gehrig disease" because this famous baseball player succumbed to this dreadful illness. Neurologists call ALS the quintessential *motor neuron disease* because both upper and lower motor neurons (UMNs and LMNs) degenerate while other neurologic systems – notably mental faculties – are usually spared.

The etiology of ALS remains an enigma, but several genetic, environmental, and pathologic findings hold some promise. One is that 5% to 10% of patients seem to inherit ALS in an autosomal dominant pattern. Some of them – 2% of all ALS patients – carry a mutation of a gene on chromosome 21 (Cu, Zn superoxide dismutase [SOD1]) that normally assists in detoxifying superoxide free radicals. Another intriguing finding is a significantly increased incidence of ALS among US veterans of the

Persian Gulf War. If the epidemiologic studies hold up, the cause in those cases may be related to either trauma, including traumatic brain injury, or exposure to a toxin, such as a pesticide or heavy metal. Among all people, cigarette smoking poses an unequivocal risk. It carries an up to fourfold increased risk for ALS.

The pathology of ALS, degeneration of motor neurons without a surrounding cellular reaction, weighs against inflammatory and infectious etiologies. Many ALS patients do respond, albeit modestly, to blocking glutamate, the excitatory neurotransmitter (see Chapter 21). Putting together these clues – the lack of a cellular response and a beneficial response to glutamate blocking – suggests that *glutamate excitotoxicity* leads to cell death from *apoptosis* (see Chapters 18 and 21).

Except for the veterans, patients develop ALS at a median age of 66 years. Their first symptoms usually consist of weakness, atrophy, and subcutaneous muscular twitching (*fasciculations*) – a sign of degenerating anterior horn cells – all in one arm or leg (Fig. 5.10). Surprisingly, even from these atrophic muscles, physicians can elicit brisk DTRs – a sign of upper motor degeneration – because damaged UMNs supply enough undamaged LMNs. The weakness, atrophy, and fasciculations spread asymmetrically to other limbs and also to the face, pharynx, and tongue. Dysarthria and dysphagia (bulbar palsy) eventually develop in most patients. When pseudobulbar palsy superimposes itself on bulbar palsy, patients' speech becomes unintelligible and interrupted by "demonic" or "pathologic" laughing and crying, and their behavior falls into the category of involuntary emotional expression disorder (see Chapter 4). Despite their extensive paresis, patients maintain control over their eye movements and bladder and bowel function.

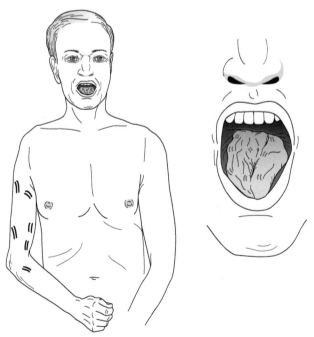

FIGURE 5.10 ■ This elderly gentleman with ALS has typical asymmetric limb atrophy, paresis, and fasciculations. His tongue, which also has fasciculations, has undergone atrophy, as indicated by clefts and furrows.

Because ALS attacks upper and lower motor neurons, cognitive impairment is not an early, pronounced, or consistent sign of the disease. However, contrary to prior thinking, up to 50% of patients with ALS may have some mild cognitive impairment, though they usually retain decisional capacity and tragically have complete awareness of their plight. A smaller group of ALS victims, about 10–20%, meet the criteria for dementia. This group generally displays some clinical and pathological features of frontotemporal dementia (FTD), in which behavioral and emotional changes accompany cognitive impairment (see Chapter 7). This so-called ALS-FTD syndrome is most commonly caused by a mutation on chromosome 9 of the C9ORF72 gene, leading to a hexanucleotide (six nucleotide) repeat expansion, though some patients with this mutation may only have symptoms of ALS *or* FTD, rather than both conditions together. This mutation is the most common identified genetic anomaly in ALS.

At present, no treatment can cure or even arrest ALS. However, riluzole (Rilutek), presumably by reducing glutamate excitotoxicity, modestly slows the illness' progression. Multidisciplinary healthcare groups, some physical therapy, nutrition supplied by gastrostomy, and noninvasive ventilation, especially at night, make ALS patients more comfortable and prolong their life. About 80% of ALS patients receiving standard or even aggressive medical care die, usually from respiratory complications or sepsis, within 5 years of the time of diagnosis.

The suicide rate among ALS patients is six times greater than controls. Suicide occurs more frequently among relatively young ALS patients and those in the early stage of their illness.

When asked to consult, psychiatrists usually find that ALS patients retain their "decisional capacity." It remains intact when, as is often the case, they refuse resuscitation measures, mechanical ventilation, and other life-support devices. Because patients remain lucid, competent, and usually free of sedating medications, but carry the burden of a relatively rapid demise from untreatable fatal disease, ALS has become the prime example for discussions concerning end-of-life care, patients' right to die, physician-assisted suicide, and euthanasia. After litigation or legislation, several patients have hastened the inevitable process of ALS. In addition, psychiatrists often find that ALS patient caregivers, just as Alzheimer disease and multiple sclerosis caregivers, have depressive symptoms.

Childhood-Onset Motor Neuron Diseases

Extensive loss of anterior horn cells with preserved cognitive function and extraocular muscle movement also characterizes several other motor neuron diseases. For example, hereditary motor neuron diseases in infants (Werdnig–Hoffmann disease) and children (Kugelberg–Welander disease) – varieties of *spinal muscular atrophy* (*SMA*) – also causes progressively severe flaccid quadriparesis with atrophic, areflexic muscles, and fasciculations. In contrast to ALS, both of these illnesses lack UMN signs. They follow an autosomal recessive pattern of inheritance due to a mutation on chromosome 5.

Poliomyelitis

Poliomyelitis (polio) had been the most frequently occurring motor neuron disease until Jonas Salk and his coworkers developed a vaccine. Mandatory poliovirus vaccination programs have almost completely eradicated the disease. However, it persists in Nigeria and the Indian subcontinent because many children in those regions receive too few or no vaccinations.

Poliovirus infects the motor neurons of the anterior horn cells of the spinal cord and lower brainstem (the bulb). Patients, who were mostly children, typically developed an acute, febrile illness with ALS-type LMN signs: asymmetric paresis with muscle fasciculations and absent DTRs. Patients with the bulbar variety of polio developed throat and chest muscle paralysis that forced them into an "iron lung" to support their respirations. The iron lung was essentially a metal tube, approximately 3 feet in diameter and 5 feet long, that extended from the patient's neck, which was sealed by a rubber ring, to the feet. A pump would suck out air from the inside of the large tube to create negative pressure that forced room air into the patient's lungs.

In polio, as in ALS, oculomotor, bladder, bowel, and sexual functions are normal (see Chapters 12 and 16). Likewise, polio patients, no matter how devastating their illness, retain normal cognitive function. For example, Franklin Roosevelt, handicapped by polio-induced paraplegia, served as president of the United States.

Some individuals who had poliomyelitis in childhood go on to develop additional weakness and fasciculations in middle age. Investigators have postulated the existence of a *post-polio syndrome* to explain the late deterioration; however, if this syndrome exists at all, it is rare. In practice, common nonneurologic conditions, such as lumbar spine degeneration, can readily account for it.

Other agents besides the poliomyelitis virus may infect motor neurons. For example, West Nile virus causes a polio-like illness. This RNA virus, which lives in birds and is transmitted by mosquitos, can also present with a polio-like illness, usually causing bilateral lower-extremity flaccid paralysis due to motor neuron dysfunction. These symptoms are usually preceded by encephalitis, with fever and confusion. Neurologists have also suspected that enterovirus 68, which is in the same family as poliovirus, similarly infects motor neurons and causes acute flaccid myelitis. These patients differ from traditional polio patients in that they do not have a preceding meningoencephalitis and pain is not always present with the onset of weakness.

BENIGN FASCICULATIONS

Fasciculations are commonplace, innocuous muscle twitches that are usually caused or precipitated by excessive physical exertion, psychological stress, excessive caffeine intake, or exposure to some insecticides. The diagnosis of benign fasciculations may be difficult because they mimic ALS-induced fasciculations and are sometimes associated with fatigue and hyperactive DTRs. A clinical guideline would be that, in contrast to ALS-induced fasciculations, benign fasciculations are unaccompanied by weakness, atrophy, or pathologic reflexes, and they usually last for only several days to weeks. Using this guideline will help calm fears of medical students and others acquainted with ALS. After all, the majority of individuals with benign fasciculations have had medical training.

Sometimes twitching, which mimics fasciculations, of the eyelid muscles (orbicularis oculi) creates annoying movements. Neurologists call them *myokymia* and blame lack of sleep, excessive caffeine, and other irritants. In a different situation – if the movements are bilateral, forceful enough to close the eyelids, or exceed a duration of 1 second – they may represent a facial dyskinesia, such as blepharospasm, hemifacial spasm, or tardive dyskinesia (see Chapter 18).

SPINE DISEASE

Cervical spondylosis is the chronic age- and occupation-related degenerative condition of the upper spine in which bony encroachment leads to stenosis of the vertebral foramina and spinal canal (Fig. 5.11). Stenosis of the neural foramina constricts cervical nerve roots, which causes neck pain with arm and hand paresis, atrophy, hypoactive DTRs, and fasciculations – signs of LMN injury. Cervical spondylosis may also create spinal canal stenosis that compresses the spinal cord to cause myelopathy with leg weakness, spasticity, hyperreflexia, and Babinski signs – signs of UMN injury.

Lumbar spondylosis, the lower spine counterpart and frequent accompaniment of cervical spondylosis, produces lumbar nerve root compression and low back pain; however, because the spinal cord descends only to the first lumbar vertebra (see Fig. 16.1), lumbar spondylosis cannot cause spinal cord compression. *Spondylolisthesis*, which may accompany spondylosis, consists of the forward slip of adjacent lumbar vertebrae or of L5 on the sacrum. Lumbar spondylosis, with or without spondylolisthesis, commonly produces chronic buttock pain that radiates down the posterior aspect of the leg (*sciatica*). Its other symptoms are leg and feet fasciculations, paresis, atrophy, and knee or ankle areflexia. Sometimes patients with lumbar stenosis have symptoms of pain and weakness in their legs only when they walk (*neurogenic claudication*).

By causing both PNS and CNS signs, cervical and lumbar spondylosis mimics ALS. The features that distinguish spondylosis from ALS are its neck or low back pain, sensory loss, and absence of abnormalities in the facial, pharyngeal, and tongue muscles.

A ramification of cervical and lumbar spondylosis is that it causes chronic pain. It deprives people of work, mobility, and leisure activities. It sometimes contributes to depression and requires strong analgesics, perhaps opioids, as well as antidepressants (see Chapter 14). Carefully selected cases of severe spondylolisthesis and lumbar spondylosis with marked, symptomatic stenosis of the spinal canal will benefit from surgery.

A related disorder is spinal intervertebral disk herniation, which neurologists abbreviate to *herniated disk*. Intervertebral disks are gelatinous shock absorbers that

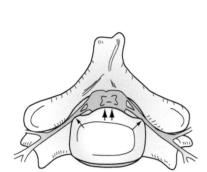

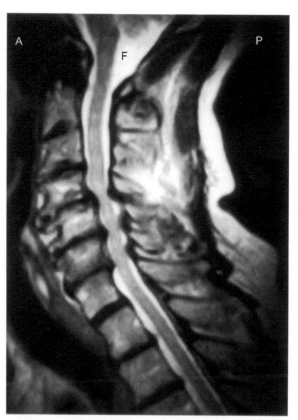

FIGURE 5.11 ■ *Left,* In cervical spondylosis, bony proliferation damages upper and lower motor neurons. Intervertebral ridges of bone (double arrows) compress the cervical spinal cord. At the same time, narrowing of the foramina (single arrows) constricts cervical nerve roots. *Right,* The MRI shows a lateral view of cervical spondylosis. The CSF in the foramen magnum (F) and surrounding the spinal cord is bright white. The spinal cord is gray. In the mid- to low cervical spine, bony protrusions and hypertrophied ligaments compress the spinal cord and its surrounding CSF.

typically herniate or bulge in the curved cervical or lumbosacral spine. When they suddenly press against nerve roots as they emerge through the spinal foramina, herniated disks produce acute neck or low back pain. The pain may radiate down the nerve root's distribution. Depending on the location and size of the herniation, sensory loss or weakness may accompany the pain.

When cervical intervertebral disks herniate and compress one or more cervical nerve roots, they typically cause neck pain that may radiate down the arm. Weakness of arm or hand muscles with loss of an upper extremity DTR sometimes accompanies the pain. Whiplash automobile injuries and other trauma may cause herniated cervical intervertebral disks. Even without trauma, probably because of degeneration, disks herniate.

More than 90% of lumbosacral disk herniations occur at either the L4–5 or L5–S1 intervertebral space. These interspaces are vulnerable because they bear the stress of the body's weight on the lumbar spine curve. Herniated lumbar disks cause low back pain that radiates into the buttock and often down one or both legs, i.e., sciatica. They may also cause weakness of the ankle and foot muscles and loss of the ankle DTR, but infrequently the knee DTR. Large lumbar disk herniations may cause compression of all the lower lumbar and sacral nerve roots, which comprise the *cauda equina* (Fig. 5.12). Such herniated disks may produce the *cauda equina syndrome*: LMN

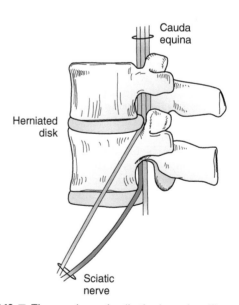

FIGURE 5.12 ■ The *cauda equina* (Latin, horse's tail) consists of the bundle of lumbar and sacral nerve roots in the lower spinal canal. The nerve roots leave the spinal canal through foramina. Herniated disks might compress the nerve roots in or near those narrow passages. Compressed nerve roots usually cause pain in the low back that radiates along the distribution of the sciatic nerve. Common movements that momentarily further protrude the disk, such as coughing, sneezing, or straining at stool, intensify the pain. Large herniated disks may compress the entire cauda equina.

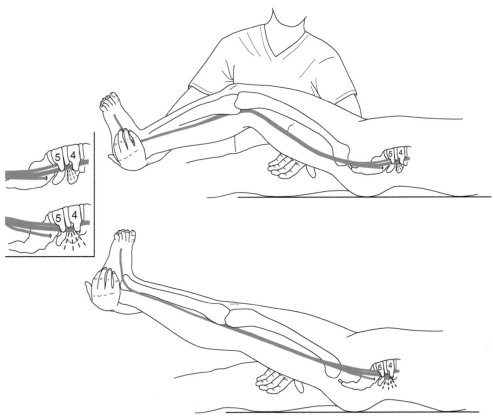

FIGURE 5.13 ■ If a patient has a herniated lumbar intervertebral disk and a physician raises the patient's straightened leg, the maneuver will probably cause low back pain to radiate to the buttocks and perhaps further down the leg (*Lasègue sign*). This position draws the nerve against the edge of a herniated disk, which leads to nerve compression and irritation.

paresis of one or both legs, perineal ("saddle area") pain and anesthesia, incontinence, and sexual dysfunction.

Poor posture and obesity, as well as the causes of cervical herniated disks, predispose individuals to lumbar herniations. Coughing, sneezing, or elevating the straightened leg – because these maneuvers press the herniated disk more forcefully against the nerve root – characteristically increase buttock and leg pain (Fig. 5.13).

Herniated disks are rarely responsible for all the chronic pain, disability, sexual dysfunction, and multitudinous other symptoms that many individuals, especially litigants, attribute to them. In fact, herniated disks are often an innocuous, chance finding. For example, MRI studies have revealed a herniated disk in 20% of asymptomatic individuals younger than 60 years. Even more so, bulging and desiccated disks, because they do not compress nerve roots, do not cause these symptoms.

Nonopioid analgesics, superficial heat, and reduction in physical activity usually alleviate acute neck or low back pain from herniated disks. Epidural injections of steroids, which often include some lidocaine, improve acute pain from lumbar herniated disks but do not alter the outcome, when compared to patients receiving just lidocaine or placebo. The popular spinal decompression machines do not help. Although 90% of acute low back pain cases resolve in 6 weeks, about 25% of patients who recover from low back pain suffer a recurrence within 1 year and about 10% devolve into a state of chronic low back pain. Surgery is indicated, most neurologists

feel, only for spinal cord compression, cauda equina syndrome, refractory objective symptoms and signs of nerve root compression, neurologic deficits, or severe disability.

WEB SITE

Agency for Toxic Substances and Disease Registry: <http://www.atsdr.cdc.gov/>.

REFERENCES

Alao, A. O., Soderberg, M. G., & Geller, G. (2004). Psychiatric symptoms in acute intermittent porphyria. *Resident and Staff Physician, 50,* 28–32.

Albert, S. M., Rabkin, J. G., Del Bene, M. L., et al. (2005). Wish to die in end-stage ALS. *Neurology, 65,* 68–74.

Armon, C., Argoff, C. E., Samuels, J., et al. (2007). Assessment: Use of epidural steroid injections to treat radicular lumbosacral pain. *Neurology, 68,* 723–729.

Aubourg, P., Adamsbaum, C., Lavallard-Rousseau, M. C., et al. (1993). A two-year trial of oleic and erucic acids ("Lorenzo's oil") as treatment for adrenomyeloneuropathy. *The New England Journal of Medicine, 329,* 745–752.

Black, D. N., Taber, K. H., & Hurley, R. A. (2003). Metachromatic leukodystrophy: A model for the study of psychosis. *The Journal of Neuropsychiatry and Clinical Neurosciences, 15,* 289–293.

Boukriche, Y., Weisser, I., Aubert, P., et al. (2000). MRI findings in a case of late onset disulfiram-induced neurotoxicity. *Journal of Neurology, 247,* 714–715.

Byrne, S., Elamin, M., Bede, P., et al. (2012). Cognitive and clinical characteristics of patients with amyotrophic lateral sclerosis carrying a C9orf72 repeat expansion: a population-based cohort study. *The Lancet Neurology, 11,* 232–240.

Clarkson, T. W., Magos, L., & Myers, G. L. (2003). The toxicology of mercury – current exposures and clinical manifestations. *The New England Journal of Medicine, 349*, 1731–1736.

Devlin, J. J., Pomerleau, A. C., Brent, J., et al. (2013). Clinical features, testing, and management of patients with suspected prosthetic hip-associated cobalt toxicity: A review of cases. *Journal of Medical Toxicology: Official Journal of the American College of Medical Toxicology, 9*, 405–415.

Elamin, M., Alderazi, Y., Mullins, G., et al. (2009). Perineuritis in acute Lyme neuroborreliosis. *Muscle and Nerve, 39*(6), 851–854.

England, J., Gronseth, G., Franklin, G., et al. (2009). Practice Parameter: Evaluation of distal symmetric polyneuropathy: Role of laboratory and genetic testing (an evidence-based review). *Neurology, 72*, 185–192.

Estrov, Y., Scaglia, F., & Bodamer, O. A. (2000). Psychiatric symptoms of inherited metabolic disease. *Journal of Inherited Metabolic Disease, 23*, 2–6.

Eyeson, J., House, I., Yang, Y. H., et al. (2010). Relationship between mercury levels in blood and urine and complaints of chronic mercury toxicity from amalgam restorations. *British Dental Journal, 208*, E7.

Fang, F., Valdimarsdottir, U., Furst, C. J., et al. (2008). Suicide among patients with amyotrophic lateral sclerosis. *Brain: A Journal of Neurology, 131*, 2729–2733.

Feder, H. M., Johnson, B., O'Connell, S., et al. (2007). A critical appraisal of chronic Lyme disease. *The New England Journal of Medicine, 357*, 1422–1430.

Filley, C. M., & Kleinschmidt-DeMasters, B. K. (2001). Toxic leukoencephalopathies. *The New England Journal of Medicine, 345*, 425–432.

Filley, C. M., Halliday, W., & Kleinschmidt-DeMasters, B. K. (2004). The effects of toluene on the central nervous system. *Journal of Neuropathology and Experimental Neurology, 63*, 1–12.

Florica, B., Aghdassi, E., Su, J., et al. (2011). Peripheral neuropathy in patients with systemic lupus erythematosus. *Seminars in Arthritis and Rheumatism, 41*, 203–211.

Friedly, J. L., Comstock, B. A., Turner, J. A., et al. (2014). A randomized trial of epidural glucocorticoid injections for spinal stenosis. *The New England Journal of Medicine, 371*, 11–21.

Gauthier, A., Vignola, A., Cavlo, A., et al. (2007). A longitudinal study on quality of life and depression in ALS patient–caregiver couples. *Neurology, 68*, 923–926.

Gonzalez-Arriaza, H. L., & Bostwick, J. M. (2003). Acute porphyrias. *The American Journal of Psychiatry, 160*, 450–458.

Herskovitz, S., Scelsa, S. N., & Schaumburg, H. H. (2010). *Peripheral Neuropathies in Clinical Practice*. New York: Oxford University Press.

Hyde, T. M., Ziegler, J. C., & Weinberger, D. R. (1992). Psychiatric disturbances in metachromatic leukodystrophy. *Archives of Neurology, 49*, 401–406.

Isbister, G., & Kiernan, M. C. (2005). Neurotoxic marine poisoning. *The Lancet Neurology, 4*, 219–228.

Katz, J. N., & Simmons, B. P. (2002). Carpal tunnel syndrome. *The New England Journal of Medicine, 346*, 1807–1812.

Khan, F. (2015). Enterovirus D68: Acute respiratory illness and the 2014 outbreak. *Emergency Medicine Clinics of North America, 33*, 319–322.

Koffman, B. M., Greenfield, L. J., & Ali, P. (2006). Neurologic complications after surgery for obesity. *Muscle and Nerve, 33*, 166–176.

Kumperscak, H. G., Plesnicar, B. K., Zalar, B., et al. (2007). Adult metachromatic leukodystrophy: A new mutation in the schizophrenia-like phenotype with early neurologic signs. *Psychiatric Genetics, 17*, 85–91.

Miller, R. G., Jackson, C. E., & Kararskis, E. J. (2009). Practice Parameter update: The care of the patient with amyotrophic lateral sclerosis: Drug, nutritional, and respiratory therapies: Report of the Quality Standards Subcommittee of the American Academy of Neurology. *Neurology, 73*, 1218–1226.

Patijn, J., Mekhail, N., Hayek, S., et al. (2011). Meralgia paresthetica. *Pain Practice, 11*, 302–308.

Peul, W. C., Houwelingen, H. C. V., & Hout, W. B. V. D. (2007). Surgery versus prolonged conservative treatment for sciatica. *The New England Journal of Medicine, 356*, 2245–2256.

Phukan, J., Pender, N. P., & Hardiman, O. (2007). Cognitive impairment in amyotrophic lateral sclerosis. *The Lancet Neurology, 6*, 994–1003.

Quecedo, E., Sanmartin, O., Febrer, M. I., et al. (1996). Mees' lines: A clue to the diagnosis of arsenic poisoning. *Archives of Dermatology, 132*, 349–350.

Research Advisory Committee on Gulf War Veterans' Illnesses. U.S. Department of Veterans Affairs. Gulf War Illness and the Health of Gulf War Veterans. <http://sph.bu.edu/insider/racreport>.

Rowland, L. P., & Shneider, N. A. (2001). Amyotrophic lateral sclerosis. *The New England Journal of Medicine, 344*, 1688–1700.

Saito, M., Kumano, H., Yoshiuchi, K., et al. (2005). Symptoms profile of multiple chemical sensitivity in actual life. *Psychosomatic Medicine, 67*, 318–325.

Schaumburg, H. H., & Albers, J. W. (2005). Pseudoneurotoxic disease. *Neurology, 65*, 22–26.

Shaibani, A. (2014). *A Video Atlas of Neuromuscular Disorders*. Oxford: Oxford University Press.

Sharief, M. K., Priddin, J., Delamont, R. S., et al. (2002). Neurophysiologic analysis of neuromuscular symptoms in UK Gulf War veterans: a controlled study. *Neurology, 59*, 1518–1525.

Simpson, D. M., Kitch, D., Evans, S. R., et al. (2006). HIV neuropathy natural history cohort study: Assessment measures and risk factors. *Neurology, 66*, 1679–1687.

Staudenmayer, H., Selner, J. C., & Buhr, M. P. (1993). Double-blind provocations chamber challenges in 20 patients presenting with "multiple chemical sensitivity". *Regulatory Toxicology and Pharmacology, 18*, 44–53.

Strong, M. J., Lomen-Hoerth, C., Caselli, R. J., et al. (2003). Cognitive impairment, frontotemporal dementia, and the motor neuron disease. *Annals of Neurology, 54*(Suppl. 5), S20–S23.

Triebig, G., Nasterlack, M., Hacke, W., et al. (2000). Neuropsychiatric symptoms in active construction painters with chronic solvent exposure. *Neurotoxicology, 21*, 791–794.

Tyler, K. L. (2014). Current developments in understanding of West Nile virus central nervous system disease. *Current Opinion in Neurology, 27*, 342–348.

Yuki, N., & Hartung, H. P. (2012). Guillain-Barré syndrome. *The New England Journal of Medicine, 366*, 2294–2304.

CHAPTER 5

QUESTIONS AND ANSWERS

1. After recovering from an overdose, a 31-year-old heroin addict has paresis of his right wrist, thumb, and finger extensor muscles. All DTRs are normal except for the right brachioradialis DTR, which is depressed. Where is the lesion?
   a. Cerebral hemisphere
   b. Spinal cord
   c. Radial nerve
   d. Median nerve

Answer: c. The patient has a wrist drop from compression of the right radial nerve as it winds around the humerus. This mononeuropathy occurs commonly among drug addicts and alcoholics who, while stuporous, are apt to lean against their arm for many hours. Drug addicts are also liable to develop brain abscesses, acquired immunodeficiency syndrome (AIDS), and cerebrovascular accidents – but these are all diseases of the CNS that cause hyperactive DTRs, a different pattern of weakness, and, usually when the dominant cerebrum is involved, aphasia.

2. An 18-year-old waiter suffered 8 days of watery diarrhea followed by the development of a Guillain–Barré syndrome. Which is the most likely cause of his illness?
   a. Lyme disease
   b. Mononucleosis
   c. A viral respiratory tract infection
   d. *Campylobacter jejuni* infection

Answer: d. All of these infectious illnesses can cause Guillain–Barré syndrome. However, *Campylobacter jejuni* infections, which cause diarrhea, characteristically lead to the most severe, extensive, and slowly resolving deficits.

3. A 24-year-old woman has the sudden onset of low back pain with inability to dorsiflex and evert her right ankle. She also has mild weakness of ankle inversion. Raising her straightened right leg produces back pain that radiates down the lateral leg. Sensation is diminished on the dorsum of her right foot. Her DTRs remain normal. Which is the most likely lesion?
   a. Fibular nerve diabetic infarction
   b. Polyneuropathy
   c. Femoral nerve compression
   d. L4-5 herniated intervertebral disk

Answer: d. The dorsiflexion and eversion paresis of her right ankle, pain on straight leg raising (Lasègue

sign), and sensory loss on the dorsum of her right foot indicate that the low back pain involves a nerve root injury rather than merely muscle strain, degenerative spine disease, or a retroperitoneal condition, such as endometriosis. Those findings indicate an L5 nerve root lesion. In view of the sudden onset and statistical likelihood in a young woman, she probably has an L4–L5 herniated intervertebral disk compressing the L5 nerve root. An injury of the fibular nerve, which neurologists and other physicians previously called the peroneal nerve, would not cause the ankle inversion weakness.

4. A 54-year-old man with pulmonary carcinoma has had 2 weeks of midthoracic back pain. He describes the sudden onset of abnormal sensation in his legs and difficulty walking. He has weakness of both legs, which are areflexic, and hypalgesia from the toes to the umbilicus. What process is evolving?
   a. Cervical spinal cord compression
   b. Thoracic spinal cord compression
   c. Lumbar spinal cord compression
   d. Guillain–Barré syndrome

Answer: b. He has acute thoracic spinal cord compression from a metastatic tumor. It is causing paraparesis, sensory loss below T10, and areflexia from "spinal shock." The pathologic process is not a neuropathy because of the absence of symptoms in the upper extremities, the presence of a sensory level (rather than a stocking-glove sensory loss), and his localized back pain.

5. After recovering consciousness, while still sitting on a toilet, a 27-year-old drug addict is unable to walk. He has paresis of the knee flexor (hamstring) muscles and all ankle and toe muscles. His knee DTRs are normal, but his ankle DTRs and plantar reflexes are absent. Sensation is absent below the knees. Where is the lesion(s)?
   a. Bilateral anterior cerebral artery occlusions
   b. Lumbar spinal cord injury
   c. Bilateral sciatic nerve compression
   d. Ankle or foot injuries

Answer: c. He has sustained a bilateral sciatic nerve compression injury, which often happens to drug addicts who take an overdose when sitting on a toilet. This injury, the "toilet seat neuropathy," is the lower-extremity counterpart of the wrist drop (see Question 1).

6. A 58-year-old carpenter reports weakness of his right arm and hand. He has fasciculations and atrophy of

the hand and triceps muscles and no triceps reflex. There is mild sensory loss along the medial surface of his right hand. What process is occurring?
a. Amyotrophic lateral sclerosis (ALS)
b. Cervical spondylosis
c. Polyneuropathy
d. Cervical spinal cord syrinx

Answer: b. He has symptoms and signs of cervical spondylosis with nerve root compression, which is an occupational hazard among laborers. Cervical spondylosis resembles ALS because of the atrophy and fasciculations, but the sensory loss precludes that diagnosis. In cervical spondylosis, depending on the degree of foraminal compression, DTRs may be either hyperactive or hypoactive. By way of contrast, the DTRs in ALS, despite the loss of anterior horn cells, remain hyperactive. A syrinx can mimic cervical spondylosis, but it causes pronounced sensory loss and, in the absence of a severe injury, develops in adolescence. Also, an MRI would easily distinguish a syrinx from spondylosis.

7. A 30-year-old computer programmer describes painful tingling in both of her palms and first three fingers on both hands that often wakes her from sleep. In addition, she reports frequently dropping small objects. She has mild paresis of her thumb (thenar) abduction and opposition muscles. Percussion of her wrists recreates the paresthesias. DTRs are normal. What is the cause?
a. Cervical spondylosis
b. Carpal tunnel syndrome
c. Toxic neuropathy
d. Fatigue

Answer: b. Her typical sensory disturbances and almost pathognomonic Tinel sign (percussion of the flexor surface of the wrist creates a tingling sensation in the median nerve distribution) indicate that she has bilateral carpal tunnel syndrome, i.e., median nerve compression at the wrist. The carpal tunnel syndrome frequently occurs when fluid accumulates in the carpal tunnel, such as during pregnancy and before menses. Acromegaly or hypothyroidism also leads to tissue or fluid accumulation in the carpal tunnel. It also occurs after trauma to the wrist, including wrist fractures and occupational "repetitive stress injuries," such as assembly-line handwork and carpentry. The clinical diagnosis in most cases can be based on the occupation, sensory symptoms, and Tinel sign. Weakness and atrophy of the thenar muscles develop inconsistently and only late in its course. Nerve conduction velocity studies demonstrating focal slowing across the wrist can confirm the diagnosis.

8. A young woman has developed marked confusion and hallucinations, flaccid paresis, and abdominal pain. Her urine has turned red. Which urine test should be performed?
a. Cocaine metabolites
b. Narcotic metabolites
c. Watson–Schwartz
d. Myoglobin

Answer: c. She has acute intermittent porphyria. Quantitative analyses for urinary and serum porphobilinogen and 5-aminolevulinic acid (ALA) have supplanted the classic Watson–Schwartz test, which is still occasionally used as a screening test. Phenothiazines, which may be safely administered, may suppress psychotic symptoms. Barbiturates and phenytoin are contraindicated because they may precipitate or worsen an attack.

9. A 31-year-old neurosurgery resident has the sudden onset of inability to elevate and evert her right ankle. She has hypalgesia on the lateral aspect of her calf and dorsum of the foot, but her ankle DTR and plantar reflexes remain normal. Which is the most likely diagnosis?
a. Spinal cord compression
b. Sciatic nerve injury
c. Fibular nerve injury
d. Polyneuropathy

Answer: c. She has had the sudden, painless onset of a fibular nerve injury. Crossing the legs, leaning against furniture, or wearing a cast commonly compresses the fibular nerve. At the lateral aspect of the knee, where nerve is covered only by skin and subcutaneous tissue, the nerve is particularly vulnerable. When patients lose weight and their subcutaneous fat is depleted, the nerve is left unprotected from compression. Sometimes diabetes, Lyme disease, or a vasculitis causes fibular nerve injury or other mononeuropathy. An L4–L5 herniated disk is unlikely because the onset of her illness was painless and her sensory loss is too lateral.

10. Several workers in a chemical factory describe tingling of their fingers and toes and weakness of their feet. Each worker has stocking-glove hypalgesia and absent ankle DTRs. Of the following, which is the most common cause of such symptoms in the industrial setting?
a. Psychogenic disturbances
b. Repetitive stress injury
c. Exposure to an industrial toxin
d. Drug abuse

Answer: c. The loss of ankle DTRs is objective. Although the hypalgesia and other symptoms and signs can be mimicked, areflexia cannot. The stocking-glove hypalgesia and absent ankle DTRs indicate a neuropathy. The lack of back pain almost entirely excludes lumbar spondylosis and other repetitive stress injuries. Heavy metals, organic solvents, n-hexane, and other hydrocarbons are industrial neurotoxins that cause neuropathies. Some individuals who crave euphoria inhale industrial chemicals that contain solvents or other neurotoxins. Not surprisingly, such abuse most commonly occurs in residents of states with heavy equipment manufacturing, particularly West Virginia, Tennessee, and Ohio. It rarely occurs among residents of the metropolitan areas of the East or West Coasts.

11. A 29-year-old woman, recently diagnosed with hypertension, rapidly develops paresis of the dorsiflexors

and evertors of the right foot, paresis of the extensors of the wrist and thumb of the left hand, and paresis of abduction of the right eye. Which is the most likely cause of her deficits?
a. Guillain–Barré syndrome
b. Alcohol abuse
c. Drug abuse
d. Mononeuritis multiplex

Answer: d. Because the illness has simultaneously struck several geographically separated nerves (the right common fibular, left radial, and right abducens), she has mononeuritis multiplex. This disorder usually results from a systemic illness, such as vasculitis. Although Wernicke–Korsakoff syndrome can cause abducens nerve palsy, it would also cause ataxia and mental status changes, but not isolated nerve injuries in the limbs. Except in extreme cases, Guillain–Barré syndrome spares pupil reflexes and extraocular function.

12. After losing a fistfight, a 17-year-old man finds that he cannot walk or feel anything below his waist. Although he has total immobility of his legs, they have retained normally active DTRs and flexor plantar responses. He has no response to noxious (pinprick) stimulation below his umbilicus, but sensation of position, vibration, and temperature is preserved. Where is the lesion?
a. Spinal cord
b. Cauda equina
c. Peripheral nerves
d. None of the above

Answer: d. He has neither a peripheral nor central nervous system lesion, such as a spinal cord lesion, because he has no objective neurologic sign, such as changes in the DTRs or the presence of Babinski signs. Moreover, he is able to feel temperature change but not pinprick, although the same neurologic pathway carries both sensations.

13. A 68-year-old diabetic man has the sudden onset of pain in the anterior right thigh. He has right-sided weakness of knee extension, absent quadriceps DTR, and hypalgesia of the anterior thigh. What is the etiology?
a. Polyneuropathy
b. Mononeuritis multiplex
c. Spinal cord injury or tumor
d. Sciatic nerve infarction
e. Femoral nerve infarction
f. Meralgia paresthetica

Answer: e. The knee weakness and especially the loss of its DTR indicate that the femoral nerve, rather than any CNS injury, has led to the pain and weakness. A sciatic nerve infarction would have led to ankle weakness and loss of the Achilles DTR. Diabetes often causes painful infarctions of the femoral, sciatic, fibular, oculomotor, or abducens nerves. When a diabetic infarction strikes the lumbosacral plexus, neurologists now may call it "*lumbosacral radiculoplexus neuropathy*," but previously

they called it "diabetic amyotrophy." Meralgia paresthetica causes sensory symptoms in the distribution of the lateral femoral cutaneous nerve but no paresis or loss of DTR.

14. A 34-year-old man with chronic low back pain experienced an exacerbation while raking leaves. He has difficulty walking and pain that radiates from the low back down the left posterior thigh to the lateral ankle. He has paresis of plantar flexion of the left ankle and an absent ankle DTR. He has an area of hypalgesia along the left lateral foot. What is the etiology of his condition?
a. Cauda equina syndrome
b. L4–L5 herniated disk
c. L5–S1 herniated disk
d. Femoral nerve infarction
e. Sciatic nerve infarction
f. None of the above

Answer: c. He probably has herniated his L5–S1 intervertebral disk, which compresses the left S1 root. The radiating pain, paresis, and loss of an ankle DTR characterize an S1 nerve root compression. In contrast to S1 compression, L5 compression does not lead to an absent ankle DTR. His symptoms and signs, although quite bothersome, are not as extensive as would be found with a cauda equina syndrome, which would cause incontinence as well as unilateral or bilateral leg weakness and areflexia.

15. A 62-year-old man has the onset over 3 months of weakness of both arms and then the left leg. He is alert and oriented but has dysarthria. His jaw jerk is hyperactive and his gag reflex is absent. The tongue is atrophic and has fasciculations. The muscles of his arms and left leg also have atrophy and fasciculations. All DTRs are hyperactive, and Babinski signs are present. Sensation is intact. What is the etiology of his illness?
a. Amyotrophic lateral sclerosis (ALS)
b. Cervical syrinx
c. Multiple sclerosis
d. Multiple strokes

Answer: a. He has a classic case of ALS with both bulbar and pseudobulbar palsy and wasting of his limb and tongue muscles. Although fasciculations are commonplace and usually benign, when they occur in multiple limbs and are associated with weakness, muscle atrophy, and hyperactive DTRs, they indicate ALS. The corticobulbar and corticospinal tracts, as well as the brainstem nuclei and spinal anterior horn cells, are all involved. He typically has normal ocular movements and mental faculties. A syrinx would have a characteristic "suspended sensory loss" (see Fig. 2.18) and absent upper extremity DTRs. Both multiple sclerosis and multiple strokes would have exclusively UMN signs.

16. A 47-year-old watchmaker has become gradually unable to move his thumbs and fingers of both hands. He has lost sensation of the fifth and medial aspect

of the fourth fingers, but has preserved reflexes. Which is the cause of his weakness?
a. Amyotrophic lateral sclerosis (ALS)
b. Syrinx
c. Cervical spondylosis
d. Ulnar nerve palsies

Answer: d. His symptoms and signs are confined to the ulnar nerves, which are vulnerable to pressure at the ulnar groove of the elbows. His diagnosis is bilateral "tardy" (late or slowly developing) ulnar nerve palsy, which is an injury caused by pressure on the ulnar nerves at the elbows. Tardy ulnar palsy is an occupational hazard of old-time watchmakers, draftsmen, and other workers who continuously lean on their elbows. (See Question 7 for occupations that predispose to median nerve compression [carpal tunnel syndrome]).

17. Which pattern would be found in autopsy of patients who die of amyotrophic lateral sclerosis (ALS)?
a. Loss of only lower motor neurons
b. Loss of only upper motor neurons
c. Loss of both upper and lower neurons
d. Loss of sensory as well as motor neurons

Answer: c. ALS, the quintessential motor disease, causes the death through apoptosis of both upper and lower motor neurons. Sensory neurons remain unaffected. While cognitive function is mildly impaired in a greater percentage of patients than previously believed, most individuals with ALS retain cognitive capacity.

18. Which one of the following is an effect of superoxide free radicals?
a. Accelerates aging and death of neurons
b. Alzheimer disease
c. Diabetes
d. Hypoxia

Answer: a. Normal metabolism produces some toxic byproducts, including superoxide free radicals. These toxins, which are usually neutralized by superoxide dismutase, accelerate aging and promote premature death of neurons. When superoxide dismutase fails, they accumulate in elderly people and those with certain diseases. Superoxide free radicals have been postulated to cause Parkinson disease and familial cases of ALS.

19. An 18-year-old high school student, awakened by his parents after he has overslept for school, finds that he cannot extend his right wrist, thumb, and fingers. He is not aphasic and has no visual field cut. His DTRs remain intact except for a depression of the right brachioradialis. What is the most likely cause of his weakness?
a. A left cerebral infarction
b. Midbrain infarction
c. Heavy metal intoxication
d. Radial nerve compression

Answer: d. He has sustained a "wrist drop" from radial nerve compression. Probably, in a deep, prolonged

sleep, he leaned his weight against his radial nerve as it winds around the humerus. Although this situation is similar to Question 1, on a deeper level, his parents or any attending physician should ask to why he had slept so soundly. Had he been drinking alcohol, perhaps to excess on a school night? Had he been using drugs?

20. Pat, a 25-year-old anxious medical student who is in psychotherapy, describes fasciculations in the limb muscles, calf cramps at night, and muscle aches during the day. A classmate found that Pat's strength was normal and that no muscle was atrophic; however, all DTRs were brisk. Pat's father, who had been a house painter, had developed arm muscle weakness and fasciculations before he died of pulmonary failure. Which is the most likely cause of Pat's fasciculations?
a. Amyotrophic lateral sclerosis (ALS)
b. Psychotropic medications
c. Anxiety and fatigue
d. Cervical spondylosis

Answer: c. In view of the lack of atrophy and weakness, the fasciculations are probably benign fasciculations. This commonly occurring disorder in young adults, which strikes fear into the heart of almost every medical student, may be accompanied by aches, cramps, and hyperactive DTRs. Also, Pat is too young to have contracted ALS. The father probably had cervical spondylosis, which is an occupational hazard of painters who must daily, for many hours, extend their head and neck. As for Pat's fasciculations, hearing a diagnosis of benign fasciculations epitomizes the medical adage that the three greatest words in the English language are not "I love you" but "It is benign."

21–25. Match the cause with the illness.

21. White lines of the nails (Mees' lines)
22. Lyme disease
23. Nitrous oxide neuropathy
24. *n*-Hexane neuropathy
25. Metachromatic leukodystrophy (MLD)
a. Genetic abnormality
b. Glue sniffing
c. Spirochete infection
d. Dental anesthetic abuse
e. Arsenic poisoning

Answers: 21–e, 22–c, 23–d, 24–b, 25–a.

26–36. For each condition, state whether it is associated with fasciculations (Yes or No).

26. Acute inflammatory demyelinating polyradiculoneuropathy (AIDP)
27. Spinal cord compression
28. Amyotrophic lateral sclerosis (ALS)
29. Insecticide poisoning
30. Spinal muscular atrophy
31. Fatigue
32. Porphyria
33. Psychologic stress
34. Cervical spondylosis

35. Post-polio syndrome
36. Poliomyelitis

Answers: 26–No, 27–No, 28–Yes, 29–Yes, 30–Yes, 31–Yes, 32–No, 33–Yes, 34–Yes, 35–Yes, 36–Yes.

37. Found with a suicide note, a 42-year-old man is brought to the hospital in a coma with cyanosis, bradycardia, and miosis; flaccid, areflexic quadriplegia; and pronounced muscle fasciculations. How had he attempted suicide?
  a. Arsenic ingestion
  b. Carbon monoxide inhalation
  c. Strangulation
  d. Insecticide ingestion

Answer: d. He has most likely swallowed a common anticholinesterase-based insecticide. Most of these interfere with neuromuscular transmission (see Chapter 6) and thereby cause an acute generalized flaccid paralysis accompanied by fasciculations. In addition, the increased parasympathetic activity causes miosis and bradycardia. The bradycardia and other manifestations of excessive parasympathetic activity can be reversed by atropine.

38. Which of the following conditions are associated with sexual dysfunction?
  a. Fibular nerve palsy
  b. Carpal tunnel syndrome
  c. Diabetes
  d. Poliomyelitis
  e. Multiple sclerosis (MS)
  f. Post-polio syndrome
  g. Amyotrophic lateral sclerosis (ALS)
  h. Myasthenia gravis

Answers: c, e.

39. A 40-year-old man with rapidly advancing Guillain–Barré syndrome develops confusion, overwhelming anxiety, and agitation. Which one of the following statements is correct?
  a. He should be treated with a benzodiazepine while further evaluation is undertaken.
  b. He may be developing hypoxia, hypercapnia, or both because of chest and diaphragm muscle paresis.
  c. He probably has "ICU psychosis."
  d. Hypokalemia, which is a frequent complication, can cause these symptoms.

Answer: b. Guillain–Barré syndrome, also called AIDP, is not associated directly with CNS dysfunction. However, respiratory insufficiency, a common complication of the illness, might cause anxiety and agitation. Other complications that can induce mental changes are metabolic aberrations, pain, sleep deprivation, or an adverse reaction to a medication. When hypokalemia occurs, which is infrequent, it does not cause mental aberrations. In contrast, severe hyponatremia often complicates Guillain–Barré syndrome and causes mental aberrations. Of course, investigations should be initiated for porphyria, Lyme disease, and other conditions that

might mimic Guillain–Barré syndrome. Treatment with a benzodiazepine for the psychosis, whatever its cause, is contraindicated because it might completely suppress respirations. The term "ICU psychosis" is a misnomer that should be avoided because it implies that psychosis results from the psychologic stress of a life-threatening illness. Instead, almost all cases of "psychosis" complicating Guillain–Barré syndrome are delirium that result from underlying life-threatening medical conditions.

40. Two days after admission to the hospital for several months of weight loss and neuropathy, a 43-year-old man suddenly developed belligerence and physical agitation. Then he developed a seizure. Of the following, which was the most likely cause of his illness?
  a. Guillain–Barré syndrome
  b. B_{12} deficiency
  c. Nutritional deficiency
  d. Leprosy

Answer: c. Alcoholic neuropathy, which is probably due to thiamine deficiency, is associated with delirium tremens (DTs) when hospitalized alcoholic patients are deprived of their usual alcohol consumption. DTs are often complicated by alcohol withdrawal seizures.

41. Which structure comprises the roof of the carpal tunnel?
  a. The median nerve
  b. The ulnar nerve
  c. Transverse carpal ligament
  d. Plantar fascia

Answer: c. The transverse carpal ligament, which underlies the skin of the palmar (flexor) surface of the wrist, forms the roof of the carpal tunnel. The median nerve passes through the carpal tunnel, but the ulnar nerve passes above and medial to it (see Fig. 5.3).

42–45. A 60-year-old man who has had mitral valve stenosis and atrial fibrillation suddenly developed quadriplegia with impaired swallowing, breathing, and speaking. He required tracheostomy and a nasogastric feeding tube during the initial part of his hospitalization. Four weeks after the onset of the illness, he remains quadriplegic with oculomotor pareses, hyperactive DTRs, and Babinski signs. Nevertheless, he appears alert and blinks appropriately to questions. Also, his vision is intact when each eye is tested separately.

42. What findings indicate that the problem is caused by CNS injury?
43. Is the lesion within the cerebral cortex or the brainstem?
44. Does the localization make a difference?
45. Which neurologic tests would help distinguish brainstem from extensive cerebral lesions?

Answers:
42. His hyperactive DTRs and Babinski signs indicate that he sustained CNS rather than PNS damage.

43. Although his quadriparesis might have several explanations, the oculomotor pareses and apnea indicate a brainstem injury. The lesion spared his cerebral functions, such as mentation and vision, as well as his upper brainstem functions, such as blinking. He exists in the well-known "locked-in syndrome" (see Chapter 11). Physicians should not misdiagnose him as being comatose, demented, or vegetative.

44. Of course, localization makes a difference. Neurologists often say, "Location, location, location … is destiny." With lesion confined to the brainstem, as in this case, intellectual function is preserved. On the other hand, extensive cerebral damage causes dementia.

45. Although CT might be performed to detect or exclude a cerebral lesion, only an MRI would be sensitive enough to detect his brainstem lesion. An EEG in this case would be a valuable test because, with his cerebral hemispheres intact, it would show a relatively normal electrical pattern. Visual evoked responses (VERs) would determine the integrity of the entire visual system, which is not part of the brainstem. Brainstem auditory evoked responses (BAERs) would determine the integrity of the auditory circuits, which are predominantly based in the brainstem.

46–60. For each feature (46–60), state whether it is associated with multiple sclerosis, Guillain–Barré syndrome, both, or neither (a–d).
  a. Multiple sclerosis
  b. Guillain-Barré syndrome
  c. Both
  d. Neither

46. Areflexic DTRs
47. Typically follows an upper respiratory tract infection
48. Unilateral visual loss
49. Paresthesias
50. Internuclear ophthalmoplegia
51. Paraparesis
52. Cognitive impairment early in the course of the illness
53. Triggered by bacterial infection
54. A demyelinating polyneuropathy
55. Recurrent optic neuritis
56. Leads to pseudobulbar palsy
57. Leads to bulbar palsy
58. An axonal polyneuropathy
59. A monophasic illness that typically peaks in several weeks and last several months
60. Sexual dysfunction can be the only or primary persistent deficit

Answers: 46–b, 47–b, 48–a, 49–c, 50–a, 51–c, 52–d, 53–b, 54–b, 55–a, 56–a, 57–b, 58–d, 59–b, 60–a.

61. A 19-year-old waitress, who describes subsisting on minimal quantities of food and megavitamin treatments, develops paresthesias of her fingers and toes. She is gaunt and pale. She has marked sensory loss and areflexia of her distal limbs. Which is the least likely cause of her symptoms?
  a. Nutritional deficiency
  b. Multiple sclerosis
  c. Substance abuse
  d. Nutritional supplement toxicity

Answer: b. In view of the distal limb sensory symptoms and areflexia, the problem is not a CNS disorder, such as multiple sclerosis, but a neuropathy. In teenagers who develop a neuropathy, neurologists give special consideration to certain conditions. Lyme disease and mononucleosis may be complicated by neuropathy. Abuse of alcohol, glue, paint thinners, or nitrous oxide (N_2O) might also be responsible, particularly when neuropathy develops concurrently in a group of risk-taking friends. Even abuse of supposedly nutritious foods, such as pyridoxine (vitamin B_6), may cause a sensory neuropathy. Also, teenagers sometimes develop alcoholism and suffer its complications.

62. One year after otherwise successful bariatric surgery, a 30-year-old man seems depressed and has symptoms and signs of neuropathy. Which condition is least likely to be responsible?
  a. Thiamine deficiency
  b. Vitamin B_{12} deficiency
  c. Toxic neuropathy

Answer: c. Thiamine deficiency, vitamin B_{12} deficiency, and electrolyte imbalance may complicate surgical resection of the stomach or duodenum, whether for morbid obesity or peptic ulcer disease. Especially if patients are noncompliant with vitamin and nutritional supplements or if they have persistent vomiting, they may develop combined system degeneration. Thus, a change in mental status following gastric surgery may be a manifestation of a potentially fatal metabolic aberration.

63. A 29-year-old lifeguard at Cape Cod developed profound malaise, an expanding rash, and then bilateral facial weakness (facial diplegia). Blood tests for Lyme disease, mononucleosis, AIDS, and other infective illnesses were negative. Of the following, which should be ordered?
  a. Lumbar puncture
  b. MRI of the head
  c. MRI of the spine
  d. Electrophysiologic studies, e.g., nerve conduction velocities and EMGs

Answer: a. The patient has a typical history, dermatologic signature (erythema migrans), and neurologic findings for Lyme disease, which is endemic on Cape Cod and other regions of the Northeast coast. Serologic tests are notoriously inaccurate for Lyme disease. Blood tests are frequently negative early in the illness and even throughout its course. Another possibility is that she has Guillain–Barré syndrome that began, as in a small fraction of cases, with involvement of the cranial nerves rather than with the lower spinal nerves. Myasthenia gravis is a possibility, but it is unlikely because of the absence of oculomotor paresis. Sarcoidosis is a rare cause of facial diplegia. The next step would be to perform a lumbar puncture to test the CSF. In Guillain–Barré syndrome, the CSF protein is characteristically elevated and the cell count has little or no increase. However, when Lyme disease causes a Guillain–Barré-like syndrome, the CSF has increased cells as well as an elevated protein concentration. MRI studies will not help in cases of PNS disease. Electrophysiologic studies might only indicate a demyelinating rather than an axonal neuropathy. If the diagnosis remains unclear, the best course might be to treat for Lyme disease.

64. In which aspects are CNS and PNS myelin similar?
    a. The same cells produce CNS and PNS myelin.
    b. CNS and PNS myelin possess the same antigens.
    c. CNS and PNS myelin insulate electrochemical transmissions in the brain and peripheral nerves, respectively.
    d. They are both affected by the same illnesses.

    Answer: c.

65. Which is the correct relationship?
    a. Oligodendrocytes are to glia cells as CNS is to PNS.
    b. Oligodendrocytes are to Schwann cells as PNS is to CNS.
    c. Oligodendrocytes are to Schwann cells as CNS is to PNS.
    d. Oligodendrocytes are to neurons as CNS is to PNS.

    Answer: c.

66. Which of the following statements is *false* concerning the neuropathy that affects otherwise normal people older than 75 years?
    a. It includes loss of ankle DTRs.
    b. It contributes to their tendency to fall.
    c. Position sensation is lost more than vibration sensation.
    d. The peripheral nerves' sensory loss is greater than their motor loss.

    Answer: c. The normal elderly often develop a subtle neuropathy that causes loss of ankle DTRs and impairs vibration sensation to a greater degree than position sensation. The neuropathy contributes to elderly individuals' gait impairment and lack of stability. Nevertheless, the neuropathy does not reduce their strength. As a practical matter, physicians should not expect elderly people to retain their ability to walk heel-to-toe (perform tandem gait).

67–70. Match the illness (a–d) with the skin lesion (67–70):
    a. Pellagra
    b. Lyme disease
    c. Herpes zoster
    d. Leprosy

67. Erythema migrans
68. Dermatitis
69. Depigmented anesthetic areas on ears, fingers, and toes
70. Vesicular eruptions in the first division of the trigeminal nerve

    Answers: 67–b, 68–a, 69–d, 70–c.

71. The wife of a homicidal neurologist enters psychotherapy because of several months of fatigue and painful paresthesias. She also describes numbness in a stocking-glove distribution, darkening of her skin, and the appearance of white lines across her nails. In addition to a general medical evaluation, which specific test should be performed?
    a. Thyroid function and other endocrinology tests
    b. Mononucleosis
    c. Lyme titer
    d. Heavy metal blood levels

    Answer: d. The astute psychiatrist suspected arsenic poisoning and ordered analysis of hair and nail samples. While many illnesses induce fatigue, the white lines across her nails (Mees' lines) pointed to the correct diagnosis.

72. Which is the most common PNS manifestation of AIDS?
    a. Guillain–Barré syndrome
    b. Myopathy
    c. Neuropathy
    d. Myelopathy

    Answer: c. Although neuropathy is the most common complication of AIDS, the other conditions frequently occur in AIDS patients.

73. Regarding low back pain, which one of the following statements is true?
    a. If an MRI shows a herniated disk, the patient should have surgery.
    b. Results of screening for depression will be a reliable guide to recommending surgery.
    c. Work-related low back pain is relatively resistant to treatment.
    d. A traditional 7- to 10-day course of bed rest, despite its simplicity, is more effective than a 2-day course.

    Answer: c. In about 20% of asymptomatic individuals, an MRI will show a herniated disk. Most patients with a herniated disk will improve spontaneously with conservative treatment. Although surgery will improve patients in the immediate postoperative period, at 4 years and longer, patients who have surgery and those who have had conservative treatment will have a similar status. Work-related and litigation-related low back pain is resistant to both conservative and surgical treatment. Psychologic evaluation and testing does not provide a reliable prediction as to the benefits of surgery. A 2-day course of bed rest is beneficial, but longer periods of bed rest are not more effective. In fact, merely continuing with a modified schedule may be the best treatment in most cases of low back pain.

74–77. Match the vitamin deficiency (a–e) with the illness that it causes (74–77):
   a. Ascorbic acid (vitamin C)
   b. Cobalamin (vitamin B₁₂)
   c. Niacin (vitamin B₃)
   d. Thiamine (vitamin B₁)
   e. Riboflavin

74. Wernicke-Korsakoff syndrome
75. Pellagra
76. Combined system degeneration
77. Scurvy

Answers: 74–d, 75–c, 76–b, 77–a.

78. A 35-year-old man with AIDS reports painful burning sensations of his feet. Although he has no significant weakness, he has lost his ankle DTRs. He has no history of diabetes, use of medications, exposure to chemicals, or other illness. Which of the following is least likely to be present?
   a. Loss of sensation on his soles
   b. High viral load
   c. High CD4 count
   d. Depression and functional impairment

Answer: c. This patient has the typical, symmetric, predominantly sensory neuropathy that complicates the late stages of AIDS. Because the sensory neuropathy occurs in the late stages of AIDS, he is likely also to have a high viral load, a low CD4 count, depression, and limited functional ability.

79. In the previous question, which medication would be least likely to relieve the abnormal sensations?
   a. Isoniazid (INH)
   b. Nortriptyline
   c. Gabapentin
   d. A long-acting morphine preparation
   e. Capsaicin cream

Answer: a. Except for isoniazid (INH), which is an antituberculosis (TB) drug, all the medicines listed represent classes of medicines useful in painful neuropathies, such as tricyclic antidepressants, antiepileptics, narcotics, and topically applied substance P depletors. INH, which is an antituberculous drug, interferes with pyridoxine (B₆) metabolism. Excessive INH treatment can lead to seizures and psychosis.

80–82. For each of the following illnesses, indicate whether it is associated with autosomal dominant (AD), autosomal recessive (AR), or sex-linked (SL) inheritance?

80. Acute intermittent porphyria (AIP)
81. Metachromatic leukodystrophy (MLD)
82. ALS with the superoxide dismutase [SOD1] gene abnormality

Answers: 80–AD, 81–AR, 82–AD.

83–85. Match the dermatologic abnormality found with neuropathy with its cause:

83. Alopecia
84. Mees' lines
85. Dark blue gum line
   a. Arsenic poisoning
   b. Lead poisoning
   c. Thallium poisoning
   d. Mercury poisoning

Answers: 83–c, 84–a, 85–d.

86. Which of the following statements is *false*?
   a. Ethyl mercury is a major component of thimerosal.
   b. Thimerosal had been used as a vaccine preservative.
   c. Organic mercury poisoning causes ataxia, dysarthria, and cognitive impairments.
   d. Childhood vaccines have been proven to cause autism.

Answer: d. Large-scale, statistically powerful studies have disproved the widespread suggestion that the thimerosal (ethyl mercury), which had been used as a vaccine preservative, caused autism. Although ingestion of organic mercury poisoning can cause ataxia, dysarthria, and cognitive impairments, far insufficient amounts are absorbed from the vaccines to cause such problems. Mercury-based dental fillings were similarly accused of causing various neurologic illnesses, but no causal association was ever established. Nevertheless, manufacturers have largely discontinued using mercury in vaccines and dental fillings.

87. Two physician vacationers in a Caribbean restaurant enjoyed what they thought was a wonderful fish dinner of shrimp, barracuda, and, for dessert, rum ice cream. However, severely painful abdominal cramps, unremitting nausea, protracted vomiting, and intense diarrhea awoke both of them later that night. After they self-medicated with antibiotic, antiemetics, and antidiarrheals, and caught several hours of sleep, the pair of physicians improved enough to catch their flight back to their teaching hospital. Never fully recovering their strength, 2 days later they began to have weakness, clumsiness, and numbness of the fingers, hands, and feet. A striking feature of their sensory loss was that all cold objects felt burning hot to the touch. Moreover, cold drinks seemed to burn their mouth and throat. A neurologic examination showed generalized mild weakness, hypoactive DTRs, and diminished sensation to pin and light touch in their distal extremities. They also displayed a Romberg sign. Given the obvious diagnosis of food poisoning, which is the most likely agent?
   a. Ciguatera
   b. *Salmonella*
   c. *Staphylococcus*
   d. Helminth

Answer: a. The diners' initial symptoms, while severe, were nonspecific for the particular etiology of the food poisoning. However, they subsequently showed evidence not only of peripheral neuropathy – distal sensory loss and hypoactive reflexes – they also reported the reversal of hot–cold sensations. Peripheral neuropathy with temperature "inversion" or "reversal" characterizes ciguatera poisoning. Reef-dwelling algae, which produce this toxin, enter the food chain in tropical waters. Reef fish, such as the barracuda, eventually accumulate enough of the odorless, colorless and heat-resistant toxin to poison diners. The other infective agents do not cause peripheral neuropathy. The patients had Romberg signs because of a distal lower extremity mild sensory loss; peripheral neuropathy, as well as posterior column disease, causes a Romberg sign.

88. In which *two* conditions do patients have the Romberg sign?
    a. Diabetic neuropathy
    b. Combined system degeneration
    c. Amyotrophic lateral sclerosis (ALS)
    d. Cerebellar atrophy
    e. Frontal lobe dysfunction

Answer: a, b. Maintenance of posture with closed eyes requires intact joint proprioception. In neuropathies where sensation is impaired, such as diabetic neuropathy, and in damage to the spinal cord's posterior columns, as occurs in B_{12} deficiency (combined system degeneration) and tabes dorsalis, patients cannot maintain their posture without visual sensory feedback.

89. A community hospital transferred a 23-year-old waitress with suspected Guillain–Barré syndrome after she developed areflexic quadriparesis. Neurologists at the tertiary center requested a psychiatry consultation because the patient demanded narcotics for abdominal pain, which they explained would not constitute a symptom of Guillain–Barré syndrome. The psychiatrist found her disoriented and inattentive. When alert, she insisted on narcotics. She had a low-grade fever but otherwise her vital signs were normal. Her oxygen saturation, blood glucose, and electrolytes were normal. Her urine tests were normal, but the urine darkened in the sunlight of the laboratory. Which test would probably clinch the diagnosis?
    a. Urine pregnancy test
    b. Pelvic ultrasound for an ectopic pregnancy
    c. Urine for toxicology
    d. Serum or urine for porphobilinogen and 5-aminolevulinic acid (ALA)

Answer: d. This patient, who presents with areflexic quadriparesis, abdominal pain, and delirium, probably has acute intermittent porphyria (AIP). This is a classic disorder in the differential diagnosis of delirium in the setting of abdominal pain and acute quadriparesis. Although physicians should consider an ectopic pregnancy and other causes of an "acute abdomen," the best test in this case would be determination of serum or urine porphobilinogen and ALA. While the testing is underway, physicians should expose the patient's urine to sunlight. Urine obtained during an attack of AIP will turn dark red. Medications that induce CYP450, such as phenobarbital and phenytoin, may precipitate or worsen an AIP attack.

90. A 45-year-old physician slipped and fell on his buttocks. As soon as he hit the pavement, he had excruciating low lumbar pain. On attempting to arise, he found that both legs were weak. In the emergency room, a neurologist confirmed that he had paraparesis and was unable to elicit DTRs or plantar reflexes. Not only did the neurologist detect a distended bladder, he found that the patient had no perception of it and that he also had perineal ("saddle") anesthesia. What is the most likely cause of the pain and neurologic deficits?
    a. Fractured femurs
    b. Herniated lumbar disk with L5 radiculopathy
    c. Herniated lumbar disk with S1 radiculopathy
    d. Cauda equina syndrome from a herniated lumbar disk

Answer: d. Acute areflexic paraparesis with loss of function in lumbar and sacral nerve roots with perineal anesthesia, which causes urinary retention or incontinence, constitutes the cauda equina syndrome. When it follows buttock trauma, the most likely cause is a large herniated low lumbar herniated disk. A diagnosis of bilateral lumbosacral plexus lesions would be a credible alternative, but they are rare and usually slowly growing malignancies.

91. A construction worker, who has gained 20 pounds over the past 2 years, presents with 2 months of numbness and pain of the right lateral thigh. He found that when his clothing rubbed against his thigh, that neutral stimulation felt painful (*allodynia*). For years, he has had dull lumbar pain when he carries heavy objects. However, he has no symptoms below the knee and he denies bowel or bladder incontinence. On examination, in the right lateral thigh, he has decreased sensation to touch and pinprick (hypalgesia), but no weakness. His DTRs are normal. Injury to which structure is causing the right thigh pain, hypalgesia, and allodynia?
    a. L4 nerve root
    b. L5 nerve root
    c. Anterior femoral cutaneous nerve
    d. Lateral femoral cutaneous nerve
    e. Sciatic nerve

Answer: d. This patient has an injury of the lateral femoral cutaneous nerve (LFCN) that is causing meralgia paresthetica, which is also known as lateral femoral cutaneous neuropathy. This painful disorder results from compression of the LFCN at the anterior superior iliac spine, which is essentially the lateral groin. Frequent causes are obesity, patients wearing pants or other garments that are too tight, and heavy or sharp objects, such as a tool belt, pressing into their groin. Unlike the anterior femoral cutaneous nerve, the LFCN is not a branch of the femoral nerve, but instead originates directly from the L2 and L3 nerve roots. Patients with L4 radiculopathy would likely have a diminished patellar (knee) DTR and weakness of the quadriceps muscle as well as numbness of the medial thigh and leg. This patient's symptoms are not in the L5 or the sciatic nerve distribution, which consists of the posterior thigh and lateral calf.

92. A 35-year-old, previously healthy woman, presents to the emergency room in southern California with high fever, lethargy, and confusion that developed over 2 days. On examination, her physical findings are weakness, diminished muscle tone, and absent reflexes in both legs. Which of the following is the most likely infectious agent?
   a. Poliovirus
   b. West Nile virus
   c. Cytomegalovirus (CMV)
   d. Herpes simplex virus (HSV)
   e. Human T-lymphotrophic virus 1 (HTLV 1)

Answer: b. West Nile virus is associated with onset of an acute flaccid paralysis, usually following onset of a meningoencephalitis. The delay in onset of weakness is usually a few days, but may be up to 1–2 weeks in atypical cases. While the virus was first identified on the East Coast of the United States, it has spread across the country, and some of the largest pockets of disease are now seen in the southwestern part of the United States. While poliovirus, an enterovirus, may cause the same presentation, the vaccination campaign eradicated poliomyelitis in the United States by the late 1970s. However, a non-polio virus, enterovirus 68, has recently probably caused small polio-like epidemics of flaccid paraparesis. CMV polyradiculitis would not be seen in an immune-competent patient, and HSV and HTLV-1 do not cause this clinical picture.

93. Is it true or false that the side effects of disulfiram occur only with concomitant alcohol ingestion?

Answer: False. While the main side effects of disulfiram, nausea and vomiting, occur only with concomitant alcohol ingestion, an axonal neuropathy is associated with disulfiram toxicity. In severe cases, patients may present with seizures, psychosis, or a movement disorder.

CHAPTER 6

MUSCLE DISORDERS

The clinical evaluation can usually distinguish disorders of muscle from those of the central nervous system (CNS) and peripheral nervous system (PNS) (Table 6.1). It can then divide muscle disorders into those of the neuromuscular junction and those of the muscles themselves, *myopathies* (Box 6.1). Surprisingly, considering their physiologic distance from the brain, several muscle disorders are associated with mental retardation, cognitive decline, personality changes, or use of psychotropic medications.

NEUROMUSCULAR JUNCTION DISORDERS

Myasthenia Gravis

Neuromuscular Transmission Impairment

Normally, the presynaptic neuron at the neuromuscular junction releases discrete amounts – packets or *quanta* – of *acetylcholine* (*ACh*) across the neuromuscular junction to trigger a muscle contraction (Fig. 6.1). After the muscle contraction, acetylcholinesterase (*AChE*) (or simply "cholinesterase") metabolizes ACh.

In myasthenia gravis (MG), the classic neuromuscular junction disorder, antibodies to the ACh receptor block binding of ACh to the receptor, leading to the development of weakness and respiratory difficulty. Other illnesses and some medications may also impair ACh transmission at the neuromuscular junction, although through different mechanisms, and cause the same problems. For example, *botulinum toxin*, as both a naturally occurring food poison and a medication, blocks the release of ACh packets from the presynaptic membrane and causes paresis (see later).

At the postsynaptic side of the neuromuscular junction, the muscle relaxant *succinylcholine* binds to the ACh receptors. With their ACh receptors inactivated, muscles weaken to the point of flaccid paralysis. Succinylcholine, which resists cholinesterases, has a paralyzing effect that lasts for hours. It facilitates major surgery and electroconvulsive therapy (ECT).

ACh, unlike dopamine and serotonin, serves as a transmitter both at the neuromuscular junction and the CNS. Also, metabolism rather than reuptake almost entirely terminates its action. Antibodies associated with MG impair neuromuscular junction but not CNS ACh transmission: one reason is that neuromuscular ACh receptors are nicotinic and cerebral ACh receptors are mostly muscarinic (see Chapter 21).

Physicians caring for MG patients who have almost complete paralysis but normal cognitive status see the stark contrast between impaired neuromuscular junction

activity and preserved CNS ACh activity. Similarly, most anticholinesterase medications have no effect on cognitive status or other CNS function because they do not penetrate the blood–brain barrier. One of the few exceptions, physostigmine, penetrates into the CNS where it preserves ACh concentrations. Thus, researchers proposed physostigmine as a treatment for conditions with low CNS ACh levels, such as Alzheimer disease. However, in various experiments with Alzheimer disease, despite increasing cerebral ACh concentrations, physostigmine produced no clinical benefit (see Chapter 7).

In MG, ACh receptor antibodies block, impair, or actually destroy ACh receptors (Fig. 6.2). These antibodies predominantly attack ACh receptors located in the extraocular, facial, neck and proximal limb muscles. When binding to antibody-inactivated receptors, ACh produces only weak, unsustained muscle contractions. Another characteristic of the ACh receptor antibodies is that they attack only *nicotinic ACh* – not muscarinic ACh – receptors. Moreover, they do not penetrate the blood–brain barrier and do not interfere with CNS function. In contrast, they readily pass through the placenta and cause transient MG symptoms in neonates of mothers with MG.

In approximately 80% of MG cases, the serum contains ACh receptor antibodies. In one-half of the remainder, the serum has antibodies to *mu*scle-*s*pecific *k*inase (MuSK).

Clinical Features

MG has a signature: weakness of the ocular motility (oculomotor), facial, and bulbar muscles that is asymmetric and fluctuating. Neurologists always suspect neuromuscular junction disease when they elicit a history of this "fatiguing" weakness and they frequently find it on physical examination. The susceptibility of those muscles and the asymmetry remain unexplained. However, the weakness, at least in the initial months of the illness, varies in almost a diurnal pattern because exertion weakens muscles and thus symptoms appear predominantly in the late afternoon or early evening as well as after vigorous activities. Rest and sleep temporarily restore strength.

As their first symptom, almost 90% of patients, typically young women or older men, develop diplopia and ptosis. When facial and neck muscle weakness emerges, a nasal tone suffuses patients' speech and they grimace when attempting to smile (Fig. 6.3). These patients have significant trouble whistling and chewing. Neck, shoulder, and swallowing and respiratory muscles weaken as the disease progresses, i.e., MG causes bulbar palsy (see Chapter 4). In severe cases, patients suffer respiratory

TABLE 6.1 **Signs of CNS, Nerve, and Muscle Disorders**

	CNS	Nerve	Muscle
Paresis	Pattern*	Distal	Proximal
Muscle tone	Spastic	Flaccid	Sometimes tender or dystrophic
DTRs	Hyperactive	Hypoactive	Normal or hypoactive
Babinski signs	Yes	No	No
Sensory loss	Hemisensory or sensory level	Stocking-glove	None

DTRs, Deep tendon reflexes
*Hemiparesis, paraparesis, etc.

BOX 6.1 **Common Neuromuscular Junction and Muscle Disorders**

NEUROMUSCULAR JUNCTION DISORDERS

  Myasthenia gravis
  Lambert–Eaton syndrome
  Botulism
  Nerve gas poisoning
  Black widow spider bite

MUSCLE DISORDERS (MYOPATHIES)

  Inherited dystrophies
    Duchenne muscular dystrophy
    Myotonic dystrophy
  Inflammatory, infectious, and toxic myopathies
    Polymyositis
    Dermatomyositis
    Eosinophilia-myalgia syndrome
    Trichinosis
    AIDS myopathy
  Metabolic myopathies
    Steroid myopathy
    Hypokalemic myopathy
    Alcohol myopathy
  Mitochondrial myopathies
    Primary mitochondrial myopathies
    Progressive ophthalmoplegia
    MELAS and MERRF
  Neuroleptic malignant syndrome

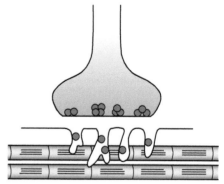

FIGURE 6.1 ■ At the neuromuscular junction, the motor nerve endings contain discrete *packets* or *quanta* of acetylcholine (ACh). In response to stimulation, the presynaptic neuron releases about 200 ACh packets. They cross the synaptic cleft of the neuromuscular junction to reach ACh receptor binding sites, situated deeply in convolutions of the postsynaptic membrane. ACh-receptor interactions open cation channels, thereby inducing an *end-plate potential*. If this potential reaches a certain magnitude, it triggers an *action potential* along the muscle fiber. Action potentials open calcium storage sites, which produce muscle contractions.

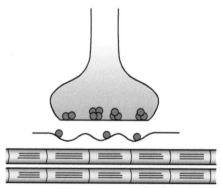

FIGURE 6.2 ■ In MG, the folds in the muscle become abnormally shallow and lose many of the ACh binding sites. The synaptic cleft widens, which further impedes neuromuscular transmission.

Although exacerbations of MG usually occur spontaneously, intercurrent illnesses such as pneumonia or psychologic stress may precipitate them. In addition, about 40% of pregnant women with MG undergo exacerbations, which occur with equal frequency during each trimester. On the other hand, about 30% of pregnant women with MG enjoy a remission.

Neurologists may confirm a clinical diagnosis of myasthenia by performing a Tensilon (edrophonium) test (Fig. 6.3, Top). Alternatively, they perform the ice pack test, which presumably slows the kinetics of acetylcholinesterase and thus improves neuromuscular transmission (Fig. 6.3, Bottom). Like the Tensilon test, the ice pack test briefly reverses ptosis. They test for serum antibodies to ACh receptors and, in certain circumstances, antibodies to MuSK. They may also perform repeated motor nerve stimulations at low frequency and after exercise (*repetitive stimulation testing*). In MG patients, affected muscles contract less and less, showing a decremental response.

Differential Diagnosis

Lesions of the oculomotor nerve (cranial nerve III), which may be a sign of a midbrain infarction (see

distress, quadriplegia, and an inability to speak (anarthria). Paralysis can spread and worsen so much that patients reach a "locked-in" state (see Chapter 11).

Absence of certain findings is equally important. Again, in contrast to the physical incapacity, neither the disease nor the medications directly produces changes in mentation or level of consciousness. In addition, although extraocular muscles weaken, intraocular muscles remain strong. Thus, patients may have complete ptosis and no eyeball movement, but their pupils are normal in size and reactivity to light. Another oddity is that even though patients may develop quadriparesis, their bladder and bowel sphincters' strength remains normal. Of course, as in muscle disorders, MG does not impair sensation.

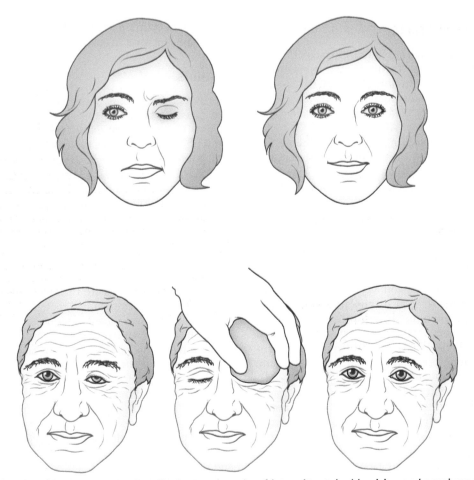

FIGURE 6.3 ■ *Top, Left,* This young woman described several weeks of intermittent double vision and nasal speech. She had left-sided ptosis and bilateral, asymmetric facial muscle weakness evident in the loss of the contour of the right nasolabial fold and sagging lower lip. *Right,* Intravenous administration of the cholinesterase inhibitor edrophonium (Tensilon) 10 mg – the Tensilon test – produces a 60-second restoration of eyelid, ocular, and facial strength. This typically brief but dramatic restoration of her strength resulted from edrophonium transiently inhibiting cholinesterase to increase ACh activity. *Bottom, Left,* A 65-year-old man presents with 2 months of fluctuating facial weakness and left eyelid ptosis. *Middle,* in performing the ice pack test, the neurologist holds a small ice pack over the eye for 1–2 minutes to cool the eyelid muscles. *Right,* immediately after removing the ice pack, the ptosis has nearly resolved. Over the next few minutes, however, the ptosis will slowly return.

Fig. 4.9) or nerve compression by a posterior communicating artery aneurysm, also cause extraocular muscle paresis. In addition to their usually having an abrupt and painful onset, these lesions are identifiable by a subtle finding: the pupil will be widely dilated and unreactive to light because of intraocular (pupillary) muscle paresis (see Fig. 4.6). In addition, many other neurologic illnesses cause facial and bulbar palsy: amyotrophic lateral sclerosis (ALS), botulism, Guillain–Barré syndrome, Lambert–Eaton syndrome, and Lyme disease. Finally, from time to time, a patient will report the sudden onset of dysarthria, dysphagia, and diplopia – and ultimately receive the diagnosis of conversion disorder.

Treatment

Standard treatments for MG attempt to either increase ACh concentration at the neuromuscular junction or restore the integrity of ACh receptors. To increase ACh concentration by slowing its metabolism, neurologists typically prescribe *cholinesterase inhibitors* (or simply, *anticholinesterases*), such as pyridostigmine (Mestinon). If patients cannot swallow, neurologists usually order intravenous or intramuscular neostigmine (Prostigmin). By increasing ACh activity, these medicines increase muscle strength.

In the other therapeutic strategy – restoring the integrity of ACh receptors – neurologists administer steroids, other immunosuppressive medications, plasmapheresis, or intravenous infusions of immunoglobulins (IVIG). In refractory cases of MG, neurologists also use the synthetic monoclonal antibody rituximab (Rituxan), which binds to the CD20 antigen on B-cells. Rituximab depletes these cells and thereby suppresses the hyperimmune response that caused the patient's symptoms. Neurologists also infuse IVIG in Guillain–Barré syndrome and rituximab in refractory forms of chronic inflammatory demyelinating polyneuropathy (CIDP) (see Chapter 5).

About 5% of patients have underlying hyperthyroidism and 10% have a mediastinal thymoma. If these conditions are present and respond to treatment, MG will usually improve.

Lambert–Eaton Syndrome

As in myasthenia, impaired ACh neuromuscular transmission causes weakness in Lambert–Eaton syndrome and botulism. The major physiologic distinction is that myasthenia results from a disorder of *postsynaptic* receptors, but Lambert–Eaton and botulism result from impaired release of *presynaptic* ACh packets.

Lambert–Eaton and botulism also differ in their etiology and, to a certain extent, their clinical manifestations. A toxin causes botulism, but an autoimmune disorder associated with serum voltage-gated calcium channel (VGCC) antibodies, causes Lambert–Eaton (see Chapter 19). This autoimmune disorder, in turn, is frequently an expression of small cell carcinoma of the lung and occasionally a component of a rheumatologic illness. When associated with any cancer, neurologists consider Lambert–Eaton a paraneoplastic syndrome (see Chapter 19).

Although Lambert–Eaton and MG both cause weakness, Lambert–Eaton usually first causes weakness of the limbs while MG most commonly first causes extraocular, head, and neck weakness. Moreover, repetitive exertion temporarily corrects weakness in Lambert–Eaton, presumably by provoking presynaptic ACh release, but any exertion exacerbates myasthenia-induced weakness. In addition, Lambert–Eaton, unlike MG, causes autonomic nervous system dysfunction. Because of Lambert–Eaton patients' autonomic dysfunction, they may also have a sluggish or absent pupillary light reflex, which would unequivocally set them apart from MG patients.

Botulism

Unlike Lambert–Eaton, botulism is an infectious illness that usually results from eating contaminated food. Most often, improperly preserved food has allowed the growth of *Clostridium botulinum* spores that elaborate a toxin with a predilection for the presynaptic neuromuscular membrane. (Experts fear that terrorists might inject these spores into commercial food manufacturing processes, such as milk pasteurizing, to create mass poisonings.)

Botulism victims develop oculomotor, bulbar, and respiratory paralyses that resemble Guillain–Barré syndrome as well as MG. However, in contrast to the course of these illnesses, botulism symptoms arise explosively and include dilated unreactive pupils.

A unique feature of botulism, which may prompt a life-saving diagnosis, is that several family members often simultaneously develop constipation, nausea, vomiting, diarrhea, and fever, and then the distinctive weakness with fixed pupils 18–36 hours after sharing a meal. Botulism, as well as tetanus (see later), may also complicate drug abuse that involves shared, contaminated needles. It develops in infants fed unpasteurized (raw) honey or corn syrup that harbor the infective spores. Treatment often requires intubation and ventilatory support.

Ironically, neurologists now routinely turn botulinum-induced paresis to an advantage. They inject pharmaceutically prepared botulinum toxin to alleviate focal dystonias and dyskinesias, such as blepharospasm, spasmodic torticollis, and writer's cramp (see Chapter 18). Even more ironically, physicians routinely inject pharmaceutically prepared botulinum toxin into the paper-thin muscles underlying furrows to smooth patients' skin.

Tetanus

A different *Clostridium* species elaborates the neurotoxin that causes tetanus. In this illness, the toxin from *Clostridium tetani* predominantly blocks presynaptic release – not of ACh – but of the CNS inhibitory neurotransmitters, gamma-aminobutyric acid (GABA) and glycine (see Chapter 21). The disease deprives patients of the normal inhibitory influence on their brain and spinal cord motor neurons. Uninhibited muscle contractions cause trismus ("lockjaw"), facial grimacing, an odd but characteristic smile ("risus sardonicus"), and muscle spasms in the limbs. The muscle contractions may be so violent that bursts of spasms mimic seizures, which neurologists term "tetanic convulsions."

Drug addicts who share infected needles and workers in farming and scrap metal recovery contract tetanus. When abortion was illegal, tetanus as well as other often-fatal infections frequently complicated the procedure.

Although acute development of facial, jaw, trunk, and limb spasms is indicative of tetanus, dopamine-blocking medications commonly produce similarly appearing dystonic reactions. Thus, physicians must not blindly attribute all facial and jaw spasms to medication-induced dystonic reactions. The differential diagnosis of these muscle spasms includes strychnine poisoning, rabies, heat stroke, and head and neck infections, as well as tetanus and dystonic reactions.

In fact, strychnine poisoning allows for an interesting comparison to tetanus. Lack of inhibitory neurotransmitter activity in both conditions underlies muscle spasms. One minor difference is that strychnine does not lead to trismus. The major difference is that tetanus results from impaired presynaptic release of the inhibitory neurotransmitters GABA and glycine, but strychnine antagonizes these same inhibitory neurotransmitters at their postsynaptic receptors.

Nerve Gas and Other Wartime Issues

Most common insecticides are organophosphates that bind and inactivate AChE. With inactivation of its metabolic enzyme, ACh accumulates and irreversibly depolarizes postsynaptic neuromuscular junctions. After insecticides cause initial muscle contractions and fasciculations, they lead to paralysis of respiratory and other muscles. For example, malathion (Ovide), the common shampoo for head lice, irreversibly inhibits AChE. It is safe as a shampoo because so little penetrates through the skin.

On the other hand, people committing suicide, especially in India, often deliberately drink organophosphate pesticides. Similarly, the *nerve gases* that threatened soldiers from World War I through the Persian Gulf War bind and inactivate AChE. The common ones – GA, GB, GD, and VX – affect both the CNS and PNS. Some are gaseous, but others, such as sarin (GB), the poison used in the Tokyo subway terrorist attack, are liquid. Several investigators postulated that pyridostigmine caused neurologic symptoms of the "Gulf War syndrome" (see

Chapter 5); however, they provided no direct evidence and patients with myasthenia have taken pyridostigmine for decades with no such untoward effects.

Accumulation of ACh from poison gas or excessive pyridostigmine treatment in MG patients causes a *cholinergic crisis*. Its initial features – tearing, pulmonary secretions, and miosis – reflect excessive cholinergic (parasympathetic) activity. If the poisons penetrate the CNS, further excess ACh causes convulsions, rapidly developing unconsciousness, and respiratory depression.

Medical personnel will ideally receive a warning and be able to provide pretreatment. They might administer pyridostigmine, which is a *reversible* AChE inhibitor, as a prophylactic agent, because it occupies the vulnerable site on AChE and thereby protects it from *irreversible* inhibition by the toxin. After nerve gas exposure or liquid ingestion, first aid consists of washing exposed skin with dilute bleach (hypochlorite). Also after exposure, field forces administer *pralidoxime* because it reactivates AChE and detoxifies organophosphates, and atropine because it is a competitive inhibitor of ACh and blocks the excessive cholinergic activity. In view of a high incidence of seizures, depending on the exposure, field forces also often administer a benzodiazepine. Other antiepileptic drugs are ineffective in this situation.

Survivors of nerve gas poisonings often report developing headaches, personality changes, and cognitive impairment, especially affecting memory. Their symptoms often mimic those of posttraumatic stress disorder. Experience has also shown that individuals in the vicinity of nerve gas poisonings, but who were not exposed and remain entirely well, i.e., the "worried well," overwhelm emergency rooms.

Agent Orange, the herbicide sprayed extensively in Southeast Asia during the Vietnam War, allegedly produced cognitive impairment, psychiatric disturbances, and brain tumors. Although large scientific reviews found no evidence that it actually caused any of those problems, advocacy groups have prodded Congress into accepting a causal relationship.

Veterans with the recent counterpart, *Persian Gulf War syndrome*, also described varied symptoms, including fatigue, weakness, and myalgias (painful muscle aches). Again, exhaustive studies have found no consistent, significant clinical sign or laboratory evidence of any neurologic sequelae. One theory had been that in anticipation of a nerve gas attack, soldiers had been ordered to take a "neurotoxic" antidote (pyridostigmine); however, numerous MG patients have taken it for decades with no such adverse effects.

The notion that silicone toxicity from breast implants causes a neuromuscular disorder and other neurologic illness, which is also unfounded, is discussed in the differential diagnosis of multiple sclerosis (see Chapter 15).

Chronic Fatigue Syndrome and Fibromyalgia

Myasthenia gravis and other neurologic disorders are sometimes unconvincingly invoked as an explanation of one of the most puzzling clinical problems: *chronic fatigue syndrome*. Individuals with this condition typically describe not only a generalized sense of weakness, sometimes preceded by myalgias and other flu-like symptoms, but also impaired memory and inability to concentrate. Patients diagnosed with chronic fatigue syndrome do not have the usual criteria of a neurologic illness: consistent symptoms, objective findings, laboratory or imaging abnormalities, or benefit from treatment. For physicians familiar with classic psychosomatic illnesses, chronic fatigue syndrome harkens back to *asthenia*, which involves chronic weakness and dyspnea but no objective findings. Some physicians who support the idea of chronic fatigue syndrome as a unique diagnosis have lobbied for a change in terminology to myalgic encephalomyelitis, while others argue that these are either two distinct conditions or two overlapping ones.

Regardless of whether chronic fatigue syndrome constitutes a distinct entity, several well-established illnesses may induce fatigue sometimes accompanied by cognitive impairment: Lyme disease, acquired immunodeficiency syndrome (AIDS), mononucleosis, multiple sclerosis, sleep apnea and other sleep disturbances, and eosinophilia-myalgia syndrome. In addition, simple deconditioning from limited physical activity, including weightless space travel and confinement to a hospital bed, frequently causes weakness and loss of muscle bulk.

Fibromyalgia, a cousin of chronic fatigue syndrome, consists of entirely subjective symptoms: chronic widespread pain, sleep dysfunction, and multiple tender points. Despite patients having prominent myalgia, they have no objective evidence of muscle inflammation (*myositis*) or any other specific abnormality. Some physicians postulate that fibromyalgia arises as the combination of a neuropathy and enhanced pain sensitization in the central nervous system. Numerous individuals fulfilling the criteria for fibromyalgia also have equally amorphous disorders, such as irritable bowel syndrome, atypical chest pain, and myofascial pain.

MUSCLE DISEASE (MYOPATHY)

Myopathies – disorders of muscle – have a predilection for the shoulder and hip girdle muscles. They strike these large, proximal muscles earliest most severely, and often exclusively. Patients have difficulty performing tasks that require these muscles, such as standing, walking, climbing stairs, combing their hair, and reaching upward. Most common myopathies spare the oculomotor, sphincter, and hand and feet muscles. (Hand and feet muscles are "distal" and more subject to neuropathies than myopathies.)

Acute myositis leads to myalgias and tenderness. Eventually in the course of their illnesses, both inflammatory and noninflammatory myopathies cause muscle weakness and atrophy (*dystrophy*). DTRs may remain normal, but usually lose reactivity roughly in proportion to their weakness. Patients show no Babinski signs or sensory loss because the corticospinal and sensory tracts remain uninvolved. With most myopathies, serum concentrations of muscle-based enzymes, such as creatine kinase (CK), which neurologists previously called creatine phosphokinase (CPK), and aldolase rise and the electromyogram (EMG) shows abnormalities. Finally, with a few exceptions (see later), myopathies do not induce mental disorders.

Steroids are helpful and probably remain the first choice in treatment of inflammatory myopathies. Other nonspecific immunosuppressants, such as azathioprine, are the second-line therapy. However, monoclonal antibody medications, such as rituximab (see above), promise to revolutionize the treatment of myositis and other inflammatory conditions.

Inherited Dystrophies

Duchenne Muscular Dystrophy

Duchenne muscular dystrophy (DMD) is the most frequent childhood-onset myopathy. Beginning in childhood, the illness follows a chronic, progressively incapacitating, and ultimately fatal course. It is an X-linked genetic illness, but about 30% of cases represent a de novo mutation. Although women who carry the abnormal gene may have some subtle findings and laboratory abnormalities, for practical purposes, DMD is restricted to boys.

DMD typically first affects boys' thighs and shoulders. The first symptom to emerge is their struggle to stand and walk. Unless they receive treatment, they never gain the strength to skip, hop, or run. Even though drastically weak, muscles paradoxically increase in size because fat cells and connective tissue infiltrate them (*muscle pseudo-hypertrophy*, Fig. 6.4, top). Instinctively learning *Gowers' maneuver* (Fig. 6.4, bottom), boys with the illness arise from sitting only by pulling or pushing themselves upward on their own legs. Usually by age 12 years, when their musculature can no longer support their maturing frame, adolescent boys become wheelchair-bound and eventually develop respiratory insufficiency.

Psychomotor retardation and an average IQ approximately one standard deviation below normal typically accompany DMD. This intellectual impairment is greater than that of comparable chronic illnesses and often overshadows the weakness. Of course, isolation, lack of education, and being afflicted with a progressively severe handicap account for psychologic, social, and cognitive deficits. Depression typically begins when a boy's illness first confines him to a wheelchair.

No cure is available, but experimental treatments include gene therapy. Steroids slow the inevitable march towards immobility. This treatment may delay the illness's progression for as long as 10 years.

Genetics. Because the absence or dysfunction of a crucial muscle cell membrane protein, *dystrophin*, causes DMD, neurologists refer to this illness as a *dystrophinopathy*. About 75% of patients carry a mutation in the dystrophin gene – one of the largest genes in the human genome – located on the short arm of the X chromosome. In many cases, the illness arises from a new mutation rather than from an inherited one. Unlike the excessive trinucleotide repeat mutation underlying myotonic dystrophy and several other neurologic disorders (see later), the DMD mutation usually consists of a DNA deletion. Genetic testing of blood samples for mutations in the dystrophin gene can diagnose not only individuals with signs of the illness but also affected fetuses, females who carry the mutation (carriers), and young male carriers destined to develop the illness.

A diagnosis of DMD can also be based on a muscle biopsy that shows little or no staining for dystrophin (the *dystrophin test*). With modern technology, needle biopsies rather than open surgical procedures provide sufficient tissue, but the procedure still involves injections, pain, and anxiety – especially for a child. The advent of DNA testing has rendered muscle biopsy largely obsolete for diagnosis of DMD.

Becker Dystrophy

A relatively benign variant of Duchenne dystrophy, *Becker dystrophy*, results from a different mutation in the same gene. This mutation causes the production of dystrophin that is abnormal but retains some function. Individuals with Becker dystrophy, which is also a dystrophinopathy, have weakness that begins in their second decade and follows a slowly progressive course that is uncomplicated by cognitive impairment.

Myotonic Dystrophy

The most frequently occurring myopathy in adults is *myotonic dystrophy*. Although also an inherited muscle disorder, myotonic dystrophy differs in several respects from DMD. The symptoms usually appear when individuals are young adults – 20 to 25 years – and both sexes are equally affected. Also, rather than having proximal muscle weakness and pseudohypertrophy, myotonic dystrophy patients develop facial and distal limb muscle weakness and atrophy. This pattern of dystrophy, while characteristic, is not unique.

Myotonic dystrophy is named for its clinical signature, *myotonia*, which is involuntary prolonged muscle contraction. Myotonia inhibits the release of patients' grip for several seconds after shaking hands, grasping, or turning a doorknob. Neurologists elicit this phenomenon by asking patients to make a fist and then rapidly release it. In addition, if the physician lightly taps a patient's thenar (thumb base) muscles with a reflex hammer, myotonia causes a prolonged, visible contraction that moves the thumb medially (Fig. 6.5).

Another feature, caused by facial and temple muscle atrophy, is a sunken and elongated face, ptosis, and a prominent forehead. This distortion forms the distinctive "hatchet face" (Fig. 6.5). Additional neurologic and nonneurologic manifestations vary. Patients often develop cataracts, cardiac conduction system disturbances, and endocrine organ failure, such as testicular atrophy, diabetes, and infertility. Treatment is limited to reducing myotonia by giving phenytoin, quinine, or other medicines, and providing hormone replacements for endocrine deficiencies.

Contrasting somewhat with the nonprogressive cognitive impairment of DMD, patients with myotonic dystrophy almost uniformly show cognitive impairment that increases with age. In addition, lack of initiative and progressive blandness characterize patients' personality.

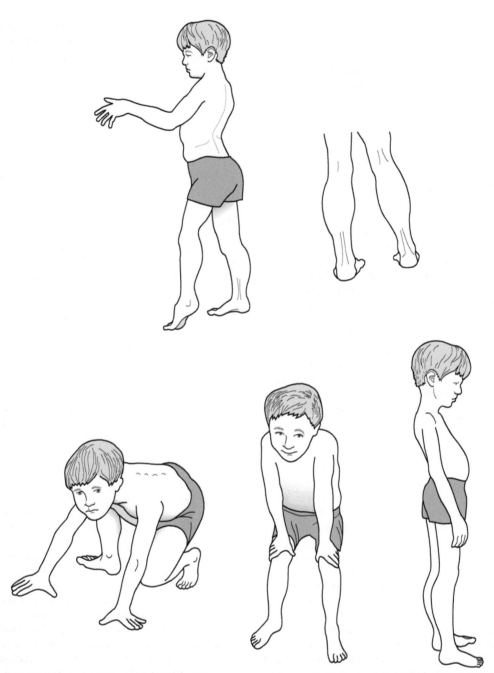

FIGURE 6.4 ■ *Top,* This 10-year-old boy with typical Duchenne muscular dystrophy has a waddling gait and inability to raise his arms above his head because of weakness of his shoulder and pelvic girdle muscles, i.e., his proximal muscles. His weakened calf muscles show enlargement (*pseudohypertrophy*) not from exercise but from fat and connective tissue infiltration. He also has exaggeration of the normal inward curve of the lumbar spine, *hyperlordosis. Bottom, Gowers' maneuver,* an early sign of Duchenne muscular dystrophy, consists of a boy's pushing his hands against his knees then thighs to reach a standing position. He must use his arms and hands because the disease primarily weakens hip and thigh muscles that normally would be sufficient to allow him to stand.

Genetics. The genetic basis of myotonic dystrophy, as well as several other neurologic illnesses, is a mutation consisting of excessive repetition of a particular nucleotide base triplet (*trinucleotide repeat*) in a particular gene. In the case of myotonic dystrophy, the trinucleotide base CTG is excessively repeated in the *DMPK* gene on chromosome 19. The mutation leads to myotonic dystrophy's transmission as an autosomal dominant genetic disorder. In addition, because the mutation alters ion channels in the membranes of muscle and other organ cells, neurologists refer to myotonic dystrophy as a *channelopathy.*

Other disorders that result from different excessive trinucleotide repeats include ones that are inherited in an autosomal recessive pattern (Friedreich ataxia), autosomal dominant pattern (spinocerebellar atrophies and Huntington disease), or sex-linked pattern (fragile X syndrome) (see Chapters 2, 13, and 18, and Appendix 3C). Whichever the particular trinucleotide base repeat and

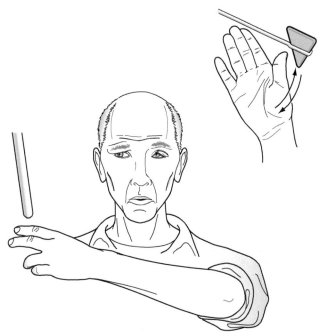

FIGURE 6.5 ■ This 25-year-old man with myotonic dystrophy has the typically elongated, "hatchet" face caused by temporal and facial muscle wasting, frontal baldness, and ptosis. Because of myotonia, a percussion hammer striking his thenar eminence muscles precipitates a forceful, sustained contraction that draws in the thumb for 3–10 seconds. Myotonia also prevents him from rapidly releasing his grasp.

pattern of inheritance, physicians can easily and reliably diagnose these illnesses in symptomatic and asymptomatic individuals by testing their DNA.

Illnesses in this group have several features that stem from the expanded trinucleotide repeats. The severity of the symptoms is roughly proportional to the length of the repeats. For example, myotonic dystrophy patients with 50 to 100 trinucleotide repeats have mild and incomplete manifestations of the disorder; those with 100 to 1000 have, to a greater or lesser degree, all the manifestations; and those with more than 2000 show florid involvement that is often obvious in infancy.

Another characteristic of trinucleotide repeat disorders is that sperm are more likely than eggs to increase their DNA repeats – as if sperm DNA were more genetically unstable than egg DNA. Thus, in these illnesses, children who have inherited the abnormal gene from their father, rather than from their mother, develop symptoms at a younger age and eventually in a more severe form. Similarly, fathers are more apt than mothers to pass along severe forms of the illness.

In addition, when transmitted from parent to child, trinucleotide repeat sequences tend to expand further instead of self-correcting. Neurologists term this tendency toward greater genetic abnormality and more pronounced symptoms *amplification*.

A clinical counterpart of amplification is *anticipation*: successive generations of individuals who inherit the abnormal gene show signs of the illness at a progressively younger age. For example, a grandfather may not have been diagnosed with myotonic dystrophy until he was 38 years old. At that age, he already had an asymptomatic boy and girl who both carried the gene. The son and daughter typically would not show signs of the illness until they reach 26 years; however, by then, they might each have several of their own children. Anticipation would be further apparent when affected grandchildren show signs in their teenage years. In the classic example, Huntington disease, dementia appears earlier in life and more severely in successive generations, especially when the father has transmitted the abnormal gene (see Chapter 18).

A less frequently occurring variety of myotonic dystrophy, *myotonic dystrophy type 2* or *proximal myotonic myopathy* (*PROMM*), has a phenotype that differs only slightly from the common myotonic dystrophy type 1. However, it has several unique genetic features: the mutation consists of a four-nucleotide repeat (a "quad" repeat), the genotype and phenotype do not correlate, and anticipation does not occur.

Inflammatory and Infectious Myopathies

Some infectious and inflammatory illnesses attack only muscles. These illnesses typically cause weakness and myalgias, as in the common "flu," but rarely alter patients' mental status.

Polymyositis is a nonspecific, generalized, inflammatory myopathy characterized by weakness, myalgias, and systemic symptoms, such as fever, and malaise. A related disorder, *dermatomyositis*, causes similar symptoms preceded or accompanied by a rash – usually on the face and extensor surfaces of the elbows and knees. In children and many adults, a benign, self-limited systemic viral illness usually causes polymyositis. In other adults, polymyositis may be a manifestation of inflammatory diseases, such as polymyalgia rheumatica and polyarteritis nodosa.

A *Trichinella* infection of muscles, *trichinosis*, causes an infectious rather than a purely inflammatory myopathy. Victims usually develop this illness from eating undercooked pork or wild game. Thus, in the United States, hunters and recent immigrants from South and Central America are most liable to have ingested *Trichinella* and develop the characteristic muscle pains, fevers, and heliotrope rash.

The *eosinophilia-myalgia syndrome*, more of a toxic than an inflammatory disorder, results from ingesting tryptophan or tryptophan-containing products, which are usually taken by insomniacs and health-food devotees. The eosinophilia-myalgia syndrome usually consists of several days of severe myalgias and a markedly elevated number and proportion of eosinophils in the blood. Patients often suffer from fatigue, rash, neuropathy, and cardiopulmonary impairments as well as from myalgias.

More than half the patients with eosinophilia-myalgia syndrome display mild depressive symptoms that cannot be correlated with their physical impairments, eosinophil concentration, or concurrent psychiatric disorders. Physicians may mislabel these patients as having chronic fatigue syndrome because of their variable symptoms and, except for the eosinophilia, lack of objective findings.

AIDS myopathy, associated with human immunodeficiency virus (HIV), also causes myalgia, weakness, weight loss, and fatigue. In most patients, the myopathy results from an infection with HIV. However, in some patients, moderate to large doses of zidovudine (popularly known as AZT) seem to be partly or totally responsible for the myopathy. In these cases, muscle biopsies often disclose abnormalities in mitochondria and withdrawing the offending medicine usually leads to at least partial improvement.

Metabolic Myopathies

With the major exception of mitochondrial myopathies' inducing combinations of muscle and cerebral impairments (see later), muscle metabolism is usually independent of cerebral metabolism. For example, prolonged steroid treatment frequently produces proximal muscle weakness and wasting (*steroid myopathy*). It also causes a round face, acne, and an obese body with spindly limbs ("cushingoid" appearance). However, only in high doses do steroids routinely cause mood changes, agitation, and irrational behavior – loosely termed "steroid psychosis." Patients with cerebral vasculitis, a brain tumor, or other disorder that compromises the CNS are particularly susceptible to steroid-induced mental changes.

Testosterone and other anabolic steroids, when taken in conjunction with exercising, can increase muscle size and strength. Athletes and body-builders use this regimen to enhance their power and appearance. While deriving obvious benefits from the steroids these individuals risk steroid myopathy, frequent depression, and occasionally steroid psychosis. Illicit steroid use is also associated with physical abuse of women.

An example of the delicate nature of muscle metabolism being notably independent of cerebral metabolism is that a low serum potassium concentration (hypokalemia) leads to profound weakness, *hypokalemic myopathy*, and cardiac arrhythmias, but not to mental status changes. Hypokalemic myopathy is often an iatrogenic condition caused by administration of diuretics or steroids, which are sometimes surreptitiously self-administered. Psychiatrists are apt to encounter hypokalemia in patients with laxative abuse or alcoholic cirrhosis.

In contrast to hypokalemia, hyponatremia (sodium depletion) causes confusion, agitation, stupor, and seizures. Psychiatrists might encounter patients with hyponatremia and its complications because it results from compulsive water drinking; use of psychotropics, such as carbamazepine (Tegretol), oxcarbazepine (Trileptal), lithium, and selective serotonin reuptake inhibitors (SSRIs); traumatic brain injury; and numerous medical conditions.

A different disorder involving potassium metabolism is *hypokalemic periodic paralysis*, in which patients have dramatic attacks, lasting several hours to 2 days, of areflexic quadriparesis. During attacks of hypokalemia, patients remain alert and fully cognizant, breathing normally, and purposefully moving their eyes despite the widespread areflexic paralysis. Contrary to its label, periodic paralysis is irregular and not "periodic." The attacks tend to occur spontaneously every few weeks, but exercise, sleep, or large carbohydrate meals often precipitate them. Although attacks resemble sleep paralysis and cataplexy (see Chapter 17), they are differentiated by a longer duration and hypokalemia. Hypokalemic periodic

paralysis, sleep paralysis, and cataplexy all differ from psychogenic episodes by their areflexia.

Usually transmitted in an autosomal dominant pattern, hypokalemic periodic paralysis becomes apparent in adolescent boys. In most cases, it stems from a mutation in the calcium ion channel gene and represents another channelopathy. An adult-onset variety is associated with hyperthyroidism.

Other common metabolic myopathies are sometimes associated with mental status changes. For example, alcoholism leads to limb and cardiac muscle wasting (alcohol cardiomyopathy). In *hyperthyroid myopathy*, weakness develops as part of hyperthyroidism. Although the hyperthyroidism usually causes heat intolerance and hyperactivity, older individuals may have *apathetic hyperthyroidism*, in which signs of overactivity are remarkably absent. As a general rule, metabolic myopathies resolve when normal metabolism is restored.

Administration of atypical neuroleptics, particularly clozapine, as well as typical dopamine receptor-blocking ones causes a mostly asymptomatic elevation of CK serum concentrations. In as many as 10% of patients with acute psychosis, the CK concentration increases to five-fold or greater levels. Physicians might find that medication injections, excessive physical activity, or subclinical neuroleptic-induced parkinsonism or dystonia (see Chapter 18) is responsible for this elevation. An asymptomatic, isolated, mild-to-moderate CK elevation should not automatically trigger a diagnosis of neuroleptic-malignant syndrome (see later); however, physicians should assess the patient for other parameters of muscle breakdown and repeat the CK determination after 48 hours.

Antidepressants and amphetamines may also cause an innocuous increase in the serum CK concentration. Similarly, about 10% of individuals taking cholesterol-lowering statins have myalgia and modest elevations in serum CK concentrations. In a more serious adverse reaction, these medicines occasionally and unpredictably cause acute, catastrophic muscle breakdown and marked elevation in serum CK concentrations (*cholesterol-lowering agent myopathy* [*CLAM*]). Patients with hypercholesterolemia must take a statin for an average of 6 months before this more severe myopathy may appear.

Mitochondrial Myopathies

Mitochondria utilize cytochrome c oxidase and related enzymes for oxidative phosphorylation (in the respiratory, aerobic chain). This metabolic system supplies about 90% of the body's energy requirement, mostly in the form of adenosine triphosphate (ATP). In turn, the brain is the body's greatest energy consumer. Other high-energy consumers are cardiac, skeletal, and extraocular muscles.

As they generate energy, mitochondria constantly remove *free radicals*, which are highly toxic metabolic by-products. Failure to remove them may lead to Parkinson disease and other illnesses (see Chapter 18).

Although vital, mitochondria's energy-producing enzymes are delicate and easily poisoned. For example, cyanide rapidly and irreversibly inactivates the respiratory enzymes. With loss of aerobic metabolism in the brain, as well as in other organs, individuals exposed to cyanide almost immediately lose consciousness and then succumb to brain death. Cyanide has been used for executions in gas chambers and taken by individuals committing suicide, including the several hundred cultists in the murder-suicide massacre in Jonestown, Guyana, in 1978. Also, certain medications, through a side effect, damage mitochondria. For example, nucleoside analogues used to treat HIV infection interfere with the mitochondria's enzyme chain and thus may cause weakness and lactic acidosis.

In a group of illnesses, inherited abnormalities in the DNA of mitochondria disrupt their function. Mitochondrial DNA (mtDNA) differs significantly from chromosomal DNA (nuclear DNA [nDNA]). In contrast to nDNA, which is derived equally from each parent and arranged in familiar pairs, mtDNA is derived entirely from the mother, double-stranded but ring-shaped, and able to carry only 37 genes. It comprises 1% of total cellular DNA. As normal individuals age, they accumulate mutations in mtDNA that are responsible for some age-related changes in the muscles and brain.

Another difference between nDNA and mtDNA is that mtDNA is passed to daughter cells' mitochondria in random, variable mixtures. The daughter cells' mitochondria inherit variable proportions of normal and abnormal mtDNA. When the proportion of abnormal mtDNA reaches a certain level, the *threshold effect*, ATP production becomes insufficient for cellular function and symptoms ensue. The variable proportion of normal and abnormal mtDNA in single cells, *heteroplasmy* (Fig. 6.6), explains why organs typically have differing proportions of abnormal cells and accounts for the illnesses' inconstant age of onset and clinical features.

A different cause of mitochondria dysfunction is that mutations and other abnormalities in nDNA can impair mtDNA. For example, mutations in nDNA that influence mtDNA probably account for many of the problems underlying Wilson disease (see Chapter 18) and Friedreich ataxia (see Chapter 2). The influence of nDNA on mtDNA can explain why paternally inherited abnormal nDNA can cause malfunction of mtDNA. Moreover, it can explain how a father might transmit an illness characterized by mitochondrial dysfunction to his child.

When they occur, mtDNA abnormalities often produce *mitochondrial myopathies*, which are inherited illnesses characterized by combinations of impaired muscle metabolism, brain damage, other organ system impairment, and abnormal lipid storage. Muscles, which are almost always included in the multisystem pathology, are filled by a vastly increased number of mitochondria. With special histologic stains, clumps of abnormal mitochondria appear as *ragged-red fibers*. In addition, normal respiratory enzymes, such as cytochrome c oxidase (COX), are absent in many cells. The inheritance patterns of the mitochondrial myopathies do not follow Mendelian patterns, such as autosomal dominance, but reflect the vagaries of mtDNA's maternal transmission, nDNA influence, heteroplasmy, and the threshold effect.

The *primary mitochondrial myopathies*, which result from mitochondria having deficiencies in cytochrome oxidase or other enzymes, cause weakness and exercise intolerance,

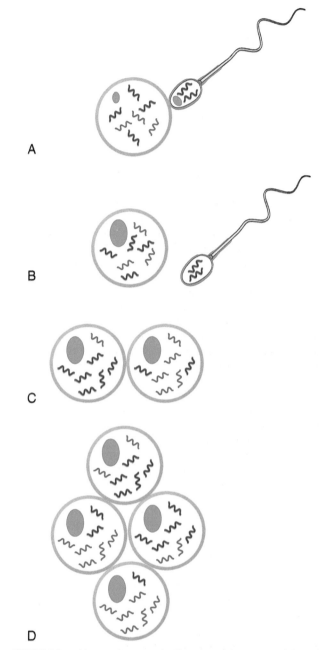

FIGURE 6.6 ■ Heteroplasmy. *A*, Sperm and egg nuclei each contain an equal complement of chromosomal DNA (nDNA). Sperm mitochondria, containing DNA (mtDNA), power the flagella. *B*, After fertilizing an egg and transferring their nDNA to the egg's nucleus, sperm drop away with their mitochondria and mtDNA intact. Thus sperm mtDNA, whether mutant or wild (normal), does not enter the fertilized egg. The fertilized egg's chromosomes undergo mitosis resulting in equal distribution of nDNA into the two daughter cells. *C*, Chromosomes divide and distribute nDNA, with or without mutations, equally to daughter cells. In contrast, although mitochondria also duplicate, they do not segregate equally. If mtDNA contains mutations, daughter cells receive unequal distributions of mutant mtDNA. *D*, The nonrandom, non-Mendelian distribution of mitochondria and their mtDNA in daughter cells ultimately gives different organs variable proportions of mtDNA. Heteroplasmy is the mixture of mutant and normal mtDNA in a single cell.

short stature, epilepsy, deafness, and episodes of lactic acidosis. Another group of mitochondrial myopathies, progressive ophthalmoplegia and its related disorders, cause ptosis and other extraocular muscle palsies along with numerous nonneurologic manifestations, such as retinitis pigmentosa, short stature, cardiomyopathy, and endocrine abnormalities. One mitochondrial DNA disorder, *Leber optic atrophy*, causes hereditary optic atrophy mostly affecting young males (see Chapter 12).

The best-known subgroup of mtDNA disorders, *mitochondrial encephalopathies*, typically causes progressive or intermittent mental abnormalities that usually appear between infancy and 12 years. Children with one of these illnesses typically have mental retardation, progressive cognitive impairment, or episodes of confusion leading to stupor. In other words, mitochondrial disorders cause dementia or intermittent delirium in children. They can also cause paresis of extraocular muscles, psychomotor retardation or regression, migraine-like headaches, and optic atrophy. Neurologists are increasingly noting the association between mitochondrial disorders and psychiatric disorders, particularly mood disorders and, less commonly, psychosis. The psychiatric diagnosis can predate the onset of neurological symptoms by more than a decade, making it harder to connect the clinical clues.

Dysfunction of mitochondrial respiration characteristically leads to lactic acidosis either constantly or only during attacks. (Cyanide poisoning, because it poisons mitochondria, also leads to lactic acidosis.) In patients with mitochondrial encephalopathy, muscle biopsies show ragged red fibers, which represent accumulation of massive numbers of mitochondria, and a checkerboard pattern of cells that fail to stain for cytochrome c oxidase.

Mitochondrial encephalopathies include two important varieties known best by their colorful acronyms:
- *MELAS*: *m*itochondrial *e*ncephalomyelopathy, *l*actic *a*cidosis, and *s*trokelike episodes.
- *MERRF*: *m*yoclonic *e*pilepsy and *r*agged-*r*ed *f*ibers

Potential therapies for the mitochondrial disorders include co-enzyme CoQ10, bone-marrow transplantation, and, for affected women who wish to conceive, cytoplasmic transfer.

Neuroleptic Malignant Syndrome

Neurologists and psychiatrists have classically attributed neuroleptic malignant syndrome (NMS) to dopamine receptor-blocking antipsychotic agents (neuroleptics), but because neuroleptics are not its sole cause, some physicians have sought to change its name to *Parkinson-hyperpyrexia* syndrome or *central dopaminergic syndrome*. By any name, this syndrome consists of three elements:
1. Delirium and decreased level of consciousness
2. Extrapyramidal signs, especially muscle rigidity, tremors, and/or dystonic posturing
3. Autonomic hyperactivity with prominent tachycardia and, although not the first sign, high fever.

The muscle rigidity, which affects the trunk and appendicular muscles, is so powerful that muscles crush themselves. The crushing causes muscle necrosis (*rhabdomyolysis*) that liberates muscle protein (*myoglobin*) into the blood (*myoglobinemia*) and allows myoglobin to appear in the urine (*myoglobinuria*). With pronounced myoglobinemia, especially in dehydrated patients, myoglobin precipitates in the renal tubules and impairs kidney function.

Laboratory tests reflect this series of events. An elevated concentration of serum CK, myoglobinemia, and myoglobinuria indicates rhabdomyolysis. If present, elevated blood urea nitrogen (BUN) and creatinine concentrations indicate renal insufficiency, not just dehydration.

NMS typically also causes autonomic dysfunction that appears as tachycardia and cardiovascular instability. NMS typically raises body temperature, sometimes to levels that damage the cerebral cortex. The mortality rate of NMS, not surprisingly, had been as high as 15% to 20%. However, with use of second- rather than first-generation antipsychotic agents, judicious use of all psychotropics, and awareness of this complication, the frequency, severity, and mortality of NMS have fallen.

Descriptions have usually portrayed NMS in agitated, dehydrated young men, but the syndrome has also occurred in children. Patients have most often received large doses of conventional, powerful first-generation antipsychotic agents that block dopamine D2 receptors. Use of second-generation antipsychotic agents has led, less frequently, to essentially the same syndrome. Case reports have linked NMS to nonpsychotropic dopamine-blocking medications, such as metoclopramide (Reglan), and medications not known primarily as dopamine-blocking agents, such as fluoxetine and lithium.

Not only does actively blocking dopamine at its receptors cause NMS, but failing to maintain dopamine treatment or depleting dopamine storage granules also causes it. All these mechanisms halt dopamine activity. For example, abruptly withholding the dopamine precursor levodopa has precipitated NMS in Parkinson disease patients. Similarly, treatment with tetrabenazine, which depletes dopamine, has rarely caused it.

Recommended treatment, aimed at restoring dopamine activity, has included administering levodopa; dopamine agonists, such as bromocriptine and apomorphine; or amantadine, which enhances dopamine activity (see Chapter 18). A complementary approach has been to administer dantrolene (Dantrium), which restores a normal intracellular calcium distribution. Several articles have proposed administering ECT, but the rationale and results have been unclear. In any case, physicians must provide fluids, antipyretics, and other supportive measures.

Other Causes of Rhabdomyolysis, Hyperthermia, and Altered Mental States

Serotonin Syndrome

The serotonin syndrome and NMS are both usually medication-induced and their primary features include delirium, often with agitation, and autonomic hyperactivity. By way of contrast, the serotonin syndrome characteristically presents with myoclonus, although sometimes tremulousness and clonus. In another difference, the serotonin syndrome causes only mild elevations in body temperature and CK serum concentration. Its features tend to be protean, variable in severity, and delayed in onset.

Physicians usually attribute the serotonin syndrome to an excess of one or more serotoninergic medicines. Potential causes all increase serotonin or serotonin-like substances at the synapse through various mechanisms: serotonin precursors (such as tryptophan); provokers of serotonin release (ecstasy, amphetamine, and cocaine); serotonin reuptake inhibitors and tricyclic antidepressants; inhibitors of serotonin metabolism (monoamine oxidase inhibitors); and serotonin agonists (sumatriptan and other triptans). Even cough suppressants, dietary supplements, and St. John's wort increase serotonin concentrations enough to cause it.

Although large enough doses of one of these medicines may alone cause the syndrome, taking them in combination more frequently precipitates the syndrome. Because serotoninergic medicines are so commonplace, the serotonin syndrome might follow use of serotonin reuptake inhibitors in a variety of neurologic illnesses with comorbid depression, such as Parkinson disease, migraines, and chronic pain. In particular, use of selegiline or rasagiline, which are MAOIs, will theoretically place a depressed Parkinson disease patient given an SSRI at risk of developing the serotonin syndrome. Use of a triptan, which is a serotonin agonist for migraine treatment, in conjunction with an SSRI or MAOI, similarly raises that possibility. However, even though the coadministration of a triptan and SSRI potentially causing the serotonin syndrome has been the subject of a Food and Drug Administration warning and the gist of many examination questions, prescribing triptans to patients taking an SSRI or SSRI at standard doses generally does not lead to significant problems.

After removing the responsible medicines, initial treatment for the serotonin syndrome should support vital functions and reduce agitation with benzodiazepines. Physicians might reverse some of the excessive CNS serotonin activity by using the serotonin 5-HT$_{2A}$ antagonist, cyproheptadine. As a last resort, some authors have recommended chlorpromazine, which is also a serotonin antagonist.

Malignant Hyperthermia

Malignant hyperthermia (MH), another disorder often compared to NMS, also leads to rhabdomyolysis, hyperthermia, brain damage, and death. In contrast to NMS, MH is precipitated by inhaled general anesthesia, such as halothane or sevoflurane, or the muscle relaxant succinylcholine. Its underlying cause is excessive calcium release by calcium channels. A vulnerability to MH is inherited as an autosomal disorder carried on chromosome 19. Thus, psychiatrists should review the family history of patients before they administer succinylcholine prior to ECT. If MH were to develop, dantrolene may be an effective treatment.

Other Causes

Although its mechanism of action probably differs, the main features of phencyclidine (*PCP*) *intoxication* – muscle rigidity, high fevers, and confusion – closely mimic NMS.

Physicians also often include *anticholinergic poisoning*, along with NMS and the serotonin syndrome, in the differential diagnosis of patients with fever and agitated delirium. In addition, anticholinergic poisoning from medications, such as scopolamine, usually produces signs of excessive sympathetic activity, including mydriasis, dry skin, urinary retention, and absent bowel sounds. Physicians faced with a febrile, agitated patient may eliminate anticholinergic poisoning from consideration if the patient has either increased muscle tone or bladder and bowel hyperactivity.

At times, distinguishing between NMS and meningitis can be difficult because both conditions cause delirium, fever, and nuchal rigidity. Finally, sometimes neurologists consider catatonia in the differential diagnosis of NMS because of the psychiatric setting and increased muscle tone; however, its course and lack of major autonomic dysfunction set it apart (see Chapter 18).

LABORATORY TESTS

Nerve Conduction Studies

Nerve conduction studies (NCS) (Fig. 6.7) can determine the site of nerve damage, confirm a clinical diagnosis of neuropathy, and distinguish polyneuropathy from myopathy. In addition, they can help separate neuropathies that have resulted from loss of myelin (demyelination), such as Guillain–Barré syndrome, in which the conduction velocities slow, from those that have resulted from axon damage, such as with chemotherapy, in which the amplitude is reduced. Myopathies, in contrast, do not slow conduction velocity, though amplitudes in motor NCS are often lowered in weak muscles.

Electromyography

Neurologists perform EMGs by inserting fine needles into selected muscles and recording the consequent electrical discharges during muscle rest and voluntary muscle contractions. In a myopathy, muscles produce characteristic EMG abnormalities. Several diseases – myasthenia gravis, ALS, and myotonic dystrophy – produce distinct EMG patterns.

Mononeuropathies and peripheral neuropathies also produce abnormal EMG patterns because, in these conditions, improperly innervated muscles malfunction and deteriorate. In other words, the EMG can detect denervated muscles and help determine which peripheral nerve

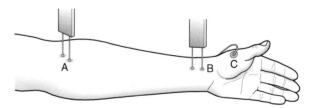

FIGURE 6.7 ■ To determine nerve conduction velocity (NCV), a stimulating electrode excites a motor nerve at two points (*A* and *B*) and a response is recorded from the appropriate muscle (*C*). The distance between A and B, divided by the time interval, determines the NCV. In the upper extremities, NCV is approximately 50 to 60 m/s, and in the lower extremities, 40 to 50 m/s.

or nerve root is damaged. Neurologists frequently use EMG in cases of cervical or lumbar pain when attempting to document or exclude radiculopathy.

Serum Enzyme Determinations

Lactic dehydrogenase (LDH), aspartate amino transferase (AST), aldolase, and CK are enzymes concentrated within muscle cells. When illnesses injure muscles, those enzymes escape into the bloodstream. Their serum concentrations rise in rough proportion to the severity of muscle damage. Of the various common conditions, NMS produces the greatest increase in CK. It is also characteristically elevated in DMD patients, affected fetuses, and women carriers; metabolic muscle diseases; and inflammatory myopathies, such as polymyositis. Therefore, for patients with unexplained, ill-defined weakness, as well as those with myopathy or NMS, one of the first laboratory tests should be a determination of the serum CK concentration.

Muscle Biopsy

In expert hands, microscopic examination of muscle may help make a diagnosis of certain myopathies or neuropathy. The muscle disorders that might be diagnosed in this way include DMD, polymyositis, trichinosis, collagenvascular diseases, mitochondrial myopathies, and several rare glycogen-storage diseases. Electron microscopy as well as routine light microscopy is required to diagnose the mitochondrial myopathies. In many of these disorders, such as MERRF, pathologists stain tissue for the respiratory enzymes and the concentration and morphology of mitochondria. However, in inherited conditions for which it is available, such as DMD and myotonic dystrophy, genetic testing usually is easier, more sensitive, and more specific.

REFERENCES

Anglin, R. E., Tamopolsky, M., Mazurek, M., et al. (2012). The psychiatric presentation of mitochondrial disorders in adults. *The Journal of Neuropsychiatry and Clinical Neurosciences, 24*(4), 394–409.

Boyer, E. W., & Shannon, M. (2005). The serotonin syndrome. *The New England Journal of Medicine, 352,* 1112–1120.

Chalk, C., Benstead, T. J., & Keezer, M. (2011). Medical treatment for botulism. *The Cochrane Database of Systematic Reviews,* (3), CD008123.

Diaz-Manera, J., Martinez-Hernandez, E., Querol, L., et al. (2012). Long-lasting treatment effect of rituximab in MuSK myasthenia. *Neurology, 78,* 189–193.

Dimauro, S. (2013). Mitochondrial encephalomyopathies – fifty years on. *Neurology, 81,* 281–291.

Ferro, S., Esposito, F., Biamonti, M., et al. (2008). Myasthenia gravis during pregnancy. *Expert Review of Neurotherapeutics, 8,* 979–988.

Gary, J. W., & Barkin, R. L. (2015). Fibromyalgia. *Disease-A-Month, 61,* 66–111.

Gervais, R. O., Russell, A. S., Green, P., et al. (2001). Effort testing in patients with fibromyalgia and disability incentives. *The Journal of Rheumatology, 28,* 1892–1899.

Gilman, P. K. (2010). Triptans, serotonin agonists, and serotonin syndrome (serotonin toxicity): A review. *Headache, 50,* 264–272.

Goetz, C. G., Bolla, K. I., & Rogers, S. M. (1994). Neurologic health outcomes and Agent Orange: Institute of Medicine report. *Neurology, 44,* 801–809.

Haney, E., Smith, M. E. B., McDonagh, M., et al. (2015). Diagnostic methods for myalgic encephalomyelitis/chronic fatigue syndrome: a systematic review for a National Institutes of Health Pathways to Prevention workshop. *Annals of Internal Medicine, 162,* 834–840.

Hassani, A., Horvath, R., & Chinnery, P. F. (2010). Mitochondrial myopathies. Developments in treatment. *Current Opinion in Neurology, 23,* 459–465.

Hyams, K. C., Wignall, F. S., & Roswell, R. (1996). War syndromes and their evaluation: From the U.S. Civil War to the Persian Gulf War. *Annals of Internal Medicine, 125,* 398–405.

Krup, L. B., Masur, D. M., & Kaufman, L. D. (1993). Neurocognitive dysfunction in the eosinophilia-myalgia syndrome. *Neurology, 43,* 931–936.

Manzur, A. Y., Kuntzer, T., Pike, M., et al. (2009). Glucocorticoid corticosteroids for Duchenne muscular dystrophy. *The Cochrane Library, 3,* 1–71.

Martin, C. O., & Adams, H. P. (2003). Neurologic aspects of biological and chemical terrorism. *Archives of Neurology, 60,* 21–25.

Melkersson, K. (2006). Serum creatine kinase levels in chronic psychosis patients – a comparison between atypical and conventional antipsychotics. *Progress in Neuro-Psychopharmacology and Biological Psychiatry, 30*(7), 1277–1282.

Meola, G., Sansone, V., Perani, D., et al. (2003). Executive dysfunction and avoidant personality trait in myotonic dystrophy type 1 (DM-1) and proximal myotonic myopathy. *Neuromuscular Disorders: NMD, 13,* 813–821.

Morse, C. G., & Kovacs, J. (2006). Metabolic and skeletal complications of HIV infection. *JAMA: The Journal of the American Medical Association, 296,* 844–854.

Shapiro, R. L., Hatheway, C., & Swerdlow, D. L. (1998). Botulism in the United States: A clinical and epidemiologic review. *Annals of Internal Medicine, 129,* 221–228.

Turner, C., & Hilton-Jones, D. (2010). The myotonic dystrophies: Diagnosis and management. *Journal of Neurology, Neurosurgery, and Psychiatry, 81,* 358–367.

CHAPTER 6

QUESTIONS AND ANSWERS

1–3. Upon looking to the left for longer than 1 minute, a 17-year-old woman has intermittent double vision. In each eye alone, her visual acuity is normal. Her examination reveals that she has right-sided ptosis and difficulty keeping her right eye adducted. Her pupils are 4 mm, round, and reactive. Her speech is nasal and her neck flexor muscles are weak. Her strength and deep tendon reflexes (DTRs) are normal.

1. Which disease most likely explains her intermittent diplopia?
a. Multiple sclerosis (MS)
b. Psychogenic weakness
c. Myasthenia gravis
d. Right posterior communicating artery aneurysm

Answer: c. This is a classic case of myasthenia gravis with ocular, pharyngeal, and neck flexor paresis but no pupil abnormality. She develops diplopia when one or more ocular muscles fatigue. By way of contrast, this pattern of neck flexor paresis, ocular muscle weakness, and ptosis does not occur in MS. Although internuclear ophthalmoplegia (INO) frequently occurs in MS, it causes nystagmus in the abducting eye as well as paresis of the adducting eye (see Chapters 12 and 15). As for psychogenic disturbances, people cannot mimic either paresis of one ocular muscle or ptosis. Compression of the third cranial nerve by an expanding aneurysm also produces ptosis and paresis of adduction. However, compression of the third cranial nerve differs from myasthenia because it has a painful onset, and the pupil dilates and loses its reactivity to light. Furthermore, such an aneurysm cannot explain the bulbar palsy.

2. Which test would most likely confirm the diagnosis of myasthenia gravis?
a. ACh receptor antibodies
b. Muscle biopsy
c. Spine MRI
d. Muscle enzymes: CK, LDH, AST

Answer: a. More than 80% of patients with generalized myasthenia have detectable serum antibodies to ACh receptor, but their concentration does not correlate with the severity of the illness. Of myasthenia patients without detectable ACh antibodies, about 50% of them will have MuSK antibodies (antibodies to anti*muscle-specific kinase*). The ice-pack test, which has replaced the Tensilon test, is usually positive in patients with ptosis.

3. Which condition is sometimes comorbid with myasthenia gravis?
a. Hypothyroidism
b. Hyperthyroidism
c. Systemic lupus erythematosus
d. Rheumatoid arthritis

Answer: b. Correction of coexistent hyperthyroidism or thymoma should improve or eliminate the illness.

4–5. During the previous week, an 18-year-old dancer began to develop progressively severe weakness of her toes and ankles. On examination, she has loss of her ankle reflexes, unresponsive plantar reflexes, and, in her toes and feet, decreased sensation.

4. Which *two* diseases are the most likely cause of her symptoms and signs?
a. Myasthenia gravis
b. Toxic polyneuropathy
c. Polymyositis
d. Guillain–Barré syndrome
e. Thoracic spinal cord tumor

Answer: b, d. She has signs of a polyneuropathy: distal lower extremity paresis, areflexia, and hypalgesia. Common causes of a polyneuropathy are alcohol abuse, chemicals, chemotherapy, and inflammatory illnesses, such as Guillain–Barré syndrome (acute inflammatory demyelinating polyradiculoneuropathy [AIDP]). Myasthenia rarely affects the legs alone and does not impair sensation. Likewise, the sensory loss and pattern of distal paresis preclude a diagnosis of muscle disease. A spinal cord tumor is unlikely because her ankle reflexes are unreactive, Babinski signs are not present, and she has no "sensory level" or urinary incontinence.

5. Which single test would be most helpful in making a diagnosis in the previous question?
a. Electroencephalogram (EEG)
b. Nerve conduction study (NCS)
c. Electromyography (EMG)
d. Tensilon test
e. Muscle enzymes: CK, LDH, AST
f. Positron emission tomography (PET)

Answer: b. NCV will probably be able to confirm the presence of a peripheral neuropathy and suggest that it is a demyelinating process. CSF analysis in cases of Guillain–Barré syndrome will usually show increased protein and normal or near-normal cell count, i.e., the "albumino-cytologic disassociation."

6–11. During the previous 6 months, a 5-year-old boy began to struggle when standing upright. He has had to push himself up on his legs in order to stand. He can no longer run. A cousin of the same age has a similar problem. The patient seems to be unusually muscular and has mild weakness of his upper leg muscles and decreased quadriceps (knee) reflexes.

6. Which single disease is he most likely to have?
 a. Porphyria
 b. Peripheral neuropathy
 c. Spinal cord tumor
 d. Duchenne muscular dystrophy
 e. A psychogenic disorder
 f. Myotonic dystrophy

 Answer: d. The boy and his cousin probably have Duchenne muscular dystrophy because he has the typical findings: Gower sign (children pushing against their own legs to stand), muscle pseudohypertrophy, and areflexia of weak muscles.

7. Which *three* tests would probably help diagnose this boy?
 a. Muscle dystrophin test
 b. NCS
 c. EMG
 d. Tensilon test
 e. Muscle enzymes
 f. CSF analysis

 Answer: a, c, e. In cases of Duchenne muscular dystrophy, muscle dystrophin will be absent on examination of a muscle biopsy. In its variant, Becker dystrophy, dystrophin will be present but abnormal. In addition, in Duchenne muscular dystrophy, EMGs will show abnormal (myopathic potential) patterns and the CK will be markedly elevated. Genetic analysis, the best test for Duchenne muscular dystrophy, will show mutations on the dystrophin gene, which is located on the X chromosome.

8. What is the sex of his cousin?
 a. Male
 b. Female
 c. Either

 Answer: a. Duchenne muscular dystrophy is a sex-linked trait transmitted disease. In contrast, myotonic dystrophy is an autosomal dominant trait inherited in a classic Mendelian pattern of transmission through chromosomes.

9. Who is the carrier of this condition?
 a. Father
 b. Mother
 c. Either
 d. Both

 Answer: b.

10. Tests show that the sister of the boy with Duchenne dystrophy is a carrier of the illness. Tests also show that her husband does not have the illness. What percent of their female children (girls) will be carriers of Duchenne dystrophy?
 a. 0%
 b. 25%
 c. 50%
 d. 75%
 e. 100%

 Answer: c.

11. As in the previous question, if a sister of the boy is a carrier and her husband does not have the illness, what percent of all her children will develop Duchenne dystrophy?
 a. 0%
 b. 25%
 c. 50%
 d. 75%
 e. 100%

 Answer: b. One half of the boys and one half of the girls will inherit the abnormal gene. The boys who inherit it will develop the disease, but the girls who inherit it will only be carriers. Therefore, 25% of the children (one half of the boys) will have the disease.

12–15. A 68-year-old man has had 2 weeks of aches and tenderness of his shoulder muscles. He is unable to lift his arms above his head. He has a persistent temperature of 99° to 100.5° in the afternoons and evenings. A blotchy red rash covers his head, neck, and upper torso.

12. Which *two* diseases should be considered most likely?
 a. Steroid myopathy
 b. Dermatomyositis
 c. Statin-induced myopathy
 d. Mitochondrial myopathy
 e. Polymyalgia rheumatica
 f. Trichinosis

 Answer: b, f. His main symptoms are proximal muscle pain and weakness combined with systemic signs of low-grade fever and a rash. The combination indicates a myopathy that is either inflammatory, such as dermatomyositis, or infectious, such as trichinosis. In each of those cases, the sedimentation rate would be elevated. Polymyalgia rheumatica, in contrast, does not cause a rash. Similarly, the cholesterol-lowering statin drugs may produce muscle pain and weakness, but not a rash. Steroid myopathy and most other metabolic myopathies are painless and not associated with a rash. Mitochondrial myopathies develop in infants and children.

13. Which *two* tests are most likely to confirm the diagnosis?
 a. EEG
 b. NCV
 c. EMG

d. Tensilon test
e. Muscle enzymes
f. Skin and muscle biopsy
g. Nerve biopsy

Answer: e, f. Laboratory tests in dermatomyositis show a marked elevation in serum CK concentration and an elevated sedimentation rate. A muscle biopsy will permit the diagnosis of dermatomyositis, vasculitis, and trichinosis. The best test for polymyalgia rheumatica is a therapeutic trial of small doses of prednisone.

14. Which *three* conditions are associated with dermatomyositis in the adult?
a. Dementia
b. Pulmonary malignancies
c. Diabetes mellitus
d. Gastrointestinal malignancies
e. Delirium
f. Polyarteritis nodosa

Answer: b, d, f.

15. Which of the above conditions are associated with polymyositis in children?

Answer: None. In children, polymyositis is associated with viral illnesses. If an adult develops dermatomyositis, physicians should search for an underlying, occult malignancy.

16–24. For each medication, state whether it is associated with a neuropathy (a), a myopathy (b), both (c), or neither (d)?

16. Disulfiram
17. Chlorpromazine
18. Nitrofurantoin
19. Isoniazid (INH)
20. Atorvastatin
21. Amitriptyline
22. Zidovudine (AZT)
23. Lithium carbonate
24. Vitamin B_6

Answers: 16–a, 17–c, 18–a, 19–a, 20–b, 21–d, 22–b, 23–d, 24–a.

25–27. A 50-year-old man has developed low thoracic back pain and difficulty walking. He has mild paraparesis, a distended bladder, diminished sensation to pinprick below the umbilicus, and equivocal plantar and DTRs. He has tenderness of the midthoracic spine.

25. Which single condition do his symptoms most clearly indicate?
a. Polymyositis
b. Herniated lumbar intervertebral disk
c. Idiopathic polyneuropathy
d. Thoracic spinal cord compression

Answer: d. The patient has spinal cord compression at T10 or slightly higher. The reflexes are equivocal because in acute spinal cord compression reflexes are diminished in a phenomenon called "spinal shock." The T10 level is indicated by the sensory change at the umbilicus. Metastatic tumors are the most frequent cause of spinal cord compression, but herniated intervertebral thoracic disks, multiple sclerosis, tuberculous abscesses, and trauma are often responsible. In contrast, polymyositis affects the arms as well as the legs and does not involve the bladder control, produce loss of sensation, or cause spine pain or tenderness.

26. If the routine history, physical examination, and laboratory tests, including a chest CT (computed tomography), were normal, which of the following tests should be performed next?
a. CT of the spine
b. X-rays of the lumbosacral spine
c. NCS
d. Tensilon test
e. MRI of the spine

Answer: e. MRI is usually the next test because it is noninvasive and readily able to detect soft tissue masses. However, if an MRI is not readily available, CT of the spine is still likely to make the diagnosis.

27. The MRI of the spine confirms the clinical diagnosis. If the paraparesis does not receive prompt, effective treatment, which complications might ensue?
a. Progression of paraparesis to paraplegia
b. Urinary incontinence
c. Sacral decubitus ulcers
d. Hydronephrosis and urosepsis
e. All of the above

Answer: e.

28. Which of the following are potential complications of prolonged use of steroids?
a. Obesity, especially of the face and trunk
b. Steroid myopathy
c. Compression fractures of the lumbar spine
d. Opportunistic lung and CNS infections
e. Gastrointestinal bleeding
f. Opportunistic oral and vaginal infections
g. All of the above

Answer: g.

29. For each of the following illnesses that cause weakness, label it as a dystrophinopathy (a), channelopathy (b), both (c), or neither (d)?
1. Duchenne dystrophy
2. Becker dystrophy
3. Myotonic dystrophy
4. Periodic paralysis
5. Lambert–Eaton syndrome

Answers: 1–a, 2–a, 3–b, 4–b, 5–b.

30. After diagnosing a 75-year-old woman with congestive heart failure, her physician placed her on a low-salt diet and began her on a potent diuretic. Although

the congestive heart failure resolves, she develops somnolence, disorientation, and generalized weakness. Which of the following is the most likely cause of her mental status change?
a. Hypokalemia
b. A cerebrovascular infarction
c. A subdural hematoma
d. Cerebral hypoxia from congestive heart failure
e. Dehydration and hyponatremia

Answer: e. Administration of potent diuretics to patients on low-salt diets eventually leads to hypokalemia, hyponatremia, and dehydration. Prolonged use of diuretics tends to cause obtundation and confusion in the elderly because of hyponatremia and dehydration. Hypokalemia alone, however, does not cause mental abnormalities. In cases of extreme hyponatremia, physicians should replete sodium slowly because too rapid correction occasionally produces a demyelinating injury of the pons (central pontine myelinolysis).

31. Which *two* myopathies are associated with cognitive impairment?
a. Polymyositis
b. Duchenne muscular dystrophy
c. Carpal tunnel syndrome
d. Myotonic dystrophy
e. Periodic paralysis
f. Trichinosis

Answer: b, d. Duchenne muscular dystrophy and myotonic dystrophy are associated with cognitive impairment. In addition, myotonic dystrophy is associated with personality changes.

32–37. Match the illness with its probable or usual cause:

32. MERRF
33. Myotonic dystrophy
34. Hypokalemic myopathy
35. Cytochrome oxidase deficiency
36. Progressive ophthalmoplegia
37. Periodic paralysis
a. Autosomal inheritance
b. Sex-linked inheritance
c. mtDNA mutation
d. Viral illness
e. Underlying malignancy
f. ACh receptor antibodies
g. Medications

Answers: 32–c, 33–a, 34–g, 35–c, 36–c, 37–a.

38. Which of the following illnesses is not transmitted by excessive trinucleotide repeats?
a. Huntington disease
b. Myotonic dystrophy
c. Duchenne muscular dystrophy
d. Spinocerebellar ataxia (type 1)
e. Friedreich ataxia
f. Fragile X

Answer: c.

39. Which pattern of inheritance precludes transmission by excessive trinucleotide repeats?
a. Autosomal dominant
b. Autosomal recessive
c. Sex-linked
d. None of the above

Answer: d. Illnesses transmitted by excessive trinucleotide repeats include autosomal dominant (Huntington disease and most spinocerebellar ataxias), autosomal recessive (Friedreich ataxia), and sex-linked disorders (fragile X syndrome).

40. What is the role of edrophonium in the Tensilon test?
a. Edrophonium inhibits cholinesterase to prolong ACh activity.
b. Edrophonium inhibits cholinesterase to shorten ACh activity.
c. Edrophonium inhibits choline acetyltransferase (CAT) to prolong ACh activity.
d. Edrophonium inhibits choline acetyltransferase (CAT) to shorten ACh activity.

Answer: a. Edrophonium (Tensilon) prolongs ACh activity by inhibiting cholinesterase (AChE), the enzyme that metabolizes it. The enzyme choline acetyltransferase (CAT) catalyzes the synthesis of ACh. Although the Tensilon test is useful in diagnosing myasthenia gravis, the ice cube test may replace it because edrophonium may produce excessive ACh activity, and because ice cubes are far more readily available than edrophonium.

41. Why does strychnine cause uninhibited muscle contractions?
a. It impairs the presynaptic release of ACh.
b. It impairs the presynaptic release of GABA and glycine.
c. It blocks the reuptake of the excitatory neurotransmitter glutamate.
d. It competes with GABA and glycine at their postsynaptic receptor.

Answer: d. Strychnine competes with GABA and glycine at their postsynaptic receptors.

42. Which *two* of the following conditions might explain an illness becoming apparent at an earlier age in successive generations?
a. Ascertainment bias
b. Age-related vulnerability
c. Mitochondria DNA inheritance
d. Anticipation

Answer: a, d. Ascertainment bias is an apparently greater increase in incidence arising from heightened vigilance for a condition. Anticipation is an actual earlier appearance of an illness' manifestations, usually because of expansion of an abnormal DNA segment in successive generations.

43. For which *three* of the following conditions is plasmapheresis therapeutic?
a. Alzheimer disease
b. Barbiturate overdose

c. Manic depressive illness
d. Guillain–Barré illness
e. Myasthenia gravis

Answer: b, d, e.

44. Which family of medicines is most apt, when given in toxic doses, to cause agitated delirium, mydriasis, dry and hot skin, urinary retention, and absent bowel activity?
    a. Anticholinergic
    b. SSRI
    c. Dopaminergic
    d. Opioid

Answer: a. These symptoms, which reflect parasympathetic paralysis, are classic manifestations of anticholinergic toxicity.

45. Which type of ACh receptors predominate in the cerebral cortex?
    a. Nicotinic
    b. Muscarinic
    c. Both
    d. Neither

Answer. b. Muscarinic receptors predominate in the cerebral cortex. They are depleted in Alzheimer disease. Antibodies directed against nicotinic receptors, which predominate in neuromuscular junctions, characterize myasthenia gravis.

46. Which one of the following is not a characteristic of Lambert–Eaton syndrome?
    a. Because Lambert–Eaton syndrome is typically found in conjunction with small cell lung carcinoma and other forms of cancer, it is considered a paraneoplastic syndrome.
    b. The syndrome is also associated with rheumatologic diseases.
    c. It results from deactivation of ACh at the postsynaptic neuromuscular junction ACh receptor.
    d. The weakness in Lambert–Eaton syndrome primarily involves the limbs. The disorder also causes autonomic nervous system dysfunction.

Answer: c. Lambert–Eaton syndrome is similar to myasthenia in that both cause weakness and are due to an autoimmune disorder involving the neuromuscular junction; however, Lambert–Eaton syndrome produces primarily limb weakness and dysfunction of the autonomic nervous system. In many cases it is a manifestation of small cell lung cancer or rheumatologic disorders, which presumably elicit antibodies directed against presynaptic voltage-gated calcium channels. The antibody–receptor interaction impairs ACh release.

47. Which neurotransmitter system does common nerve gases poison?
    a. Glycine
    b. Gamma aminobutyric acid (GABA)
    c. Serotonin
    d. Acetylcholine

Answer: d. Nerve gases, which are typically organophosphorus agents, inactivate acetylcholinesterase (AChE). The loss of AChE leads to excessive ACh activity. Tetanus blocks the release of the inhibitory neurotransmitters, particularly glycine and GABA, in the spinal cord and elsewhere in the CNS. Botulinum toxin blocks the release of acetylcholine at the neuromuscular junctions.

48. Called to a subway station because of a terrorist attack, a physician is confronted with dozens of passengers in a state of panic who all have abdominal cramps, dyspnea, miosis, weakness, and fasciculations. Many passengers are unconscious and several are having seizures. Which medication should she first administer?
    a. Large doses of a minor tranquilizer
    b. Small doses of a major tranquilizer
    c. Atropine
    d. Naloxone

Answer: c. A terrorist nerve gas poison has produced PNS dysfunction from excessive ACh activity in the affected passengers. The nerve gas also has penetrated into the CNS to impair consciousness and provoked seizures. The first antidote to excessive ACh activity is atropine. It penetrates the blood–brain barrier and thus restores CNS as well as PNS ACh activity. Emergency workers also administer an oxime because it restores AChE activity and deactivates the organophosphate poison. In addition, emergency workers often prophylactically administer a benzodiazepine or possibly phenobarbital for their antiepileptic effects. Other antiepileptic drugs are ineffective in this situation.

49. A friend brings a 52-year-old woman with a history of several episodes of psychosis to the emergency room because she is agitated and confused. She has muscle rigidity and tremulousness, but her neck is supple. Her temperature is 105°F and white blood count 18,000. Her friend said that her medications had been changed, but he could provide no other useful information. A head CT and lumbar puncture revealed no abnormalities. Her urine was dark brown. Of the following tests, which one should be performed next?
    a. Urine analysis
    b. An MRI of the brain
    c. An EEG
    d. An HIV test

Answer: a. The key to the case is the nature of the urinary pigment. Is it myoglobin or hemoglobin? Are there signs of renal damage? In addition to the standard analysis, the urine should be tested for metabolites of cocaine, PCP, and other intoxicants, as well as signs of a urinary tract infection. The other tests are too time-consuming or nonspecific to be helpful for this desperately ill woman. Although meningitis is unlikely in view of the supple neck and normal CSF, many clinicians would administer antibiotics while further evaluation is undertaken. Similarly, whatever the cause, her temperature should be lowered to avoid brain damage. Individuals with a chronic neurologic illness, such as myasthenia, multiple sclerosis, or epilepsy, or a chronic psychiatric illness often have an exacerbation if they develop a systemic illness, such as sepsis.

50. Concerning the preceding question, which *two* conditions might cause myoglobinuria?
   a. Neuroleptic malignant syndrome
   b. Porphyria
   c. Serotonin syndrome
   d. Glomerular nephritis
   e. Malaria

Answer: a, c. All these conditions (a–e) can be associated with psychosis and dark urine, but several different pigments may darken urine. Neuroleptic malignant syndrome (NMS) (also known as the hyperpyrexia-rigidity syndrome) and the serotonin syndrome cause myoglobinuria because of muscle breakdown. However, NMS increases CK and release of myoglobin to a greater degree than the serotonin syndrome. Acute intermittent porphyria leads to porphyrins in the urine. Glomerular nephritis and falciparum malaria produce hemoglobinuria.

51–56. Match the disorder with the phenomenon:

51. Unilateral ptosis
52. Facial rash
53. Waddling gait
54. Inability to release a fist
55. Pseudohypertrophy of calf muscles
56. Premature balding and cataracts
   a. Myasthenia gravis
   b. Duchenne dystrophy
   c. Myotonic dystrophy
   d. Dermatomyositis

Answers: 51–a, 52–d, 53–b, 54–c, 55–b, 56–c.

57. An 8-year-old girl has episodes of confusion and headaches lasting between 1 and 3 days. Between attacks, she has a normal neurologic examination and unremarkable blood tests, head CT, and head MRI. Also, an EEG during attacks shows no epileptiform discharges and between attacks it shows normal alpha rhythm. Eventually, a physician determines that the serum lactic acid concentration rises markedly during every attack and is normal between them. Which should be the next diagnostic test?
   a. Lumbar puncture
   b. Chromosome analysis for trinucleotide repeats
   c. DNA testing
   a. Anticardiolipin antibody determination
   b. Polysomnography

Answer c. This child most likely has MELAS (*m*itochondrial *e*ncephalopathy, *l*actic *a*cidosis, and *s*troke-like episodes). Genetic testing would show a mutation in her mitochondrial DNA. A muscle biopsy, if done, should show proliferation of mitochondria, ragged red fibers, and absence of respiratory enzymes. Although the other causes of episodic confusion that the answers suggest – migraines,

epilepsy, TIAs, sleep disorders – are reasonable alternatives, the repeated elevation of the lactic acid suggests only a mitochondrial encephalopathy.

58. A 45-year-old scrap-metal worker, who was an illegal immigrant from an underdeveloped country, came to the hospital because of stiffness and spasms of his right leg that had begun 1 week before. While at work 10 days before coming to the hospital, he had sustained a laceration, which remained infected. During the 2 days before he came to the hospital, the stiffness and spasms spread to his lower back and other leg. The spasms came in waves. They followed loud sound, light touch, and his own movements. Despite the spasms, his strength and DTRs were normal. A psychiatry consult was solicited because the spasms seemed voluntary to the housestaff, he had excessive response to stimulation, and the disability potentially offered great secondary gain. Which is the most likely diagnosis?
   a. Malingering
   b. Conversion disorder
   c. Drug-induced dystonia
   d. Tetanus
   e. Spinal cord compression

Answer: d. Tetanus is an occupational hazard of farming and scrap-metal work. It also occurs in drug addicts who share dirty needles. Most individuals in the United States receive vaccinations in school, the military, or certain occupations, including health care. Although vaccination-induced immunity wears off over decades, individuals vaccinated in childhood retain partial immunity and, if infected, develop only a limited form of the illness. This man has "regional tetanus" causing stimulus-sensitive tetanic contractions.

59. A corporation's chief executive officer develops amyotrophic lateral sclerosis (ALS). His left arm begins to weaken. Then a multinational conglomerate that claims the executive is losing his mental capabilities initiates a hostile takeover bid. Can the stockholders be sure that ALS is causing his cognitive decline and apparently abnormal behavior?
   a. Yes
   b. No

Answer: b. ALS is a motor neuron disease, and the majority of patients do not have cognitive impairment or behavioral abnormality. However, some studies have shown that about 10% of ALS patients develop a frontotemporal type dementia and some mild cognitive impairment in an even larger minority.

60. A psychiatrist has been called to evaluate a 30-year-old woman for agitation and bizarre behavior. She had been admitted to an intensive care unit for exacerbation of myasthenia gravis and treated with high-dose anticholinesterase medications, such as pyridostigmine [Mestinon] and neostigmine. When no substantial improvement occurred, she was given plasmapheresis. The next day she had regained strength, but was confused and agitated. Which is the most likely cause of her mental status change?

a. Anticholinesterase medications
b. Plasmapheresis
c. Cerebral hypoxia
d. CNS depletion of ACh

Answer: c. Mental status abnormalities are a relatively common neurologic problem in severe, poorly controlled myasthenia gravis, Guillain–Barré syndrome, and other neuromuscular diseases – even though they do not directly involve the CNS. Mental status abnormalities in myasthenia gravis are not directly attributable to the illness, routine anticholinesterase medications, or plasmapheresis. Instead, generalized weakness, extreme fatigue, or respiratory insufficiency can cause cerebral hypoxia, and high-dose steroids can produce psychotic behavior and thought disorder. In addition, being hospitalized in an intensive care unit with a life-threatening illness creates a psychologically stressful situation that, superimposed on medical illnesses and sleep deprivation, can precipitate hallucinations, delusions, and mental and physical agitation.

61. The family of a 45-year-old man, who had a history of depressive illness, brings him and his girlfriend to the emergency room. Both are comatose and apneic. Their pupils are mid-sized and reactive. Extraocular movements are normal. The head CT, illicit drug screening, blood glucose, and other blood tests are all normal except for an anion gap that proves to be due to a markedly elevated lactic acid concentration. Of the following, which is the most likely intoxicant?

a. Botulinum
b. Heroin
c. Cyanide
d. Barbiturates

Answer: c. All of these intoxicants are potential suicide and murder instruments that depress respiration, but only cyanide causes pronounced lactic acidosis. Because cyanide destroys mitochondrial respiratory enzymes, it leads to pronounced lactic acidosis reflected in an anion gap. Botulinum causes dilated pupils and ophthalmoplegia. A heroin or barbiturate overdose causes miosis and, in the case of heroin, pulmonary edema.

62. An impressionable health and wellness faddist presents for evaluation for weakness. For several weeks he has been giving himself high colonic enemas two or three times a day. Which will be the most pronounced disturbance in his electrolyte determination?

a. Hyponatremia
b. Hypernatremia
c. Hypokalemia
d. Hyperkalemia

Answer: c. The loss of colonic fluid, which is relatively high in potassium, leads to hypokalemia that can be so pronounced that it causes hypokalemic myopathy.

Steroids and thiazide diuretics, as well as laxative abuse, also cause weakness from hypokalemia.

63. Why does tetanus cause uninhibited muscle contractions?

a. It impairs the presynaptic release of ACh.
b. It impairs the presynaptic release of GABA and glycine.
c. It blocks the reuptake of the excitatory neurotransmitter glutamate.
d. It competes with GABA and glycine at their postsynaptic receptors.

Answer: b. Tetanus results from the toxin impairing the presynaptic release of the inhibitory neurotransmitters, GABA and glycine.

64. Which of the following is deactivated more by extracellular metabolism than reuptake?

a. Dopamine
b. Serotonin
c. Acetylcholine

Answer: c.

65. A 35-year-old woman, who has had myasthenia for 15 years, has been stable on pyridostigmine (Mestinon) 120 mg four times daily. After a psychologically stressful situation developed, she began to have cramping abdominal pains, diarrhea, rhinorrhea, and excessive pulmonary secretions. Her face, jaw, and neck muscles weakened. Then her limb muscles weakened. Which of the following is most likely to have developed?

a. Psychogenic fatigue
b. Cholinergic toxicity
c. Relapse of her myasthenia
d. Nerve gas poisoning
e. Acute dystonic reaction

Answer: b. Pyridostigmine, which enhances ACh activity at the neuromuscular junction by inactivating cholinesterase, has led to a medication-induced cholinergic crisis. Its symptoms mimic those of an organophosphate nerve poison. Reducing the pyridostigmine dose will probably reverse the symptoms.

66. Which of the following treatments is not associated with the development of the NMS?

a. Metoclopramide
b. Levodopa withdrawal
c. Haloperidol
d. Risperidone
e. None of the above

Answer: e. This syndrome is generally attributable to sudden deprivation of dopamine activity. Almost all cases are caused by dopamine receptor-blocking antipsychotic medications. However, occasionally nonpsychiatric dopamine receptor-blocking agents, such as metoclopramide, cause it. Similarly, sudden withdrawal of dopaminergic precursor therapy, such as abruptly stopping levodopa treatment in Parkinson disease patients, may cause the syndrome.

67. Which are characteristics of myotonic dystrophy but not of Duchenne dystrophy?
    a. Muscle weakness
    b. Cataracts
    c. Baldness
    d. Myotonia
    e. Infertility
    f. Autosomal inheritance
    g. Cognitive dysfunction
    h. Distal muscle weakness
    i. Pseudohypertrophy

Answer: b–f, h. Weakness and cognitive dysfunction are typical of both. Calf pseudohypertrophy is present in Duchenne muscular dystrophy, but not in myotonic dystrophy.

68. Which conditions are associated with episodic quadriparesis in teenage boys?
    a. Low potassium
    b. REM activity
    c. Hypnopompic hallucinations
    d. Hypnagogic hallucinations
    e. Hyponatremia
    f. 3-Hz spike-and-wave EEG discharges

Answer: a–d. Hypokalemic periodic paralysis and narcolepsy-cataplexy syndrome cause episodic quadriparesis. Hypokalemia causes episodes lasting many hours to days rather than a few minutes. Hyponatremia, when severe, causes stupor and seizures but not quadriparesis. 3-Hz spike-and-wave EEG discharges are associated with absence or petit mal seizures, which do not cause episodic quadriparesis.

69. Which statement concerning mitochondria is *false*?
    a. They produce energy mostly in the form of adenosine triphosphate (ATP).
    b. Their DNA is inherited exclusively from the mother.
    c. Their DNA is in a circular pattern.
    d. They generate but remove toxic free radicals.
    e. Compared to the massive energy consumption of the heart and voluntary muscles, the brain's consumption is low.

Answer: e. The brain has the body's greatest energy consumption. The heart and voluntary muscles have the next greatest energy consumption.

70. Which one of the following is not a characteristic of MERRF?
    a. Ragged red fibers in muscle biopsy
    b. Lactic acidosis
    c. Greatly increased numbers of mitochondria in muscle
    d. Uneven staining for cytochrome oxidase enzyme in muscle cells
    e. Absence of dystrophin
    f. Reduced ATP in muscle cells

Answer: e. Absence of dystrophin characterizes Duchenne muscular dystrophy. The other abnormalities characterize MERRF and, to a certain extent, other mitochondrial myopathies. Uneven staining for respiratory enzymes reflects the threshold effect and heteroplasmy of mtDNA.

71. Which of the following statements regarding dystrophin is *false*?
    a. Dystrophin is located in the muscle surface membrane.
    b. Dystrophin is absent in muscles affected in Duchenne dystrophy.
    c. Dystrophin is absent in myotonic dystrophy.
    d. Dystrophin absence in voluntary muscle is a marker of Duchenne dystrophy.
    e. Dystrophin is present but abnormal in Becker dystrophy, which results from a different mutation of the same gene as Duchenne dystrophy.

Answer: c. Absence of dystrophin in voluntary muscle characterizes Duchenne dystrophy.

72. In regard to the genetics of myotonic dystrophy, which are *three* consequences of its particularly unstable gene?
    a. Males are more likely than females to inherit the illness.
    b. Mitochondrial DNA might be affected.
    c. In successive generations the disease becomes apparent at an earlier age, i.e., offspring often show anticipation.
    d. In successive generations, the disease is progressively more severe.
    e. When the illness is transmitted by the father rather than the mother, its symptoms are more pronounced.

Answer: c, d, e. The excessive trinucleotide repeat's instability leads to the illness becoming apparent at an earlier age with more severe symptoms in successive generations, i.e., anticipation. In addition, as in other conditions that result from excessive trinucleotide repeats, when the illness is inherited from the father, its symptoms are more severe because the DNA in sperm is less stable than the DNA in eggs.

73. Which statement concerning mitochondrial abnormalities is *false*?
    a. Abnormalities affect the brain, muscles, and retinae in various combinations.
    b. Abnormalities typically produce combinations of myopathy, lactic acidosis, and epilepsy.
    c. Ragged red fibers characterize mitochondrial myopathies.
    d. Mitochondrial encephalopathies can cause mental retardation or dementia.
    e. Specific neuropsychologic deficits characterize the dementia induced by mitochondrial encephalopathies.

Answer: e. Although dementia may be superimposed on mental retardation, it is often severe and accompanied by numerous physical deficits but nonspecific in its characteristics.

74. Which of the following may be the result of body-builders' taking steroids?
    a. Muscle atrophy
    b. Muscle development
    c. Mood change
    d. Euphoria
    e. Depression
    f. Acne
    g. Compression fractures in the spine
    h. Oral and vaginal infections

Answer: a–h. If taken in excess, steroids produce myopathy, mental changes, susceptibility infections, and a Cushing disease appearance.

75–79. Match the etiology (75–79) with the illness (a–e):

75. Steroid abuse
76. HIV infection
77. Tryptophan-containing products
78. Alcohol
79. Trichinella
    a. Trichinosis
    b. Eosinophilia-myalgia syndrome
    c. AIDS-associated myopathy
    d. Osteoporosis
    e. Cardiac myopathy

Answers: 75–d, 76–c, 77–b, 78–e, 79–a.

80. Which of the following is *true* about myotonic dystrophy Type 2?
    a. It presents with distal limb weakness.
    b. The genetic abnormality consists of increased quad-nucleotide repeats.
    c. The genetic abnormality consists of increased tri-nucleotide repeats.
    d. Patients are more severely affected than myotonic dystrophy Type 1.

Answer: b. Myotonic dystrophy Type 2 (also known as proximal myotonic myopathy, or PROMM) is character-ized by proximal muscle weakness. The genetic abnormal-ity causing this disease is an abnormal number of repeats of the same four nucleotides (CCTG). Unlike myotonic dystrophy Type 1, which is caused by an abnormal number of trinucleotide repeats (CTG), there is no genetic antici-pation from generation to generation and patients have fewer cognitive deficits and cardiac conduction problems.

81. An 80-year-old shoe salesman has had Parkinson disease for 12 years. For the past several years he has become progressively incapacitated and bed-ridden. His medication regimen consists only of levodopa-carbidopa and antihypertensive medications. About 1 week before the visit, he began to have weakness and lack of appetite. His neurologist, diagnosing progression of his Parkinson disease, added a low dose of selegiline to the regimen. Over the next several days, he became confused and febrile. His rigidity increased. Which is the most likely cause of his immediate deterioration?
    a. Pneumonia
    b. NMS
    c. Serotonin syndrome
    d. Depression

Answer: a. In advanced Parkinson disease, the most likely cause of physical deterioration, confusion, and fever is pneumonia. In this circumstance, it is often fatal. Depression is also common. Although depression may cause anorexia and increased immobility in advanced Par-kinson disease, it does not cause fever or rigidity. The initial symptoms of his deterioration and medication regimen would not suggest NMS. Finally, toxic accumu-lations of serotonin would be unexpected because sero-tonin is metabolized by MAO-A and selegiline is an inhibitor of MAO-B. On the other hand, simultaneously administering a selective serotonin reuptake inhibitor (SSRI) and selegiline might, at least theoretically, lead to the serotonin syndrome.

82. A 25-year-old woman under the care of a psycho-therapist for mild depression reported that she has recently developed weakness and fatigue but not sleepiness or change in mood. She mentioned that while she had begun to drink "gallons" of water and various beverages, she felt that she was urinating even more fluid than she was drinking. She denied bulimia and purging. She has lost 10 lbs. With the weakness being her primary symptoms, which would be the next test?
    a. Serum electrolytes and glucose
    b. MRI of the brain
    c. Serum prolactin level
    d. Prescription of antidepressants

Answer: a. In view of polyuria, polydipsia, and weight loss, the most likely diagnosis is diabetes mellitus. An elevated serum prolactin level and certain abnormali-ties on the MRI may indicate some pituitary tumors; however, the clinician should first investigate the diagno-sis of diabetes because it is more common and more likely to be immediately life-threatening. Moreover, the poly-uria and polydipsia are more indicative of diabetes than pituitary insufficiency and are harbingers of diabetic ketoacidosis.

MAJOR NEUROLOGIC SYMPTOMS

INTRODUCTION

The second section of this book focuses on neurologic conditions that are common, illustrate neurologic principles, or indicate serious illnesses. It stresses ones that cause cognitive impairment with comorbid psychiatric disturbances. In addition, it discusses several specifically because, possibly contrary to expectations, they do not cause cognitive impairment or psychiatric symptoms.

Each chapter reviews these conditions' essential neurologic symptoms and signs, psychiatric comorbidity, appropriate laboratory tests, differential diagnoses, and treatment options. When pertinent, the chapters compare these features to definitions in the *Diagnostic and Statistical Manual of Mental Disorder*, 5th edition (DSM-5). Psychiatrists familiar with this material will be able to perform reliable and effective evaluations that will help their patients and colleagues.

At the same time, this section intentionally does not offer an encyclopedic review. It presents high-yield discussions of material relevant to practicing psychiatry and preparing for standard tests. For textbooks containing detailed information, particularly about the underlying basic science, please see "Notes About References" (in the Preface).

Questions and answers at the ends of chapters recapitulate the important elements of the discussions. A section on questions and answers at the end of the book compares conditions contained in different chapters. In keeping with the current problem-based method of teaching medicine, this question and answer approach allows readers to deduce neurologic principles from individual cases and gain some indirect clinical experience.

For reference, Appendix 1 lists self-help groups for each illness; Appendix 2, the costs of diagnostic tests, which can be considerable; Appendix 3, the genetics – chromosomal and mitochondrial – of inherited illnesses; and Appendix 4, chemical and biological neurotoxins. Readers should heed the warnings, reservations, and precautions described in "Physician-Readers, Please Note" (in the Preface).

DEMENTIA

Physicians have long used the term *dementia* to refer to a progressive decline in cognitive function that impairs daily activities. Criteria for this diagnosis include memory impairment plus one or more of the following: aphasia, apraxia, agnosia, or disturbance in executive function (see Chapter 8). Because this definition requires deficits in two domains, it excludes both isolated *amnesia* (Greek, forgetfulness) and *aphasia* (Greek, speechlessness).

The authors of the *Diagnostic and Statistical Manual of Mental Disorders, 5th Edition* (DSM-5) have largely eschewed the term *dementia* (which literally means "without a mind") and in its stead introduced the concept of Neurocognitive Disorder (NCD), with subtypes *mild* and *major*. The criteria for both mild and major neurocognitive disorders require impairments that represent a decline from a previous level of performance in one or more cognitive domains. (An exception is Major NCD due to Alzheimer disease, which requires decline in memory and learning, and at least one other cognitive domain.) This decline must be of "significant" magnitude for Major NCD and of "modest" magnitude for Mild NCD. Mild neurocognitive disorder by definition must not interfere with independence, but major neurocognitive disorder is sufficiently severe to interfere with independence. Neither occurs exclusively in the context of delirium nor is attributable to another mental disorder, such as major depressive disorder.

Before the etiology is known, psychiatrists may simply apply the label of Major or Mild NCD. However, when the underlying diagnosis is clear, they may associate the Neurocognitive Disorder with a specific etiology, e.g., *Neurocognitive Disorder Due to Alzheimer's Disease*. The DSM-5 recognizes 10 specific etiologies that can underlie NCD, as well as NCD due to another medical condition, NCD due to multiple etiologies, and unspecified NCD (Box 7.1).

In this book we shall continue to use the traditional term *dementia* as it captures a useful and well-defined neuropsychiatric clinical entity and denotes a concept well entrenched in the neurologic and general medical communities. When discussing specific diagnoses, we shall note the DSM-5 nomenclature alongside the traditional neurologic terminology.

DISORDERS RELATED TO DEMENTIA

Congenital Cognitive Impairment

Physicians and the public – but not the federal government – loosely refer to *stable* cognitive impairment since infancy or childhood as "mental retardation" or "developmental delay." The DSM-5 equivalent is Intellectual Developmental Disorder. Its diagnosis requires significant impairment in adaptive function and onset during the "developmental period."

Physical manifestations of congenital cerebral injury, such as seizures and hemiparesis ("cerebral palsy," see Chapter 13), frequently accompany intellectual developmental disorder. In cases of genetic abnormalities, distinctive behavioral disturbances and anomalies of non-neurologic organs – the face, skin, ocular lenses, kidneys, and skeleton – often combine in patterned ways to constitute syndromes.

Whatever the basic condition, children with intellectual developmental disorder may develop dementia later in life. A commonly cited example is the almost universal tendency for individuals with trisomy 21 (Down syndrome) to develop an Alzheimer disease-like dementia by their fifth or sixth decades (see later).

Amnesia

Memory loss with otherwise preserved intellectual function constitutes *amnesia*. Individuals with *retrograde amnesia* typically cannot recall previously presented information, while those with *anterograde amnesia* do not retain newly presented information; patients with both deficits suffer from *global amnesia*. Although amnesia may occur as an isolated deficit, it appears more often as one of two or more components of dementia. In fact, amnesia is a requirement for the diagnosis of dementia.

Various neuropsychologic and physical abnormalities usually accompany amnesia resulting from neurologic conditions. For example, behavioral disturbances, depression, and headache are comorbid with posttraumatic amnesia. With severe traumatic brain injury (TBI, see Chapter 22), hemiparesis, ataxia, pseudobulbar palsy, or epilepsy often accompany posttraumatic amnesia. Similarly, in addition to its characteristic anterograde amnesia, the Wernicke–Korsakoff syndrome comprises ataxia and eye movement abnormalities

In another example, herpes simplex encephalitis causes amnesia accompanied by personality changes, complex partial seizures, and the Klüver–Bucy syndrome (see Chapters 12 and 16) because the virus typically enters the undersurface of the brain through the nasopharynx and preferentially attacks the temporal lobes. This condition occurs relatively frequently because herpes simplex is the most common cause of sporadically occurring (nonepidemic) viral encephalitis. (*Human immunodeficiency virus* [*HIV*] *encephalitis*, which does not cause this scenario, is epidemic.)

Conversely, apparent memory impairment may also appear as an aspect of several psychiatric disorders (see later, Dissociative Amnesia). In general, individuals with amnesia from psychiatric illness or malingering (non-neurologic amnesia) lose memory for personal identity or

BOX 7.1	Etiologies of Mild and Major Neurocognitive Disorders as Specified in the DSM-5

- Alzheimer disease
- Frontotemporal lobar degeneration
- HIV infection
- Huntington disease
- Lewy bodies disease
- Parkinson disease
- Prion disease
- Substance/medication use
- Traumatic brain injury
- Vascular disease
- Another medical condition
- Multiple etiologies
- Unspecified

BOX 7.2	Commonly Cited Causes of Transient Amnesia

Alcohol abuse
   Wernicke–Korsakoff syndrome
   Alcoholic blackouts
Electroconvulsive therapy (ECT)
Head trauma
Medications
   Gamma hydroxybutyrate (GHB)*
   Zolpidem (Ambien),
   Scopolamine, other anticholinergic medications
   Benzodiazepines
   Sildenafil (Viagra), tadalafil (Cialis)?
   Pramipexole (Mirapex)?
   Statins?
Complex partial seizures (see Chapter 10)
Transient global amnesia

*When used illicitly, people call GHB the "date-rape drug." Under carefully controlled conditions, neurologists prescribe GHB as oxybate (Xyrem) to treat cataplexy (see Chapter 17).

emotionally laden events rather than recently acquired information. For example, a criminal deeply in debt may travel to another city and "forget" his debts, wife, and past associates, but he would retain his ability to recall people, events, and day-to-day transactions in his new life. Nonneurologic amnesia also characteristically produces inconsistent results on formal memory testing. Also, amytal infusions may temporarily restore memories in individuals with nonneurologic amnesia, but not in those with brain damage.

Transient amnesia that occurs suddenly and lasts several minutes to several hours has several potential medical and neurologic explanations (Box 7.2). One of them, electroconvulsive therapy (ECT), routinely induces both anterograde and retrograde amnesia; the retrograde amnesia, especially for autobiographical information, tends to persist longer than the anterograde amnesia. ECT-induced amnesia is more likely to occur or to be more pronounced following treatment with high electrical dosage, with bilateral rather than unilateral electrode placement, with use of alternating current, and with greater frequency of administration (e.g., three times weekly rather than two times weekly). Without a pretreatment assessment of a patient's memory and other aspects of cognitive function, clinicians may have problems separating ECT-induced amnesia from memory difficulties reflecting underlying depression, medication effects, and, especially in the elderly, pre-existing cognitive impairment.

Transient Global Amnesia

One of the most dramatic disorders that neurologists and psychiatrists encounter is *transient global amnesia* (*TGA*) because it causes acute onset of anterograde amnesia. The etiology of TGA is not well understood. Some neurologists conceive of TGA as a TIA in the posterior cerebral arteries, affecting blood flow to the medial temporal lobes (Fig. 11.2) and thereby disrupting the hippocampi (see Fig. 16.5). Other theories view TGA as a form of migraine, a type of seizure, or the result of impaired outflow of blood in the venous system of the brain. It is likely that different mechanisms lead to TGA in different patients.

TGA typically occurs in middle-aged and older individuals who may have cerebrovascular disease. These attacks typically develop in the midst of frightening events or physical exertion, particularly sexual activity – a coincidence that might lead physicians to misinterpret them as a psychiatric phenomenon.

The fundamental clinical feature of TGA is the acute onset of amnesia. During an attack, patients cannot memorize or learn new information, i.e., they have anterograde amnesia. They also cannot recall information acquired very recently, such as the events of the last several hours or days, i.e., they also have retrograde amnesia. Usually the anterograde amnesia is more profound, has a greater duration, causes the greater disability and creates more distress than the retrograde amnesia. As examples of their anterograde amnesia, patients typically do not know how they came to the physician's office or the emergency room. Once there, they lose track of their conversations, and an examining physician may require reintroduction several times during the visit.

In the midst of TGA, individuals may perform rote but relatively complex activities competently, such as driving a well-known route or preparing dinner. However, unable to comprehend their situation, some individuals become distraught, agitated, or panicked. Some, as if recoiling, appear apathetic and immobile. Most, however, seem calm but bewildered.

In contrast to their amnesia for new facts, TGA patients characteristically retain their general knowledge and fundamental personal information. For example, they remain able to recite their name, address, telephone number, and occupation. (All this preserved memory contradicts the adjective *global* in TGA.)

TGA lasts for 3 to 24 hours, but is most severe during the initial 1 to 2 hours. By definition, the total duration must not exceed 24 hours. The recurrence rate is approximately 10% and TGA does not represent a risk factor for stroke.

Even in the absence of a confirmatory laboratory test for TGA, its clinical features differentiate it from other neurologic conditions. TGA patients' preserved intellect and general knowledge, as well as their remaining fully conscious, distinguish them from patients in delirium. TGA patients, despite their amnesia, also do not confabulate in the manner of Wernicke–Korsakoff patients. Unlike TGA, focal seizures with alteration in awareness are associated with dulling of the sensorium, simple repetitive actions, paroxysmal or other epileptiform EEG changes, and a high rate of recurrence (see Chapter 10).

Physicians using the DSM-5 might be tempted to diagnose a patient with no recall of recent events as having Dissociative Amnesia, which it defines primarily as "inability to recall important autobiographical information, usually of a traumatic or stressful nature" and requires that, presumably over time, patients experience "significant distress or impairment in social, occupational, or other important areas of functioning." That definition would exclude TGA patients because they retain fundamental personal information. The DSM-5 also notes a subtype of Dissociative Amnesia, termed Dissociative Fugue (previously, Psychogenic Fugue) in which individuals purposefully travel or show "bewildered wandering." Presumably, after establishing a new location, these individuals function there without recalling their previous life's crucial aspects, such as a spouse, debts, or crimes. In other words, unlike TGA patients, these patients' anterograde memory remains normal, but their retrograde amnesia persists, and the disorder lasts for months, years, or possibly indefinitely.

Neuropsychologic Conditions

Confabulation is a neuropsychologic condition in which patients offer explanations in a sincere and forthcoming manner despite being unaware of the truth. Confabulating patients do not intend to deceive. Confabulation is a well-known aspect of Wernicke–Korsakoff syndrome, Anton syndrome (see Cortical Blindness, Chapter 12), and anosognosia (see Chapter 8). As these conditions are referable to entirely different regions of the brain, confabulation lacks consistent anatomic correlations and associated physical features.

Discrete neuropsychologic disorders – aphasia, anosognosia, and apraxia – may occur alone, in various combinations, or as comorbidities of dementia (see Chapter 8). If one or more of these occurs together with dementia, the implication is that the dementia originates in "cortical" rather than "subcortical" dysfunction (see later). These disorders, unlike dementia, are attributable to discrete cerebral lesions. When mild, sometimes formal neuropsychologic testing is needed to detect these disorders and tease them apart from dementia.

NORMAL AGING

Beginning at about age 50 years, people are subject to a variety of natural, age-related changes. Many neurologic functions resist age-related changes, but some are especially vulnerable. Those that decline do so at different rates and with unpredictable trajectories.

Memory and Other Neuropsychologic Functions

Compared to young adults, older well-functioning adults have impaired recall of newly learned lists, but given enough time, they are able to retrieve the new material. Other age-related losses include shortened attention span, slowed learning, and decreased ability to perform complex tasks.

On the other hand, several cognitive processes normally withstand aging. For example, older people have little or no loss of vocabulary, language ability, reading comprehension, or fund of knowledge. Well-spoken, well-read, and knowledgeable individuals remain so. In addition, as measured by the *Wechsler Adult Intelligence Scale – Revised* (*WAIS-R*), older adults' general intelligence declines only slightly.

Sleep

In the elderly, sleep becomes fragmented, the absolute and relative amount of slow-wave sleep both decline, and times of falling asleep and awakening both phase advance (move earlier). In addition, restless legs syndrome and REM sleep behavior disorder commonly disrupt their sleep (see Chapter 17). All these changes may occur with or without dementia.

Motor and Gait

As most older people recognize, loss of muscle mass and strength accompanies aging. They tend to lose vibration sensation in their legs and deep tendon reflexes (DTRs) in their ankles become diminished. They also have impaired postural reflexes and loss of balance. A standard, simple test will show that most cannot stand on one foot with eyes closed.

When combined with age-related skeletal changes, these motor and sensory impairments lead to the common walking pattern of older individuals, "senile gait." This pattern is characterized by increased flexion of the trunk and limbs, diminished arm swing, and shorter steps. Slowing of gait and shortening of stride length commonly accompany dementia and often precede cognitive dysfunction.

Age-related neurologic and skeletal changes predispose individuals to falls, which carry significant morbidity and mortality. Additional risk factors for falls include neurologic disorders, prior falls, visual impairment, cognitive impairment, and use of medications, including antihypertensives, sedatives, and antidepressants. Among antidepressants, selective serotonin reuptake inhibitors (SSRIs) confer the same degree of risk as tricyclic antidepressants.

Special Senses

Age-related deterioration of sensory organs impairs hearing and vision (see Chapter 12). Older individuals typically have smaller, less reactive pupils and some retinal degeneration. They require greater light, more contrast, and sharper focusing to be able to read and drive. Their hearing tends to be poorer, especially for speech discrimination. Their senses of taste and smell also deteriorate.

Physicians or other professionals should regularly test vision and hearing in elderly patients because loss of these senses magnifies cognitive and physical impairments. As a practical matter, many elderly individuals insist on driving, which requires full ability in all these skills. Deprivation of the special senses can cause or worsen depression, sleep impairment, and perceptual disturbances, including hallucinations.

EEG and Imaging Changes

As individuals age, the electroencephalogram (EEG) background alpha activity slows to the lower end of the normal 8–12-Hz alpha range. Computed tomography (CT) and magnetic resonance imaging (MRI) often reveal decreased volume of the frontal and parietal lobes, atrophy of the cerebral cortex, expansion of the Sylvian fissure, and concomitantly increased volume of the lateral and third ventricles (see Figs. 20.2, 20.3, and 20.18). In addition, MRI reveals white matter hyperintensities ("white dots"). Although striking, these abnormalities are usually innocuous and, by themselves, do not reflect the onset of dementia.

Macroscopic and Microscopic Changes

With advancing age, brain weight decreases to about 85% of normal. Age-associated histologic changes include granulovacuolar degeneration of neurons and the accumulation of amyloid-containing senile plaques and neurofibrillary tangles. These changes affect the frontal and temporal lobes more than the parietal lobes. In addition, advancing age leads to loss of neurons in many important deeply situated structures, including the locus ceruleus, suprachiasmatic nucleus, substantia nigra, and nucleus basalis of Meynert. In contrast, the mammillary bodies remain unaffected.

DEMENTIA

Classifications and Causes

When neurologists or psychiatrists are confronted with a patient with dementia, one of their primary questions is that of etiology: What is the cause of the patient's dementia? The DSM-5 division of NCDs into 12 etiological subtypes (see Box 7.1) reflects the importance of this question. Some of the clinical features that clinicians find practical and useful in seeking to identify the cause of a patient's dementia are the following:

- *Prevalence*: Studies reporting on the epidemiology of dementia-producing illnesses vary by whether cases are defined clinically or postmortem, drawn from primary or tertiary care settings, or reported by their incidence or prevalence. By any measure, Alzheimer disease is the most prevalent cause of dementia not only because its incidence is so high, but also because its victims live with it for a

| BOX 7.3 | Causes of Dementia in Adolescents |

Autoimmune or inflammatory diseases
   Paraneoplastic syndromes, including NMDA antibody encephalitis
   Vasculitis
Cerebral and noncerebral neoplasms
   Chemotherapy (intrathecal)
   Radiotherapy treatment
Drug, inhalant, and alcohol abuse, including overdose
Head trauma, including child abuse
Infections
   HIV-associated dementia
   Variant Creutzfeldt–Jakob disease (vCJD)
   Subacute sclerosing panencephalitis (SSPE)
Metabolic abnormalities
   Adrenoleukodystrophy
   Wilson disease
Neurodegenerative illnesses
   Huntington disease
   Metachromatic leukodystrophy
   Other rare, usually genetically transmitted, illnesses

relatively long time. A typical breakdown of the prevalence of dementia-producing illnesses would list Alzheimer disease 70%, dementia with Lewy bodies (DLB) 15%, vascular cognitive impairment (VCI – or, in DSM-5 terminology, Vascular Neurocognitive Disorder) 10%, frontotemporal dementia 5%–10%, and all others, in total, 5%–10%.

- *Patient's age at the onset of dementia*: Similarly, beginning at age 65 years, those same illnesses cause almost all cases of dementia. However, individuals between 21 to 65 years are more likely to suffer from different dementia-producing illnesses: HIV, substance abuse, severe TBI, end-stage multiple sclerosis (MS) (see Chapter 15), frontotemporal dementia, and VCI. In adolescence, the causes are different and even more numerous (Box 7.3).

- *Accompanying physical manifestations*: Distinctive physical neurologic abnormalities that may accompany dementia and allow for a diagnosis by inspection. They include ocular motility impairments, gait apraxia (see later), myoclonus (see later and Chapter 18), peripheral neuropathy (see Box 5.1), chorea, other involuntary movement disorders (see Box 18.4), and lateralized signs such as hemiparesis.

- *Genetics*: Of frequently occurring illnesses, Huntington disease, frontotemporal dementia, some prion illnesses, and, in a minority of families, Alzheimer disease follow an autosomal dominant pattern. Wilson disease follows an autosomal recessive pattern.

- *Rapidity of onset*: In patients with Alzheimer disease, dementia evolves over a period of many years to a decade. In contrast, several diseases produce dementia within 6 to 12 months of onset. These "rapidly progressive dementias" include HIV-associated dementia, frontotemporal dementia, dementia with Lewy bodies, paraneoplastic limbic encephalitis (Chapter 19), other autoimmune encephalopathies, and, perhaps most notoriously, Creutzfeldt–Jakob disease.

- *Reversibility*: The most common conditions that neurologists usually list as "reversible causes of dementia" are depression, over-medication, hypothyroidism, vitamin B_{12} deficiency, other metabolic abnormalities, subdural hematomas, normal-pressure hydrocephalus, and frequent focal seizures with dyscognition. Although reversible dementias are rightfully sought, the results of this approach are discouraging. Only about 9% of dementia cases are potentially reversible and physicians actually partially or fully reverse less than 1%.
- *Cortical and subcortical dementias*: According to this classic distinction, cortical dementias consist of illnesses in which neuropsychologic signs of cortical dysfunction – typically aphasia, agnosia, and apraxia – accompany dementia. Because the brain's subcortical areas are relatively untouched, patients remain alert, attentive, and ambulatory. Alzheimer disease serves as the prime example of a cortical dementia.

In contrast, subcortical dementias are typified by apathy, affective change, and slowed mental processing, which overshadow cognitive impairment. Gait abnormalities constitute the other core feature. Autopsies in subcortical dementia usually show damage in the white matter, basal ganglia, or subcortical structures. Prime examples are Parkinson disease, normal-pressure hydrocephalus, HIV-associated dementia, VCI, and MS.

Although the cortical–subcortical distinction persists, it has slipped into disuse because of several problems. The presence or absence of aphasia, agnosia, and apraxia does not reliably predict the etiology of dementia. In addition, this classification cannot account for the prominent exceptions inherent in several illnesses, including subcortical pathology in Alzheimer disease or the mixed clinical picture in frontotemporal dementia.

Large epidemiologic studies conducted in the United States and in various European countries in recent decades, have found a decrease in the prevalence and incidence of dementia. Researchers attribute this improvement to improved recognition and more prompt and effective treatment of vascular risk factors, such as hypertension, diabetes, hypercholesterolemia, and tobacco use.

Mental Status Testing

Screening Tests

Several screening tests are widely used, standardized, and have foreign language versions. However, they also carry several inherent warnings. Unless these tests are carefully considered, they tend to overestimate cognitive impairment in the elderly, individuals with minimal education (8 years or less of school), and ethnic minorities. In addition, they may fail to detect cognitive impairment in a highly educated person. Screening tests are not specific for etiology and cannot distinguish between dementia produced by Alzheimer disease, dementia from other illnesses, or depression-induced cognitive dysfunction.

Mini-Mental State Examination (Fig. 7.1). Physicians so regularly administer the Mini-Mental State Examination (MMSE) that it has risen to the level of the standard screening test. Its results are reproducible and correlate with histologic changes in Alzheimer disease. In addition to detecting cognitive impairment, the MMSE has predictive value. For example, among well-educated individuals with borderline scores, as many as 10% to 25% may develop dementia in the next 2 years. The MMSE can also cast doubt on a diagnosis of Alzheimer disease as the cause of dementia under the certain circumstances: (1) if scores on successive tests remain stable for 2 years, the diagnosis should be reconsidered because Alzheimer disease almost always causes a progressive decline, and (2) if scores decline precipitously, illnesses that cause a rapidly progressive dementia become more likely diagnoses (see later).

Critics attack the MMSE for being "too easy." It permits mild cognitive impairment and even early dementia to escape detection. Age, education, and language skills influence the score. The MMSE may also fail to test adequately for executive function and thereby miss cases of frontotemporal dementia. Also, because the MMSE depends so heavily on language function, it may be inadequate in conditions such as MS and toluene abuse, where the subcortical white matter receives the brunt of the damage.

Alzheimer Disease Assessment Scale. The Alzheimer Disease Assessment Scale (ADAS) consists of cognitive and noncognitive sections. Its cognitive section (*ADAS-Cog*) (Fig. 7.2) includes not only standard tests of language, comprehension, memory, and orientation, but also tests of visual-spatial ability, such as drawing geometric figures, and physical tasks that reflect ideational praxis, such as folding a paper into an envelope. Patients obtain scores of 0 to 70; higher scores indicate poorer performance.

Compared to the MMSE, the ADAS-Cog is more sensitive, reliable, and less influenced by educational level and language skills. However, it is more complex and subjective. Test-givers need not be physicians but must undergo special training. The testing usually requires 45 to 60 minutes. Alzheimer disease researchers, especially those involved in pharmaceutical trials, routinely use the ADAS-Cog to monitor the course of Alzheimer disease and measure the effect of medication.

Montreal Cognitive Assessment (Fig. 7.3). The Montreal Cognitive Assessment (MoCA), which has greater sensitivity than the MMSE, readily detects mild impairment. It is useful when a patient's only symptom is memory impairment or there is concern for cognitive impairment despite a high score on the MMSE. The MoCA is used widely in patients with neurodegenerative illness – a category that includes Alzheimer disease, Parkinson disease, dementia with Lewy bodies, and frontotemporal dementia. In Parkinson disease, the MoCA is more sensitive than the MMSE in detecting early cognitive impairment (see Chapter 18).

Further Testing

If a screening test yields borderline or otherwise indefinite results, formal neuropsychologic testing may help

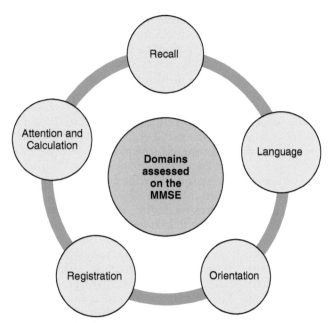

FIGURE 7.1 ■ The Mini-Mental State Examination (MMSE), developed by Folstein et al. (see References), tests five domains of cognition. The examiner assigns points for correct answers, with a maximum score of 30. Scores of 20 points or less indicate dementia, delirium, schizophrenia, or affective disorders – alone or in combination. However, such low scores are not found in normal elderly people or in those with neuroses or personality disorders. MMSE scores fall in proportion to dementia-induced impairments in daily living as well as cognitive decline. For example, scores of 20 correlate with inability to keep appointments or use a telephone. Scores of 15 correlate with inability to dress or groom.

clarify the diagnosis. These tests, which usually require at least 3 hours, assess the major realms of cognitive function, including language (which the examiner should test first to assure the validity of the entire test), memory, calculations, judgment, perception, and construction. Neuropsychologic testing is not required for a diagnosis of dementia and is not part of a standard evaluation, but it can help in several situations:

- For very intelligent, well-educated, or highly functional individuals with symptoms compatible with dementia whose screening tests fail to show a cognitive impairment;
- For individuals whose ability to execute critical occupational or personal decisions, including legal competency, must be assured;
- For assessing individuals with confounding deficits, such as intellectual development disorder, learning disabilities, minimal education, deafness, or aphasia;
- In distinguishing dementia from depression, other psychiatric disturbances, and malingering;
- In distinguishing Alzheimer disease from frontotemporal dementia.

Laboratory Evaluation in Dementia. Depending on the clinical evaluation, neurologists generally request a series of laboratory tests (Box 7.4) in patients with suspected dementia. Although testing is expensive (Appendix 2), it may allow a firm diagnosis or even detect a potentially

---

ALZHEIMER'S DISEASE ASSESSMENT SCALE COGNITIVE ITEMS (ADAS-COG)

1. Spoken language ability ____
2. Comprehension of spoken language ____
3. Recall of test instructions ____
4. Word-finding difficulty ____
5. Following commands ____
6. Naming objects, fingers ____

Naming:	Objects		Fingers		
High:	1	2	3	4	Fingers: Thumb
Medium:	1	2	3	4	Pinky Index
Low:	1	2	3	4	Middle Ring

7. Constructions: drawings ____
   Figures correct: 1   2   3   4
   Closing in: Yes ____ No ____
8. Ideational praxis ____
   Step correct:
   1   2   3   4
9. Orientation ____
   Day ____   Year ____   Person ____   Time of day ____
   Date ____   Month ____   Season ____   Place ____
10. Word recall: mean error score ____
11. Word recognition: mean error score ____
    Cognition total

FIGURE 7.2 ■ The cognitive section of the Alzheimer Disease Assessment Scale (ADAS-Cog), the standard test for assessing pharmacologic intervention, has been designed to measure many important aspects of cognitive function that are liable to deteriorate in Alzheimer disease. The noncognitive section (not shown) measures mood, attention, delusions, and motor activity, such as pacing and tremors. As dementia begins or worsens, patients' responses change from no impairment (where the patient receives 0 points) to severe cognitive impairment (5 points). In other words, as dementia worsens, patients accumulate points. Total ADAS-Cog scores for patients with mild-to-moderate Alzheimer disease range from 15 to 25 and, as cognitive function declines, scores increase by 6 to 12 points yearly. (From Rosen WG, Mohs RC, Davis KL. A new rating scale for Alzheimer's disease. Am J Psychiatry. 1984, 141, 1356-1364. Reprinted with permission from the American Journal of Psychiatry, Copyright 1984. American Psychiatric Association.)

BOX 7.4	**Screening Laboratory Tests for Dementia**

Routine tests
   Chemistry profile: electrolytes, glucose, liver function, renal function
   Complete blood count
Specific blood tests
   B[12] level, with homocysteine and methylmalonic acid levels if equivocal
   Human immunodeficiency virus (HIV) antibodies[+]
   Lyme immunoassay and Western blot[+]
   Syphilis test[*+]
   Thyroid function
   Apolipoprotein E (ApoE)[+]
Physiologic test
   Electroencephalogram (EEG)[+]
Imaging tests
   Computed tomography (CT)
   Magnetic resonance imaging (MRI)

---

*See text for current recommendations regarding role of treponemal and nontreponemal tests in evaluation for possible neurosyphilis.
[+]For individuals in risk groups (see text).

MONTREAL COGNITIVE ASSESSMENT (MOCA)

NAME:
Education:
Sex:

Date of birth:
DATE:

VISUOSPATIAL / EXECUTIVE				Points

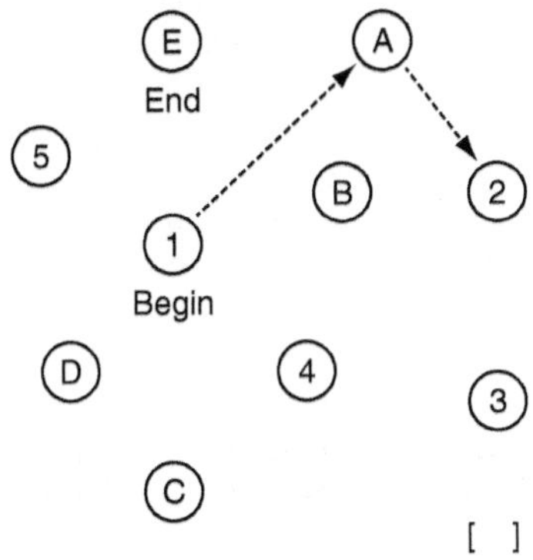

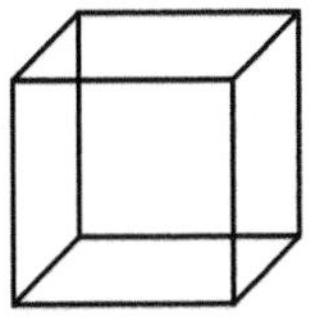

Copy cube

Draw CLOCK (Ten past eleven) (3 points)

E
End

A

5

1
Begin

B

2

D

4

3

C

[ ]

[ ]

[ ] [ ] [ ]
Contour Numbers Hands

__/5

NAMING

[ ] [ ] [ ]

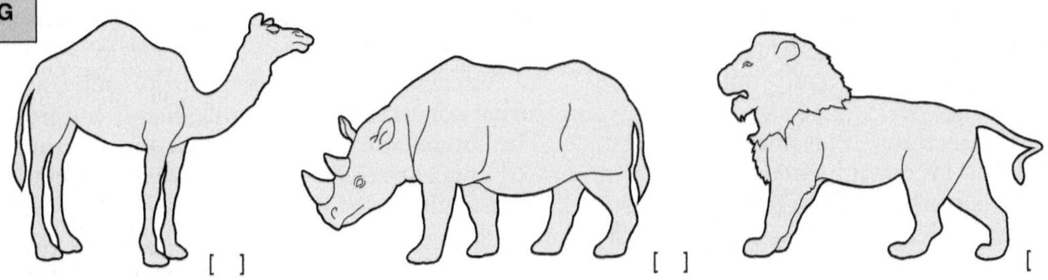

__/3

MEMORY	Read list of words, subject must repeat them. Do 2 trials, even if 1st trial is successful. Do a recall after 5 minutes.		FACE	VELVET	CHURCH	DAISY	RED	No points
		1st trial						
		2nd trial						

ATTENTION	Read list of digits (1 digit/sec.).	Subject has to repeat them in the forward order [ ] 2 1 8 5 4 Subject has to repeat them in the backward order [ ] 7 4 2	__/2

Read list of letters. The subject must tap with his hand at each letter A. No points if 2 errors
[ ] FBACMNAAJKLBAFAKDEAAAJAMOFAAB __/1

Serial 7 subtraction starting at 100   [ ] 93   [ ] 86   [ ] 79   [ ] 72   [ ] 65
4 or 5 correct subtractions: **3 pts**, 2 or 3 correct: **2 pts**, 1 correct: **1 pt**, 0 correct: **0 pt** __/3

LANGUAGE	Repeat: I only know that John is the one to help today. [ ] The cat always hid under the couch when dogs were in the room. [ ]	__/2

Fluency/Name maximum number of words in one minute that begin with the letter F   [ ] ____(N 11 words) __/1

ABSTRACTION	Similarity between e.g. banana - orange = fruit [ ] train - bicycle [ ] watch - ruler	__/2

DELAYED RECALL	Has to recall words WITH NO CUE	FACE [ ]	VELVET [ ]	CHURCH [ ]	DAISY [ ]	RED [ ]	Points for UNCUED recall only	__/5
Optional	Category cue							
	Multiple choice cue							

ORIENTATION	[ ] Date [ ] Month [ ] Year [ ] Day [ ] Place [ ] City	__/6

Normal 26 / 30   **TOTAL**   __/30

Add 1 point if 12 yr edu

Administered by: _____

FIGURE 7.3 ■ The Montreal Cognitive Assessment (MoCA). This assessment includes eight cognitive domains. As with the MMSE, the total score reaches 30 and values lower than 26 indicate cognitive impairment. However, some authors found that a cutoff of 23 yields a sensitivity and specificity of at least 95%. (Copyright Z. Nasreddine M.D. Reproduced with permission. The test and instructions may be accessed at www.mocatest.org.)

correctable cause of dementia. In addition, certain tests may reveal the illness before individuals manifest cognitive impairment, i.e., in their preclinical or presymptomatic state. Neurologists modify the testing protocol based on clinical features – such as dementia in an adolescent (see Box 7.3) or dementia that has progressed rapidly.

Head CT can detect most structural abnormalities associated with dementia, such as hydrocephalus or subdural hematomas. However, MRI is superior because it is better able to diagnose multiple infarctions, white matter diseases, and small lesions.

An EEG is not indicated for routine evaluation of dementia because the common dementia-producing illnesses cause only slowing or other minor, nonspecific abnormalities. Moreover, those EEG abnormalities are often indistinguishable from normal age-related changes. On the other hand, EEG abnormalities can be specific for certain conditions, such as Creutzfeldt–Jakob disease, subacute sclerosing panencephalitis (SSPE), or delirium (see later). Therefore, physicians should consider ordering it in patients who have shown certain clinical features, such as seizures, myoclonus, rapidly progressive dementia, or stupor. An EEG can also contribute to a diagnosis of depression-induced cognitive impairment, in which the EEG will be normal or show only mildly slowed background activity.

Likewise, a lumbar puncture (LP) is not a routine test, but possibly is helpful in certain circumstances. For example, neurologists perform an LP to test the cerebrospinal fluid (CSF) when patients with dementia have indications of infectious illnesses, such as neurosyphilis, SSPE, or Creutzfeldt–Jakob disease. They also perform it to measure the pressure and withdraw CSF in cases of suspected normal-pressure hydrocephalus.

Physicians should reserve other tests for particular indications. For instance, if adolescents or young adults develop dementia, an evaluation might include serum ceruloplasmin determination and slit-lamp examination for Wilson disease; urine toxicology screens for drug abuse; and perhaps urine analysis for metachromatic granules and arylsulfatase A activity to assess for metachromatic leukodystrophy (see Chapter 5). Likewise, physicians should judiciously request serologic tests for autoimmune or inflammatory disease, serum Lyme disease titer determinations, and other tests for systemic illnesses.

ALZHEIMER DISEASE

The DSM-5 defines Mild and Major subtypes of Neurocognitive Disorder Due to Alzheimer Disease. The definition of the Major subtype requires decline in memory and learning and at least one other cognitive domain, while in the Mild subtype only memory and learning need be affected. The DSM-5 recognizes both probable and possible Alzheimer disease as causes of Major and Mild NCD.

Modern concepts of Alzheimer disease in the neurologic literature identify three stages of the disease, which are not analogous to those in the DSM-5:

- Preclinical (presymptomatic)
- Mild cognitive impairment
- Dementia

Preclinical Alzheimer Disease

Neurologists no longer require any cognitive deficit, much less a disabling one, for a diagnosis of Alzheimer disease. They refer to asymptomatic individuals who have certain laboratory evidence as being in the preclinical or presymptomatic stage of the disease. Because Alzheimer disease causes no symptoms at the preclinical stage, patients in this stage do not seek neurological or psychiatric attention, and therefore this stage is more a theoretical construct than a practical clinical condition at this time. In the future, identifying patients in the presymptomatic stage of Alzheimer disease should allow earlier therapeutic intervention compared to the current situation where physicians offer treatment to patients only in later stages of the disease.

Researchers have sought to identify biomarkers that allow for the diagnosis of Alzheimer disease in its asymptomatic as well as its overt state. One approach uses positron emission tomography (PET) scans in conjunction with ligands – including Pittsburgh compound B, florbetapir, and flumetamol – that can localize and quantify an individual's cerebral amyloid burden. Accumulation of amyloid in the cortex, especially in the frontal and parietal lobes and less in the sensory-motor strip, serves as a marker for Alzheimer disease. Another approach consists of measuring concentrations of amyloid and tau protein in CSF. The combination of low amyloid and elevated tau protein CSF concentrations serves as another marker for Alzheimer disease, although neither of these findings is specific for that diagnosis. A recent analysis suggested that a combination of variables from multiple domains – ApoE4 positivity (a genetic variable), scores on the digits symbol substitution test and the paired associates immediate recall test (cognitive variables), level of phosphorylated tau in CSF (a biochemical variable), and right entorhinal cortex thickness and right hippocampal volume on MRI (radiographic variables) – taken together could reliably predict a patient's progression to MCI due to Alzheimer disease.

Mild Cognitive Impairment

Neurologists consider mild cognitive impairment (MCI) as consisting of impairment predominantly in either memory (amnestic) or in nonmemory (nonamnestic) domains, such as executive ability or language function. Unlike individuals with dementia, those with MCI continue to work, socialize, maintain their hobbies, and function independently. Physicians assessing the situation might compare patients' cognitive functions to their peers'.

Individuals with MCI progress to dementia at a rate of 10% yearly, but their unaffected peers develop dementia at a rate of only 1% to 2% yearly. Risk factors for progression of MCI to dementia include the severity of cognitive impairment (particularly memory impairment) at the time of diagnosis and the standard risk factors for Alzheimer disease (see later). Cholinesterase inhibitors do not slow the deterioration of MCI to dementia.

Although the major implication of a diagnosis of MCI is that many cases progress to dementia, the cognitive impairment reverts to normal in as many as 30%. Researchers attribute this group's improvement to treatment of psychiatric illnesses or reversible toxic-metabolic disturbances.

Dementia

Alzheimer disease eventually produces dementia, but at different rates and in uneven trajectories for different patients. *Cognitive reserve* potentially explains some of the differences. In this explanation, education, occupation, and leisure-time activities protect the brain. Well-educated individuals, for example, continue to maintain an intellectual perspective and employ alternate psychologic strategies that allow them to compensate for decline in certain domains.

In the dementia stage, patients may remain superficially conversant, sociable, able to perform routine tasks, and physically intact. Nevertheless, a spouse or caregiver will report that they suffer from incapacitating memory impairment and inability to cope with new situations. Patients' language changes typically include a decrease in spontaneous verbal output, an inability to find words (*anomia*), use of incorrect words (*paraphasic errors*), and a tendency for circumlocution to avoid forgotten words (see Chapter 8).

Several other symptoms stem from deterioration in visual-spatial abilities. This impairment explains why patients lose their way in familiar surroundings. It also explains *constructional apraxia*, the inability to translate an idea into use of a physical object or to integrate visual and motor functions.

Neuropsychiatric Manifestations

The majority of Alzheimer disease patients with dementia demonstrate apathy or agitation. In addition, many demonstrate dysphoria and abnormal behavior. Delusions, which emerge in about 20% to 40% of patients, are usually relatively simple, but often incorporate paranoid ideation.

Occurring about half as frequently as delusions, hallucinations are usually visual, but sometimes auditory or even olfactory. Whatever their form, hallucinations portend behavioral disturbances, rapidly progressive dementia, an unequivocally abnormal EEG, and a poor prognosis. However, their presence carries several important clinical caveats. An underlying toxic-metabolic disturbance, such as pneumonia or urinary tract infection, rather than progression of dementia, is often the cause of hallucinations. In another caveat, the presence of visual hallucinations early in the course of dementia, particularly if the patient has a parkinson-like gait, suggests a different diagnosis – namely, DLB (see later).

Disruptive behavior – wandering, verbal outbursts, physical agitation, and restlessness – occurs in almost 50% of Alzheimer disease patients and increases in frequency as cognition and function deteriorate. It prompts institutionalization and the problematic use of antipsychotics. Despite its dangerous aspects and association with deterioration, disruptive behavior does not increase the mortality rate.

Wandering constitutes a particularly troublesome, although not unique, manifestation of Alzheimer disease. It may originate in any combination of numerous disturbances, including memory impairment, visual-spatial perceptual difficulties, delusions and hallucinations, akathisia (see Chapter 18), and mundane activities such as looking for food.

Alzheimer patients also lose their normal circadian sleep–wake pattern to a greater degree than cognitively intact elderly people (see Chapter 17). Their sleep becomes fragmented throughout the day and night. The disruption of their sleep parallels the severity of their dementia.

Alzheimer patients' motor vehicle crashes rate is greater than comparably aged individuals, and it increases with the duration of their illness. Clues to unsafe driving include missing exits, under- or over-turning, inability to parallel park, and delayed braking. Accidents are more apt to occur on local streets than on the highway. (Still, 16- to 24-year-old men have a higher rate of motor vehicle crashes than Alzheimer patients!) Several states require that physicians report patients with medical impairments that interfere with safe driving, presumably including Alzheimer disease.

Physical Signs

Patients with Alzheimer disease characteristically have no physical impairment except for one small but intriguing finding – anosmia (see Chapter 4). Even before the onset of dementia, Alzheimer disease patients require high concentrations of a volatile substance to detect and identify it by smell. Neurologists also find anosmia in patients with Parkinson disease and dementia with Lewy bodies, but not in those with VCI or depression. Patients with TBI with or without dementia also have anosmia because the trauma results in shearing of the olfactory nerve fibers traversing the cribriform plate (see Chapter 22).

Until Alzheimer disease advances to unequivocal dementia, patients usually remain ambulatory and able to feed themselves. The image of an Alzheimer disease patient walking steadily but aimlessly through a neighborhood characterizes the disparity between intellectual and motor deficits. When patients reach advanced stages of the illness, physicians can elicit frontal release signs (Fig. 7.4) and perhaps a jaw jerk reflex (see Fig. 4.13) and/or Babinski signs. Unlike patients with VCI, those with Alzheimer disease do not have lateralized signs. They eventually become mute, fail to respond to verbal requests, remain confined to bed, and frequently slip into a persistent vegetative state (see Chapter 11).

Laboratory Tests

When neurologists suspect Alzheimer disease, they order testing primarily to exclude other causes. The earliest change in the EEG is usually slowing of background activity; however, this change is not universal and overlaps with the expected age-related slowing. In advanced disease, the EEG usually shows disorganized and slow background activity, which is diagnostically helpful but still nonspecific.

CT shows cerebral atrophy and a widened third ventricle, which is also suggestive but nonspecific. MRI shows sequential, progressive atrophy: first the hippocampus, then the temporal and parietal lobes, and eventually the frontal lobes. As with CT, MRI shows widening of the third ventricle as well as cerebral atrophy. Although CT and MRI are both useful and in practice at

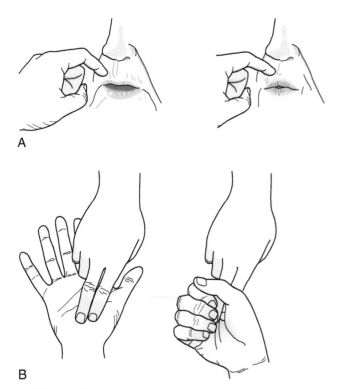

FIGURE 7.4 ■ The snout and grasp reflexes – frontal lobe release reflexes – are frequently present in individuals with severe dementia. *A,* Physicians elicit the snout reflex by tapping the patient's upper lip with a finger or a percussion hammer. This reflex causes the patient's lips to purse and lower facial muscles to pout. *B,* Physicians elicit the grasp reflex by stroking the patient's palm crosswise or the fingers lengthwise. The reflex causes the patient to grasp the physician's fingers and fail to release despite requests.

least one should be performed, neither can diagnose Alzheimer disease with high specificity because its most consistently visible abnormalities – cerebral atrophy, hippocampal atrophy, and an enlarged third ventricle – are also present in people with normal age-related changes and numerous illnesses, including trisomy 21, alcoholic dementia, HIV-associated dementia, and some varieties of schizophrenia.

In about one-half of Alzheimer patients, PET shows areas of decreased glucose metabolism in the bilateral parietal and temporal association cortex (see Fig. 20.29). These hypometabolic areas are indistinct at first, but as the disease progresses, hypometabolism spreads to the frontal lobe cortex and becomes more pronounced. PET with radiolabeled glucose remains unsuitable for routine testing mainly because of its low sensitivity and specificity as well as its cost. The changes are more specific and more cost-effective in frontotemporal dementia (see later). PET for amyloid accumulation is useful in the diagnosis of the preclinical stage of Alzheimer disease, but may be unnecessary in the symptomatic stage. Similarly, CSF analysis for reduced concentration of amyloid and elevated concentration of tau may be helpful in the preclinical stage, but perhaps is superfluous in the symptomatic stage. Neurologists have

not yet defined the role of PET and advanced CSF analysis in MCI.

Neurologists almost never request cerebral cortex biopsies for diagnostic purposes – chiefly because of the invasive nature of this procedure and the sensitivity and specificity of only approximately 90%.

$$\text{Sensitivity} = \frac{\text{true positives}}{(\text{true positives} + \text{false negatives})}$$
$$\text{Specificity} = \frac{\text{true negatives}}{(\text{true negatives} + \text{false positives})}$$

In addition, histologic findings of Alzheimer disease mainly differ quantitatively, rather than qualitatively, from age-related changes. As a last resort, cerebral cortex biopsies can help establish a diagnosis of herpes simplex encephalitis, familial Alzheimer disease, and Creutzfeldt–Jakob disease or its variant.

Pathology

Compared to age-matched controls, the brains of Alzheimer disease patients are more atrophic. The cerebral atrophy in Alzheimer disease, although generalized, primarily affects the cortical association areas, such as the parietal–temporal junction, and the limbic system. It particularly strikes the hippocampus and prominently involves the locus ceruleus and olfactory nerve. The atrophy spares the cerebral regions governing primary motor, sensory, and visual functions, thus explaining the absence of paresis, sensory loss, and blindness in Alzheimer disease.

Cerebral atrophy naturally leads to compensatory dilation of the lateral and third ventricles. Of these, the temporal horns of the lateral ventricles expand the most. Nevertheless, in Alzheimer disease and most other illnesses that cause dementia, the anterior horns of the lateral ventricles maintain their concave (bowed inward) shape because of the indentation on their lateral border by the head of the preserved caudate nucleus (see Figs. 20.3 and 20.18). The exception is Huntington disease, where atrophy of the head of the caudate nucleus permits the ventricle to expand laterally and assume a convex (bowed outward) shape (see Fig. 20.5).

On a histologic level, "plaques and tangles" remain the most conspicuous feature of Alzheimer disease. Although also present in normal aging and several other illnesses, in Alzheimer disease the plaques and tangles are more plentiful. Moreover, they do not distribute themselves randomly, but congregate, like the atrophy, in the cortical association areas, limbic system, and hippocampus.

The plaques, technically *neuritic plaques* or *senile plaques,* consist of an amyloid core surrounded by abnormal axons and dendrites. They deposit in the neuropil of the brain – not actually inside neurons – and look like burned-out campfires. Up to 50% of the amyloid core contains an insoluble, 42-amino-acid peptide, *beta-amyloid* (*Aβ*) (see later). Accumulation of Aβ is necessary, but alone is insufficient for the development of Alzheimer disease.

The tangles, *neurofibrillary tangles,* are also necessary but insufficient. They follow a somewhat different geographic distribution than plaques. They cluster within hippocampus neurons. The tangles appear as paired helical filaments within neurons and disrupt the normal cytoskeletal architecture. They consist mostly of hyperphosphorylated forms of *tau protein*, which is a microtubule binding protein that undergoes conformational changes. In other words, an abnormal intraneuronal protein – *tau* – aggregates in Alzheimer disease and contributes to the death of critical neurons. Although the concentration of plaques correlates with dementia, the correlation between neurofibrillary tangles and dementia is stronger. On the other hand, neurofibrillary tangles occur in other conditions, including progressive supranuclear palsy, frontotemporal dementia, and TBI.

Another histologic feature of Alzheimer disease is the *loss of neurons* in the frontal and temporal lobes. Neuron loss in the *nucleus basalis of Meynert*, which is a group of large neurons located in the *substantia innominata* near the septal region beneath the globus pallidus (see Fig. 21.4), constitutes the most distinctive change. Their loss depletes the neurotransmitter acetylcholine from the cerebral cortex (see later). Of all these histologic features, loss of neuron synapses correlates most closely with dementia.

Histologic examination of Alzheimer disease brains also reveals coexistent vascular disease in the majority. The reverse is also true: the brains of many VCI patients also show the histologic hallmarks of Alzheimer disease. In other words, many cases of dementia have a combination of both pathologies.

Amyloid Deposits

In Alzheimer disease, Aβ accumulates early and permanently in the cerebral cortex and vital subcortical regions. Aβ is formed when *secretase* enzymes cleave *amyloid precursor protein (APP)*, a large protein encoded by a gene on chromosome 21, into insoluble 42-amino-acid Aβ fragments that precipitate in plaques (Fig. 7.5). Aβ differs from amyloid deposited in viscera as part of various systemic illnesses, such as multiple myeloma and amyloidosis.

Several lines of evidence have given rise to the *amyloid cascade hypothesis* (or simply the *amyloid hypothesis*) as the critical mechanism in Alzheimer disease. This hypothesis proposes that the accumulation of Aβ causes inflammatory and oxidative cerebral damage. Evidence for this theory includes several powerful observations:

- All known genetic mutations associated with Alzheimer disease increase Aβ production (chromosomes 1, 14, 21) or Aβ aggregation (chromosome 19).
- The most powerful established genetic risk factor, which involves *apolipoprotein E (ApoE)*, promotes Aβ deposition.
- Aβ is toxic in vitro (probably because it binds to cerebral acetylcholine [ACh] receptors and poisons cerebral mitochondria).
- At least in some nonhuman studies, antibodies to Aβ reduce clinical and pathologic aspects of Alzheimer disease.

For several reasons, the amyloid hypothesis has lost traction in recent years. The advent of in vitro amyloid imaging techniques has demonstrated that amyloid deposition is present in the brains of many individuals with no evidence of dementia. Conversely, some patients who meet clinical criteria for Alzheimer disease have scans that do not show significant amyloid burden. Most importantly, numerous large clinical trials of monoclonal anti-Aβ antibodies designed to clear amyloid plaques from the brain or secretase inhibitors to prevent Aβ formation have yielded disappointing results. Some authorities feel that it is time to abandon the amyloid hypothesis and focus on other processes, such as the role of tau or ApoE, in the pathogenesis of Alzheimer disease. Others continue to view amyloid deposition as a necessary and causative factor, and advocate trials in which anti-amyloid treatments are begun earlier in the disease process – perhaps at the preclinical stage – in hopes of intervening before amyloid deposition causes irreversible damage.

Biochemical Abnormalities

Under normal circumstances, neurons in the basal nucleus of Meynert synthesize ACh. Using the enzyme *choline acetyltransferase (ChAT)*, these neurons convert acetylcoenzyme-A (acetyl-CoA) and choline to ACh:

$$Acetyl\text{-}CoA + Choline \xrightarrow{\text{ChAT}} ACh$$

Normally, neurons in the basal nucleus of Meynert send axonal projections throughout the entire cerebral cortex and the limbic system to provide cholinergic (i.e., acetylcholine [ACh]) innervation. Loss of neurons in the basal nucleus of Meynert characterizes Alzheimer disease. Their loss leads to a marked reduction in ChAT activity, then in cerebral cortex ACh concentrations, and finally in cerebral cholinergic activity. As with the distribution of the macroscopic and microscopic changes in Alzheimer disease, ACh activity is particularly reduced in the cortical association areas and limbic system.

Alzheimer disease is also associated with reduced concentrations of other established or putative neurotransmitters: somatostatin, substance P, norepinephrine (noradrenaline), vasopressin, and several other polypeptides. However, compared to the ACh loss, their concentrations are not decreased profoundly or consistently, and do not correlate with dementia.

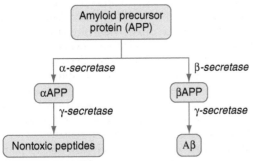

FIGURE 7.5 ■ The amyloid precursor protein (APP) consists of 770 amino acids. Three secretase enzymes (α-, β-, and γ-) cleave it into polypeptide fragments. In one pathway, α-secretase cleaves APP to form the polypeptide αAPP. Then γ-secretase cleaves αAPP into soluble, nontoxic polypeptides. In the other pathway, β-secretase cleaves APP into a different polypeptide, βAPP. Then γ-secretase cleaves βAPP to form Aβ peptides of varying lengths, including the insoluble, toxic 42-amino-acid polypeptide.

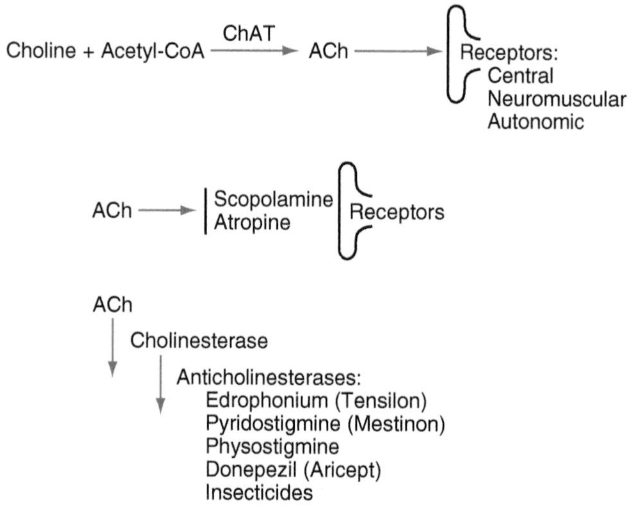

Choline + Acetyl-CoA $\xrightarrow{\text{ChAT}}$ ACh $\longrightarrow$ Receptors:
Central
Neuromuscular
Autonomic

ACh $\longrightarrow$ Scopolamine
Atropine $\Big\}$ Receptors

ACh
$\downarrow$ Cholinesterase

Anticholinesterases:
Edrophonium (Tensilon)
Pyridostigmine (Mestinon)
Physostigmine
Donepezil (Aricept)
Insecticides

FIGURE 7.6 ■ *Top,* The enzyme *choline acetyltransferase (ChAT)* catalyzes the reaction of choline and acetyl-coenzyme A to form acetylcholine (ACh) in neurons of the CNS, PNS, and autonomic nervous system. When released from its presynaptic neurons, ACh interacts with postsynaptic ACh receptors. *Middle,* Various anticholinergic substances block ACh from interacting with its receptors. For example, scopolamine, which readily crosses the blood–brain barrier, blocks ACh from binding with its receptors in the CNS. Likewise, atropine blocks ACh receptors, but predominantly those in the autonomic nervous system. (Unless its concentration is great, atropine does not cross the blood–brain barrier.) Substances like curare and pancuronium block ACh receptors at the neuromuscular junction and cause paralysis. *Bottom,* Cholinesterase metabolizes ACh and terminates ACh activity. (In contrast, most dopamine and serotonin activity is terminated by reuptake.) Anticholinesterases – or cholinesterase inhibitors – block cholinesterase and raise ACh concentrations. Donepezil, rivastigmine, and galantamine make use of this strategy. Using cholinesterase inhibitors is also applicable to PNS disorders. For example, edrophonium (Tensilon) and pyridostigmine (Mestinon) are anticholinesterases that restore neuromuscular junction ACh activity in myasthenia gravis (see Fig. 6.2).

The *cholinergic hypothesis,* drawn from these biochemical observations, postulates that reduced cholinergic activity causes the dementia of Alzheimer disease. In addition to the histologic and biochemical data, supporting evidence includes the finding that even in normal individuals, blocking cerebral ACh receptors causes profound memory impairments. For example, an injection of scopolamine, which has central anticholinergic activity, induces a several-minute episode of cognitive impairment which can be reversed with physostigmine (Fig. 7.6). The cholinergic hypothesis led to the introduction of cholinesterase inhibitors as therapies intended to preserve ACh activity by inactivating its metabolic enzyme, cholinesterase (see Fig. 7.6) (see later).

Although the ChAT deficiency in Alzheimer disease is striking, it is not unique. Pronounced, widespread ChAT deficiencies are also present in the cortex of brains in trisomy 21, Parkinson disease, and DLB, but not in those of Huntington disease.

Risk Factors and Genetic Causes

Researchers have established several risk factors for Alzheimer disease. Living longer than 65 years is the most statistically powerful risk factor for Alzheimer disease because, beginning at that age, its incidence doubles every 5 years. Thus, the prevalence rises from 10% among individuals aged 65 years to almost 40% among individuals over 85 years.

Family history of Alzheimer disease is another well-established risk factor. Although most cases of Alzheimer disease occur sporadically, the disease develops in about 20% of patients' offspring and 10% of second-degree relatives, but in only 5% of age-matched controls. Other risk factors include trisomy 21, several genetic mutations, and possessing ApoE 3/4 or 4/4 allele pairs (see later). Studies have found other potential risk factors, but with influences that remain weak, inconsistent, or as yet unproven, such as myocardial infarction, elevated homocysteine levels, TBI, hypertension, hyperthyroidism, and exposure to aluminum.

Certain allele combinations of the gene coding for ApoE, a cholesterol-carrying serum protein, confer substantial risk. Synthesized in the liver and brain, serum ApoE binds to Aβ and degenerating nerve ends, glia, and other cellular debris, forming neuritic plaques. Chromosome 19 encodes the gene for ApoE, which occurs in three alleles: ApoE2, ApoE3, and ApoE4. Everyone inherits one of these three alleles from each parent, giving each person an allele pair. Approximately 10% to 20% of the population inherits E3-E4 or E4-E4, which are the pairs most closely associated with Alzheimer disease.

Having two E4 alleles (being homozygous for E4) – and to a lesser degree having one E4 allele (being heterozygous for E4) – significantly increases the risk of developing Alzheimer disease. Of individuals carrying no E4 alleles, only about 20% develop Alzheimer disease; of those carrying one E4 allele, 50% develop the disease; and of those carrying two E4 alleles, 90% develop it. Overall, more than 50% of Alzheimer disease patients carry one E4 allele. Not only does the E4 allele put the individual at risk for developing the disease, it also hastens the appearance of the symptoms. For example, compared to individuals carrying no E4 alleles, those carrying one E4 allele show Alzheimer disease symptoms 5 to 10 years earlier, and those with two E4 alleles show the symptoms 10 to 20 years earlier.

On the other hand, having one or even two E4 alleles is neither necessary nor sufficient for developing Alzheimer disease. Because E4 alleles remain a powerful risk factor and not a cause, neurologists refer to the ApoE4 gene as a "susceptibility" gene. Inheriting an ApoE4 allele also serves as a marker for rapid progression from mild cognitive impairment to dementia in HIV disease, in Parkinson disease, and after severe TBI. Studies investigating whether ApoE4 influences the development of cognitive impairment in MS have yielded inconsistent results.

Physicians can order a blood test to determine a patient's ApoE status in order to try to clarify patient's diagnosis and prognosis, but this information generally is less useful than the clinical evaluation and other testing. When the testing is performed, patients learning that they carry ApoE4 alleles show no significant short-term psychological risks.

In contrast to these risk factors for Alzheimer disease, several factors in addition to cognitive reserve offer a

TABLE 7.1 Genetic Abnormalities Associated With Alzheimer Disease

Chromosome	Gene	Percent of Cases	Age at Onset (years)
1	Presenilin 2	<1%	50–65
14	Presenilin 1	1–5%	30–60
19	Apolipoprotein E (ApoE)	50–60%	>60
21	Amyloid precursor protein (APP)	<1%	45–60

decreased incidence or postponed onset of symptoms. Studies have shown that certain leisure activities – playing board games, reading, playing musical instruments, and ballroom dancing – provide some protection against dementia. Individuals who speak two or more languages appear to enjoy delayed onset of dementia irrespective of education level. Regular strenuous exercise, a healthy diet, and other nonpharmacologic interventions also are associated with lower risk of cognitive decline. Control of hypertension, hyperlipidemia, and diabetes reduces the incidence of dementia, probably because they reduce VCI. Some studies have shown that certain genes may confer longevity and relative freedom from Alzheimer disease.

Genetic Causes

Unlike the gene on chromosome 19, which codes for ApoE alleles, mutations on at least three other chromosomes – 1, 14, and 21 – perforce cause Alzheimer disease (Table 7.1). In other words, while the ApoE gene confers susceptibility, these mutations – "obligate genes" – actually cause the illness. All of them usually transmit Alzheimer disease in an autosomal dominant pattern, promote Aβ production, and lead to Aβ deposition in plaques. Although mutations account for only 5% to 10% of all cases, they determine the fate of many individuals, provide a window into the pathogenesis of sporadic Alzheimer disease, and probably account for the vast majority of cases of "early-onset Alzheimer disease" (symptoms appearing before 60 years of age).

Treatment of Dementia

Physicians from time immemorial have attempted to enhance memory and other cognitive function in normal and overachieving as well as impaired individuals by prescribing *nootropics* (Greek, *nous*, intellect; *tropos*, to turn). Aside from stimulants, which can improve attentiveness and thus academic performance, purported nootropics have produced at most only modest improvements for limited periods.

In light of the plausibility of the cholinergic hypothesis and the finding that postsynaptic cholinergic receptors remain relatively intact, several widely prescribed nootropics aim at restoring ACh activity in Alzheimer disease patients. In attempting to replicate the strategy of administering the dopamine precursor levodopa (L-dopa) to Parkinson disease patients, Alzheimer disease researchers have administered ACh precursors, such as choline and lecithin (phosphatidyl choline), to drive the synthesis of ACh. Similarly, to reach the same end, they administered ACh agonists, such as arecoline, oxotremorine, acetyl-L-carnitine, and bethanechol. Whether given by intraventricular or traditional routes, none of these strategies produces a consistent, significant benefit.

A complementary strategy, similar to maintaining ACh neuromuscular junction activity in myasthenia (see Chapter 6), attempts to preserve or increase cerebral ACh concentration by reducing ACh breakdown by cholinesterases. In Alzheimer disease treatment, several commercially available cholinesterase inhibitors that penetrate the blood–brain barrier – donepezil, rivastigmine, and galantamine – produce modest, temporary (approximately 9–12 months) improvement in cognitive tests, "global evaluations," and measurements of quality of life. They may either reduce certain troublesome symptoms, such as depression, psychosis, and anxiety, or make them amenable to psychotropics. The cholinesterase inhibitor donepezil reduces the risk of progression of dementia for as long as 1 year; however, by 36 months it has little or no effect. Cholinesterase inhibitors may also slow the progression of dementia in Parkinson disease and DLB, which are also characterized by an ACh deficit (see later), but not in other neurodegenerative illnesses, MCI, pure VCI, TBI, or delirium.

Whatever their indication, cholinesterase inhibitors increase cholinergic (parasympathetic) activity – occasionally to the point of toxicity. Even routine doses increase intestinal activity and trigger unpleasant abdominal cramps. Patients have accidentally poisoned themselves by taking too many cholinesterase inhibitor pills or applying the medicated patches without removing expired ones. An overdose produces delirium in a patient with dementia and causes all the physical manifestations of a cholinergic crisis: nausea and vomiting; excessive salivation and sweating; bradycardia, hypotension, and lightheadedness. In extreme cases, an overdose can lead to respiratory depression, collapse, and convulsions.

Another nootropic strategy involves blocking toxic glutamate excitatory neurotransmission, a mechanism employed by the N-methyl-D-aspartate (NMDA) receptor antagonist memantine (Namenda). This medicine, in combination with donepezil or used alone, produces modest improvement in memory and learning for several months in patients with moderate-to-severe Alzheimer disease. It also transiently suppresses agitation or aggression.

Seeking a different approach, some therapeutic trials attempted to replenish other deficient presynaptic neurotransmitters, such as somatostatin and vasopressin. Despite their promise, these attempts were unsuccessful.

Another theory postulated that cholesterol-lowering medicines, commonly known as statins, would leach cholesterol from plaques and reduce the amyloid burden. Rigorous analysis showed that statin treatment failed to protect against, reverse, or even slow the progression of Alzheimer disease. On the other hand, statins reduce the risk of stroke and VCI, and thereby may slow the progression of cognitive impairment.

Researchers initially expected that estrogen replacement therapy (ERT), which suppresses menopausal symptoms, would also reduce the risk or delay the onset of Alzheimer disease. However, women taking ERT still developed the disease at the same rate and followed the same or a more accelerated course.

Although reduced cerebral blood flow is a result, not a cause, of Alzheimer disease, researchers attempted to improve blood flow with cyclandelate (Cyclospasmol), a vasodilator. Studies found that the minimal improvement that followed this treatment was attributable to its antidepressant properties.

A completely different approach is immunization against amyloid. The expectation was that antibodies would attack and destroy amyloid plaques. Researchers first administered an anti-amyloid vaccine to mice with an experimental Alzheimer-like illness and then to patients with Alzheimer disease and presymptomatic individuals destined to develop the disease because they were carrying mutations that doomed them to the illness. Although the vaccination program was successful in the mice, human volunteers derived no benefit or suffered inflammatory encephalitis. Looking toward a different method of reducing the amyloid burden, researchers have attempted to interrupt the synthesis of Aβ by administering inhibitors of β-secretase or γ-secretase, enzymes that play a key role in the formation of Aβ (see Fig. 7.5). However, a large clinical trial of a γ-secretase inhibitor exacerbated rather than helped the problem.

Studies have shown no benefit from a host of foodstuffs, additives, and complementary therapies, including tocopherol (vitamin E) and other antioxidants, gingko biloba, piracetam, acetyl-L-carnitine, folic acid, and omega-3 fatty acids. On the other hand, medium-chain triglycerides did improve ADAS-Cog scores – but only in patients negative for the ApoE4 allele.

Treatment of Neuropsychiatric Symptoms

Because depression may complicate Alzheimer disease and even cause or worsen cognitive impairment, neurologists often prescribe antidepressants. However, in view of the ACh deficiency in Alzheimer disease, neurologists avoid prescribing antidepressants with anticholinergic activity, particularly tricyclic antidepressants. Instead, prescribing serotonin and possibly norepinephrine reuptake inhibitors may alleviate depression as much or more than tricyclic antidepressants, and produce fewer side effects.

Neurologists often prescribe antipsychotic agents for an episode of acute agitation, but usually only if it exhausts the patient or caregiver (see later) or represents a danger. Regarding long-term relief, the Clinical Antipsychotic Trials of Intervention Effectiveness – Alzheimer's Disease (CATIE–AD) showed no significant differences between atypical antipsychotics and placebo on cognition, functioning, care needs, or quality of life. Antipsychotics may alleviate a particular disruptive symptom or improve one measure. For example, only some of these antipsychotics (olanzapine and risperidone) improved the Neuropsychiatric Inventory total score and the hostile suspiciousness

factor of the Brief Psychiatric Rating Scale, and only one (risperidone) produced improvement in the Clinical Global Impression of Change and the psychosis factor of the Brief Psychiatric Rating Scale. Antipsychotics do not eliminate wandering and other dangerous behavior. Moreover, analyses of multiple studies suggest that both conventional and atypical antipsychotics are associated with a slightly increased risk of stroke and death in elderly patients treated for dementia-related psychosis; in 2008 the Food and Drug Administration (FDA) issued a black box warning to this effect. Physicians must weigh the limited benefits of antipsychotics against their carrying this small but significant risk of stroke and death.

"Behavior management techniques," such as removing doorknobs and constructing large indoor and outdoor "safe zones," may painlessly confine the patient. Also, scheduling frequent snacks and trips to the toilet may reduce wandering.

Alzheimer disease-induced sleep disruptions often pose caregivers' greatest burden. Caregivers' may reduce mild sleep disturbances by providing daytime exercise, exposure to sunlight, and restricted naps. Otherwise, for everybody's benefit, dangerous and disruptive sleep disturbances usually merit preemptive, early evening administration of hypnotic, anxiolytic, or antipsychotic agents.

In general, neurologists treating a patient with Alzheimer disease target one symptom and begin treatment with a low dose of a single medicine and then gradually proceed to an effective dose. They avoid confounding medication side effects, especially sedation, with disease progression. Before adding new medicines or increasing the dose of current ones, they assess the patient's entire medication regimen. Because many elderly patients are over-medicated rather than under-medicated, the first strategy often entails subtracting rather than adding medicines. They periodically re-assess the need for psychotropics because, as the disease progresses, symptoms change or even disappear. Also, if agitation or another behavioral disturbance comes to dominate the clinical picture, neurologists may reconsider the diagnosis of Alzheimer disease and see if the patient's underlying problem is actually frontotemporal dementia or DLB.

Caregiver Stress

Although the patient always remains the focus of attention, physicians caring for Alzheimer disease patients must consider the spouse or other caregiver who is often old and infirm. Physicians sometimes prescribe medicines to a patient to ease a caregiver's duties. If the burdens threaten the caregiver's well-being, physicians might advise that keeping the patient at home is in neither the patient's nor the caregiver's best interest. Inability to walk, incontinence, highly demanding nursing requirements, nighttime outbursts, and other disruptive behavior – not cognitive decline – eventually compel caregivers to place these patients in nursing homes. Physicians can help caregivers by keeping their expectations realistic, preserving their financial and emotional resources, securing help from social service agencies, and preventing a hopeless situation from dominating family life.

RELATED DISORDERS

Trisomy 21

Almost all individuals with trisomy 21, if they live to 50 years of age, develop an Alzheimer-like dementia superimposed on their Intellectual Developmental Disorder. All their ancillary tests – CT, MRI, PET, and amyloid-binding studies – show Alzheimer-like changes. At autopsy, their brains show the pathologic findings of Alzheimer disease. Even women who give birth to a child with trisomy 21 have a five-fold increase in risk of Alzheimer disease.

Dementia With Lewy Bodies

Dementia with Lewy bodies (DLB), previously called Lewy bodies disease or diffuse Lewy bodies disease, accounts for approximately 15% of cases of dementia. The DSM-5 includes it within Neurocognitive Disorder with Lewy Bodies.

Neurologists named DLB for its histologic signature, cortical Lewy bodies. These histologic abnormalities are spherical intracytoplasmic inclusions, each composed of a dense circular eosinophilic core surrounded by loose fibrils. Their core contains mostly aggregates of α-synuclein – a 140-amino-acid protein encoded on chromosome 4 – and a less specific substance, *ubiquitin*. The concentration of the Lewy bodies correlates with the severity of dementia. (Lewy bodies are widely known as a marker for Parkinson disease, where they primarily populate the substantia nigra in the basal ganglia rather than the cerebral cortex [Chapter 18].)

Alzheimer disease and DLB share several features. Both are neurodegenerative illnesses, arise in older individuals, and cause dementia. Also in both diseases, the brain concentrations of ChAT and acetylcholine are diminished and these reductions correlate with the degree of cognitive impairment. Although the loss of ChAT is greater in DLB than in Alzheimer disease, cholinesterase inhibitors transiently slow cognitive decline in both diseases. While tau accumulates in neurons in Alzheimer disease, α-synuclein accumulates in neurons in DLB. In addition, compared to individuals with Alzheimer disease, patients with DLB are more likely to be younger, to be male, to have a history of depression, to have attained a higher level of education, to have a family history of Parkinson disease, and to have no ApoE4 allele.

DLB also shares many features with Parkinson disease. The histology of both, of course, features Lewy bodies. Patents with DLB exhibit *parkinsonism* – a masked face, bradykinesia, rigidity, and gait impairment – but little or no tremor. However, in contrast to Parkinson disease, where cognitive impairment usually does not arise until 5 years into the illness, cognitive impairment, if not dementia, is characteristically present within a year of onset of DLB. In addition, PET shows widespread, profound cholinesterase deficiency in patients with DLB and Parkinson disease with dementia.

Visual hallucinations also plague DLB patients, and begin early after the onset of their illness. Hallucinations correlate with Lewy bodies in the temporal lobes. In DLB, visions of people or animals and other hallucinations often appear so detailed and vivid that they provoke fear and precipitate confusion. A classic symptom of DLB is Capgras syndrome in which patients believe that an "impostor" has replaced a close friend or relative.

Another common symptom, which ultimately occurs in about 50% of DLB patients as well as many Parkinson disease patients, is *rapid eye movement (REM) sleep behavior disorder* (see Chapter 17). Normal individuals during REM sleep lose tone in their muscles except for those that control respiratory and ocular movement. In contrast, individuals with REM sleep behavior disorder, whether idiopathic or from DLB or Parkinson disease, do not experience the usual REM-induced atonia and appear to enact their dreams. For example, they make running, punching, and similar movements while dreaming. The long-acting benzodiazepine clonazepam effectively suppresses REM sleep behavior disorder in DLB as well as in its other causes.

DLB also typically causes sudden, unexpected changes in cognition, attentiveness, and alertness. These fluctuations in mental status may mimic episodes of delirium. Depression is another very common characteristic of DLB.

Physicians should be aware of several pitfalls in treating DLB patients. Although the extrapyramidal signs suggest Parkinson disease, levodopa and similar Parkinson disease medicines provide little or no benefit in correcting these motor disturbances and, at the same time, often exacerbate the visual hallucinations. Another potential iatrogenic problem is that visual hallucinations might prompt a physician to administer dopamine-blocking antipsychotic agents; however, even small amounts of antipsychotic agents cause parkinsonism with severe akinesia and rigidity.

The aforementioned aspects of DLB, which accompany the dementia, are so pronounced and distinctive that they serve as the basis for diagnosis. Neurologists usually diagnose DLB based on three core features and two suggestive features:

Three Core Features:

1. Parkinsonism
2. Visual hallucinations
3. Fluctuating cognition.

Two Suggestive Features:

1. REM behavior disorder
2. Antipsychotic hypersensitivity.

FRONTAL LOBE DISORDERS

Injuries

The frontal lobes contain the main centers for personality, emotion, and executive decisions. They also integrate cognitive functions, consider potential solutions, weigh probable outcomes, and initiate responses. Equally important, the frontal lobes also inhibit instinctive behaviors. Thus, individuals with frontal lobe damage from physical injury or disease characteristically display uninhibited physical, emotional, and behavioral disturbances.

Neuropsychologists and behavioral neurologists tend to describe at least three syndromes of frontal lobe dysfunction: *dorsolateral*, *orbitofrontal*, and *mediofrontal*. However, practicing neurologists rarely see these syndromes as discrete or readily diagnosable entities; rather, they tend to overlap considerably and occur in combination. Typically, patients with frontal lobe dysfunction are apathetic and indifferent to their surroundings, ongoing events, and underlying illness. They also have slowness of cognitive processing. Their impairments prevent them from making transitions, changing sets, and adopting alternate strategies. Patients also have slowed thinking (*bradyphrenia*), lack of emotion, and a paucity of speech that can range from reticence to silence (*abulia*). In addition, if an illness or injury damages their dominant frontal lobe's language center, patients will have impaired verbal output and other signs of aphasia (see Chapter 8).

Their movements tend to be slow (*bradykinetic*), repetitive (*perseverative*), reduced, or absent (*akinetic*). Walking becomes clumsy and uncertain (*apraxic*). Absence of voluntary movement can accompany an absence of speaking and expression (*akinetic mutism*). Viscous thinking and bradykinesia combine to cause *psychomotor retardation*.

Patients' impaired inhibitory systems allow flighty ideas, inappropriate comments, and unrestrained expression of sexual urges. In extreme cases, impaired inhibition causes bladder or bowel incontinence. Because patients cannot suppress a natural tendency to attend to new stimuli, they are easily distracted from their tasks. They may be so incapable of disregarding new stimuli that physicians describe them as "stimulus-bound." For example, people entering a room, a soft noise, or an unrelated idea easily pulls their attention from an assigned task. Also, patients who have lost inhibition characteristically display a superficial, odd jocularity with uncontrollable, facetious laughter (*Witzelsucht*).

Despite all its attendant neuropsychologic abnormalities, frontal lobe damage does not necessarily cause dementia. Patients with limited frontal lobe damage tend to retain memory, simple calculation ability, and visual-spatial perception because these cognitive domains are either based largely in the parietal and temporal lobes or distributed throughout the cerebral cortex. Indeed, IQ tests and the MMSE often yield normal results. The MoCA is more reliable than the MMSE in detecting frontal lobe damage.

Slowly growing frontal lesions, especially when in the nondominant hemisphere, may reach enormous size before producing any signs of frontal lobe dysfunction. At the onset, only subtle physical signs accompany these neuropsychologic abnormalities, but sooner or later, expanding frontal lobe lesions may cause pseudobulbar palsy, nonfluent aphasia, and frontal release reflexes (see later). Also, because of the olfactory nerves' location on the undersurface of the frontal lobes, patients with frontal lobe injuries often have anosmia.

Causes of bilateral frontal lobe damage include TBI, glioblastoma, metastatic tumors, MS, ruptured anterior cerebral artery aneurysm, infarction of both anterior cerebral arteries, and rare metabolic disorders such as metachromatic leukodystrophy. In the *frontal lobotomy*, a largely abandoned procedure which physicians had introduced to control psychotic thought and behavior long before the first-generation antipsychotic agents, neurosurgeons injected sclerosing agents into the frontal lobe or severed its underlying large white matter tracts (see Fig. 20.23). Patients who underwent the procedure showed less agitation, but usually at the expense of developing apathy, restricted spontaneous verbal output, indifference to social conventions, and impaired abstract reasoning.

In contrast to bilateral frontal lobe injury producing neuropsychologic impairments, modern-day surgical removal of the anterior, nondominant frontal lobe causes little if any impairment. For example, neurosurgeons routinely remove this "silent area" of the brain in cases of tumor, arteriovenous malformation, or seizure focus refractory to antiepileptic drugs (AEDs) (see Chapter 10).

Frontotemporal Dementia or Frontotemporal Degeneration

Frontotemporal dementia or frontotemporal degeneration (*FTD*) *consists of an insidious onset of dementia greatly overshadowed by personality and behavioral disturbances and/or language impairment.* Occurring twice as frequently in men as in women, this illness has an average age of onset of 53 years and follows a fatal course lasting less than 4 years. Its DSM-5 equivalent is Frontotemporal Neurocognitive Disorder, which can be major or mild.

Subtypes of FTD include one characterized by behavioral disturbances and others with progressive aphasia (see Chapter 8). The *behavioral variant*, which is especially important to psychiatrists, reflects degeneration primarily of the frontal rather than the temporal lobes. As with other disorders resulting from frontal lobe degeneration, patients with the behavioral variant show a broad decline in affect and behavior. In fact, physicians may reasonably initially misdiagnose FTD as major depression, bipolar disorder, obsessive-compulsive disorder, or other psychiatric illnesses. Neurologic criteria for a "possible" diagnosis specifically require that patients show three of six disturbances:

1. Disinhibition
2. Apathy
3. Loss of sympathy
4. Perseverative or compulsive behaviors
5. Hyperorality (excessive – sometime compulsive – talking, eating, or cigarette smoking)
6. Impaired executive ability.

A "probable" diagnosis requires only the addition of compatible imaging studies (see later). A "definite" diagnosis requires histologic confirmation or presence of one of the mutations known to cause FTD on genetic testing.

Other variants of FTD include two forms of *primary progressive aphasia* (*PPA*). Patients with the nonfluent/agrammatic subtype exhibit marked difficulty with speech production, with apraxia of speech and impaired prosody; the posterior left frontal lobe is most involved in this variant. The semantic variant of PPA robs patients of their ability to comprehend sentences and even single words, with dysfunction most prominent in the left anterior temporal lobe. (A third form of PPA, known as the logopenic variant, impairs repetition severely but is considered a form of Alzheimer disease based on the pathologic finding of plaques and tangles.)

Notably, these criteria do not fulfill the definition of dementia, as memory may not be affected in patients with FTD. Some authors – as well as patients – prefer the term frontotemporal *degeneration* rather than *dementia*. (Fortunately, the abbreviation is the same for both.) Astute clinicians usually are able to differentiate FTD from dementias, such as Alzheimer disease (Table 7.2), but neuropsychological testing can be invaluable in making this distinction

Despite their impairments, patients with FTD characteristically retain their visual-spatial ability – a function governed largely by the parietal lobes. For example, patients can copy a picture but cannot draw one from memory, i.e., they do not show constructional apraxia. Also, they do not lose their sense of direction, even in new surroundings.

Neuropathologists named DLB for the intraneuronal inclusions visible under the microscope, but they named frontotemporal dementia for the brain's gross appearance: the frontal and anterior temporal lobes are atrophic, but the parietal and occipital lobes are preserved. Plaques and tangles are uncommon and acetylcholine concentrations are normal – in marked contrast to Alzheimer disease. In some cases of FTD, neurons contain argentophilic (silver-staining) inclusions known as *Pick bodies*, echoing the name "Pick disease," an older term for FTD.

FTD may account for only 5% to 10% of all cases of dementia, but, with a mean age of onset of 53 years, it accounts for about 50% of individuals younger than 60 years. Many of them – 40% – have a family history of the same disease and they mostly follow an autosomal dominant pattern.

In many cases FTD is linked with a mutant gene on chromosome 17, which codes for the protein tau. Another genetic mutation linked to FTD is the expansion of the GGGGCC repeat in the C9ORF72 gene on chromosome 9. This mutation can also be detected in patients with motor neuron disease/amyotrophic lateral sclerosis (see Chapter 5), and frequently causes the two conditions in combination, especially in familial cases.

FTD also can overlap with a number of other neurodegenerative disorders, including progressive supranuclear palsy (see Chapter 18) and corticobasal degeneration (an atypical parkinsonian disorder whose features include asymmetric dystonia, apraxia, cortical sensory loss, and myoclonus). Current conceptions view the primary neuropathologic process in these conditions as an abnormality in tau metabolism. Thus, neuropathologists have found it useful to group FTD, progressive supranuclear palsy, and corticobasal degeneration – as well as Alzheimer disease - into a single family of *tauopathies*, and DLB and Parkinson disease into *synucleinopathies* (Table 7.3).

PET scans in FTD patients often show readily identifiable hypometabolism in frontal lobes but relatively normal metabolism in parietal and occipital lobes. Probably because acetylcholine levels are normal, cholinesterase inhibitors provide no benefit for either its cognitive or behavioral impairments.

TABLE 7.2 Features Distinguishing Alzheimer Disease and Frontotemporal Dementia

Feature	Alzheimer Disease	Frontotemporal Dementia
Age at onset (years)	> 65	53 (mean)
Memory impairments	Early, pronounced	Subtle, at least initially, with preserved visual-spatial ability
Behavior abnormalities	None until middle or late stage	Early and prominent perseverative and compulsive behavior; hyperorality; impaired executive ability
Language impairment	Except for anomia, none until late stage	Paraphasias, anomia, decreased fluency
CT/MRI* appearance	General atrophy, but especially parietal and temporal lobes	Frontal and temporal lobe atrophy
Histologic marker	Aβ accumulation	Tau accumulation

*CT, computed tomography; MRI, magnetic resonance imaging

TABLE 7.3 Neurodegenerative Diseases and the Corresponding Proteins That Accumulate in Neurons

Disease	Protein
Creutzfeldt–Jakob disease	PrP^{Sc}
Dementia with Lewy bodies	α-synuclein
Parkinson disease	α-synuclein
Alzheimer disease	Tau (Aβ is extracellular)
Frontotemporal dementia	Tau
Progressive supranuclear palsy	Tau
Huntington's disease	Huntingtin

OTHER DEMENTIAS

Vascular Cognitive Impairment

Previously known as "multi-infarct dementia" or "vascular dementia" and currently labeled as Vascular Neurocognitive Disorder according to DSM-5, vascular cognitive impairment (VCI) is essentially the dementia that results from cerebral infarctions (strokes) or other cerebral vascular insults (see Chapter 11). VCI patients may have any combination of amnesia, aphasia, dyscalculia, anosognosia, or other neuropsychologic disorders depending on the location of underlying strokes. VCI's primary distinction is that the underlying strokes also cause abnormal physical findings, such as hemiparesis, hemianopia, dysarthria, ataxia, and pseudobulbar palsy, and gait impairment. In VCI – unlike in Alzheimer disease, DLB, and FTD – these physical signs overshadow the cognitive impairments. Finally, unlike those other dementia-producing illnesses, VCI typically follows a step-wise deterioration that presumably reflects the accumulation of strokes over time.

Imaging studies usually can confirm a clinical diagnosis of VCI. CT or MRI shows evidence of strokes, small (0.5–1.5-cm) lacunar infarcts, or more confluent ischemic changes in the white matter of the cerebral hemispheres. MRI is more sensitive than CT in milder cases. Although rarely necessary, PET shows multiple hypometabolic regions.

Strokes that obliterate 50 g or more of brain tissue may lead to VCI regardless of the extent or location of the destruction. Alternatively, small strokes may lead to VCI by striking strategic regions of the brain, particularly the limbic system. Another common mechanism consists of multiple lacunar infarcts predominantly in the subcortical white matter, primarily due to hypertension. These insults produce the histologic condition *état lacunaire* (French, lacunar state) or *Binswanger disease*.

As mentioned earlier, histologic studies in VCI have shown that the majority of patients with VCI have concomitant Alzheimer disease pathology. These findings indicate that most patients who clinically appear to have VCI actually have a mixture of Alzheimer disease and VCI.

Among risk factors for VCI, pre-existing cognitive impairment – especially from Alzheimer disease – exerts the greatest influence. Risk factors for stroke are naturally risk factors for VCI (see Chapter 11). Even vascular disease in other organs, such as coronary artery disease, increases the risk for VCI. However, despite its importance in other circumstances, ApoE4 is not a risk factor for VCI.

Cholinesterase inhibitors, according to some reports, retard the progression of VCI. However, their benefit might be attributable to their effect on the portion of the dementia that represents comorbid Alzheimer disease. Another therapeutic strategy is to assess and possibly treat VCI patients for depression, which is frequently comorbid.

Wernicke–Korsakoff Syndrome

Chronic alcohol consumption may lead to *Wernicke–Korsakoff syndrome*, in which amnesia is a prominent feature. This disorder falls into the DSM-5 category of Substance-Induced Neurocognitive Disorder.

The cognitive impairment develops in proportion to the lifetime consumption of alcohol. It occurs in about 50% of all chronic alcoholics and characteristically begins with a *global confusional state*. However, alcoholism does not equally impair all cognitive domains. It mostly impairs short-term memory, abstract reasoning, and visual and psychomotor dexterity. In contrast, it impairs long-term memory and language function so little that without formal testing, alcoholics sometimes appear to have normal intellect.

Wernicke–Korsakoff syndrome includes retrograde amnesia, but its hallmark is anterograde amnesia. By itself, amnesia – like aphasia and the frontal lobe syndrome – does not constitute dementia. If the amnesia worsens, however, it interferes with various memory-based cognitive functions, especially learning, and eventually evolves into an Alzheimer-like dementia. Contrary to classic descriptions, confabulation is usually absent or inconspicuous.

In its acute stages, Wernicke–Korsakoff syndrome comprises a triad of amnesia, ataxia, and ocular motility abnormalities, including conjugate gaze paresis and nystagmus. However, fewer than 20% of patients display all these abnormalities. With or without Wernicke–Korsakoff syndrome, patients with alcoholism develop a peripheral neuropathy and cerebellar degeneration particularly affecting the vermis (see Chapter 2), with consequent development of an ataxic gait (see Fig. 2.13).

CT and MRI may be normal or show cerebral and cerebellar atrophy. In acute Wernicke–Korsakoff syndrome, distinctive and potentially fatal petechial hemorrhages develop in the mammillary bodies, thalamus, and periaqueductal gray matter (see Fig. 18.2). The damage to these structures, which are elements of the limbic system (see Fig. 16.5), explains the amnesia. Also, because the periaqueductal gray matter is immediately adjacent to the nuclei of the third and sixth cranial nerves and the medial longitudinal fasciculus, damage to this region causes ocular motility abnormalities (see Chapters 4 and 12).

Wernicke–Korsakoff syndrome does not develop only in alcoholics. Similar clinical and pathologic changes have also occurred in nonalcoholic individuals who have undergone starvation, dialysis, chemotherapy, or gastric or bariatric surgery. On rare occasion, anorexia nervosa, prolonged vomiting, and self-induced fasting have led to Wernicke–Korsakoff syndrome.

These observations and others demonstrate that Wernicke–Korsakoff syndrome is not solely the result of alcohol toxicity. In fact, it probably results primarily from a nutritional deficiency of thiamine (vitamin B_1), an essential co-enzyme in carbohydrate metabolism. Thiamine administration can prevent or even partially reverse Wernicke–Korsakoff syndrome. Keeping in mind that only a minority of patients present with all three components of the disorder, most neurologists immediately administer thiamine in equivocal as well as clear-cut cases of Wernicke–Korsakoff syndrome. Although thiamine treatment may reverse acute Wernicke–Korsakoff syndrome, only 25% of patients recover from chronic alcohol-induced dementia.

Other Causes of Dementia in Alcoholics

Alcoholics are prone to motor vehicle crashes because of impaired judgment, slowed physical responses, and a tendency to fall asleep while driving. In addition, because of repeated falls, alcoholics suffer head trauma sufficient to cause contusions and subdural hematomas, which in turn can lead to epilepsy. They are also susceptible to seizures from either excessive alcohol use or alcohol withdrawal, and because the underlying problem is a metabolic derangement, the seizures are more likely to be generalized tonic-clonic rather than focal. Another complication of alcoholism, gastrointestinal bleeding, especially with underlying Laennec cirrhosis, causes hepatic encephalopathy. Rarely, but interestingly, they can develop *Marchiafava–Bignami* syndrome, degeneration of the corpus callosum that causes a "split brain syndrome" (see Chapter 8).

Infants of severely alcoholic mothers are often born with the *fetal alcohol syndrome*, which includes facial anomalies, low birth weight, microcephaly, tremor, and intellectual developmental disorder.

Medication-Induced Cognitive Deficits

Medication effects remain one of the few commonly occurring correctable causes of cognitive impairment. Neurologists themselves prescribe many medicines – opioids, AEDs, antiparkinson agents, steroids, and psychotropics – that routinely produce cognitive impairment and other neuropsychologic side effects. Even medicated eye drops may seep into the systemic circulation and cause symptoms. Also, seemingly innocuous over-the-counter medicines, such as St. John's wort, may directly produce a side effect or cause an adverse drug–drug interaction.

Normal-Pressure Hydrocephalus

Normal-pressure hydrocephalus (NPH) is celebrated as a correctable cause of dementia. Most cases of NPH are idiopathic, but meningitis or subarachnoid hemorrhage often precedes it. In those cases, inflammatory material or blood probably clogs the arachnoid villi overlying the brain and obstructs reabsorption of CSF. As CSF production continues despite inadequate reabsorption, excessive CSF accumulates in the ventricles and expands them to the point of producing hydrocephalus (Fig. 7.7).

NPH consists of three elements: dementia, urinary incontinence, and gait apraxia. The dementia conforms to the subcortical classification because it entails slowing of thought and gait, but spares language skills. Abulia is commonly present. Although the dementia may bring the patient to a psychiatrist's attention, gait apraxia is generally the initial, most consistent, and most prominent feature of NPH (Fig. 7.8). It is also the first to improve with treatment (see later). If dementia precedes the gait dysfunction, a diagnosis of NPH is less likely. Urinary incontinence consists of urgency and frequency which progress to incontinence, and it also improves with treatment. The physical features of NPH easily separate it from Alzheimer disease and other dementia-producing illnesses.

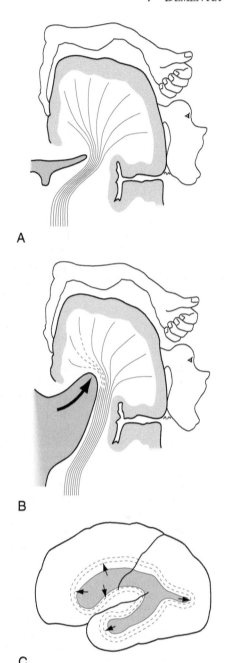

A

B

C

FIGURE 7.7 ■ *A*, and *B*, Ventricular expansion, as in normal pressure hydrocephalus (NPH), results in compression of brain parenchyma and stretching of the corticospinal and other tracts of the internal capsule (see Fig. 18.1). Gait impairment (apraxia) and urinary incontinence are prominent symptoms of NPH because the ventricular enlargement predominantly disrupts the most medial fibers, which innervate the legs and the voluntary muscles of the bladder. *C*, Also, internal pressure on the frontal lobes leads to cognitive impairment and psychomotor retardation.

In NPH, CT and MRI show ventricular dilation, particularly of the temporal horns (see Figs. 20.7 and 20.19), and sometimes signs of CSF reabsorption across ventricular surfaces. Nevertheless, diagnosing NPH exclusively by CT and MRI is unreliable because the findings

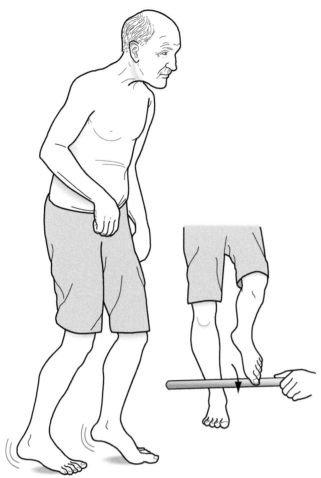

FIGURE 7.8 ■ Gait apraxia, the hallmark of NPH, appears in several aspects of gait testing. Patients with gait apraxia fail to alternate their leg movements and do not shift their weight to their forward foot. They tend to pick up the same leg twice and attempt to elevate their weight-bearing foot. When their weight remains on the foot that they attempt to raise, that foot trembles and appears to be stuck or "magnetized" to the floor. Patients demonstrate a magnetic gait when they require multiple steps to complete a turn. Despite being unable to walk, they can typically step over a stick because their stepping reflex is relatively preserved.

are nonspecific, particularly because they resemble cerebral atrophy with resultant hydrocephalus (*hydrocephalus ex vacuo*, see Fig. 20.3). The CSF pressure and its protein and glucose concentrations are normal.

One worthwhile test is simply to withdraw large volumes (30–60 ml) of CSF by LP or to perform a series of three LPs. Following the removal of large volumes of CSF, which presumably reduces hydrocephalus, improvement in the patient's gait – not necessarily the dementia – indicates NPH and predicts a benefit from permanent CSF drainage. A negative test, however, does not preclude the diagnosis.

NPH can be relieved by neurosurgical insertion of a shunt into a lateral ventricle to drain CSF into the chest or abdominal cavity. However, a clinically beneficial response is difficult to predict and surgical complications, which can be serious, occur in up to 30% of cases.

INFECTIONS

Neurosyphilis

Caused by persistent *Treponema pallidum* infection, neurosyphilis had been largely of historic interest until the start of the acquired immunodeficiency syndrome (AIDS) epidemic. Not only do most cases of syphilis now occur in HIV-infected patients, syphilis infections follow an unusually aggressive course in such patients because they lack the immunologic capacity to fight it.

Neurologists may care for patients with *acute syphilitic meningitis*, which causes the usual symptoms and signs of meningitis, such as headache, fever, and nuchal rigidity. This presentation overlaps with *meningovascular syphilis*, which causes stroke-like insults to the spinal cord or brain.

Both neurologists and psychiatrists encounter patients with syphilis if the infection has spread to the CNS, when the term "parenchymatous syphilis" is appropriate. Infection of the brain leads to "general paresis," and spinal cord involvement causes "tabes dorsalis" (see Chapter 2).

General paresis, the brain infection, initially causes the insidious onset of nonspecific cognitive impairments and personality changes. If the infection remains untreated, patients progress to develop dementia, hallucinations, and disordered thinking. However, delusions of grandeur, despite their notoriety, rarely arise. The cognitive impairments are often accompanied by any of a wide variety of physical abnormalities, including dysarthria, tremors, Argyll–Robertson pupils (see Chapter 12), or loss of hearing or vision.

Imaging studies do not help in the diagnosis of neurosyphilis because they reveal only nonspecific cerebral atrophy, although perhaps mostly of the frontal lobe. Serologic tests for syphilis include treponemal tests – which detect antibodies to *T. pallidum* – and nontreponemal tests. The approach to testing for neurosyphilis has changed in recent years, thanks largely to improvements in treponemal tests. One current recommendation for neurosyphilis testing in the work-up of dementia involves first screening with a treponemal test, such as the *fluorescent treponemal antibody absorption* (*FTA-ABS*) or the *treponemal microhemagglutination assay* (*MHA-TP*). If this test is negative, syphilis is very unlikely, though repeat testing is warranted if recent exposure is possible and the first sample may have been drawn prior to seroconversion. If the treponemal test is positive, a nontreponemal test should be performed. If this is negative, neurosyphilis is unlikely (though latent syphilis may be present). If the nontreponemal test is positive, the physician should perform an LP for CSF analysis. A positive *venereal disease research laboratory* (*VDRL*) test in CSF confirms neurosyphilis but false-negative results occur. Therefore, in the appropriate clinical setting, with a supportive CSF profile – including an elevated protein concentration (45–100 mg/dl) and a lymphocytic pleocytosis (5–200 cells/ml) – physicians can presumptively diagnose neurosyphilis and institute treatment. The threshold for initiating treatment should be low in patients infected with HIV.

Subacute Sclerosing Panencephalitis

Subacute sclerosing panencephalitis (SSPE) is a rare, predominantly childhood-onset neurologic illness that probably results from a latent or mutant measles (rubella) virus infection of neurons. Alternatively, the body's aberrant response to this infection causes the illness. About 85% of patients with SSPE develop it at a mean of 12 years, but 15% develop it as adults. In most children and adolescents, routine measles precedes SSPE by about 6 years. Less than 10% of them had received a measles vaccination in childhood. In adults, measles precedes SSPE by about 20 years.

Symptoms and signs develop gradually. Early manifestations include poor schoolwork, nonspecific behavioral disturbances, restlessness, and personality changes. Over weeks, cognition deteriorates into dementia and weakness in one limb evolves into complete paralysis. Patients may have partial or generalized seizures, but the hallmark of SSPE is myoclonus (see Chapter 18).

After lingering in a state of akinetic mutism, most patients succumb in 1–2 years and 95% within 5 years. Although antiviral treatment may slow or arrest its course, survivors usually remain in a vegetative state.

Clinicians can confirm a diagnosis of SSPE by finding an elevated measles antibody titer in the CSF. An EEG is also diagnostically helpful: It shows periodic sharp-wave complexes or a burst-suppression pattern (see Fig. 10.6). (The EEG pattern in Creutzfeldt–Jakob disease also shows periodic discharges.) Histologic examination of the brain in SSPE reveals intra*nuclear* eosinophilic inclusions (Cowdry bodies). By way of contrast, Lewy bodies are intra*cytoplasmic* eosinophilic inclusions.

Creutzfeldt–Jakob and Related Diseases

Creutzfeldt–Jakob disease causes a constellation of dementia, myoclonus, ataxia, and periodic EEG patterns. Compared to Alzheimer disease, Creutzfeldt–Jakob disease appears at a younger age (50–64 years) and causes death much more rapidly (in about 6 months). The DSM-5 includes Creutzfeldt–Jakob disease as Neurocognitive Disorder Due to Prion Disease (see later).

Although the dementia of Creutzfeldt–Jakob disease lacks specific qualities, myoclonus almost always accompanies it at some time during the course of the illness. In addition, patients frequently have pyramidal, extrapyramidal, or cerebellar signs. Special laboratory tests and cerebral histology can confirm a clinical diagnosis.

While researchers cannot transmit Alzheimer disease, DLB, or VCI from patients to animals, they can transmit Creutzfeldt–Jakob disease to primates by inoculating their brains with brain tissue from affected patients. Transmitting the illness to laboratory animals demonstrates that the illness is infectious and that *inter*species transmission can occur. Although most cases have been sporadic, accidents involving corneal transplantation, intracerebral EEG electrodes, and neurosurgery specimens have transmitted the disease between humans, i.e., *intra*species transmission. For example, in a well-known tragedy, growth hormone extracted from human cadaver pituitary glands once transmitted the illness to a group of children undergoing treatment for short stature because of pituitary insufficiency.

Prions

In work for which they were honored with the Nobel Prize, Drs. D. Carleton Gajdusek and Stanley Prusiner showed that a novel group of pathogens, *prions* (*prote*in*aceous *infective agents), composed entirely or almost entirely of protein and completely lacking DNA and RNA, cause Creutzfeldt–Jakob disease and related illnesses. Prions remain the only known infectious agents lacking nucleic acid. Also unlike conventional infectious agents, prions resist routine sterilization, heat, formaldehyde, and treatments that hydrolyze nucleic acids. However, because they are protein-based, prions are susceptible to procedures that denature proteins, such as exposure to proteases.

Prion protein (*PrP*), an amyloid protein encoded on chromosome 20, is the predominant or sole constituent of prions. It probably has a role in the formation of synapses, signaling between cells, and copper transportation. Normally, PrP exists in a PrP^c isoform, which is folded in a certain configuration, soluble, and easily digested by proteases. In Creutzfeldt–Jakob disease and related illnesses, PrP^c is transformed to the PrP^{Sc} isoform, which is folded differently, insoluble in most detergents, and considered to be pathogenic. Although PrP^{Sc} does not reproduce in the conventional sense, it continuously reconfigures PrP^c into PrP^{Sc}, which aggregates in neurons. As PrP^{Sc}-induced changes accumulate, the cerebral cortex takes on a distinctive microscopic, vacuolar (sponge-like) appearance (*spongiform encephalopathy*). Special histologic stains can detect PrP^{Sc}.

Although Creutzfeldt–Jakob disease meets the criteria for an infectious illness, histologic CNS specimens lack the inflammatory cells normally seen in infections. Creutzfeldt–Jakob disease nevertheless serves as the primary example of a *prion infection* causing a *transmissible spongiform encephalopathy*.

During the course of Creutzfeldt–Jakob disease, the EEG usually shows periodic sharp-wave complexes that can confirm a clinical impression (see Fig. 10.6). Brain MRI in Creutzfeldt–Jakob disease typically shows hyperintensities in cerebral cortex and deep nuclei. As additional evidence, the CSF in Creutzfeldt–Jakob disease usually contains elevated concentrations of markers of rapid neuronal injury, including total tau protein, 14-3-3 protein, and neuron-specific enolase, but none of these is entirely specific and they can be present in other illnesses characterized by acute neuronal death such as encephalitis, hypoxia, and tumors. Some studies have tentatively diagnosed Creutzfeldt–Jakob disease by locating PrP^{Sc} deposits in olfactory nerves and even in extraneural organs, such as the spleen and muscle.

If all else fails, neurologists consider a brain biopsy. In Creutzfeldt–Jakob disease cerebral tissue shows spongiform changes. However, because of the dangers in obtaining and processing the tissue, and the absence of effective treatment, neurosurgeons usually perform cerebral biopsies only if treatable alternative diagnoses, such as vasculitis or lymphoma, are reasonably likely. Although researchers have deciphered the pathophysiology, neurologists cannot offer effective treatment.

Other Spongiform Encephalopathies

Several other spongiform encephalopathies occasionally develop in humans or animals. In general, their symptoms do not appear until after an incubation period of many years and reflect only CNS involvement. As with Creutzfeldt–Jakob disease, their symptoms consist primarily of mental deterioration accompanied by myoclonus and ataxia, and their course is relentlessly progressive and ultimately fatal.

Several spongiform encephalopathies remain confined to animals. For example, *scrapie* causes sheep and goats to scrape against walls so forcefully and repeatedly that they rub off patches of their coat. (PrP^{Sc} is named after the "scrapie prion.") In *transmissible mink encephalopathy*, infected mink show vicious behavior and then progressive deterioration of their motor function.

Bovine spongiform encephalopathy (*BSE*), commonly known as "mad cow disease," is the notorious veterinary spongiform encephalopathy that struck 180,000 British cattle in the late 1980s and early 1990s. BSE caused belligerence and apprehension and then tremulousness and ataxia in affected animals. Although its origin remains a mystery, the subsequent intraspecies transmission of BSE probably resulted from slaughterhouses' incorporating scraps of infected brain and spinal cord into animal feed (offal). The wholesale slaughter of almost 4 million cattle halted the epidemic in Britain; however, isolated animals with the disease have appeared in the United States, Canada, Japan, and Western Europe.

In an American counterpart of BSE, which also was brought under control through draconian methods, *chronic wasting disease* (*CWD*) of deer and elk arose in these species living in the Rocky Mountain States and adjacent provinces of Canada. Infected animals lost muscle, strength, and vitality before succumbing. Because elk and deer are not carnivorous, exchange of bodily fluids probably transmitted this illness.

Among prion diseases affecting humans, *kuru*, characterized by dementia, tremulousness, dysarthria, and ataxia, plagued members of the Fore Tribe of New Guinea during the mid-20th century. Until Australian and American health officials discovered and stopped their cannibalism, tribe members, most often women and their children preparing ritual meals, evidently inoculated themselves with infected brain tissue. The health officials found that an asymptomatic incubation period was 4 years to 30 years, but once victims showed symptoms, they usually died within the year.

Some spongiform encephalopathies appear to affect only individuals with a genetic susceptibility. *Gerstmann–Sträussler–Scheinker* (*GSS*) disease causes dysarthria, ataxia, and dementia and follows an autosomal dominant pattern. GSS is rarer than Creutzfeldt–Jakob disease, has an earlier age of onset, and progresses more slowly. Most GSS patients have a mutation on the PrP gene situated on chromosome 20, which presumably confers genetic susceptibility. *Fatal familial insomnia* is a sleep disorder that also depends on a genetic vulnerability.

Variant Creutzfeldt–Jakob Disease

An alarm arose in the 1990s when many people in Great Britain succumbed to the human counterpart of BSE, *variant Creutzfeldt–Jakob disease* (*vCJD*). Their illness probably represented an interspecies transfer of a prion illness. Victims were usually young adults (mean age 27 years) who developed psychiatric disturbances, then painful paresthesias, and lastly neurologic dysfunction. The initial symptoms consisted of dysphoria, withdrawal, and anxiety. Subsequently patients developed more substantial disturbances – memory impairment, inattention, aggression, and disordered thinking. Dementia, accompanied in many cases by myoclonus and decorticate posture, eventually supervened.

Victims died after an approximately 14-month course. About 200 individuals died – almost all of them British citizens, visitors, or individuals who ate meat exported from Britain. The widespread slaughter of infected and potentially infected cattle ended the epidemics of both BSE and vCJD.

Physicians should note two aspects of vCJD. It was a cause of dementia in adolescents and young adults (Box 7.3). Its initial symptoms were largely psychiatric and unaccompanied by objective physical neurologic correlates.

The EEG in vCJD shows nonspecific slowing rather than the characteristic periodic pattern of Creutzfeldt–Jakob disease. As in Creutzfeldt–Jakob disease, the MRI has characteristic abnormalities. Pharyngeal tonsil biopsy tissue in vCJD cases contained evidence of prion infection. Genetic testing found at least one gene that was a risk factor for vCJD.

Several conditions mimic Creutzfeldt–Jakob disease and vCJD. Lithium or bismuth intoxication or Hashimoto encephalopathy may produce myoclonus with dementia; however, these conditions usually cause more of a delirium than dementia, and all are readily diagnosable with specific blood tests. Paraneoplastic syndromes also might produce wasting, myoclonus, ataxia, and dementia (see Chapter 19).

Lyme Disease

Acute *Lyme disease* (*neuroborreliosis*), which involves the nervous system in less than 15% of cases, may cause facial palsy (cranial neuritis), headache, peripheral neuropathy or radiculopathy, meningitis, or encephalitis. With an acute CNS infection, patients may be delirious, but their serum and CSF tests are usually positive. The typical CSF profile consists of lymphocytic pleocytosis, elevated protein concentration, reduced glucose concentration, and positive Lyme serologies.

A standard 2- to 4-week course of antibiotics cures almost every patient with an acute CNS infection. However, despite thorough treatment and resolution of CSF and serologic abnormalities, approximately 15% of patients remain with numerous and variable symptoms, particularly muscle and joint pain, sleep disturbances, fatigue, inattention, memory impairment, and depressed mood. Patients, much more often than physicians, attribute their symptoms to "chronic Lyme disease," implying persistence of the infection.

Studies have shown that many of these patients do not have a persistently positive serum Lyme titer. Even if their titer were persistently positive, the persistence would be analogous to life-long abnormal serologies after successful syphilis treatment. Moreover, when Lyme tests are positive, the titers do not correlate with memory impairments. Confusing matters somewhat, because the infectious agent, *Borrelia burgdorferi*, is a spirochete as is *T. pallidum*, the causative agent of syphilis, serum FTA-ABS and VDRL tests may turn positive in Lyme disease. Chronic Lyme disease patients often report that repeated courses of antibiotics or other nontraditional treatments reduce their symptoms, but large-scale studies do not support such claims. Nevertheless, the nature of chronic Lyme symptoms remains enigmatic. Some symptoms fall into the realm of depression or chronic fatigue syndrome (see Chapter 6).

Human Immunodeficiency Virus-Associated Dementia

After a long evolution, current terminology among neurologists recognizes a spectrum of *HIV-associated neurocognitive disorder* (*HAND*) divided into three subtypes ranging from asymptomatic neurocognitive impairment (mildest) to mild NCD to HIV-associated dementia (human immunodeficiency virus-associated dementia [HAD], most severe). All of these are subsumed under the DSM-5 category of Neurocognitive Disorder Due to HIV Infection. The advent of highly-active antiretroviral therapy (HAART) has reduced the prevalence of the severe HIV-associated dementia, but the overall prevalence of HAND remains largely unchanged at 44%.

In the brain, HIV primarily infects macrophages and microglia rather than neurons. The infection involves the subcortical as well as cortical structures. The duration of HIV infection and the progression from uncomplicated HIV infection to AIDS correlate most closely with the onset of HAD. Other risk factors for HAD are the nadir CD4 count, advanced age, ApoE4 alleles, anemia, low platelet count, substance abuse, TBI, coinfection with hepatitis C, and depression.

In untreated patients, low CD4 counts (usually below 200 cells/ml) and high plasma viral loads also correlate with the onset of HAD. However, in HIV patients receiving antiretroviral medications, HAD may complicate their illness without the usual markers of susceptibility. In other words, occasionally HIV patients develop HAD despite relatively high CD4 counts and low plasma and CSF viral loads. As a practical matter, if an HIV-positive patient receiving antiretroviral therapy shows signs of HAND, physicians should check for the patient's compliance with the medication regimen and be sure that all components of the regimen cross the blood–brain barrier.

Manifestations

Because HAD develops rapidly – over several weeks to a few months – neurologists include it as a "rapidly progressive dementia." Impairments arise in four domains: memory, attention, psychomotor speed, and construction.

HAD patients initially remain verbal and articulate. Later, reticence, apathy, and withdrawal predominate.

Psychomotor retardation, loss of dexterity, and gait impairment, which reflect infection of deep cerebral structures, are so characteristic that neurologists consider HAD a prime example of subcortical dementia. Even in the elderly, the rapidity of onset and presence of psychomotor retardation and gait impairment readily separate the clinical picture of HAD from Alzheimer disease.

Patients eventually decline into a persistent vegetative state (see Chapter 11). Myoclonus, extrapyramidal signs, and slowed ocular saccades and pursuits (see Chapter 12) – signs of basal ganglia and brainstem impairment – may also complicate this phase.

Treatment

HAART improves cognitive function in HAD patients and reduces the systemic complications of HIV infection. Instituting HAART as early as possible may decrease the risk of developing HAND. However, HAART is not a panacea or even easy to take. Patients must strictly adhere to a demanding multidrug schedule. Many patients, especially those with denial, depression, or dementia, have difficulty adhering to it. Several agents, such as efavirenz and zidovudine, can cause cognitive impairment or even psychosis. Components that rely on the cytochrome P450 enzyme system for metabolism potentially create adverse drug–drug interactions. Furthermore, some produce neuropathy, interfere with methadone and precipitate opiate withdrawal, or, because they interfere with mitochondrial metabolism, cause myopathy (see Chapters 5 and 6).

Most concerning, some research has suggested that HAART drugs with superior CNS penetration are actually correlated with higher risk of HAD. The reasons for this association are unclear, but could include poorer compliance with these medications, direct toxicity to the brain, or the effect of complications, such as the immune reconstitution inflammatory syndrome (IRIS).

In addition to antiviral therapy, other therapies that may be useful include stimulants such as dextroamphetamine and methylphenidate, which may ameliorate fatigue, psychomotor retardation, and depressed mood. Depression is prevalent in AIDS patients and particularly in those with HAD. It interferes with medication adherence, which exacerbates the illnesses and worsens cognitive impairment, allows rapid progression of the illness, and increases mortality. Physicians should prescribe antidepressants not only for the usual indications, but also to increase compliance with HAART and other medical regimens.

Testing

In HAD, both CT and MRI show cerebral atrophy with enlarged ventricles and basal ganglia abnormalities. MRI may, in addition, show nonspecific scattered white matter abnormalities. CSF typically reveals a mild lymphocytic pleocytosis, normal or slightly elevated protein concentration, and, as a nonspecific reflection of inflammation, oligoclonal bands. Physicians routinely measure the CD4 count and viral load in the blood. Depending on the circumstance, they might order additional tests for other illnesses that are associated with drug abuse or unsafe sex, such as hepatitis, syphilis, and bacterial endocarditis.

At autopsy, the brain is atrophic and pale. Changes are most apparent in the frontal lobes and basal ganglia. Microscopic examination shows perivascular infiltrates, gliosis of the cerebral cortex, demyelination, microglial nodules, and multinucleated giant cells. Evidence of HIV is detectable in the brains and CSF of almost all HAD patients.

AIDS-Induced Cerebral Lesions

Infectious or neoplastic AIDS-induced cerebral lesions, like other cerebral lesions, cause headache, focal seizures, lateralized signs, and increased intracranial pressure. Moreover, they can exacerbate cognitive, personality, and mood disorders.

A pitfall for physicians is attributing headaches to depression in AIDS patients. In this setting, headaches actually represent a particularly ominous symptom. They may signal serious underlying pathology, such as cryptococcal meningitis or cerebral toxoplasmosis.

Second to HIV itself, *Toxoplasma gondii* causes the most common AIDS-related CNS infection, *cerebral toxoplasmosis*. This protozoan typically produces multiple ring-shaped enhancing lesions that are readily detectable by CT or MRI (see Fig. 20.11). Serologic testing is available and this infection readily responds to antibiotics. Neurologists recommend a cerebral biopsy for patients who do not improve after several weeks of antibiotic treatment.

Progressive multifocal leukoencephalopathy (PML), one of the most commonly occurring brain lesions in AIDS patients, complicates the latter stages of the illness. The *JC virus* causes this illness by infecting oligodendroglia, which generate and maintain the CNS myelin. ("JC" are the initials of the patient from whom the virus was first isolated and identified as a human polyomavirus. Do not confuse JC with Jakob–Creutzfeldt, the prion disease.) PML also complicates other conditions that impair immunity, such as leukemia and lymphoma, and may occur with immunosuppressive therapy, including treatment for MS and organ transplantation.

Through damage to oligodendroglia, the infection leads to demyelination in the white (Greek, *leuko*) matter of the brain and spinal cord (see Fig. 15.11). As its name implies, PML produces multiple, widespread, and often confluent white matter lesions.

PML patients show combinations of cognitive impairment, hemiparesis, spasticity, blindness, and ataxia. These deficits accumulate insidiously and irreversibly. Two tests may confirm a clinical impression of PML. MRI typically shows characteristic multiple areas of demyelination without mass effect that slowly become confluent. Polymerase chain reaction (PCR) techniques detect JC virus DNA in the CSF.

Other infections that cause cerebral lesions in AIDS patients include fungi, such as *Candida*, and *Aspergillus*, and other viruses, such as cytomegalovirus (CMV).

Although actually rare in the HAART era, the most common cerebral neoplasm complicating HIV disease remains *primary central nervous system lymphoma* (see Chapter 19). This lymphoma, unlike toxoplasmosis, usually presents as a solitary lesion. In cases of AIDS-associated CNS lymphoma, spinal fluid testing usually detects Epstein–Barr virus DNA.

Other AIDS-Related Conditions

All components of the nervous system are vulnerable to infection. Patients can contract HIV encephalitis, myelitis, meningitis, neuropathy, and myopathy. All CNS tissue, especially CSF, is infectious.

The spinal cord is subject to HIV infection as well as lymphoma. HIV infection of the spinal cord causes *vacuolar myelopathy* that results in paraparesis, the Romberg sign, and other indications of spinal cord injury. The damage is located predominantly in the posterior columns (the fasciculi gracilis and cuneatus [see Chapter 2]). Although this pattern resembles subacute combined degeneration, vitamin B_{12} treatment does not alleviate the problem.

A virus related to HIV, the *human T-cell lymphotrophic virus type 1* (*HTLV-1*) similarly infects the spinal cord and causes paraparesis; however, it does not lead to cognitive impairment. Like HIV, HTLV-1 is transmitted sexually and by blood transfusion. Because HTLV-1 infection of the spinal cord, *HTLV-1 myelopathy*, is endemic in the Caribbean region and Africa, neurologists have called it "tropical spastic paraparesis." HTLV-1 can also affect muscle and nerve, causing myopathy and neuropathy, respectively.

Nutritional deficiencies are prevalent among patients with HIV and AIDS. Clinicians should consider looking for evidence of malnutrition, such as a deficiency of vitamins B_1 and B_{12}, in patients with HAND.

PSEUDODEMENTIA

When a psychiatric disturbance produces or mimics cognitive dysfunction, physicians call the apparent cognitive impairment *pseudodementia*. Depression is most often responsible, but anxiety, psychosis, and other psychiatric conditions may produce the same problem.

Despite the overlapping symptoms of dementia and depression, physicians should attempt to separate them. Depression does not significantly impair performance on cognitive testing if testers provide enough time and encouragement. On the other hand, clinicians biased toward diagnosing Alzheimer disease may err if they fail to appreciate a patient's mood. They may compound that error by overestimating the significance of age-related neurologic test results, such as mild EEG slowing and cerebral atrophy on CT or MRI.

Although the immediate diagnosis may appear to be depression, studies have shown that patients who seem to have depression-induced cognitive impairment develop Alzheimer disease dementia almost six times more frequently than their age-adjusted counterparts. Some studies have found that depression – especially recurrent depression – is a risk factor for dementia. Contrary to classic literature citing pseudodementia as the most frequent "correctable cause of dementia," pseudodementia is often a harbinger of dementia.

DELIRIUM/TOXIC-METABOLIC ENCEPHALOPATHY

The core characteristics of *delirium* (Latin, derangement) are an altered level of awareness and inability to maintain attention. While the DSM-5 uses the term "delirium," neurologists usually call the same condition *toxic-metabolic encephalopathy*, which is cumbersome but valid. When apparent, neurologists specify the cause, such as uremic or hepatic encephalopathy.

By anyone's terminology, delirium is one of the most commonly occurring and deadliest disturbances in neurology. Among hospital patients 65 years or older, delirium occurs in approximately 20%, and in 75% of patients in intensive care units. Delirium is a powerful risk factor for death. For example, in this group of patients, delirium carries a mortality rate of greater than 33%. Its duration correlates with the mortality rate and with worse cognition when assessed months later.

Characteristics

Neurologists, like psychiatrists, initially diagnose delirium when patients have depressed or otherwise altered levels of consciousness, disorientation, and inattention – usually in the context of a medical illness or intoxication. Patients are typically amnestic and beset by perceptual disorders. They usually have autonomic system hyperactivity. However, some patients exhibit a hyperactive and hypervigilant state with fixed, undivided attention. Depending on the underlying illness, seizures may complicate the condition.

Symptoms arise over several hours to several days and then fluctuate hourly to daily; often they are worse at night. They usually resolve with successful treatment of the underlying medical problem, but improvement occasionally lags (Fig. 7.9).

Delirium in children and adolescents typically causes sleep disturbances and disorientation. In the majority of them, delirium also causes inattention, short-term amnesia, and agitation.

Some signs allow a bedside diagnosis of a specific underlying illness. For example, patients with Wernicke–Korsakoff syndrome typically have oculomotor palsies, nystagmus, ataxia, and polyneuropathy. Those with hepatic or uremic encephalopathy have *asterixis* (Fig. 7.10). Those with uremia, penicillin or bismuth intoxication, meperidine (Demerol) treatment, and several other metabolic encephalopathies have myoclonus. Narcotic or barbiturate intoxication causes constricted pupils, but amphetamine, atropine, or sympathomimetic drug intoxication causes dilated pupils.

EEG typically shows background slowing and disorganization (see Chapter 10); however, numerous conditions cause the same alterations. Some EEG findings suggest a specific etiology. For example, triphasic waves often indicate hepatic or uremic encephalopathy (see Fig. 10.5). The clinical abnormalities and EEG findings

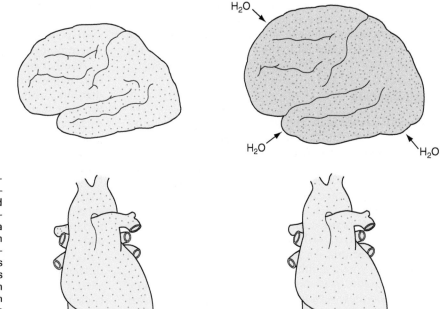

FIGURE 7.9 ■ A distressing clinical situation occurs when patients deteriorate – become confused, lethargic, and agitated – after apparent correction of certain metabolic abnormalities. *A*, In cases of uremia or hyperglycemia, the brain and serum contain an approximately equal concentration of solute (dots). *B*, Overly vigorous dialysis or insulin administration clears solute more rapidly from the serum than the brain, leaving solute concentration in the brain much greater than in the serum. The concentration gradient causes free water to move into the brain, which produces cerebral edema.

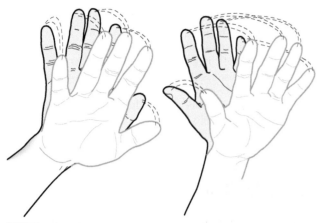

FIGURE 7.10 ■ Neurologists elicit asterixis by having patients extend their arms and hands as though they were stopping traffic. Their hands intermittently quickly fall forward and slowly return, as though flapping or waving good-bye.

chiefly reflect dysfunction of the cerebral hemispheres, but dysfunction of the reticular activating system also may be responsible.

CT and MRI frequently show cerebral atrophy because of age-related atrophy or comorbid dementia-producing illness. Neurologists routinely order a scan to exclude a structural lesion as either a cause or complication of delirium. For example, they might order a CT to exclude an acute subdural hematoma in an alcoholic patient with falls.

Most patients recover from delirium if the underlying illness responds to treatment, but sometimes, as in anoxic encephalopathy, patients are left with permanent cognitive impairment. Physicians must bear in mind that overly rapid correction of metabolic derangements, such as hyponatremia, can lead to *central pontine myelinolysis*, a prime example of the *osmotic demyelination syndrome*. Vulnerable patients, such as alcoholics with malnutrition, liver transplant recipients, and pregnant women with hyperemesis, lose myelin in their pons and are often left with permanent nystagmus, quadriparesis, and ataxia.

Risk Factors

Dementia represents the most powerful and most common risk factor for delirium. It may also explain why patients' confusion sometimes persists – perhaps indefinitely – after medical treatment has corrected the underlying disorder. In actuality, delirium in a patient with dementia often precedes accelerated cognitive decline or imminent death.

In general, brain damage from any cause, including congenital injuries, TBI, and Alzheimer disease, is a risk factor for delirium. An immature as well as a damaged brain leaves young children especially susceptible.

Hearing and visual impairments are also risk factors. Not only do these sensory deprivations frequently coexist with dementia in the elderly, they also intensify the symptoms. As survivors of torture attest, sensory deprivation even in healthy young adults may cause disturbances akin to delirium.

BOX 7.5	Commonly Cited Causes of Delirium

Dementia
Fluid or electrolyte imbalance, especially dehydration
Hepatic or uremic encephalopathy, and other organ failure
Medications
Narcotics or alcohol
Sensory deprivation
Pain
Pneumonia, urinary tract infections, and other nonneurologic infections
Sepsis
Sleep disturbance
Immobility
Constipation

Causes

Innumerable disorders, alone or in combination, may cause delirium; however, relatively few account for the majority of cases in acute care hospitals and nursing homes (Box 7.5). Medicines are a frequent cause of delirium. Even when administered in a low dose, medications may have this unintended effect when given to a previously unexposed patient. Medicine-related problems also include the build-up of toxic concentrations because of inadequate hepatic metabolism or renal clearance, drug–drug interactions, or absorption of ocular or topical medicines. Ironically, medicines for psychiatric and neurologic disorders – including anticholinergics, AEDs, antiparkinson agents, opioids, and serotonin agents – readily cross the blood–brain barrier and can produce delirium. In a surprising and paradoxical example, intramuscular injections of olanzapine administered for schizophrenia may produce confusion, agitation, anxiety, sedation, and more severely depressed levels of consciousness rather than calming the patient. Researchers have labeled this reaction the *post-injection delirium/sedation syndrome* (*PDSS*) and attribute it to the medicine seeping into the vasculature.

Another consideration is medicine withdrawal. Unlike the depressed sensorium typically associated with delirium, withdrawal from benzodiazepines, opioids, or nicotine may cause an agitated delirium. In addition, withdrawal from alcohol, barbiturates, and benzodiazepines – but not nicotine – routinely causes seizures.

General Treatments

Even before arriving at an exact diagnosis or instituting specific treatment, physicians must ascertain that the patient has adequate cerebral oxygen, blood glucose, fluid and electrolytes, nutrition, and other necessities. Pain, infection, constipation, and disordered sleep are other factors that physicians can usually treat. Physicians should minimize polypharmacy, and avoidance of psychoactive drugs is particularly crucial. Other nonpharmacologic measures consist of providing orientation cues, such as illumination, clocks, and calendars, and promoting a familiar environment by surrounding the patient with objects from home and minimizing changes in hospital personnel. Assigning the patient to a bed with a window can help with orientation to time of day.

When pharmacotherapy for delirium is considered, antipsychotics can reduce dangerous and exhausting activity, hallucinations, and disordered thinking. Physicians should hesitate before prescribing antipsychotics or benzodiazepines to avoid respiratory depression. Sometimes physicians can calm a dangerously disruptive patient by restoring a missing substance or providing a reasonable alternative, such as methadone or a nicotine patch.

Hepatic Encephalopathy

A particularly interesting and frequently occurring example of delirium is *hepatic encephalopathy*. With hepatic insufficiency, mental function and consciousness steadily decline. Mild confusion with either lethargy or, less frequently, agitation may precede coma and overtly abnormal liver function tests. In classic cases, the neurologic examination demonstrates asterixis and the EEG shows triphasic waves.

Neurologists traditionally attribute hepatic encephalopathy to an elevated serum concentration of ammonia (NH_3). This mechanism occurs in the common scenario of gastrointestinal bleeding or high-protein meals in patients with cirrhosis. In these situations, cirrhosis-induced portal hypertension shunts NH_3 released from protein in blood or food directly into the systemic circulation. Because NH_3 is a small and nonionic (uncharged) molecule, it readily penetrates the blood–brain barrier. As a treatment of hepatic encephalopathy, physicians often administer lactulose in an attempt to acidify the gastrointestinal tract. This strategy promotes conversion of ammonia (NH_3) to ammonium (NH_4^+), which is ionic and unable to penetrate the blood–brain barrier.

An alternative explanation for hepatic encephalopathy emphasizes the production of false neurotransmitters that bind to benzodiazepine–gamma amino butyric acid (GABA) receptors and increase GABA activity. Thus, giving flumazenil, a benzodiazepine antagonist that interferes with benzodiazepine-GABA receptors (but carries some risk of precipitating seizures) temporarily reduces hepatic encephalopathy symptoms.

PRECAUTIONS IN DIAGNOSING ALZHEIMER DISEASE

Even though this and other chapters have presented numerous causes of dementia and delirium, Alzheimer disease occupies the preeminent position in the diagnosis of dementia, especially in the elderly. Physicians should maintain vigilance and recall the "red flags" that warn against its diagnosis (Box 7.6). Although they certainly do not preclude a diagnosis of Alzheimer disease, these red flags will help prevent a misdiagnosis in cases of toxic-metabolic encephalopathy, psychiatric disorders, dementia in young adults (see Box 7.3), and neurodegenerative illnesses that strike at more than the brain's cognitive centers.

REFERENCES

Age-Related Changes

Alladi, S., Bak, T. H., Duggirala, V., et al. (2013). Bilingualism delays age at onset of dementia, independent of education and immigration status. *Neurology, 81,* 1938–1944.

Clarfield, A. M. (2003). The decreasing prevalence of reversible dementias. *Archives of Internal Medicine, 163,* 2219–2229.

Folstein, M. R., Folstein, S. E., & McHugh, P. R. (1975). "Mini-Mental State:" A practical method for grading the cognitive state of patients for the clinician. *Journal of Psychiatric Research, 12,* 189–198.

Iverson, D. J., Groseth, G. S., Reger, M. A., et al. (2010). Practice parameter: Evaluation and management of driving risk in dementia. Report of the Quality Standards Subcommittee of the American Academy of Neurology. *Neurology, 74,* 1316–1324.

Larson, E. B., Yaffe, K., & Langa, K. (2013). New insights into the dementia epidemic. *The New England Journal of Medicine, 369*(24), 2275–2277.

Luis, C. A., Keegan, A. P., & Mullan, M. (2009). Cross validation of the Montreal Cognitive Assessment in community dwelling older adults residing in the Southeastern US. *International Journal of Geriatric Psychiatry, 24,* 197–201.

Nasreddine, Z. S., Phillips, N. A., Bedirian, V., et al. (2005). The Montreal Cognitive Assessment, MoCA: A brief screening tool for mild cognitive impairment. *Journal of the American Geriatrics Society, 53,* 695–699.

Smyth, A., Dehghan, M., O'Donnell, M., et al. (2015). Healthy eating and reduced risk of cognitive decline: A cohort from 40 countries. *Neurology, 84,* 2258–2265.

Thurman, D. J., Stevens, J. A., & Rao, J. K. (2008). Practice parameter: Assessing patients in neurologic practice for risk of falls. Report of the Quality Standards Subcommittee of the American Academy of Neurology. *Neurology, 70,* 473–479.

Verghese, J., Annweiler, C., Ayers, E., et al. (2014). Motoric cognitive risk syndrome: Multicountry prevalence and dementia risk. *Neurology, 83-718,* 726.

Alzheimer Disease

Albert, M., Soldan, A., Selnes, O., et al. Using combinations of variables to identify individuals with preclinical AD. Abstract #1540. Presented at: Alzheimer's Association International Conference 2015; July 18–23, 2015; Washington, DC.

Allan, L. M., Ballard, C. G., Burn, D. J., et al. (2005). Prevalence and severity of gait disorders in Alzheimer's and non-Alzheimer's dementias. *Journal of the American Geriatrics Society, 53*, 1681–1687.

Ballard, C., Hanney, M. L., Theodoulou, M., et al. (2009). The dementia antipsychotic withdrawal trial (DART-AD): Long-term follow-up of a randomized placebo-controlled trial. *The Lancet. Neurology, 8*, 151–157.

Green, R. C., Roberts, J. S., Cupples, L. A., et al. (2009). Disclosure of APOE genotype for risk of Alzheimer's disease. *The New England Journal of Medicine, 361*, 245–254.

Larner, A. J. (2010). Cholinesterase inhibitors. *Expert Review of Neurotherapeutics, 10*, 1699–1705.

Mayeux, R. (2010). Early Alzheimer's disease. *The New England Journal of Medicine, 362*, 2194–2201.

Meyer, G. D., Shapiro, F., Vanderstichele, H., et al. (2010). Diagnosis-independent Alzheimer disease biomarker signature in cognitively normal elderly people. *Archives of Neurology, 67*, 949–956.

Ott, B. R., Heindel, W. C., & Papandonatos, G. D. (2003). A survey of voter participation by cognitively impaired elderly patients. *Neurology, 60*, 1546–1548.

Petersen, R. C. (2011). Mild cognitive impairment. *The New England Journal of Medicine, 364*, 2227–2234.

Rossetti, H. C., Lacritz, L. H., & Weiner, M. F. (2011). Normative data for the Montreal Cognitive Assessment (MoCA) in a population-based sample. *Neurology, 77*, 1272–1275.

Querfurth, H. W., & LaFeria, F. M. (2010). Alzheimer's disease. *The New England Journal of Medicine, 362*, 329–344.

Schneider, L. S., Tariot, P. N., Dagerman, K. S., et al. (2006). Effectiveness of atypical antipsychotic drugs in patients with Alzheimer's disease. *The New England Journal of Medicine, 355*, 1525–1538.

Shi, J., Han, P., & Kuniyoshi, S. (2014). Cognitive impairment in neurological diseases: lessons from apolipoprotein E. *Journal of Alzheimer's Disease, 38*, 1–9.

Sperling, R. A., Aisen, P. S., Beckett, L. A., et al. (2011). Toward defining the preclinical stages of Alzheimer's disease: Recommendations from the National Institute on Aging-Alzheimer's Association workgroups on diagnostic guidelines for Alzheimer's disease. *Alzheimer's & Dementia, 7*, 280–292.

Sultzer, D. L., Davis, S. M., Tariot, P. N., et al. (2008). Clinical symptom responses to atypical antipsychotic medications in Alzheimer's disease: Phase 1 outcomes from the CATIE–AD Effectiveness Trial. *The American Journal of Psychiatry, 165*, 844–854.

Yaffe, K., Weston, A., Graff-Radford, N. R., et al. (2011). Association of plasma beta-amyloid and cognitive reserve with subsequent cognitive decline. *JAMA: The Journal of the American Medical Association, 305*, 261–266.

HIV-Associated Dementia

Cohen, R. A., & Gongvatana, A. (2010). The persistence of HIV-associated neurocognitive dysfunction and the effects of comorbidities. *Neurology, 75*, 2052–2053.

Elbirt, D., Mahlab-Guri, K., Bezalel-Rosenberg, S., et al. (2015). HIV-associated neurocognitive disorders (HAND). *The Israel Medical Association Journal, 17*, 54–59.

Heaton, R. K., Clifford, D. B., Franklin, D. R., et al. (2010). HIV-associated neurocognitive disorders persist in the era of potent antiretroviral therapy: CHARTER Study. *Neurology, 75*, 2087–2096.

Rackstraw, S. (2011). HIV-related neurocognitive impairment – a review. *Psychology, Health and Medicine, 16*, 548–563.

Dementia With Lewy Bodies

Boot, B. P., Orr, C. F., Ahlskog, J. E., et al. (2013). Risk factors for dementia with Lewy bodies: A case-control study. *Neurology, 81*, 833–840.

Devinsky, O. (2008). The neurology of Capgras syndrome. *Reviews in Neurological Diseases, 5*, 97–100.

Geser, F., Wenning, G. K., Poewe, W., et al. (2005). How to diagnose dementia with Lewy bodies: State of the art. *Movement Disorders: Official Journal of the Movement Disorder Society, 12*(Suppl. 12), S11–S20.

Goldman, J. G., Goetz, C. G., Brandabur, M., et al. (2008). Effects of dopaminergic medications on psychosis and motor function in dementia with Lewy bodies. *Movement Disorders: Official Journal of the Movement Disorder Society, 23*, 2248–2250.

McKeith, I. G., Dickson, D. W., Lowe, J., et al. (2005). Diagnosis and management of dementia with Lewy bodies: Third report of the DLB consortium. *Neurology, 65*, 1863–1872.

Nagahma, Y., Okina, T., Suzuki, N., et al. (2010). Neural correlates of psychiatric symptoms in dementia with Lewy bodies. *Brain: A Journal of Neurology, 133*, 557–567.

Depression and Pseudodementia

Dotosn, V. M., Beydoun, M. A., & Zonderman, A. B. (2010). Recurrent depressive symptoms and the incidence of dementia and mild cognitive impairment. *Neurology, 75*, 27–34.

Goodman, W. K. (2011). Electroconvulsive therapy in the spotlight. *The New England Journal of Medicine, 364*, 1785–1789.

Saczynski, J. S., Beiser, A., Seshadri, S., et al. (2010). Depressive symptoms and risk of dementia: The Framingham Heart Study. *Neurology, 75*, 35–41.

Taylor, W. D. (2014). Depression in the elderly. *The New England Journal of Medicine, 371*, 1228–1236.

Frontotemporal Dementia

Boeve, B. F., Boylan, K. B., Graff-Redford, N. R., et al. (2012). Characterization of frontotemporal dementia and/or amyotrophic lateral sclerosis associated with the GGGGCC repeat expansion in C9ORF72. *Brain: A Journal of Neurology, 135*, 765–783.

Kertesz, A., Blair, M., McMonagle, P., et al. (2007). The diagnosis and course of frontotemporal dementia. *Alzheimer Disease and Associated Disorders, 21*, 155–163.

Kucharski, A. (1984). History of frontal lobotomy in the United States, 1935–1955. *Neurosurgery, 14*, 762–772.

Rascovsky, K., Hodges, J. R., & Knopman, D. (2011). Sensitivity of revised diagnostic criteria for the behavioral variant of frontotemporal dementia. *Brain: A Journal of Neurology, 134*, 2456–2477.

Lyme Disease

Feder, H. M., Johnson, B. J. B., O'Connell, S., et al. (2007). A critical appraisal of "chronic Lyme disease." *The New England Journal of Medicine, 357*, 1422–1430.

Halperin, J. J. (2011). Neurologic manifestations of Lyme disease. *Current Infectious Disease Reports, 13*, 360–366.

Creutzfeldt–Jakob Disease and Related Illnesses

Binelli, S., Agazzi, P., Canafoglia, L., et al. (2010). Myoclonus in Creutzfeldt-Jakob disease. *Movement Disorders, 25*, 2818–2827.

Heath, C. A., Cooper, S. A., Murray, K., et al. (2010). Validation of diagnostic criteria for variant Creutzfeldt-Jakob disease. *Annals of Neurology, 67*, 761–770.

Heath, C. A., Cooper, S. A., Murray, K., et al. (2011). Diagnosing variant Creutzfeldt-Jakob disease: A retrospective analysis of the first 150 cases in the UK. *Journal of Neurology, Neurosurgery, and Psychiatry, 82*, 646–651.

Paterson, R. W., Takada, L. T., & Geschwind, M. D. (2012). Diagnosis and treatment of rapidly progressive dementias. *Neurology Clinical Practice, 2*, 187–200.

Prusiner, S. B. (2001). Neurodegenerative diseases and prions. *The New England Journal of Medicine, 344*, 1516–1526.

Rabinovici, G. D., Wang, P. N., Levin, J., et al. (2006). First symptom in sporadic Creutzfeldt-Jakob disease. *Neurology, 66*, 286–287.

Schott, J. M., Reiniger, L., Thom, M., et al. (2010). Brain biopsy in dementia: Clinical indications and diagnostic approach. *Acta Neuropathologica, 120*, 327–341.

Williams, E. S., & Miller, M. W. (2002). Chronic wasting disease in deer and elk. *Revue Scientifique et Technique, 1*, 305–316.

Zerr, I., Kallenberg, K., Summers, D. M., et al. (2009). Updated clinical diagnostic criteria for sporadic Creutzfeldt-Jakob disease. *Brain: A Journal of Neurology, 132*, 2659–2668.

Delirium (Toxic-Metabolic Encephalopathy)

Detke, H. C., McDonnell, D. P., Brunner, E., et al. (2010). Post-injection delirium/sedation syndrome in patients with schizophrenia treated with olanzapine long-acting injection: Analysis of cases. *BMC Psychiatry, 10*, 43.

Grover, S., Malhotra, S., Bharadwaj, R., et al. (2009). Delirium in children and adolescents. *International Journal of Psychiatry in Medicine, 39*, 179–187.

Grover, S., Mattoo, S. K., & Gupta, N. (2011). Usefulness of atypical antipsychotics and choline esterase inhibitors in delirium: A review. *Pharmacopsychiatry, 44*, 43–54.

Inouye, S. K. (2006). Delirium in older persons. *The New England Journal of Medicine, 354*, 1157–1165.

Lonergan, E., Luxenberg, J., Areosa-Sastre, A., et al. (2009). Benzodiazepines for delirium. *The Cochrane Database of Systematic Reviews*, (1), CD006397.

Meagher, D. J., Leonard, M., Donnelly, S., et al. (2010). A comparison of neuropsychiatric and cognitive profiles in delirium, dementia, comorbid delirium-dementia and cognitively intact controls. *Journal of Neurology, Neurosurgery, and Psychiatry*, *81*, 876–881.

O'Mahony, R., Murthy, L., Akunne, A., et al. (2011). Synopsis of the National Institute for Health and Clinical Excellence guideline for prevention of delirium. *Annals of Internal Medicine*, *154*, 746–751.

Ozbolt, L. B., Paniagua, M. A., & Kaiser, R. M. (2008). Atypical antipsychotics for the treatment of delirious elders. *Journal of the American Medical Directors Association*, *9*, 18–28.

Pandharipande, P. P., Girard, T. D., Jackson, J. C., et al. (2013). Long-term cognitive impairment after critical illness. *The New England Journal of Medicine*, *369*, 1306–1316.

Wong, C. L., Holyroyd-Leduc, J., Simel, D. L., et al. (2010). Does this patient have delirium? Value of bedside instruments. *JAMA: The Journal of the American Medical Association*, *304*, 779–786.

Vascular Cognitive Impairment

Gorelick, P. B., Scuteri, A., Black, S. E., et al. (2011). Vascular contributions to cognitive impairment and dementia: A statement for healthcare professionals from the American Heart Association/American Stroke Association. *Stroke; a Journal of Cerebral Circulation*, *42*, 2672–2713.

Malouf, R., & Birks, J. (2004). Donepezil for vascular cognitive impairment. *The Cochrane Database of Systematic Reviews*, (1), CD004395.

Sachdev, P. S., Brodaty, H., Valenzuela, M. J., et al. (2004). The neuropsychological profile of vascular cognitive impairment in stroke and TIA patients. *Neurology*, *62*, 912–919.

Solfrizzi, V., Scafato, E., Capurso, C., et al. (2010). Metabolic syndrome and the risk of vascular dementia: The Italian Longitudinal Study on Ageing. *Journal of Neurology, Neurosurgery, and Psychiatry*, *81*, 433–440.

Other Illnesses That Cause Dementia

Centers for Disease Control and Prevention. (2008). Syphilis testing algorithms using treponemal for initial screening: Four laboratories, New York City, 2005–2006. *Morbidity and Mortality Weekly Report*, *57*, 872–875.

Chahine, L. M., Khoriaty, R. N., Tomford, W. J., et al. (2011). The changing face of neurosyphilis. *International Journal of Stroke*, *6*, 136–143.

Ghanem, K. G. (2010). Neurosyphilis: A historical perspective and review. *CNS Neuroscience & Therapeutics*, *16*, e157–e168.

Gutierrez, J., Issacson, R. S., & Koppel, B. S. (2010). Subacute sclerosing panencephalitis: An update. *Developmental Medicine and Child Neurology*, *52*, 901–907.

Halperin, J. J., Kurlan, R., Schwalb, J. M., et al. (2015). Practice guidelines: Idiopathic normal pressure hydrocephalus: Response to shunting and predictors of response. *Neurology*, *85*, 2063–2071.

Henao-Martinez, A. F., & Johnson, S. C. (2014). Diagnostic tests for syphilis: New tests and new algorithms. *Neurology Clinical Practice*, *4*, 114–122.

Sonia, M., Lalit, D., Shobha, B., et al. (2009). Subacute sclerosing panencephalitis in a tertiary care centre in post measles vaccination era. *The Journal of Communicable Diseases*, *41*, 161–167.

Yatabe, Y., Hashimoto, M., Kaneda, K., et al. (2011). Neuropsychiatric symptoms of progressive supranuclear palsy in a dementia clinic. *Psychogeriatrics*, *11*, 54–59.

CHAPTER 7

QUESTIONS AND ANSWERS

1. Which of the following statements is *true* regarding individuals with mild cognitive impairment (MCI)?
   a. They have impairment of their social or occupational activities.
   b. As with Alzheimer disease, cholinesterase inhibitors slow the cognitive decline in MCI.
   c. Approximately 10% progress from MCI to dementia disease annually.
   d. The risk factors associated with progression of MCI to dementia differ from those for developing Alzheimer disease.

Answer: c. Mild cognitive impairment is most often the first clinical sign of Alzheimer disease. Because individuals with MCI maintain their social and occupational activities, neurologists cannot diagnose them as having dementia. However, each year approximately 10% of them progress from that stage to the next, dementia. The risk factors associated with progression of MCI to dementia are similar to those for individuals developing Alzheimer disease, including carrying the ApoE4 allele and having a family history of Alzheimer disease. Physicians should test MCI patients for correctable causes of dementia. Cholinesterase inhibitors do not slow the cognitive decline or reduce the risk of deterioration of MCI into dementia.

2. Advancing age leads to loss of neurons in the cerebral cortex and many deep structures. Which of the following structures is *not* subject to age-related neuron loss?
   a. Locus coeruleus
   b. Suprachiasmatic nucleus
   c. Substantia nigra
   d. Nucleus basalis of Meynert
   e. Mammillary bodies

Answer: e. The mammillary bodies resist age-related changes. In contrast, age-related changes in the other structures contribute to disturbances in affect (locus coeruleus), sleep (locus coeruleus and suprachiasmatic nucleus), and locomotion (substantia nigra).

3. In a 70-year-old man who has normal cognitive and physical function, which sensation is most likely to be lost?
   a. Joint position
   b. Vibration
   c. Pain
   d. Temperature

Answer: b. In normal individuals older than 65 years, vibration sensation declines to a greater degree than other sensations. Although loss of position sense is less

pronounced than diminution of vibration sense, the former is more troublesome because it leads to gait impairment and falls. In contrast, pain and temperature sensations remain relatively well preserved. Preservation of pain sensation is well known to physicians who care for elderly patients who describe painful feet from osteoarthritis, peripheral vascular disease, and diabetic neuropathy.

4. The diagnosis of normal-pressure hydrocephalus (NPH) has received much attention because installation of a ventricular-peritoneal shunt may correct the dementia. Most cases are idiopathic. Which condition predisposes a patient to NPH?
   a. Hypothyroidism
   b. Meningitis
   c. Cysticercosis
   d. Tuberous sclerosis

Answer: b. Both meningitis and subarachnoid hemorrhage can cause communicating hydrocephalus that sometimes leads to NPH. Cysticercosis and tuberous sclerosis cause obstructive hydrocephalus. Nevertheless, most cases of NPH are idiopathic.

5. *True* or *false*? A cerebral cortex biopsy is appropriate for the diagnosis of Alzheimer disease.

Answer: False. Although a definitive diagnosis is desirable, a single cerebral cortex biopsy cannot provide it because the histologic changes are quantitative rather than qualitative. For example, normal-aged brains contain the characteristic plaques and tangles – although in lesser concentrations and different distributions. Neurologists also do not request a cerebral biopsy for the diagnosis of frontotemporal dementia, dementia with Lewy bodies, or vascular cognitive impairment (VCI), which the *Diagnostic and Statistical Manual of Mental Disorders, 5th Edition*, (DSM-5) calls Vascular Neurocognitive Disorder. All these diseases are incurable and a brain biopsy carries risks of hemorrhage and seizures. On the other hand, a biopsy may have benefits that outweigh the risks in the diagnosis of Creutzfeldt–Jakob disease, variant Creutzfeldt–Jakob disease (vCJD), other infections, and neoplasms.

6. With which histologic feature is the severity of Alzheimer disease dementia most closely correlated?
   a. Accumulation of tau
   b. Increased concentration of plaques
   c. Increased concentration of tangles
   d. Degree of synapse loss

Answer: d. Although neurofibrillary tangles and, to a lesser extent, tau accumulation and plaques are associated with Alzheimer disease, loss of synapses is most closely correlated with the severity of dementia. Tau characteristically accumulates in frontotemporal dementia. On a macroscopic level, atrophy of the hippocampus is most closely associated with Alzheimer disease.

7. Which of the following types of medication is *least* likely to be helpful in treating Alzheimer disease?
   a. A β-secretase inhibitor
   b. A γ-secretase inhibitor
   c. A cholinesterase inhibitor
   d. An NMDA receptor antagonist
   e. An anticholinergic medication
   f. A monoclonal antibody directed against beta-amyloid

Answer: e. Scientists believe that a cholinergic deficit is responsible, at least in part, for the cognitive dysfunction in Alzheimer disease. Medications that enhance cholinergic stimulation (like cholinesterase inhibitors) may be helpful, and three are approved for this use (donepezil, rivastigmine, galantamine); conversely, anticholinergic medication should be avoided. An NMDA receptor antagonist, memantine, is approved for moderate to severe Alzheimer dementia. β-Secretase and γ-secretase are proteolytic enzymes that are critical to formation of beta-amyloid; inhibiting their activity might prevent its deposition. Research into immunologic therapies to clear amyloid plaques is ongoing.

8–11. What is the pattern of inheritance (a–d) of the following diseases?

8. Wilson disease
9. Huntington disease
10. Familial Creutzfeldt–Jakob disease
11. Familial Alzheimer disease
    a. Sex-linked recessive
    b. Autosomal recessive
    c. Autosomal dominant
    d. None of the above

Answer: 8–b, 9–c, 10–c, 11–c.

12–14. For each structure important in Alzheimer disease, match the name with its description (a–c).
12. Neurofibrillary tangles
13. Neuritic plaque
14. Nucleus basalis of Meynert
    a. Paired, hyperphosphorylated helical filaments
    b. Cluster of degenerating nerve terminals surrounding an amyloid core
    c. Group of neurons beneath the globus pallidus

Answer: 12–a, 13–b, 14–c.

15. Which findings are present on computed tomography (CT) or magnetic resonance imaging (MRI) in Alzheimer disease?
    a. Enlarged third ventricle and atrophy of the hippocampus
    b. Atrophy of the head of the caudate nuclei
    c. Atrophy of the cerebellar vermis

    d. Petechial hemorrhages in the mammillary bodies and periaqueductal gray matter

Answer: a. Imaging studies usually show an enlarged third ventricle and atrophy of the hippocampus in Alzheimer disease. They show atrophy of the head of the caudate nuclei in Huntington disease, atrophy of the cerebellar vermis in chronic alcoholism, and petechial hemorrhages in the mammillary bodies and periaqueductal gray matter in Wernicke–Korsakoff disease.

16. Which *two* conditions feature α-synuclein?
    a. Alzheimer disease
    b. Parkinson disease
    c. Dementia with Lewy bodies
    d. Frontotemporal dementia
    e. Huntington disease

Answer: b, c. Neurons in the basal ganglia in Parkinson disease and the cerebral cortex in dementia with Lewy bodies contain Lewy bodies – eosinophilic, intracytoplasmic inclusions that stain for α-synuclein. In other words, α-synuclein is the intraneuronal protein aggregate common to Parkinson disease and dementia with Lewy bodies. Therefore, neurologists refer to these illnesses as "synucleinopathies."

17. Which *three* conditions feature intraneuronal tau proteins?
    a. Alzheimer disease
    b. Parkinson disease
    c. Dementia with Lewy bodies
    d. Frontotemporal dementia
    e. Huntington disease
    f. Progressive supranuclear palsy (PSP)

Answer: a, d, f. Tau – a microtubule-associated protein – is the intraneuronal protein that aggregates in Alzheimer disease, frontotemporal dementia, and PSP. Thus, neurologists refer to these illnesses as "tauopathies."

18. From which area of the brain does cholinergic stimulation of the cerebral cortex predominantly originate?
    a. Hippocampus
    b. Basal ganglia
    c. Frontal lobe
    d. Nucleus basalis of Meynert

Answer: d.

19–22. What is the effect of the following substances on cerebral acetylcholine (ACh) activity?

19. Cholinesterase inhibitors that penetrate the blood–brain barrier
20. Scopolamine
21. Organic phosphate insecticides
22. Physostigmine
    a. Increases ACh activity
    b. Decreases ACh activity
    c. Does not change ACh activity

Answers:

19–a. Centrally acting cholinesterase inhibitors, such as donepezil, rivastigmine, and galantamine, increase cerebral ACh activity. In contrast, peripherally acting anticholinesterases, such as pyridostigmine (Mestinon), correct the neuromuscular junction ACh activity deficit in myasthenia, but because they do not penetrate the blood–brain barrier they have no effect on cognition or other cerebral function.

20–b. Scopolamine, like atropine, is a peripherally acting anticholinergic medication. In routine pharmacologic doses, neither scopolamine nor atropine crosses the blood–brain barrier; however, in high doses both penetrate the blood–brain barrier and may cause a toxic psychosis.

21–a. Organic phosphate insecticides usually contain anticholinesterases. They produce an abundance of ACh that overwhelms the neuromuscular junction and the autonomic nervous system.

22–a. Physostigmine is a centrally acting anticholinesterase that can penetrate the blood–brain barrier but has a short half-life.

23. Which of the following statements is *false* regarding the cognitive subsection of the Alzheimer Disease Assessment Scale (ADAS-Cog)?
  a. The testing requires about 45 minutes.
  b. The testing, including scoring, must be performed by a trained individual.
  c. The scores of patients with Alzheimer disease typically increase by 9 points yearly.
  d. Despite the advantages of the ADAS-Cog, the Mini-Mental State Examination (MMSE) is the standard test in assessing pharmacologic treatment in Alzheimer disease.

Answer: d. The ADAS, which has noncognitive as well as cognitive sections, is a standard measure in clinical trials.

24. Of the following, which is the most common risk factor for delirium?
  a. Use of multiple medications
  b. Age older than 65 years
  c. Preexisting psychosis
  d. Preexisting dementia
  e. Sensory deprivation
  f. Pain and analgesic use

Answer: d. All of these conditions are risk factors for delirium, but preexisting dementia is the most common and the most powerful. It underlies almost two-thirds of cases in the acute care hospital. Moreover, in hospital settings, delirium superimposed on dementia nearly doubles the mortality of delirium occurring without underlying dementia. In hospitalized patients 65 years or older, delirium carries a mortality rate of greater than 33%.

25. Which CNS cells does human immunodeficiency virus (HIV) primarily infect?
  a. Neurons
  b. Macrophages and microglia
  c. Ependymal cells
  d. Oligodendroglia

Answer: b.

26. A test for Alzheimer disease purportedly has high sensitivity but low specificity. In a revision of the test, what would be the most likely effect of reducing the proportion of false-positive results?
  a. The sensitivity would increase.
  b. The specificity would increase.
  c. Both the sensitivity and specificity would increase.
  d. Neither the sensitivity nor specificity would increase.

Answer: b. Specificity would increase because it is calculated by dividing the true-negatives by the sum of true-negatives and false-positives. In simple terms, with fewer false-positives, the results would be more specific because a greater percentage of individuals without disease would correctly test negative.

27. A man with no neurologic symptoms requests DNA testing of his ApoE status, and finds out that he has two ApoE4 alleles. What is the most likely consequence of his learning this result?
  a. Onset of depressive symptoms
  b. Onset of anxiety
  c. Increased suicide ideation
  d. No significant short-term psychological risks

Answer: d. Neurologists discourage individuals, even those with early dementia, from undergoing ApoE testing because no preventative or curative treatments are available for Alzheimer disease. Many neurologists had forecast that patients receiving such results would develop anxiety, depression, and suicidality. However, studies show that patients learning that they carry ApoE4 alleles demonstrate no significant short-term psychological risks.

28. Two 70-year-old individuals with the clinical diagnosis of Alzheimer disease for the same duration have similar patterns of amyloid accumulation on Pittsburgh Compound B positron emission tomography (PET) studies. One of these individuals attended college, spent his professional life as a university professor, and always had been an avid tennis player: he scores 23 on the MMSE. The other was uneducated, had few friends, and worked in menial jobs: he scores 18 on the MMSE. Which is the explanation that neurologists apply to the discrepancy of cognitive impairment despite similar laboratory studies?
  a. Lack of correlation between cognitive function and Pittsburgh Compound B PET studies
  b. Cognitive reserve
  c. Bias of the MMSE and other neuropsychologic testing in favor of well-educated individuals

Answer: b. Education, vocation, and leisure-time activities give individuals a storehouse of knowledge, intellectual abilities, and problem-solving capabilities – "cognitive reserve" – that allow them to ward off declining cognitive function, at least temporarily. Neuropsychologic tests are sophisticated enough to correct for education, language, and other characteristics of test subjects.

29. Which one of the following conditions is *not* a complication of professional boxing?
    a. Dementia pugilistica
    b. Intracranial hemorrhage
    c. Parkinsonism
    d. Slowed reaction times
    e. Progression of dementia, even after retirement
    f. Peripheral neuropathy

Answer: f. Unless trauma injures individual nerves, boxers do not develop a peripheral neuropathy. However, repeated blows to the head cause chronic cognitive impairment, deterioration of motor skills, and extrapyramidal signs (dementia pugilistica).

30. A volunteer in a pharmaceutical study inadvertently receives an overdose of scopolamine. Of the following, which would be the best antidote?
    a. Atropine
    b. Edrophonium
    c. Neostigmine
    d. Physostigmine

Answer: d. Scopolamine, like atropine, blocks acetylcholine receptors. When excessive, their anticholinergic activity can mimic the cognitive changes of Alzheimer disease. Cholinesterase medications that cross the blood–brain barrier would be the antidote. Although edrophonium, neostigmine, and physostigmine all inhibit cholinesterase and thus enhance cholinergic activity, only physostigmine readily crosses the blood–brain barrier.

31. The family of a previously healthy 65-year-old bartender who has suffered repeated falls during the previous several months brings him to a neurologist for evaluation. The neurologist encounters a dull man who is slow to speak and very slow in moving about. He has a facial grimace, but denies anger and all other emotions. He is oriented and eventually recalls 4 of 6 digits. His muscle strength and deep tendon reflexes are normal, but his muscle tone is increased. The patient, despite having postural instability, walks erect with short steps and appropriate stance. He cannot look upward or downward. Which is the most likely diagnosis?
    a. Alzheimer disease
    b. Parkinson disease
    c. PSP
    d. VCI
    e. Wernicke–Korsakoff disease

Answer: c. The neurologist should flex and extend the patient's neck. That oculocephalic maneuver will overcome a patient's inability to voluntarily move his eyes up and down and will elicit reflex vertical eye movements.

This patient's vertical ocular movement impairment indicates PSP. His falls probably resulted from both his inability to look downward and postural instability. His apathy and slowed cognitive and physical function, all characteristics of PSP, reflect frontal lobe dysfunction. Although the neurologist might reasonably first consider Wernicke–Korsakoff disease, the patient has no clear-cut amnesia, nystagmus, or ataxia. Dementia complicates Parkinson disease, but usually not until at least 5 years after the diagnosis.

32. Which substance accumulates in the brain of patients like the one described in the previous question?
    a. Amyloid
    b. Tau
    c. Prions
    d. Argentophilic bodies
    e. Lewy bodies

Answer: b. Tau-containing neurofibrillary tangles accumulate in PSP. They also accumulate in frontotemporal dementia and, less so, in Alzheimer disease.

33–35. Match the following conditions which produce confabulation (33–35) with the location of the usual underlying brain damage (a–d):

33. Wernicke–Korsakoff syndrome
34. Anton syndrome
35. Anosognosia for left hemiparesis
    a. Right parietal lobe
    b. Periventricular gray matter, mammillary bodies
    c. Bilateral occipital lobes
    d. Left parietal lobe

Answers: 33–b, 34–c, 35–a.

36. According to his coworkers, a 59-year-old bank manager has lost his ability to complete financing arrangements. Although he seems to know the individual facts of each deal, he fails to follow the sequence of the established procedures. In addition, his wife reported that, in a change of character, he has begun to tell off-color jokes. Otherwise, he is apathetic and speaks only when prodded for a response. His MMSE score was 25. A general neurologic examination revealed no myoclonus, hemiparesis, or ataxia. Which is the most likely cause of his deterioration?
    a. Alzheimer disease
    b. Depression
    c. Frontotemporal dementia
    d. Dementia with Lewy bodies disease

Answer: c. His problem at work consists mostly of a failure to execute the proper sequence of steps, i.e., "ideational apraxia" (see Chapter 8), rather than a memory impairment or general cognitive ability. The combination of his apathy, lack of inhibition (seen in his joke-telling), and his executive impairment supports a diagnosis of frontotemporal dementia. As in this case, frontotemporal degeneration typically causes neurobehavioral changes that are more pronounced than the dementia.

Another important aspect of this case is that, perhaps more so than in other varieties of dementia, the physician must speak with a collateral historian, such as a spouse or coworker. To make a diagnosis of frontotemporal dementia, neurologists usually require three of the following six symptoms: disinhibition, apathy, loss of sympathy, perseverative or compulsive behaviors, hyperorality, and impaired executive ability.

37. A 35-year-old man with HIV disease for 17 years and a CD4 count of 190 cells/ml presents with left hemiparesis and bilateral ataxia that have evolved over several weeks. His cognitive function is within normal limits. His MRI shows several large areas of demyelination, without mass effect, in the cerebral hemispheres. Which test would most likely indicate the diagnosis?
    a. CSF analysis for JC virus
    b. CSF analysis for oligoclonal bands
    c. Brain biopsy for toxoplasmosis
    d. Brain biopsy for lymphoma

Answer: a. He probably has developed progressive multifocal leukoencephalopathy (PML), in which case CSF would contain JC virus nucleic acid demonstrable with polymerase chain reaction. PML usually develops only in patients with CD4 counts below 200 cells/ml. However, HIV patients receiving antiretroviral therapy (ART) have developed PML despite CD4 counts substantially above that level. Inflammatory neurologic illnesses, particularly multiple sclerosis (MS), result in areas of demyelination visible on MRI and oligoclonal bands in CSF. Both toxoplasmosis and lymphoma are lesions that would have caused headaches from increased intracranial pressure. They would also have produced mass effect on CT or MRI. PML causes neither headaches nor mass effect on imaging studies. Cerebral lymphomas are usually solitary lesions in HIV patients.

38. Which variety of amnesia is typically accompanied by a peripheral neuropathy?
    a. Wernicke–Korsakoff syndrome
    b. Alzheimer disease
    c. Vascular cognitive impairment
    d. TBI

Answer: a. Wernicke–Korsakoff syndrome is more likely the result of thiamine deficiency rather than direct toxicity from alcohol. At its onset, Wernicke–Korsakoff syndrome consists of amnesia (especially anterograde amnesia) accompanied by oculomotor gaze palsy, nystagmus, ataxia, and neuropathy. In time, alcoholism leads to dementia. Certain toxins – such as solvents, heavy metals, and porphyrins – may also attack the peripheral as well as the central nervous system and cause the combination of neuropathy and dementia.

39. Which skin lesion is most closely associated with AIDS?
    a. Lymphoma
    b. Herpes simplex
    c. Kaposi sarcoma
    d. Chancre
    e. Herpes zoster

Answer: c. Kaposi sarcoma is so closely linked to AIDS that it is an AIDS-defining condition. Herpes zoster is an infection of the dorsal root ganglia. It occurs commonly in individuals with immunologic compromise, including normal older adults. The infection leads to zoster of the skin ("shingles") and, in many cases, postherpetic neuralgia.

40. A physician suspects that a retired college professor has the onset of Alzheimer disease. However, after she scored 27 on the MMSE, the physician sought another screening instrument to measure her cognitive function. Which of the following tests would best serve that purpose?
    a. MoCA
    b. A repeat MMSE
    c. ADAS-Cog
    d. Graduate Record Examination (GRE)

Answer: a. The MoCA is a good screening test for individuals who score above the cut-off on the MMSE and for a well-educated person who complains only of memory impairment. It is also useful as a screen for Parkinson disease dementia and frontotemporal dementia. The ADAS-Cog and the GRE require expertise to administer and interpret.

41. Which diagnosis will be supported by detecting the 14-3-3 protein in the CSF?
    a. Alzheimer
    b. Parkinson
    c. Dementia with Lewy bodies
    d. Creutzfeldt–Jakob

Answer: d. In the setting of compatible clinical and electroencephalography (EEG) findings, detecting 14-3-3 protein in the CSF supports a diagnosis of Creutzfeldt–Jakob disease. In encephalitis and tumors CSF may also contain 14-3-3 protein, but their clinical presentation and MRI appearance are, of course, entirely different.

42. Which is the most common cause of multiple discrete cerebral lesions in AIDS patients?
    a. Lymphoma
    b. Cysticercosis
    c. *Cryptococcus*
    d. Toxoplasmosis
    e. Tuberculosis

Answer: d. Of the cerebral mass lesions that potentially complicate AIDS, toxoplasmosis is the most common. It characteristically produces multiple ring-enhancing masses. Lymphoma, the second most common, causes single lesions. Cysticercosis is the most common cause of multiple, discrete cerebral lesions in South and Central American citizens. Tuberculosis is the most common cause of single or multiple lesions in citizens of the Indian subcontinent.

43. Which is the most frequently occurring nonepidemic form of encephalitis?
    a. HIV encephalitis
    b. Herpes simplex encephalitis
    c. Herpes zoster encephalitis
    d. Meningococcal encephalitis

Answer: b. Herpes simplex is the most common nonepidemic infectious agent that causes encephalitis. This virus typically invades via the temporal lobes and attacks the limbic system. Thus, herpes simplex encephalitis causes seizures, amnesia, and the Klüver–Bucy syndrome. In contrast, HIV and meningococcus occur in epidemic patterns. Herpes zoster rarely invades the brain.

44. Which CSF pattern is a marker for Alzheimer disease?
    a. Low Aβ and low tau protein concentrations
    b. High Aβ and high tau protein concentrations
    c. Low Aβ and high tau protein concentrations
    d. High Aβ and low tau protein concentrations

Answer: c. Asymptomatic as well as symptomatic individuals with Alzheimer disease show low Aβ and high tau protein CSF concentrations. Detection of the illness in an early stage may allow medical intervention to prevent the onset of dementia. In the proper clinical setting, neurologists could diagnose the presymptomatic stage of Alzheimer disease on the basis of these and other laboratory findings.

45. Which feature distinguishes cases of Alzheimer dementia attributable to trisomy 21 from those associated with the apolipoprotein E4 allele on chromosome 19?
    a. Onset in the fourth and fifth decades
    b. Low concentrations of cerebral choline acetyltransferase
    c. Reduced amyloid precursor protein (APP)
    d. Low concentrations of cerebral acetylcholine
    e. Abundant plaques and tangles

Answer: a. Alzheimer disease dementia attributable to trisomy 21 usually appears when patients are relatively young (fourth or fifth decade). Because a gene on chromosome 21 codes for APP, trisomy 21 leads to excess APP and thus excessive insoluble β-amyloid (Aβ). Cases related to apolipoprotein E4 (ApoE4) alleles show dementia after age 65 years. Otherwise, the histology of Alzheimer disease dementia in trisomy 21 and with ApoE4 is indistinguishable.

46. Amnesia in Alzheimer disease may be most closely associated with deficiency of which of the following substances?
    a. Dopamine
    b. Norepinephrine
    c. Somatostatin
    d. Acetylcholine
    e. Serotonin

Answer: d. Although studies have shown a deficiency of each of these transmitters to a greater or lesser extent in Alzheimer disease, the acetylcholine deficit is greatest and most closely associated with memory impairment.

47. Which group of drivers has the highest rate of motor vehicle crashes (MVCs)?
    a. Healthy individuals older than 65 years
    b. Alzheimer disease patients older than 65 years
    c. Teenagers
    d. 16–24 year old men

Answer: d. Individuals older than 65 years have a higher rate of MVCs than the average driver's rate. Those with Alzheimer disease have a higher rate than same-aged drivers and their rate increases with the duration and severity of their illness. Factors that explain their high rate include poor judgment, impaired eye–hand–foot coordination, slowed reaction time, diminished vision and hearing, and excessive daytime sleepiness. Teenagers have a high rate, with young adult men (ages 16–24 years old) having the highest. In addition to lacking judgment and experience, they often abuse alcohol.

48. Of the following, which is most often cited as the reason for placing Alzheimer patients in nursing homes?
    a. Dementia
    b. Incontinence
    c. Hallucinations
    d. Disruptive behavior

Answer: d. Disruptive behaviors – agitation, the interruption of the family's sleep, dangerous activities, and wandering – are the most common reason for families to place Alzheimer patients in a nursing home. Other important ones are incontinence, requiring help with bathing and toileting, and the development of a medical illness. All these problems place tremendous stress on the spouse or other caregiver. Alternatively, the death or disability of the caregiver forces the patient into a nursing home.

49. Which region of the brain is most affected by toxic-metabolic encephalopathy?
    a. Frontal lobes
    b. Reticular activating system
    c. Hippocampus
    d. Limbic system

Answer: b. Reticular activating system dysfunction leads to depressed level of consciousness and inattention – two hallmarks of toxic-metabolic encephalopathy (delirium).

50. Which of the following medicines used in the treatment of Alzheimer disease blocks N-methyl-D-aspartate (NMDA) receptors?
    a. Donepezil
    b. Rivastigmine
    c. Galantamine
    d. Memantine

Answer: d. Memantine (Namenda) blocks or antagonizes NMDA receptors. It is indicated for moderate-to-severe dementia. In contrast to memantine, the other three medications are cholinesterase inhibitors, which are indicated for mild-to-moderate Alzheimer disease dementia.

51. Which neurocognitive disorder will result from infections, trauma, or posterior cerebral artery strokes that damage the mesial portion of both temporal lobes?
    a. Amnesia
    b. Anosognosia
    c. Ideational apraxia
    d. Ideomotor apraxia
    e. Abulia

Answer: a. Bilateral mesial temporal injury characteristically produces amnesia predominantly in an anterograde pattern. Anosognosia is the inability to appreciate an illness or deficit, typically a left hemiparesis, with a right parietal lesion. Ideomotor apraxia, essentially impaired conversion of an idea into an action, is usually the result of a left-sided frontal or parietal lobe infarction (see Chapter 8). Ideational apraxia, impairment of an individual's ability to perform a sequence of steps requiring a simple plan and continual monitoring, usually reflects either frontal lobe injury or diffuse cerebral disease (see Chapter 8). Abulia, complete or nearly complete loss of spontaneous speech and other expression, results from extensive lateral or bifrontal frontal lobe injury (see Chapter 8).

52. Regarding the association between ApoE and Alzheimer disease, which one of the following statements is *false*?
    a. Because people inherit 1 of 3 alleles (E2, E3, E4) from each parent, everyone has two alleles, forming one pair, such as E2–E3, E2–E4, E2–E2, etc.
    b. Aβ binds to apolipoprotein and forms neuritic plaques.
    c. Inheriting the E4–E4 pair causes Alzheimer disease.
    d. Approximately 10% to 20% of the population has the pair E3–E4 or E4–E4, which is closely associated with Alzheimer disease.

Answer: c. Although inheriting the E4–E4 pair increases the risk of developed Alzheimer disease by approximately eight-fold, it does not cause Alzheimer disease. Many individuals carrying that pair have not developed Alzheimer disease. In contrast, the presenillin and APP mutations are obligate genes and cause the illness. Not only do ApoE4 alleles, which are carried on chromosome 19, increase the risk of Alzheimer disease, they advance, by as much as 20 years, the appearance of the first symptoms.

53. Through which structure is CSF normally absorbed?
    a. Cerebral ventricles
    b. The brain parenchyma
    c. Choroid plexus
    d. Arachnoid villi

Answer: d. CSF is secreted through the choroid plexus, which is located mostly in the lateral ventricles. CSF circulates through all the ventricles and then over and around the brain and spinal cord. The arachnoid villi absorb CSF and allow it to enter the venous circulation. Sometimes following subarachnoid hemorrhage or meningitis, blocked arachnoid villi lead to communicating hydrocephalus.

54. Which is a cause of obstructive hydrocephalus?
    a. Aqueductal stenosis
    b. Chronic meningitis
    c. Subarachnoid hemorrhage
    d. Hydrocephalus ex vacuo

Answer: a. Stenosis of the aqueduct of Sylvius blocks the CSF passage from the third to the fourth ventricle and causes obstructive hydrocephalus. In infants, whose cranial sutures have not yet fused, untreated hydrocephalus expands the skull, causing macrocephaly. Cerebral atrophy leads to ventricular expansion, *hydrocephalus ex vacuo*. As noted in the previous question, subarachnoid hemorrhage and meningitis block arachnoid villi and lead to communicating hydrocephalus.

55. Which statement is *false* regarding the gait of the normal elderly?
    a. It is characterized by a short stride.
    b. It frequently leads to falls.
    c. Orthopedic changes are as important as most neurologic illness in causing it.
    d. It is characterized by apraxia.
    e. Peripheral nerve changes are an important component.

Answer: d. Gait apraxia, an abnormality at any age, has several components. Patients with gait apraxia fail to alternate their leg movements and do not shift their weight to their forward foot. They also attempt to elevate their weight-bearing foot, but because their weight remains on that foot, they seem stuck or "magnetized" to the floor.

56. Of the following risk factors for falls in the elderly, which is most statistically powerful?
    a. Use of sedatives
    b. Transient ischemic attacks
    c. Neuropathy
    d. History of a stroke

Answer: a. Of these choices, use of sedatives is the most powerful risk factor for falls in the elderly. Additional ones include cognitive impairment, musculoskeletal changes, and a history of a fall.

57. Which feature is usually *absent* in Creutzfeldt–Jakob disease?
    a. Inflammatory cells in cerebral cortex biopsies
    b. Dementia
    c. Burst suppression pattern or periodic sharp-wave EEG changes
    d. Survival less than 1 year
    e. Spongiform changes in cerebral cortex biopsies
    f. PrP^{Sc} in cerebral tissue
    g. Myoclonus

Answer: a. Even though Creutzfeldt–Jakob disease is an infectious illness, transmitted by prions, brain biopsies fail to reveal inflammatory cells, which would be a typical response to an infective agent. Biopsies show spongiform changes and, with special stains, PrP^{Sc} (scrapie protein).

58. Which statement is *false* regarding the infective agent in spongiform encephalopathies?
    a. It is largely, if not totally, composed of protein.
    b. It is resistant to formalin fixation and conventional sterilization techniques.
    c. Interspecies transfer is rare but occurs.
    d. Similar agents cause subacute sclerosing panencephalitis (SSPE)

Answer: d. Prions cause spongiform encephalopathies: Creutzfeldt–Jakob disease, variant Creutzfeldt–Jakob disease (vCJD), its familial variant, Gerstmann–Sträussler–Scheinker disease, kuru, and fatal familial insomnia. However, a mutant measles virus probably causes SSPE. Prions also cause spongiform diseases in animals, including bovine encephalopathy ("mad cow disease"), wasting disease of elk and deer, scrapie, and mink encephalopathy. Interspecies transfer, which requires a large inoculum but a short incubation time, probably gave rise to vCJD.

59. What is the effect of ART on HIV-associated dementia (HAD) and longevity?
    a. ART improves cognitive function and increases longevity in patients with HAD.
    b. Although ART improves longevity, it has no demonstrable effect on cognitive function.
    c. Although ART improves cognitive function, it has no demonstrable effect of longevity.
    d. ART causes no interaction with medications that AIDS patients are likely to take.

Answer: a. ART improves cognitive function and increases longevity in patients with HAD. Its benefits correlate with low serum and CSF viral loads. However, because ART medications are metabolized by the cytochrome P450 system, drug–drug interactions, including ones with antidepressants, may occur. ART medications may compete with methadone and, when added to a methadone regimen, precipitate opiate-withdrawal symptoms.

60. In which condition are the anterior horns of the lateral ventricles convex (bowed outward)?
    a. Alzheimer disease
    b. Parkinson disease
    c. Dementia with Lewy bodies
    d. Frontotemporal dementia
    e. Huntington disease

Answer: e. Atrophy of the head of the caudate nucleus allows the anterior horns of the lateral ventricles to bow outward. Although the ventricles expand in the other conditions, their configuration is preserved.

61. Which of the following are risk factors for HIV-associated dementia (HAD) in AIDS patients?
    a. Anemia
    b. Weight loss
    c. Late stages of AIDS
    d. High viral load
    e. All of the above

Answer: e. Since the widespread use of ART, the incidence of HIV dementia has declined. Before the introduction of ART, HAD would almost always develop only if CD4 counts fell below 200 cells/ml. Nevertheless, AIDS patients receiving ART with higher CD4 counts have still developed HAD. To be fair, some of them have been unable to maintain their medication regimen, which is onerous and likely to counteract methadone and other medicines. Noncompliance is one of the most powerful risk factors for HIV dementia.

62. Of the following, with which illness are visual hallucinations most closely associated?
    a. Alzheimer disease
    b. Dementia with Lewy bodies
    c. Vascular cognitive impairment (VCI)
    d. Frontotemporal dementia

Answer: b. Visual hallucinations are characteristic of dementia with Lewy bodies. In addition, they are associated with Parkinson disease dementia and use of dopaminergic medications. Visual hallucinations are relatively infrequent in Alzheimer disease, especially during its early stages. When visual hallucinations occur in Alzheimer disease, they often develop in the context of delirium. In general, physicians should look for the development of pneumonia, urinary tract infection, or other new illness when dementia patients develop hallucinations.

63. After being given a medication, a 66-year-old man developed forgetfulness, dry mouth, blurred vision, and urinary retention. Which was the most likely type of medication?
    a. Anticholinergic
    b. β-Blocker
    c. Cholinesterase inhibitor
    d. Dopamine agonist

Answer: a. He has developed classic anticholinergic side effects. Patients older than 65 years and those of any age with dementia are particularly vulnerable to anticholinergic side effects.

64. According to the cortical–subcortical classification of dementia, which of the following illnesses would produce cortical dementia, and which would result in subcortical dementia?
    a. Cerebral anoxia
    b. Parkinson disease
    c. Huntington disease
    d. Normal-pressure hydrocephalus
    e. Alzheimer disease
    f. HIV-associated dementia (HAD)

Answers: Cerebral anoxia – cortical; Parkinson disease – subcortical; Huntington disease – subcortical; normal pressure hydrocephalus – subcortical; Alzheimer disease – cortical; HAD – subcortical.

65. Which statement is *false* concerning hepatic encephalopathy?

a. Ammonia (NH₃) crosses the blood–brain barrier more readily than ammonium (NH₄⁺).
b. Toxins bind to benzodiazepine-GABA ion channels and increase GABA activity.
c. Ammonia (NH₃) is the primary cause of hepatic encephalopathy, and the concentration of NH₃ directly correlates with its severity.
d. Benzodiazepine receptor antagonists, such as flumazenil, can briefly reverse hepatic encephalopathy.

Answer: c. Although therapy usually aims at reducing NH_3, its concentration correlates poorly with the severity of hepatic encephalopathy. NH_3 crosses the blood–brain barrier much more readily than ammonium, NH_4^+.

66. In the Clinical Antipsychotic Trials of Intervention Effectiveness – Alzheimer Disease (CATIE–AD) study, atypical antipsychotic agents improved which measure relative to placebo?

a. Cognition
b. Functioning
c. Care needs
d. Quality of life
e. Neuropsychiatric Inventory total score

Answer: e. In this landmark study, atypical antipsychotic agents improved only the hostile suspiciousness factor of the Brief Psychiatric Rating Scale and Neuropsychiatric Inventory total score. It showed that some atypical antipsychotics, particularly risperidone, compared to a placebo, may reduce aggression and improve psychosis.

67. A physician asks a 76-year-old right-handed man who had developed confusion to draw a clock. The drawing is shown in the figure. What problem does his drawing most likely represent?

a. Alzheimer disease
b. Normal aging
c. A dominant frontal lobe infarction
d. A nondominant frontal lobe infarction
e. A dominant parietal lobe infarction
f. A nondominant parietal lobe infarction

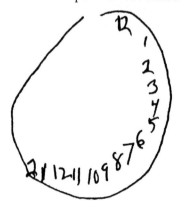

Answer: f. The drawing shows a neglect of the left field and constructional apraxia. The clock is an incomplete, poorly drawn circle with uneven spacing between the digits and the circle. There is also perseveration of the digits. Constructional apraxia can be a manifestation of dementia and injuries of either parietal lobe; however, it is most closely associated with nondominant parietal lobe lesions. The left-sided neglect is also referable to a nondominant parietal lobe lesion.

68. A family brings a 58-year-old woman for medical evaluation of depression after she has lost interest in them and has given up her job. Family members report that she dresses too lightly for the winter weather and she is reluctant to participate in conversations. Other than scoring 24 in the MMSE, her neurologic examination shows no abnormalities. Her general medical evaluation, including routine blood tests, shows no abnormalities. CT shows atrophy of the frontal lobes. After the psychiatrist informs the patient's sister, who is the health-care proxy, that the problem is dementia rather than depression, she reveals for the first time that their father had developed the same problem at the same age. Which is the most likely diagnosis?

a. Alzheimer disease
b. Frontotemporal dementia
c. Dementia with Lewy bodies
d. Neurosyphilis

Answer: b. She most likely has frontotemporal dementia. This neurodegenerative illness, which has a strong genetic influence, often presents with apathy, loss of initiative, and reticence as a manifestation of apathy. Alternatively, frontotemporal dementia may present with verbosity, hyperorality, inappropriate or disinhibited behavior, or progressive aphasia.

69. Which of the following statements concerning the MMSE is *false*?

a. Compared to the Montreal Cognitive Assessment (MoCA), the MMSE is less sensitive in detecting MCI and early dementia.
b. Unlike the ADAS-Cog, the MMSE can be administered without special training.
c. It reliably distinguishes Alzheimer dementia from VCI.
d. Educational levels influence the MMSE more than the ADAS-Cog.
e. Low scores can reflect metabolic aberrations, thought disorders, or mood disorders, as well as dementia.

Answer: c. Although the MMSE will identify most cases of dementia, it cannot determine the etiology. Moreover, it gives some false-positive results. ADAS-Cog testing is more complicated than MMSE testing. ADAS-Cog testing requires about 1 hour to complete and a trained person to administer and score it. Nevertheless, the ADAS-Cog is the standard in Alzheimer disease pharmaceutical trials.

70. Which of the following is *least* likely to unfavorably impact an individual's score on the MMSE?

a. Gender
b. Less than an 8th grade education

c. Being an ethnic minority
d. Being over 75 years of age

Answer: a. An individual's gender has almost no effect on the MMSE score. However, limited education, being a member of a minority group, and advancing age all reduce the score. Correction factors can reduce the adverse influence of age and limited education. Spanish-language versions of the test are available.

71. A 45-year-old man with AIDS and a CD4 count of 50 cells/ml reports slowly developing a generalized, dull headache and inability to concentrate. An examination reveals a temperature of 101°F, but no focal findings or indication of increased intracranial pressure. An MRI shows no intracranial pathology. Which of the following would be the best diagnostic test?
a. A lumbar puncture
b. Determining serum toxoplasmosis titers
c. A therapeutic trial of an antidepressant
d. A therapeutic trial of a serotonin agonist

Answer: a. About 85% of AIDS patients with headaches have serious intracranial pathology rather than a tension-type headache, migraine, or depression. Almost one-half of them have cryptococcal meningitis or cerebral toxoplasmosis. As in this case, the normal neurologic examination and head MRI almost completely exclude toxoplasmosis and other mass lesions.

72. The family of a 45-year-old waiter brings him to the emergency room because he had been confused and behaving strangely during the previous day. They state that the patient has not experienced any unusual event, stress, or trauma. A neurologist found no physical abnormalities and extensive testing, including toxicology, EEG, MRI, and LP, showed no abnormality. The patient cannot state his name, birthday, or address. He cannot recall any personal events of the previous 6 months or any current political events. His affect is constricted but his language function is normal. Which of the following is the most likely diagnosis?
a. Transient global amnesia
b. Dissociative amnesia
c. Wernicke–Korsakoff syndrome
d. Frontal lobe dysfunction

Answer: b. Personal identification – name, birthday, address, and telephone number – is deeply embedded in our memory. Only an extensive, devastating brain injury, such as advanced Alzheimer disease or major head trauma, would uproot this information, but those conditions would also impair his affect, language, and motor function. This man's amnesia most likely does not have a neurologic basis.

73. Which of the following is usually *not* considered a domain of cognitive function?
a. Language
b. Mood

c. Complex attention
d. Perceptual motor

Answer: b. The six neurocognitive domains recognized in DSM-5 are complex attention, executive function, learning and memory, language, perceptual-motor, and social cognition. Each subsumes several cognitive abilities. Mood, affect, and emotion, although they originate in cerebral function, are not domains of cognitive function.

74. What percent of Alzheimer disease cases are attributable to genes coding for APP (chromosome 21), presenillin 1 (chromosome 14), and presenillin 2 (chromosome 1)?
a. 5%
b. 10%
c. 25%
d. 50%

Answer: a. Despite their importance, this group of genes determines 5% or less of Alzheimer disease cases. When they cause Alzheimer disease, it usually follows an autosomal dominant pattern and becomes symptomatic at a relatively young age (30 to 60 years).

75. As part of an evaluation for dementia, an examiner asks a 77-year-old retired minor league baseball player to copy a sequence of four sets of three squares followed by a circle. Almost immediately after beginning the task, he begins to tell the examiner a nonsensical joke with sexual innuendo. After briefly returning to the task, he is distracted first by a small defect in the paper and then by soft noise outside the room. Finally, he excuses himself to go to the men's room, but only after he lets some urine escape onto his pants. Upon returning, he recounts a similar joke and says he could not concentrate because of all the distractions. He scores 22 on the MMSE. He has no lateralized neurologic findings. Which area of this man's brain is responsible for his behavior?
a. The cortical association areas, as in Alzheimer disease
b. The parietal lobe, as in hemi-inattention
c. The frontal lobe
d. The temporal lobe, as in Klüver–Bucy syndrome

Answer: c. He has easy distractibility, marked disinhibition, inappropriate jocularity, and a suggestion of urinary incontinence, in the absence of frank dementia. The distractibility is a manifestation of inability to suppress attentiveness to new stimuli, another form of disinhibition. He was unable to inhibit shifting his attention to new stimuli as they appeared, i.e., he was "stimulus-bound." All these phenomena reflect frontal lobe damage. Some elements of frontal lobe damage are similar to limbic system damage largely because the limbic system is closely connected with the frontal lobes. Moreover, as is probably the diagnosis is this case, frontotemporal dementia causes all these symptoms.

In contrast, Alzheimer disease particularly strikes cerebral cortical association areas. While causing dementia, it usually produces apathy. Its behavioral abnormalities are less severe and less predictable than those of frontotemporal dementia. Damage to the nondominant parietal lobe typically causes hemi-inattention and related symptoms. Damage to the temporal lobe, which may be a component of frontotemporal dementia, typically disrupts the limbic system, causing amnesia and Klüver–Bucy syndrome.

76. In an attempt to commit suicide, an elderly man swallows an entire bottle of donepezil. He becomes unconscious, hypotensive, and markedly bradycardiac. Which medication should be administered?
    a. A mild cholinesterase inhibitor PO
    b. Pyridostigmine IV
    c. Atropine IV
    d. Edrophonium (Tensilon) IV

Answer: c. The overdose of donepezil, which is a cholinesterase inhibitor, caused increases in ACh concentrations that reached toxic levels. The excessive cholinergic (parasympathetic) activity led to the bradycardia. Atropine, an anticholinergic agent, given intravenously counteracts the cholinergic-induced bradycardia. Pyridostigmine and edrophonium, like donepezil, increase ACh activity and would worsen bradycardia.

77. A 19-year-old exchange student from Britain began to have deterioration in her personality, cognitive impairment, painful burning sensations in her feet, and myoclonic jerks. There was no family history of neurologic or psychiatric illness. Results of the following tests were normal: CT, MRI, B_{12}, TSH, T_4, RPR, CSF protein and glucose, CSF protein and glucose, CSF measles antibodies, serum ceruloplasmin, urine for metachromatic granules, heavy metal screening, toxicology, porphyrin screening, HIV, Lyme titer, and DNA testing for excessive trinucleotide repeats. The EEG showed disorganization and a slow background, but no distinctive abnormal features. After exhaustive noninvasive testing, a neurosurgeon performed a cerebral biopsy. The cerebral cortex showed microscopic vacuoles. She died after a 1-year course. Which is the most likely etiology of her neurologic illness?
    a. Retrovirus infection
    b. Prion infection
    c. Drug or alcohol abuse
    d. A psychiatric illness

Answer: b. The clinical presentation of progressive, fatal mental deterioration with burning paresthesias and myoclonus is consistent with several illnesses, but the biopsy showing spongiform changes (microscopic vacuoles) indicates a diagnosis of vCJD. This illness represents an interspecies transmission of bovine spongiform encephalopathy (BSE). Unlike classic Creutzfeldt–Jakob disease, vCJD occurred almost exclusively in British teenagers and young adults, and their EEG lacked characteristic changes, such as periodic sharp-wave complexes. Moreover, vCJD caused prominent psychiatric symptoms and sensory disturbances. The majority of initial vCJD victims, in fact, first consulted a psychiatrist.

78. An 80-year-old retired janitor who has developed mild forgetfulness scores 19 on the MMSE. The physical portion of the neurologic examination discloses no abnormalities. The standard blood tests and head CT are unremarkable; however, the ApoE test shows an E4 allele. Which statement is the most valid in this case?
    a. Neurologists routinely recommend ApoE screening of individuals at risk for dementia, as well as those already afflicted with dementia.
    b. A single ApoE4 determination, in the context of dementia, is diagnostic of Alzheimer disease.
    c. Little or no education and ApoE4 alleles are each risk factors for Alzheimer disease.
    d. Determining ApoE4 alleles never has a role in cases of Alzheimer disease.

Answer: c. Being uneducated and having one or two ApoE4 alleles are risk factors for Alzheimer disease; however, neither causes the illness. ApoE determination plays a role in investigations of multiple family members with early-onset Alzheimer disease; however, neurologists do not usually order this test as a screening procedure for individuals with or without dementia.

79. What do the following conditions have in common: toluene abuse, multiple sclerosis (MS), progressive multifocal leukoencephalopathy (PML), metachromatic leukodystrophy, and adrenoleukodystrophy?
    a. All are commonly associated with seizures.
    b. All are infectious illnesses.
    c. All affect cerebral white matter.
    d. All cause dementia early in their course

Answer: c. All these conditions primarily injure CNS white matter, i.e., each of them causes leukoencephalopathy. PML is an opportunistic infection due to the JC virus. MS is considered an autoimmune illness. Metachromatic leukodystrophy and adrenoleukodystrophy are considered inherited enzyme-deficiency diseases. Most importantly, because these illnesses spare cerebral cortex gray matter, they usually cause dementia only in their late stages.

80. In Alzheimer disease, which region of the brain contains the greatest concentration of amyloid plaques?
    a. Frontal lobe
    b. Parietal lobe
    c. Hippocampus
    d. Nucleus basalis
    e. Caudate nuclei

Answer: c. In Alzheimer disease, the concentration of plaques and neurofibrillary tangles is greatest in the hippocampus. Other sites of high concentrations are the cerebral cortex association areas, such as the frontal and parietal lobes.

81–84. At the risk of oversimplification, match each dementia-producing illness (81–84) with its characteristic presenting feature(s) (a–e). More than one answer may be correct.

81. Alzheimer disease
82. Dementia with Lewy bodies
83. Frontotemporal dementia
84. Vascular cognitive impairment (VCI)
   a. Aggressiveness and other behavioral disturbances
   b. Memory impairment
   c. Parkinsonism
   d. Stepwise motor and cognitive deterioration
   e. REM sleep behavior disorder

Answers: 81–b, 82–c and e, 83–a, 84–d.

85. A hospital review board refers a 60-year-old well-respected surgeon for psychiatric evaluation in a neighboring county because several female patients have accused him of improper sexual advances. During the examination, the surgeon has good cognitive function, but he does not seem as verbal or forthcoming as the examining psychiatrist had expected. However, when he speaks, he is impetuous. He dismisses the accusations. He acknowledges several episodes of his recent uncharacteristic, public verbal attacks on junior colleagues. He has continued to work, maintain family life, and pursue his hobbies. A neurologist who previously examined the surgeon has already reported that his MMSE score was 27, physical neurologic testing showed no abnormalities, and MRI of the brain and an EEG were within normal limits. Which of the following conditions has he most likely developed?
   a. Mild cognitive impairment
   b. Dementia from Alzheimer disease
   c. Dementia from diffuse Lewy bodies disease
   d. Frontotemporal dementia

Answer: d. The surgeon has shown uninhibited behavior and impaired judgment in the inappropriate sexual advances and impetuousness. In addition, some of his behavior might have been aggressive, such as the attacks on colleagues. He does not fulfill criteria for dementia because he can still function at work and at home, and his MMSE score, while lower than expected for his education, is within normal limits. Although the surgeon does not have dementia, he is not normal. Because his abnormal behavior outstrips his cognitive impairment, the neurologist felt that the surgeon most likely has developed frontotemporal dementia. (Alternatively, in a slightly different scenario, hypomania or bipolar disorder might have been the best diagnosis.)

86. If the neurologist has made the correct diagnosis in the previous case, which abnormality would probably be found on immunologic staining?
   a. Argentophilic inclusions
   b. Tau deposits
   c. Alpha-synuclein inclusions
   d. Lewy bodies in the cortex

Answer: b. Immunologic staining consistently shows tau deposits in frontotemporal dementia and several other neurodegenerative illnesses (collectively labeled as *tauopathies*). In a minority of frontotemporal dementia cases, standard histologic staining shows argentophilic inclusions (Pick bodies). In dementia with Lewy bodies, inclusions known as Lewy bodies, which contain alpha-synuclein, are found in neurons in the cerebral cortex.

87. A wife brought her 70-year-old husband, a retired high school physics teacher, to a psychiatrist because for the previous 3 to 6 months he has suffered from increasingly vivid and frightening nocturnal hallucinations and memory problems throughout the day. During the initial evaluation, he was alert and oriented. His MMSE score was 25/30. He had reduced spontaneous movements and increased tone in his wrist and elbow muscles. His gait was shuffling, and he had a positive pull test. A CT and routine blood tests, including thyroid function and vitamin B12, revealed no abnormalities. During the follow-up evaluation, he was lethargic and scored only 20/30 on the MMSE. However, still untreated, he was alert during the next examination. The wife confirmed that he had a fluctuating sensorium. Which is the most likely disorder?
   a. Parkinson disease
   b. Side effect from a medication
   c. Alzheimer disease
   d. Dementia with Lewy bodies

Answer: d. Dementia with Lewy bodies presents with features of both Alzheimer and Parkinson diseases. In addition, with its characteristic fluctuating level of consciousness, this illness mimics delirium. The development of REM sleep behavior disorder often precedes the onset of dementia with Lewy bodies. In addition to sharing clinical features with Alzheimer disease and delirium, dementia with Lewy bodies is similar to long-standing Parkinson disease, except that rigidity and akinesia predominate over tremor. An important clinical distinction is that, at its onset, Parkinson disease causes neither cognitive impairment nor visual hallucinations, but dementia with Lewy bodies typically presents with these symptoms.

88. Which of the following structures are intranuclear inclusion bodies?
   a. Cowdry bodies
   b. Lewy bodies
   c. Pick bodies
   d. Neurofibrillary tangles

Answer: a. All of these structures are *intraneuronal* aggregates seen in illnesses that cause dementia. Cowdry bodies are *intranuclear* inclusion bodies, typically found in sclerosing panencephalitis (SSPE), that result from infection with measles virus. Lewy bodies, Pick bodies, and neurofibrillary tangles are all intracytoplasmic inclusions.

89. A 68-year-old man who had recently sustained a right cerebral infarction was asked to reproduce the physician's 10-block pyramid (left figure). He attempted four times (right figure), but it always fell before completion. (The blocks are shown from the

patient's perspective.) What is the implication of his inability to reproduce the pyramid?

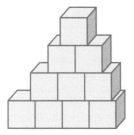 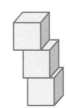

a. Dementia
b. Executive impairment
c. Left hemi-inattention
d. Left homonymous hemianopia

Answer: c. He has left hemi-inattention – not a hemianopia – in failing to appreciate both sides of the pyramid. He probably also has an element of constructional apraxia in failing to instinctively know that his unbalanced structure would topple.

90. A 40-year-old woman developed sudden paresis of her left upper and lower face. A blood test for Lyme disease was positive, and physicians treated her with intravenous antibiotics for 2 weeks. During the treatment she began to describe fatigue, irritability, memory impairment, and depression. After these symptoms persisted for 6 months and her Lyme titer remained reactive, her physician administered a second course of antibiotics. Nevertheless, her chronic fatigue and memory impairment remained so disabling that she could not work. Which statement is *true*?
a. An additional course of antibiotics would not relieve the symptoms more than a placebo.
b. An additional course of antibiotics is indicated because her Lyme serology remains positive.
c. An additional course of antibiotics is warranted whether or not her Lyme serology remains positive.
d. Her chronic symptoms are attributable to the antibiotics.

Answer: a. Several studies have shown that additional courses of antibiotics for "chronic Lyme disease" do not reverse the neurocognitive symptoms or chronic fatigue in either seropositive or seronegative patients. The antibiotics themselves do not cause these symptoms.

91. A 16-year-old rural boy loses interest in school, his farm work, and then in his friends. When he becomes apathetic, his parents bring him for a full evaluation. The neurologist detects mild but definite cognitive impairment and subtle myoclonus. An EEG shows periodic sharp-wave complexes and the CSF contains a markedly elevated level of antibodies to measles, but no cells and no 14-3-3 protein. Which illness does the evaluation indicate?
a. Variant Creutzfeldt–Jakob disease (vCJD)
b. Subacute sclerosing panencephalitis (SSPE)
c. Schizophrenia
d. Tourette syndrome

Answer: b. Antibodies to measles in CSF strongly indicate SSPE, which has a clinical profile of dementia and myoclonus in a child. SSPE is most apt to develop in rural farm boys. However, SSPE may occur in adults. Unlike conventional Creutzfeldt–Jakob disease, vCJD typically affects teens and young adults, and the EEG lacks periodic complexes. In schizophrenia and Tourette syndrome, neither the EEG nor CSF contains any consistent reliable abnormality.

92. In which condition will anosmia most likely develop?
a. Alzheimer disease
b. Vascular cognitive impairment
c. Depression
d. Multiple sclerosis (MS)

Answer: a. In neurodegenerative diseases, particularly Alzheimer and Parkinson diseases, the olfactory apparatus degenerates and anosmia develops. In addition, simply because of trauma to the olfactory nerve fibers as they pass through the cribriform plate, patients with head trauma, with or without TBI, often have anosmia. In contrast, patients with depression and those with VCI have preserved olfactory nerves and sense of smell.

93. Four months ago, a neurologist evaluated a 70-year-old retired restaurant owner and found mild cognitive impairment and early signs of Parkinson disease, but wanted to reevaluate him before prescribing any medicines. His daughter now brings him for a psychiatric consultation. The patient reports hallucinations that occur during the daytime as well as during sleep and last many minutes. They are vivid and vary in content, but often threaten him and disrupt his sleep and daytime activities. The patient claims that the woman who brought him is actually an impostor of his 40-year-old daughter. The psychiatrist sees no sign of a mood disorder. His MMSE score is 24. The psychiatrist, like the neurologist, detects a paucity of speech and slowness of movement. In particular, he has reduced arm swing when walking and he turns en bloc. Which is the most likely cause of the hallucinations and delusion?
a. Dementia with Lewy bodies disease
b. Parkinson-induced dementia
c. Bipolar disorder
d. Alzheimer disease

Answer: a. In view of his parkinsonism and cognitive impairment, the patient probably has dementia with Lewy bodies. In addition to parkinsonism and dementia, characteristic symptoms of this illness are hallucinations and delusions, including, as in this case, Capgras syndrome. Although Alzheimer and Parkinson diseases – and the medicines used to treat Parkinson disease – may also cause visual hallucinations, that complication usually occurs relatively late in the course of those illnesses and only when patients have unequivocal dementia. In this case, atypical antipsychotic agents that do not block dopamine receptors may suppress the hallucinations without exacerbating his bradykinesia. Some neurologists would add a cholinesterase inhibitor in an effort to preserve his cognitive function. (Chapter 12 discusses other causes of visual hallucinations.)

94. Which clinical feature argues against a diagnosis of Alzheimer disease?
    a. A strong family history of the disorder
    b. Evolution of dementia over 5 years
    c. Behavioral and emotional changes more pronounced than cognitive impairment
    d. Stable level of consciousness

Answer: c. In frontotemporal dementia, but not in Alzheimer disease, changes in behavior and emotion are more prominent than cognitive impairment. See Box 7.6 for "red flags" in the diagnosis of Alzheimer disease.

95. In individuals with Wernicke–Korsakoff syndrome, which cognitive domain is most severely impaired?
    a. Memory
    b. Visual-spatial function
    c. Language function
    d. General intelligence

Answer: a. Chronic alcoholism does not equally impair all cognitive domains. Its hallmark is anterograde amnesia, but it also may impair abstract reasoning and visual and psychomotor dexterity.

96. Several neighbors bring an elderly retired waitress, who lives alone, to the psychiatry clinic, where she is a longstanding patient because of Alzheimer disease. Her neighbors tell the psychiatry resident that during the previous 2 days she has been unable to find her apartment, or cook or dress appropriately. The patient is disoriented, and says that she is nauseated and light-headed. The resident finds that she has drooling, sweating, and miosis, and that her blood pressure is 95/50, pulse 48, and temperature 98.6°F. Which is the most likely cause of the patient's symptoms?
    a. A sudden advance in Alzheimer disease
    b. An intercurrent illness, such as pneumonia, causing delirium
    c. Excessive cholinergic activity
    d. Excessive anticholinergic activity

Answer: c. Bradycardia (which has led to hypotension and lightheadedness), miosis, and excessive salivation and sweating all reflect excessive cholinergic activity. As a result of her dementia, the patient took too many donepezil pills. At toxic doses, their anticholinesterase activity led to excessive cholinergic activity, which in turn caused parasympathetic overactivity, with bradycardia, hypotension, salivation, miosis, and confusion.

97. The police brought a young adult man, who had a history of schizophrenia, to the psychiatric emergency room because he had been ranting, raving, and throwing bricks at children. His treatment regimen was based on olanzapine, but his outpatient psychiatrist suspected that he was noncompliant. In the emergency room, a neurologist and internist each conducted a thorough evaluation and found no underlying disorder in their fields. The psychiatrist, concluding that the patient was an immediate danger to himself and others, ordered an intramuscular injection of long-acting olanzapine. Soon after receiving it, the patient became disoriented, confused, and more agitated. Then he lapsed into coma. However, his muscle tone was normal and he had no myoclonus. His vital signs, including his temperature, remained normal. His CK, CBC, and other blood test results were also normal. Which is the best description of this iatrogenic reaction?
    a. Neuroleptic malignant syndrome (NMS)
    b. Serotonin syndrome
    c. Postinjection delirium/sedation syndrome (PDSS)
    d. Cholinergic crisis

Answer: c. Small amounts of long-acting olanzapine probably seeped into the vascular system and caused delirium and then coma.

98. The geriatric service solicits a psychiatry consultation for a 70-year-old retired physician who has become intermittently withdrawn and apathetic during the course of his hospitalization for a myocardial infarction. He has a history of depression and mild cognitive impairment. Other than a low-grade fever, his medical and neurologic examinations show no abnormalities. His head CT and CSF analysis are normal for his age. During the psychiatric evaluation, he fails to establish eye contact and seems to have trouble attending to the mental status test. He scores 20 on the MMSE before falling asleep. When conversing, his output is spare but correct. During the interview he tugs on his bedclothes. Which is the most likely explanation for his having become withdrawn and apathetic?
    a. Dementia
    b. Aphasia
    c. Anosognosia
    d. Delirium
    e. Depression

Answer: d. The characteristic feature of his mental status impairment is his impaired and fluctuating level of consciousness, which indicates delirium. Cognitive impairment predisposes patients to delirium.

99. Which of the following conditions most often persists after electroconvulsive therapy (ECT)?
    a. Disorientation
    b. Retrograde amnesia
    c. Anterograde amnesia
    d. General confusion

Answer: b. Retrograde amnesia, perhaps particularly for autobiographical information, is the most persistent complication of ECT. Disorientation and general confusion usually clear within a day or two. Anterograde amnesia usually resolves within several weeks.

100. After a 72-year-old retired high school teacher reported developing forgetfulness and irritability, his physician performed a full evaluation, ordered routine blood tests, and obtained a head CT. The examination found an MMSE of 22, but no abnormal physical findings. All his blood tests, including a B$_{12}$ level, thyroid function panel, and syphilis test, were within normal limits. A head CT showed a 1 cm x 1 cm calcified mass over the right cerebral convexity. Which approach should the physician recommend?

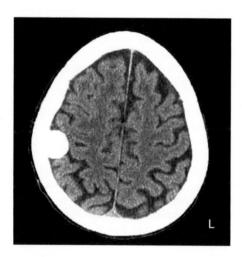

a. Refer the patient to a neurosurgeon for biopsy and removal of the lesion.
b. Refer the patient to an oncologist for radiotherapy, chemotherapy, or both.
c. Begin the patient on an antiepileptic drug.
d. Evaluate the patient for Alzheimer disease.

Answer: d. The CT shows a small, dural-based, densely calcified lesion that produces no surrounding edema, compression or invasion of adjacent cerebral tissue, or midline shift. In all probability, it is a meningioma. Meningiomas such as this one are prevalent, benign, and slowly growing. They rarely produce cognitive impairment, mood change, or thought disorder. Although neurologists may repeat a CT in 6 months, they would further evaluate and treat this patient for the most likely cause of his cognitive impairment, Alzheimer disease.

101. A 27-year-old male prostitute with AIDS has been receiving ART therapy for 5 years. His friends bring him for an evaluation of memory impairment. An examination finds that he has psychomotor retardation, generalized cognitive impairment, tremulousness, and a slow unsteady gait, but no lateralized

neurologic signs or indication of increased intracranial pressure. His hematocrit is 37%, white blood cell count 2100 cells/μl, and CD4 count 150 cells/ml. A brain MRI shows only mild atrophy and CSF analysis reveals no significant abnormality. Given all this information, which of the following is the most likely explanation for the memory impairment?
a. Progressive multifocal leukoencephalopathy (PML)
b. Toxoplasmosis
c. HIV-associated dementia (HAD)
d. Depression

Answer: c. He has the typical symptoms and signs of HAD, including gait abnormality and memory impairment. Although depression may cause psychomotor retardation and noncompliance with his medical regimen, it would not cause tremulousness or abnormal gait. The MRI and CSF analysis, which are largely unremarkable, excludes several frequent causes of cognitive impairment, such as PML, toxoplasmosis, and cryptococcal meningitis. Instead, his low CD4 count indicates that the HIV infection remains active, perhaps because he is noncompliant with his medical regimen.

102. A malnourished man with a history of chronic alcohol abuse was admitted with seizures and postictal delirium. His physicians had treated him with antiepileptic drugs, thiamine, niacin, glucose, and, because his serum sodium was 119 mEq/L, a rapid infusion of hypertonic saline. When the delirium persisted for several days, his physicians solicited a neurology consultant who found nystagmus, dysarthria, quadriparesis, and ataxia, as well as confusion and disorientation. CT of the head and routine blood tests showed no significant abnormalities. Which is the most likely explanation of his physical findings?
a. Wernicke–Korsakoff syndrome
b. Pellagra
c. Osmotic demyelination syndrome
d. Subdural hematoma

Answer: c. Alcoholics, especially those who are malnourished, are vulnerable to all of these conditions, but the rapid correction of hyponatremia and the localization of this patient's findings to the pons suggest central pontine myelinolysis, the classic presentation of the osmotic demyelination syndrome. Those at risk of this disorder also include liver transplant recipients, pregnant women with hyperemesis gravidarum, and others prone to hyponatremia. The generally accepted explanation is that too rapid correction of hyponatremia (>12 mEq/L/day), not the hyponatremia itself, leads to myelin breakdown in the pons.

103. Which test will best reveal the abnormalities in central pontine myelinolysis?
a. CT
b. MRI
c. PET
d. EEG

Answer: b. This disorder presumably involves lysis of oligodendrocytes, which leads to demyelination. MRI is the best test because it can visualize myelin-containing structures and those that are relatively small or located in the posterior fossa.

104–110. Match the histologic finding with the disease (a–g). More than one answer may be appropriate.

104. Argentophilic intraneuronal inclusions
105. Cowdry bodies
106. Lewy bodies
107. Neurofibrillary tangles
108. Spongiform encephalopathy
109. Staining with α-synuclein antibodies
110. Accumulation of tau
  a. Creutzfeldt–Jakob disease
  b. Wilson disease
  c. Frontotemporal dementia
  d. Dementia with Lewy bodies
  e. Parkinson disease
  f. Alzheimer disease
  g. Subacute sclerosing panencephalitis (SSPE)

Answers:
104–c (in cases of Pick disease)
105–g
106–d, e
107–f, g and chronic traumatic encephalopathy (dementia pugilistica)
108–a and variant Creutzfeldt–Jakob disease, kuru, fatal familial insomnia, scrapie, and other animal spongiform encephalopathies
109–d, e
110–c, f.

APHASIA AND ANOSOGNOSIA

Since the inception of the discipline of neurology in the 19th century, neurologists have studied language, language impairment (*aphasia*), and related disorders to deduce how the normal brain functions and to advance linguistics studies. In practice, they test for language-related disorders, often quite striking in their presentation, to help localize and diagnose neurologic disease.

Aphasia appears prominently in many neurologic and psychiatric disorders, and can disrupt cognition and halt fundamental mental functions. Nevertheless, it does not have a separate category in the *Diagnostic and Statistical Manual of Mental Disorders, 5th Edition* (DSM-5). The DSM-5 only includes Language Disorder as one of the Neurodevelopmental Disorder and Aphasia as a potential component of Neurocognitive Disorders.

LANGUAGE AND DOMINANCE

The *dominant hemisphere*, by definition, governs language function and houses the brain's language centers. The dominant hemisphere's *perisylvian language arc* (see later) processes the most basic aspects of language, including language production and comprehension, reading, and writing. In its *association areas*, the dominant hemisphere also integrates language with intellect, emotion, and somatic, auditory, and visual sensations. Because of these crucial roles, the dominant hemisphere serves as the brain's main portal for comprehension and expression of cognitive activity and emotions.

Language development begins in infancy, which is also the period of greatest brain *plasticity* (ability to undergo remodeling). By 5 years of age, the brain establishes dominance for language. Afterwards, as vocabulary, verbal nuance, and intellectual complexity increase, plasticity declines. For example, once past puberty, children usually cannot learn a new (second) language without preserving traces of their native (primary) language. Also once a person has reached this stage, the nondominant hemisphere can no longer assume a meaningful role in language recovery following injury of the dominant hemisphere.

The dominant hemisphere controls languages learned in infancy, but it does not necessarily control those learned as adults, including a second language. Nor does it monitor obscenities, which are usually expressions of emotion. The *nondominant* hemisphere governs *prosody*, which consists of speech's inflection, rhythm, and tone. Prosody is closely related to speech's affective component (see later). Interestingly, certain prosodic and visual-spatial aspects of language, which are critical in tone-dependent languages (such as many East Asian and African languages) and sign language, respectively, depend on the dominant hemisphere.

For most people, cerebral hemisphere dominance extends to control of fine, precise, rapid hand movements (handedness) and, to a lesser degree, reception of vision and hearing. For example, right-handed people not only use their right hand for writing and throwing a ball, they use their right foot for kicking, right eye when peering through a telescope, and right ear for listening to words spoken simultaneously in both ears (*dichotic listening*).

The superior temporal gyrus – the planum temporale – is distinctive in its exception to the general left–right anatomic symmetry of the brain. Its cortex in the dominant hemisphere has a much greater area than its nondominant counterpart because it has more gyri and deeper sulci. The relatively large cortical area of the dominant planum temporale provides greater language capacity. It probably also allows for greater musical ability because it is larger in musicians than nonmusicians, and largest in musicians with perfect pitch. However, this normal asymmetry is lacking or even reversed in many individuals with dyslexia, autism, Tourette disorder, and chronic schizophrenia – conditions with prominent language abnormalities.

HANDEDNESS

About 85% of all people are right-handed and correspondingly left hemisphere-dominant. In addition, most left-handed people are actually left hemisphere-dominant or have mixed dominance.

Of people who are left-handed (old English *lyft*, weak, foolish; compare Latin *sinister* and French *gauche*), some have sustained an often undiagnosed congenital injury to their left hemisphere that forced their right hemisphere to assume dominance. Compared to right-handed people, left-handed ones are over-represented among individuals with overt neurologic impairment, such as *intellectual disability* and epilepsy, and certain major psychiatric disorders, such as *schizophrenia* and *autism spectrum disorder*. Moreover, left-handed children are over-represented among those with many neuropsychologic abnormalities, including dyslexia, other learning disabilities, and stuttering. Economic studies have found that left-handed workers earn approximately 10% less than right-handed ones. Psychologic studies have found that left-handed compared to right-handed individuals scored approximately 10% lower on cognitive testing except if the individual's mother was also left-handed, in which case the left-handed ones showed no difference.

However, in certain endeavors, being left-handed seems to confer some advantages. Left-handed people are disproportionately over-represented among musicians, artists, mathematicians, athletes, and recent US presidents. In the last several decades, left-handed presidents have included

Gerald Ford, George H. Bush, Bill Clinton, Barack Obama, and, on most occasions, Ronald Reagan. In contrast, Jimmy Carter and George W. Bush were right-handed. Also, left-handed athletes tend to perform better than right-handed ones in sports involving direct confrontation, such as baseball, tennis, table tennis, fencing, and boxing. Only a small fraction of their benefit comes from tactical advantages, such as a left-handed batter standing one or two steps closer to first base. However, left-handed athletes achieve no greater success in sports without direct confrontation, such as swimming and running.

Unlike right-handed individuals, left-handed ones can develop aphasia after injury to either cerebral hemisphere. In addition, if left-handed individuals develop aphasia, its subtype relates less closely to the specific injury site (see later), and their prognosis is better than if right-handed individuals develop a comparable aphasia. These observations support the idea of mixed hemispheric dominance in left-handed individuals.

Ambidextrous individuals, who presumably have mixed dominance and are endowed with language, music, and motor skill function in both hemispheres, tend to excel in sports and performing with musical instruments.

Sometimes neurologists need to determine a patient's cerebral dominance. For example, when neurosurgeons must resect a portion of the dominant temporal lobe because it houses a tumor or generates focal seizures (see Chapter 10), they must avoid resecting language and memory areas. A devastating aphasia or memory impairment may complicate resection of an incorrect or too large an area. Using the *Wada test* – essentially injections of amobarbital directly into a carotid artery – neurologists can establish which hemisphere is dominant. When the amobarbital perfuses the dominant hemisphere, it renders the patient temporarily aphasic. Similarly, perfusion of one temporal lobe may cause temporary amnesia if the other temporal lobe is already damaged. A more recent alternative, functional magnetic resonance imaging (fMRI), which uses MRI to detect blood flow to a particular brain area while subjects perform a linguistic task, may indicate which hemisphere is dominant. The rest of this chapter assumes that the left hemisphere is dominant.

MUSIC

Musically gifted people generally tend to process music, like language, in their dominant hemisphere. Those having perfect pitch – the ability to identify a tone in the absence of a reference tone – display distinctive fMRI patterns when listening to music. If these people develop aphasia, they also lose a great deal of their musical ability.

In contrast, the great majority of individuals possessing no particular musical ability rely on their nondominant hemisphere to carry a tune. The proximity of their musical and emotional systems, both in the nondominant hemisphere, may explain the emotional effects music has on them. The primary location of music in the nondominant hemisphere for most people may also explain why many aphasic individuals, handicapped in language, often retain their ability to recognize music and to sing,

an observation that has been utilized in approaches to rehabilitation of aphasia (*melodic intonation therapy*).

APHASIA

The Perisylvian Language Arc

Impulses conveying speech, music, and other sounds travel from the ears along the acoustic (eighth cranial) nerves into the brainstem where they synapse in the medial geniculate body. Crossed and uncrossed brainstem tracts bring the postsynaptic impulses to the primary auditory cortex, *Heschl's gyri*, in each temporal lobe (see Fig. 4.16). Most music and some other sounds are processed in the nondominant hemisphere. In contrast, the brain transmits language impulses to *Wernicke's* area, which is situated in the dominant temporal lobe. From there, they travel in the *arcuate fasciculus*, coursing posteriorly through the temporal and parietal lobes, and then anteriorly to *Broca's area* in the frontal lobe. During its loop, the arcuate fasciculus allows communication with areas of the brain involved in all other functions. Broca's area, its terminus, is a vital language center located immediately anterior to the motor center cortex representing the right face, larynx, pharynx, and arm (Fig. 8.1). It receives processed, integrated language impulses, converts them to speech, and activates the adjacent motor cortex. Wernicke's area, the arcuate fasciculus, and Broca's area form a horseshoe-shaped region of cerebral cortex surrounding the Sylvian fissure that neurologists call the *perisylvian language arc*.

Using the perisylvian language arc model, researchers have established normal and abnormal language patterns. Under normal circumstances, when people repeat aloud what they hear, auditory impulses go first to Wernicke's area, then pass through the arcuate fasciculus, and finally arrive in Broca's area for speech production (Fig. 8.2A). Reading aloud is a complicated variation of repeating aloud because it requires both hemispheres and a learned system of transforming written symbols into sounds. As people read, their visual pathways transmit impulses to the calcarine (visual) cortex in both the left and right occipital lobes (see Fig. 4.1). Impulses from the left visual field go to the right occipital cortex. Then those impulses must travel through the posterior corpus callosum to reach the left (dominant) cerebral hemisphere. The impulses that have crossed from the right visual cortex merge with those already in the left hemisphere's parietal lobe. Decoded, coherent language information then travels from the left parietal lobe via the arcuate fasciculus to Broca's area for articulation (Fig. 8.2B).

All along its path, the language arc maintains reciprocal connections with cerebral cortical areas for memory, emotion, and other neuropsychologic domains. It also has strong connections with the thalamus, basal ganglia, and other subcortical structures.

Clinical Evaluation

Before diagnosing aphasia, the clinician must keep in mind normal language variations when examining a

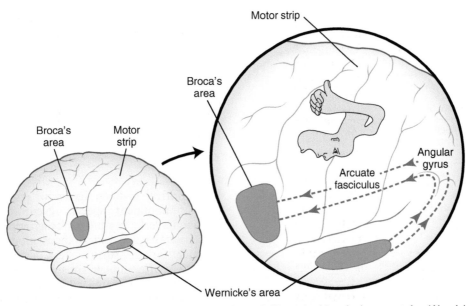

FIGURE 8.1 ■ In the standard model of language function, the dominant (left) cerebral hemisphere contains *Wernicke's area* in the temporal lobe and *Broca's area* in the frontal lobe. The *arcuate fasciculus*, the "language superhighway," which connects these areas, curves posteriorly from the temporal lobe to the parietal lobe. It then passes through the angular gyrus and anteriorly to the frontal lobe. These structures surrounding the Sylvian fissure, which comprise the *perisylvian language arc*, form the central processing unit of the language system. Note the proximity of Broca's area to the motor strip that innervates the muscles of the face, throat, arm, and hand.

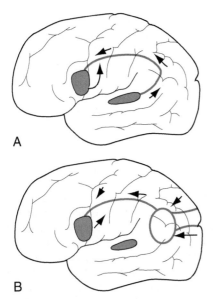

FIGURE 8.2 ■ *A,* When people repeat words aloud, language signals arrive in Wernicke's area, located adjacent to Heschl's gyrus (see Fig. 4.16), and then travel through the parietal lobe in the arcuate fasciculus to Broca's area. This area innervates the adjacent cerebral cortex for the tongue, lips, larynx, and pharynx. *B,* When people *read aloud,* visual signals travel to the left and right occipital visual cortex regions. Both regions send signals to a left parietal lobe association region (the oval), which converts text to language. Signals from the left visual field, which have initially traveled to the right cortex, must pass through the posterior corpus callosum to reach the language centers (see Fig. 8.4).

patient. Normal individuals may struggle and stammer when confronted with a novel experience, particularly a neurologic examination. Many people have their own style and rhythm of speaking. Some may be reticent, uneducated, intimidated, or hostile. Others, before speaking, consider each word and formulate every phrase as though carefully considering which item to choose from a menu, but some blurt out the first thing that comes to their mind.

In diagnosing aphasia, the clinician can use various classifications. One distinguishes *receptive (sensory)* from *expressive (motor)* aphasia based on relative impairment of language production versus comprehension. However, a major drawback of that classification is that most aphasic patients display a mixture of impairments that does not permit a strict classification.

The most useful classification of the aphasias, *nonfluent* versus *fluent*, rests on the quantity and grammatical correctness of the patient's verbal output (Table 8.1A). It suffices for clinical evaluations and roughly correlates with imaging studies. Aphasia pundits subdivide nonfluent aphasia and fluent aphasia each into four categories based primarily on the patient's ability to comprehend, repeat, and name objects. When repetition ability remains intact in either nonfluent or fluent category, neurologists add the designation *transcortical*.

Clinicians usually detect aphasia in a patient during the introductory conversation, history taking, or mental status examination. They then perform a standard series of simple verbal tests to identify and classify the aphasia. The tests systematically evaluate *three basic language functions*: *comprehension*, *naming*, and *repetition* (Box 8.1). Mildly affected patients may perform well with simple items but show difficulty with comprehension of more demanding materials, naming more uncommon objects, or repeating more complicated phrases. The examiner may also perform the same testing with written requests and responses; however, with one notable exception, alexia without agraphia (see later), defects in written communication generally parallel those in verbal communication.

TABLE 8.1A   Salient Features of the Nonfluent and Fluent Aphasias

Feature	Nonfluent	Fluent
Other terms	Expressive Motor Broca's	Receptive Sensory Wernicke's
Content	Paucity of words, mostly nouns and verbs	Complete sentences with normal syntax
Articulation	Dysarthric, slow, stuttering	Good
Errors	Telegraphic speech	Paraphasic errors, circumlocutions, tangentialities, clang associations
Associated deficits	Right hemiparesis (arm, face>leg)	Hemianopia, hemisensory loss
Localization of lesion	Frontal lobe	Temporal or parietal lobe Occasionally diffuse

TABLE 8.1B   Nonfluent Aphasias

	Comprehension	Repetition
Broca's	Intact	Lost
Transcortical motor	Intact	Intact
Mixed transcortical (Isolation)	Lost	Intact
Global	Lost	Lost

BOX 8.1   Clinical Evaluation for Aphasia

Spontaneous speech: fluent versus nonfluent
Verbal tests
  Comprehension
    Ability to follow simple requests, "Please pick up your hand."
    Ability to follow complex requests, "Please show me your left ring finger and stick out your tongue."
  Naming
    Common objects: tie, keys, pen
    Uncommon objects: watchband, belt buckle
  Repetition
    Simple phrases: "The boy went to the store."
    Complex phrases: "No ifs, ands, or buts"
Reading and writing tests

Nonfluent Aphasia

Characteristics

Paucity of speech characterizes nonfluent aphasia. Patients say little and usually only speak in response to direct questions. Whatever speech they produce consists almost exclusively of single words and short phrases. They rely on basic words, particularly nouns and verbs without proper conjugation. They cannot use the connective tissue of language, such as adjectives, adverbs, and conjunctions. Their longer phrases typically consist of stock phrases or sound bites, such as, "Not so bad" or "Get out of here." Synonyms for nonfluent aphasia include "expressive" or "motor" aphasia because of the prominent impairment in language production.

Patients' speech typically contains fewer than 50 words-per-minute, which is much slower than the normal 100 to 150 words-per-minute, and they produce it in a slow, effortful manner. Excessive pauses interrupt the flow of nonfluent speech. Neurologists sometimes describe its jerky rhythm as "telegraphic." For example, in response to a question about food, a patient might stammer "fork . . . steak . . . eat . . . no." Depending on the variety of nonfluent aphasia, patients cannot repeat simple phrases or name common objects. In contrast, most patients with nonfluent aphasia retain relatively normal comprehension that can be illustrated by their ability to follow simple verbal requests, such as "Please close your eyes" or "Raise your left hand, please."

Nonfluent aphasia's four major subdivisions are the following (Table 8.1B):

- *Broca's aphasia*: commonly occurring, classic nonfluent aphasia with comprehension intact and repetition lost
- *Transcortical motor aphasia*: similar to Broca's, but repetition remains intact
- *Mixed transcortical* or *isolation aphasia*: with loss of comprehension but repetition remains intact
- *Global aphasia*: devastating, with loss of both comprehension and repetition (see later).

Localization and Etiology

Lesions responsible for nonfluent aphasias usually encompass, surround, or sit near Broca's area (Fig. 8.3A). Their etiology is usually a middle cerebral artery stroke or another discrete structural lesion. Their location, not their pathology, produces the aphasia. Whatever the etiology, these lesions tend to be so extensive that they damage neighboring structures, particularly the motor cortex and posterior sensory cortex. Moreover, because the lesions are usually spherical or conical, rather than superficial and two-dimensional, they damage underlying white matter tracts, including the visual pathway. Diffuse cerebral injuries, such as anoxia, metabolic disturbances, or Alzheimer disease, rarely cause nonfluent aphasia.

Associated Deficits

Because the lesion causing nonfluent aphasia usually damages the adjacent motor cortex, right hemiparesis usually accompanies this aphasia. In such cases, the hemiparesis predominately affects the arm and lower face, and causes poor articulation (dysarthria). Deeper lesions also sever the visual pathway and can cause a right homonymous hemianopia (see Chapter 12). One of the most common syndromes in neurology is an occlusion of the left middle cerebral artery producing the combination of

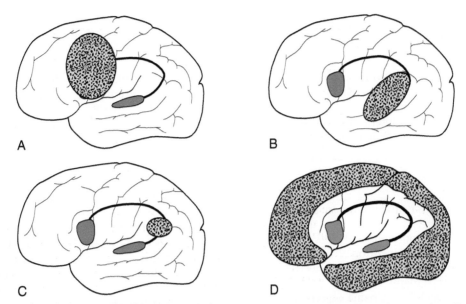

FIGURE 8.3 ■ *A*, Lesions causing nonfluent aphasia are typically located in the frontal lobe and encompass Broca's area and the adjacent cortex motor strip. *B*, Those causing *fluent aphasia* are in the temporoparietal region. Neurodegenerative illnesses may damage Wernicke's areas and more posterior regions and cause fluent aphasia. *C*, Lesions causing *conduction aphasia*, which are relatively small, interrupt the arcuate fasciculus in the parietal or posterior temporal lobe. *D*, Those causing *mixed transcortical (isolation) aphasia* involve the watershed region, which encircles the perisylvian language arc.

nonfluent aphasia and right-sided hemiparesis and homonymous hemianopia.

Another nonlanguage consequence of the lesions is buccofacial apraxia, also called "oral apraxia." This apraxia consists of the inability to execute normal voluntary movements of the face, lip, and tongue. When buccofacial apraxia occurs in conjunction with nonfluent aphasia, it adds to the dysarthria.

To test for buccofacial apraxia, the clinician might ask patients to say, "La . . Pa . . La . . Pa . . La . . Pa"; protrude their tongue in different directions and pretend to blow out a match and suck through a straw. Patients with buccofacial apraxia will be unable to comply, but they may be able to use the same muscles reflexively or when provided with cues. For example, patients who cannot speak might sing, and those who cannot pretend to use a straw might be able to suck water through an actual one.

Patients who suffer aphasia due to stroke or traumatic brain injury (TBI) generally improve to some extent. Presumably, at least some ischemic areas of the brain recover and surviving neurons form new connections.

Mixed Transcortical or Isolation Aphasia

Some lesions, which must be diffuse and extensive, damage the cerebral cortex surrounding the language arc. By sparing the language pathway, these lesions leave basic language function intact but removed from other cognitive functions. In *mixed transcortical* or *isolation* aphasia, which stems from such a cerebral injury, patients retain their ability to repeat whatever they hear; however, they cannot interact in a conversation, follow requests, or name objects. Because these patients can characteristically only duplicate long strings of syllables, neurologists consider them to have nonfluent aphasia.

The signature of isolation aphasia is this disparity between patients' seeming muteness and their preserved ability to repeat long and complex sentences. Patients who display such repetition, *echolalia*, mindlessly reiterate visitors' words readily, involuntarily, and sometimes compulsively. A cursory evaluation could understandably confuse this disturbance with irrational jargon.

This aphasia usually stems from the loss of the precarious blood supply of the cerebral cortex. While major branches of left middle cerebral artery perfuse the perisylvian arc, only thin, fragile, distal branches of middle, anterior, and posterior cerebral arteries perfuse its border with the surrounding cortex (watershed area). When these vessels deliver insufficient blood to this portion of the cortex, it suffers a *watershed infarction* (Fig. 8.3D). Thus, cardiac or respiratory arrest, suicide attempts using carbon monoxide, and hypoxic episodes cause isolation aphasia.

Damage to the entire remaining cortex usually causes cognitive impairment, usually to the point of dementia. It also usually causes decorticate posture (see Fig. 11.5).

Global Aphasia

Extensive dominant hemisphere damage abolishes so much language function that it results in an extreme form of nonfluent aphasia, known as global aphasia. Aside from uttering some unintelligible sounds, patients with global aphasia remain mute. Although they can follow some gestured requests, which bypass the language arc, they cannot comply with verbal ones. They also lack emotional responsiveness.

Comparably severe physical deficits – right hemiplegia, right homonymous hemianopia, and conjugate deviation of the eyes toward the left – parallel the extensive language deficits. Causes frequently include internal carotid artery occlusions with extensive cerebral ischemia, dominant hemisphere tumors, cerebral hemorrhages, and gun-shot wounds.

Global aphasia patients can sometimes express themselves with left-hand gestures and shoulder shrugs. They may even be able to comply with some nonverbal requests, such as gestures. Their communication, albeit limited and silent, distinguishes them from patients with psychogenic mutism.

Fluent Aphasia

Fluent aphasia's four major subdivisions are the following (Table 8.1C):

- *Wernicke's aphasia*: common, with loss of comprehension, naming, and repetition
- *Transcortical sensory aphasia*: similar to *Wernicke's* except repetition remains intact
- *Anomic aphasia*: inability to name objects
- *Conduction aphasia*: inability to repeat.

Of them, *Wernicke's* aphasia is the epitome and most common subdivision. Its characteristic is *paraphasic errors* or *paraphasias*, which are incorrect, meaningless, or even nonsensical words. Patients insert paraphasias into relatively complete, well-articulated, grammatically correct sentences that are spoken at a normal rate. However, paraphasias may render their conversation unintelligible. Moreover, patients typically cannot fully comprehend language nor repeat simple phrases. Patients with its less severe variant, *transcortical sensory aphasia*, can repeat phrases, but otherwise their language impediments are similar.

Paraphasias most often consist of a word substitution, such as "clock" for "watch" or "spoon" for "fork" (*related or semantic paraphasia*), in which the substitute word arises from the same category. Less commonly, the words involved have little relation, such as "glove" for "knife" (*unrelated paraphasia*); or a nonspecific relation, such as "that" for any object (*generic substitution*). Paraphasias may also consist of altered words, such as "bed" for "bread" (*phonemic paraphasia*).

Furthermore, paraphasias may include nonsensical coinages (*neologisms*), such as "I want to fin the gunt in the fark." Patients can bounce from one word to another with a similar sound, but one with little or no shared meaning (*clang associations*, from the German *klang*, sound). For example, a patient making a clang association might ask, "What's for dinner, diner, slimmer, thinner?"

As if to circumvent their word-finding difficulty, fluent aphasia patients often speak in *circumlocutions*. They also tend toward *tangential diversions* or *tangentialities*, as though once having spoken the wrong word, they pursue the idea triggered by their error. These patients, caught in a tangentiality, may string together meaningfully related words until they reach an absurd point. For example, when attempting to name a pencil, the patient may say, "pen … pence … paper … papal …"

Despite their loss of verbal communication, patients' nonverbal expressions are preserved because nondominant hemisphere functions remain unaffected. For example, patients' prosody remains consistent with their mood. Patients continue to express their feelings through facial gestures, body movements, and cursing. Similarly, most patients retain their ability to produce a melody even though they may be unable to repeat the lyrics. For example, patients might hum a tune, such as "Jingle Bells," but if they attempt to sing it, paraphasias crop up in the middle of the lyrics.

Associated Deficits

Unlike in nonfluent aphasia, hemiparesis and other corticospinal tract signs do not accompany fluent aphasia because the responsible lesion is distant from the cerebral cortex motor strip. For example, neurologists typically elicit right-sided hyperactive deep tendon reflexes (DTRs) and a Babinski sign, but not hemiparesis, in fluent aphasia patients. However, they may detect a right-sided sensory impairment or visual field cut because the underlying lesions often interrupt sensory or visual cerebral pathways in the parietal lobe.

Fluent aphasia patients are often strikingly unaware of their paraphasias, unable to edit them, and oblivious to their listener's consternation. Sometimes these patients, frustrated by their inability to communicate, develop anxiety, agitation, or paranoia. Clinicians not finding any hemiparesis and unable to capture the patient's attention for sensory or visual field testing often do not appreciate the neurologic basis of their patient's abnormal language, thought, or behavior. For many psychiatry liaison consultations, the sudden onset of fluent aphasia often explains a patient's anger, acute psychosis, consternation, change in behavior, or management confrontations. Conversely, the "gibberish" of fluent aphasia may mimic the speech of a psychotic patient (see later).

Localization and Etiology

Small discrete structural lesions, such as strokes, in the temporoparietal region are the usual cause of Wernicke aphasia and fluent aphasias in general (see Figs. 8.3B and 20.16). In addition, neurodegenerative illnesses, particularly Alzheimer disease and *neurocognitive disorder* due to *frontotemporal lobar degeneration* (frontotemporal dementia, see Chapter 7), often cause fluent aphasia among other symptoms.

Anomic Aphasia

A variety of fluent aphasia, *anomic aphasia* or *anomia*, is simply inability to name objects. Patients often cannot name objects, but at times, using a paraphasia, they offer substitutes and they usually can demonstrate the function

TABLE 8.1C **Fluent Aphasias**		
	Comprehension	**Repetition**
Wernicke's	Lost	Lost
Transcortical sensory	Lost	Intact
Conduction	Intact	Lost
Anomic	Intact	Intact

of the object. For example, they can use a pencil or a comb, but cannot say that it is a pencil or a comb. Comprehension and repetition remain intact.

Small strokes, because they are so common, are the most frequent causes of anomic aphasia. Less often, neurodegenerative illnesses cause it. For patients with neurodegenerative illnesses, anomic aphasia rather than dementia or simply memory impairment sometimes explains inability to name the current month or familiar places, objects, and people. Thus, these patients may perform poorly on a mental status test because of aphasia rather than dementia.

Conduction Aphasia

In contrast to lesions that damage Broca's or Wernicke's areas, lesions occasionally damage only the tract – the arcuate fasciculus – that connects them. Such a critically situated lesion interrupts the language arc and produces *conduction aphasia*. (Neurologists consider conduction aphasia as one of the *disconnection syndromes* [see later].)

Conduction aphasia patients, who remain fluent and retain comprehension, cannot repeat short sentences or even short phrases. Their deficit is the opposite of patients with isolation aphasia.

The most frequent cause of conduction aphasia is an embolic stroke in the parietal or posterior temporal lobe (Fig. 8.3C). Infarctions that cause conduction aphasia are usually so small that they produce little or no physical deficit. At worst, patients show right lower facial weakness.

MENTAL ABNORMALITIES WITH LANGUAGE IMPAIRMENT

Comorbid Depression

Psychiatrists face obstacles when assessing the mood of aphasic patients because they tend to appear apathetic, cannot freely communicate, and offer potentially misleading facial expressions. Aphasic patients who appear depressed may actually be manifesting underlying dementia or pseudobulbar palsy. For example, following one or more strokes, patients may have aphasia along with dementia or poststroke depression (see Chapter 11). In another example, lesions damaging both frontal lobes reduce patients' expression to a paucity of speech, emotion, and responsiveness.

However, physicians cannot attribute depression with comorbid aphasia entirely to brain damage. Most nonfluent aphasia patients remain aware of their impairments. They have suddenly lost their ability to communicate – a major loss. They naturally feel sad, hopeless, and frustrated. Treatment of depression comorbid with aphasia should follow the same strategies as treatment of depression without the comorbidity.

Dementia

Although aphasia is not equivalent to dementia, it can mimic dementia. For example, when aphasia impairs routine communications – saying the date and place, repeating a series of numbers, and following requests – it mimics dementia. At times, patients with aphasia seem so bizarre that they appear incoherent. Because people think in words, aphasia also clouds cognition and memory.

Dementia and aphasia also differ in their time course. Dementia develops slowly, but aphasia begins abruptly, except in the infrequent case when it heralds a neurodegenerative illness. Nonfluent aphasia further differs from dementia in its accompanying physical aspects: dysarthria and obvious lateralized signs, such as a right-sided hemiparesis and homonymous hemianopia. Moreover, paraphasias occur frequently in fluent aphasia but rarely in dementia.

Nevertheless, patients occasionally have both aphasia and dementia. This combination occurs with one or more strokes superimposed on *neurocognitive disorder due to Alzheimer disease*. It routinely develops in *frontotemporal lobar degeneration*. These situations defy classification because aphasia usually invalidates standard cognitive testing.

Distinguishing aphasia from dementia and recognizing when the two conditions coexist are more than academic exercises. A diagnosis of aphasia usually suggests that a patient has had a discrete dominant cerebral hemisphere injury. Because a stroke or other structural lesion would be the most likely cause, the appropriate evaluation would include a computed tomography (CT) or magnetic resonance imaging (MRI). In contrast, a diagnosis of dementia suggests that the most likely cause would be a neurodegenerative illness and the evaluation would include various blood tests as well as a CT or MRI.

Schizophrenia

Distinguishing fluent aphasia from schizophrenic speech can, theoretically at least, prove even more troublesome. Circumlocutions, tangential diversions, clang associations, and neologisms are common manifestations. As the thought disorder of schizophrenia develops, its language abnormalities increase in frequency and similarity to aphasia. In a different situation, previously healthy people suddenly developing aphasia can be so frightened and confused that they become agitated and irrational.

Despite these confounding elements, clinicians can discern many differences. Schizophrenic speech generally develops gradually in patients who are usually in their third through fifth decades and have had long-standing psychiatric illness. Their neologisms and other paraphasias occur infrequently and tend toward the inconspicuous. Unlike most patients with fluent aphasia, those with schizophrenia can repeat polysyllabic words and complex phrases.

In contrast, aphasia usually appears suddenly in individuals in their seventh or eighth decade, often with other risk factors for stroke. Except for some patients with fluent aphasia, most patients with aphasia retain awareness that they cannot communicate and they very often request help. Also, possibly because of self-monitoring, patients with aphasia keep their responses short and pointed. Any right-sided hemiparesis or hemianopia clinches the diagnosis.

Other Disorders

Children with autism may demonstrate language impairment – not only in their verbal expression, but also in their facial and bodily communication, such as failure to point. In many cases, nonsensical repetitions (stereotypies), idiosyncrasies, and echolalia overwhelm their speech. Also, they often fail to appreciate the nuance and affective components of language.

Several clear-cut pediatric neurologic illnesses may present with language impairment in children and must be considered when assessing children for autism. In girls with Rett syndrome, language characteristically regresses after several years of normal development (see Chapter 13). Similarly, language regression accompanied by seizures characterizes Landau–Kleffner syndrome (see Chapter 13).

Mutism and other apparent language abnormalities are frequently manifestations of conversion disorder and related disturbances (see Chapter 3). In these cases, the apparent language impairment is usually inconsistent and amenable to suggestion. Acquired stuttering also often indicates a psychogenic disturbance. For example, a patient with psychogenic aphasia might stutter and seem to be at a loss for words, but communicate normally by writing. An amobarbital interview might reveal perfectly intact language function.

A common psychogenic aphasia-like condition is the sudden, unexpected difficulty in recalling the name (blocking) of someone who triggers a strong emotional response. The classic aphasia-like condition remains the *Freudian slip*, originally known as a *parapraxis*. Freud's work on aphasia, which presaged his exploration of the unconscious, described his view of language circuitry and then words spoken "in error" actually as a manifestation of a repressed wish or conflict. Depending on their viewpoint, clinicians who assess everyday word substitutions may term them either paraphasias or insights into the unconscious. For example, when a physician's former secretary, suspected of harboring a neurologic disorder, says that she has been Dr. So-and-So's "medical cemetery," a clinician could interpret the comment as either her feelings about the competence of the doctor, an indication of the patient's own fears of death, or a paraphasia referable to a dominant hemisphere lesion.

DISORDERS RELATED TO APHASIA

Dyslexia

In most cases, reading impairment despite normal or near-normal intelligence and education represents a developmental disorder, Developmental Dyslexia (Greek, *lexis*, word or phrase), which falls into the DSM-5 category of Specific Learning Disorders. When tested, approximately 10% of all United States schoolchildren display some developmental dyslexia. Languages with more complexities (irregular verbs, multiple tenses) produce the greatest prevalence of dyslexia. Therefore, developmental dyslexia is most prevalent in English-speaking children, less prevalent in French-speaking children, and even less so in Italian-speaking children.

Moreover, developmental dyslexia occurs in 80% of all children with learning disabilities. Teachers usually detect it when children first try to read, but mild forms may escape detection until high school or college when students confront complicated reading tasks. In up to about 25% of children and, to a lesser extent, in some adults, developmental dyslexia is co-morbid with attention-deficit/hyperactivity disorder (*ADHD*). Developmental dyslexia persists throughout life, but some strategies ameliorate or circumvent the problem.

Developmental dyslexia affects boys with disproportionate severity and frequency, such that the boy:girl ratio lies between 2:1 and 5:1. Most dyslexic children come from families where other members also have the disorder. In general, the incidence of dyslexia in children is 25% if a sibling has the disorder, 50% if one parent has it, and 75% if both parents have it. Studies have implicated autosomal dominant and sex-linked genes. Imaging and pathologic studies reveal that the brains of some dyslexic individuals, especially boys, lack the normal planum temporale asymmetry. In other words, their brains are symmetric, which is abnormal.

In older children and adults, strokes, trauma, or other lesions of the dominant hemisphere may suddenly impair reading ability. Neurologists call this condition *acquired dyslexia*. In contrast to developmental dyslexia, acquired dyslexia is usually a component of aphasia. Thus, right-sided motor deficits including *agraphia* (inability to write) accompany acquired dyslexia (but see the next section for an important exception). Also, schizophrenic patients have a significant incidence of dyslexia.

Alexia and Agraphia

In the exception, *alexia without agraphia* (Fig. 8.4), patients suddenly find that they can no longer read. Despite this deficit, they have little or no impairment in comprehending speech or expressing themselves verbally or by writing. They can transcribe another person's dictation and write their own thoughts, but then they cannot read their own handwriting. Alexia without agraphia (which should be called "alexia with intact graphia" to avoid the double negative) usually results from a stroke or other destructive lesion encompassing the dominant (left) occipital lobe and adjacent posterior corpus callosum (the splenium). Aside from having a right homonymous hemianopia, patients remain physically intact. In contrast, agraphia almost always accompanies alexia in developmental dyslexia.

Gerstmann Syndrome

Gerstmann syndrome, a classic disorder that may appear in children and adults, consists of four neuropsychologic disturbances: *acalculia* (impaired arithmetic skills), *finger agnosia* (inability to identify fingers), *left/right confusion*,

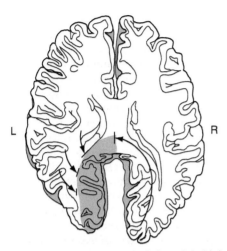

FIGURE 8.4 ■ Lesions that damage the left occipital lobe and the posterior corpus callosum (the splenium) cause *alexia without agraphia*. Patients are unable to see anything in their right visual field because of the left occipital cortex damage. Images in their left visual field still reach their right cortex, but their signals cannot reach the left cerebral language centers because the damaged splenium blocks neurotransmission. With obstacles in both information routes (the right visual field cut and transfer of information to the dominant hemisphere), patients cannot read written material presented to either visual field. In contrast, they can still write full sentences from memory, imagination, or dictation because these forms of information still reach the language centers.

TABLE 8.2 Testing for Ideomotor Apraxia

	Gesture*	Action Imagined	Action Real
Buccofacial	Kiss the air	Pretend to blow out a match	Blow out a match
	Repeat "Pa"	Pretend to suck on a straw	Drink water through a straw
Limb	Salute	Pretend to use a comb	Comb the hair
	Stop traffic	Pretend to write	Write with a pencil or pen

*Symbolic acts

and agraphia. When all four elements occur, neurologists usually attribute the syndrome to a stroke or other lesion in the *angular gyrus* of the dominant parietal lobe (see Fig. 8.1).

Some neurologists question the existence of this syndrome as a distinct clinical entity, because patients rarely display all of its components and those with three or all four components usually also have aphasia or other neuropsychologic impairment. Nevertheless, even if the four elements do not constitute a syndrome, they are frequently comorbid with each other and with subtle physical signs of dominant hemisphere injury, such as right-sided hyperactive DTRs and a Babinski sign.

Apraxia

Apraxia, the motor system's rough equivalent of aphasia, is inability to execute learned actions despite normal strength, sensation, and coordination. Neurologists attribute apraxia to disruption of links between the cerebrum's motor and neuropsychologic centers, particularly the perisylvian language arc and frontal lobe executive centers.

Although apraxia can be readily differentiated from simple paresis, it is often comorbid with aphasia or dementia. In fact, apraxia often appears as a symptom of Alzheimer disease and other cortical dementias (see Chapter 7).

In assessing patients for apraxia, the examiner usually first tests their buccofacial (lips, face, tongue) and limb movements when they attempt to make gestures or perform "symbolic acts" (Table 8.2). Next, the examiner asks them to perform certain actions, first on pretend objects (pantomime) and then on actual ones. After seeing the examiner perform an action, patients with apraxia typically can copy it. For example, a patient with apraxia might be unable to follow the request, "Please pretend to salute an officer," but after the examiner demonstrates the salute, the patient will duplicate it. Similarly, when patients with apraxia are handed an actual object, which gives them a cue, they can often perform the object's intended action. For example, a patient with apraxia might be unable to pretend to use a comb, but when presented with one, the patient will readily comb his hair.

As a general rule, inability to use a common tool, such as a comb or spoon, most reliably demonstrates apraxia. Further testing, depending on circumstances, includes performing a series of steps, copying figures, arranging matchsticks, walking, or dressing.

Patients typically remain unaware of their apraxia because they usually do not spontaneously attempt the various tests, such as saluting an unseen officer or using an imaginary screwdriver. Moreover, an unsophisticated clinician might incorrectly attribute the impairment to paresis, incoordination, or dementia.

Despite its complexity, neurologists designate several clinically useful categories of apraxia. *Ideomotor apraxia*, the most common category, consists essentially of the inability to convert an idea into an action. For example, patients with ideomotor apraxia cannot pantomime despite possessing a clear understanding and retaining the physical ability to comply. Clinicians might envision ideomotor apraxia as the result of a disconnection between cognitive or language regions and motor regions (Fig. 8.5). Almost invariably, a left-sided frontal or parietal lobe lesion is responsible for this variety of apraxia. Thus, ideomotor apraxia often coexists with aphasia, particularly nonfluent aphasia, and inability of the right hand to pantomime.

Another variety, *buccofacial apraxia*, as previously discussed, is a feature of nonfluent aphasia. In *limb apraxia*, patients cannot execute simple requests usually involving their right arm or leg. They cannot pretend to brush their teeth, turn a key, comb their hair, or kick a ball. When asked to pretend to *use* an object, these patients characteristically use their hand as though it *were* the actual object. For example, they will brush their teeth with their forefinger instead of pretending to hold a toothbrush.

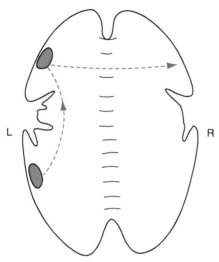

FIGURE 8.5 ■ In a schematic axial view, requests for normal movements travel to Wernicke's area in the left posterior temporal lobe. They then travel anteriorly to the motor regions and, through the anterior corpus callosum, to the contralateral motor strip. Interruptions of the path within the left cerebral hemisphere result in bilateral ideomotor limb apraxia. Lesions in the anterior corpus callosum interrupt only those signals destined to control left arm and leg movements, which causes unilateral left arm and leg ideomotor apraxia.

In *ideational apraxia*, patients cannot conceive and then perform a sequence of steps. For example, they cannot pretend to fold a letter, place it into an envelope, address the envelope, and then affix a stamp. In contrast to ideomotor apraxia, which is associated with nonfluent aphasia, ideational apraxia is almost inseparable from dementia. In particular, ideational apraxia is a hallmark of *frontotemporal lobar degeneration* where it reflects executive dysfunction. Alzheimer disease and multiple strokes, because they lead to dementia and impaired planning and execution, typically cause ideational apraxia.

In the next section of this chapter, this book covers *construction apraxia* and *dressing apraxia*, which are typically manifestations of nondominant hemisphere lesions. It has already covered *gait apraxia* in the discussion of normal-pressure hydrocephalus (see Fig. 7.8).

NONDOMINANT HEMISPHERE SYNDROMES

Symptoms arising from nondominant hemisphere injury tend to be subtle, predominantly neuropsychologic, and apparent in several well-known syndromes. Detecting them requires considerable clinical acumen and gentle probing. Physicians confronting patients risk precipitating a catastrophic reaction.

The cause is almost always a structural lesion, such as trauma, stroke, or malignant tumor that has rapidly developed in the nondominant parietal or frontal lobe cortex, underlying thalamus, and reticular activating system. Corticobasal degeneration, a rare neurodegenerative illness, also may attack these regions and cause the symptoms. Alternatively, corpus callosum lesions may produce some symptoms. Whatever the pathology, it impairs spatial attention.

The onset of nondominant hemisphere syndromes often leaves patients perplexed because they cannot appreciate their situation. More than with other cerebral injuries, patients with nondominant hemisphere lesions turn to classic defense mechanisms. Most often, they deny – implicitly or explicitly – that they have hemiparesis, visual loss, or other neurologic deficit. For example, patients who have just developed left hemiplegia will continue to use their left hand despite its uselessness and either say that they do not know why their actions are not producing any effect or claim that they are performing the task. Using projection in a conflict between their own self-image and the reality of having a brain tumor-induced hemiparesis, such patients may declare that their deficit is really a roommate's who sustained a stroke. Patients may also rationalize their problem. For example, when asked why he did not move his left arm, one patient stated, "I don't want to. If I wanted to move it, I would." Another stroke victim explained that she did not move her arm because of pain, not paresis, and that if her doctors gave her adequate pain relief, she would be able to move it. Sometimes laughing off the deficit, patients dispassionately avoid dealing with their loss of body function and its implications.

Whatever the reason that patients cannot accept a neurologic deficit, their misperceptions prevent them from complying with hospital routines. Patients with nondominant hemisphere syndromes frequently refuse to participate in rehabilitation programs because they feel no need for them and participating would force them to confront their deficits. Implicitly or explicitly denying their deficits also leads to potentially dangerous behavior, such as when patients with a left homonymous hemianopia plan to drive home. Patients often refuse to make realistic discharge plans and insist on premature hospital discharge. Even if encounters with medical staff and family do not precipitate a catastrophic reaction, patients with nondominant disorders tend to be bellicose when conversations address their illness, deficit, and need for realistic plans.

Hemi-Inattention

A patient with nondominant hemisphere damage may ignore visual, tactile, and other sensory stimuli that originate from their left side (Fig. 8.6). For example, *visual inattention*, a variety of hemi-inattention or hemineglect, occurs when patients disregard, fail to perceive, or misinterpret objects in their left visual field (Fig. 8.7). Sometimes people leave food on the left side of plates, and men with this condition leave the left side of their face unshaven. A patient asked to draw a clock may place all 12 numerals on the right side (see Chapter 7, Questions and Answer, Question 67). In contrast, patients with homonymous hemianopia usually develop some awareness of their deficit and make compensatory eye movements to keep objects in the preserved visual field.

Another manifestation of hemi-inattention – *extinction on double simultaneous stimulation (DSS)* – occurs when an examiner touches both sides of a patient's body, but the patient pays no attention to the left-sided stimulation. For example, when the examiner touches the left arm, the

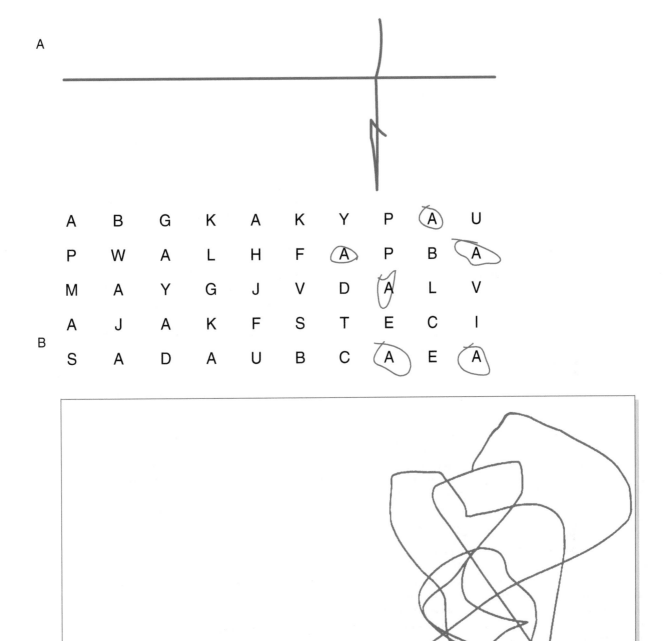

FIGURE 8.6 ■ Simple bedside tests for hemi-inattention. *A*, The examiner has asked the patient, who has just sustained a right middle cerebral infarction, to bisect a horizontal line. The patient, neglecting a portion of the line's left side, draws the vertical line off-center to the right and bisects only the line's perceived segment. *B*, Then the examiner asks the patient to circle all the "A"s on the page. Again neglecting the left side of the page, the patient circles only those on the right. *C*, An examiner has asked a 4-year-old boy, recovering from right parietal trauma, to draw a man. Because of a combination of hemi-inattention and constructional apraxia (see later), he merely scribbles on the right side of the paper. (A normal 4-year-old's drawing of a man is expected to a have a head, eyes, arms, and legs.)

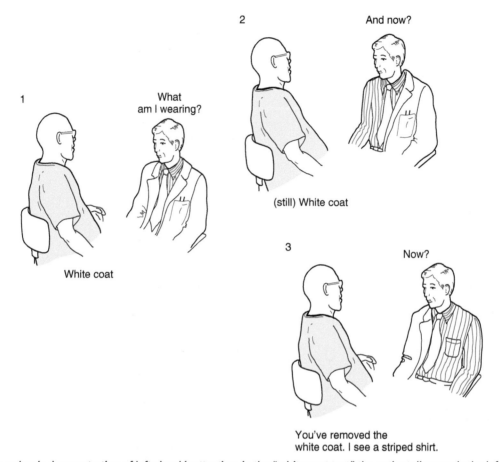

FIGURE 8.7 ■ In a classic demonstration of left visual inattention, in the "white coat test" the patient disregards the left-sided stimulation and perceives only the examiner's clothing in his right visual field. If the patient's problem were simply a left homonymous hemianopia, he still would have explored and discovered, with his intact right visual field, that the examiner was half-dressed.

patient correctly reports that it was touched, but when the examiner touches both arms, the patient reports that only the right one was touched. Another example of DSS can occur with visual stimulation. A patient might correctly perceive hand movement in the left visual field, but when the examiner simultaneously waves hands in both visual fields, the patient would report seeing it only in the right-sided field.

Constructional Apraxia

Another frequently occurring manifestation of nondominant hemisphere injury is *constructional apraxia*, which is a *visual-spatial* perceptual impairment. Patients with this disorder cannot organize visual information and integrate it with fine motor skills. For example, they cannot copy simple figures or arrange matchsticks in patterns (Fig. 8.8). However, clinicians cannot always attribute constructional apraxia to a nondominant lesion. It also appears in tests of patients with *intellectual disability*, diffuse cerebral dysfunction, and executive impairment from frontal lobe disease.

Dressing Apraxia

In *dressing apraxia* (impaired ability to dress), patients characteristically leave their left side partly or entirely

undressed. In extreme cases, they completely fail to dress. Patients may not merely leave their left limbs out of their shirts and pants, they may put both hands into one sleeve, misalign buttons, and become befuddled when presented with their clothing turned inside out (see Additional Review Questions and Answers, Question 299). Moreover, patients remain unaware that their clothing is disheveled. Even though their dressing apraxia includes hemi-inattention and other perceptual impairments, neurologists label it an apraxia because of the initial, obvious problem with skilled movements.

Alien Hand Syndrome

A remarkable form of hemi-inattention occurs in the *alien hand (alien limb) syndrome*. In this disorder, a patient's left hand usually retains at least rudimentary motor and sensory functions, but the patient cannot control its movements or appreciate its sensations. In classic cases, the hand moves semipurposefully, independently making autonomous explorations and performing simple tasks, such as scratching or unbuttoning pajamas without the patient's awareness. It sometimes fondles the patient or reaches out to the examiner. It may counteract the right hand's actions (inter-manual conflict) or make uncharacteristic movements. In an often-quoted example, a patient reported that her left hand intermittently attempted to

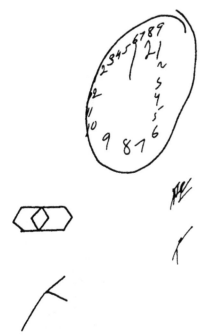

FIGURE 8.8 ■ When asked to draw a clock, a patient with *constructional apraxia* drew an incomplete circle, repeated (perseverated) the numerals, and placed them unevenly. When attempting to copy the top left figure, the patient only repeated several lines. The patient also misplaced and rotated the position of the bottom left figure (see also Fig. 2.8). Such abnormalities also may be detected with instruments such as the WAIS and Bender–Gestalt tests.

choke her. Patients may treat the hand as though it were an errant child and rebuke, slap, or chastise it.

The alien hand syndrome definition technically requires that the patient reveal two misperceptions: (1) the patient does not possess the hand and (2) because the hand's movements take place without the patient's knowledge and control, another person (the alien) governs the hand. Most patients simply feel estranged from their hand or accept only a tenuous relationship with it. For those patients who develop the alien hand syndrome following a corpus callosum injury, their situation is akin to their right hand not knowing what their left hand is doing.

Anosognosia

Anosognosia – a term constructed by Babinski (Greek, *a*, without; *noso*, disease; *gnosis*, knowledge) – has come to describe patients' inability to acknowledge a physical deficit or their denial of it. The classic example is anosognosia for a left hemiparesis. Patients with anosognosia typically cannot identify the affected part of their own body (*somatotopagnosia* or *autotopagnosia*). For example, they might claim that the examiner's limb is really theirs; fail to recognize their own paretic limb; or refuse to accept that the obviously paralyzed limb is even weak (denial). Sometimes they attribute the weakened limb to a third person, such as another patient (projection). This ploy holds instant appeal if that person has an immobilized limb from a stroke or fracture. Alternatively, even while accepting their hand's weakness, patients might offer an

improbable explanation, such as that they merely fell asleep on it and its strength will return in a few hours, or that they simply do not wish to move it (rationalization).

Anosognosia holds more than academic interest. It complicates and delays recovery from right hemisphere strokes and TBI. Physicians caring for patients with left hemiparesis and anosognosia for their deficit might tentatively introduce the idea that the patient has limitations, but with participation in rehabilitation and the passage of time, improvement will occur. The patient's realization will follow.

Loss of afferent sensory input, particularly proprioception, is invariably present in anosognosia but is not sufficient to produce it. For example, patients with a thoracic spinal cord transection lose feeling in their lower trunk and legs, but they remain acutely aware of their paraparesis and sensory loss. Another theory attributes nondominant symptoms to disordered attentiveness and arousal stemming from damage of the underlying thalamus and reticular activating system. In any case, patients' premorbid personality and emotional state have no bearing on development of this condition.

Aprosody

Prosody is the melodic contour of speech. Loss of prosody, *aprosody* or *aprosodia*, results in the inability to produce emotional or affective qualities in one's speech or to recognize them in the speech of others. Thus, nondominant hemisphere lesions interfere with patients' capacity to sense emotions in a speaker's tone of voice. For example, a patient with aprosody would be unable to appreciate the contrasting feelings in the question "Are you going home?" asked first by a jealous hospital roommate and then by a gleeful child. In addition, aprosody restricts the ability to impart emotional qualities to speech. With no inflection or style, patients' speech sounds bland and unfeeling.

To assess prosody, the examiner should note the patient's variations in volume, pitch, and emphasis during casual conversation. The examiner might then have the patient ask a question, such as "May I have the ball?" in the manner of a friend and then a stern schoolteacher using appropriate vocal and facial expressions. The examiner then may ask the same question while the patient tries to identify the different tones.

Loss of nonverbal communication tends to accompany aprosody. In particular, patients lose access to meaningful face and limb expressions, popularly called "body language" or technically called speech's *paralinguistic component*. These physical aspects of communication lend conviction, emphasis, and affect to spoken words. Indeed, such physical expressions seem independent and sometimes more credible than speech. Well-known examples are children crossing their fingers when promising, adults who wink while they are telling an incredible story, and people who smile while relating sad events.

DISCONNECTION SYNDROMES

Injuries that sever communication pathways between cortical centers cause uncommon but interesting

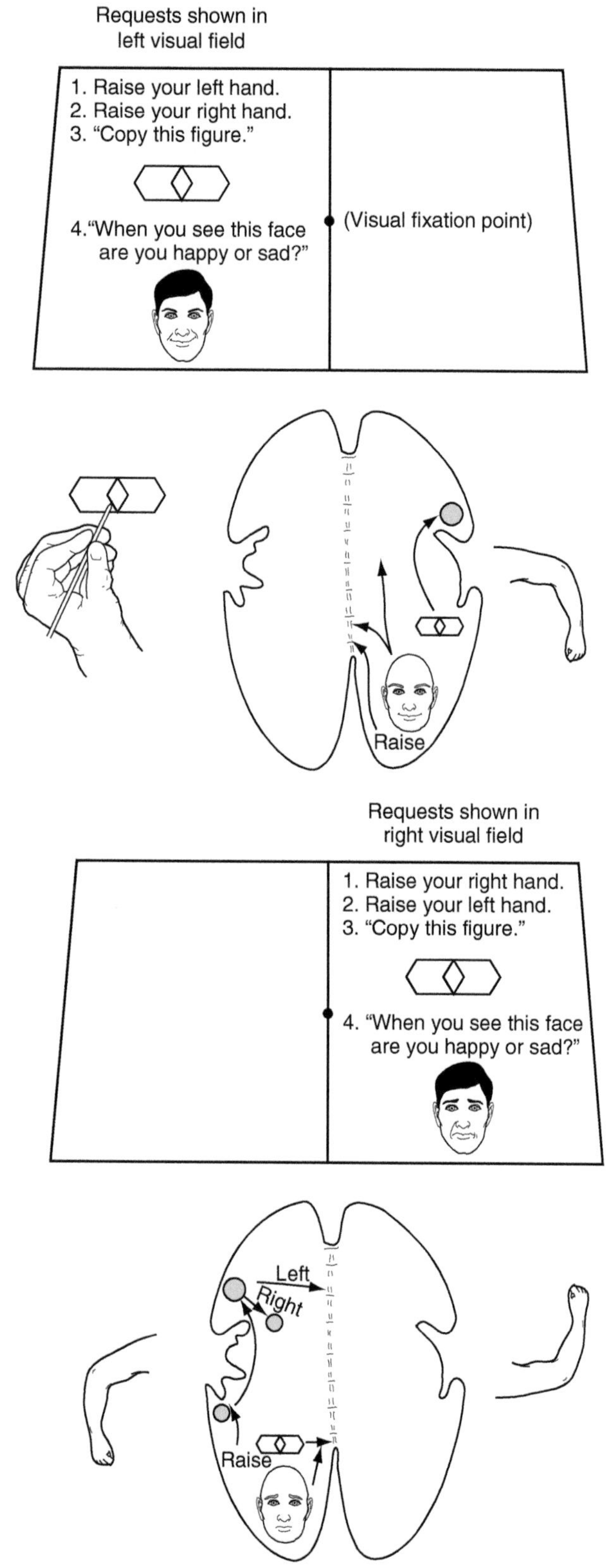

Requests shown in left visual field

1. Raise your left hand.
2. Raise your right hand.
3. "Copy this figure."

4. "When you see this face are you happy or sad?"

(Visual fixation point)

Raise

Requests shown in right visual field

1. Raise your right hand.
2. Raise your left hand.
3. "Copy this figure."

4. "When you see this face are you happy or sad?"

Left
Right

Raise

FIGURE 8.9 ■ A commissurotomy typically leaves patients with the *split-brain syndrome*. Each of their hemispheres can be tested individually by showing requests, objects, and pictures in the contralateral visual field. *Top,* Objects and written requests shown in the left visual field are perceived by the right visual field. Since connections to the ipsilateral motor area are intact, the left hand can copy figures. However, since the right hemisphere is unable to transmit information through the corpus callosum to the dominant left cerebral hemisphere, which

phenomena that neurologists call *disconnection syndromes*. Neurologists had predicted the existence of such syndromes before verifying them in patients, much as physicists have predicted certain subatomic particles before demonstrating them. This chapter has already discussed several disconnection syndromes: (1) alexia without agraphia; (2) conduction aphasia; and (3) ideomotor apraxia with its varieties, buccofacial and limb apraxia. Subsequent chapters will present other disconnection syndromes, including the medial longitudinal fasciculus (MLF) syndrome, also known as internuclear ophthalmoplegia (INO) (see Chapters 12 and 15).

Another disconnection syndrome, the *anterior cerebral artery syndrome*, results from an occlusion of both anterior cerebral arteries that causes an infarction of both frontal lobes and the anterior corpus callosum (the genu). In this syndrome, information cannot pass between the left hemisphere language centers and the right hemisphere motor centers. Although the patient's left arm and leg will have normal spontaneous movement, those limbs fail to follow an examiner's verbal or written requests to move them. In other words, the patient will have unilateral (left-sided) limb apraxia (see Fig. 8.5).

Other injuries of the corpus callosum may surprisingly not produce disconnection syndromes. For example, individuals with a congenital absence of the corpus callosum may show no overt impairment. In *Marchiafava–Bignami syndrome*, which has been attributed in a minority of cases to excessive consumption of Italian red wine, patients show disconnection signs, but only as part of extensive cerebral dysfunction.

Split-Brain Syndrome

The most important disconnection syndrome referable to the corpus callosum is the *split-brain syndrome*. This condition most often results from a longitudinal surgical division of the corpus callosum (commissurotomy) performed by neurosurgeons in an effort to control intractable epilepsy (see Chapter 10). Rarely performed nowadays, the commissurotomy almost completely isolates each cerebral hemisphere. This isolation permits examiners to present information to only a single, isolated hemisphere. For example, examiners can show pictures, writing, and other visual information in one of the patient's visual fields, presenting information only to the contralateral hemisphere (Fig. 8.9). Likewise, by having a blindfolded patient touch objects with the one hand, examiners can present tactile information to only one hemisphere.

governs language function, patients cannot read the requests or describe the objects. Although patients cannot speak of the feelings evoked by emotionally laden pictures shown in their left visual field, they have sympathetic nonverbal responses. *Bottom,* The left hemisphere perceives written requests and objects shown in the right visual field. Patients can read those written requests, copy those objects with the right hand, and comply with the requests; however, because the language areas cannot send information through the corpus callosum, the left hand cannot comply. When patients describe emotions portrayed in a picture, their language lacks affect, derived from the nondominant hemisphere.

For example, if an object is placed in a blindfolded patient's left hand, the patient cannot name or describe it (because the information does not reach the dominant hemisphere), and the right hand cannot choose an identical object. Similarly, if one hand learns to follow a maze, the other hand will have to be taught separately.

However, auditory information cannot be presented exclusively – only predominantly – to one hemisphere. (Because pathways are duplicated in the brainstem [see Fig. 4.16], sounds presented to one ear travel, after the medial geniculate synapse, to both hemispheres, but predominantly to the contralateral one.)

The interruption of the corpus callosum prevents the right hemisphere from sharing most information with the entire brain, particularly the left hemisphere's language centers. Thus, the right hemisphere's information, experience, and emotion cannot reach the patients' consciousness at the level of verbal expression. For example, if a humorous picture were shown to the right visual field, a patient might laugh and be able to describe the picture's humorous content; however, if the same picture were shown to the patient's left visual field, it might provoke an amused response but one that the patient could not verbalize or even fully comprehend.

Split-brain studies have suggested that normal people have, in their two hemispheres, neuropsychologic systems that are independent, parallel, and capable of simultaneous reasoning. Although the systems usually complement each other, they potentially conflict. For example, if a sad picture were shown in the left visual field and a humorous one in the right, the patient would probably display a bewildered response because of the discrepancy.

REFERENCES

Benton, A. L. (1992). Gerstmann's syndrome. *Archives of Neurology, 49*, 445–447.

Besson, M., & Schon, D. (2001). Comparison between language and music. *Annals of the New York Academy of Sciences, 930*, 232–358.

Binder, J. R. (2015). The Wernicke area: Modern evidence and a reinterpretation. *Neurology, 85*, 2170–2175.

Brust, J. C. (2001). Music and the neurologist. *Annals of the New York Academy of Sciences, 930*, 143–152.

Buxbaum, L. J., Ferraro, M. K., Veramonti, T., et al. (2004). Hemispatial neglect. *Neurology, 62*, 749–756.

Croquelois, A., & Bogousslavsky, J. (2011). Stroke aphasia. *Cerebrovascular Diseases, 31*, 392–399.

Faber, R., Abrams, R., Taylor, M. A., et al. (1983). Comparison of schizophrenic patients with formal thought disorder and neurologically impaired patients with aphasia. *The American Journal of Psychiatry, 140*, 1348–1351.

Gokhale, S., Lahoti, S., & Caplan, L. R. (2013). The neglected neglect: Auditory neglect. *Journal of the American Medical Association Neurology, 70*, 1065–1069.

Goodman, J. (2014). The wages of sinistrality: Handedness, brain structure, and human capital accumulation. *Journal of Economic Perspectives*, 193–212.

Greenberg, V. D. (1998). *Freud and His Aphasia Book: Language and the Sources of Psychoanalysis*. Ithaca, New York.: Cornell University Press.

Hemenway, D. (1983). Bimanual dexterity in baseball players. *The New England Journal of Medicine, 309*, 1587.

Hickok, G., Bellugi, U., & Klima, E. S. (2001). Sign language in the brain. *Scientific American*, 59–65.

Hills, A. E. (2007). Aphasia: Progress in the last quarter of a century. *Neurology, 69*, 200–213.

Kikkert, M. A., Ribbers, G. M., & Koudstaal, P. J. (2006). Alien hand syndrome in stroke: A report of 2 cases and review of the literature. *Archives of Physical Medicine and Rehabilitation, 87*, 728–732.

Laurent-Vannier, A., Pradat-Diehl, P., Chevignard, M., et al. (2003). Spatial and motor neglect in children. *Neurology, 60*, 202–207.

Motley, M. T. (1985). Slips of the tongue. *Scientific American, 253*, 116–125.

Newlands, F., Shrewsbury, D., & Robson, J. (2015). Foundation doctors and dyslexia: A qualitative study of their experiences and coping strategies. *Postgraduate Medical Journal, 91*, 121–126.

Paulesu, E., Démonet, J. F., Fazio, F., et al. (2001). Dyslexia: Cultural diversity and biological unity. *Science, 291*, 2165–2167.

Portal, J. M., & Romano, P. E. (1988). Patterns of eye–hand dominance in baseball players. *The New England Journal of Medicine, 319*, 655.

Revheim, M., Corcoran, C. M., Dias, E., et al. (2014). Reading deficits in schizophrenia and individuals at high clinical risk. *The American Journal of Psychiatry, 171*, 949–959.

Ringman, J. M., Saver, J. L., Woolson, R. F., et al. (2004). Frequency, risk factors, anatomy, and course of unilateral neglect in an acute stroke cohort. *Neurology, 63*, 468–474.

Vocat, R., Staub, F., Stroppni, T., et al. (2010). Anosognosia for hemiplegia: A clinical-anatomic prospective study. *Brain: A Journal of Neurology, 133*, 3578–3597.

QUESTIONS AND ANSWERS

1–5. For each of these patients, diagnose the language disorder, if any:
   a. Nonfluent aphasia
   b. Fluent aphasia
   c. Mild neurocognitive disorder
   d. Major neurocognitive disorder
   e. Delirium

Case 1

A 68-year-old retired waiter suddenly developed right hemiparesis. On examination, he only utters "Oh, Oh!" when stimulated. He remains impassive, mute to questions, and unresponsive when asked to move. Although his palpebral fissures are symmetric and he spontaneously closes his eyelids, his right lower face sags downward, flattening his nasolabial fold, and his right arm and leg have no muscle tone or movement. He makes no response to objects placed in his right visual field.

Case 2

A 70-year-old retired high-school science teacher, since suffering a stroke the previous year, can only say "weak, arm," "go away," and "give… supper me." His speech is slurred. When requested by an examiner, he can raise his left arm, protrude his tongue, and close his eyes. However, he cannot name objects or repeat phrases. His right arm is paretic, but he can walk.

Case 3

Over a period of 6 weeks, a previously healthy 64-year-old state senator has developed headaches, progressively severe difficulty in finding words, and confusion. She speaks continuously and incoherently: "Go to the warb," "I can't hear," "My heat hurts." When asked to repeat the phrase, "Four score and seven years ago," she says, "Four sevenths and many years before." She is unable to follow requests or name objects. When tested, she displays pronation of the outstretched right arm, but no frank weakness. The examiner elicits a right Babinski sign and finds papilledema.

Case 4

A 34-year-old taxi cab driver with mitral stenosis had the sudden onset of aphasia after an unusually severe transient left-sided headache. Although conversant, articulate, and able to follow requests and repeat phrases, he has difficulty naming objects. For example, when the examiner holds up in succession a pen, pin, and penny, the patient substitutes the name of one for the other and often repeats the name of the preceding object; however, when the examiner places these objects in front of him, the patient correctly points to the "money," "sharp object," and "writing instrument." A neurologic examination discloses no abnormal physical signs.

Case 5

A 54-year-old salesman, over the course of 8 months, has developed difficulty closing sales and memory impairment particularly for words and customers' names. He has difficulty completing his paperwork, but he has remained friendly, fully conversant, and articulate. He is able to name six objects, follow double requests, and repeat complex phrases; however, he has difficulty recalling six digits and three objects after 3 minutes, and recent events.

Answers: 1–5.
Case 1: a. He has loss of expressive language function accompanied by right hemiplegia and homonymous hemianopia. The language loss is so severe and extensive that many neurologists would describe it as a variety of nonfluent aphasia known as *global aphasia*. In this man's case, an occlusion of the left internal carotid artery probably caused an infarction of the entire left hemisphere.
Case 2: a. This man can say only a few phrases or several words in a telegraphic pattern, but he is able to comply with verbal requests, which indicates that his comprehension is intact. Although neurologists can neatly characterize only about one-third of cases of aphasia, this man has a textbook case of the Broca's variety of nonfluent aphasia. A right hemiparesis, in which the arm is more paretic than the leg, as in this case, typically accompanies his aphasia. An occlusion of the left middle cerebral artery and resulting cerebral infarction is the usual cause of this syndrome. The infarction would encompass Broca's area and the adjacent cortical motor region but spare the cortical fibers for the leg, which are supplied by the anterior cerebral artery.
Case 3: b. She has a normal quantity of speech; however, impaired comprehension and repetition and prominent paraphasic errors make her language unintelligible. She has a fluent aphasia that falls into the subdivision of Wernicke's aphasia. Only subtle right-sided corticospinal tract abnormalities – a pronator drift without frank paresis and a Babinski sign – accompany her aphasia. She probably has a lesion

in the left parietal or posterior temporal lobe. The headaches, papilledema, and relatively slow development indicate that the cause is a mass lesion, such as a glioblastoma.

Case 4: b. Because this man's impairment consists exclusively of improper identification of objects, he has a variety of fluent aphasia, known as anomic aphasia. Although anomic aphasia and other fluent aphasias may result from a neurodegenerative illness, they usually result from strokes or other small structural lesions in the temporal or parietal lobes. In his case, the mitral stenosis and headache indicate that the origin was probably an embolus (see Chapter 11).

Case 5: c. Although he has naming problems, his diagnosis is primarily mild neurocognitive disorder. Judging from the rapidity of onset, he may soon transition into major neurocognitive disorder.

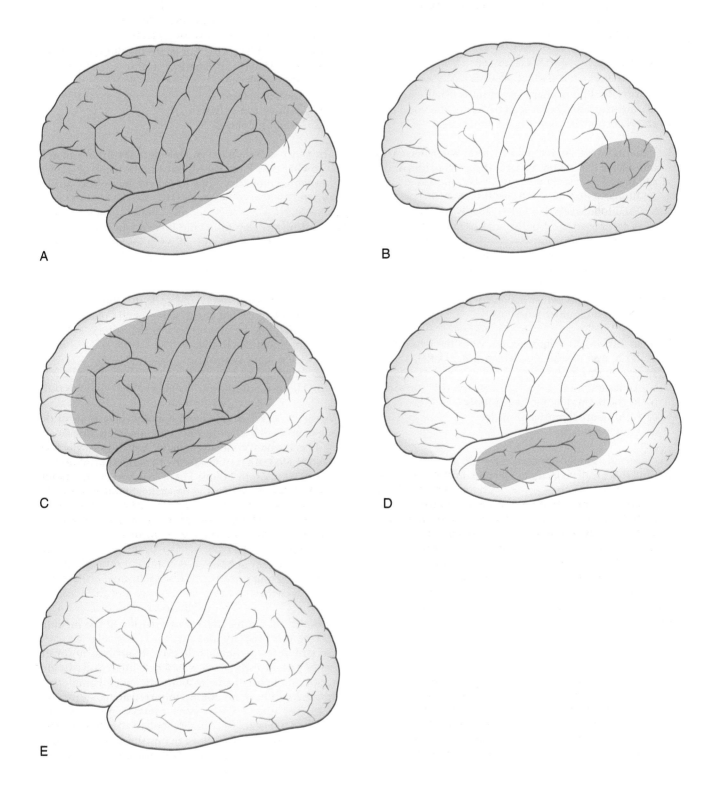

A

B

C

D

E

6–10. Match the lesions that are pictured schematically with those expected in cases 1–5.

Answers: *Case 1*, drawing A; *Case 2*, drawing C; *Case 3*, drawing D; *Case 4*, drawing B or D; *Case 5*, drawing E.

11. Various surgical procedures involving the neck, including thyroidectomy, placement of a vagus nerve stimulator, and cancer surgery, risk damaging the recurrent laryngeal nerve. What is the primary symptom of recurrent laryngeal nerve damage?
a. Aphasia
b. Dysarthria
c. Bulbar palsy
d. Dysphagia

Answer: b. The primary symptom is usually a hypophonic, breathy voice because of paresis of the vocal cord that the recurrent laryngeal nerve innervates.

12. Patients with amyotrophic lateral sclerosis (ALS) often have dysarthria. What is the usual origin of this symptom?
a. Bulbar palsy
b. Pseudobulbar palsy
c. A combination of bulbar and pseudobulbar palsy
d. Vocal cord atrophy

Answer: c. ALS is the quintessential motor neuron disease. It leads to death by apoptosis of both upper and lower motor neurons. Most patients with ALS have both bulbar and pseudobulbar palsy.

13. If an individual demonstrates right-left confusion, dyslexia, and dyscalculia, which other deficit should an examiner seek?
a. Aphasia
b. Right homonymous hemianopia
c. Mild neurocognitive disorder
d. Finger agnosia

Answer: d. Finger agnosia, right-left confusion, dyslexia, and dyscalculia constitute Gerstmann syndrome.

14. To which area of the brain do neurologists localize the damage that causes Gerstmann syndrome?
a. Dominant frontal lobe
b. Nondominant parietal lobe
c. Dominant parietal lobe
d. Left occipital lobe and adjacent splenium

Answer: c. Neurologists usually attribute Gerstmann syndrome to damage in the dominant parietal lobe's angular gyrus.

15. Which condition results from damage to the left occipital lobe and the adjacent splenium?
a. Alexia without agraphia
b. Klüver–Bucy syndrome
c. Anosognosia
d. Developmental dyslexia

Answer: a.

16. Which condition results from lesions that interrupt the dominant hemisphere's arcuate fasciculus?
a. Fluent aphasia
b. Anomic aphasia
c. Conduction aphasia
d. Isolation aphasia

Answer: c. Individuals with conduction aphasia cannot repeat what they have heard, but can name objects and follow verbal requests.

17. Which condition results from insults, such as cerebral anoxia, that are severe enough to damage the entire cerebral cortex but spare the dominant hemisphere's perisylvian language arc?
a. Fluent aphasia
b. Anomic aphasia
c. Conduction aphasia
d. Isolation aphasia

Answer: d. Individuals with isolation aphasia can only repeat what they have heard, but cannot name objects or follow verbal requests. They have a major neurocognitive disorder.

18. During the day following a stroke in his nondominant parietal lobe and adjacent corpus callosum, a 68-year-old man found that as he closed the buttons on his shirt with his right hand, his left hand would open them. When he was trying to eat, the left hand would also push away the fork that his right hand was holding. What is the name of the phenomenon in which one hand counteracts the other?
a. Intermanual conflict
b. Alien hand syndrome
c. Anosognosia
d. Hemi-inattention

Answer: a. When one hand opposes the actions of the other, neurologists label the phenomenon intermanual conflict. This counterproductive activity, which is usually subconscious, is often a manifestation of a nondominant parietal and corpus callosum lesion. Hemi-inattention, anosognosia, and alien hand syndrome typically accompany it.

19. Which of the following problems is a lateral medullary infarction most likely to cause?
a. Fluent aphasia
b. Nonfluent aphasia
c. Dementia
d. Dysarthria

Answer: d. Cranial nerves originating in the medulla innervate the pharynx and larynx. If a stroke weakens those structures, patients will have dysarthria; however, as with patients who have sustained infarctions in the pons or midbrain, patients with the lateral medullary syndrome will have no cognitive impairment.

20. When neurologists qualify aphasia with the term "transcortical," what does the qualification indicate?
a. The aphasic patient cannot repeat.
b. The aphasic patient can repeat.

c. The responsible cerebral lesion spans two or more regions of the cerebral cortex.

d. The underlying cause involves both cerebral hemispheres.

Answer: b. The term "transcortical" in the context of aphasia means that the patient's ability to repeat remains intact. Transcortical aphasia is a subtype of both nonfluent and fluent aphasias. The most dramatic form of transcortical aphasia is *isolation aphasia*, in which patients deprived of all other language and cognitive function are only able to repeat.

21. Which historical figure performed seminal work on language and its abnormalities?
    a. Alfred Adler
    b. Anna Freud
    c. Sigmund Freud
    d. Carl Jung

Answer: c. Sigmund Freud studied the neuroanatomy underlying language before he explored the potential for parapraxis (Freudian slips) to offer insights into the unconscious.

22. Which of the following causes of major neurocognitive disorder is most closely associated with aphasia?
    a. Alzheimer disease
    b. Frontotemporal dementia
    c. Huntington disease
    d. Human immunodeficiency virus

Answer: b. Frontotemporal dementia routinely has a component of language impairment. Aphasia may also complicate Alzheimer disease, but it is usually limited to anomic aphasia. Illnesses that attack predominantly subcortical structures, such as Huntington disease and human immunodeficiency virus (HIV), impair language function late in their course.

23. A woman brings her 74-year-old father, from whom she has been estranged for 10 years, for an urgent evaluation after a neighbor called and told her that he suddenly became confused. The daughter had little information, but she said that her father probably had been developing dementia for years. When asked about the date and place, the patient offered incoherent answers and was unable to follow verbal requests or repeat simple phrases. The patient showed no abnormal physical findings. Which test would diagnose dementia in the setting of aphasia?
    a. Mini-Mental State Examination (MMSE)
    b. Alzheimer's Disease Assessment Scale Cognitive Items (ADAS-COG)
    c. Montreal Cognitive Assessment (MOCA)
    d. None of the above

Answer: d. Although sections of each of these tests might help detect dementia in the setting of aphasia, none would be reliable. Collateral history regarding his functional state before the onset of aphasia would be helpful. Neuropsychologists recommend nonverbal testing of cognitive function referable to the nondominant hemisphere

using Raven's Progressive Matrices (Raven's Matrices), Reyes Complex Figure Tests, and the Wisconsin Card Sorting Test, which is now performed on a computer rather than with actual cards.

24. During an evaluation of a retired policeman's declining cognitive function, the neurologist asked him to pretend to use a broom to sweep the floor. He then used his hand as the broom itself. What would be the best term for his substituting his own hand for doing this?
    a. Dementia
    b. Ideational apraxia
    c. Ideomotor apraxia
    d. Concrete conceptualization

Answer: c. The policeman substituted his body part for the object that he should have been able to imagine. Ideational apraxia generally pertains to impairment in conceiving and executing a sequence of steps.

25. Which of the following statements regarding children with developmental dyslexia is *false*?
    a. Children with developmental dyslexia are as likely to have parents that are college professor parents as they are to have ones in any other occupation.
    b. Children with developmental dyslexia, especially boys, usually lack the normal asymmetry of the planum temporale.
    c. Dyscalculia, poor penmanship, and attention-deficit/hyperactivity disorder (ADHD) are comorbid with developmental dyslexia.
    d. Neurologists can frequently detect subtle right-sided motor impairments in individuals with dyslexia.

Answer: a. Because most cases of developmental dyslexia have a genetic basis, college professors are less likely to have a child with dyslexia. Dyslexic boys and to a lesser extent dyslexic girls lack the normally greater convolutions of their left compared to their right superior surface of the temporal lobe, the planum temporale. Other learning disabilities, poor handwriting, ADHD, and subtle right-sided motor impairments tend to accompany developmental dyslexia.

26. Which of the following statements regarding children with developmental dyslexia is *true*?
    a. The incidence of developmental dyslexia in children is equal in those who speak English, French, and Italian.
    b. The DSM-5 includes Developmental Dyslexia as a Neurocognitive Disorder.
    c. The DSM-5 includes Developmental Dyslexia as a Specific Learning Disorder.
    d. Developmental dyslexia is a lifelong impediment to success.

Answer: c. The DSM-5 subsumes Developmental Dyslexia, like Dyscalculia, into Specific Learning Disorder, which falls under the heading of Neurodevelopmental Disorders. Neurocognitive disorder generally refers to adult-onset, progressive intellectual deterioration. Children who speak English have twice the incidence of developmental dyslexia as those who speak Italian. Some investigators have attributed the greater incidence of dyslexia in English-speaking children to the relative complexity of English compared to Romance languages.

27. Paramedics revived a 34-year-old man who had attempted suicide inside a garage by sitting in a car with the motor running. During the next week, the man sat in bed and looked out of the window. He displayed no emotion and did not respond to requests. Although he was otherwise mute, he seemed to repeat in intricate detail whatever he was asked and whatever was spoken on TV shows he was watching. Physicians found brisk deep tendon reflexes, bilateral palmomental reflexes, and extensor plantar reflexes, i.e., Babinski signs. Which of the following is the most likely explanation of his inability to converse?
a. Persistent vegetative state
b. Nonfluent aphasia
c. Major neurocognitive disorder
d. Isolation aphasia

Answer: d. Whether or not the patient has major depressive disorder, he has isolation aphasia (transcortical aphasia). In this condition, which is a type of transcortical aphasia, the patient retains the ability to speak, which sometimes becomes irrepressible, but otherwise remains mute. In addition to losing conversational language, patients lose cognitive ability. In this patient's case, carbon monoxide led to generalized cerebral anoxia except that the perisylvian arc, being well perfused, escaped damage. Language processes continue within the perisylvian arc, but it receives no input from other regions of the cerebral cortex.

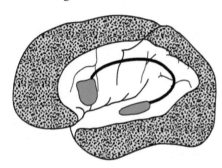

28. A left-handed 64-year-old schoolteacher sustained a thrombosis of the right middle cerebral artery. What might be predicted regarding his language function?
a. He will certainly develop aphasia.
b. He will have left hemiparesis and aphasia.
c. If he develops aphasia, his prognosis is relatively good compared to a right-handed person with a left middle cerebral artery thrombosis.
d. He will have a homonymous hemianopia only if he has aphasia.

Answer: c. Most left-handed individuals with normal intelligence remain either predominantly left-hemisphere dominant or mixed cerebral dominant. If left-handed individuals suffer an infarction of the right cerebral hemisphere, they do not necessarily develop aphasia. In fact,

they may develop aphasia if they have an infarction in the left cerebral hemisphere. Most important, left-handed individuals, compared to right-handed ones, have a better prognosis for the resolution of aphasia.

29. How do neurologists establish cerebral dominance for language function before cerebral cortex resection for epilepsy surgery?
a. MRI
b. CT
c. Wada test
d. PET

Answer: c. In the Wada test, infusion of barbiturates directly into the carotid artery ipsilateral to the dominant hemisphere produces aphasia. It is performed to establish which cerebral hemisphere is dominant before removal of a seizure focus. PET scans are difficult to perform because they require short-lived cyclotron-generated substrates and their spatial resolution is inadequate. Neither the CT nor MRI will reliably determine the dominant hemisphere. Functional MRI (fMRI, see Chapter 20), a noninvasive test, will probably replace the Wada test in locating the language regions, i.e., correlating anatomy and function.

30. In which condition is confabulation *not* found?
a. Anton's syndrome
b. Gerstmann syndrome
c. Anosognosia
d. Wernicke–Korsakoff syndrome

Answer: b. Gerstmann syndrome consists of the combination of right and left confusion, dyslexia, dyscalculia, and finger agnosia, but not confabulation. By way of contrast, in denying their blindness (Anton's syndrome), patients typically confabulate about the appearance of objects presented to them. Anosognosia often provokes confabulation, denial, and other defense mechanisms. Wernicke–Korsakoff syndrome is characterized by marked memory impairment, but confabulations also occur.

31. A 45-year-old man was driving slowly through normal city traffic when his car was struck in the rear by another car. Because he had been wearing his seatbelt, he sustained no direct head trauma, but he said that he was dazed. When evaluated 1 month later he seemed to have developed stuttering speech. MRIs of the head and cervical spine showed no pathology. Which is the most likely cause of his stuttering speech?
a. Subclinical aphasia
b. Dysarthria
c. A *contracoup* frontotemporal lobe injury
d. Psychogenic disturbance

Answer: d. Head trauma or other cerebral insult may reactivate childhood stuttering. In rare instances, frontal or temporal insults have caused stuttering. However, acquired stuttering, especially in the absence of major direct head trauma, is extraordinarily rare. Low-impact, rear-end motor vehicle crashes notoriously produce symptoms far in excess of actual bodily injury. Neurologists, closing their eyes to the distinction between unconscious and conscious processes, usually consider all symptoms without a physiologic basis to be psychogenic.

32. Which condition *routinely* causes aphasia?
    a. Chronic subdural hematomas
    b. Myasthenia gravis
    c. Multiple sclerosis (MS)
    d. Parkinsonism
    e. None of the above

Answer: e. Although chronic subdural hematomas may cause headaches and dementia, they usually do not cause aphasia or other neuropsychologic symptoms. Myasthenia typically causes dysarthria, but not cerebral impairment. When MS affects large regions of the cerebrum, it causes dementia. However, like other white matter diseases, MS rarely causes aphasia or other disorders of cortical function. Parkinsonism causes a hypophonic and tremulous voice and, late in the illness, dementia; however, it rarely causes aphasia.

33. A 25-year-old graduate student reported that when she awoke earlier in the morning, for approximately 5 minutes she had "expressive aphasia," by which she meant that she was unable to speak, but she understood the news on the radio. Then she developed a throbbing, unilateral headache and right-sided hemiparesis that lasted 1 hour. Which of the following conditions is the most likely reasonable explanation for her episode?
    a. Seizure
    b. Transient ischemic attack (TIA)
    c. Migraine
    d. Cocaine intoxication

Answer: c. In this patient migraine is the most likely, but the other conditions are possible in the appropriate conditions. A seizure originating in the left frontal lobe could lead to transient, postictal aphasia. A TIA in the distribution of the left carotid artery might cause aphasia with right hemiparesis, but probably not a headache. Cocaine may cause headache, aphasia, and lateralized neurologic deficits because it induces vasospasm, ischemic stroke, or cerebral hemorrhage. Incidentally, the potential etiologies of transient hemiparesis and transient aphasia are similar (see Hemiplegic Migraines, Chapter 9, and Carotid Artery TIAs, Chapter 11).

34. A 70-year-old newspaper reporter suddenly developed inability to read. Although he can write his name and most sentences that are dictated to him, he cannot read aloud or copy written material. His speech is fluent and contains no paraphasic errors. He can see objects only in his left visual field. He remains articulate and has no paresis. Which is the most appropriate term for his impairment?
    a. Alexia without agraphia
    b. Cortical blindness
    c. Psychogenic impairments
    d. Receptive aphasia

Answer: a. He clearly has alexia, as demonstrated by his inability to read, and a right homonymous hemianopia. Because he can transcribe dictation and write words from memory, he does not have agraphia. He does not have any aphasia. Because memory and auditory circuits, as well as the corticospinal system, are intact, he can write words that he hears or remembers. A stroke or tumor, such as a glioblastoma, that destroys the left occipital lobe and posterior corpus callosum, causes most cases of alexia without agraphia (see Fig. 8.4).

35. A 68-year-old taxicab driver had an accident after he drifted into oncoming traffic. The emergency room physician finds that he has a left homonymous hemianopia and a mild left hemiparesis, which the patient did not appreciate. Which neuropsychologic problem describes his denying his left arm weakness?
    a. Anosognosia
    b. Aphasia
    c. Anton's syndrome
    d. Alexia

Answer: a. After having the accident because a left homonymous hemianopia prevented him from seeing oncoming traffic, the patient remained oblivious to his deficits, which qualifies as anosognosia.

36. Which one of the following statements concerning Heschl's gyrus is *false*?
    a. Heschl's gyrus is bilateral and located adjacent to the planum temporale.
    b. Words and sound heard in the right ear are transmitted mainly to the right cerebral cortex.
    c. Each Heschl's gyrus reflects auditory stimulation predominantly from the contralateral ear.
    d. Heschl's gyrus sorts auditory stimuli for direction, pitch, loudness, and other acoustic properties.

Answer: b. Each hemisphere's Heschl's gyrus processes the auditory qualities of sound (see Fig. 4.16); however, words and sound heard in the right ear are transmitted to both the right and, more so, left cerebral cortex. The dominant hemisphere planum temporale, which is integral to language function, has greater surface area than the nondominant one.

37. Patients with nondominant hemisphere lesions are reported to have loss of the normal inflections of speech and diminished associated facial and limb gestures. What are the technical terms used to describe these findings?
    a. Limb apraxia
    b. Buccolingual apraxia
    c. Hypophonia
    d. Aprosody and loss of paralinguistic components of speech

Answer: d. Aprosody is the loss of the normal inflections of speech and emotional content. Diminished facial and limb gestures – body language – constitute loss of paralinguistic components of speech.

38. A man has undergone a commissurotomy for intractable seizures. His physicians show him a written request to raise both arms. How will he respond when the request is shown in his left visual field?
    a. He will raise only his left arm.
    b. He will raise only his right arm.
    c. He will raise both arms.
    d. He will raise neither arm.

Answer: d. When the examiner shows the request in the patient's left visual field, he will not raise either arm because the written visual information does not reach the left hemisphere language centers. In contrast, when the examiner shows the request in the patient's right visual field, the information reaches the language centers and he will raise his right hand.

39. With which condition is gait apraxia associated?
    a. Incontinence
    b. Dressing apraxia
    c. Limb apraxia
    d. Aphasia

Answer: a. Gait apraxia, incontinence, and dementia constitute classic manifestations of normal-pressure hydrocephalus (NPH).

40. With which condition is dressing apraxia associated?
    a. Limb apraxia
    b. Hemi-inattention
    c. Ideational apraxia
    d. Aprosody

Answer: b. Dressing apraxia, hemi-inattention, neglect, and constructional apraxia are all associated with nondominant parietal dysfunction.

41. With which condition is buccofacial apraxia associated?
    a. Nonfluent aphasia
    b. Fluent aphasia
    c. Limb apraxia
    d. Aprosody

Answer: a. Buccofacial apraxia and nonfluent aphasia both originate in left frontal lobe dysfunction.

42. In the middle of the night, an intern calls because a patient insists on leaving the hospital. This patient, a 72-year-old retired priest, had been admitted against his will for left hemiparesis. Earlier in the day, he had refused rehabilitation and further testing. Although unable to walk, the patient demands his clothing so that he may return home. He has become agitated, argumentative, and hostile, and even threatened physical violence. Aside from neurologic and psychiatric disorders, his general medical evaluation, including blood tests, showed no abnormality. Which would be the best management of this situation?
    a. Allow him to depart against medical advice.
    b. Administer a parenteral antipsychotic medicine.

    c. Explain that he had a stroke that gave him paralysis, which would prevent his walking safely.
    d. Administer intravenous glucose.

Answer: b. He is displaying dangerous reasoning and behavior characteristic of anosognosia. A careful explanation is sometimes helpful, but he has become irrational and sometimes frank explanations precipitate a catastrophic reaction. Administering a parenteral antipsychotic medicine would tide him over for the night. Once calmer and rational, he might accept the idea that, although he is paralyzed, he would improve with time and rehabilitation.

43. Which is the most powerful risk factor for the development of anosognosia for left-hemiparesis following a stroke?
    a. Loss of proprioception
    b. The degree of left hemiparesis
    c. Premorbid personality
    d. Premorbid emotional status

Answer: a. Loss of proprioception is almost a prerequisite, but it alone does not cause the condition.

44. How do patients typically respond to a stroke that causes left hemiparesis, hemianopia, and hemisensory loss?
    a. They stoically grin and bear these deficits.
    b. They employ defense mechanisms.
    c. They look toward the side of their deficits.
    d. Because they have aphasia, they do not discuss their response.

Answer: b. After sustaining a nondominant hemisphere stroke or other acute structural lesion, patients typically employ denial, projection, humor, and other defense mechanisms.

45. Which answer is incorrect in response to the question, "How does aphasia in left-handed people differ from aphasia in right-handed people?"
    a. Aphasia can result from lesions in either hemisphere.
    b. The variety of aphasia is less clearly related to the site of cerebral injury.
    c. The prognosis is better.
    d. The etiologies are different.

Answer: d.

46. Which of the following is *not* a disconnection syndrome?
    a. Internuclear ophthalmoplegia
    b. Conduction aphasia
    c. Split-brain syndrome
    d. Isolation aphasia

Answer: d. Disconnection syndromes refer to disorders in which lesions sever connections between primary centers. Although not a neuropsychologic disorder, neurologists consider internuclear ophthalmoplegia a disconnection syndrome because it results from damage to the pathway that connects brainstem nuclei, the medial longitudinal fasciculus.

47. Which artery supplies most of the perisylvian language arc?
    a. Anterior cerebral artery
    b. Middle cerebral artery
    c. Posterior cerebral artery
    d. Vertebrobasilar artery system

Answer: b.

48. Which term do neurologists apply to the area of the cerebral cortex located between branches of the major cerebral arteries?
    a. Watershed area
    b. Limbic system
    c. Cornea
    d. Arcuate fasciculus

Answer: a. People call the geographic region that a river or stream drains a "watershed." To neurologists, the term means areas of the cerebral cortex that are perfused by the terminal branches of arteries. During hypotension or anoxia, the already tenuous blood supply of a watershed cerebral region falls to an insufficient level.

49. Which is *true* regarding sign language?
    a. In congenitally deaf individuals, sign language, like spoken language, is based in the dominant hemisphere.
    b. Occlusion of the middle cerebral artery in the dominant hemisphere typically causes aphasia in users of sign language.
    c. Sign language relies on visual rather than auditory input.
    d. American Sign Language (ASL) is the proper name for the common, gesture-based sign language in the United States.
    e. All of the above

Answer: e.

50. In nonfluent aphasia, why is the arm typically more paretic than the leg?
    a. The middle cerebral artery, which is usually occluded in strokes that cause nonfluent aphasia, supplies the motor cortex for the arm but not the leg.
    b. The arm has a larger cortical representation.
    c. The infarct occurs in the internal capsule.
    d. The anterior cerebral artery, which is usually occluded in strokes that cause nonfluent aphasia, supplies the motor cortex for the arm but not the leg.

Answer: a. The anterior cerebral artery, which is usually spared in strokes that cause nonfluent aphasia (except for global aphasia), supplies the motor cortex for the leg.

51. An intern summons a psychiatry consultant to assess the decisional capacity of a 78-year-old woman who insists on leaving the hospital against advice despite having had a series of strokes that caused blindness but no paresis. The woman, who has walked to the nursing station in her hospital gown, has remained oblivious to her physicians' explanations of her condition and states that she is not blind. Not only does she insist on leaving, she wants to drive home. Although she cannot find it, she says she still has her driver's license and that is "all I need." She also states that she does not have Alzheimer disease because she knows the date and place. Which is the best diagnosis?
    a. Anton's syndrome
    b. Cortical blindness
    c. Dementia
    d. Optic ataxia

Answer: a. This woman has Anton's syndrome. She not only explicitly denies her blindness; she implicitly denies it by behaving as though she has full sight. In a variation of the syndrome, patients may concede that they are blind but behave as though they have full sight. Anton's syndrome patients frequently confabulate. Denial of blindness or other deficit typically leads to poor compliance with hospital regimens, demands for early discharge, and potentially dangerous behavior. In this case, physicians should not allow her to leave because she would be a danger to herself and others.

52. Which statement is *false* regarding gait apraxia as a manifestation of normal-pressure hydrocephalus (NPH)?
    a. Gait apraxia is the most distinctive sign of NPH.
    b. Gait apraxia resolves first with successful treatment of NPH.
    c. Taking an excessive number of steps to turn, failure to alternate weight-bearing, and seeming to be stuck to the floor characterize gait apraxia.
    d. Gait apraxia consists of many short, shuffling, and accelerating steps.

Answer: d. Short, shuffling, and accelerating steps characterize the festinating gait of Parkinson disease.

53. In which disorder(s) is echolalia a symptom?
    a. Autism
    b. Isolation aphasia
    c. Dementia
    d. Tourette's syndrome
    e. All of the above

Answer: e. Echolalia, the involuntary repetition of another person's words, is a manifestation of several different neurologic conditions.

54. An aging retired salesman has developed a slovenly appearance. He remains well-spoken, oriented, and has retained his good mood, memory, and judgment. The physician notes that the patient is unshaven, his belt does not go through the loops on his pants, and the buttons on his shirt are not aligned. The neurologic examination detects a left homonymous

hemianopia and a mild left hemiparesis. Which is the most precise term for his slovenly appearance?
a. Aphasia
b. Dementia
c. Depression
d. Dressing apraxia

Answer: d. He has lost the ability to manipulate his clothing, dress himself, and appreciate his appearance. Although the term dressing apraxia refers to the physical inability to dress, most patients also fail to perceive their state of partial undress in the largest sense of the word. Thus, closer examination may reveal that he fails to shave the left side of his face, does not comb the left side of his hair, and disregards his left sleeve and pants leg.

55. Which conclusion has stemmed from studies of patients who have undergone a commissurotomy?
a. The corpus callosum is vital to the auditory system.
b. Patients with the split brain have gross, readily identifiable physical and cognitive abnormalities.
c. Emotions generated in the right hemisphere are not as readily described as those generated in the left hemisphere.
d. Emotions generated in the left hemisphere are not as readily described as those in the right hemisphere.

Answer: c.

56. As part of a research project, a 60-year-old man who has undergone a commissurotomy placed his hands in a closed box containing many objects. A researcher put a set of keys in his left hand. By voice and gesture, the researcher asked the man to identify the keys. Which would be the subject's most likely response?
a. He would say, "A set of keys."
b. With his right hand, he would write, "A set of keys."

c. Although unable to say, "A set of keys," he would, if requested, be able to pick another set of keys from the various objects.
d. He would be unable to comply with the request under any circumstance.

Answer: c. Although the commissurotomy has severed the language center from his right hemisphere, he is still capable of comprehending the request, especially if it is gestured. In this case, at a nonverbal level, the man can identify the keys, but he is unable to formulate their name.

57. A psychiatrist is called to see a 74-year-old woman (See figure) at a nursing home because she constantly makes false reports of intruders in her nursing home room. Her family had placed her in the facility following partial recovery from a right-sided parietal stroke. Its residual deficits were a mild left hemiparesis and hemisensory impairment but no dementia. The psychiatrist finds that the woman has a tenuous relationship to her hand, which moves freely and, without her knowledge, pulls at her clothing. The woman does not deny that she had a stroke, but disclaims the hand at the end of her arm. "I am not moving it. Who is?" she finally asks the psychiatrist. Which is the most likely description for her perception?
a. Delusions or hallucinations associated with a nondominant hemisphere infarction
b. Alien hand syndrome
c. Anosognosia
d. Dementia

Answer: b. She has alien hand syndrome due to a nondominant hemisphere stroke. As is typical, she reports that the autonomously moving hand, which she does not fully feel, belongs to someone else. A patient often attributes deficits in the affected hand, such as

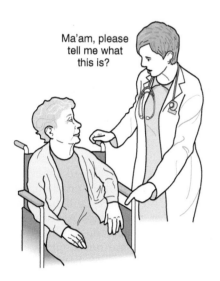

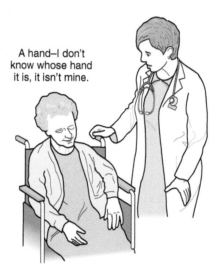

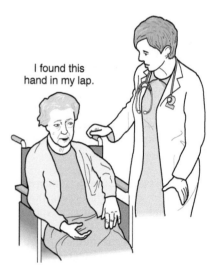

numbness or weakness, to another person. Such cases exemplify patients' use of defense mechanisms to cope with nondominant syndromes.

58. Which structure relays visual information from the lateral geniculate body to the visual cortex?
    a. The medial geniculate body
    b. The optic radiations
    c. The optic chiasm
    d. The Edinger–Westphal nucleus

Answer: b. The optic tract transmits visual information to the lateral geniculate body. After the synapse, the information passes via the optic radiations (geniculocalcarine tract) to the occipital lobe's visual cortex. The Edinger–Westphal nucleus relays information regarding light intensity to adjust pupil size.

59. Which structure relays auditory information from the brainstem to the auditory cortex?
    a. The medial geniculate body
    b. The lateral geniculate body
    c. The optic chiasm
    d. The Edinger–Westphal nucleus

Answer: a. The medial geniculate body receives auditory information from ipsilateral and contralateral brainstem auditory tracts. After the synapse, the medial geniculate sends the information to the temporal lobe's auditory cortex. Unlike transmission of visual information equally but exclusively to the contralateral visual cortex, both ears transmit auditory information to both auditory cortices; however, each ear's signals go predominantly to the contralateral one. Almost all auditory signals regarding language go to the dominant hemisphere cortex.

60. When asked to identify a tie, an aphasic patient said, "Fly, sigh, my, my, my, bye …" Which term best describes the response?
    a. Paraphasias
    b. Tangentialities
    c. Clang associations
    d. Jargon speech

Answer: c. The string of words is associated by sound rather than meaning, which constitutes clang associations. If the patient had associated the words with their meaning, neurologists would have described the string as a tangentiality. Both clang associations and tangentialities occur in aphasia as well as psychiatric disturbances.

61. When the ER resident asked a 68-year-old retired US Navy captain why he had come to the ER, he responded, "Get lost. Need assistance." When asked his location, the captain replied, "Sick bay." He complied with requests to pick up his left hand and then to stick out his tongue. He did not even begin to respond to requests to repeat phrases. He could not name the month and year, or spell the word "world" backward. All of his speech was dysarthric but comprehensible. Which of the following conditions does the examination indicate?
    a. Jargon speech of schizophrenia
    b. Nonfluent aphasia
    c. Fluent aphasia
    d. Dementia

Answer: b. This is a straightforward case of Broca's nonfluent aphasia. He has a paucity of speech, which is dysarthric. Moreover, it contains almost exclusively nouns and verbs. He can comprehend, but he cannot repeat. His use of naval jargon, such as "sick bay," does not constitute use of paraphasias.

62. In the preceding case, where would the abnormality most likely be identifiable?
    a. Left frontal lobe
    b. Left temporal lobe
    c. Entire cerebrum
    d. Bilateral frontal lobes

Answer: a. Immediately after a stroke, CT may not reveal changes of a stroke; however, diffusion weighted sequences on the MRI will show abnormalities. In any case, the clinical examination indicates that the lesion is probably in his left frontal lobe.

63. One week after surviving a cardiac arrest, a 50-year-old retired baseball player remained mute and apathetic. He assumed a fetal position. Although his pupils reacted to light and he had roving eye movements, he failed to establish eye contact with his examiners or family members and did not fixate on objects. Whether or not examiners spoke directly to him, he repeated long phrases he heard. He failed to respond to questions and requests, but instead would often repeat the sentence. His vital signs, general medical function, and routine laboratory tests were normal. The MRI showed changes indicative of diffuse cerebral ischemia, except around the perisylvian area, which appeared normal. Which is the most likely location of the responsible lesion?
    a. Most of the cerebral cortex
    b. Left frontal lobe
    c. Left parietal
    d. Both frontal lobes

Answer: a. Both clinical and MRI examinations indicate that he has sustained a severe and extensive, although incomplete, cerebral cortical anoxic insult. Survivors of cardiac arrest and those who have attempted suicide by hanging or carbon monoxide poisoning often suffer a similar injury. In such cases, patients may have preservation of the well-perfused language arc, but destruction of almost the entirety of other cortical regions.

64. In the previous question, in view of the patient's limited abilities, which is the best description of his language impairment?
    a. Nonfluent aphasia
    b. Conduction aphasia

c. Isolation aphasia
d. Dementia

Answer: c. His language capacity is limited to repetition. Although he probably has dementia, his language impairment is best termed isolation aphasia.

65. In the same question, which is the explanation for his being unable to see objects and family members?
    a. Psychogenic blindness
    b. Ocular ischemia
    c. Cortical blindness
    d. Anton's syndrome

Answer: c. The diffuse cerebral cortical damage included the occipital lobe. The pupillary light reflex depends only on the optic and oculomotor cranial nerves and the midbrain. Thus, the pupillary light reflex remains intact even with massive cerebral damage unless it causes cerebral herniation. Anton's syndrome is a perceptual problem in which blind individuals implicitly or explicitly deny that they are blind.

66. The children of a 60-year-old man have brought their father for psychiatric evaluation because during the previous year he has become loud and unrestrained, and he has made unwise investments. Although he has no history of depressive symptoms, they have suggested a diagnosis of bipolar disorder. His children also report that in his late 50s his own father – their paternal grandfather – had developed similar behavior and died several years later of Alzheimer disease.

    During a routine mental status examination, the psychiatrist notes that the patient is unable to name infrequently occurring objects, such as the knot of his tie, stem of his watch, and buckle of his belt. Also, he recalls only four or five of six digits. However, he remains able to follow two-step requests and repeat complicated phrases. The psychiatrist sees no paresis, gait impairment, or other physical deficit. Which of the following conditions is most likely responsible for the patient's behavior?
    a. Alzheimer disease
    b. Frontotemporal dementia
    c. Bipolar disorder
    d. Vascular dementia

Answer: b. The patient has mild but definite anomic aphasia, which is a fluent aphasia, as well as dementia, which is probably inherited. While a structural lesion produces most cases of aphasia, the cause here, as in many cases of anomic aphasia, is probably frontotemporal dementia. This neurodegenerative illness develops earlier and progresses more rapidly than Alzheimer disease. Moreover, even though Alzheimer disease follows a genetic pattern in many families, frontotemporal dementia more frequently follows one. With this disorder, behavioral changes or language deficits accompany or overshadow cognitive impairment.

67. Neurologists have been caring for an elderly man who sustained a nondominant hemisphere stroke that caused left-sided hemiparesis and sensory loss. He has been uncooperative with hospital routine and insisted on being discharged to his apartment. When they show him an American flag, he reports seeing only red stripes.

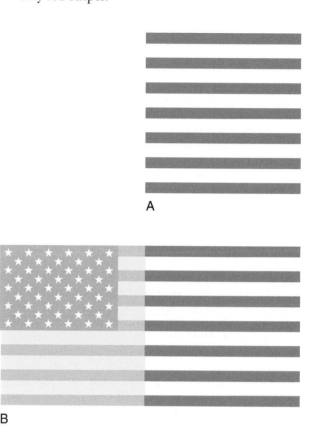

Even when the neurologists ask him to look all around and fully examine the fabric, the man maintains it is only striped cloth and probably part of a prisoner's striped shirt. Which is the most likely explanation of his misperception?
    a. He has a left homonymous hemianopia.
    b. He has left-sided neglect or hemi-inattention.
    c. He has left-right confusion.
    d. He has dementia.

Answer: b. Although he may have left homonymous hemianopia, his problem extends beyond a simple lack of vision on his left side. Someone with a left homonymous hemianopia, especially when asked to look all around and fully examine something, would notice all its elements. He would have brought the star-filled rectangle into his right visual field. Instead, he neglected or remained inattentive to it.

Moreover, his misinterpreting the flag as a prisoner's shirt may represent a reworking of his feeling of being kept against his will in the hospital.

HEADACHES

In the most widely accepted categorization, the International Headache Society (IHS) recognizes three major categories: primary headaches, secondary headaches, and cranial neuralgias. Primary headaches include *tension-type*, *migraine*, and *cluster headaches*. Although not life-threatening, primary headaches may create excruciating pain, incapacitate patients, and, with frequent attacks, reduce a patient's quality of life. Neurologists diagnose these headaches not by physical findings or laboratory tests, which are characteristically normal, but by their distinctive symptoms.

Secondary headaches, on the other hand, are often manifestations of an underlying serious, sometimes life-threatening, illness. This category includes *temporal arteritis*, *intracranial mass lesions*, *idiopathic intracranial hypertension* (*pseudotumor cerebri*), meningitis, subarachnoid hemorrhage, and *postconcussion headaches* (see Chapter 22). Unlike the diagnosis of primary headaches, the diagnosis of secondary headaches typically rests on their clinical context, physical exam and radiographic findings, or laboratory abnormalities.

PRIMARY HEADACHES

Tension-Type Headache

Tension-type headache (TTH), previously called "tension headache," is the most common primary headache. TTH is characterized by intermittent dull pain, lasting between 30 minutes and 7 days, usually located bilaterally in the frontal or cervical regions. Patients have only pain. They do not have other symptoms that typify migraine, such as photophobia, hyperacusis, phonophobia, nausea, vomiting, or other autonomic disturbance. This headache plagues women more than men and often affects multiple family members. Patients with TTH tolerate their pain and usually go about their daily activities without interruption. (In contrast, patients who have activity-related headache exacerbation probably have migraine.)

TTH has traditionally been attributed to contraction of the scalp, neck, and face muscles (Fig. 9.1), as well as emotional "tension." Fatigue, cervical spondylosis, bright light, loud noise, and, at some level, emotional factors allegedly produce or precipitate TTH. However, because studies have demonstrated that this headache results from neither muscle contractions nor psychological tension, the designation "muscle contraction" or "tension" probably represents a misnomer. The term "tension-type" headache is more appropriate. In fact, many neurologists place this headache at the opposite end of a headache spectrum from migraine, where both result from a common, but unknown, physiological disorder.

Treatment

Neurologists generally first assure themselves and their patients that the headache does not represent a brain tumor or other potentially fatal illness, which is frequently an unspoken fear. On the other hand, these headaches are liable to become a chronic, intractable, demoralizing painful condition. Risk factors for chronicity or other poor outcome include comorbid migraine or sleep disorders and being unmarried.

For headaches that occur less than twice a week, neurologists usually suggest "acute therapy" – medicines taken at the headache's onset to abort an incipient attack or reverse a full-blown one. Over-the-counter medicines such as aspirin, aspirin-caffeine compounds, acetaminophen, and nonsteroidal anti-inflammatory drugs (NSAIDs) usually suffice. Patients keep these medicines readily available in the car, at work, and in pocketbooks to take at the first sign of a headache. However, physicians should be mindful that daily use often leads to *chronic daily headache* (see later).

Neurologists often recommend "preventive therapy" – prophylactic medicines taken daily – under several circumstances: if headaches occur more frequently than two or three times per week, acute therapy is ineffective, or analgesic consumption becomes excessive. Even if patients have no history of depression or epilepsy, neurologists often prescribe small nighttime doses of a tricyclic antidepressant (TCA) or certain antiepileptic drugs (AEDs), such as valproate/divalproex (Depakote) or topiramate (Topamax). However, they usually avoid prescribing older antiepileptics, such as benzodiazepines or phenobarbital. As if to confirm that muscle contraction does not cause TTH, botulinum toxin injections into scalp and cervical muscles, even though they reduce muscle spasm, fail to alleviate these headaches. Similarly, other "muscle relaxants," such as cyclobenzaprine (Flexeril), are ineffective in the treatment of episodic and chronic TTH.

In children and adolescents, relaxation and cognitive-behavioral therapy (CBT) reduce the frequency and severity of chronic headache. In adults, insight-oriented psychotherapy and psychoanalysis do not alleviate headaches, but may provide insight, reduce anxiety, treat depression, and offer other benefits. Stress management therapy, especially when combined with a TCA, provides modest help.

Migraine

Neurologists have said, "Whereas tension-type headaches are boring in their sameness, migraine headaches are typically rich in symptoms." In clinical practice, the core criteria for migraine consist of episodic, disabling

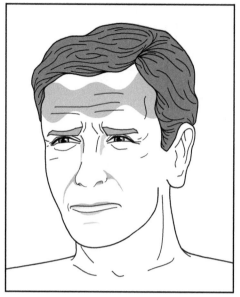

FIGURE 9.1 ■ Tension-type headaches produce a bandlike, squeezing, symmetric pressure at the neck, temples, or forehead.

BOX 9.1	Criteria for Migraine*

Recurrent (≥5) attacks of headache each with a duration of 4–72 hours (untreated or unsuccessfully treated)
At least two of the following characteristics:
a. Unilateral location
b. Pulsating quality (throbbing pain)
c. Moderate or severe in intensity
d. Aggravation by routine physical activity
The headache is accompanied by at least one of the following symptoms:
a. Nausea and/or vomiting
b. Photophobia and phonophobia

*Essential features of the International Headache Society (IHS) classification

BOX 9.2	Auras of Migraine

Sensory phenomena
  Special senses
    Visual, olfactory, auditory, gustatory
  Paresthesias, especially lips and hand
Motor deficits
  Hemiparesis, hemiplegia
Neuropsychologic changes
  Aphasia
  Perceptual impairment, especially for size, shape, and time
Emotional and behavioral
  Anxiety, depression, irritability, (rarely) hyperactivity

headaches associated with nausea and photophobia. The nonheadache symptoms, in fact, often overshadow or replace the headache (see later). The headaches' qualities – throbbing pain and unilateral location – are typical and included in the IHS criteria (Box 9.1).

Approximately 12% of all Americans suffer from migraine. Not only do women suffer from migraine three times more frequently than men, but their migraines are also more severe. Migraine may first appear in childhood, but most often not until adolescence or early adulthood. The prevalence increases until age 40. Although migraine symptoms are complex and variable, they are usually consistent from attack to attack for the individual patient.

Neurologists grossly divide episodic migraine into two subtypes – defined primarily by the presence or absence of an *aura*.

Migraine With Aura

Migraine with aura, previously labeled *classic migraine*, affects only about 20–30% of migraine patients. The aura, which can represent almost any symptom of cortex or brain dysfunction, typically precedes or accompanies the headache (Box 9.2). The headache itself is similar to the headache in *migraine without aura* (see later).

Auras usually appear gradually and then evolve over 5 to 20 minutes, persist for less than 1 hour, and evaporate with the onset of the headache. They characteristically consist of a transient visual phenomenon, but sometimes a simple olfactory hallucination. Instead of a disturbance in one of the special senses, aura occasionally consists of language impairment similar to aphasia, sensory misperception, or personality change. In children, but not adults, recurrent colic or "cyclic abdominal pain" with nausea and vomiting may constitute a migraine variant, but not technically an aura.

By far, the commonest migraine auras are visual hallucinations (see Chapter 12). They usually consist of a graying of a region of the visual field (*scotoma*) (Fig. 9.2A), flashing zigzag lines (*scintillating* or *fortification scotomata*) (Fig. 9.2B), crescents of brilliant colors (Fig. 9.2C), tubular vision, or distortion of objects (*metamorphopsia*). Unlike visual auras that represent other neurologic conditions (see Box 12.1), migraine auras most often involve the simultaneous appearance of positive phenomena, such as scintillations, and negative ones, such as opaque areas. Finally, instead of sensory auras, some migraineurs experience premonitory somatic symptoms, such as fatigue, stiff neck, yawning, hunger, and thirst. These patients can frequently predict their impending migraine hours to days before onset.

Migraine Without Aura

Previously labeled *common migraine*, migraine without aura affects about 75% of migraine patients. In other words, most individuals with migraine do not have an aura. Arising without warning, their headaches are initially throbbing and located predominantly behind a temple (temporal) or around or behind one eye (periorbital or retro-orbital), but usually on only one side of the head (hemicranial) (Fig. 9.3). In the majority of cases, the side of the headache switches within and between attacks. Individual attacks usually occur episodically and last 4 to 72 hours. Frequent attacks may transform into a dull, symmetric, and continual pain – chronic daily headache – that mimics TTH.

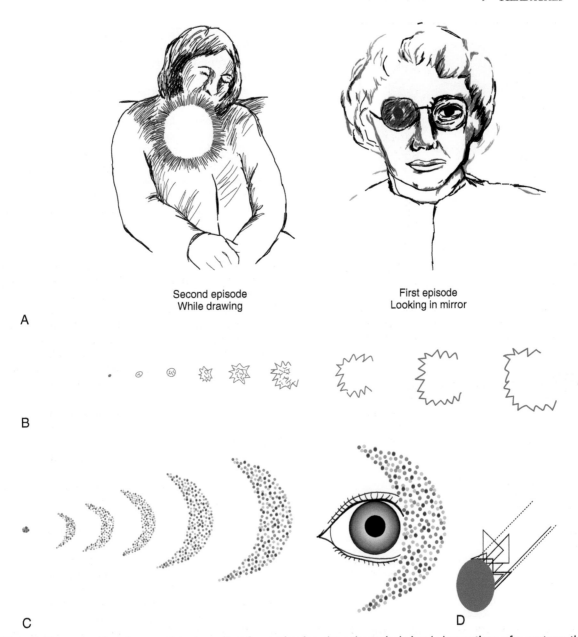

Second episode
While drawing

A

First episode
Looking in mirror

B

C

D

FIGURE 9.2 ■ *A,* These drawings by an artist who suffers from migraine show the typical visual obscurations of a *scotoma* that precedes the headache phase of her migraines. In both cases, she loses a small circular area near the center of vision. As occurs with most migraineurs, she says that although the aura is only gray and has a simple shape, it mesmerizes her. *B,* The patient who drew this aura, a *scintillating scotoma,* wrote, "In the early stages, the area within the lights is somewhat shaded. Later, as the figure widens, you can peer right through the area. Eventually, it gets so wide that it disappears." This typical scotoma consists of an angular, brightly lit margin and an opaque interior that begins as a star and expands into a crescent. She somehow calculated that it scintillated at 8 to 12 Hz. Neurologists refer to auras with angular edges as *fortification scotomas* because of their similarity to medieval military fortresses. *C,* A 30-year-old female artist in her first trimester of pregnancy had several migraine headaches that were heralded by this scotoma. Each began as a blue dot and, over 20 minutes, enlarged to a crescent of brightly shimmering, multicolored dots. When the crescent's intensity peaked, she was so dazzled that she lost her vision and was unable to think clearly. *D,* Having patients, especially children, draw what they "see" before a headache has great diagnostic value. One adolescent reconstructed this "visual hallucination" using his computer.

For patients and neurologists, what clearly distinguishes migraine from TTH are migraine's nonheadache symptoms, including sensory hypersensitivity (photophobia and phonophobia), autonomic dysfunction (nausea and vomiting), and disability. In common terms, people with migraine typically have episodes of moderately severe headaches accompanied by nausea and during a painful attack, they gravitate to dark, quiet places.

During migraine attacks, patients often have dysphoria and inattentiveness that can mimic depression, seizures, and other neurologic disturbances (Box 9.3). Most patients withdraw during an attack, but some become feverishly active. Many tend to drink large quantities of water or crave certain foods or sweets, particularly chocolate. Children often become confused and overactive. After an attack clears, especially when it ends with sleep,

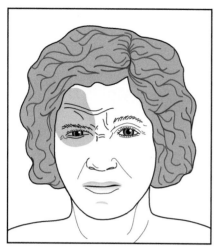

FIGURE 9.3 ■ Patients with migraine usually have throbbing hemicranial headaches that may either move to the other side of the head or become generalized.

BOX 9.3	**Common Neurologic Causes of Transient Mood Disturbance or Altered Mental Status**

Drugs
    Illicit
    Medicinal
Metabolic aberrations
    Hypoglycemia
    Hepatic encephalopathy
Migraine
Mitochondrial encephalopathy
Seizures (see Chapter 10)
    Absence
    Complex partial
    Frontal lobe
Sleep attacks (e.g., narcolepsy, sleep apnea naps [see Chapter 17])
Transient global amnesia (see Chapter 11)
Transient ischemic attacks (see Chapter 11)

---

migraine sufferers may experience a sense of tranquility or even euphoria.

An additional point of contrast to TTH is that migraine attacks typically begin in the early morning rather than the afternoon. In fact, they often have their onset during rapid eye movement (REM) sleep, which predominates in the several hours before awakening (see Chapter 17). Sometimes migraines begin exclusively during sleep – neurologists use the term "nocturnal migraines" though this term is no longer included in IHS classification. No matter when a migraine attack has begun, naturally occurring or medication-induced sleep characteristically cures it.

In women, migraine often first develops at menarche, recurs premenstrually, and is aggravated by some oral contraceptives. Most women with migraine report that their attacks are most likely to occur immediately before or at the beginning of their menses, and about 10% of them suffer migraines exclusively at this time. During pregnancy, about 70% of women with migraine experience dramatic relief, but usually only during their second or third trimesters. However, pregnancy can also have adverse effects. About 10% of women with migraine experience their first attack during pregnancy. Furthermore, 10% to 20% of pregnant women with migraine have more frequent or more severe attacks than usual. Nevertheless, pregnant women beset by migraine are no more likely than ones free of migraine to suffer miscarriage, eclampsia, or fetal malformations. That being said, the features of new headaches in a pregnant woman may not be specific enough to exclude secondary causes of headache, and prompt evaluation is warranted. Additionally, though postpartum headaches may represent a recurrence of migraine, they may instead represent more serious conditions, such as cortical vein thrombosis, complication of epidural anesthesia, or pituitary infarction. Postmenopausal women usually enjoy improvement in their migraine frequency and severity.

Another important characteristic of migraine is that it can be precipitated – in susceptible individuals – by certain factors or "triggers," such as skipping meals or fasting on religious holidays, too little or excessive sleep, menses, psychologic or occupational stress, overexertion, head trauma, and alcoholic drinks. (Alcohol can also provoke attacks of cluster headaches [see later].) Red wine and brandy are the alcoholic drinks most likely to trigger an attack, with vodka and white wine the least likely.

To the chagrin of many patients, migraine attacks often coincide with weekends and the start of a vacation. Many of the factors associated with these holidays likely contribute to this paradox: withdrawal from work-related stress, anxieties associated with leisure periods, too little sleep, sleeping later than usual (which extends REM periods and does not allow the customary morning cup of coffee [see later]), and lavish meals, which typically include wine as well as foods spiced with monosodium glutamate (MSG).

Psychiatric Comorbidity

Contrary to old views, migraine is not restricted to individuals in upper-income brackets or more prevalent among those who are rigid, perfectionist, and competitive. Neurologists consider "migraine personality" an outmoded concept.

Depression is strongly comorbid with migraine and the conditions appear reciprocal. Major depression increases the risk of migraine but not of other severe headaches. Similarly, unlike other headache disorders, migraine increases the risk of major depression up to four times. Migraineurs are also more likely to carry the diagnosis of generalized anxiety disorder, panic disorder, and bipolar disorder. Studies differ as to the effect of comorbid depression on the frequency or disability of migraine. In an effect that seems to be restricted to women, adverse life events increase headache frequency. Regardless of the causal relationship, neurologists and psychiatrists must pay close attention to mood disorders in patients with migraine headaches. One large study showed that patients with migraine have increased rates of lifetime suicidal ideation and attempts in comparison to the general population. In the subset of patients who had concomitant migraine headache and fibromyalgia, another chronic pain syndrome (see Chapter 6), rates of suicidal ideation were almost 60% and rates of suicide attempt were 15–20%, significantly higher than rates in the migraine-only group and the general population.

Therapy for patients with migraine and comorbid depression should start with simple behavioral advice, such as getting sufficient sleep on a regular schedule, exercising moderately, avoiding alcohol and drugs, and keeping a "headache diary" (see later). CBT and biofeedback, as an adjunct to medication, may be helpful.

TCAs are effective for treating migraine comorbid with depression, and are more effective than selective serotonin or norepinephrine reuptake inhibitors (SSRIs or SNRIs) for treating migraine with or without comorbid depression. However, when administered concurrently with one of the popular antimigraine serotonin (5-hydroxytryptamine [5HT]) agonists, such as a "triptan" (see later) or dihydroergotamine (DHE), SSRIs and SNRIs carry a low but often-cited risk of producing the serotonin syndrome (see Chapter 6).

The *Diagnostic and Statistical Manual of Mental Disorders-5* (DSM-5) places headache as a diagnostic modifier. For example, a patient with depression triggered by severe headaches would be diagnosed with Depressive Disorder due to Another Medical Condition. However, as depression and migraines are highly comorbid, it is often difficult for neurologists and psychiatrists to prove this causal relationship. If patients fabricate reports of migraine to obtain opioids or other tangible benefit, the diagnosis would be Factitious Disorder Imposed on Self or Malingering.

Other Subtypes of Migraine

Childhood migraine is not simply migraine in "little adults." Compared to migraine in adults, children with migraines have a headache that is more severe, but briefer (frequently less than 2 hours) and less likely to be unilateral (only one-third of cases). However, as with migraine in adults, the nonheadache components may overshadow the headache. For example, childhood migraine often produces episodes of confusion, incoherence, or agitation. In addition, it frequently leaves children incapacitated by nausea and vomiting. Physicians caring for children with such episodes may consider mitochondrial encephalopathy as an alternative, although rare, diagnosis (see Chapter 6). Pediatric neurologists also consider mitochondrial encephalopathy as well as hemiplegic migraine (see later) in the differential diagnosis of transient hemiparesis in a child with headaches.

Children are particularly susceptible to migraine variants. In *basilar-type migraine*, the headache is accompanied or even overshadowed by ataxia, vertigo, dysarthria, or diplopia – symptoms that reflect brain dysfunction in the basilar artery distribution (the cerebellum, brainstem, and posterior cerebrum [see Fig. 11.2]). In addition, when basilar migraine impairs the temporal lobes, children as well as adults may experience temporary generalized memory impairment, reminiscent of transient global amnesia (see Chapter 7). Children may also have syndromes such as cyclic vomiting and recurrent benign paroxysmal positional vertigo, which can precede the diagnosis of migraine headaches by many years. *Hemiplegic migraine*, another variant, is defined by hemiparesis of various grades often accompanied by hemiparesthesia, aphasia, or other cortical symptoms. All these symptoms usually precede or occur with an otherwise typical migraine headache, but they may also develop without any headache or other migraine symptom. Thus, in evaluating a patient who has had transient hemiparesis, the physician might consider hemiplegic migraine along with transient ischemic attacks (TIAs), stroke, postictal (Todd's) hemiparesis, and conversion disorder.

In *familial hemiplegic migraine* (*FHM-1*), patients develop transient hemiparesis before or during the headache. This variant of migraine is transmitted in an autosomal dominant pattern by a genetic abnormality on chromosome 19. The basic mechanism is a calcium channel abnormality – a "channelopathy." Other channelopathies include myotonic dystrophy (see Chapter 6), spinocerebellar ataxia type 6 (also transmitted by a mutation on chromosome 19), and varieties of epilepsy.

Stroke occasionally complicates migraine. Of its variants, migraine with aura serves as the most powerful risk factor for stroke. Female migraine patients who both smoke cigarettes and use oral contraceptives are particularly at risk of stroke.

Migraine-Like Conditions: Food-Induced Headaches

Neurologists look at certain foods and medications as both a cause of nonspecific headache and a trigger of migraine. However, other than alcohol, the role of food is overemphasized. It precipitates migraine or other headache in only about 15% of patients.

The two clearest examples of foods precipitating headaches occur in the *Chinese restaurant syndrome*, where the offending agent is MSG, and the *hot dog headache*, where nitrites, used in many processed meats, are the offending agent. A different situation is the *ice cream headache*, where any very cold food that touches the pharynx triggers a headache, though this does not usually have the features of migraine. Some people – but fewer than generally assumed – develop migraine-like headaches after eating foods containing tyramine, such as ripened cheese, or ones containing phenylethylamine, such as chocolate. In view of chocolate's tendency in some individuals to precipitate attacks, it is ironic that many migraine sufferers crave chocolate before an attack. Nevertheless, migraine sufferers should probably avoid the "Four 'C's": chocolate, cheese, Chinese food, and alcohol (C_2H_5OH).

On the other hand, people who miss their customary morning coffee typically develop the *caffeine-withdrawal syndrome* that consists of moderate-to-severe headache often accompanied by anxiety and depression. Although this syndrome is almost synonymous with coffee deprivation, withdrawal of other caffeine-containing beverages or caffeine-containing medications can precipitate it (see Chapter 17). Herein lies a dilemma: sudden withdrawal of caffeine can cause the withdrawal syndrome, but excessive caffeine leads to irritability, palpitations, and gastric acidity. Moreover, excessive caffeine also is a risk factor for transforming migraine to chronic daily headache.

Medication-Induced Headaches

Similarly, neurologists look at certain medications as playing both roles. Antianginal medicines, such as nitroglycerin or isosorbide (Isordil), perhaps because they contain nitrites that dilate cerebral as well as cardiac arteries, cause headaches. Elderly patients who have cerebrovascular atherosclerosis are particularly vulnerable. Curiously, whereas some calcium channel blockers, such as nifedipine (Procardia), trigger headaches, others, such as verapamil (Calan), may prevent them. For the psychiatrist, the most notorious iatrogenic headache, which is often complicated by cerebral hemorrhage, is produced by the interaction of monoamine oxidase inhibitor (MAOI) antidepressants with other medications or foods (see later).

Sex-Related Headaches

Sexual intercourse or masturbation, with or without orgasm, may trigger a severe headache. Currently termed *primary headache associated with sexual activity*, these headaches were previously termed *coital cephalgia* or *orgasmic headache*, depending on the circumstances. Sex-related headaches, which are especially common in individuals with migraine, typically last for several minutes to several hours. The pain may be severe and incapacitating, but the neurologic problem is almost always benign. Nevertheless, in assessing headaches occurring during sex, physicians might consider intracerebral or subarachnoid hemorrhage (see later). When the diagnosis of sex-related headaches is secure, taking propranolol or indometacin before sex usually prevents an ensuing headache.

Proposed Causes of Migraine

A once popular theory postulated that constriction of muscles of the cerebral arteries first caused an aura and then, when the muscles fatigued, the arteries dilated and allowed pulsations to pound the interior of the arterial walls. In this theory, the unsuppressed pounding produced the typical throbbing headache.

A current, more credible theory attributes migraine to "spreading neuronal depression." This theory postulates that impaired metabolism of cerebral neurons spreads – first as increased neuronal activity and then as inhibited neuronal activity – from the posterior to anterior cerebral cortex. The impaired metabolism, according to the theory, produces the aura and activates the trigeminal nucleus, which innervates the meninges and triggers the release of vasoactive neuropeptides, including serotonin, substance P, and neurokinin. Then these neuropeptides incite painful vasodilation and perivascular inflammation. Related theories propose that the relationship between serotonin and migraine headaches explains why migraineurs have relatively high rates of epilepsy, major depression, and anxiety.

Other theories postulate faulty serotonin neurotransmission because several serotonin-related observations stand out. For example, at the onset of migraine, platelet serotonin concentration falls. Triptans, which are an effective and specific treatment for migraine, act primarily as serotonin $5HT_{1B}$ and $5HT_{1D}$ receptor agonists in the cerebral vessels' trigeminal nerve endings. They most likely relieve migraine by blocking the release of the vasoactive neuropeptides.

Whatever the biochemical mechanism, a genetic abnormality predisposes certain individuals to migraine. About 70% of migraine patients have a close relative with the disorder, and studies of twins show a high concordance. The risk of migraine is 50% or greater in relatives of an individual with migraine, and this risk increases with the severity of attacks. In the case of hemiplegic migraine, the genetic basis is well established.

Acute Treatment

In attempting to identify triggers, neurologists usually suggest that patients create a headache diary to note associations with particular days and note potential precipitants or triggers, such as alcohol consumption, meals, menses, and stressful episodes. Migraine sufferers may download any of several computer and smart phone applications that allow them to perform these functions and review the information with their physician. If migraine sufferers cannot avoid triggers, they should at least anticipate attacks.

For treatment of migraine, relaxation techniques or other forms of CBT may be helpful. In contrast, scientific studies have not documented benefits from hypnosis, acupuncture, transcutaneous electrical stimulation, or spinal manipulation. Successful treatment usually requires medications to dampen the headache and ameliorate the accompanying nausea and vomiting. Treatment regimens for children and adolescents differ from those for adults. As with TTH, patients take medications on an acute basis to abort an incipient migraine or to reverse one that has already reached peak intensity. For acute treatment of occasional mild attacks, simple analgesics, NSAIDs, and other over-the-counter medicines may suffice.

Although opioids may suppress headaches, neurologists have remained wary of their leading to drug-seeking behavior (see Chapter 14). In the majority of patients receiving opioid treatment, emergency room visits and hospitalizations decrease, but their headaches and disability persist. Nevertheless, neurologists often prescribe them in limited, controlled doses when vasoactive or serotoninergic medications carry too many risks, such as for pregnant or elderly patients.

Triptans, the $5HT_{1B/1D}$ serotonin receptor agonists, include, among others, frovatriptan (Frova), naratriptan (Amerge), rizatriptan (Maxalt), sumatriptan (Imitrex), and zolmitriptan (Zomig). They are rapidly effective for moderate-to-severe migraine and some are available as injections, sublingual wafers, and nasal sprays. The variety of forms allows patients to administer their medicines without delay, even when in public or beset by nausea. Women with menstrually related, or *catamenial*, migraine might suppress attacks by taking a triptan or NSAID for the several days before menses commence or during the days of their cycle when their headaches occur.

Ergotamine and dihydroergotamine, which are primarily vasoconstrictors, are also rapidly effective. Although widely used decades ago, triptans largely have supplanted them. Excessive use of the vasoconstrictors may lead to persistent, excessive vasoconstriction (*ergotism*) in the coronary arteries, digits, and elsewhere. In another caveat, because vasoconstrictors might precipitate a miscarriage or cause fetal malformations, ergotamine and dihydroergotamine, unlike triptans, are unequivocally contraindicated in pregnant women. Finally, administration of either a triptan or vasoconstrictor to patients already under treatment with an SSRI or SNRI potentially risks causing the serotonin syndrome.

Many of these migraine medications have the same worrisome side effect as those used to treat TTH. Their frequent use – as little as two to three times a week – may lead not to cure but to chronic daily headache.

Nausea and vomiting not only constitute symptoms of migraine, but they also may be side effects of DHE or another antimigraine medicine. Whatever their cause or severity, nausea and vomiting prevent gastric absorption of orally administered medicines. Many migraine sufferers thus require a parenterally administered antiemetic, such as metoclopramide (Reglan). One caveat remains: dopamine-receptor-blocking antiemetics may cause dystonic reactions identical to those induced by dopamine-receptor-blocking antipsychotics (see Chapter 18). Thus, neurologists often prophylactically administer diphenhydramine (Benadryl) along with those antiemetics.

Migraine attacks lasting more than 3 days (*status migrainosus*) usually lead to prostration, prolonged painful distress, and dehydration. Patients suffering from such prolonged, refractory illness benefit substantially from parenteral medication, intravenous fluids, antiemetics, and a quiet, dark refuge. Neurologists must often hospitalize patients in status migrainosus. Medically supervised withdrawal from over-the-counter medications, opioids, or even excessive conventional antimigraine medicines may also require hospitalization.

Preventative Treatment

Neurologists prescribe preventative treatment under several circumstances: migraine occurring more than four times a month; migraine causing 3 to 4 days of disability per month; acute medicines losing their effectiveness; or patients taking excessive medications. For realistic purposes, neurologists expect to decrease their patients' migraine frequency and intensity by 50%. Most preventative medicines fall into three classes: antidepressants, antihypertensives, and antiepileptics.

TCAs, particularly amitriptyline and nortriptyline, reduce the severity, frequency, and duration of migraine. Apart from their mood-elevating effect, TCAs may ameliorate migraine because they suppress REM sleep, which is the phase when migraine attacks tend to develop. In addition, because TCAs enhance serotonin, they are analgesic (see Chapter 14). As most migraine patients are young and require only small doses of TCAs compared to those used to treat depression, the side effects of TCAs in this situation are rarely a problem. Interestingly, for preventing migraine, SSRIs are ineffective compared to TCAs.

Neurologists often prescribe β-blockers for migraine prophylaxis, as well as for treatment of essential tremor (see Chapter 18). However, they avoid prescribing β-blockers to migraine patients with comorbid depression because of their tendency to precipitate or exacerbate mood disorders.

Certain AEDs, such as topiramate and valproate, offer preventative treatment for migraine, as well as for neuropathic pain and epilepsy. Valproate is suitable for migraine sufferers with or without mood disorders. It may suppress migraine by reducing 5-HT neurons firing in the dorsal raphe nucleus or by altering trigeminal $GABA_A$ receptors in the meningeal blood vessels. However, its side effects, especially weight gain and the risk of fetal teratogenicity, often preclude its use.

Numerous medications in other categories show some benefit for chronic migraine. Among them, botulinum toxin injections reduce the frequency or severity of migraines that both last 4 hours or longer and occur at least 15 times a month. Indeed, botulinum toxin injections reduce the impact of migraines and improve a patient's quality of life.

Neurologists also employ nonpharmacologic interventions for the prevention and reduction in frequency of migraines. Cognitive-behavioral therapy and biofeedback are both successful adjunctive treatment strategies. The FDA approved use of a transcutaneous electrical nerve stimulation (TENS) device and a transcranial magnetic stimulation (TMS) device for the reduction of migraine frequency. Similar devices have been used in other chronic pain conditions (see Chapter 14). Finally, naturopaths have long hailed acupuncture as a successful preventative treatment for migraines. While there is no difference between the efficacies of "true" acupuncture in comparison to a "sham" acupuncture control group, up to 50% of patients in both groups can have improvement in their headache frequency and severity.

Chronic Daily Headache

When patients report headaches lasting 4 hours or longer for at least 15 days each month for at least 3 months, neurologists diagnose chronic daily headache. Patients may arrive at this state via several different routes. For years, they may have had migraine or THH – to the extent that they can be differentiated (Table 9.1) – that transformed from episodes to a daily or nearly every-day affliction. Alternatively, individuals, especially children, may develop chronic daily headache after a lifetime of having few headaches or no headaches at all, a situation that neurologists label *new daily persistent headache* (NDPH). Specific conditions, such as a posttraumatic syndrome or psychiatric disturbances, may also lead or contribute to daily headache. Moreover, whatever the route, overuse of analgesics or other medicines often paves the way to chronic daily headache.

Patients with chronic daily headache typically describe generalized, waxing and waning, dull, pressing, and nonpulsatile pain, which is usually only mild-to-moderate in

TABLE 9.1 **Comparison of Tension-Type and Migraine Headaches**

	Tension-Type	Migraine
Location	Bilateral	Hemicranial*
Nature	Dull ache	Throbbing*
Severity	Slight–moderate	Moderate–severe
Associated symptoms	None	Nausea, hyperacusis, photophobia
Behavior	Continues working	Seeks seclusion
Effect of alcohol	Reduces headache	Worsens headache

*In approximately half of patients, at least at onset

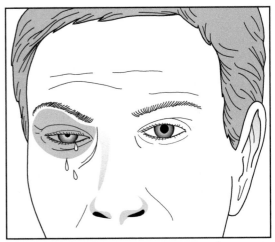

FIGURE 9.4 ■ This 43-year-old man with cluster headaches suffers from nightly right-sided unrelenting severe, stabbing unilateral periorbital pain for 45 minutes to 3 hours accompanied by ipsilateral tearing and nasal discharge, along with ptosis and miosis (a partial Horner syndrome). Note that the ptosis prompts compensatory elevation of the eyebrow.

severity. Nevertheless, the discomfort, if not the pain, is incapacitating. Headaches that transform from episodic to chronic not only lose any distinctive pain qualities, they shed associated features, such as scotoma and autonomic dysfunction. The headaches, which blend, vary, and recur, have lost their punch.

Children and adolescents with chronic daily headaches usually have had no history of medication overuse, but otherwise medication overuse is overwhelmingly the most powerful risk factor. The medicines most commonly implicated are aspirin-butalbital-caffeine compounds (e.g., Fiorinal*), triptans, NSAIDs, benzodiazepines, and opioids. Some medicines are more dangerous than others. For example, use of triptans or opioids more frequently than 10 days a month leads to these headaches in less than 2 years, but frequent use of nonopioid analgesics requires almost 5 years.

Other risk factors include obesity, head trauma, low socioeconomic status, disability, major stressful life-events, and several psychiatric conditions, particularly depression and anxiety. Risk factors for adolescents are primarily depression and anxiety.

In terms of treatment, all of a patient's physicians must work together to prevent medication overuse and look for underlying psychiatric disorders – some obvious, some not. Injection of botulinum toxin into the head and neck muscles has a therapeutic role (see Chapter 18), and TCAs, valproate, and topiramate may help; however, chronic daily headache generally resists treatment. Non-pharmacologic treatments of this disorder, which are of unproven benefit, include modification of lifestyle, behavior therapy, and elimination of precipitating factors.

When they attribute chronic daily headache to a medication overuse, neurologists attempt to eliminate the culprit. However, abruptly stopping a headache medicine may lead to withdrawal symptoms that can be as troublesome as opioid withdrawal. Neurologists often hospitalize chronic daily headache patients with comorbid

depression and those who have a history of excessive use of any medicine.

Cluster Headaches

An individual cluster headache consists of searing pain in one eye and its adjacent periorbital region. Ipsilateral eye tearing, conjunctival injection, nasal congestion and a partial Horner syndrome are often present (Figs. 9.4 and 12.16). Thus, neurologists sometimes classify this headache as *trigeminal autonomic cephalalgia* (TAC). Each headache lasts only 45 to 90 minutes, but to the patient, the attack seems interminable. The pain's severity often drives patients to agitation, restlessness, and thoughts of suicide.

The appellation "cluster headaches" derives from the tendency of these headaches to strike in groups (clusters) that consist of one to eight attacks daily for several months. The demography of cluster headache patients is unique: compared to patients with other primary headache disorders, cluster headaches affect men, typically between the ages of 20 to 40 years, six to eight times more frequently than women.

Most cluster attacks have a predictable, cyclic pattern. For example, some patients develop attacks every spring or fall. During clusters, headaches do not occur randomly throughout the day. Most strike between 9:00 pm and 9:00 am and one-half of them develop during REM sleep. Alcohol characteristically precipitates an attack. While cluster headaches respond to calcium-channel blockers and triptans, inhaling 100% high-flow oxygen will abort them. Thus, administering oxygen can be diagnostic as well as therapeutic.

Compared to migraines, cluster headaches are more predictable and briefer, but more intense. Also, unlike migraine, only local autonomic signs accompany cluster headaches. The headaches are not preceded by an aura, have no accompanying systemic autonomic signs, and are not alleviated by sleep, quiet, darkness, or seclusion. Like migraine, cluster has a familial tendency, but it is weak.

---

*Fiorinal and Fioricet were developed at and named for Montefiore Medical Center, which offered the country's first headache center and has been the employer of this book's authors for decades.

Treatment

Orally administered acute migraine medications are ineffective mostly because each cluster headache's abrupt, unexpected onset and relatively short duration does not allow enough time for the patient to swallow a medicine and absorb it. However, injections of sumatriptan or dihydroergotamine injections and oxygen inhalation at 8 to 10 L/minute may abort them. Preventative medicines include lithium, steroids, verapamil, and valproic acid. (Neurologists introduced lithium treatment for cluster headaches because these headaches, like bipolar disease, follow a cyclic pattern and affect middle-aged individuals.)

SECONDARY HEADACHES

Temporal Arteritis/Giant Cell Arteritis

Temporal arteritis (giant cell arteritis) is a disease of unknown etiology in which the temporal arteries, other cranial arteries, and often also medium-sized arteries throughout the body develop overt inflammation. Because the disease is systemic and histologic examination of affected arteries reveals giant cells, the term *giant cell arteritis* is more appropriate than the restrictive common designation of *temporal arteritis*.

Because patients are almost always older than 55 years, temporal arteritis is one of the several headache conditions that predominantly affect the elderly (Box 9.4). The headache itself usually consists of dull and continual pain located in one or both temples. Jaw pain on chewing ("jaw claudication") is frequent and almost pathognomonic. In advanced cases, the temporal arteries are tender and red from induration. Signs of systemic illness, such as malaise, myalgias, arthralgias, low-grade fever, and weight loss, characteristically accompany the headache and reflect the systemic nature of the illness. In fact, polymyalgia rheumatica or another rheumatologic disorder occurs concurrently in about 25% of cases of giant cell arteritis.

Because untreated arterial inflammation leads to arterial occlusion, serious complications may develop if the diagnosis of giant cell arteritis were delayed. Two dreaded complications, which stem from occlusions of the ophthalmic, ciliary, and cerebral arteries, are blindness and stroke.

In over 90% of cases, the erythrocyte sedimentation rate (ESR) rises above 40 mm/hour. C-reactive protein (CRP), a more sensitive indicator for this diagnosis, may be abnormally elevated in patients with normal ESR. A temporal artery biopsy remains the definitive test, but it is sometimes hazardous or impractical. Timely treatment with high-dose steroids will relieve the headaches, alleviate systemic symptoms, and prevent the complications.

Intracranial Mass Lesions

The first symptom of brain tumors and chronic subdural hematomas – common mass lesions (see Chapters 19 and 20) – is most often headaches. However, the headaches' qualities are nonspecific and potentially misleading. For example, brain tumor headaches usually mimic TTH. Also, when headaches are unilateral, they are on the side opposite the tumor in 20% of cases. Even though brain tumor headaches notoriously begin during early morning REM sleep and awaken patients, that pattern develops in less than half of cases. Moreover, numerous other headaches display the same early-morning onset, including migraine, cluster, carbon dioxide retention, sleep apnea, and caffeine withdrawal.

At least subtle cognitive and personality changes accompany headaches from mass lesions. Even if not present initially, lateralized signs usually develop within 8 weeks. However, overt signs of increased intracranial pressure – papilledema and stupor – usually do not develop until late in the course, if at all.

To avoid missing a diagnosis of brain tumor and to calm the often-unstated fears of patients, their families, and medical colleagues, neurologists readily order computed tomography (CT) or magnetic resonance imaging (MRI). In addition, for patients with headaches beginning after 55 years, they order an ESR.

Idiopathic Intracranial Hypertension (Pseudotumor Cerebri)

Neurologists have begun to change the popular terms "pseudotumor cerebri" and "benign intracranial hypertension" to *idiopathic intracranial hypertension*. This term better acknowledges the unknown etiology and serious nature of this condition.

Idiopathic intracranial hypertension develops predominantly in young, obese women who have menstrual irregularity. Although reports from several decades ago reported consumption of excessive vitamin A, outdated tetracycline, or polar bear meat as the cause of several cases, recent studies found that the cause in many cases is elevated intracranial venous sinus pressure – often from venous sinus occlusion or stenosis. In some patients, a venous sinus thrombosis has triggered their symptoms. Neurologists say that these patients, however, have secondary intracranial hypertension.

Whatever its etiology, idiopathic intracranial hypertension gives rise, as in so many other conditions, to a dull, generalized headache that is often associated with pulsatile tinnitus and/or transient episodes of blackening of vision, known as *visual obscurations*. This condition's distinctive feature is papilledema. If untreated, the papilledema leads to an enlarged blind spot within each visual field and eventually blindness from optic atrophy (see Chapter 12).

BOX 9.4	Causes of Headaches Predominantly in the Elderly

Brain tumors: glioblastoma, metastases
Cervical spondylosis
Vasodilators and other medications
Postherpetic neuralgia
Subdural hematomas after little or no trauma
Temporal arteritis (giant cell arteritis)
Trigeminal neuralgia

Increased intracranial pressure also sometimes stretches and then damages one or both of the abducens (sixth) cranial nerves. The abducens nerve palsy leads, in turn, to unilateral or bilateral inward eye deviation because of the unopposed action of the intact third cranial nerves (see Chapter 4).

Although many patients with idiopathic intracranial hypertension suffer from severe headaches and have florid papilledema, their neurologic examination is otherwise surprisingly normal. In fact, idiopathic intracranial hypertension is one of the most common causes of papilledema.

Neurologists, aware of potential causes of headaches and papilledema, routinely order not only MRI, but also MR studies of the intracranial veins (MRV). If there is no contraindication, such as kidney failure, the addition of gadolinium to an MRI can help illustrate flow (or its absence) in the venous sinuses. In pseudotumor cerebri, CT and MRI typically show cerebral swelling and compressed, small ventricles that neurologists label "slit-like." MRV may show slowing or occlusion of intracranial venous drainage.

With a lumbar puncture (LP), the CSF pressure is typically greater than 300 mm H_2O, and often reaches levels greater than 400 mm. The CSF protein concentration may be low; however, the CSF glucose concentration remains normal and no cells are present. Treatment usually consists of carbonic anhydrase inhibitors and diuretics – first-line treatment is acetazolamide (Diamox). Neurologists frequently monitor treatment with repeated LPs to measure the pressure and drain CSF. In refractory cases, neurosurgeons can decompress the ventricular system by installing CSF shunts or decompress the optic nerve by performing an optic nerve sheath fenestration, thus preventing or slowing vision loss.

Post-Dural Puncture Headache

Headache is a common complication of LP or "dural puncture" and may appear up to 5 days following the procedure. It probably originates in continued leakage of CSF through a tear in the lumbar dura and subsequently low intracranial pressure. Neurologists usually refer to the condition as "post-LP headache," but the term *post-dural puncture headache* (PDPH), while wordier, is more accurate and inclusive.

As though withdrawal of CSF lets the brain rest unprotected against the inside of the skull, sitting upright or even rapidly turning the head and neck can exacerbate the headache. Neck stiffness or tinnitus often accompanies the headache and prostration.

Surprisingly, patient rehydration and prolonged post-LP bedrest do not lower rates of PDPH. While neurologists traditionally prescribe bed rest, fluids, and caffeine, the best treatment is an epidural "blood patch" that consists of 20–30 mL of the patient's own blood injected into the epidural space to seal the tear in the dura.

Bacterial Meningitis, Herpes Encephalitis, and Subarachnoid Hemorrhage

Bacterial meningitis and subarachnoid hemorrhage produce commonly occurring, life-threatening illnesses characterized initially by headache. *Meningococcus* and *Pneumococcus*, the most common causes of bacterial meningitis, often spread in a small epidemic pattern among children and young adults in confined areas, such as college dormitories and military training camps. In addition, pneumococcal meningitis has a predilection for older, debilitated individuals in whom meningitis and many other infectious illnesses have an insidious onset and subtle signs. Whichever the infectious agent, meningitis usually causes the development, over several hours to several days, of malaise, fever, photophobia, nuchal rigidity, and moderate-to-severe headache. The headaches are usually generalized, but sometimes they are retro-orbital or nuchal. When physicians suspect bacterial meningitis, they routinely examine the CSF (see Table 20.1) and, if indicated, intravenously administer penicillin or other antibiotic. Vaccinations against meningococcal and pneumococcal infections provide a great deal of protection to students, recruits, and nursing home residents.

Viral infections of the brain (*viral encephalitis*) also cause headaches. With a few exceptions, these headaches and other symptoms are usually nonspecific and run a more benign course than bacterial infections. However, in contrast to almost all other forms of encephalitis that develop in the United States, herpes simplex encephalitis has distinct clinical features. The herpes simplex-1 virus (HSV-1) is the most frequent cause of serious, nonepidemic viral encephalitis. It has a remarkable predilection for the frontal inferior surface of the brain and attacks the undersurface of both the frontal and temporal lobes. Like most other viral infections, herpes simplex encephalitis causes fever, somnolence, and delirium. In addition, because the virus attacks the temporal lobes and thus damages the limbic system, it routinely causes complex partial seizures and memory impairment (amnesia). Bilateral temporal lobe damage in some patients may lead to the human variety of the Klüver–Bucy syndrome (see Chapter 16). Frontal and temporal lobe damage may lead to language impairment (aphasia) and frontal lobe behavioral disorders (see Chapter 7). In herpes simplex and other forms of encephalitis, a LP, CT, MRI, and sometimes an electroencephalogram (EEG) are the most useful diagnostic tests.

Another cause of severe, acutely occurring headache is *subarachnoid hemorrhage*, which usually results from a ruptured cerebral aneurysm. Cerebral artery aneurysms – often shaped like "berries" (*berry aneurysms*) – usually develop in the arteries that comprise the circle of Willis (see Fig. 11.2 and Chapter 20). If the arteries fuse incompletely in utero, weak junctions may eventually form an aneurysm. When an aneurysm ruptures, blood shoots into the subarachnoid space, which surrounds the brainstem and cerebral hemispheres and contains CSF, which is normally crystal clear. Depending on the aneurysm's location and size, it may also send a jet of blood into the brain. Beginning almost immediately after a subarachnoid hemorrhage, a CT usually reveals blood in the subarachnoid space. Several hours after the hemorrhage, the CSF color turns from red to yellow (xanthochromic).

Subarachnoid hemorrhages often occur during exertion, including exercise, straining at stool, and sexual intercourse. Whether or not preceded by exertion, subarachnoid hemorrhages typically cause severe headache, prostration, and nuchal rigidity – symptoms similar to those of bacterial meningitis. Although most patients with a subarachnoid hemorrhage have symptoms that indicate serious intracranial pathology, sentinel bleeds ("leaks") or otherwise atypical subarachnoid hemorrhages are not as dramatic and often escape detection. For example, physicians may reasonably misdiagnose them as migraine headache.

Chronic Meningitis

Chronic meningitis, like mass lesions, produces weeks of a dull, continual headache accompanied by progressive cognitive impairment and personality changes. However, with chronic meningitis, symptoms and signs of systemic infectious illness may predominate. Meningeal inflammation at the base of the brain causes additional, distinctive features. The inflammation chokes various cranial nerves, leading to facial palsy (from seventh cranial nerve injury), hearing impairment (eighth nerve), or extraocular muscle palsy (third, fourth, or sixth nerves).

A variety of infectious agents can cause chronic meningitis, but generally only in susceptible individuals. For example, *Cryptococcus* commonly causes meningitis in patients who have an impaired immune system, but very uncommonly in others. With almost any variety of chronic meningitis, CT or MRI typically reveals enlargement of all four ventricles because impaired reabsorption of cerebrospinal fluid (CSF) through the arachnoid villa leads to communicating hydrocephalus. The CSF pressure is elevated and its analysis shows lymphocytic pleocytosis, low glucose concentration, and elevated protein concentration (see Table 20.1).

MAOIs and the Hypertensive Crisis

MAOIs occasionally react with tyramine-rich foods or a variety of other medicines to cause severe hypertension, excruciating headache, and sometimes a subarachnoid or intracerebral hemorrhage – a hypertensive crisis. This iatrogenic catastrophe, classically associated with MAOI antidepressants, is not peculiar to their use. For example, MAOIs used in Parkinson disease treatment, such as selegiline and rasagiline (see Chapter 18), may cause it. However, the potential for this adverse side effect is low with Parkinson disease medications at recommended doses because they selectively inhibit MAO-B. In contrast, when selegiline is used as an antidepressant (as a patch in Emsam) at doses greater than 12 mg/day, it inhibits MAO-A as well as MAO-B and leaves the patient vulnerable to the reaction.

Neurologists often prescribe other medicines that might adversely interact in this way with MAOIs, including triptans, meperidine (Demerol), sympathomimetics, such as amphetamines and the entire class of dibenzepin derivatives, including carbamazepine and TCAs. Once a hypertensive reaction develops, phentolamine (Regitine), which is an α-adrenergic blocking agent, chlorpromazine, or propranolol may attenuate or abort it.

Given that the causes of secondary headaches are diverse in etiology, treatment strategy, and potential risk

BOX 9.5	Secondary Causes of Headache

"SNOOP⁵"
S – Systemic symptoms/signs
N – Neurologic symptoms/signs
O – Onset sudden (thunderclap headache)
O – Onset after age 50
P – Progressive headache
P – Precipitated by Valsalva maneuver
P – Postural worsening (upright or supine)
P – Papilledema
P – Pregnancy

Adapted from Dodick, D. W. (2010). Pearls: Headache. *Seminars in Neurology, 30,* 74–81.

to the patient, many neurologists use the acronym SNOOP⁵ to remember the "red flags" which might point away from a primary headache diagnosis (Box 9.5). For example, the presence of fever and nuchal rigidity (**S**ystemic signs and **N**eurologic signs) might point to bacterial meningitis, whereas worsening headache in a 60-year-old man with blurred disc margins (**O**nset after 50, **P**rogressive headache, **P**ostural aggravation, and **P**apilledema) might suggest an intracranial mass.

CRANIAL NEURALGIAS

Trigeminal Neuralgia

Of conditions in which pain originates in a cranial nerve – cranial neuralgias – the most clinically important one is *trigeminal neuralgia*. Formerly called *tic douloureux*, trigeminal neuralgia is a chronic, recurring disorder consisting of dozens of 20- to 30-second jabs daily of agonizing, sharp pain extending along one or more of the three divisions of the trigeminal nerve. Trigeminal neuralgia most commonly affects the V_2 division of the trigeminal nerve (see Fig. 4.12). Unlike the other headaches, touching the affected area can provoke the pain. Stimulating these sensitive areas or trigger zones – by eating, brushing one's teeth, or drinking cold water as well as by touching – evokes a dreadful shock. Thus, patients in the midst of an attack hesitate to eat, brush their teeth, or speak. They tend to become reclusive. Fortunately, in a characteristic reprise, trigeminal neuralgia abates at night, allowing the patient a full night's sleep. Trigeminal neuralgia develops in women more often than men and typically only after age 60 years, making it one of the most important causes of headache in the elderly (see Box 9.4).

Cause and Treatment

In most cases, an aberrant superior cerebellar artery or other cerebral blood vessel compressing the trigeminal nerve root as it emerges from the brainstem is the most common cause of trigeminal neuralgia. Tumors of the cerebellopontine angle may have the same effect. When trigeminal neuralgia develops in young adults, a multiple sclerosis plaque that irritates the trigeminal nerve nucleus may be responsible.

Neurologists usually begin treatment with carbamazepine (Tegretol) or oxcarbazepine (Trileptal). If the pain does not subside, they may prescribe gabapentin (Neurontin), pregabalin (Lyrica), or occasionally lamotrigine (Lamictal). Refractory cases may require a glycerol injection, radiofrequency ablation, or gamma knife surgery directed at the root of the trigeminal nerve. In patients with an aberrant vessel, neurosurgical placement of a barrier between the vessel and trigeminal nerve (*microvascular decompression*) is effective, but risky.

REFERENCES

Abramowicz, M. (Ed.), (2011). Drugs for Migraine. *Medical Letter, 9*, 7–12.

Allais, G., Gabellari, I. C., Airola, G., et al. (2009). Headache induced by the use of combined oral contraceptives. *Neurological Sciences, 30*(Suppl. 1), S15–S17.

Bigal, M. E., Liberman, J. N., & Lipton, R. B. (2006). Obesity and migraine: a population study. *Neurology, 66*, 545–550.

Bigal, M. E., & Lipton, R. B. (2007). The differential diagnosis of chronic daily headaches: An algorithm-based approach. *The Journal of Headache and Pain, 8*, 263–272.

Bigal, M. E., & Lipton, R. B. (2008). Excessive acute migraine medication use and migraine progression. *Neurology, 71*, 1821–1828.

Breslau, N., Lipton, R., Stewart, W., et al. (2003). Comorbidity of migraine and depression: investigating potential etiology and prognosis. *Neurology, 60*, 1308–1312.

Chronicle, E., & Mulleners, W. (2004). Anticonvulsant drugs for migraine prophylaxis. *The Cochrane Database of Systematic Reviews, (3)*, CD003226.

Dodick, D. W. (2006). Chronic daily headache. *The New England Journal of Medicine, 354*, 158–165.

Dodick, D. W. (2010). Pearls: Headache. *Seminars in Neurology, 30*, 74–81.

Eccleston, C., Yorke, L., Morley, S., et al. (2003). Psychological therapies for the management of chronic and recurrent pain in children and adolescents. *The Cochrane Database of Systematic Reviews, (1)*, CD003968.

Evers, S., & Marziniak, M. (2010). Clinical features, pathophysiology, and treatment of medication-overuse headache. *The Lancet. Neurology, 9*, 391–401.

Francis, G. J., Becker, W. J., & Pringsheim, T. (2010). Acute and preventative pharmacologic treatment of cluster headache. *Neurology, 75*, 463–473.

Frese, A., Eikermann, A., Frese, K., et al. (2003). Headache associated with sexual activity. *Neurology, 61*, 796–800.

Gronseth, G., Cruccu, G., Alksne, J., et al. (2008). Practice parameter: The diagnostic evaluation and treatment of trigeminal neuralgia (an evidence-based review): Report of the Quality Standards Subcommittee of the American Academy of Neurology and the European Federation of Neurologic Societies. *Neurology, 71*, 1183–1190.

Hamelsky, S. W., & Lipton, R. B. (2006). Psychiatric comorbidity of migraine. *Headache, 46*, 1327–1333.

Headache Classification Committee of the International Headache Society. (2004). The International Classification of Headache Disorders (2nd Edition). *Cephalalgia: An International Journal of Headache, 24*, 1–160.

Hershey, A. D., & Lipton, R. B. (2010). Lifestyles of the young and migrainous. *Neurology, 75*, 680–681.

Kirchmann, M., Thomsen, L. L., & Olesen, J. (2006). Basilar-type migraine: clinical, epidemiologic, and genetic factors. *Neurology, 66*, 880–886.

Lewis, D., Ashwal, S., Hershey, A., et al. (2004). Practice Parameter: Pharmacological treatment of migraine headache in children and adolescents. Report of the American Academy of Neurology Quality Standards Subcommittee and the Practice Committee of the Child Neurology Society. *Neurology, 63*, 2215–2224.

Linde, K., & Rossnagel, K. (2004). Propranolol for migraine prophylaxis. *The Cochrane Database of Systematic Reviews, (2)*, CD003225.

Lipton, R. B., Varon, S. F., Grosberg, B., et al. (2011). OnabotulinumtoxinA improves quality of life and reduces impact of chronic migraine. *Neurology, 77*, 1465–1472.

Lipton, R. B., Buse, D. C., Hall, C. B., et al. (2014). Reduction in perceived stress as a migraine trigger. *Neurology, 82*, 1395–1401.

Liu, H.-Y., Fuh, J.-L., Lin, Y.-Y., et al. (2015). Suicide risk in patients with migraine and comorbid fibromyalgia. *Neurology, 85*, 1017–1023.

Loder, E. (2010). Triptan therapy in migraine. *The New England Journal of Medicine, 363*, 63–70.

Lyngberg, A. C., Rasmussen, B. K., Jørgensen, T., et al. (2005). Prognosis of migraine and tension-type headache: A population-based follow-up study. *Neurology, 65*, 580–585.

Mallery, R. M., Friedman, D. I., & Liu, G. T. (2014). Headache and the pseudotumor cerebri syndrome. *Current Pain and Headache Reports, 18*, 446–453.

Meng, F. G., Zhang, J. G., Schoenen, J., et al. (2013). Migraine prevention with a supraorbital transcutaneous stimulator: a randomized controlled trial. *Neurology, 81*, 1102–1103.

Nierenburg, H., Ailani, J., Malloy, M., et al. (2015). Systematic review of preventive and acute treatment of menstrual migraine. *Headache, 55*, 1052–1071.

Pringsheim, T., Davenport, W. J., & Dodick, D. (2008). Acute treatment and prevention of menstrually related migraine headache. *Neurology, 70*, 1555–1563.

Robbins, M. S., Farmakidis, C., Dayal, A. K., et al. (2015). Acute headache diagnosis in pregnant women. *Neurology, 85*, 1024–1030.

Saper, J. R., Lake, A. E., Hamel, R. L., et al. (2004). Daily scheduled opioids for intractable head pain. Long-term observations of treatment program. *Neurology, 62*, 1687–1694.

Wang, S. J., Fuh, J. L., & Lu, S. R. (2009). Chronic daily headache in adolescents. *Neurology, 73*, 416–422.

Winawer, M. R., & Hesdorffer, D. C. (2010). Migraine, epilepsy, and psychiatric comorbidity. *Neurology, 74*, 1166–1168.

Zakrswska, J. M., & Linsky, M. E. (2015). Trigeminal neuralgia. *BMJ (Clinical Research Ed.), 350*, h1238.

CHAPTER 9

QUESTIONS AND ANSWERS

1. Over the previous 6 hours, a 17-year-old Marine recruit has developed a severe generalized headache, lethargy, nuchal rigidity, and fever. Which should be considered first?
   a. Acute bacterial meningitis
   b. Subarachnoid hemorrhage
   c. Migraine headache
   d. Encephalitis

Answer: a. Bacterial meningitis frequently develops – often in mini-epidemics – among military recruits, high school and college students, and other young people brought into confined areas from diverse backgrounds. This is a classic case where acute onset of headache, fever, and meningeal signs (nuchal rigidity) indicate acute bacterial meningitis. An alternative diagnosis is subarachnoid hemorrhage, which also presents with headache, lethargy, and nuchal rigidity. However, in minor clinical differences, the subarachnoid hemorrhage headache has a cataclysmic onset and the fever is less pronounced than in meningitis. Nevertheless, even when these symptoms and signs are mild or not all present, prudent physicians often test further for bacterial meningitis and subarachnoid hemorrhage. Migraine, which is a chronic and recurrent rather than a one-time problem, causes headache, prostration, and a tendency for sufferers to seek seclusion, but it does not cause nuchal rigidity and fever. Encephalitis less commonly develops in an epidemic fashion and does not cause nuchal rigidity.

Given the differential diagnosis of an acutely occurring severe headache, neurologists, after obtaining computed tomography (CT) or magnetic resonance imaging (MRI), perform a lumbar puncture (LP) for cerebrospinal fluid (CSF) analysis (see Table 20.1). High-dose intravenous antibiotics remain the standard treatment in cases of established or suspected bacterial meningitis. Vaccinations will greatly reduce the incidence of meningococcal meningitis.

2. Following 5 days of moderate bitemporal headaches, a woman brought her 45-year-old husband for psychiatric evaluation because he began to develop episodes of purposeless, repetitive behavior. On examination, he was febrile, disoriented, inattentive, and unable to recall any recent or past events. CT revealed no abnormalities in the brain or sinuses. His CSF contained three red blood cells (RBCs), 89 white blood cells (WBCs), of which 90% were lymphocytes; 45 mg/dL glucose; and 80 mg/dL protein. An electroencephalogram (EEG) showed spikes overlying both temporal lobes. Which is the most likely diagnosis?
   a. Acute bacterial meningitis
   b. Subarachnoid hemorrhage
   c. Migraine headache
   d. Encephalitis

Answer: d. His complex partial seizures and amnesia reflect temporal lobe dysfunction. In view of the delirium, fever, and the CSF profile, the underling illness is most likely an infectious process. Herpes simplex encephalitis, the most common nonepidemic encephalitis, has a predilection for the temporal lobes, which house major portions of the limbic system, and the undersurface of the frontal lobes. Herpes simplex encephalitis typically produces this picture of fever, delirium, complex partial seizures, and amnesia. Severe cases cause temporal lobe hemorrhagic infarctions, which allow some blood to seep into the CSF. Because of the bilateral temporal lobe damage, herpes simplex encephalitis survivors may exhibit the human form of the Klüver–Bucy syndrome (see Chapter 16).

3. Which symptoms most accurately differentiate migraine from other forms of headache?
   a. Headaches that are unilateral and throbbing
   b. Headaches that are exacerbated by physical activity
   c. Headaches that respond only to opioids for relief
   d. Headaches accompanied by nausea, vomiting, and photophobia

Answer: d. Autonomic and other associated symptoms typify migraines. The quality, severity, and location of the headache, although important, are less specific and less consistent.

4. In which age group does migraine most often first develop?
   a. Childhood
   b. Adolescence
   c. Young adult years
   d. Middle age

Answer: b. The peak incidence of the first migraine attack is in adolescence. The prevalence continues to rise until approximately age 40 years. Women are affected more than men (at a ratio of almost 3:1).

5. Which of the following statements about migraine during pregnancy is *true*?
   a. Pregnancy usually increases the frequency and severity of attacks.
   b. Migraine during pregnancy is associated with complications.
   c. In almost 10% of cases, women with migraine had their first attack during pregnancy.

189

d. In women who have migraine, postpartum headaches usually represent depression.

Answer: c. Almost 10% of women with migraine had their first attack during pregnancy. At least during the second and third trimesters, pregnancy reduces the frequency and intensity of migraine attacks in about 70% of women who suffered from migraine before conceiving. Even if migraine attacks persist throughout pregnancy, they are not associated with miscarriage, eclampsia, or fetal malformations. Postpartum depression may intensify postpartum headaches, which usually represent a recurrence of migraine. Depending on the circumstances, physicians might evaluate pregnant or postpartum women with headaches for other obstetric neurologic complications, such as preeclampsia, pituitary necrosis (Sheehan's syndrome), intracranial hypotension, or cortical vein thrombosis.

6. A 4-year-old boy has had several headaches with incapacitating nausea and vomiting complicated by confusion, incoherence, and agitation, but no paresis or nuchal rigidity. Serum lactate and pyruvate levels rise to very high levels during these attacks. Between attacks, he is clinically normal. Which of the following is the most likely explanation for the child's episodes?
   a. Migraines
   b. Brain tumor
   c. Diabetes
   d. Mitochondrial encephalopathy

Answer: d. Although the history has features of migraine, the elevated serum lactate and pyruvate levels suggest a mitochondrial encephalopathy.

7. Which of the following is the least significant risk factor for chronic daily headache?
   a. Frequent if not daily use of headache medicines
   b. History of tension-type headache
   c. History of migraine
   d. History of cluster headache
   e. Depression
   f. Head trauma

Answer: d. Tension-type and migraine headaches, but not cluster headaches, are significant headache risk factors for chronic daily headache. Compared to pediatric patients, adults with daily headaches usually have had prolonged treatment with headache medications. Depression is a comorbidity if not a cause of daily headache. Head trauma often precedes chronic daily headache. In this case, other symptoms of postconcussion syndrome typically accompany the headache.

8. If a patient with major depression were treated with a selective serotonin reuptake inhibitor (SSRI) or selective norepinephrine reuptake inhibitor (SNRI), what would be the risk of administering a triptan for migraine?
   a. Eruptions at the mucocutaneous border
   b. Hypertension leading to a cerebral hemorrhage

c. Delirium, fever, myoclonus
d. Muscle rigidity, rhabdomyolysis, fever, and renal failure

Answer: c. If physicians prescribe triptans, which are serotonin agonists, in conjunction with an SSRI or SNRI, patients may at least theoretically develop the serotonin syndrome. Eruptions at the mucocutaneous border are a manifestation of the Steven–Johnson syndrome. Hypertension leading to a cerebral hemorrhage may complicate treatment with a monamine oxidase inhibitor (MAOI). Muscle rigidity, rhabdomyolysis, fever, and renal failure are manifestations of the neuroleptic malignant syndrome.

9. Which is the cause of hemiplegic migraine?
   a. Mitochondrial DNA abnormality
   b. Excessive use of headache medications
   c. Mutation of a gene coding for a calcium channel
   d. Excessive trinucleotide repeats on chromosome 4

Answer: c. A mutation of a gene on chromosome 19, which codes for a calcium channel, has been implicated in hemiplegic migraine. Other disorders attributable to calcium channel abnormalities are myotonic dystrophy, spinocerebellar ataxia type 6, and several varieties of epilepsy. Excessive CAG trinucleotide repeats on chromosome 4 are present in patients with Huntington disease.

10. A young hypertensive woman suddenly developed severe right periorbital pain; prostration; ptosis, pupil dilation, and lateral eye deviation on the right; and nuchal rigidity. What is the most likely explanation?
    a. Rupture of an aneurysm in the circle of Willis
    b. Myasthenia gravis
    c. Acute angle-closure glaucoma
    d. None of the above

Answer: a. Although several illnesses may cause severe periorbital pain, the third nerve palsy indicates that a right posterior communicating artery aneurysm has ruptured and caused a subarachnoid hemorrhage. Myasthenia gravis may cause extraocular muscle weakness that can mimic a third nerve palsy; however, because myasthenia gravis spares the pupillary muscles, pupils remain round, equal, and reactive to light. Also, myasthenia gravis does not cause either pain or nuchal rigidity. Acute angle-closure glaucoma may cause the abrupt onset of severe pain in and around the eye and a dilated, unreactive pupil, but vision in the affected eye is markedly impaired and nuchal rigidity does not develop.

11. While watching television, a middle-aged hypertensive man has the sudden onset of the worst headache of his life. On examination, he is able to speak coherently, but has nausea and vomiting. Of the following, which is the most likely cause?
    a. An intracranial hemorrhage
    b. Migraine
    c. Seizure
    d. Brain tumor

Answer: a. The description "worst headache of my life" is a "red flag" for a cerebral or subarachnoid hemorrhage. Physicians may consider migraine or cluster headache as the cause, but they should entertain those diagnoses when headaches are a chronic, recurrent problem, which often requires months of observation, and after they have excluded potentially fatal conditions. Thus, when a patient offers this complaint, neurologists generally order a CT or MRI and, if unrevealing, possibly perform an LP.

12. An elderly depressed man develops a continual, moderately severe, generalized headache. He has a decreased attention span and a short-stepped gait. Which illness is least likely to be present?
    a. Giant cell arteritis
    b. Subdural hematoma
    c. Brain tumor
    d. Dementia with Lewy bodies
    e. Depression

Answer: d. Elderly individuals are particularly vulnerable to giant cell arteritis, trigeminal neuralgia, subdural hematomas that develop either spontaneously or following trivial injuries, primary or metastatic brain tumors, depression, and side effects of medications. Dementia with Lewy bodies does not cause headache. To a certain extent, a short-stepped gait and decreased attention span normally develop as individuals age.

13. Which two of the following headache varieties are unilateral and repeatedly strike the same side?
    a. Migraine
    b. Trigeminal neuralgia
    c. Cluster
    d. Idiopathic intracranial hypertension

Answer: b, c. Trigeminal neuralgia and cluster headaches are almost always unilateral and almost never switch sides. Although migraine headaches are frequently unilateral, they often switch sides or generalize. Idiopathic intracranial hypertension, which neurologists previously called pseudotumor cerebri, causes a generalized headache.

14–25. Match the condition (Questions 14–25) with the characteristic symptoms (a–m). Some questions may have more than one answer:

14. Trigeminal neuralgia
15. Bell's palsy
16. Idiopathic intracranial hypertension
17. Basilar migraine
18. Subarachnoid hemorrhage
19. Temporal arteritis
20. Angle-closure glaucoma
21. Subdural hematoma
22. Postconcussion headache
23. Medulloblastoma
24. Viral meningitis
25. Hemiplegic migraine
    a. Severe ocular pain, conjunctival injection ("red eye"), markedly decreased vision
    b. Papilledema, generalized headache, obesity, and menstrual irregularity
    c. Mastoid pain followed by facial palsy
    d. Lancinating pain on one side of the jaw
    e. Moderate headache, focal seizures, and fever
    f. Mild headache and hemiparesis after a fortification scotoma
    g. Chronic pain, depressed sensorium
    h. Unilateral forehead pain, malaise, jaw claudication, high sedimentation rate
    i. Daily dull headaches, inattention, insomnia, depression, and anxiety
    j. Apoplectic headache, nuchal rigidity
    k. Horner syndrome
    l. Headache, nausea, vomiting, diplopia, and ataxia
    m. Several days of headache, fever, and photophobia, with CSF lymphocytic pleocytosis

Answers: 14–d; 15–c; 16–b; 17–l; 18–j; 19–h; 20–a; 21–g, i, or l; 22–i; 23–l; 24–m; 25–f.

26. Which of the following is not an indication for changing from acute to preventative therapy for migraine?
    a. More than four migraines every month
    b. Once-monthly migraine with aura
    c. Ergotism
    d. Habitual narcotic use

Answer: b. Indications for using preventative migraine medicines include suffering a migraine more frequently than once a week, having side effects from abortive medicines, and overuse or other abuse of acute medications.

27. Which one of the following is not a common trigger of migraine?
    a. Menses
    b. Glare
    c. Alcohol consumption
    d. Non-REM sleep
    e. Relief from stress

Answer: d. Menses, glare, alcohol, missing meals, too much or too little sleep, and relief from stress may precipitate migraine attacks. REM sleep is also a trigger, but it is more closely associated with the development of cluster headaches.

28. Which of the following statements describes the difference between migraine headaches in children and adults?
    a. Basilar-type migraines are more common in adults.
    b. Conjunctival injection, tearing, and nasal stuffiness are often the sole manifestation of migraine headaches in adults.
    c. Children are likely to have abdominal pain as a migraine manifestation.
    d. Adults have behavioral changes associated with migraine headaches more frequently than do children.

Answer: c. Although autonomic dysfunction occurs in all migraine patients, children are particularly prone to cyclic vomiting, abdominal pain, and autonomic dysfunction as their primary or exclusive symptom. Children are also more likely than adults to develop basilar-type migraine and have behavioral disturbances, such as agitation or withdrawal, as prominent migraine symptoms.

29. Which of the following neurologic disorders does not cause visual hallucinations?
    a. Brown–Séquard syndrome
    b. Migraine
    c. Seizures
    d. Narcolepsy
    e. Dementia with Lewy bodies

Answer: a. Brown–Séquard syndrome, a partial or complete hemisection of the spinal cord, does not cause visual hallucinations. Causes of visual hallucinations include migraine, seizures originating in the temporal or occipital lobes, narcolepsy (hypnopompic or hypnagogic hallucinations), hallucinogens (such as LSD), alcohol withdrawal (delirium tremens), and dementia with Lewy bodies.

30. In which part of the brain are serotonin-containing neurons concentrated?
    a. Limbic system
    b. Frontal lobes
    c. Dorsal raphe nucleus
    d. Cerebellum

Answer: c.

31. Concerning migraine, to which process does "spreading neuronal depression" refer?
    a. The organically based changes in affect that accompany migraine
    b. The wave of neuronal hypometabolism that precedes and may cause the migraine
    c. The inability of the cortex to respond to the migraine
    d. The comorbid depressive disorder

Answer: b. Spreading neuronal depression refers to hypometabolism of cerebral neurons that spreads – first as increased neuronal activity and then as inhibited neuronal activity – posteriorly to anteriorly over the cerebral cortex. It precedes and may cause the migraine. This phenomenon leads to the aura and, through activation of the trigeminal ganglia, the headache.

32. Which statement is *false* concerning xanthochromic CSF?
    a. The CSF is yellow.
    b. Subarachnoid bleeding probably occurred within several hours to several days.
    c. Elevated serum bilirubin concentration or CSF protein concentration causes xanthochromic CSF.
    d. The CSF is opaque.

Answer: d.

33. Which type of headache do brain tumors most often mimic?
    a. Tension-type
    b. Migraine
    c. Cluster
    d. Subarachnoid hemorrhage
    e. Trigeminal neuralgia

Answer: a.

34–37. For each of the following headache types, state whether sleep ameliorates it (Yes/No).

34. Migraine with aura
35. Trigeminal neuralgia
36. Cluster
37. Temporal arteritis

Answers: 34–Yes: Although REM sleep may actually trigger migraine, sleep typically relieves it. 35–No: Trigeminal neuralgia does not interrupt sleep, but sleep does not alleviate trigeminal neuralgia. 36–No: REM sleep typically precipitates cluster headaches. 37–No: Temporal arteritis and sleep have no relationship.

38. Which one of these conditions does not awaken patients from sleep?
    a. Migraine
    b. Sleep apnea
    c. Brain tumor
    d. Subdural hematoma
    e. Tension-type headaches
    f. Cluster headaches
    g. Chronic obstructive pulmonary disease

Answer: e.

39. During which stage of sleep do migraine and cluster headaches begin?
    a. REM
    b. NREM
    c. Slow-wave
    d. None of the above

Answer: a.

40. The diagnosis of chronic migraine includes all of the following except:
    a. Headaches lasting longer than 4 hours
    b. Medication overuse
    c. Headaches more than 15 days/month
    d. Headaches for more than 3 months

Answer: b. The diagnosis of chronic migraine requires 15 or more days each month of headache, each lasting 4 hours or longer, without indication of medication overuse and at least 3 months of headaches.

41. An adolescent schoolgirl drew this sketch (see figure) of what she sees immediately before her headaches, which are accompanied by nausea and vomiting. The

headaches prevent her from attending school or cause her teacher to send her to the nurse's office. Of the following, which is the most plausible interpretation of her visions?

a. They indicate child abuse.
b. A food or industrial toxin has been causing her visual hallucinations, headaches, and nausea and vomiting.
c. The visual hallucinations are an aura of a partial seizure.
d. She has been suffering from migraine with aura.

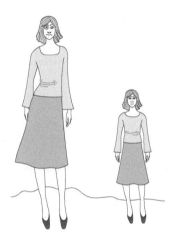

Answer: d. Some migraine sufferers, especially children, perceive distortions of themselves, other people, or their environment as a prelude (aura) to the headache phase of an attack. One example, as in this figure, consists of a parent shrinking (*micropsia*) or growing (*macropsia*). Some patients have likened the symptom to looking in a "fun-house mirror without the fun." Neurologists have termed the micropsia–macropsia phenomenon the "*Alice in Wonderland*" syndrome because of its similarity to Alice's experience after she drinks the potion in the famous novel (also see Table 12.1).

42. A graduate student develops severe periorbital headaches every winter when he goes to Miami. Which two varieties of headache does this pattern suggest?

a. Depression-induced
b. Tension-type
c. Migraine
d. Cluster
e. Trigeminal neuralgia
f. Giant cell arteritis

Answer: c or d. Going on vacation, especially when it entails psychologic stress, disrupted sleep, or alcohol consumption, may precipitate migraines. Alternatively, cluster headaches are characterized by, and named for, their temporal grouping, which usually occurs around predictable events.

43. Which two of the following conditions cost industry the largest number of lost work-hours?

a. Low back pain
b. Epilepsy
c. Headache
d. Cerebrovascular disease
e. Brain tumors
f. Neck pain

Answer: a, c.

44–46. For each of the following headaches, state whether it runs in families (Yes/No).

44. Migraine
45. Cluster
46. Tension-type

Answers: 44–Yes, 45–Yes, 46–Yes.

47. A 35-year-old man who suffers several migraine attacks a year developed a uniquely severe headache during sexual intercourse. He described it as "the worst headache of his life." Two evenings later, this headache recurred during masturbation. Which condition is he most likely experiencing?

a. Psychogenic disturbance
b. Cluster headache
c. Coital cephalgia
d. Tension-type headache

Answer: c. Most likely, he has been experiencing coital cephalgia, i.e., sex-induced benign headaches. This variety of headache is common and falls under the rubric of "primary headache associated with sexual activity." Before considering it completely benign, neurologists usually order a CT or MRI and possibly an LP to exclude a subarachnoid hemorrhage.

48. When may a woman's migraine attacks be particularly severe or frequent?

a. Premenstrual days
b. During menopause
c. When taking oral contraceptives
d. Menarche
e. All of the above

Answer: e.

49. With which headache is depression least closely associated?

a. Chronic daily headache
b. Migraine
c. Tension-type
d. Trigeminal neuralgia

Answer: d. Depression is comorbid with chronic daily headache, migraine, and tension-type headache, but not with trigeminal neuralgia or the other secondary headache syndromes.

50. Which cranial nerve innervates the meninges?

a. Olfactory
b. Oculomotor

c. Trigeminal
d. Facial
e. Vagus

Answer: c.

51. Which of the following statements concerning serotonin (5HT) is *false*?
    a. Serotonin is metabolized to 5-hydroxyindolacetic acid (5HIAA).
    b. At the onset of migraine attacks, platelet serotonin concentration falls.
    c. Sumatriptan, dihydroergotamine, and ergotamine all act on serotonin receptors.
    d. Serotonin-containing neurons are concentrated in the dorsal raphe.
    e. During a migraine, urinary serotonin and 5-HIAA concentrations fall.

Answer: e.

52–55. Match each medication (52–55) with its potential adverse effect (a–e):

52. SSRI combined with a triptan
53. Propranolol
54. Cafergot (ergotamine/caffeine)
55. Aspirin
    a. Vascular spasm, claudication, muscle cramps (with prolonged use)
    b. Myoclonus, fever
    c. Gastric distress and bleeding, easy bruisability
    d. Bradycardia, asthma, fatigue
    e. None of the above

Answers: 52–b (serotonin syndrome), 53–d, 54–a (ergotism), 55–c.

56. Which condition is usually cyclic or periodic, develops predominantly in men, and responds to lithium?
    a. Migraine
    b. Cluster headaches
    c. Trigeminal neuralgia
    d. Giant cell arteritis

Answer: b. The similarities of cluster headache and bipolar disorder prompted investigators to perform clinical trials with lithium. Neurologists currently prescribe verapamil, valproate, or lithium to prevent cluster headaches.

57. A 40-year-old woman has had migraine since adolescence and depression for the previous 10 years. Her psychiatrist changed her antidepressant to an SSRI, which initially seemed to reduce her headaches and improve her mood. However, after 1 month her headaches returned with much greater severity. Her family brought her to the emergency room when she developed agitated confusion and tremulousness. Her blood pressure is 110/70 and her temperature, 100°F. Her urine contains a small quantity of myoglobin. Which of the following is the most likely cause of her condition?
    a. Neuroleptic malignant syndrome
    b. SSRI overdose
    c. Serotonin syndrome
    d. An MAOI crisis

Answer: c. She has the serotonin syndrome because she apparently took an antimigraine serotonin agonist, such as a triptan, in combination with the SSRI. She lacks the muscle rigidity and high temperature of neuroleptic malignant syndrome. A MAOI–tyramine interaction would almost invariably cause hypertension.

58. Which of the following headache varieties is most often associated with a mood change?
    a. Idiopathic intracranial hypertension
    b. Trigeminal neuralgia
    c. Giant cell arteritis
    d. Migraine

Answer: d.

59. Which of the following headache varieties occurs more often in men than women?
    a. Migraine with aura
    b. Migraine without aura
    c. Idiopathic intracranial hypertension
    d. Trigeminal neuralgia
    e. Tension-type
    f. Cluster

Answer: f.

60. Which two CNS structures are pain-sensitive?
    a. Optic nerves
    b. Meninges
    c. Cerebral neurons
    d. Ventricles

Answer: a, b.

61–68. Match the headache (61–68) with one or more of its causes or precipitants (a–k):

61. Trigeminal neuralgia
62. Hot-dog headache
63. Sinusitis with seizures
64. Idiopathic intracranial hypertension
65. Giant cell arteritis
66. Chinese restaurant syndrome
67. Nocturnal migraine
68. Antianginal medication-induced headaches
    a. Inflammation of extracranial and intracranial arteries
    b. Autonomic nervous system dysfunction
    c. Vascular compression of the trigeminal nerve
    d. Nitrites
    e. Monosodium glutamate (MSG)
    f. Cerebral edema
    g. Nightmares
    h. REM sleep

i. NREM sleep
j. Infection causing meningitis or a brain abscess
k. Cerebral artery dilation

Answers: 61–c, 62–d or e, 63–j, 64–f, 65–a, 66–e, 67–h, 68–k.

69. Which of the following measures reduces the incidence of a patient developing a postdural puncture headache (PDPH)?
a. Aggressive hydration
b. Reduction of CSF removed during lumbar puncture
c. Keeping the patient supine for extended time post dural puncture
d. None of the above

Answer: d. None of these measures, despite their continued use, have shown a significant effect on reducing the incidence of PDPH.

70. Which of the following complications is more likely to develop in pregnant women with migraine than in pregnant women without migraine?
a. Miscarriage
b. Eclampsia
c. Fetal malformations
d. All of the above
e. None of the above

Answer: e. Pregnant women beset by migraine are not at increased risk of miscarriage, eclampsia, or fetal malformations.

71. A 23-year-old woman told her physician that beginning about 10 minutes before most of her headaches, which are usually one-sided and throbbing, she develops jagged lines and surrounding a blurred region in the corner of her left eye. The visual distortion expands to fill most of that eye and then flickers. Over several minutes, it expands beyond both eyes. She said, "It engulfs everything. I am mesmerized." Then suddenly it shrinks to a small area in the lower outside corner of her left eye and disappears. She sketched this picture that shows the visual distortion from her perspective (see figure). Which is the most likely variety of her headaches?

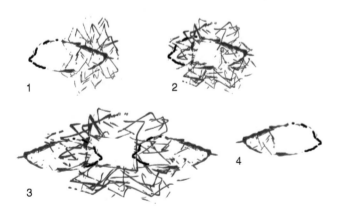

a. Migraine with aura
b. Migraine without aura
c. Status migrainosus
d. None of the above

Answer: a. She has auras of scintillating fortification spectra preceding hemicranial pulsatile headaches. This is a classic history for migraine with aura.

72. A 26-year-old waitress reports 6 weeks of a progressively severe, dull headache. Aside from her optic disks (see figure) and enlarged bind spots on formal visual field determination, her neurologic examination discloses no abnormalities. Her CT and MRI show small ventricles, but no mass lesions, hydrocephalus, or other abnormality. Which is the most likely diagnosis?

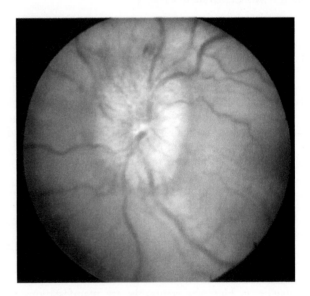

a. Idiopathic intracranial hypertension
b. Bilateral subdural hematomas
c. Obstructive hydrocephalus
d. Papillitis

Answer: a. This fundoscopy photograph shows swelling of the optic nerve head, indistinct border of the nerve head, and vessels draped over its edge, which define papilledema. All of the choices may produce this appearance. However, given her headache, enlarged blind spots (without blindness), normal examination, and reports of her imaging, she most likely has idiopathic intracranial hypertension (pseudotumor cerebri). Suddenly developing, severe increased pressure in this condition may lead to stretching of one or both sixth cranial nerves and thus lateral rectus palsy as well as papilledema. In some cases of idiopathic intracranial hypertension, appropriate imaging studies reveal an occlusion of an intracranial venous sinus in some cases.

73. In the case described in Question 72, a lumbar puncture showed that the opening pressure was 350 mm H_2O, but the CSF was acellular and had normal glucose and protein. The patient had

menstrual irregularity and her body mass index (BMI) was calculated to be 48 kg/m². Which is the best initial treatment?
a. A steroid
b. A carbonic anhydrase inhibitor
c. A diuretic
d. Restricted calorie diet

Answer: b. Carbonic anhydrase inhibitors, such as acetazolamide (Diamox), will reduce intracranial pressure and alleviate her symptoms. If her intracranial pressure remains elevated, it may lead to optic atrophy and blindness. Other diuretics and steroids will also reduce intracranial pressure, but their benefit-to-adverse effect ratio is not as favorable as with carbonic anhydrase inhibitors. In addition, because she is morbidly obese, she should begin a stringent diet. If that strategy is unsuccessful, she should consider bariatric surgery.

74. A 28-year-old surgical intern, fighting off the effects of sleep-deprivation, drinks at least three cups of coffee each day. Her strategy allows her to work, sleep, and socialize. Various professional and social stressors eventually drive her to psychiatric counseling. A psychiatrist begins psychotherapy and prescribes fluvoxamine. Rather than improving, the intern develops anxiety, palpitations, insomnia, and sometimes a fine tremor. Which is the most likely explanation of her new symptoms?
a. The fluvoxamine causes panic attacks.
b. The fluvoxamine and psychotherapy cannot overcome her professional and social stressors.
c. The addition of fluvoxamine to her caffeine-fueled existence led to caffeinism.
d. She has developed exhaustion from physical and psychologic stress.

Answer: c. Her new symptoms are manifestations of caffeine intoxication, which developed because fluvoxamine inhibited the enzymes that metabolize caffeine. In other words, the inhibition of the metabolizers increased the substrate. Many other SSRIs and SNRIs do not pose this risk.

75. A pregnant 24-year-old woman with a history of episodic migraine headaches presents to her neurologist with 4 days of progressive throbbing headache. She is in her third trimester, and has had no migraine headaches during her pregnancy. The headache originated from the right occiput but has been progressive and is now bilateral. She denies photophobia, phonophobia, or vomiting, though she does have mild nausea. The headache was severe enough to wake her from sleep the morning of presentation. What test or treatment is indicated as the best next step in evaluation?
a. STAT MRI brain
b. Reassurance and more acetaminophen as needed
c. Blood pressure assessment and urinalysis
d. Administration of sumatriptan 50 mg PO
e. Fundoscopic evaluation

Answer: c. Assessment for possible preeclampsia, including blood pressure measurement and urinalysis for proteinuria, should always be the first consideration in a patient with a progressive headache while in her third trimester. Neuroimaging (MRI) should be considered next, given the increased risk of cerebral venous sinus thrombosis in late pregnancy and the early postpartum period. Fundoscopy is an important part of the neurological exam in a headache patient, but would not be the most critical step. This headache does not have the features of a typical migraine, and so conservative management should only come once emergent etiologies have been ruled out. Additionally, sumatriptan use is contraindicated in pregnancy, so this would not be the appropriate treatment even if she were having a migraine headache.

EPILEPSY

Epilepsy, defined as the tendency to have recurrent unprovoked seizures, affects about six of every 1000 individuals in the United States. For a number of reasons, it is important for psychiatrists to be familiar with this condition. Seizures can mimic psychiatric disturbances and vice versa. Epilepsy is often comorbid with cognitive impairment, depression, and other psychiatric illnesses. Moreover, many antiepileptic drugs (AEDs), which also are used to treat migraine and other types of neuropathic pain, tend to induce cognitive impairment and mood changes.

ELECTROENCEPHALOGRAM

Normal and Abnormal

Invented in the first half of the 20th century by a psychiatrist (Hans Berger) and improved by computerization and correlation with patient videos, the electroencephalogram (EEG) remains the most useful test for investigating the possibility of seizures. In addition, it helps in the diagnosis of several other neurologic conditions. Neurologists consider the EEG to be a painless, harmless, relatively inexpensive, and potentially very helpful diagnostic test.

The routine EEG uses "surface" or "scalp" electrodes to record cerebral electrical activity (Fig. 10.1). EEG readers first ascertain the patient's age and level of consciousness. They also determine the arrangement of the electrodes (the *montage*) and note the time scale, which is demarcated by vertical lines on the EEG paper or displayed as 1-second horizontal bars. Although approaches vary, most readers then determine the EEG's *background* or *dominant rhythm* (see later), organization, and symmetry. EEG readers accord special attention to unusually pointed single discharges, which are either *sharp waves* or *spikes*, and abnormal patterns, especially if they occur in *paroxysms*. Video monitoring concurrent with the EEG recording enhances characterization of episodes that may be seizures.

EEG activity varies in frequency, with the frequency range divided into four bands represented by Greek letters (Table 10.1). The normal background rhythm in an awake adult consists of waves of activity in the *alpha* range of 8 to 13 cycles per second (Hertz [Hz]) detectable mostly over the occipital region (Fig. 10.2). Neurologists refer to this pattern as the *posterior dominant rhythm*. It is prominent when individuals are relaxed with their eyes closed, but disappears if they open their eyes, concentrate, or are anxious. When people undergoing an EEG merely fix their gaze on a clock or add two single-digit numbers, faster rhythms replace alpha activity. Alpha activity also disappears when people fall asleep or take psychotropic medicines. Because alpha activity reflects an anxiety-free state, it represents an important parameter in "alpha training," biofeedback, and other behavior modification techniques.

With aging, the background rhythm typically slows slightly but remains within or just below the alpha range. In the early stages of Alzheimer disease, the background activity also is slower than normal. In more advanced stages of Alzheimer disease, as well as in many other neurologic illnesses, the background EEG activity not only slows well below the alpha range, but also loses its organization.

Beta activity consists of high (> 13 Hz)-frequency, low-voltage activity located maximally overlying the frontal region. It replaces alpha activity when people concentrate, become anxious, or take various hypnotics or sedatives, including benzodiazepines. Beta activity usually inserts itself into the background EEG activity of most adults.

Theta (4 to 7 Hz) and *delta* (< 4 Hz) activity occurs normally in children and in everyone during deep sleep, but is usually absent in healthy adults when alert. If present over the entire brain, theta or delta activity in wakefulness often indicates a neurodegenerative illness, such as Alzheimer disease, or a metabolic derangement. Slow activity, especially when continuous, focal, and associated with *phase reversal* in bipolar montages (Fig. 10.3), suggests an underlying cerebral lesion; however, the absence of theta or delta activity certainly does not exclude one.

Spikes, sharp waves, and slowing are nonspecific changes and occur in about 3% to 15% of the general, healthy population. When they are isolated and asymptomatic, these anomalies have no clinical significance and require no further investigation. However, when spikes and sharp waves are repetitive and phase-reversed, they are an indication of an irritative cerebral focus with potential to produce seizures.

Seizures

During a seizure (*ictus*), the EEG reveals paroxysmal activity usually consisting of bursts of spikes, slow waves, or complexes of spike-and-waves or polyspike-and-waves. Although ictal EEG abnormalities are distinct when captured, muscle or movement artifacts may obscure them. After the seizure, in the *postictal period*, EEGs commonly show only slow low-voltage activity, *postictal depression*, often followed by diffuse high-voltage slowing.

In most patients, EEGs obtained between seizures, in the *interictal period*, contain abnormalities that support (but do not prove) a diagnosis of epilepsy. On the other

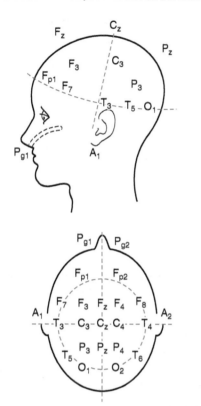

FIGURE 10.1 ■ In the standard array of scalp electrodes, most are named for the underlying cerebral region (e.g., frontal, temporal, central, parietal, and occipital). Odd-numbered ones are on the left, and even-numbered ones on the right. The P_g electrodes attach to nasopharyngeal leads and the A electrodes to the ears (aural leads).

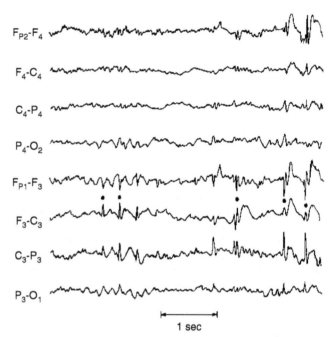

FIGURE 10.3 ■ This bipolar *montage* shows four channels from the right side (upper four) and four from the left (lower four). Each side progresses from the frontal to the occipital region. On at least five occasions (marked by dots), sharp waves and spikes, in *phase reversal*, appear to point toward each other. These sharp waves and spikes originate from the common electrode, F_3, situated over the left frontal lobe. Such isolated, phase-reversed sharp waves are associated with seizures, but, without additional clinical or EEG evidence, they are insufficient for a diagnosis of seizures.

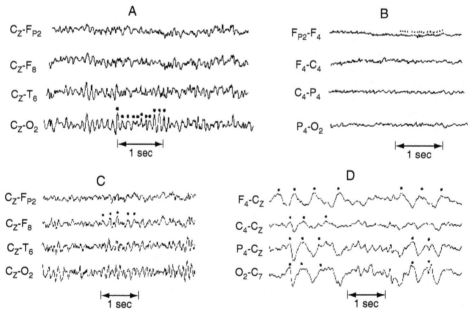

FIGURE 10.2 ■ *A*, Alpha rhythm of regular 8–13 Hz activity overlying the occipital lobe. *B*, Beta rhythm of low voltage, irregular >13 Hz activity overlying the frontal lobe. *C*, Theta rhythm of 4–7 Hz activity overlying the right frontal lobe. *D*, Delta activity of high-voltage <4 Hz activity present over the entire hemisphere.

TABLE 10.1 Common EEG Rhythms

Activity	Hz (Cycles/Second)	Usual Location
Alpha	8–13	Posterior
Beta	> 13	Anterior
Theta	4–7	Generalized or focal
Delta	< 4	Generalized or focal

hand, because many epilepsy patients have no abnormalities on interictal EEG, a normal interictal EEG cannot exclude a diagnosis.

EEG technicians employ certain maneuvers to provoke EEG abnormalities in patients suspected of having primary generalized epilepsy (see later). For example, hyperventilation or looking at a stroboscopic light may elicit discharges during the test that can be diagnostic. If these strategies fail to yield diagnostic EEG patterns and a strong suspicion of seizures persists, neurologists might repeat an EEG following sleep deprivation. In about 30% of epileptic patients, a *sleep-deprived EEG* reveals abnormalities not apparent in routine studies.

In some epilepsy patients, specially placed electrodes reveal abnormalities undetectable by ordinary scalp electrodes. For example, anterior temporal scalp, nasopharyngeal, or sphenoidal electrodes can detect discharges from the inferior-medial surface of the temporal lobe (Fig. 10.4).

Another diagnostic strategy, *continuous EEG-video monitoring*, consists of several days of video recordings of clinical activity and EEG usually undertaken in hospital epilepsy units. The monitoring system records any seizures, changes in behavior, and effects of sleep. During the admission, physicians usually check serum AED concentrations and various physiologic data. Continuous EEG-video monitoring has become the gold standard for many epilepsy studies, including diagnosing, classifying, and determining the frequency of seizures, evaluating patients for epilepsy surgery, treating patients who seem to suffer from *refractory seizures* (frequent seizures that do not respond to AEDs), and identifying disorders that mimic epilepsy, particularly psychogenic nonepileptic seizures (see later). For example, continuous EEG-video monitoring would be the ideal test for a child who exhibits discrete periods of abnormal repetitive behavior in whom the routine EEG has shown only a few spikes that did not occur in paroxysms and were not temporally associated with the questionable behavior. It would also be the ideal test for an adolescent who has developed a new pattern of seizures superimposed on the usual seizure pattern in whom routine EEGs never captured a seizure.

Finally, electrodes surgically implanted in the dura or subdural space, or on the cerebral cortex can localize an epileptic focus when conventional tests are inconclusive. Neurologists may use these to pinpoint a seizure focus prior to surgery (see later).

Quantitative EEG analysis (QEEG) or *EEG brain mapping* involves topographic displays and comparisons of a patient's EEG to standard results. This technique,

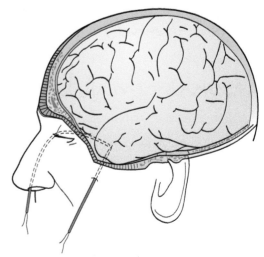

FIGURE 10.4 ■ *Nasopharyngeal electrodes*, which are inserted through the nostrils, reach the posterior pharynx. There, separated by the thin sphenoid bone, they are adjacent to the temporal lobe's medial surface, which is the focus (origin) of about 80% of complex partial seizures. (Figures in Chapter 20 show the relatively large distance between the temporal lobe's medial surface and the scalp, and the closeness of the temporal lobe to the sphenoid bone.) *Sphenoidal* electrodes are inserted through the skin to reach the lateral surface of the sphenoid wing. Electrodes in this location are near the temporal lobe's inferior surface. (Although nasopharyngeal and sphenoidal electrodes are valuable, specially placed scalp electrodes, new arrays, electronic filters, and critical reading of the EEG may be just as accurate and less invasive.) To pinpoint a seizure focus in anticipation of its surgical removal, neurosurgeons place a grid of electrodes in the subdural space.

which is still essentially a research tool, remains too unreliable for clinical application to patients with neurologic conditions, including epilepsy, minor and moderate head injury, and postconcussive syndrome. Its uncertain status precludes its credibility in litigation.

With children, an evaluation could actually begin with parents making videos of episodic disturbances that might be seizures but could also turn out to be temper tantrums, breath-holding spells, night terrors, other parasomnias (see Chapter 17), dopamine responsive dystonia, or other paroxysmal movement disorders (see Chapter 18).

Toxic-Metabolic Encephalopathy

During the initial phase of toxic-metabolic encephalopathy (delirium), when patients have only subtle behavioral or cognitive disturbances, theta and delta activity replace alpha activity. The EEG in toxic-metabolic encephalopathy almost always shows generalized slowing and disorganization. Additional EEG changes point to specific diagnoses. Hepatic and uremic encephalopathies characteristically produce *triphasic waves* (Fig. 10.5). In fact, with hepatic failure, triphasic waves usually appear before bilirubin levels rise. While metabolic derangements are the most common cause of triphasic waves, this EEG finding may also be seen with toxic levels of several medications, including lithium. Benzodiazepine use produces beta-activity, most prominent frontally. Herpes simplex

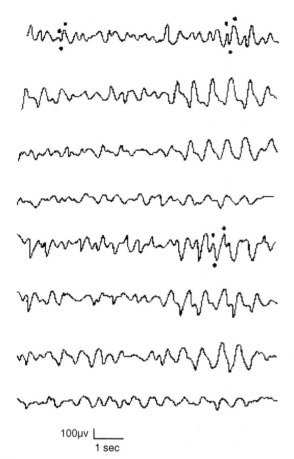

100µv ⌐
1 sec

FIGURE 10.5 ■ This EEG obtained from a patient with hepatic encephalopathy reveals characteristic *triphasic waves* overlying the frontal lobes (the 1st and 5th channels in this montage). In addition to the presence of triphasic waves, the EEG lacks the normal, organized alpha activity over the occipital lobes (the 4th and 8th channels).

encephalitis produces spikes and periodic lateralized epileptiform discharges (PLEDs) over the temporal lobes.

Just as a toxic-metabolic encephalopathy almost always produces EEG abnormalities, the converse holds equal weight: a normal EEG reliably excludes a toxic-metabolic encephalopathy.

Dementia

In early Alzheimer disease, the background activity usually slows to below 8 Hz, while in late Alzheimer disease, the background is universally slow and often disorganized. Vascular dementia also induces EEG abnormalities. However, these changes cannot reliably differentiate vascular dementia from Alzheimer disease dementia (see Chapters 7 and 11).

In contrast, the EEG is quite definitive in diagnosing subacute sclerosing panencephalitis (SSPE) and sporadic Creutzfeldt–Jakob disease (see Chapter 7). In these conditions – characterized clinically by dementia and myoclonus – the EEG shows *periodic sharp-wave complexes* (Fig. 10.6). (*Variant* Creutzfeldt–Jakob disease – "mad cow disease" – does not produce these EEG changes [see Chapter 7].)

The EEG can also help distinguish between *pseudodementia* and dementia – to the extent that they constitute

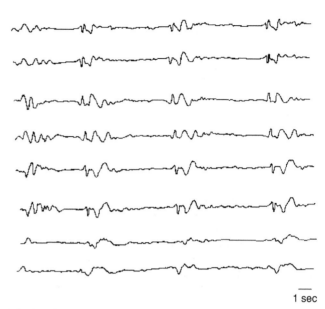

⌐
1 sec

FIGURE 10.6 ■ *Periodic sharp-wave complexes* classically appear all in channels as fairly regular, 1–3-second, bursts of electrical activity followed by minimal activity. Neurologists often describe this EEG pattern as "burst-suppression." Myoclonic jerks represent the clinical counterpart of the periodic complexes. Together myoclonic jerks and periodic complexes are cardinal features of two illnesses characterized by dementia: SSPE and Creutzfeldt–Jakob disease (see Chapter 7).

separate entities (see Chapter 7). In pseudodementia the EEG theoretically should remain normal, but in dementia from almost any cause, it should show slowing. For the many patients with a mixture of depression and mild dementia, the EEG cannot measure each condition's relative contribution to cognitive impairment.

Even though EEGs are relatively inexpensive and carry no risk, neurologists do not routinely order them in the evaluation of a patient with dementia except when the clinical presentation suggests an alternative diagnosis – such as depression, toxic-metabolic encephalopathy, or nonconvulsive seizures – or if a dementia with a specific EEG pattern (like Creutzfeldt–Jakob disease) is suspected.

Structural Lesions

The EEG does not reliably detect or exclude structural lesions, even those that frequently cause seizures, such as brain tumors and cysticercosis. In fact, the EEG is normal in many of these conditions and, when abnormal, does not distinguish among them. Neuroimaging with computed tomography (CT) or magnetic resonance imaging (MRI) is standard and, despite their expense, cost-effective for detecting structural lesions (see Chapter 20). Although CT may suffice, MRI better detects small lesions. More important, MRI is especially effective in detecting mesial temporal sclerosis, which underlies many seizures (see later).

Altered States of Awareness

The EEG shows distinctive changes during normal stages of sleep and during dreaming. Coupled with monitors of ocular movement and muscle activity in the polysomnogram (PSG), the EEG is critical in diagnosing sleep disturbances (see Chapter 17), which can include sleep-related behavioral disturbances and involuntary movement disorders, as well as seizures.

The EEG is also useful in diagnosing the *locked-in syndrome*, a condition in which patients cannot speak or move their trunk or limbs and may appear to be comatose or demented, but remain fully alert and in possession of their cognitive capacity (see Chapter 11). The locked-in syndrome most commonly results from either an infarction in the base of the lower brainstem or extensive cranial and peripheral nerve disruption. With their cerebral hemispheres and thalamus intact, patients retain normal cortical function and normal EEG activity.

Physicians must differentiate the locked-in syndrome from the *persistent vegetative state* (*PVS*), which also is characterized by patients' inability to speak. PVS typically follows cerebral cortex anoxia from cardiac arrest, drug overdose, carbon monoxide poisoning, or traumatic brain injury (TBI) (see Chapter 22). Because patients in a PVS have sustained extensive cerebral cortex injury, they have profound cognitive impairment. Nevertheless, their vegetative functions, such as respiration and digestion, continue. In addition, their eyes continue to open and close, but mostly randomly or in response to light. As would be predicted, the extensive cerebral cortical damage leads to slow and disorganized EEG activity.

Finally, EEG activity is completely absent (*electrocerebral silence*) in brain death, in which – by definition – brain function is utterly abolished. Making the determination of brain death before the heart stops beating permits procurement of organs for transplantation. Certain conditions – such as hypothermia, drug overdose, or metabolic derangement – can suppress cortical activity and mimic brain death on EEG; therefore, reversible conditions must be considered before diagnosing brain death, even when EEG activity is absent. For example, people may fully recover from either barbiturate overdose or drowning in icy water that initially left them with no obvious signs of life and a "flat" EEG. In most cases, obtaining an EEG is not necessary in order to declare brain death, but any EEG pattern other than electrocerebral silence is incompatible with a diagnosis of brain death.

Psychiatric Disturbances and Psychotropics

Because the EEG does not consistently show abnormalities indicative of psychiatric illnesses, obtaining EEGs on a routine basis for psychiatric patients remains unwarranted. EEGs in uncomplicated psychiatric illness show either normal patterns or minor, nonspecific abnormalities, such as excessive beta or theta activity, a few sharp waves or spikes, or mild disorganization.

As a confounding factor, psychotropic medications induce EEG changes. Although these changes are usually minor and nonspecific, some are prominent and can persist for up to 2 months after medications are withdrawn. Most common is background slowing into the theta (but sometimes delta) range. Benzodiazepines and barbiturates typically produce beta activity, which may be

a telltale sign of surreptitious drug use. Phencyclidine (PCP) and other excitatory drugs cause generalized, paroxysmal discharges. Phenothiazines, even at therapeutic serum concentrations, also produce sharp waves. Lithium at toxic levels, clozapine, and tricyclic antidepressants (TCAs) can cause spikes and sharp waves. As described previously, lithium toxicity may induce triphasic waves on EEG monitoring. Among the antipsychotics, clozapine, olanzapine, and trifluoperazine generally produce the most EEG changes, and quetiapine, loxapine, and haloperidol the least.

Electroconvulsive therapy (ECT) also induces EEG changes. During and immediately after ECT, EEG changes resemble those of a generalized tonic-clonic seizure and its aftermath. Subsequently, EEG slow-wave activity develops over the frontal lobes or the entire cerebrum and persists for up to 3 months. When ECT is unilateral, EEG slowing may be restricted to the treated side. Although ECT-induced EEG slowing is associated with memory impairment, it is also associated with effective treatment of depression.

SEIZURE TYPES

A *seizure* is a transient episode causing symptoms and/or signs – commonly, abnormal movements and/or changes in behavior – due to abnormal electrical discharges in the brain. In 2010 the International League Against Epilepsy revised the classification of seizure types; we will use the current terminology while mentioning the familiar older terms for reference. Neurologists classify seizures on the basis of how they originate in the brain. The two major seizure categories are *focal* (formerly *partial*) *seizures*, which begin in one hemisphere, and *generalized seizures*, which originate in both cerebral hemispheres. Focal seizures previously were classified as *complex partial* if they were associated with change in consciousness or awareness, *simple partial* if awareness was unaffected, and *secondarily generalized* if they spread to involve both hemispheres. However, the current scheme eliminates these terms and encourages use of descriptors to characterize focal seizures (see below). Important subcategories of generalized seizures include *tonic-clonic seizures* and *absence seizures* (Box 10.1).

BOX 10.1	**Classification of Seizure Descriptions (International League Against Epilepsy, 2010 Revision, Modified)**

Focal seizures
  Without impairment of consciousness or awareness
  With impairment of consciousness or awareness
  Evolving to a bilateral convulsive seizure
Generalized epilepsies
  Tonic-clonic (grand mal)
  Myoclonic
  Absence

Focal seizures exhibit different manifestations depending upon where in the cerebral cortex the *focus* – the region where the abnormal electrical discharges arise – is located. Seizures with cognitive or behavioral alterations are often attributable to a focus in the temporal cortex but sometimes to one in the frontal cortex. Seizures with motor symptoms usually arise from a focus in the contralateral frontal cortex, and those with visual symptoms from one in the contralateral occipital cortex. Most focal seizures last between several seconds and several minutes.

As a general rule, for a given epilepsy patient, seizures consist of similar, stereotyped symptoms in almost every episode. Conversely, highly variable symptoms suggest a psychogenic disorder.

Although seizure discharges may remain confined to their original cerebral cortex focus, sometimes they spread slowly to adjacent cortical areas. Once the spread occurs, additional symptoms arise. Discharges may eventually spread over the entire cortex or travel directly through the corpus callosum to the contralateral cerebral hemisphere. If the discharges involve both hemispheres, patients lose consciousness, develop bilateral motor activity, and show generalized EEG abnormalities.

In contrast to focal seizures, primary generalized seizures occur when the thalamus or other subcortical structures generate discharges that immediately spread upward to excite the entire cerebral cortex simultaneously. In *tonic-clonic seizures*, patients exhibit bilateral, symmetric, and violent movements, while in an *absence seizure*, a type of generalized seizure which occurs predominantly in children, awareness is impaired but no such movements occur. Just as generalized seizures do not produce focal clinical manifestations, they likewise cause widespread EEG findings but not focal abnormalities.

Generalized seizures usually last a few seconds to several minutes. However, both tonic-clonic seizures and absence seizures may persist with little or no interruption for many hours, i.e., *status epilepticus*.

FOCAL SEIZURES

During a focal seizure patients may be able to continue performing routine activities, such as driving familiar routes, dressing in their usual clothing, and eating. Focal seizures that do not impair consciousness or awareness may be associated with observable motor or autonomic features, or less often with purely subjective sensory or psychic phenomena. Those associated with purely *motor* symptoms, formerly called *simple partial* or *focal motor seizures*, typically consist of rhythmic jerking (clonic movement) of a body region that may be limited to one finger or extend to an entire side of the body (Fig. 10.7). These seizures may evolve into status epilepticus or develop into a bilateral convulsive seizure (formerly termed secondary generalization). Besides elementary movements like tonic stiffening or clonic contractions, motor manifestations may be negative with loss of muscle tone or quite complex and resembling voluntary movements (formerly called *automatisms*). Sometimes, a seizure discharge spreads along the motor cortex in a "Jacksonian march," such that the movements begin in one anatomic

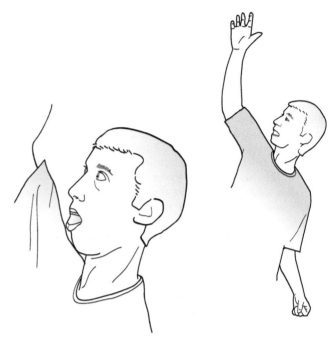

FIGURE 10.7 ■ In this patient having a focal seizure with motor symptoms, his head, neck, and eyes deviate toward the right, his right arm extends, and his left arm flexes. A focal epileptic discharge in the contralateral left frontal lobe is producing this typical "adversive posture."

region and subsequently extend to body parts represented by adjacent areas of motor cortex.

After a focal motor seizure, affected limbs may remain temporarily weak. This transient postictal monoparesis or hemiparesis, *Todd's paralysis*, usually lasts minutes to hours, but may persist for days in a debilitated patient. Thus, the differential diagnosis of transient hemiparesis includes Todd's paralysis along with hemiplegic migraine, transient ischemic attack (TIA), and conversion disorder.

Some patients have seizures with observable autonomic manifestations, including tachycardia, goose bumps, sweating, drooling, pallor, nausea, and vomiting, or respiratory difficulty. Such seizures may localize to the medial temporal lobe, and are likely to have associated emotional symptoms when the seizure focus is on the left.

Focal seizures can be associated with phenomena from any sensory modality, including auditory, visual, olfactory, gustatory, somatosensory, and pain sensations. Seizures with auditory symptoms arise from a seizure focus in the temporal lobe. Patients frequently report hearing repetitive noises, musical notes, or single meaningless words. Visual symptoms, which are attributable to occipital lesions, usually consist of bright lights. Sometimes though, these seizures may produce lines, spots, or splotches of color that move slowly across the visual field or, like a view through a kaleidoscope, rotate around the center of vision. Physicians must distinguish elaborate visual seizure phenomena from visual hallucinations due to other causes (see Box 12.1).

Olfactory symptoms classically consist of perceiving vaguely recognizable odors, such as the frequently cited one of burning rubber. However, contrary to popular belief, these odors are not necessarily repugnant. Because olfactory hallucinations usually result from discharges in the amygdala or the *uncus* (the anterior medial tip of the temporal lobe), focal seizures with olfactory symptoms are sometimes called *uncinate fits*. If discharges spread from sensory regions to engulf a larger area of the temporal lobe, they often evolve to impair consciousness.

Seizures with somatosensory symptoms typically arise from a focus in the parietal lobe's sensory cortex, and most frequently consist of tingling or burning paresthesias in body regions with extensive cortical representation, such as the face and thumb. Very rarely, sensory loss, a "negative symptom," might be a seizure's only manifestation.

Another sensory experience classically associated with seizure activity is the *rising epigastric sensation*. This symptom consists of a sensation of swelling in the abdomen that, as if progressing upward within the chest, turns into tightness of the throat and then a sensation of suffocation. Although it could be an ictal phenomenon, a rising epigastric sensation may also represent a panic attack or *globus hystericus*, a commonly occurring psychogenic disturbance that causes a similar tightening of the throat and an inability to breathe.

EEG and Etiology

During a focal seizure, the EEG shows spikes, sharp or slow waves, or spike–wave complexes overlying the seizure focus. For example, during seizures with motor symptoms, EEG abnormalities are usually detectable in channels overlying motor cortex in the frontal lobe (Fig. 10.8). Interictally, EEGs may still show occasional spikes in the same channels.

In trying to establish the cause of focal seizures, the patient's age at the onset of seizures is one of the most important factors. For example, when young children

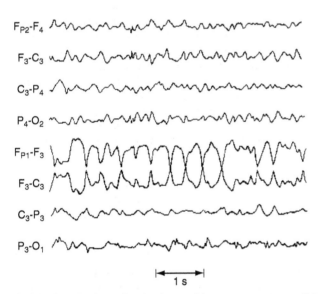

FIGURE 10.8 ■ During a focal seizure with motor symptoms, this EEG contains a paroxysm of 4-Hz sharp wave activity with phase reversals referable to the F_3 electrode. Because the F_3 electrode overlies the left frontal region, the seizure probably consists of right face or arm motor activity and, very likely, a deviation of the head and eyes to the right.

develop focal seizures, typical causes are congenital cerebral malformations, such as cortical dysgenesis, and neurocutaneous disorders (see Chapter 13). In young adults, common causes of focal seizures are head trauma, arteriovenous malformations (AVMs), and previously asymptomatic congenital lesions. However, posttraumatic seizures are not associated with trivial head injuries, but follow serious trauma, such as that causing more than 30 minutes of unconsciousness, depressed (not just linear) skull fractures, intracranial hematomas, and penetrating head wounds (see Chapter 22).

Young adults with major psychiatric and neuropsychiatric disorders are prone to seizures. For example, about 30% of autistic individuals and 70–90% of those with Rett syndrome develop epilepsy by the time they are adults. Also, genetic abnormalities in sodium or calcium channels or the GABA$_A$-receptor subunit can cause both focal and generalized seizures. Such genetically determined epilepsy syndromes generally arise between infancy and adolescence. Also, in these syndromes, other stigmata of neurologic disease such as myoclonus and mental retardation often accompany the epilepsy.

Because drug and alcohol abuse carries multiple neurologic ramifications, neurologists often consider substance abuse in young adults presenting with seizures. Profound alcohol intoxication or alcohol-induced hypoglycemia can precipitate seizures. Also, 1 to 3 days of abstinence from chronic, excessive alcohol consumption produces seizures (see later). Although the clinical and EEG manifestations of these seizures resemble those of genetically determined seizures, the interictal EEG is normal. Withdrawal from daily use of benzodiazepines (especially alprazolam) is similar and these withdrawal seizures often evolve into *status epilepticus*. Most cases of benzodiazepine-withdrawal seizures are associated with prescription medicines rather than "street" drugs.

Especially when seizures are accompanied by psychotic or otherwise abnormal behavior, physicians should suspect use of cocaine, PCP, synthetic marijuana (K2 or spice), or amphetamines. (Cocaine leads to seizures not only by reducing the seizure threshold, but also by disrupting sleep, interfering with AED compliance, and causing strokes.) However, although neonates may develop seizures during opiate withdrawal, adult drug addicts generally do not develop seizures during heroin use, withdrawal, or detoxification. Also, marijuana does not lead to seizures and actually has a mild antiepileptic effect.

A seizure associated with drug or alcohol abuse may represent a provoked seizure; it does not necessarily constitute epilepsy, which requires recurrent unprovoked seizures. Moreover, a neurologic complication of substance abuse, rather than withdrawal, may be the cause of the seizure. For example, cocaine routinely causes vasoconstriction or cerebral hemorrhage, which in turn causes seizures. Similarly, although heroin may not directly produce seizures, its intravenous use can lead to bacterial endocarditis, episodes of cerebral anoxia, acquired immune deficiency syndrome (AIDS), hepatitis, and vasculitis, which all can cause seizures.

Adults aged 40 to 60 years most often develop seizures because of a structural lesion, such as a primary or metastatic brain tumor. Patients older than 60 years are more likely to have a stroke rather than a tumor. In young adults with AIDS, cerebral toxoplasmosis must be considered. The patient's geographic origin also suggests the cause. For example, in South and Central America, cerebral cysticercosis is the most common cause of seizures. In the Indian subcontinent, tuberculomas are one of the most common causes. By extension, those infections may very well underlie the development of epilepsy in recent immigrants to the Unites States.

FOCAL SEIZURES WITH IMPAIRED CONSCIOUSNESS OR AWARENESS (COMPLEX PARTIAL SEIZURES)

Focal seizures that impair cognition most often begin in late childhood or early adulthood. Affecting about 65% of epilepsy patients, they are the most common seizure type. Neurologists and patients themselves solicit psychiatry consultation because of these seizures' variable and often ambiguous ictal manifestations, interictal and postictal symptoms, and comorbid psychiatric conditions. Physicians and epilepsy patients may ask psychiatrists about indications for antidepressants and antipsychotics and potential adverse reactions.

Etiology

Focal seizures with impaired awareness most often arise from the temporal lobe, though the frontal lobe also can harbor the seizure focus. The most common cause is mesial temporal sclerosis, which is characterized by sclerosis of the hippocampus and atrophy of the temporal lobe. Although anoxia at birth, other perinatal insults, and prolonged febrile seizures – but not brief, occasional febrile seizures – lead to most cases of mesial temporal sclerosis, some studies suggest that temporal lobe infections (such as with a herpes virus) can lead to this type of epilepsy. Mass lesions in the temporal lobe – such as hamartomas or astrocytomas – can cause focal seizures with impaired consciousness. Any of the lesions mentioned above may also produce focal seizures without altered consciousness.

Menses, intercurrent illness, or subtherapeutic AED serum concentrations may precipitate seizures of any variety. For example, up to 80% of women with epilepsy report an increase in seizure frequency around the time of their menses. Lack of sleep and self-reported stress and anxiety often predate seizures.

Ictal Symptoms

In 20% to 80% of patients, focal seizures begin with a characteristic premonitory sensation, called an *aura* (Greek for breeze or soft wind). Not merely a warning, the aura constitutes the first portion of the seizure.

During a focal seizure with impaired consciousness, patients usually display a blank stare and are inattentive and uncommunicative. In most cases, they also have partial or complete memory loss, *amnesia*, presumably because seizure discharges disrupt the limbic system in the temporal lobe. The amnesia is so striking that it may appear to be a patient's only symptom. (For this reason, physicians should strongly consider seizures among the neurologic causes of the *acute amnestic syndrome* [see Box 7.2].)

Physical manifestations of focal seizures with impaired cognition usually consist of only simple, repetitive, purposeless movements (*automatisms*) of the face and hands. Present in about 80% of seizures originating in the temporal lobe, common automatisms include repetitive licking or smacking the lips, swallowing, or kissing – *oral automatisms* – or fumbling with clothing, scratching, rubbing the abdomen, or fidgeting – *manual automatisms* (Fig. 10.9). Other physical manifestations are simple actions, such as standing, walking, pacing, or even driving; however, sometimes these actions are simply ingrained tasks that continue despite the seizure. In addition, more than 25% of patients utter brief phrases or unintelligible sounds. Facial expressions suggesting strong emotion (such as fear) or bursts of crying also may occur.

Many times the environment triggers actions and words. For example, a child may clutch and continually stroke a nearby stuffed animal while repeating a familiar phrase. Impaired consciousness, apparent self-absorption, and subsequent failure to recall the event would separate these activities from normal behavior.

A variety of psychic-experiential phenomena has been reported to occur as ictal phenomena, including *déjà vu* (French, previously seen or experienced), *jamais vu* (French, never seen or experienced), confusion, detachment, and depersonalization. Such phenomena are not highly reliable for accurate localization, diagnosis, or prognosis.

A possible exception may be seizures that originate in the amygdala, which are said to cause overwhelming fear as the primary or only symptom. However, the medical literature does not support strongly the notion of pronounced fear, as an isolated sensation, as a seizure manifestation. It is more likely to represent a panic attack.

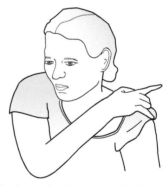

FIGURE 10.9 ■ During a focal seizure with impaired consciousness, patients typically appear dazed. They perform only rudimentary, purposeless actions, such as pulling on their clothing, and pay little or no attention to their surroundings or examiners. Their hands and fingers move in clumsy and misdirected patterns. Repetitive, simple oral, limb, or body movements, *automatisms*, such as lip smacking, occur in approximately 80% of cases with a temporal lobe focus and the majority of those with absence seizures.

Any focal seizure may evolve to a bilateral convulsive seizure, previously termed *secondary generalization*. In contrast, in *focal status epilepticus*, seizures emanating from a single brain region persist or wax and wane in quick succession. In *nonconvulsive status epilepticus*, patients demonstrate neuropsychological aberrations – such as thought disorder, language impairment, or change in sensorium – which can last hours to days. Patients' behavior may be so bizarre that it merits the label *ictal psychosis*. It often mimics delirium, TBI, and numerous other neurologic disorders as well as an acute psychotic episode. Neurologists encounter nonconvulsive status epilepticus most often in patients known to have epilepsy, particularly those who have been noncompliant with their AEDs. They also see it in critically ill patients who have sustained cerebral injury or anoxia. EEG readily makes the diagnosis of nonconvulsive status epilepticus, and first-line therapy is intravenous administration of a benzodiazepine, which will usually abort status epilepticus and awaken the patient.

Sex, Violence, and Aggression

During seizures, patients sometimes fumble with buttons, tug at their clothing, or make rudimentary masturbatory movements. They may even seem to undress partially. However, these patients are not deliberately exposing themselves or attempting to engage in sexual activities.

Continuous EEG-video monitoring has demonstrated that *ictal violence*, with rare exception, consists only of random shoving, pushing, kicking, or screaming. This behavior is fragmented, unsustained, ineffectual, and, most important, unaccompanied by rage or anger. Moreover, violence, which occurs in less than 0.1% of cases, is virtually never the sole manifestation of any type of seizure.

Belligerence or *resistive violence*, a different form of seizure-related violence, occurs when patients fight against restraints during their ictal or postictal period. Occurring much more frequently than ictal violence, resistive violence stems largely from patients' fighting off health-care workers or family members who attempt to restrain them or administer injections.

Physicians must distinguish ictal violence, with its lack of aggression, from both criminal violence, which is characterized by aggression, and episodic dyscontrol syndrome (see later). For physicians to consider it aggression, the behavior must be directed, have a conscious or unconscious rationale, and be accompanied by a consistent affect. Although aggression may consist only of threats or taking control, it often leads to deliberate personal and property damage.

During seizures, patients cannot engage in sequential activities, premeditated actions, or meaningful interactions with other people – all requirements for criminality. Interictally, patients also lack the cognitive ability to operate mechanical devices. These limitations preclude violent crimes either in the midst of a seizure or as a manifestation of a seizure. Consequently, most neurologists accept violence, but neither aggression nor criminal acts, as a rare manifestation of seizures.

Immediate Postictal Symptoms

Immediately after a focal seizure, which has an average duration of 2 to 3 minutes, patients characteristically experience confusion, clouding of mentation, disorientation, flat affect, and sleepiness. However, seizures occasionally lead not to somnolence, inactivity, and withdrawal, but rather to agitation, i.e., *postictal agitation*. If seizures involve the brain's language region and cause transient aphasia (see Chapter 8), postictal symptoms may be more pronounced. Similarly, if the seizure focus includes the cortical areas involved with motor function, patients may have a Todd's hemiparesis. For 15 to 40 minutes after a seizure, many patients have measurable physiologic changes: Approximately 40% of them have an elevated serum prolactin concentration and focal EEG depression.

Astute physicians are unlikely to mistake seizures for psychotic episodes. Focal seizures with altered consciousness usually last only a few minutes, consist of stereotyped symptoms, necessarily include impaired consciousness, and usually have dramatic postictal manifestations. After recovering from a seizure and its aftermath, patients gradually return to their interictal personality, which admittedly might be abnormal. In contrast, psychotic episodes, which are frequently triggered by factors in the environment, typically last at least several days. Also, the manifestations of the psychosis vary greatly from episode to episode and often include hypervigilance.

Frontal Lobe Seizures

Named for the region of the brain where they originate, *frontal lobe seizures* constitute a distinct, important variety of focal seizures. Their manifestations consist of abrupt onset of vocalizations and bilateral complex movements lasting for a relatively short time (less than 1 minute). There is no premonitory aura and the seizure is followed by little or no postictal confusion. Frontal lobe seizures tend to begin in the adult years, occur relatively frequently (several times a month), develop predominantly during sleep, and produce paroxysmal EEG discharges that are difficult to detect by conventional EEG studies.

Frontal lobe seizures, even compared to seizures of temporal lobe origin, are most apt to cause bizarre behavior and the rare instances of aggressive violence. With their behavioral manifestations and EEG changes usually undetectable, frontal lobe seizures mimic psychogenic nonepileptic seizures. In addition, when frontal lobe seizures arise exclusively during sleep, they mimic sleep disorders (see Chapter 17).

Rolandic Epilepsy

Rolandic epilepsy (childhood epilepsy with centrotemporal spikes), the most common form of focal epilepsy in childhood, almost always begins between ages 5 and 9 years, occurs mostly in boys, and remits by puberty. The seizures consist of unilateral paresthesias, movements of the face, and speech arrest. They tend to undergo secondary generalization during sleep. Interictal EEG changes consist of high-voltage spikes in the central temporal region (*Rolandic spikes*) during sleep. AEDs usually suppress the seizures, though many neurologists favor a nonpharmacologic approach to this self-limited epilepsy syndrome.

Unlike other epilepsies with focal seizures, Rolandic seizures are restricted to childhood, are not associated with an underlying structural lesion, and are inherited (in an autosomal dominant pattern). In contrast to children with absence seizures (see later), those with Rolandic epilepsy are not at risk of later developing other varieties of epilepsy.

Testing During and Between Focal Seizures

EEG

During a focal seizure, the EEG most often shows paroxysms of spikes, slow waves, or other abnormalities in leads overlying the temporal or frontotemporal region. Even though a seizure focus may be unilateral, bilateral EEG abnormalities appear because of additional foci, interhemispheric projections, or "reflections." Nasopharyngeal and other specially placed leads may capture temporal lobe discharges that routine scalp electrodes fail to detect (Fig. 10.10).

In the interictal period, the routine EEG contains spikes or spike-and-wave complexes over the temporal lobes in about 40% of cases. When accompanied by an appropriate history, these EEG abnormalities are specific enough to corroborate the diagnosis. Looking at the situation in reverse, about 90% of persons with anterior temporal spikes on the EEG will have temporal lobe seizures. Nevertheless, a diagnosis of seizures should not be based entirely on EEG spikes, but rather requires correlation of EEG abnormalities with symptoms and signs.

If the diagnosis remains unclear after a routine EEG, especially where episodic behavioral abnormalities are believed to result from seizures, physicians should arrange for continuous EEG-video monitoring. EEG corroboration of focal seizures might begin with a routine EEG, but it has only a 40% yield. Although EEGs performed during sleep and wakefulness or following sleep deprivation might improve sensitivity, EEG-video monitoring offers virtually a 100% yield when an event is captured.

Other Tests

Because focal seizures usually originate from a structural brain lesion, neurologists routinely order MRI of the brain to investigate seizure etiology (unless the patient has a contraindication – see Chapter 20). With even greater resolution than CT and freedom from artifacts produced by the bones surrounding the middle fossa, MRI reveals mesial temporal lobe sclerosis, tuberous sclerosis nodules, small strokes, and cryptic AVMs, as well as more overt lesions (see Fig. 20.26). (MRI with thin "cuts" through the temporal lobes is often required to detect mesial temporal lobe sclerosis.)

Neurologists also order MRI for tonic-clonic seizures because clinical and EEG data may not distinguish primary generalized seizures from focal seizures that generalize rapidly. With drug- or alcohol-withdrawal seizures and absence seizures (see later), these scans may add little or no information.

Functional neuroimaging with *positron emission tomography* (PET) or *single-photon emission computed tomography* (SPECT) helps in the planning of epilepsy surgery. On PET scanning, which images cerebral metabolism, a seizure focus may show hypometabolism interictally, but due to technical requirements, obtaining PET during the seizure remains difficult. Because SPECT, which images cerebral blood flow, is less technically demanding, it often can be obtained intraictally, when it will show hyperemia in the region of the seizure focus.

COMORBID CONDITIONS AND THEIR TREATMENT

Depression

Depression is more prevalent in epilepsy than in other chronic neurologic illnesses, including Alzheimer and Parkinson diseases. With prevalence in epilepsy patients ranging from approximately 7.5 to 55% (with higher prevalence in intractable seizure patients), depression is epilepsy's most common psychiatric comorbidity. Given those rates, many authors assert that physicians under-diagnose and under-treat depression in epilepsy patients.

Risk factors for comorbid depression include seizures with cognitive impairment, onset of epilepsy in late-adult years, and, in most studies, frequent seizures. Several AEDs – levetiracetam, tiagabine, topiramate, and vigabatrin – carry a risk for depression and self-destructive behavior (see later). In contrast, a long history of epilepsy and the laterality of the seizure focus are weak risk factors. Perhaps surprisingly, some studies associate depression with a failure of focal seizures to undergo secondary generalization – as though experiencing a generalized seizure ameliorates underlying depression. This observation led to the development of electroconvulsive therapy for depression (see later).

Once depression complicates epilepsy, seizure frequency increases. For example, depression-associated behavior – such as sleep deprivation, noncompliance with an AED regimen, or substance abuse – precipitates seizures. Depressed patients may also consciously or unconsciously develop psychogenic nonepileptic seizures in addition to epileptic ones. Additionally, depressed

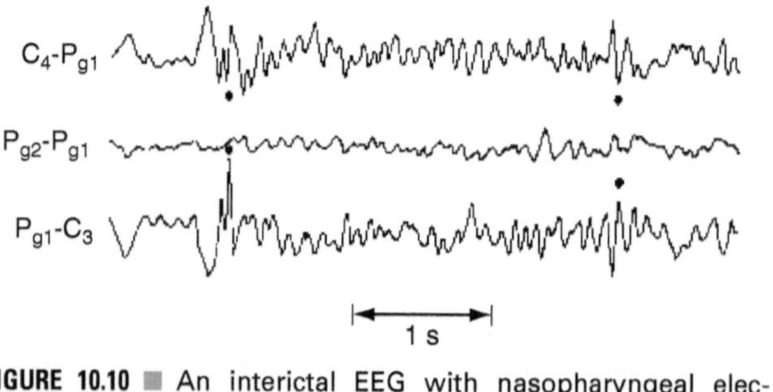

FIGURE 10.10 ■ An interictal EEG with nasopharyngeal electrodes (P_{g1} and P_{g2}) shows phase-reversed spikes that routine scalp electrodes may not detect.

epilepsy patients are more likely to require hospitalization than patients suffering from epilepsy or depression alone.

Whatever the cause, comorbid depression worsens epilepsy patients' quality of life. It exerts a more powerful effect than the frequency of seizures, variety of seizures, use of AEDs, or toxicity of AEDs. It is also one of several risk factors for suicide (see later).

Physicians should direct initial therapy of comorbid depression not necessarily toward depression, but toward better seizure control. Seizure control will probably improve patients' mood, reduce behavioral disturbances, and restore some cognitive function. Fortunately, several AEDs possess mood-stabilizing as well as anticonvulsant properties: carbamazepine (which bears a structural similarity to TCAs), lamotrigine, and valproate (valproic acid/divalproex). These AEDs raise serotonin levels.

Once patients and physicians achieve optimum seizure control, they may add antidepressants to their AED regimen; however, their use carries several caveats. While antidepressants improve patients' mood, they will probably not further reduce the frequency of seizures. Because of their effect on cytochrome P450 enzymes, psychotropic drugs may render certain AEDs less effective on one hand or toxic on the other (see later). For example, prescribing an enzyme-inhibiting antidepressant such as fluoxetine to an AED regimen of carbamazepine or phenytoin may lead to toxic levels of the AED. Even some apparently benign, readily available substances may alter AED serum concentrations. For example, grapefruit juice can increase concentrations of carbamazepine and zonisamide, and St. John's wort can decrease their concentrations. Moreover, AEDs alone or in combination with other medicines may induce mental status changes (see later).

Most importantly, psychotropics, perhaps more than any other class of medication, precipitate seizures in epilepsy patients. Rarely, they even cause seizures in patients with no history of epilepsy. Risk factors for psychotropic-induced seizures generally include a history of epilepsy, other neurologic disorders, including Alzheimer disease and TBI, prior ECT, and drug or alcohol abuse.

Psychotropic-induced seizures, in general, most often occur during the first week of treatment, following sudden large increases in dose, or with regimens involving multiple medicines. With routine antidepressant treatment, the risk of seizures is typically dose-dependent. For example, the incidence of seizures with bupropion immediate-release formulations at up to 400 mg daily is less than 1%, but at higher doses, the incidence rises to unacceptable levels. In an exception, clomipramine led to seizures in 1.5% of patients taking 300 mg or less per day. This relatively high rate represents clomipramine's most significant adverse reaction. Moreover, this risk does not diminish over time, as is the case with most other antidepressants.

In contrast to the relatively high rates of seizures associated with tricyclic and heterocyclic antidepressants, monamine oxidase inhibitors, selective serotonin reuptake inhibitors (SSRIs), and serotonin-norepinephrine reuptake inhibitors produce seizures in less than 0.3% of cases.

Overall, most cases of antidepressant-induced seizures result from overdose. TCAs lead to seizures in approximately 5% to 25% of overdose cases, and the incidence following overdose of amoxapine and maprotiline is even greater. Overdose-induced seizures most often appear within 3 to 6 hours, but almost never after 24 hours.

As an adjunct or an alternative to antidepressants, use of ECT in epilepsy patients is safe provided that their seizures are under control. For depressed patients taking AEDs, physicians sometimes must reduce the AED regimen before ECT. Although prolonged seizures may unexpectedly follow ECT, this complication is rare and readily responds to AEDs. (As mentioned above, ECT originated in the observation that depressed epileptic patients' mood improved after a seizure. This benefit led to physicians' inducing hypoglycemic seizures by injections of large amounts of insulin. Use of electricity was a later innovation.) Seizures have also complicated treatment with transcranial magnetic stimulation (TMS) administered for medication-resistant depression.

Even though most psychotropic medicines in epileptic patients are generally safe, some words of warning are required. Despite all precautions, adding any psychotropic may increase seizure frequency. Physicians can reduce the risk by slowly introducing psychotropics, attempting to use low doses of a single medicine, checking for paradoxical effects and drug–drug interactions, and monitoring serum concentrations of medicines.

On the other hand, if a patient taking a psychotropic were to develop a seizure, physicians must guard against reflexively assigning the blame to the medication. For example, a brain tumor might be the cause of both the seizure and symptoms of depression. Similarly, a seizure in depressed patients may result from a deliberate medicine overdose or failure to take prescribed AEDs.

Not only is depression a comorbidity of epilepsy, it is a consideration in various epilepsy-related situations. For example, seizure-like episodes are occasionally a manifestation of depression or other psychiatric conditions (see later, psychogenic nonepileptic seizures). Also, chronic depression is a risk factor for a suboptimal outcome from epilepsy surgery.

Bipolar Disorder

Bipolar symptoms in epilepsy patients are relatively uncommon, but occur more frequently than in either the general population or individuals with other medical disorders. When mania develops in epilepsy patients, they frequently display childish behavior, fluctuating moods, and rapid cycling. In addition to epilepsy patients who have comorbid bipolar disorder, epilepsy patients postoperative from temporal lobectomy, particularly right-sided procedures, and those with preoperative bilateral EEG abnormalities may develop mania.

Anxiety

Various studies suggest that anxiety is comorbid with epilepsy in 20% to more than 60% of cases. Variation in patients' reports and physicians' interpretation of the symptoms may help explain the wide range in frequency. For example, in the face of an impending seizure, many patients are reasonably fearful and may panic. Additionally, a seizure's aura may have anxiety-like components.

In other cases, anxiety may be a manifestation of a generalized anxiety or panic disorder. Physicians may freely treat anxiety comorbid with epilepsy with benzodiazepines because these have antiepileptic effects. Conversely, abrupt withdrawal from benzodiazepines may precipitate seizures that lead to status epilepticus.

Psychosis

Besides being susceptible to postictal confusion, patients may develop a frank *postictal psychosis*. This thought disorder characteristically emerges after several hours to several days of clear sensorium and minimal symptoms (a "lucid interval") following one or usually more seizures. It consists of hours to 2 weeks of hallucinations, delusions, agitation, and occasionally violence. Depending on its severity, patients usually require administration of benzodiazepines or antipsychotics.

The greatest risk factor for postictal psychosis is a preceding flurry of seizures in patients with chronic epilepsy. Up to 7% of focal seizures with altered awareness refractory to AEDs lead to postictal psychosis. Other risk factors include low intelligence, bilateral seizure foci, and a family history of psychiatric illness. Episodes of postictal psychosis, in turn, represent a risk factor for cognitive decline and interictal psychosis.

Unlike postictal psychosis, *interictal psychosis*, sometimes loosely called "schizophreniform psychosis" or "schizophrenia-like psychosis of epilepsy," is a chronic condition. It generally arises in patients 30 to 40 years of age whose epilepsy began in childhood, especially between 5 and 10 years of age. In other words, interictal psychosis develops decades after the onset of epilepsy. Its symptoms include persistent hallucinations, paranoia, and social isolation. Unlike typical schizophrenia patients, epilepsy patients with interictal psychosis retain a relatively normal affect, do not deteriorate, and do not have an increased incidence of schizophrenia in their families.

Risk factors for interictal psychosis are childhood onset of epilepsy, physical neurological abnormalities, low intelligence, frequent seizures, multiple seizure types, seizures that require multiple AEDs, and episodes of postictal psychosis.

Patients with interictal psychosis also have neuropathological as well as clinical signs of brain damage. Their brains have large cerebral ventricles, periventricular gliosis, and focal damage. In an interesting comparison, multiple sclerosis (MS) patients, despite having equally extensive cerebral damage, rarely have these symptoms.

A related condition, which neurologists originally called *forced normalization*, followed a change in a patient's AED regimen that completely suppressed abnormal EEG activity and eliminated long-standing seizures. Patients, suddenly seizure-free, occasionally developed either psychosis or depression. Some researchers propose that the seizures, while troublesome, had suppressed a thought or mood disorder, perhaps through an ECT-like mechanism. Although the mechanisms surrounding forced normalization remain unclear, physicians should monitor patients who rapidly achieve complete seizure control. This caveat applies to epilepsy patients whose seizures suddenly come under control following epilepsy surgery or changes in their AED regimen.

In the opposite scenario, *withdrawal-emergent psychopathology*, psychiatric disorders – particularly anxiety or depression – appear upon abrupt discontinuation of AEDs. (Although withdrawal-emergent psychopathology is a risk of suddenly stopping AEDs, status epilepticus is a much more frequent and life-threatening risk of doing so.) Neurologists have postulated that in patients with withdrawal-emergent psychopathology, the AEDs had suppressed a latent psychiatric disorder along with the epilepsy. Withdrawal-emergent psychopathology may also appear after epilepsy surgery – in this case because it allows patients to curtail if not eliminate their AED regimen.

In the *Diagnostic and Statistical Manual of Mental Disorders, 5th Edition* (DSM-5) classification scheme, psychoses that occur during, immediately afterwards, or interictally would all fall into the category of Psychotic Disorder due to Another Medical Condition (epilepsy).

Many of the rules governing treatment of depression complicating epilepsy also apply to treating psychosis complicating epilepsy. Foremost, AEDs should remain the mainstay of treatment, but if they alone are ineffective, neurologists or psychiatrists should add an antipsychotic. Another rule is that an overdose of an antipsychotic, just like an overdose of antidepressant, can lead to seizures. Among antipsychotics, an overdose of chlorpromazine is more likely than one of haloperidol, thioridazine, fluphenazine, or the newer atypical agents to cause seizures.

In therapeutic doses, antipsychotic-induced seizures are usually dose-dependent, occur with large dose increases, and develop more frequently in patients with epilepsy or underlying brain damage. In the therapeutic as well as the overdose range, chlorpromazine again remains most apt to provoke seizures. Except for clozapine, which leads to seizures in 4% of patients taking more than 600 mg daily, atypical antipsychotics carry a seizure risk of less than 1%.

Physicians forced to restart an antipsychotic following a medication-induced seizure should, while excluding other causes of psychosis and seizures, prescribe a different antipsychotic or slowly reintroduce the original one. If the patient requires clozapine or another seizure-inducing antipsychotic, physicians may offer some protection by simultaneously adding an AED.

Cognitive Impairment

Of individuals with either a congenital intellectual disability or cerebral palsy, 10% to 20% have comorbid epilepsy (see Chapter 13). In these patients, epilepsy usually appears before age 5 years and its incidence increases in proportion to their physical and intellectual impairments. Of individuals institutionalized because of these disorders, 40% have epilepsy. Also, children with autism symptoms, particularly Rett syndrome, are susceptible to seizures (see earlier). Among survivors of fetal alcohol syndrome, 18% develop epilepsy.

When brain damage underlying seizures is progressive – as in tuberous sclerosis, inherited metabolic diseases, mitochondrial encephalopathies, and some neurodegenerative illnesses – seizure control, cognitive capacity, and motor function all decline. Conversely, progressive cognitive decline or increasingly refractory seizures suggests a progressive rather than a congenital static neurologic disorder. As with interictal psychosis, many risk factors for cognitive decline in epilepsy reflect underlying brain damage.

Many patients beset with focal seizures associated with impaired consciousness suffer increasingly severe cognitive impairment. Risk factors include longer duration of epilepsy, older age, and premorbid intellectual impairment. Possible explanations for this progressive cognitive decline include spread of damage from mesial temporal sclerosis to the surrounding limbic system, brief interictal EEG discharges in the temporal lobes that disrupt memory and other cognitive processes, and cognitive side effects of AEDs. If epilepsy surgery or adjustment of AEDs controls the seizures, the cognitive decline may stop and partly reverse. However, if surgery does not arrest the seizures, the cognitive decline may accelerate. Moreover, unsuccessful surgery may lead to depression and other psychiatric disorders.

Destructive Behavior

Suicide

Suicide occurs four to five times more frequently in all epilepsy patients and 25 times more frequently in those with focal seizures with altered consciousness than in the general population. Risk factors for suicide in epilepsy are psychotic disturbances, borderline personality disorder, and other interictal psychopathology, as well as those risk factors present in the general population, including depression, poor physical health, life stress, previous suicide attempts, and access to firearms. As in other neurologic illnesses, such as Huntington disease, impaired judgment and poor impulse control, rather than deliberate planning, may precipitate suicide.

A landmark 2008 meta-analysis of clinical trials involving AEDs found that among epilepsy patients, AED use was linked with an almost two-fold risk for "suicidality" (suicide acts or ideation). Suicidality was greater in patients taking AEDs for epilepsy than for other indications, including mood stabilization, and among individuals taking multiple AEDs rather than a single AED. Subsequent studies found that only certain AEDs, such as those associated with causing depressive symptoms, placed patients at risk. In contrast to the 2008 study, Arana et al. (see References) reported in 2010 that AEDs posed no risk of suicidality in patients with epilepsy. In a 2010 British case-control study, use of an AED associated in clinical trials with a risk of depression greater than 1% (levetiracetam, tiagabine, topiramate, vigabatrin) was associated with a three-fold increased risk of self-harm or suicidal behavior, while no such association was seen with other AEDs.

Crime and Interictal Violence

The consensus among neurologists is that criminal violence cannot be a manifestation of a seizure. However, epilepsy-related factors – intellectual deficits, poor impulse control, and lower socioeconomic status – can steer people toward crime but not specific acts of violence. Studies have found that, although the incidence of epilepsy is at least four times greater among men in prison than in the general population, crimes of prisoners with epilepsy are no more violent than those with psychogenic nonepileptic seizures. Similarly, the prevalence of epilepsy is the same in nonviolent criminals as violent ones. Also, EEG abnormalities do not correlate with violent offenses.

Interictal violence rather than ictal violence, which was discussed previously, usually consists of only verbal and minor physical acts. It occurs predominantly in epilepsy patients who are antisocial, schizophrenic, or mentally retarded. Epilepsy patients with interictal violence, show no differences in the variety or frequency of seizures, EEG abnormalities, or AED treatment compared to patients who are not violent.

In general, behavioral changes tend to develop in individuals with a history of epilepsy that had an early onset, seizures that undergo secondary generalization, and EEGs showing bilateral changes. Epilepsy patients with comorbid psychosis or mood disorders are particularly prone to show behavioral abnormalities.

Personality Traits

Classic studies, such as those by Bear and Fedio (see References), described "temporal lobe epilepsy" patients as distinctively circumstantial in thinking, hyposexual, humorless, "sticky" in interpersonal relations, and overly concerned with general philosophic and religious questions. These patients showed excessive and compulsive writing (*hypergraphia*). Supporting studies suggested that the presence of these abnormal traits depended on whether the seizure focus was in the right or left temporal lobe. Right-sided foci supposedly predisposed patients to anger, sadness, and elation, but left-sided ones to ruminative and intellectual tendencies.

More contemporary studies based on continuous EEG-video monitoring and strict methodology have either not corroborated the presence of those personality traits or found them in a small minority of patients. In fact, the same traits and others, such as dysphoria, occurred in patients with other diseases, such as migraine. In particular, hypergraphia can be a symptom of schizophrenia or bipolar disorder. The studies also found no difference in personality traits when foci are in different temporal lobes or even other brain areas, and no difference in personality traits among patients with different varieties of epilepsy. As a general rule, personality changes and cognitive impairment in epilepsy patients serve only as clinical markers of brain damage. They do not fit into any distinct personality disorders in the DSM-5.

Delirium

Sometimes epilepsy patients present for medical care in a stuporous, disoriented, confused, or amnestic state. Their behavior, which may be irrational, agitated, and belligerent, can preclude a complete mental status examination.

Most frequently, such patients are simply delirious because they are in the midst of a prolonged postictal period.

Another common scenario involving delirium is iatrogenic. When a physician prescribes an additional medicine the combination results in the inhibition or induction of the metabolism of the preexisting AED or the new medicine. The number of potential adverse interactions is enormous. In one well-known example, adding valproate to lamotrigine increases lamotrigine concentrations, sometimes to toxic levels.

Nonconvulsive status epilepticus or absence status epilepticus may present with delirium. Because those seizure varieties may cause cognitive changes without overt physical abnormalities, a diagnosis based solely on clinical grounds without a corroborating EEG is unreliable.

When seizures lead to head trauma, patients may develop intracerebral or subdural hematomas that lead to acutely or permanently altered mental states. Of course, the reverse pathway also occurs: head trauma leads to seizures and epilepsy.

TREATMENT

AEDs

Neurologists routinely prescribe AEDs as the primary treatment for epilepsy (Table 10.2). They generally prefer AED monotherapy to polytherapy (polypharmacy) because it minimizes side effects, noncompliance, and cost. However, when epilepsy remains refractory to monotherapy, neurologists usually add a second AED. Nevertheless, only a minority of patients benefits from the addition of a second AED, and less than 5% benefit from the addition of a third one.

Neurologists typically refrain from instituting AED therapy following a first idiopathic seizure, which itself does not constitute epilepsy. In some circumstances, such as status epilepticus or other emergency situations, neurologists quickly initiate AED therapy, while in other settings, such as use of lamotrigine, which can produce Stevens–Johnson syndrome, the AED dose is titrated very slowly.

Paradoxically, AEDs can sometimes cause seizures. For example, carbamazepine and oxcarbazepine may induce hyponatremia severe enough to cause seizures. Also, AEDs at toxic levels may cause seizures.

AEDs and Hepatic Enzymes

Several "older" AEDs, particularly phenytoin, carbamazepine, and phenobarbital, induce cytochrome P450 hepatic enzymes that increase the metabolism of concurrently administered medicines. For example, phenytoin or carbamazepine – administered either as a mood stabilizer or AED – may increase the clearance and reduce the serum concentration of many benzodiazepines, typical and atypical antipsychotics, tricyclics, and SSRIs. This AED-induced change in metabolism is more than a pharmacologic observation. It often lowers the effectiveness of these psychotropics and allows the reemergence of anxiety, depression, or psychosis.

Likewise, phenytoin's enzyme-inducing effect reduces methadone activity. The reduction may be so great that administering phenytoin to a patient enrolled in a methadone program may precipitate narcotic withdrawal. (To prevent the withdrawal symptoms and noncompliance that would ensue from this interaction, physicians can increase the daily dose of methadone before prescribing an enzyme-inducing AED.)

Another example of enhanced metabolism of a medicine due to concomitant use of an enzyme-inducing AED is reduced efficacy of oral contraceptives. Women relying on oral contraceptives who begin taking these AEDs may conceive. In that case, as an added consequence, these AEDs potentially expose the fetus to teratogenic effects.

Moreover, because many AEDs themselves undergo hepatic metabolism, alcohol, erythromycin, and various psychotropics alter their metabolism. For example, if an individual with epilepsy that was well-controlled with carbamazepine were to begin erythromycin treatment, the serum concentration of carbamazepine might rise. If the carbamazepine concentration were to reach a toxic level, the patient likely would have ataxia, nystagmus, diplopia, or headache. Similarly, various antidepressants can increase the serum concentration of phenytoin or carbamazepine by interfering with hepatic metabolism.

In contrast, valproate *inhibits* the hepatic metabolic enzymes. Thus, valproate may reduce the clearance and increase the serum concentration of several concomitantly

TABLE 10.2	Commonly Used AEDs	
AED	Usual Daily Dose (mg)	Therapeutic Serum Concentration (μ/ml)*
Carbamazepine (Tegretol)†	600–1200	5–12
Divalproex (Depakote)	1500–2000	50–100
Ethosuximide (Zarontin)	2000	40–100
Gabapentin (Neurontin)	900–1800	
Lamotrigine (Lamictal)	100–500	
Levetiracetam (Keppra)	1500–3000	
Phenytoin (Dilantin)	300–400	10–20
Topiramate (Topamax)	400	

†To reach a steady state, five "half-lives" are required (e.g., carbamazepine 4–6 days; phenytoin 5–10 days; and valproate 3–6 days).

*Recommended concentrations vary and should be altered depending on the clinical situation. Often a "subtherapeutic level" is sufficient, and increasing the dose will create side effects without improving seizure control.

N.B.: These AEDs have mostly replaced phenobarbital and its closely related AED, primidone (Mysoline), both of which cause sedation, cognitive impairment, and depression. Also, barbiturates, particularly when used in children and adults with brain damage, may produce a "paradoxical reaction" of excitement and hyperactivity rather than sedation. On the other hand, most children with epilepsy and comorbid hyperactivity may safely use stimulants.

administered medicines. It increases the concentration, effect, and side effects of some benzodiazepines, tricyclics, SSRIs, and other AEDs, particularly lamotrigine.

The "newer" AEDs, particularly lamotrigine, topiramate, and levetiracetam, exert little or no effect on hepatic enzymes. These AEDs are cleared primarily or exclusively through the kidneys. Physicians should prescribe them at lower doses in patients with renal impairment.

Another major effect of the AEDs that induce cytochrome P450 hepatic enzymes – phenobarbital, carbamazepine, and especially phenytoin– is their tendency to reduce bone density and cause osteopenia (moderately decreased bone loss). This adverse effect occurs in men as well as women taking these AEDs, and partly explains their two- to seven-fold greater incidence of hip fracture.

In addition, although valproate does not induce these enzymes, it causes bone loss by acting on osteoblasts. The newer AEDs have little or no effect on bone.

Use of enzyme-inducing AEDs and valproate entails determining patients' liver function tests, serum concentrations of calcium and AEDs, and concomitantly administered medicines. For patients taking these AEDs, neurologists also often monitor their patients with bone density studies, and prescribe calcium and vitamin D and advise weight-bearing exercises.

Cognitive and Related Side Effects

AED-induced cognitive impairment develops most often following rapid introduction, high doses, elevated serum concentrations, and a regimen with more than one AED. Even at therapeutic levels, AEDs may decrease processing speed and impair attention as their first and most common adverse cognitive side effect. Toxic levels, in general, cause memory difficulties, intellectual dulling, and inattention. Some AEDs, particularly lamotrigine, levetiracetam, phenobarbital, and topiramate (in moderate to high doses), adversely affect cognition. Topiramate also impairs attention and word fluency.

In contrast, when physicians prescribe AEDs for conditions other than epilepsy, such as migraines, neuropathic pain, or psychiatric disorders, neuropsychologic side effects develop infrequently.

Sometimes AEDs lead to psychotic or depressive symptoms, exacerbation of pre-existing psychiatric disorders, and suicidality. For example, levetiracetam, topiramate, and zonisamide can cause psychotic symptoms. Almost the same group (levetiracetam, tiagabine, topiramate, and vigabatrin) causes depression and suicidal ideation (see earlier). In addition, AED-induced forced normalization may lead to psychiatric disturbances (see earlier).

Physical Side Effects

As with other classes of medications, AEDs as a group tend to cause particular side effects. For example, AEDs may cause a potentially fatal mucocutaneous allergic reaction, the *Stevens–Johnson syndrome*. This condition, which begins as a rash, consists of blisters on the mucous membranes around the mouth, eyes, and other areas of the skin. The blisters often weep and become confluent.

Disrupted skin and mucous membranes leak serum, fluid, and electrolytes. In severe cases, bacteria can invade the blood stream. Although almost any AED, even at a therapeutic level, can cause Stevens–Johnson syndrome, administration of carbamazepine to patients of Asian ancestry who carry the HLA-B 1502 allele is particularly apt to cause the disorder. Before prescribing carbamazepine to Asian patients, physicians should first test them for this allele; however, if they have been taking carbamazepine for longer than several months without this adverse reaction, their risk of subsequently developing it is low. Overly rapid introduction of lamotrigine not only causes a transient rash, it also increases the risk of Stevens–Johnson syndrome.

Similarly, most AEDs may cause hepatic abnormalities and bone marrow suppression. Several accelerate age-related osteoporosis and leave epilepsy patients with increased vulnerability to hip fractures from falls. Women older than 65 years, individuals confined to wheelchairs or bed, and those receiving little sunlight are particularly susceptible to osteoporosis.

As mentioned previously, individual AEDs may have drug-specific side effects. For example, valproate increases patients' weight; lamotrigine and levetiracetam have little effect on weight; and topiramate and zonisamide reduce weight – although not to the degree or with the safety required in a weight-loss program.

Phenytoin, carbamazepine, and other AED intoxications cause a well-known constellation of nystagmus, ataxia, and dysarthria. These signs, however, are not diagnostic of AED overtreatment. Alcohol intoxication or use of phencyclidine (PCP) may cause them. Fortunately, serum drug levels are readily available for many AEDs, as are serum and urine toxicological screening for a variety of other intoxicants.

Other drug-specific side effects are topiramate's occasionally causing acute glaucoma and calcium phosphate renal stones. These side effects may stem from its inhibition of carbonic anhydrase.

AEDs and Pregnancy

As previous discussed, several AEDs, through their effect on hepatic enzymes, increase the metabolism and thereby decrease the effectiveness of oral contraceptives. Other AEDs may interfere through different mechanisms. Frequently prescribed AEDs that decrease the effectiveness of oral contraceptives include phenytoin, carbamazepine, phenobarbital, and topiramate. In a related side effect, valproate induces polycystic ovarian syndrome, in which women develop one or more of the following: obesity, thinning of hair, hyperandrogenism, and polycystic ovaries.

Apart from the possibility of fetal exposure to AEDs, epilepsy itself carries a considerable teratogenic risk. For mothers with epilepsy, the rate of fetal malformations – exclusive of AED-induced malformations – is 4% to 8%. In comparison, the rate for nonepileptic mothers is lower – 2% to 4% – but still substantial. If only the father has epilepsy, an increased but lesser teratogenic risk is present.

Fetal exposure to AEDs increases the rate of malformations, some of which are devastating. The malformation rate is increased if the mother takes an AED during the first trimester, requires AED polypharmacy, or has a low serum folate level. No AED is risk-free and none exclusively induces a particular malformation. The Food and Drug Administration (FDA) has placed carbamazepine and valproate in Category D ("dangerous" because of evidence of human fetal risk), but lamotrigine, levetiracetam, oxcarbazepine, and topiramate in the somewhat safer Category C ("caution" because animal studies show adverse fetal effect).

Malformations associated with AEDs are probably induced during the first trimester when the CNS forms. The most serious – *meningomyelocele* and other *neural tube defects* (see Chapter 13) – have been closely, but not exclusively, associated with both carbamazepine (0.5%) and valproate (1%). In addition, AEDs increase the rate of cleft lip, cleft palate, and ventricular septal defect.

Less severe fetal malformations are likewise not exclusively associated with any specific AED. In particular, the *fetal hydantoin (phenytoin) syndrome*, which consists of craniofacial abnormalities and limb defects, is not peculiar to prenatal phenytoin therapy.

Notwithstanding the risks associated with taking AEDs, tonic-clonic seizures in a pregnant woman pose a substantial threat to both the mother and fetus. Several strategies may reduce AEDs' teratogenic potential. Physicians should review both prospective parents' family histories for congenital malformations, epilepsy, and other neurologic problems. If possible, physicians ideally should taper if not discontinue AEDs before conception through at least the first trimester. If patients must continue an AED, they should take a single AED as monotherapy, avoiding valproate, carbamazepine, and phenobarbital. Because serum AED concentrations tend to fall during pregnancy, physicians should frequently check blood levels.

Neonatologists, neurologists, and psychiatrists should be mindful that many AEDs cross into breast milk. Ethosuximide, lamotrigine, phenobarbital, and topiramate concentrations may reach therapeutic levels in breastfeeding neonates. However, aside from sleepiness, symptoms of toxicity rarely develop. In contrast, carbamazepine, phenytoin, and valproate are relatively safe in the postpartum period. An important consequence of transplacental transfer of medications occurs when pregnant women taking phenobarbital or opioids, including methadone, induce dependence in the fetus. During the first several postpartum days, unless neonatologists replace these medicines, the baby may experience withdrawal symptoms including seizures.

In addition, women – whether or not they are taking AEDs – should take folic acid or folate before conception and throughout the pregnancy, particularly to reduce the risk of neural tube defects. Physicians should avoid prescribing carbamazepine and valproate during this period because of their association with neural tube defects. Once pregnant, women should undergo a serum α-fetoprotein measurement, an ultrasound examination, and possibly other obstetrical tests to detect fetal neural tube defects.

Another potential problem is that some AEDs (including phenobarbital, primidone, phenytoin, and carbamazepine) deplete vitamin-K-dependent clotting factors. Because the resulting anticoagulant effect may lead to

intracerebral hemorrhage in the fetus, obstetricians administer vitamin K.

AEDs may also induce CNS and cognitive abnormalities later in life. For example, phenytoin therapy initiated before puberty may retard normal cerebellar growth. Also, carbamazepine, phenytoin, topiramate, and oxcarbazepine elevate the serum homocysteine level, which is a risk factor for strokes and heart attacks. Reports have linked valproate exposure in utero to decreased verbal intelligence and memory impairment as well as increased risk of autism.

Vagus Nerve Stimulation

Vagus nerve stimulation (VNS), a technique for reducing refractory seizures, consists of an implanted pacemaker-like device that stimulates the cervical portion of the left vagus nerve (cranial nerve X). VNS sends impulses upward along the vagus nerve's afferent fibers to synapse in the medulla's solitary nucleus, which projects to upper brainstem, hypothalamus, limbic system, and cortex (see Chapters 4 and 16). The vagus nerve seems the most appropriate conduit to the brain because it is readily accessible in its cervical portion, contains almost entirely afferent fibers but few pain-conveying ones, and carries, on the left side, few efferent cardiac fibers.

The VNS device regularly generates electric impulses, such as for 30 seconds every 5 minutes, which suppress seizures. In addition, when sensing an aura, the patient can activate the device and interrupt the seizure.

To a certain extent, VNS suppresses generalized and partial seizures in children and adults. Over 5 years, it reduces the mean seizure frequency by about 30%. In addition, VNS decreases AED requirements, but it does not eliminate them. Neurologists suggest the procedure in a patient who has failed trials of multiple oral AEDs and for whom surgery would be inappropriate. Although VNS remains a credible therapy, patients must continue at least one AED and surgical resection remains more effective than VNS for seizures emanating from a single focus. VNS also reduces depression and anxiety comorbid with epilepsy.

Despite its benefits, VNS causes expectable side effects. In its most prominent one, the electrical stimulation briefly impairs the vagus nerve's function. Thus, during activation, VNS often causes hoarseness and dyspnea.

A newer device is the responsive neurostimulator system (RNS), in which electrical leads are implanted in the brain near the seizure focus or foci. The stimulator delivers electrical stimulation as needed to prevent seizures. The FDA has approved this approach in patients with focal-onset seizures originating from one or two foci that are not controlled with oral AEDs.

In Europe, but not in the United States, deep brain stimulation (DBS) is approved for the treatment of epilepsy. In the United States it is approved for treatment of essential tremor, Parkinson disease, dystonia, and obsessive-compulsive disorder.

Brain Resection Surgery

Under the appropriate circumstances, surgical removal of a cortical seizure focus with or without a surrounding portion of the brain has risen to the level of standard treatment. Although most patients who undergo surgery must continue taking an AED, approximately two-thirds of them enjoy a significant reduction in their seizure frequency if not their complete cessation. The surgical success rate is greatest for seizures emanating from mesial temporal sclerosis.

Neurologists have warned that the goal of epilepsy surgery is not to prevent the brain from generating seizures, but to allow AEDs to suppress seizures. If only by reducing the need for multiple or high doses of AEDs, surgery also often improves cognitive function and reduces comorbid depression and anxiety experience. When surgery controls epilepsy, patients enjoy great neuropsychologic benefits. Overall, surgery improves most patients' quality of life.

With proper preoperative planning, surgeons can remove large areas of the temporal cortex and underlying hippocampus and amygdala unilaterally without producing either language or memory impairment. Even with extensive resections, the surgical morbidity and mortality remain very low.

If epilepsy patients undergo three trials of appropriate AEDs at therapeutic doses that fail to suppress seizures, neurologists consider their epilepsy to be refractory. Children, adolescents, and adults who suffer from refractory epilepsy become candidates for surgery. For many refractory epilepsy patients with focal seizures associated with dyscognition, surgery offers unequivocal advantages over prolonged AED therapy even if it suppresses seizures.

Another surgical requirement for patients with refractory seizures is a single frontal or temporal lobe lesion clearly identifiable on clinical, EEG, and radiographic testing. In addition, if the lesion is located in their dominant hemisphere, patients often must also undergo a Wada test, functional MRI, or similar testing to avoid removal of a portion of the cerebral cortex that would lead to aphasia, amnesia, or other neuropsychologic problems (see Chapter 8). If both temporal lobes were injured from birth or during surgery, patients undergoing even a unilateral temporal lobectomy may suffer permanent amnesia or the Klüver–Bucy syndrome (see Chapters 12 and 16).

Despite the substantial benefits that epilepsy surgery offers, patients risk several postoperative complications. During the first two postoperative months, many patients experience depression, mania, and personality changes. The depression persists well beyond the postoperative period in about 10% of patients. It occasionally complicates surgery that completely eliminates seizures as well as less successful surgery. The depression's origin remains speculative. Some investigators attribute it to the discontinuation of AEDs that had been suppressing psychiatric symptoms as well as seizures, or the sudden complete seizure control causing forced normalization (see above). Also, loss of ECT-like effects of seizures may play a role. Psychologically oriented investigators note that the "cure" of patients' chronic illness deprives them of their family's attention and ability or "excuse" to avoid various obligations.

A different and more invasive procedure may rarely be indicated in individuals with intractable bilateral frontal seizures or infants with atonic seizures ("drop attacks") who have no readily resectable seizure focus. In a *commissurotomy* or *corpus callosotomy*, a neurosurgeon longitudinally severs the anterior two-thirds or entire corpus callosum, interrupting the spread of discharges between cerebral hemispheres. Because it "splits" apart the cerebral hemispheres, this procedure may cause the *split-brain syndrome* (see Fig. 8.9).

GENERALIZED SEIZURES

Immediate loss of consciousness accompanied by bilateral, symmetric, synchronous, paroxysmal EEG discharges characterizes generalized seizures. These seizures may result from an autosomal dominant genetic disorder, a physiologic disturbance, or a metabolic aberration, including drug and alcohol withdrawal. In contrast to focal seizures, generalized seizures lack lateralized motor or sensory disturbances and focal EEG abnormalities. Also, seizures that are generalized at onset, as opposed to focal-onset seizures that evolve to bilateral convulsions, almost never result from brain tumors, cerebral infarctions, or other structural lesions. Most generalized seizures are of either the absence (previously called *petit mal*) or tonic-clonic (*grand mal*) variety.

Absence Seizures

Absence seizures usually begin between ages 4 and 10 years and disappear in early adulthood. The seizures, which may occur many times daily, consist of 2- to 10-second lapses in attention often accompanied by automatisms, subtle clonic limb movements, or blinking (Fig. 10.11). The blinking sometimes occurs rhythmically at 3 Hz, which is the frequency of the associated EEG abnormality. During the seizure, children maintain muscle tone and bladder control; however, they cannot

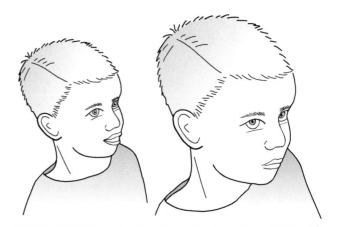

FIGURE 10.11 ■ Seen in the midst of an absence seizure, this 8-year-old boy has staring that has suddenly and unexpectedly interrupted his playing with a friend. He has become glassy-eyed and mute, his eyes have rolled upward, and he blinks at 3 Hz. Although he has lost consciousness, he maintains bodily tone and does not become incontinent. At the end of his seizure, which will last for only 2 to 10 seconds, he will resume playing and be unaware of the pause.

carry on mental and physical activities. If they suffer from frequent seizures, children may appear inattentive, dull, or even mentally retarded. After a seizure, as though it had never occurred, children have no retrograde amnesia, confusion, agitation, or sleepiness.

Absence status epilepticus typically leads to a several-hour episode of apathy, psychomotor retardation, and confusion. Such an attack usually develops in children or young adults with a history of absence or other seizures who suddenly stop taking their AEDs. Absence status epilepticus in any age group mimics acute psychosis. If an EEG confirms a clinical diagnosis of absence status epilepticus, intravenous administration of a benzodiazepine will usually abort it.

EEG, Etiology, and Treatment

During an absence seizure, the EEG shows synchronous 3-Hz spike-and-wave complexes in all channels (Fig. 10.12). Even in the interictal period, an EEG reveals occasional asymptomatic bursts of 3-Hz spike-and-wave complexes lasting 1 to 1.5 seconds. This discharge reflects an underlying abnormality in the reciprocal circuits between the thalamus and the cerebral cortex.

In patients with absence, either hyperventilation or photic stimulation can precipitate the characteristic clinical and EEG abnormalities. Just as the EEG abnormality reflects generalized cerebral dysfunction, PET scans performed during absence seizures show increased metabolism in the thalamus and the entire cortex.

Patients' relatives often also have absence seizures or 3-Hz spike-and-wave complexes that can be precipitated by hyperventilation. This finding supports the hypothesis that patients inherit a predisposition in an autosomal dominant pattern. In contrast to tonic-clonic seizures,

absence seizures are not associated with drug withdrawal, metabolic aberrations, or structural lesions. Therefore, as a general rule, CTs and MRIs are not indicated in evaluating children with absence seizures.

Neurologists usually prescribe ethosuximide for absence seizures in children. About two-thirds of them enjoy a permanent remission during adolescence. In the others, tonic-clonic seizures frequently replace absence seizures.

Although absence seizures bear a superficial resemblance to focal seizures with altered awareness, physicians should distinguish the two conditions by their different manifestations, EEG abnormalities, prognoses, and treatments (Table 10.3).

Tonic-Clonic Seizures

Even though they are both varieties of generalized seizures and share, at their onset, the characteristic loss of consciousness and generalized EEG abnormalities, tonic-clonic and absence seizures have completely different clinical manifestations, treatment, and prognosis. Tonic-clonic seizures begin at any age after infancy, persist through adult life, and cause massive motor activity and profound postictal residua. Although patients may have a prodrome of malaise or a depressed mood, tonic-clonic seizures usually arise as an unheralded event. In the initial tonic phase, patients lose consciousness, roll their eyes upward, and, as if to form a back-bending arch, extend their neck, trunk, and limbs. Immediately afterwards, in a dramatic clonic phase, patients violently and rhythmically jerk their limbs, neck, and trunk (Fig. 10.13).

It can be difficult to differentiate a primary generalized tonic-clonic seizure from a focal-onset seizure that has quickly undergone secondary generalization. Often an

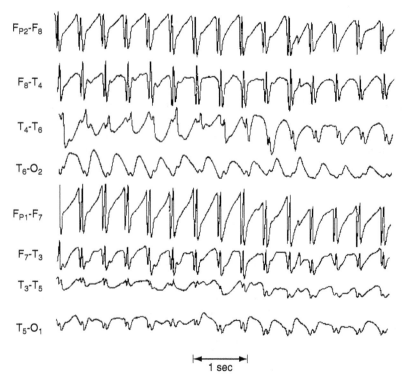

F_{P2}-F_8

F_8-T_4

T_4-T_6

T_6-O_2

F_{P1}-F_7

F_7-T_3

T_3-T_5

T_5-O_1

1 sec

FIGURE 10.12 ■ Absence seizures are often so brief and liable to be confused with either inattention or focal seizures that neurologists often attempt to precipitate them for diagnostic purposes in an EEG laboratory. One common practice consists of asking a child to count numbers slowly while hyperventilating. An absence seizure would be evident when the counting pauses and the EEG shows regular, symmetric, and synchronous 3-Hz spike-and-wave complexes arising from and returning to a normal EEG background.

TABLE 10.3 **Comparison of Focal Seizures With Altered Consciousness and Absence Seizures**

Feature	Focal Seizure With Altered Consciousness	Absence
Aura	Often	Never
Consciousness	Impaired	Lost at onset
Movements	Usually simple, repetitive but may include complex	Blinking and facial and finger automatism activity
Postictal behavior	Amnesia, confusion, and tendency to sleep	No abnormality, except amnesia for ictus
Frequency	1–2 per week	Several daily
Duration	2–3 minutes	1–10 seconds
Precipitants		Hyperventilation, photic stimulation
EEG	Spikes and poly spike and waves, usually over one or both temporal regions	Generalized 3-Hz spike-and-wave complexes
Treatment	Carbamazepine, phenytoin	Ethosuximide, valproate

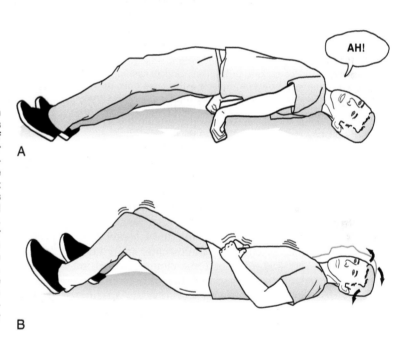

FIGURE 10.13 ■ *A*, This man in the tonic phase of a tonic-clonic seizure arches his torso and extends his arms and legs. He assumes this position because of the relatively greater strength of the extensor muscles compared to the flexor muscles. Simultaneous diaphragm, chest wall, and laryngeal muscle contractions force air through his tightened larynx to produce the shrill "epileptic cry." During this phase, he may also bite his tongue and lose control of his urine. *B*, In the clonic phase, his head, neck, and legs contract symmetrically and forcefully for about 10–20 seconds. Saliva, aerated and often blood-tinged from tongue lacerations, froths from his mouth. His pupils dilate and he sweats profusely. Finally, his muscular contractions lose strength. The seizure usually ends with stertorous breathing. In the immediate postictal period, he remains unresponsive. Before regaining consciousness, he may pass through a state of confusion and agitation.

intraictal EEG can help distinguish between them, but in some cases the secondary generalization can be so rapid that even the EEG is misleading.

If electronic filters could eliminate the superimposed muscle electric artifact during the tonic phase, the EEG would show repetitive, increasingly higher-amplitude spikes occurring with increasing frequency in all channels. Then, in the clonic phase, slow waves would interrupt the spikes, which usually decrease in frequency (Fig. 10.14).

After the clonic phase, the EEG shows postictal depression. The postictal EEG is often the only one available, but it can support the diagnosis. Similarly, after ECT, EEG activity slows. After most tonic-clonic or ECT-induced seizures, as well as after approximately 40% of focal seizures, the serum prolactin concentration rises for 10 to 20 minutes. Importantly, absence of prolactin elevation after an apparent tonic-clonic seizure casts doubt on its having been an epileptic event.

About 50% of patients with tonic-clonic seizures have interictal asymptomatic brief bursts of spikes, polyspikes, or slow waves on the EEG. Photic stimulation or hyperventilation may precipitate seizures and accompanying EEG abnormalities.

Etiology

Many cases of tonic-clonic epilepsy result from an autosomal dominant trait expressed between the ages of 5 and 30 years. Patients often have a history of childhood absence. Various factors, such as sleep deprivation, can precipitate these seizures in susceptible individuals. Medical house officers who have worked all night are susceptible to tonic-clonic seizures the following day.

Most seizures arising in sleep emerge during nonrapid eye movement (NREM) sleep (see Chapter 17). Rapid eye movement (REM) sleep, in contrast, remains relatively seizure-free. Some epileptic patients have seizures

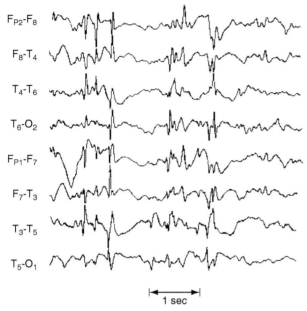

FIGURE 10.14 ■ During a tonic-clonic seizure, the EEG ideally shows paroxysms of spikes, polyspikes, and occasional slow waves in all channels; however, muscle artifact can obscure this pattern. Even during interictal periods, the EEG contains multiple bursts of generalized spikes in the background. In contrast to occasional temporal lobe spikes, this pattern confirms a diagnosis of epilepsy in patients with seizures.

predominantly or exclusively during sleep, and others experience them only on awakening. To avoid committing a diagnostic error, physicians should evaluate patients with exclusively sleep-related episodes for a sleep disorder masquerading as epilepsy (see later and Chapter 17).

A small number of children, adolescents, and adults have *reflex epilepsy* – absence or tonic-clonic seizures in response to particular sensory stimuli. In its most common form, *photosensitive* or *photoconvulsive epilepsy*, specific visual stimuli such as discotheque strobe lights, flickering television pictures, televised cartoons, or video games trigger seizures in susceptible individuals. Even stationary patterns of certain letters, words, or figures may trigger seizures. Likewise, particular musical passages may trigger seizures.

Treatment

As in their initial treatment of other seizures, neurologists attempt to suppress tonic-clonic seizures with monotherapy. Several older and newer AEDs have an indication for treatment of primary seizures.

Febrile Seizures

Febrile seizures, occurring at least once in 2% to 4% of all children, are the most common variety of childhood seizure. These seizures usually last less than 30 seconds and lack focal findings. Older literature suggested that febrile seizures often cause mesial temporal sclerosis, which in turn would lead to epilepsy. Recent studies demonstrate that children experiencing brief febrile seizures have little or no increased risk of developing epilepsy, but

having prolonged febrile seizures does constitute a risk factor for epilepsy.

In the past, pediatricians and neurologists, would routinely prescribe prophylactic phenobarbital or valproic acid for febrile seizures. However, those and other AEDs not only provided little protection, they impaired cognitive function and produced hyperactivity. Today, physicians sometimes recommend oral or rectal diazepam to be taken when fevers develop to prevent febrile seizures.

Landau–Kleffner Syndrome

A rare condition, Landau–Kleffner syndrome (LKS) is an epileptic encephalopathy causing aphasia and behavioral disturbances in children. Children tend to develop normally for the first years of life, after which their cognition (especially expressive and receptive language function) deteriorates, and many exhibit autistic features. Most patients have seizures, which can be focal, absence, or tonic-clonic. EEG during slow-wave sleep shows continuous or nearly continuous spike-and-wave discharges. Neurologists consider LKS among the neurologic causes of symptoms of autism spectrum disorder (see Chapter 13). Early management with AEDs, including possibly high-dose steroids, may reverse the regression in some patients.

NONEPILEPTIC CONDITIONS

Psychogenic Nonepileptic Seizures

"Psychogenic nonepileptic seizures" (PNES) is the currently preferred term for events formerly labeled with the terms "pseudoseizures" or "nonepileptic attacks." Under the DSM-5, psychiatrists would probably diagnose most patients with PNES as having a Conversion Disorder (Functional Neurologic Symptom Disorder) or simply a Factitious Disorder.

PNES occur 5% to 10% as frequently as epileptic seizures, most commonly in females aged 19 to 35 years, relatives of patients with epilepsy, and individuals reporting a history of abuse. On several occasions, a group of individuals – particularly families, classmates, or friends, especially female adolescents – has simultaneously or in succession developed seizure-like episodes. The neurologic literature terms small epidemics of seizure-like episodes or similar disturbances "mass hysteria" or "mass psychogenic illness."

As with epileptic seizures, PNES tend to be stereotyped for the individual. The most important difference is that, despite the apparent generalized nature of PNES, patients retain consciousness throughout them. Also, patients with PNES often demonstrate slow development of limb movements without a preceding tonic period. Once the nonepileptic seizure starts, patients frequently rock their head side-to-side or thrust their pelvis up and down. They forcefully close their eyes and, if medical personnel place them on their side, as if to prevent aspiration, they look downward. They will even look downward if rocked side-to-side. When patients speak, they often stutter or stammer.

Sometimes, as in epileptic seizures, PNES patients bite their lip or tip of their tongue, urinate on themselves, or bang their head or limbs. As fatigue ensues, the movements decline in intensity and regularity, but often resume after rest. The duration of PNES – typically 2 to 5 minutes – exceeds that of the average epileptic seizure. Studies have shown that patients bringing along a stuffed animal, particularly a teddy bear, to their continuous EEG-video monitoring, is a positive predictive indicator for PNES.

Unless they deliberately feign postictal confusion, PNES patients recover their attentiveness and motor function immediately after the cessation of the movements. Most patients have no lingering confusion, headache, retrograde amnesia, or hemiparesis. In short, postictal symptoms do not follow most PNES.

During a PNES, EEGs would ideally be normal, but muscle movement artifact obscures the recording. An EEG after the episode, which is more feasible, would lack the usual postictal depression. Also, unlike following an epileptic seizure, the serum prolactin concentration remains normal.

If routine testing fails to provide a diagnosis, continuous EEG-video monitoring usually can differentiate PNES from epileptic seizures. The portion of the monitoring obtained during sleep is especially important because epileptic seizures – but not nonepileptic ones – often arise from genuine sleep.

PNES can be quite convincing. They can include urination, tongue biting, and, in as many as 20% of cases, deliberate or inadvertent self-injury. Applying only clinical criteria, the distinction between psychogenic nonepileptic and epileptic seizures in most studies is no more than 80% to 90% accurate.

One pitfall arises because patients with PNES also can have epileptic seizures. Although only 5% to 10% of adult patients with PNES have comorbid epileptic seizures, 25% to 40% of children with PNES have comorbid epileptic seizures. In patients with both types of seizures, the psychogenic seizures so closely mimic the epileptic seizures that physicians must perform continuous EEG-video monitoring to distinguish them. The combination of psychogenic nonepileptic and epileptic seizures may occasionally explain "refractory epilepsy." Another pitfall is that some seizures (e.g., frontal lobe seizures) produce such bizarre behavior that neurologists might summarily decide that the patient has a psychiatric condition.

Compared to patients with only epileptic seizures, those with PNES, whether or not they also have epileptic ones, fare poorly. Although psychiatric intervention often helps patients with many different psychogenic neurologic symptoms, such as psychogenic hemiparesis, it provides little benefit to those with psychogenic seizures. PNES are usually refractory to psychotherapy, psychotropics, and AEDs. Potentially helpful approaches include cognitive-behavioral therapy and treatment directed at psychiatric comorbidities, such as depression, rather than the seizures themselves. In general, psychogenic nonepileptic seizure patients remain at least partially dependent on caregivers and their quality of life ratings are especially low. They remain as disabled as if they had epilepsy.

Risk factors for persistent PNES have been TBI, anxiety, depression, receiving Social Security payments, and female gender.

Intermittent Explosive Disorder

The condition listed in DSM-5 as Intermittent Explosive Disorder usually consists of violently aggressive, primitive outbursts, including screaming, punching, wrestling, and throwing objects that injure people or destroy property. Minor stimuli, such as verbal threats, anger, or frustration, especially after consuming even small amounts of alcohol, often trigger episodes (although if alcohol "fully accounts" for the episodes, the DSM-5 would not label them as Intermittent Explosive Disorder). A highly charged affect often precedes and accompanies the outburst. After it, patients typically claim justification, regret, or amnesia for the event.

In contrast to violent focal seizures (see before), which are rare, episodic dyscontrol episodes are nonstereotyped, at least momentarily purposeful, and highly emotional. Furthermore, the episodes have a clearly directed and aggressive intent. They occur predominantly in young men who have congenital malformations or TBI, borderline intelligence, and minor physical neurologic abnormalities. Many have interictal EEG abnormalities. Although the neurologic community does not equate episodes of episodic dyscontrol syndrome with seizures, physicians generally agree with the use of AEDs as mood stabilizers.

RELATED ISSUES

Driving

The motor vehicle crash rate of epilepsy patients compared with the general population is seven-fold greater. Not only might they have seizures while driving, the AEDs can make them sleepy enough to cause traffic accidents. Epilepsy patients also have increased rates of traffic violations, including driving under the influence of alcohol or drugs. As in the general population, automobile accidents are most closely associated with male drivers younger than 25 years.

Almost all states require a waiting period for a driving license or renewal after having a seizure, but modifications are sometimes allowed for seizures provoked by an isolated medical illness, such as hypoglycemia. Most states set a waiting period of 3 to 12 months, but several, including New York and California, allow some flexibility for noncommercial driving. They also require applicants to reveal any history of seizures or loss of consciousness (for any reason). In addition, several states require physicians to report drivers with seizures ("mandatory physician reporting").

Driving is not the only activity to represent a potential hazard to the epilepsy patient. Drowning is probably the most common cause of accidental death. In addition, during a seizure, patients sometimes sustain nonlethal injuries, such as head trauma, limb dislocations, lacerations, and ocular injuries.

Alcohol

Drinking alcoholic beverages in moderation should not give rise to seizures in epileptic patients, but consuming larger amounts of alcohol has been linked to greater risk of epilepsy. Acute or chronic ethanol intoxication, as well as alcohol withdrawal, can give rise to seizures via a number of mechanisms, such as modulating NMDA and GABA receptors, increasing excitotoxic compounds, altering electrolyte concentrations, and leading to multiple head traumas and cerebral hemorrhages.

AEDs generally do not prevent seizures that arise from alcohol abuse or withdrawal. In addition, alcohol can induce liver enzymes, thereby reducing AED levels. Also, alcohol can potentiate many of the side effects of AEDs. For these reasons, AEDs are usually not useful for prevention of alcohol-related seizures. When they occur, first-line treatment should be with a benzodiazepine, an effective GABA agonist. In an alcoholic patient with seizures not felt to be provoked by alcohol, use of an AED with minimal hepatic effects (such as levetiracetam, lamotrigine, or topiramate) can be considered.

Cerebrovascular Disease

TIAs resemble focal seizures because both may cause momentarily impaired consciousness and physical abnormalities (see Chapter 11). In general, however, TIAs have slower onset and rarely cause loss of consciousness.

Of the various cerebrovascular disturbances, *transient global amnesia* (*TGA*) most closely resembles a focal seizure with impaired awareness (see Chapter 7). During a TGA episode, a frequent cause of transient amnesia (see Box 7.2), patients cannot learn new information, such as the date, location, and examining physicians; however, they retain basic memories, such as their name, address, and telephone number. This discrepancy separates TGA from psychogenic amnesia, in which basic as well as new information is lost.

During TGA, EEGs may show spikes, but not paroxysmal bursts, typically emanating from the left hemisphere. MRI may show unilateral or bilateral hippocampal abnormalities indicative of ischemia, and SPECT can show reduced blood flow to one or both mesial temporal lobes. Because physicians rarely obtain diagnostic testing during the amnestic episode, they rely upon the clinical history to diagnose TGA, although with some uncertainty.

Migraines, which also partly result from vascular disturbance, may induce episodes of confusion and personality change followed by a tendency to sleep (see Chapter 9). Migraines particularly mimic seizures when they lead to transient hemiparesis and abnormal EEGs. In fact, migraine patients have a greater than usual incidence of seizures, making migraines a risk factor for epilepsy. The diagnosis of migraine relies almost entirely on the patient's history.

Sleep Disorders

Bizarre behavior during the night might represent a sleep disorder (see Chapter 17) rather than a nocturnal seizure. Some sleep disorders so closely mimic seizures that only polysomnography or continuous EEG-video monitoring can distinguish them. For example, children might have *night terrors* or another *parasomnia*, and older adults are liable to develop *REM sleep behavior disorder*. Narcolepsy can include several seizure-like features, such as momentary loss of body tone (cataplexy) and dream-like hallucinations. Unlike seizures, cataplexy has no premonitory aura, motor activity, incontinence, or subsequent symptoms. Moreover, during attacks of cataplexy, an EEG shows normal activity.

Metabolic Aberrations

Of the various metabolic aberrations that can mimic seizures, reactions to medicines are probably the most common. Many medicines, including some administered as eyedrops, produce transient mental and physical alterations; however, they almost never induce stereotyped movements or thoughts.

Hyperventilation commonly induces giddiness, confusion, and other psychologic symptoms that can be confused with seizures (see Chapter 3). When prolonged and deep, hyperventilation may precipitate seizures, but probably only in epileptic individuals.

Hypoglycemia, which can result from use of insulin or oral hypoglycemic agents, alcohol intoxication, or skipping meals, can induce anxiety and seizure-like symptoms. Similar disturbances can occur with excessive intake of stimulants such as coffee. Although the severity and frequency of these symptoms are probably overestimated, small frequent meals and reduction of caffeine consumption should remedy most cases.

Sudden Unexplained Death in Epilepsy

Neurologists define sudden unexplained death in epilepsy (SUDEP) as "sudden, unexpected, witnessed or unwitnessed, nontraumatic, and nondrowning death in epilepsy, with or without evidence for a seizure and excluding documented status epilepticus, in which postmortem examination does not show a toxicological or anatomical cause for death." Although SUDEP represents a significant mortality cause – up to 17% in one study – in this population, neurologists have a poor understanding of its mechanism. Potential factors include cardiac arrhythmia, postictal cardiomyopathy, autonomic abnormalities, and respiratory failure related to seizure activity. Risk factors for SUDEP include male gender, young age at onset and longer duration of epilepsy, frequent convulsive seizures, and use of multiple AEDs.

REFERENCES

AEDs

Andersohn, F., Schade, R., Willich, S. N., et al. (2010). Use of antiepileptic drugs in epilepsy and the risk of self-harm or suicidal behavior. *Neurology, 75*, 335–340.

Arana, A., Wentworth, C. E., Ayuso-Mateos, J. L., et al. (2010). Suicide-related events in patients treated with antiepileptic drugs. *The New England Journal of Medicine, 363*, 542–551.

Chong, D. J., & Bazil, C. W. (2010). Update on anticonvulsant drugs. *Current Neurology and Neuroscience Reports, 10*, 308–318.

Christensen, J., Gronberg, T. K., Sorensen, M. J., et al. (2013). Prenatal valproate exposure and risk of autism spectrum disorders and childhood autism. *JAMA: The Journal of the American Medical Association, 309*, 1696–1703.

Jentink, J., Loane, M. A., Dolk, H., et al. (2010). Valproic acid monotherapy in pregnancy and major congenital malformations. *The New England Journal of Medicine, 362*, 2185–2193.

Pack, A. M., Morrell, M. J., Randall, A., et al. (2008). Bone health in young women with epilepsy after one year of antiepileptic drug monotherapy. *Neurology, 70*, 1586–1593.

Patorno, E., Bohn, R. L., Wahl, P. M., et al. (2010). Anticonvulsant medications and the risk of suicide, attempted suicide, or violent death. *JAMA: The Journal of the American Medical Association, 303*, 1401–1409.

Perucca, P., Carter, J., Vahle, V., et al. (2009). Adverse antiepileptic drug effects: Towards a clinically and neurobiologically relevant taxonomy. *Neurology, 72*, 1223–1229.

Salinsky, M. C., Storzbach, D., Spencer, D. C., et al. (2005). Effects of topiramate and gabapentin on cognitive abilities in healthy volunteers. *Neurology, 64*, 792–798.

Shallcross, R., Bromley, R. L., Cheyne, C. P., et al. (2014). In utero exposure to levetiracetam vs valproate: Development and language at 3 years of age. *Neurology, 82*, 213–221.

Surgery

Devinsky, O., Barr, W. B., Vickrey, B. G., et al. (2005). Changes in depression and anxiety after resective surgery for epilepsy. *Neurology, 65*, 1744–1749.

Hemb, M., Velasco, T. R., Parnes, M. S., et al. (2010). Improved outcomes in pediatric epilepsy surgery: The UCLA experience, 1986-2008. *Neurology, 74*, 1768–1775.

Langfitt, J. T., Westerveld, M., Hamberger, M. J., et al. (2007). Worsening of quality of life after epilepsy surgery: Effect of seizures and memory decline. *Neurology, 68*, 1988–1994.

Roswall, L. A., Engman, E., Samuelsson, H., et al. (2010). Cognitive outcome 10 years after temporal lobe epilepsy surgery. *Neurology, 74*, 1977–1985.

Vagus Nerve Stimulation

Morris, G. L., Gloss, D., Buchhalter, J., et al. (2013). Evidence-based guideline update: Vagus nerve stimulation for the treatment of epilepsy: Report of the Guideline Development Subcommittee of the American Academy of Neurology. *Neurology, 81*, 1453–1459.

Interictal Comorbidities and Their Treatment

Bacon, D., Fisher, R. S., Morris, J. C., et al. (2007). American Academy of Neurology position statement on physician reporting of medical conditions that may affect driving competence. *Neurology, 68*, 1174–1177.

Bear, D. M., & Fedio, P. (1977). Quantitative analysis of interictal behavior in temporal lobe epilepsy. *Archives of Neurology, 34*, 454–467.

Devinsky, O. (2008). Postictal psychosis: Common, dangerous, and treatable. *Epilepsy Currents, 8*, 31–34.

Ettinger, A. B., & Kanner, A. M. (Eds.), (2007). *Psychiatric Issues in Epilepsy* (2nd ed.). Philadelphia: Lippincott Williams & Wilkins.

Fiest, K. M., Dykeman, J., Patten, S. B., et al. (2013). Depression in epilepsy: A systematic review and meta-analysis. *Neurology, 80*, 590–599.

Gross, A., Devinsky, O., Westbrook, L. E., et al. (2000). Psychotropic medication use in patients with epilepsy: Effect on seizure frequency. *The Journal of Neuropsychiatry and Clinical Neurosciences, 12*, 4.

Hermann, B. P., Seidenberg, M., Dow, C., et al. (2006). Cognitive prognosis in chronic temporal lobe epilepsy. *Annals of Neurology, 60*, 80–87.

Irwin, L. G., & Fortune, D. G. (2014). Risk factors for psychosis secondary to temporal lobe epilepsy: A systematic review. *The Journal of Neuropsychiatry and Clinical Neurosciences, 26*, 5–23.

Krauss, G. L., Ampaw, L., & Krumholz, A. (2001). Individual state driving restrictions for people with epilepsy in the US. *Neurology, 57*, 1780–1785.

Lee, K. C., Finley, P. R., & Alldredge, B. K. (2003). Risk of seizures associated with psychotropic medications: Emphasis on new drugs and new findings. *Expert Opinion on Drug Safety, 2*, 233–247.

Schachter, S. C. (Ed.), (2003). *Visions: Artists Living With Epilepsy*. Elsevier.

Pillmann, F., Rohde, A., Ullrich, A., et al. (1999). Violence, criminal behavior, and the EEG. *The Journal of Neuropsychiatry and Clinical Neurosciences, 11*, 454–457.

Tellez-Zenteno, J. F., Patten, S. B., Jette, N., et al. (2007). Psychiatric comorbidity in epilepsy: A population-based analysis. *Epilepsia, 48*, 2336–2344.

Tracy, J. I., Dechant, V., Sperling, M. R., et al. (2007). The association of mood with quality of life ratings in epilepsy. *Neurology, 68*, 1101–1107.

Tremont, G., Smith, M. M., Bauer, L., et al. (2012). Comparison of personality characteristics on the Bear-Fedio Inventory between patients with epilepsy and those with non-epileptic seizures. *The Journal of Neuropsychiatry and Clinical Neurosciences, 24*, 47–52.

Whitman, S., Coleman, T. E., Patmon, C., et al. (1984). Epilepsy in prison: Elevated prevalence and no relationship to violence. *Neurology, 34*, 775–782.

Psychogenic Nonepileptic Seizures

Benbadis, S., Agrawal, V., & Tatum, W. O. (2001). How many patients with psychogenic nonepileptic seizures also have epilepsy. *Neurology, 57*, 915–917.

Brigo, F., Igwe, S. C., Ausserer, H., et al. (2015). Terminology of psychogenic nonepileptic seizures. *Epilepsia, 56*, e21–e25.

Goldstein, L. H., Chalder, T., Chigwedere, C., et al. (2010). Cognitive-behavioral therapy for psychogenic nonepileptic seizures. *Neurology, 74*, 1986–1994.

McKenzie, P., Oto, M., Russell, A., et al. (2010). Early outcomes and predictors in 260 patients with psychogenic nonepileptic attacks. *Neurology, 74*, 64–69.

Marchetti, R. L., Kurcgant, D., Neto, J. G., et al. (2008). Psychiatric diagnoses of patients with psychogenic nonepileptic seizures. *Seizure: The Journal of the British Epilepsy Association, 16*, 247–253.

Martin, R., Burneo, J. G., Prasad, A., et al. (2003). Frequency of epilepsy in patients with psychogenic seizures monitored by video-EEG. *Neurology, 61*, 1791–1792.

Prasad, A., Mendez, M., & Kuzniecky, R. I. (2003). Teddy bears: An observational finding in patients with non-epileptic events. *Neurology, 61*, 714–715.

Szaflarski, J. P., Hughes, C., Szaflarski, M., et al. (2003). Quality of life in psychogenic nonepileptic seizures. *Epilepsia, 44*, 236–242.

Seizures and Epilepsy

Berg, A. T., & Millichap, J. J. (2013). The 2010 Revised Classification of Seizures and Epilepsy. *CONTINUUM: Lifelong Learning in Neurology, 19*, 571–597.

Berg, A. T., Berkovic, S. F., Brodie, M. J., et al. (2010). Revised terminology and concepts for organization of seizures and epilepsies: Report of the ILAE Commission on Classification and Terminology, 2005–2009. *Epilepsia, 51*, 676–685.

Boro, A., & Haut, S. (2003). Medical comorbidities in the treatment of epilepsy. *Epilepsy and Behavior: E&B, 4*, S2–S12.

Camfield, C. S., & Camfield, P. R. (2014). Rolandic epilepsy has little effect on adult life 30 years later: A population-based study. *Neurology, 82*, 1162–1166.

Caraballo, R. H., Cejas, N., Chamorro, N., et al. (2014). Landau-Kleffner syndrome: A study of 29 patients. *Seizure: The Journal of the British Epilepsy Association, 23*, 98–104.

Chang, B. S., & Lowenstein, D. H. (2003). Epilepsy. *The New England Journal of Medicine, 349*, 1257–1266.

Crompton, D. E., & Berkovic, S. F. (2009). The borderland of epilepsy: Clinical and molecular features of phenomena that mimic epileptic seizures. *The Lancet. Neurology, 370*, 370–381.

Hara, H. (2007). Autism and epilepsy: A retrospective follow-up study. *Brain and Development, 29*, 486–490.

Haut, S. R., Hall, C. B., Masur, J., et al. (2007). Seizure occurrence: Precipitants and prediction. *Neurology, 69*, 1905–1910.

Kwon, Y., Yang, Y., Jang, J.-W., et al. (2014). Left dominance of EEG abnormalities in patients with transient global amnesia. *Seizure: The Journal of the British Epilepsy Association, 23*, 825–829.

Leach, J. P., Mohanraj, R., & Borland, W. (2012). Alcohol and drugs in epilepsy: Pathophysiology, presentation, possibilities, and prevention. *Epilepsia, 53*, 48–57.

Mula, M., Jauch, R., Cavanna, A., et al. (2008). Clinical and psychological definition of the interictal dysphoric disorder of epilepsy. *Epilepsia, 49*, 650–656.

Samokhvalov, A. V., Irving, H., Mohapatra, S., et al. (2010). Alcohol consumption, unprovoked seizures, and epilepsy: A systematic review and meta-analysis. *Epilepsia, 51*, 1177–1184.

Surges, R., & Sander, J. W. (2012). Sudden unexpected death in epilepsy: mechanisms, prevalence, and prevention. *Current Opinion in Neurology, 25,* 201–207.

Ye, B. S., Cho, Y.-J., Jan, S. H., et al. (2012). The localizing and lateralizing value of auras in lesional partial epilepsy patients. *Yonsei Medical Journal, 53,* 477–485.

Yerby, M. S., Kaplan, P., & Tran, T. (2004). Risks and management of pregnancy in women with epilepsy. *Cleveland Clinic Journal of Medicine, 71*(Suppl. 2), S25–S37.

Testing

Coburn, K. L., Lauterbach, E. C., Boutros, N. N., et al. (2006). The value of quantitative electroencephalography in clinical psychiatry: A report by the Committee on Research of the American Neuropsychiatric Association. *The Journal of Neuropsychiatry and Clinical Neurosciences, 18,* 460–500.

Kim, S., & Mountz, J. M. (2011). SPECT imaging of epilepsy: An overview and comparison with F-18 FDG PET. *International Journal of Molecular Imaging, 2011,* 1–9.

Therapeutics and Technology Assessment Subcommittee of the American Academy of Neurology. (1997). Assessment of digital EEG, quantitative EEG, and EEG brain mapping. *Neurology, 49,* 277–292.

Therapeutics and Technology Assessment Subcommittee of the American Academy of Neurology. (1992). Assessment: Magnetoencephalography (MEG). *Neurology, 42,* 1–4.

QUESTIONS AND ANSWERS

1–4. Match the EEG abnormality with its associated seizure type:

1. Interictal temporal lobe spikes
2. Generalized 3-Hz spike-and-wave
3. Generalized spike and polyspike-and-wave
4. Occipital spike-and-wave
   a. Tonic-clonic seizures
   b. Focal seizures with visual phenomena
   c. Focal seizures with altered consciousness
   d. Absence seizures

Answers: 1–c, 2–d, 3–a, 4–b.

5–12. Match the EEG pattern with its most likely cause (more than one answer may be correct):

5. Delta activity, phase reversed over left posterior cerebrum
6. Bifrontal beta activity
7. Alpha rhythm
8. Triphasic waves
9. Rapid extraocular movement artifact
10. Periodic complexes
11. Unilateral cerebral theta and delta activity
12. Electrocerebral silence
   a. Normal resting state
   b. Hepatic encephalopathy
   c. Benzodiazepine use
   d. Occipital lobe tumor
   e. Brain death
   f. Dream-filled sleep
   g. Unilateral electroconvulsive therapy (ECT)
   h. Psychosis
   i. Creutzfeldt–Jakob disease
   j. Barbiturate overdose

Answers: 5–d, 6–c, 7–a, 8–b, 9–f (REM sleep), 10–i, 11–g, 12–e and j.

13. In which four conditions will an EEG be helpful in suggesting a specific diagnosis?
   a. Cerebral tumor
   b. Hepatic encephalopathy
   c. Neurosis
   d. Huntington disease
   e. Cerebral abscess
   f. Creutzfeldt–Jakob disease
   g. Psychogenic nonepileptic seizures (PNES)
   h. Bipolar illness
   i. Cerebellar tumor
   j. SSPE

   k. Psychosis
   l. Multiple sclerosis
   m. Early Alzheimer disease

Answers: b, f, g, j.

14–16. Match each antiepileptic drug (AED) complication with its definition:

14. Stevens–Johnson syndrome
15. Forced normalization
16. Paradoxical hyperactivity
   a. Suppression of seizure activity and conversion to a normal EEG that may trigger a psychosis
   b. Allergic reaction evident on skin that often involves the gastrointestinal mucosa
   c. Psychosis as an allergic reaction
   d. Excitement instead of sedation, especially with phenobarbital treatment of children and brain-damaged adults

Answers: 14–b, 15–a, 16–d.

17–20. Identify the following statements as *true* or *false*.

17. Psychotropic medications may confound the diagnosis of neurologic illness by altering the EEG.
18. Benzodiazepines and barbiturates induce beta EEG activity.
19. Lithium at toxic levels, clozapine, and tricyclic antidepressants may cause EEG spikes and sharp waves.
20. In terms of psychotropic-induced EEG changes, clozapine, olanzapine, and trifluoperazine produce the most, and quetiapine, loxapine, and haloperidol the least.

Answers: 17–True, 18–True, 19–True, 20–True.

21. Carbamazepine is often used in the treatment of epilepsy patients with comorbid depression. Which of the following medications has a chemical structure most similar to carbamazepine?
   a. Lithium
   b. Phenytoin
   c. Imipramine
   d. Haloperidol
   e. Phenelzine
   f. Tranylcypromine

Answer: c. Imipramine has a chemical structure most like carbamazepine.

22. Which of the following AEDs is most closely associated with medication-induced psychosis, depression, and hostility?
    a. Topiramate
    b. Lamotrigine
    c. Levetiracetam
    d. Phenytoin

Answer: c. Levetiracetam causes or precipitates these psychiatric adverse reactions, but, of course, only in a small percentage of patients. Epilepsy patients who develop psychosis may not be experiencing neurologic deterioration but an iatrogenic disturbance.

23. Which application of ECT is least likely to produce amnesia?
    a. Unilateral, nondominant hemisphere
    b. Unilateral, dominant hemisphere
    c. Bilateral
    d. Each pattern will produce similar incidence and severity of amnesia

Answer: a. Although ECT in a unilateral pattern over the nondominant hemisphere may be least effective in reversing depression, it will produce the least amnesia.

24. Which feature suggests a frontal lobe seizure rather than another form of complex partial seizure?
    a. Childhood onset
    b. Olfactory auras
    c. Absence of an aura, duration of less than 1 minute, and little postictal symptomatology
    d. The ability of sleep to suppress these seizures

Answer: c. Frontal lobe seizures, unlike other complex partial seizures, usually develop in adults and consist of numerous, relatively brief episodes of bizarre activity devoid of aura, automatisms, and postictal confusion. Frontal lobe seizures develop predominantly during sleep. Relying on their clinical manifestations, physicians are especially apt to misdiagnose them as psychogenic episodes. Also, the routine EEG is often unable to assist in the diagnosis.

25. A 28-year-old man comes to the hospital after having several seizures. Previous evaluations attributed his seizures to a congenital cerebral injury. The patient is enrolled in a methadone program for narcotic addiction and also is followed in an epilepsy clinic. After an intravenous benzodiazepine controls the seizures, physicians change his AED to phenytoin and renew his methadone. Several days later he develops agitation, anxiety to the point of incoherence, diaphoresis, and tachycardia. Which should the consulting psychiatrist prescribe?
    a. An atypical neuroleptic
    b. A typical neuroleptic
    c. A different AED
    d. An increase in his daily methadone dose
    e. A decrease in his phenytoin dose

Answer: d. Because phenytoin decreases methadone activity, it precipitates narcotic withdrawal. To avoid this problem, physicians should increase the dose of methadone when initiating therapy with phenytoin. Abruptly stopping or reducing the phenytoin could precipitate additional seizures or even cause status epilepticus, though it could be gradually tapered off and replaced with another AED over 5 to 10 days.

26. How do carbamazepine and phenytoin interact with oral contraceptives?
    a. These AEDs increase the contraceptive's effectiveness, permitting lower estrogen preparations to be effective.
    b. These AEDs decrease the contraceptive's effectiveness, risking conception.
    c. These AEDs have no effect on a contraceptive's effectiveness.
    d. In contrast to these AEDs having a teratogenic effect, other AEDs have been shown to be risk-free.

Answer: b. Several AEDs that induce enzymes, including carbamazepine, phenobarbital, and phenytoin, greatly increase the metabolism of oral contraceptives, possibly inactivating them.

27. In which phase of sleep are seizures least likely to occur?
    a. NREM
    b. REM
    c. Sleep following sleep deprivation
    d. Awakening from sleep

Answer: b. Seizures are most likely to emerge during NREM sleep and least likely during REM sleep.

28. Which statement regarding depression in epilepsy patients is *true*?
    a. Studies show that depression and suicide in epilepsy patients are unrelated to risk factors in the general population.
    b. The addition of a second or third AED to an anticonvulsant regimen is a risk factor for suicidal ideation.
    c. Compared to depression without comorbid epilepsy, depression comorbid with epilepsy is more often bipolar.
    d. ECT for depression is contraindicated in epilepsy.

Answer: b. Suicidal ideation increases following the addition of an AED to a regimen of one or more AEDs, i.e., multiple AEDs or polypharmacy. The incidence of bipolar disorder in epilepsy patients is near or only slightly higher than that of the general population. In addition to comorbid depression and risk factors in the general population, those for suicide in epilepsy are psychotic disturbances, borderline personality disorder, and other interictal psychopathology.

29. Which statement regarding Landau–Kleffner syndrome (LKS) is *false*?
    a. Patients with LKS have an increased rate of autism spectrum disorder (ASD) symptoms.
    b. Patients with LKS develop normally in the first years of life, after which they regress.

c. Antiepileptic medications are of no benefit in LKS.

d. In LKS the EEG is abnormal during sleep.

Answer: c. LKS, or acquired epileptic aphasia, causes regression in language function and usually other behavioral domains in children. The EEG characteristically shows electrical status epilepticus during sleep or continuous spike-waves during sleep. Early treatment of LKS, which may include AEDs and steroids, may prevent worsening.

30–39. The patient's age when focal seizures begin suggests the cause. Match the cause with the age(s) when associated seizures are likely to appear (the same answer may be applicable to different questions):

30. Head injury
31. Congenital cerebral malformation
32. Arteriovenous malformation
33. Glioblastoma
34. Metastatic brain tumor
35. Meningitis
36. Stroke
37. Cysticercosis
38. Mesial temporal sclerosis
39. Perinatal cerebral hypoxia
   a. Childhood
   b. Adolescence
   c. Middle age

Answers: 30–b; 31–a; 32–a and b; 33–c; 34–c; 35–a, b, and c; 36–c; 37–a, b, and c; 38–a and b; 39–a.

40. Withdrawal from daily use of which substance is unlikely to cause seizures?
   a. Alcohol
   b. Benzodiazepines
   c. Nicotine
   d. Short-acting barbiturates
   e. AEDs

Answer: c. Withdrawal from nicotine may cause an agitated delirium but it is very unlikely to cause seizures. Withdrawal from the other substances frequently causes seizures and occasionally status epilepticus.

41. Which of the following statements is *true* concerning the risk of seizures with clozapine use?
   a. The risk of seizures is independent of the dose of clozapine.
   b. With increasing dosage of clozapine, the risks of seizures and agranulocytosis both increase.
   c. With increasing dosage of clozapine, the risk of seizures increases but the risk of agranulocytosis remains constant.
   d. If seizures pose a threat during high-dose clozapine treatment, physicians should add carbamazepine.

Answer: c. Most studies have found that seizures complicate clozapine treatment in a dose-related pattern, but agranulocytosis develops independent of dosage. Adding carbamazepine in clozapine greatly increases the risk of agranulocytosis.

42. Which of the following AEDs undergoes almost complete renal clearance and would, strictly from a pharmacologic viewpoint, would be most appropriate for patients with hepatic insufficiency?
   a. Carbamazepine
   b. Valproic acid
   c. Levetiracetam
   d. Lamotrigine

Answer: c. Levetiracetam is mostly excreted unchanged by the kidneys. The others require hepatic metabolism.

43. A 6-year-old boy has absence seizures with paroxysms of 3-Hz spike-and-wave EEG activity. He was unable to tolerate ethosuximide (Zarontin). Which AED should be tried next?
   a. Phenytoin
   b. Carbamazepine
   c. Valproic acid
   d. Phenobarbital

Answer: c. Absence seizures with 3-Hz spike-and-wave activity are usually first treated with ethosuximide. Valproic acid is an alternative, especially if ethosuximide is unacceptable or if tonic-clonic seizures also occur.

44. A 23-year-old medical student was experimenting with smoking marijuana. Its effect, completely different than he anticipated, was anxiety and fear. The student was brought to the emergency room with hallucinations, agitation, fever, and nystagmus. Increasing mental and physical agitation soon developed, culminating in a seizure. Of the following, which is the most likely culprit?
   a. Marijuana
   b. Phencyclidine (PCP)
   c. Cocaine
   d. Demerol

Answer: b. PCP, even in minute amounts, can cause hallucinations, nystagmus, and seizures. Drug users or suppliers sometimes mix it with marijuana. Cocaine not only produces hallucinations and seizures, it may cause cerebral hemorrhage, ischemic stroke, or vasculitis.

45. After developing lethargy and confusion, a 30-year-old woman with a history of focal seizures is brought to the emergency room. Which of the following conditions is the most likely cause?
   a. Expansion of a temporal lobe tumor
   b. Development of a subdural hematoma from head trauma
   c. Nonconvulsive status epilepticus
   d. AED intoxication
   e. Development of a systemic disorder, such as renal failure

Answer: d. Although treating physicians might reasonably consider all these potential explanations, the usual cause in such cases is AED intoxication or prolonged postictal confusion. If AED intoxication is profound or recurs, physicians should consider the possibility that the episode was a deliberate overdose or an adverse interaction of her AED with a psychotropic or other medication.

46. Which six of the following signs may indicate phenytoin intoxication?
    a. Hemiparesis
    b. Ataxia of gait
    c. Nystagmus
    d. Aphasia
    e. Dysarthria
    f. Lethargy or stupor
    g. Dysmetria on heel–shin testing
    h. Tremor on finger–nose testing
    i. Papilledema

Answer: b, c, e, f, g, h. Phenytoin intoxication causes nystagmus, cerebellar dysfunction, and depressed sensorium.

47. In which part of the skull are the temporal lobes situated?
    a. Sella
    b. Anterior fossa
    c. Posterior fossa
    d. Middle fossa

Answer: d. The temporal lobes occupy the entire middle cranial fossae. The posterior fossa holds the cerebellum, medulla, fourth ventricle, and vertebral and basilar arteries.

48. What is the duration of the serum prolactin level elevation after a generalized tonic-clonic or complex partial seizure?
    a. 24 hours
    b. 12 hours
    c. 2 hours
    d. Less than 1 hour

Answer: d. Following a majority of tonic-clonic, most ECT-induced, and a minority of focal seizures, the serum prolactin level rises for approximately 10 to 20 minutes. It does not rise following psychogenic or most focal seizures.

49–50. Identify the following statements as *true* or *false*.

49. Epileptic individuals are more likely than others to be convicted of a crime and sent to prison.
50. Epileptic criminals are no more likely than other criminals to commit violent crimes.

Answer: 49–True, 50–True.

51. Which one of the following statements concerning neural tube defects is *false*?
    a. Meningomyeloceles may be induced by AED treatment of pregnant women.
    b. The incidence of neural tube defects is reduced by folic acid diet supplements.
    c. The neural tube is derived from the endoderm.
    d. The neural tube forms the brain and the spinal cord.

Answer: c. Soon after conception the ectodermal layer of the embryo invaginates to form the neural tube. The AEDs implicated most often in causing neural tube defects are carbamazepine and valproate. Studies have shown that pregnant women can reduce the incidence of neural tube defects by taking folic acid. However, no studies have shown that taking folic acid will prevent neural tube defects in pregnant women taking those AEDs.

52. Which of the following AEDs leads to weight loss?
    a. Valproate
    b. Levetiracetam
    c. Topiramate
    d. Phenytoin
    e. Gabapentin

Answer: c. Topiramate often leads to a small weight loss. Valproate frequently causes weight gain. The others have little or no effect on weight.

53. Which is the most frequently occurring electrolyte disturbance associated with carbamazepine or oxcarbazepine treatment?
    a. Hyponatremia
    b. Hypernatremia
    c. Hypokalemia
    d. Hyperkalemia

Answer: a. When given as either a mood-stabilizer or AED, both carbamazepine and oxcarbazepine can cause hyponatremia. The effect may be so pronounced as to cause seizures, delirium, or both. In addition, psychogenic polydipsia can cause equally serious hyponatremia.

54. If a medication that induced CYP 3A4 enzymes were administered to an individual taking carbamazepine, what would happen to the carbamazepine plasma concentration?
    a. The plasma concentration of carbamazepine would increase.
    b. The plasma concentration of carbamazepine would decrease.
    c. The plasma concentration of carbamazepine would remain unchanged.
    d. None of the above

Answer: b. Medications that induce CYP 3A4 enzymes, including phenobarbital, phenytoin, and carbamazepine itself, decrease the plasma concentration of carbamazepine, possibly to subtherapeutic levels. Thus, in the case of carbamazepine treatment, increasing doses are often required to maintain a therapeutic concentration. Moreover, carbamazepine-induced enzymes decrease plasma concentrations of alprazolam, clozapine, haloperidol, oral contraceptives, and valproate.

55. Which of the following AEDs is an inhibitor of cytochrome P450 enzymes?
a. Phenytoin
b. Phenobarbital
c. Carbamazepine
d. Valproate

Answer: d. Valproate is an inhibitor of P450 enzymes, but the others induce the enzymes.

56. Electrocerebral silence on an EEG typically indicates brain death; however, other conditions may also abolish EEG activity. Of the following, which *two* other conditions also produce electrocerebral silence?
a. Psychogenic unresponsiveness
b. Depression
c. Severe Alzheimer disease
d. Barbiturate overdose
e. Hypothermia
f. Locked-in syndrome

Answer: d, e. Before declaring brain death on the basis of an EEG, neurologists must be certain that the patient's body temperature is near normal and that blood toxicology analysis does not detect barbiturates.

57. Which is the best test for demonstrating mesial temporal sclerosis?
a. MRI of the brain
b. SPECT of the brain
c. CT of the brain
d. CT with contrast of the brain
e. EEG
f. EEG with nasopharyngeal leads

Answer: a.

58. Which one of these statements regarding epilepsy, the EEG, and ECT treatment is *false*?
a. When unilateral right-sided ECT is administered, the EEG changes are found predominantly over the right hemisphere.
b. Generalized EEG changes after ECT are associated with more successful treatment of depression.
c. Generalized EEG changes after ECT are associated with greater amnesia.
d. ECT may precipitate status epilepticus in patients with epilepsy or a structural lesion.
e. ECT is contraindicated when epilepsy is comorbid with depression.

Answer: e. ECT is an effective, safe treatment when epilepsy is comorbid with depression provided that seizures are under control. Physicians can also administer ECT and expect good results in depressed epilepsy patients who are taking AEDs, but sometimes the physicians must reduce the number or dose of AEDs prior to ECT.

59. Which statement regarding the EEG in a normal resting awake person, with eyes closed, is *false*?

a. Anxiety or concentrating on a simple problem will abolish alpha activity.
b. Hyperventilation will produce slow waves or slow the background activity.
c. The normal background rhythm is low voltage and "fast."
d. Drowsiness, as well as sleep, will slow the background activity.
e. Stroboscopic lights may induce cerebral activity.

Answer: c. The normal background rhythm of an awake person with closed eyes is alpha activity, which is 8–12 Hz and medium in voltage. By contrast, beta activity, which is faster and lower in voltage, replaces alpha when the EEG subject experiences anxiety or concentrates on mental activities. It also replaces alpha activity if the subject takes sedatives or minor tranquilizers, including benzodiazepines.

60. A man with alcoholism and epilepsy is taking phenytoin. He presents with confusion, nystagmus, and ataxia. A routine medical and neurologic evaluation reveals no abnormal findings, except that he has alcohol on his breath. What should be the *two* first steps?
a. Determine the blood alcohol and glucose concentrations
b. Obtain an EEG
c. Administer more phenytoin
d. Administer thiamine

Answer: a, d. Many alcoholic individuals have epilepsy. When inebriated, they pose several dilemmas. Wernicke–Korsakoff syndrome, hypoglycemia from liver disease, or head trauma, as well as persistent seizures (status epilepticus), could each cause confusion and obtundation. In addition, the confusion, nystagmus, and ataxia suggest phenytoin intoxication. However, AED intoxication is unlikely because alcoholics in the midst of a binge usually do not take their AEDs. Moreover, in the midst of a binge, they may omit other crucial medications, including insulin and antihypertensives.

61–62. A 32-year-old left-handed woman has had focal seizures with altered consciousness since her adolescence. Her seizures have not responded to monotherapy. When taking two or three AEDs, which were only slightly more effective in suppressing seizures than taking one, she usually developed AED intoxication. EEG-video monitoring documented continued seizures despite therapeutic AED concentrations. EEG also showed a single left anterior temporal lobe seizure focus.

61. In contemplating surgery, what test should be performed next?
a. Amobarbital interview
b. Withdrawal of AEDs
c. PET scan
d. Wada test

Answer: d. The patient, who may be right hemisphere-dominant for language, might benefit from a partial or complete left temporal lobectomy. However, if her left temporal lobe were dominant, which is usually the case, she would be able to withstand only a limited resection. In the future, functional MRI may provide as reliable guidance as the Wada test.

62. Assuming a temporal lobectomy is safely performed, what is the likelihood of complete or near-complete remission of her seizures?
    a. 25%
    b. 50%
    c. 75%
    d. Almost 100%

Answer: c. In approximately 75% of cases, epilepsy surgery completely eliminates seizures or allows their control with fewer AEDs and lower doses.

63. Which of the following statements regarding Rolandic epilepsy is *true*?
    a. It is also called childhood epilepsy with centro-temporal spikes.
    b. The most common cause is mesial temporal sclerosis.
    c. When children with the condition become adults they are prone to develop other varieties of seizures.
    d. The diagnosis often requires EEG-video monitoring, and if a single focus is identified, a partial lobectomy is indicated.

Answer: a. Rolandic epilepsy, an inherited condition, is restricted to the childhood years. EEGs performed during sleep may be necessary for diagnosis, but elaborate monitoring is rarely necessary. Once diagnosed, Rolandic epilepsy is readily responsive to AEDs. Unlike absence seizures, which lead to later development of tonic-clonic or other seizures in one-third of cases, Rolandic epilepsy usually remits in adolescence.

64–68. Match the condition with its closest description (the same answer may be applicable to different questions):

64. Nonconvulsive status epilepticus
65. Seizure-like activity under conscious control
66. Activity not under conscious control that mimics seizures
67. Withdrawal emergent psychopathology
68. Forced normalization
    a. Psychiatric disturbances, including psychotic behavior, arising after AEDs rapidly and completely suppress frequent seizures
    b. Psychiatric disturbances, especially anxiety and depression, developing after discontinuation of AEDs
    c. PNES
    d. Repetitive or prolonged seizures with mental impairment as the primary or exclusive symptom

Answers: 64–d, 65–c, 66–c, 67–b, 68–a.

69. Which *two* statements regarding the relationship of interictal violence to epilepsy are *true*?
    a. Violence is associated with epilepsy patients taking two or more AEDs.
    b. Violence tends to occur in schizophrenic or mentally retarded epilepsy patients, but rarely in other epilepsy patients.
    c. Crimes of adult epileptic incarcerated criminals are no more violent than those of nonepileptic ones.
    d. The prevalence of epilepsy is no greater in prisoners than in the general population.

Answer: b, c.

70. Which variety of seizure do physicians most often misdiagnose as a PNES?
    a. Partial complex seizure that originates in the temporal lobe
    b. Partial complex seizure that originates in the frontal lobe
    c. Febrile seizure
    d. Absence
    e. Drug withdrawal seizure

Answer: b. Physicians are most likely to misdiagnose frontal lobe seizures because they often induce bizarre behavior, such as pelvic thrusting, flailing limb movements, and alternating head movements.

71. Which of the following is associated with postictal EEG depression?
    a. Vegetative symptoms
    b. Tendency toward suicide
    c. Sleep–wake disturbances
    d. Slow, low-voltage EEG activity

Answer: d. Postictal EEG depression refers not to a mood disorder but to the slow, low-voltage EEG patterns that follow seizures, including those induced by ECT.

72. A commercial airliner from South America to New York crashed after exhausting its fuel supply. A young man who had been one of the passengers was brought to the hospital with blunt abdominal trauma. Shortly after arriving in the emergency room, he became agitated, incoherent, diaphoretic, and hypertensive. Although physicians found no sign of head injuries, he developed status epilepticus and unstable vital signs. During one seizure, several ruptured condoms passed through his rectum. Other condoms, still intact and containing a white powder, subsequently passed out of his rectum. What is the most likely cause of his seizures and unstable vital signs?
    a. Epidural hematoma
    b. Cysticercosis
    c. Subdural hematoma
    d. Cocaine overdose
    e. Hypoxia

Answer: d. Smugglers of contraband ("mules") commonly swallow condoms stuffed with cocaine. If one breaks, cocaine spills into the intestine and toxic quantities enter the systemic circulation. The resulting cocaine overdose causes psychosis, cardiac instability, and seizures. Although irrelevant in this case, the most common cause of seizures in South and Central America is cysticercosis.

73. Which AED(s) is/are associated with polycystic ovaries and hyperandrogenism?
    a. Carbamazepine
    b. Valproate
    c. Phenytoin
    d. Topiramate
    e. a and b
    f. b and c

Answer: f. Older AEDs adversely affect many endocrine-based functions in women. Carbamazepine and valproate increase the risk of neural tube defects. Valproate treatment is also associated with transient thinning of hair and obesity, as well as with polycystic ovaries and hyperandrogenism. Both phenytoin and carbamazepine reduce the effectiveness of oral contraceptives. Phenytoin also causes increased facial hair.

74. Which one of the following statements does not describe Todd's paralysis?
    a. Todd's paralysis is usually apparent only during the first 24 hours following a seizure.
    b. Todd's hemiparesis may follow any seizure.
    c. Todd's hemiparesis may be accompanied by other lateralized deficits, such as aphasia.
    d. Todd's paralysis suggests a focal, rather than a generalized, seizure disorder.

Answer: b. Todd's paralysis, typically a transient postictal hemiparesis, rather than a quadriparesis or paraparesis, usually follows focal motor seizures. It does not follow absence seizures and several other seizure varieties.

75. Valproate and carbamazepine induce neural tube closure defects. Which of the following is *not* a neural tube closure defect?
    a. Meningomyelocele
    b. Meningocele
    c. Spina bifida
    d. Encephalocele
    e. Tetralogy of Fallot

Answer: e. Meningomyelocele, meningocele, and spina bifida – in decreasing severity of malformation – are neural tube closure deficits of the lumbar spine and spinal cord. An encephalocele is the cerebral counterpart.

76. Which of the following is a *false* statement regarding EEG changes associated with bilateral ECT?
    a. During and immediately after ECT, EEG changes resemble those of a generalized tonic-clonic seizure.
    b. EEG slow-wave activity persists for up to 3 months after bilateral ECT.

c. ECT-induced EEG slowing is associated with memory impairment.
d. ECT-induced EEG slowing is associated with ineffective treatment of depression.

Answer: d. ECT-induced EEG slowing is associated with more effective treatment of depression. However, it is also associated with prolonged amnesia.

77. Which of the following conditions is *not* associated with the presence of triphasic waves on EEG?
    a. Hepatic failure
    b. Renal failure
    c. Alzheimer disease
    d. Lithium toxicity

Answer: c. Triphasic waves are most commonly seen in metabolic encephalopathies, such as hepatic and renal failure. They also occur in some cases of lithium toxicity. However, they do not result from dementia.

78. Which of the following psychotropics is most likely to cause a seizure?
    a. Clozapine
    b. Aripiprazole
    c. Olanzapine
    d. Risperidone
    e. Quetiapine
    f. Ziprasidone

Answer: a. Clozapine carries a seizure risk of approximately 4% when administered in high doses, i.e., more than 600 mg daily. In contrast, at therapeutic doses, the other antipsychotics carry a risk of less than 1%.

79. Which of the following is the greatest risk factor for depression complicating seizures?
    a. Duration of epilepsy
    b. Focal seizures with altered consciousness.
    c. Family history of epilepsy
    d. Frequent seizures

Answer: b. Among epilepsy patients, depression occurs particularly in those who have focal seizures with altered consciousness or require multiple AEDs. The duration of epilepsy, seizure frequency, and family history of depression are less significant. Epilepsy-associated depression is rarely bipolar. When depression is comorbid with epilepsy, it reduces patients' quality of life – even more than seizure frequency or severity.

80. In rating the potential teratogenic risks of AEDs, which group carries the FDA label of Category D (dangerous)?
    a. Carbamazepine and valproate
    b. Lamotrigine, levetiracetam, oxcarbazepine, and topiramate
    c. Phenobarbital and phenytoin
    d. Ethosuximide

Answer: a. Carbamazepine and valproate, which are both associated with neural tube defects, carry the FDA label Category D. The FDA has classified lamotrigine, levetiracetam, oxcarbazepine, and topiramate as Category C (caution).

81. What proportion of adults with well-documented PNES also has epileptic seizures?
    a. ≤10%
    b. 25%
    c. 50%
    d. 66%

Answer: a. Although early reports indicated that approximately 50% of adults with PNES also have epilepsy, recent studies suggest that PNES are comorbid with epilepsy in only 5% to 10% of cases. Because PNES remain refractory to neurologic and psychiatric treatments, PNES patients have a worse prognosis than those with epileptic seizures.

82. What is the effect of drinking large quantities of grapefruit juice on the serum concentration of carbamazepine?
    a. Increased concentrations
    b. Decreased concentrations
    c. No effect

Answer: a. The same liver enzymes that metabolize multiple AEDs also metabolize grapefruit juice. Thus, drinking grapefruit juice increases serum concentrations of carbamazepine and zonisamide, as well as several psychotropic medications.

83. What is the effect of pregnancy on seizure frequency?
    a. Seizures tend to decrease in frequency.
    b. Seizures tend to increase in frequency.
    c. Pregnancy has no effect on seizure frequency.

Answer: b. During pregnancy seizure frequency increases because serum AED levels drift downward as their clearance increases and the increase in the woman's body mass dilutes AED concentrations.

84. If two AEDs fail to suppress seizures, what is the likelihood that the addition of a third will be successful?
    a. ≤5%
    b. 25%
    c. 75%
    d. 100%

Answer: a. If two AEDs do not suppress seizures, the likelihood of success with the addition of a third is ≤5%. Moreover, AED polypharmacy often creates unbearable side effects. If AEDs cannot suppress seizures, physicians should reassess the diagnosis of epilepsy, variety of seizure(s), appropriate AED, and the patient's compliance (by measuring AED blood levels). If optimum medical management remains ineffective, neurologists often consider vagus nerve stimulation or neurosurgery.

85. Which of the following statements is *false* concerning suicide in epilepsy patients?
    a. The suicide rate among epilepsy patients is one- to three-fold greater than among the general population.
    b. Among epilepsy patients, the risk is greatest among those with focal seizures with altered consciousness.
    c. Epilepsy patients with psychotic disturbances or borderline personality disorder are at increased risk.
    d. The addition of a second or third AED increases rather than decreases the incidence of suicide ideation and suicide rates.

Answer: a. The suicide rate among epilepsy patients is actually four- to five-fold greater then among the general population. In addition to the usual risk factors for depression, epilepsy patients have an increased risk attributable to seizures with altered consciousness; psychopathology common among epileptics, such as psychotic disturbances and borderline personality disorder as well as depression; and use of multiple AEDs.

86. Which of the following is the LEAST significant risk factor for interictal psychosis?
    a. Early age of onset of epilepsy
    b. Low intelligence
    c. Certain EEG patterns
    d. Family history of psychosis

Answer: c. While no specific EEG abnormality predicts interictal psychosis, signs of brain damage and a family history of psychosis are risk factors for interictal psychosis.

87. Which of the following drugs crosses the placenta?
    a. Phenobarbital
    b. Methadone
    c. Carbamazepine
    d. Topiramate
    e. All of the above

Answer: e. AEDs, and many other medications and drugs of abuse cross the placenta into the fetal circulation. For example, opioids pass through and, with continued use, may lead to fetal dependency. Moreover, unless neonatologists provide a replacement at delivery, neonates with prolonged in utero opioid exposure may undergo withdrawal symptoms and experience a seizure.

88. Which of the following is/are readily transferred through breast milk?
    a. Topiramate
    b. Lamotrigine
    c. Phenobarbital
    d. Ethosuximide
    e. Zonisamide
    f. All of the above

Answer: f. Most AEDs pass into breast milk and, in breast-feeding neonates, some reach substantial serum concentrations. Although usually their only effect is sleepiness, more serious reactions may occur.

89. Which group of antidepressants has the greatest likelihood of inducing seizures?
    a. Bupropion, clomipramine
    b. Nefazodone
    c. Fluoxetine, paroxetine, sertraline

Answer: a.

90. Which group of antipsychotics has the greatest likelihood of inducing seizures?
    a. Chlorpromazine, clozapine
    b. Haloperidol
    c. Risperidone

Answer: a.

91. Which of the following AEDs is least likely to cause osteopenia?
    a. Carbamazepine
    b. Phenytoin
    c. Levetiracetam
    d. Valproate
    e. Phenobarbital

Answer: c. Unlike the other AEDs, levetiracetam is not associated with osteopenia (moderately decreased bone density). Carbamazepine, phenytoin, phenobarbital, and valproate cause bone reabsorption, which enhances age-related osteoporosis. Dual-emission X-ray absorptiometry (DEXA) scans in patients taking these AEDs show decreased mineral (calcium) density. The AEDs implicated in osteopenia, with the exception of valproate, induce cytochrome P450 enzymes. Neurologists often follow women taking these AEDs with bone scans and supplement their AED regimen with calcium and vitamin D and weight-bearing exercises. Sometimes neurologists switch patients to another AED if DEXA scans detect osteoporosis (severely decreased bone density).

92. A 52-year-old woman suffered from focal seizures with impaired consciousness that began when she was a teenager. Multiple AED regimens had produced mental dulling and other side effects, and still allowed one or two seizures each week. One year before a psychiatric consultation she underwent partial left temporal lobectomy for seizure control. Subsequently, she remained seizure-free even without any AEDs. However, she developed postoperative anxiety, fearfulness, dysphoria, and "moodiness." CCTV-EEG monitoring during this time showed no epileptic activity. Which would be the best strategy to restore her preoperative mental status?
    a. Prescribe an antidepressant
    b. Prescribe an anxiolytic
    c. Reinstitute an AED, such as valproate
    d. Install a vagus nerve stimulator

Answer: c. Following neurosurgical removal of a seizure focus in the temporal lobe, many patients experience postoperative psychiatric complications, particularly personality changes and depression. Psychosis sometimes emerges, but usually only if seizures recur. Although this patient probably is not experiencing seizures, a mood-stabilizing AED would probably reestablish her equilibrium.

93. What proportion of autism patients has seizures?
    a. 0.5%, the same as the general population
    b. 5%
    c. 33%
    d. 75%
    e. 100%

Answer: c. During the course of their lifetime, one-third of autism patients develop seizures.

94. Which of the following AEDs inhibits cytochrome P450 and readily causes toxic concentrations of lamotrigine when given in combination?
    a. Gabapentin
    b. Valproate
    c. Carbamazepine
    d. Levetiracetam

Answer: b.

95. A 25-year-old woman with epilepsy that is well controlled with carbamazepine developed pharyngitis. Because she is allergic to penicillin, her physician prescribed erythromycin. Although she initially felt that the pharyngitis subsided, she rapidly developed ataxia, nystagmus, and diplopia. In retrospect, what is the cause of her new symptoms?
    a. Allergy to erythromycin
    b. Carbamazepine toxicity
    c. Spread of the pharyngitis to her brain
    d. The development of hepatitis

Answer: b. The erythromycin inhibits hepatic cytochrome enzymes that ordinarily metabolizes her carbamazepine. With reduced metabolism, the carbamazepine rose to toxic levels and caused her new symptoms. This is a classic adverse interaction.

96. Which is the most common AED-induced cognitive adverse effect?
    a. Slowed processing speed and impaired attention
    b. Word-finding difficulty
    c. Dyscalculia
    d. Amnesia

Answer: a. In general, AEDs are most apt to decrease processing speed and impair attention. At toxic levels, they cause lethargy and amnesia. More than other AEDs, topiramate may cause word-finding difficulty.

97. Two weeks before his wife brought him to the psychiatric emergency room, a 40-year-old well-regarded high school teacher, who has had epilepsy

since childhood, had a several day cluster of eight focal seizures that sometimes underwent secondary generalization. Vigorous treatment in another emergency room controlled those seizures. Although too groggy and confused to return to work, he was free of seizures, oriented, and pleasant. However, he then began to push away his food, pace around the house, and complain about the neighbors' noise intruding into his school plans. He became verbally, although not physically, aggressive with his brother. His threats of killing a neighbor finally drove his wife to bring him to the psychiatry emergency room. He has no family history of psychiatric illness. There is no evidence of his using drugs of abuse or being noncompliant with his AEDs. Which is the most likely explanation of this patient's behavior?

a. Postictal psychosis
b. Interictal psychosis
c. Bipolar disorder
d. Drug abuse

Answer: a. In this classic scenario, following a cluster of seizures, especially complex partial and secondarily generalized ones, and then a characteristic lucid interval, the patient developed postictal psychosis. The best treatment in his case would be an antipsychotic agent, but in less severe cases, a benzodiazepine might suffice. Notably, repeated episodes of postictal psychosis are a risk factor for interictal psychosis.

98. The parents of a 5-year-old boy have noticed that for the previous 6 months their son has developed brief, completely unprovoked episodes of laughter. During the episodes, which have a duration of about 30 seconds, they cannot communicate with him or interrupt his spontaneous outburst. Also, he does not seem to be particularly happy before or during the laughter. Once the parents began to study it, they noticed that rather than laughing normally with gusto, their son seems to be saying, "Hee, hee, hee." A pediatric neurologist found that the boy was developmentally and physically normal. CCTV-EEG monitoring showed generalized spike-and-wave discharges during the events that it captured. MRI revealed a hypothalamic hamartoma. Which is the most accurate diagnosis?

a. Complex partial seizures from the temporal lobe
b. Frontal lobe seizures
c. Gelastic seizures
d. Absence seizures

Answer: c. This boy has epilepsy, whose sole manifestation consists of bouts of mirthless laughter (gelastic seizures) that are triggered by a hypothalamic hamartoma. Gelastic seizures are rare but a good example of a neurologic disorder causing, at least on a superficial level, an emotional outburst. Less frequently, frontal or temporal lobe lesions cause gelastic seizures. In those cases, patients are generally older and have other manifestations of complex partial seizures.

99. Friends bring a 45-year-old man to the emergency room after they witnessed a generalized tonic-clonic seizure. He reports daily alcohol intake of 1 pint of vodka and 6 beers. However, he has not had anything to drink in 3 days because he ran out of money. He had a similar event 2 years ago following abstinence. His physical examination shows mild generalized tremulousness and tachycardia, but no other abnormalities. His head CT shows mild cortical atrophy for age, but is otherwise normal. Which AED should his physicians start?

a. Phenytoin
b. Valproic acid
c. Levetiracetam
d. Phenobarbital
e. None of the above

Answer: e. This patient has classic alcohol withdrawal seizures. If the patient continues to drink alcohol, AEDs will not prevent further seizures. Physicians should focus their treatment strategies on alcohol cessation.

100. Which of the following conditions has the lowest incidence of epilepsy?

a. Moderate-to-severe traumatic brain injury (TBI)
b. Neurofibromatosis type 2 (NF2)
c. Autism spectrum disorders
d. Rett syndrome
e. Cerebral palsy (CP) (all forms)

Answer: b. NF2 consists of unilateral or bilateral acoustic neuromas, which rarely cause seizures. In contrast, because it may be associated with meningiomas or other intracranial neoplasms, NF1 occasionally causes seizures. ASD and Rett syndrome cause seizures in at least 33% of patients. CP is closely associated with epilepsy. Overall, the comorbidity of epilepsy and CP is high (approximately 50%), but it is reasonably low (approximately 10%) in the athetotic variety of CP.

101. For many years, a 34-year-old homeless woman with epilepsy since age 10 years has had persistent hallucinations, paranoia, and social isolation. Her seizures are usually focal with impaired consciousness, but many undergo secondary generalization, and occur frequently, in part because she is noncompliant with her AED regimen. She has low-\normal intelligence and a mild right hemiparesis. Which is the most accurate diagnosis of her condition?

a. Interictal psychosis
b. Schizophrenia
c. Vascular dementia
d. Postictal psychosis

Answer: a. She has interictal ("schizophreniform") psychosis, which is a chronic condition that develops in middle-aged epilepsy patients who have had decades of poorly controlled seizures despite regimens of multiple AEDs. Patients with this complication of epilepsy frequently have low intelligence and physical neurologic deficits. Their CTs or MRIs often show structural brain damage. Unlike postictal psychosis, interictal psychosis is a chronic disorder rather than an episodic one. Unlike patients with schizophrenia, those with interictal psychosis maintain a normal affect, do not deteriorate, and, compared to the general population, have no increased family incidence of schizophrenia.

102. Which test should a woman of Asian ancestry undergo before a physician prescribes carbamazepine?
a. Eosinophil count
b. HLA-B 1502 allele
c. Sedimentation rate
d. Complete blood count

Answer: b. Although almost any AED, even at a therapeutic level, can cause Stevens–Johnson syndrome, administration of carbamazepine to patients of Asian ancestry who carry the HLA-B 1502 allele is particularly apt to cause the disorder. If individuals have been taking carbamazepine for longer than several months and have not experienced this adverse reaction, their risk of subsequently developing it is low.

103. The police bring a teenage girl, dressed in "punk clothing," to the psychiatry emergency room because she has been found sitting alone on a park bench, confused and belligerent. On examination, she is inattentive and unable or unwilling to reveal her personal or medical history. She does not follow requests, participate in an examination, or speak, except to repeat a single, unintelligible phrase. She has loud, repetitive lip smacking. She is afebrile and normotensive, but she has tachycardia. An extensive medical and neurologic evaluation, including an MRI, discloses no other abnormalities. Repeated tests for drugs of abuse, pregnancy, and alcohol are negative. Finally, her mother arrives and explains that the patient has been epileptic but noncompliant with her AED regimen. Which procedure(s) should the prudent physician initiate?
a. Administer thiamine 50 mg IV
b. Obtain an EEG
c. Determine, if possible, the serum concentrations of her AEDs
d. All of the above

Answer: d. This patient's presentation is most consistent with focal nonconvulsive status epilepticus in that her primary symptom was a change in mental status with a stereotypy (repetitive lip-smacking) rather than tonic-clonic activity. Her episode typically followed her being noncompliant with her AED regimen. An EEG would confirm that diagnosis. Nonconvulsive status epilepticus may mimic alcohol intoxication, illicit drug use, sleep disturbances, and numerous neurologic conditions. Prudent physicians generally administer thiamine because of the comorbidity of alcohol and drug abuse. Physicians might also, after drawing the appropriate blood tests, administer glucose.

104. In the case in Question 103, the EEG shows continuous spike-and-waves and multiple spikes. Repeat evaluations find no other abnormality. Which intravenous treatment do most neurologists begin?
a. Benzodiazepine
b. Phenobarbital
c. Phenytoin
d. None of the above

Answer: a. Whether the status epilepticus is focal motor, focal with dyscognition, or tonic-clonic, most neurologists administer an intravenous benzodiazepine as the initial treatment. In a frequent dramatic response, patients in status epilepticus who receive a benzodiazepine awaken rather than sleep.

105–108. Match each EEG with the appropriate interpretation (see pages 232–233):

105. Spike and polyspike-and-wave
106. 3-Hz spike-and-wave
107. Normal
108. Temporal spike focus
a. Fig. EEG-A
b. Fig. EEG-B
c. Fig. EEG-C
d. Fig. EEG-D

Answers: 105–d, 106–c, 107–a, 108–b.

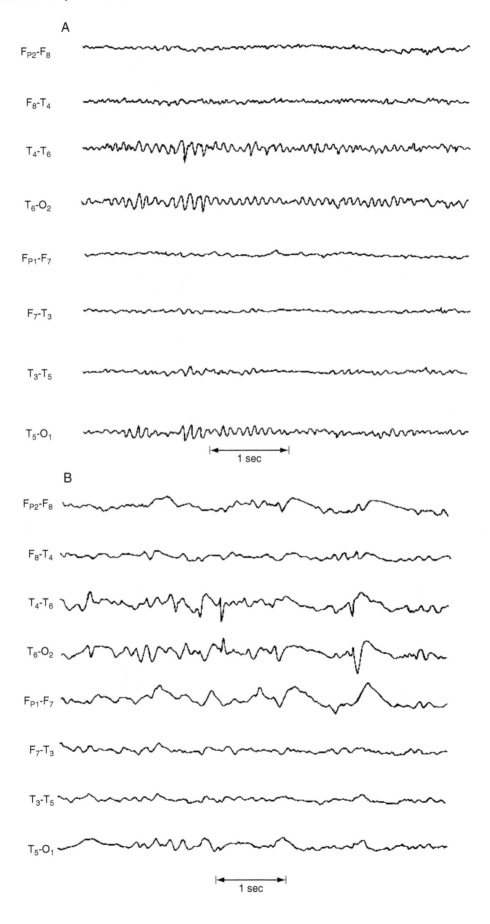

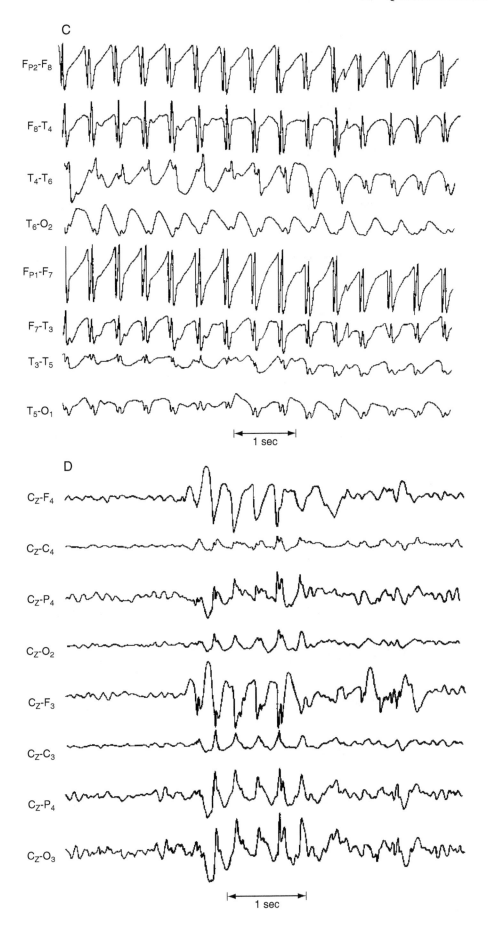

TIAs AND STROKES

Transient ischemic attacks (*TIAs*) and *strokes* cause readily recognizable constellations of transient or permanent neurologic deficits. Psychiatrists should be able to recognize their physical manifestations and anticipate their most common accompanying neuropsychologic sequelae, including amnesia, depression, and altered level of consciousness. Psychiatrists should also be able to distinguish TIAs and strokes from conditions that produce similar clinical manifestations, such as seizures and brain tumors.

TRANSIENT ISCHEMIC ATTACKS

As their name suggests, transient ischemic attacks (TIAs) are temporary interruptions in the cerebral circulation that give rise to neurologic deficits. Most TIAs resolve in 30 to 60 minutes, and only 10% last longer than 4 hours.

The traditional definition of TIA required that deficits resolve within 24 hours of onset. In 2009, the American Heart Association/American Stroke Association redefined TIA as "a transient episode of neurological dysfunction caused by focal brain, spinal cord, or retinal ischemia without infarction." Thus, regardless of symptom duration, the new definition of TIA requires the absence of infarction – if infarction is actually present, the diagnosis is stroke rather than TIA. In practice, the most efficient modality for determining whether cerebral infarction is present is magnetic resonance imaging (MRI).

The majority of TIAs result from aggregates of platelets that arise on the surface of atherosclerotic plaques that have built up on the inner wall of the *extracranial arteries*: i.e., the carotid and vertebral arteries and the aortic arch. The plaques are usually ulcerated and cause some degree of stenosis. When these platelet emboli break off, they travel distally and lodge in a cerebral artery, temporarily interrupting the local circulation and inducing a brief period of ischemia; subsequently the emboli break up and blood flow is restored. Alternatively, cardiac arrhythmias, hypotension, and other causes of cerebral hypoperfusion can produce TIAs.

TIAs cause only temporary neurologic deficits, but importantly they reflect underlying atherosclerotic cerebrovascular disease and represent a risk factor for stroke. An atherosclerotic plaque can cause a stroke by growing large enough to occlude an extracerebral vessel or by throwing off an embolus that permanently blocks a "downstream" cerebral artery. Within the first 2 days after a TIA, approximately 5% of patients suffer a stroke, and within the first month, approximately 12% develop one.

TIAs mimic other transient neurologic conditions, particularly focal seizures, postictal confusion and (Todd's) paralysis, hemiplegic migraine, metabolic derangements, adverse reactions to medicines, and, rarely, effects of cerebral mass lesions. In addition, when TIAs produce aphasia, amnesia, or another neuropsychologic deficit but no physical impairment, they can mimic psychogenic episodes.

Carotid Artery TIAs

Platelets commonly aggregate on plaques at the common carotid artery bifurcation (Fig. 11.1) and if they embolize and travel up the internal carotid artery they can lead to cerebral hemisphere TIAs. Occasionally, auscultation over the carotid artery bifurcation reveals a harsh systolic sound (*bruit*) that suggests carotid artery stenosis. In the event of a complete carotid artery occlusion, where no blood flow is present, no bruit will be audible.

Contralateral hemiparesis and/or hemisensory loss is most typical of carotid artery TIAs. A TIA also may induce neuropsychologic aberrations, the nature of which will depend upon whether the involved carotid artery irrigates the dominant or nondominant hemisphere. For example, dominant hemisphere TIAs may cause transient aphasia or apraxia, while nondominant hemisphere TIAs may cause short-lived neglect or hemi-inattention. Occasionally, TIAs cause neuropsychological manifestations unaccompanied by hemiparesis or other physical deficits.

Sometimes a TIA causes only brief visual loss in one eye, i.e., monocular blindness. Neurologists call this distinctive symptom *amaurosis fugax* (Greek, fleeting darkness). The underlying mechanism consists of emboli from the internal carotid artery traveling into the ophthalmic artery, the internal carotid artery's first branch, to induce several minutes of ischemia in the retina and optic nerve (Box 11.1). Amaurosis fugax is usually painless. Fundoscopy may demonstrate retinal emboli (Hollenhorst plaques) of atheromatous material that has embolized from the more carotid artery and traveled distally.

Laboratory Tests

When a patient experiences a transient neurologic deficit, neurologists invariably order cerebral imaging – usually computed tomography (CT) and, when possible, MRI, – to see if the patient sustained a stroke or harbors a structural lesion. When stroke or TIA is suspected they routinely request several tests in hopes of determining the specific cause: an electrocardiogram (ECG) and a 24-hour recording of the heart rhythm (Holter monitor) to look for cardiac arrhythmias, an echocardiogram to seek a cardiac source of emboli, and imaging of the intracranial and extracranial arteries with magnetic resonance imaging angiography (MRA) and/or ultrasound studies

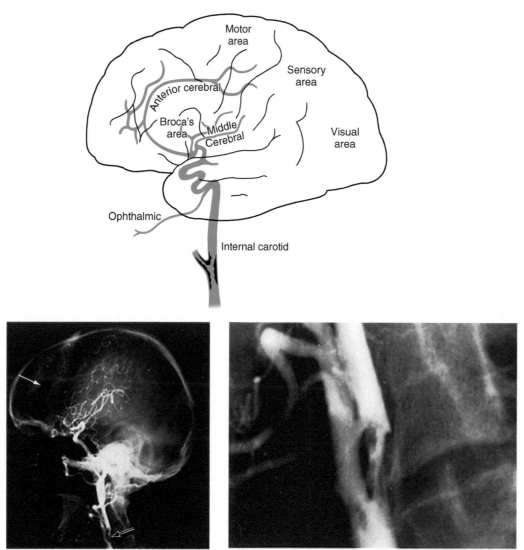

FIGURE 11.1 ■ *Top,* At its bifurcation in the neck, the common carotid artery divides to form the external and internal carotid arteries. Giving off no branches until it is within the skull, the internal carotid artery first sends off the ophthalmic artery. It then gives rise to the posterior communicating artery (not the posterior cerebral artery) and anterior choroidal artery. The internal carotid artery then divides into the anterior and middle cerebral arteries. Thus each internal carotid artery perfuses the ipsilateral eye and anterior and middle portions of the ipsilateral cerebral hemisphere. The *middle cerebral artery* supplies the deep and midsection of the hemisphere. This region contains most of the motor cortex, sensory cortex, and, in the dominant hemisphere, the perisylvian language area (see Fig. 8.1). Each *anterior cerebral artery* supplies the frontal lobe, including the medial surface of the motor cortex, which contains the motor innervation for the leg. *Bottom Left,* An arteriogram of the carotid artery and its branches prominently displays the bifurcation (*black arrow*), the typical "candelabra" of branches that comprise the middle cerebral artery, and a faint anterior cerebral artery that sweeps from anterior to posterior (*white arrow*). *Bottom Right,* A magnification of the bifurcation reveals an extensive circumferential plaque constricting the internal carotid artery. The remaining blood flow appears as an "apple core." The rough interior surface of the artery gives rise to retinal and cerebral emboli.

(carotid duplex). They also request blood tests, particularly seeking evidence of modifiable stroke risk factors such as elevated cholesterol or blood glucose levels. If seizures are possible, the physician may consider obtaining an electroencephalogram (EEG).

Preventative Measures

The goal of treatment is not merely to prevent recurrence of TIAs, but to prevent a stroke. In conjunction with the patient's internist, neurologists generally suggest lifestyle modifications to reduce stroke risk, such as smoking cessation, weight reduction, and treatment of hypertension, diabetes, and elevated cholesterol. In addition, neurologists usually suggest inhibiting platelet aggregation with aspirin (81 mg daily), clopidogrel (Plavix), or a dipyridamole–aspirin combination (Aggrenox). In many patients with atrial fibrillation, they may suggest warfarin (Coumadin) or one of the newer oral anticoagulants, dabigatran (Pradaxa), rivaroxaban (Xarelto), or apixaban (Eliquis), to prevent cardioembolism.

For TIA patients with atherosclerotic plaque causing at least 70% stenosis of the internal carotid artery, neurologists often recommend a carotid endarterectomy. This is invasive, delicate surgery in which surgeons briefly open the carotid artery to remove the plaque. Although

BOX 11.1	Carotid Artery Transient Ischemic Attacks

Symptoms
    Contralateral hemiparesis, hemianopia, hemisensory loss
    Aphasia, if dominant hemisphere
    Neglect and hemi-inattention, if nondominant hemisphere
    Ipsilateral amaurosis fugax
Associated findings
    Carotid bruit
    Retinal artery emboli
Tests
    Ultrasonography (carotid Doppler studies)
    Magnetic resonance imaging angiography (MRA)
    Cerebral arteriography
Therapy
    Medical: platelet inhibitors, e.g., aspirin
    Risk-reduction measures, e.g., control blood pressure, glucose levels, cholesterol, etc.
    Surgical: carotid endarterectomy, if stenosis >70% and symptomatic
    Endovascular: placement of stent

BOX 11.2	Vertebrobasilar Artery Transient Ischemic Attacks

Symptoms
    Vertigo, vomiting, tinnitus
    Circumoral paresthesias or numbness
    Dysarthria, dysphagia
    Drop attacks
Associated findings
    Nystagmus
    Ataxia
    Cranial nerve abnormalities
Tests
    Ultrasonography (transcranial Doppler studies)
    Magnetic resonance imaging angiography (MRA)
    Cerebral arteriography
Therapy
    Medical: platelet inhibitors*
    Risk-reduction measures*
    Surgical: none

*See Box 11.1.

effective, carotid endarterectomy carries substantial risk because it briefly interrupts the cerebral blood supply and potentially allows pieces of the plaque to enter the cerebral circulation that can embolize and cause a stroke. Carotid endarterectomy for asymptomatic individuals with comparably severe carotid stenosis may also be indicated to prevent a stroke; however, the criteria remain less clear than in patients with symptomatic stenosis. No procedure is feasible for a completely occluded artery.

For patients who cannot undergo carotid endarterectomy, an alternative is intravascular insertion of stents. These devices are essentially expandable tubes that neuroradiologists insert through a catheter into the carotid artery to widen atherosclerotic stenoses (see Fig. 20.28). They also trap underlying atheromatous debris against the inner surface of the arterial wall to reduce the likelihood of emboli. In contrast to the benefits of inserting stents into the extracranial carotid arteries, inserting stents into intracerebral arteries, such as the basilar or middle cerebral artery, carries more risk, limiting its widespread use.

Basilar Artery TIAs

The *vertebrobasilar system* – sometimes referred to simply as the *posterior circulation* – supplies the brainstem, cerebellum, occipital lobes, and medial-inferior portion of the temporal lobes (Fig. 11.2). Emboli-generating plaques tend to develop at the origin of the vertebral arteries (from the subclavian arteries) and at their junction at the base of the brain.

Symptoms and signs of basilar artery TIAs (Box 11.2), which usually reflect patchy brainstem ischemia, differ greatly from those of carotid artery TIAs. Typical basilar artery TIA symptoms include tingling around the mouth (circumoral paresthesias), dysarthria, nystagmus, diplopia, ataxia, and vertigo. On rare occasions, when all blood flow through the basilar artery momentarily stops, almost the entire brainstem suffers from ischemia. The brainstem ischemia interrupts consciousness and body tone, which causes patients to collapse suddenly and unexpectedly. (Such events, sometimes termed "drop attacks," may appear similar to cataplexy [see Chapter 17].)

Until recently, neurologists had attributed *transient global amnesia* (TGA), manifest primarily by the acute onset of anterograde amnesia for several hours, to TIA-induced ischemia of the temporal lobes. Various lines of evidence now point to other causes of TGA (see Chapter 7).

Although vertigo represents one of the most characteristic symptoms of basilar artery TIAs, disruption of the peripheral vestibular system in the inner ear can also cause it. (As a medical symptom, vertigo denotes a sensation of the patient or the surroundings revolving or otherwise moving. The thoughtful physician should label no other descriptions as vertigo. In particular, the common complaint of "dizziness" has no clinical value because patients may use the term to mean imbalance, lightheadedness, anxiety, confusion, altered vision, or almost any other ailment.)

The evaluation of basilar artery symptoms typically includes – as with assessment of carotid artery symptoms – MRI, MRA, and evaluation for cardiac and systemic illness. In addition, a transcranial Doppler examination harmlessly uses ultrasound to measure blood flow in the vertebrobasilar system. For treatment, neurologists prescribe the same medications used for carotid artery TIAs. Because the usual sites of vertebrobasilar stenosis remain shielded by the chest, vertebrae, and skull, endarterectomy is not feasible.

STROKE

Strokes cause permanent physical and neuropsychologic deficits. Most result from an arterial thrombosis, embolus, or hemorrhage. Feeling that there is nothing accidental

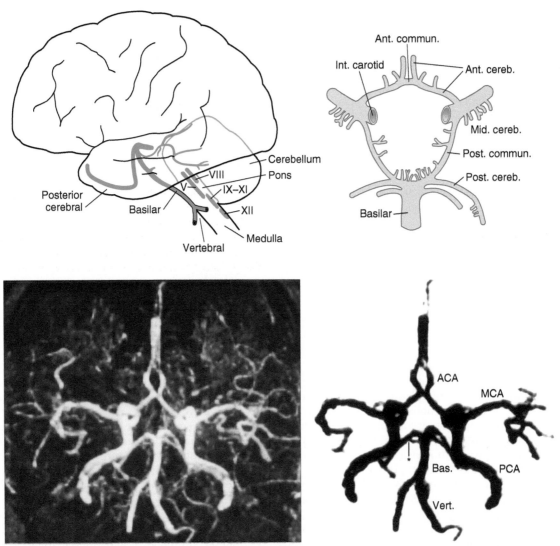

FIGURE 11.2 ■ *Top left,* After ascending, encased in the cervical vertebrae, the two vertebral arteries enter the skull. They join to form the basilar artery at the base of the brain. Small, delicate branches of the basilar artery supply the brainstem and its contents. (The Roman numerals refer to cranial nerve nuclei.) Large branches, as if wrapping their arms around the brainstem, supply the cerebellum and posterior portion of the cerebrum (i.e., the occipital lobes and inferomedial portions of the temporal lobes). The posterior cerebral arteries are the terminal branches of the basilar artery. They supply the occipital cortex and the inferior aspect of the temporal lobes. *Top right,* The circle of Willis is completely patent in only about 20% of people. Connections between the basilar and internal carotid arteries ideally form the circle, which should give off the anterior, middle, and posterior cerebral arteries. The circle should provide anastomoses between anterior–posterior and right–left cerebral circulations. Despite the advantages that the circle confers, junctions of the arteries are weak spots. Defects at the junctions may balloon outward to form berry aneurysms that rupture and produce subarachnoid hemorrhages. *Bottom left,* This axial MRA shows the major cerebral arteries that form the circle of Willis and anterior and posterior circulations. *Bottom right,* This MRA highlights the major cerebral arteries and shows the anterior and posterior circulations. The anterior circulation consists of the middle cerebral arteries (MCA), anterior cerebral (ACA) arteries, and the anterior communicating artery, which connects the ACAs. The posterior circulation consists of the two vertebral arteries (Vert.), basilar artery (Bas.), posterior cerebral arteries (PCA), and posterior communicating arteries (*), which connect the PCAs and the basilar artery.

about strokes, neurologists have largely abandoned the term "cerebrovascular accident" in order to underscore to patients and other physicians the importance of risk factor modification in reducing stroke risk.

Risk Factors

Reflecting the goal of preventing strokes, many epidemiologic studies have been performed to identify stroke risk factors, with emphasis on those that are modifiable (Box 11.3). Although physicians customarily list stroke risk factors as individual threats, the factors actually tend to cluster. For example, obesity, elevated low-density lipoprotein (LDL) cholesterol, and hypertension frequently occur together in the metabolic syndrome. Some factors by themselves have a weak correlation with stroke, but pose a synergistic risk when paired with others. For example, cigarette smoking correlates with stroke; however, with concomitant use of oral contraceptives or in sufferers of migraine with aura, it becomes a more powerful risk factor. More striking, smokers who are hypertensive have a 20-fold greater risk. Curiously, total

BOX 11.3	Risk Factors for Strokes

UNMODIFIABLE

    Age greater than 65 years
    Chromosomal and mitochondrial mutations
    Low birth weight

STRONG MODIFIABLE (RR* >4)

    Atrial fibrillation
    Cocaine and other drug abuse
    Diabetes
    Hypertension
    Sickle cell disease
    Smoking
    Transient ischemic attack

MODERATE MODIFIABLE (RR 2–4)

    Antiphospholipid syndrome
    Migraine with aura
    Obesity
    Periodontal disease
    Physical inactivity

MILD MODIFIABLE (RR 1–2)

    Alcohol abuse
    Depression
    Postmenopausal hormone replacement therapy

*Relative risk

serum cholesterol carries a strong risk for myocardial infarctions but a weak risk for stroke.

Age older than 65 years constitutes a major risk factor. Yet, about 25% of stroke victims are younger than 65 years and 12% younger than 45 years. Hypertension, a major risk factor, leads to strokes in younger individuals as well as all adults. It is also probably the most common cause of vascular dementia (see later).

Various cardiac conditions – valvular disease, prosthetic valves, acute myocardial infarction, and atrial fibrillation – constitute stroke risk factors because they tend to produce thromboses on valves and endocardial surfaces that embolize to the brain and elsewhere. Treatment with an anticoagulant greatly reduces the incidence of embolic stroke in patients with these cardiac diseases.

Diabetes mellitus and elevated total cholesterol represent powerful risk factors for myocardial infarction but less so for stroke. In fact, for individuals younger than 45 years, elevated total cholesterol carries little risk of stroke.

Cigarette smoking and inhaling second-hand smoke convey significant risk for stroke. Even former cigarette smokers retain an almost two-fold greater risk of stroke. Although judicious alcohol drinking (one drink daily to weekly) provides a slight protective effect, heavy alcohol intake poses a risk.

Drug abuse frequently causes stroke through intravenous injection of particulate material, episodes of anoxia and hypotension, cerebral vasculitis, hypertension, and vasospasm. For example, amphetamines and cocaine are sympathomimetic stimulants that routinely lead to stroke or myocardial infarction by inducing bursts of hypertension and prolonged arterial vasospasm (see Chapter 21).

In particular, cocaine alkaloid ("crack cocaine") notoriously leads to cerebral hemorrhage. By way of contrast, marijuana intoxication or even its chronic use is not associated with stroke. Studies have also implicated over-the-counter medicines, particularly phenylpropanolamine and ephedra, which are sympathomimetic ingredients of weight-loss and cough-suppressant medicines. Because of their association with stroke, the Food and Drug Administration (FDA) has banned many of these medications.

Estrogen, when used alone for post-menopausal hormone replacement, slightly increases stroke risk. The danger from oral contraceptives is probably restricted to the original, high-dose estrogen preparations. Currently available low-dose estrogen preparations confer a negligible risk for stroke.

Elevated serum concentration of homocysteine serves as a marker for an increased risk. In the autosomal recessive genetic condition *homocystinuria*, children have a Marfan-like habitus, ocular lens displacement, and other anatomic abnormalities. More importantly, they routinely suffer strokes in childhood. Elevated homocysteine levels in adults are associated with use of antiepileptic drugs and coronary artery and peripheral vascular disease, as well as stroke. Folic acid reduces elevated serum homocysteine concentrations (see Fig. 5.9), as well as reducing the incidence of fetal neural tube defects (see Chapter 13), but surprisingly it does not reduce the incidence of stroke.

Although most risk factors relate to atherosclerosis, credible data suggest that systemic infection or vascular inflammation can also give rise to strokes. For example, elevated serum concentration of C-reactive protein (CRP), a marker for inflammation, has a strong association with stroke. Other compelling data link periodontal disease and gout to subsequent stroke.

Migraine – in general – represents a minor risk factor for stroke. Any increased risk is probably restricted to migraineurs who smoke, use oral contraceptives, or have migraine with aura.

The presence of anticardiolipin antibodies is a hallmark of the *antiphospholipid syndrome*. This syndrome produces a hypercoagulable state in which mostly young women develop repeated deep vein thromboses (DVT), suffer miscarriages, and have a susceptibility to migraine and stroke. Treatment, mostly aimed at preventing thromboses, consists of anticoagulants and sometimes immunosuppressants. Although the antiphospholipid syndrome carries no specific direct psychiatric comorbidity, its associated migraines and repeated miscarriages have psychiatric repercussions. Thus, a young woman who seeks psychiatric consultation for depression following two or more miscarriages and has a history of migraine and DVT may actually have the antiphospholipid syndrome.

Examples abound of hematologic disorders causing stroke. For example, sickle cell disease and possibly sickle cell trait lead to stroke. Because pregnancy also induces a hypercoagulable state, it causes a small but significantly increased incidence of stroke during pregnancy, delivery, and the postpartum period. In addition, several obstetric problems, such as eclampsia, venous sinus thrombosis, cortical vein thrombosis, and ruptured aneurysms, lead to stroke-like brain damage.

Surgery is a risk factor. Not surprisingly, cardiac surgery is riskier than noncardiac surgery, urgent surgery is riskier than elective surgery, and older patients are more vulnerable than younger ones.

Psychiatric Risk Factors for Stroke

Various studies have concluded that depressive symptoms, major depression, anger, negative emotions, and, as determined by the Mental Health Inventory, increased psychologic distress constitute stroke risk factors. Some early studies pertaining to depression failed to adjust for stroke-inducing behavior common among depressed individuals, such as obesity, cigarette smoking, heavy alcohol consumption, lack of exercise, noncompliance with medical regimens, and use of antidepressants. However, more recent research that accounts for these potentially confounding factors supports the conclusion that depression indeed represents an independent risk factor for stroke.

In several but certainly not all studies, typical and atypical antipsychotic agents, compared to placebo, were associated with increased risk of stroke and sudden death. The conclusion most clearly applies to medicated patients with dementia displaying psychotic behavior. Atypical and typical agents pose an approximately equal risk for stroke, but a lower risk than for myocardial infarction.

In contrast to risk factors, several factors offer some protection against stroke – at least on a statistical level. For example, drinking coffee, consuming red wine, adhering to the Mediterranean diet, and regular physical activity each reduces the incidence of stroke.

Thrombosis and Embolus

Thromboses cause stroke by occluding arteries and depriving the "downstream" brain tissue of its blood flow. Similarly, emboli originating in the heart, aortic arch, cervical extracranial arteries, or intracranial arteries may travel distally to lodge in a cerebral artery and disrupt distal cerebral blood flow. Because cerebral thromboses and emboli deprive a region of the brain of its oxygen supply, they cause *ischemic infarction*. Comprising 85% of all strokes, cerebral ischemic infarctions are by far the most common form.

Other important conditions that lead to stroke include vasculitis, drug abuse, sickle-cell disease, and other blood dyscrasias. In short, the most frequent cause of stroke consists of an abnormality of the heart, blood vessels, or blood.

The time course of a stroke can suggest whether it resulted from an embolus or a thrombosis. Cerebral emboli induce infarctions suddenly when the embolus lodges in a cerebral vessel. Usually deficits are maximal at the onset of an embolic stroke and resolve to a certain extent over the next several days. Cerebral thromboses, in contrast, generally develop slowly or wax and wane and often begin during sleep.

With both embolic and thrombotic strokes, the region surrounding the infarction becomes edematous. In large strokes, edema is most severe and neurologic deficits are most pronounced during the third to fifth days. Some clinical improvement occurs as the edema resolves and ischemic areas recover; however, the infarction remains a functionless scar. In addition to creating long-lasting clinical deficits, stroke scars are potentially epileptogenic. Approximately 50% of seizures that develop in adults older than 65 years originate from these lesions (see Chapter 10). Thus, when a patient with a history of a cortical stroke develops confusion, unresponsiveness, or abnormal movements or behavior, neurologists consider the possibility of a seizure in the differential diagnosis.

Necrosis

Ischemic strokes, like brain tumors, gunshot wounds, and other destructive processes, lead to cell death by *necrosis*. Cellular necrosis requires no cellular energy to begin or progress, but the necrotic debris (dead cells) elicits a cellular inflammatory response. In contrast, *apoptosis* – which is programmed cell death – takes place in amyotrophic lateral sclerosis (ALS), Huntington disease, and many other neurodegenerative diseases. Apoptosis also serves as the mechanism for the normal involution of several organs, including the thymus gland and ductus arteriosus. Unlike necrosis, apoptosis requires cellular energy to begin and progress, and the dead cells do not evoke an inflammatory response.

Infarctions in the Carotid Artery Distribution

A cerebral artery thrombosis or embolism produces an infarction in the distribution of the occluded artery. These strokes result in well-known clinical syndromes (see Fig. 11.1 and Box 11.4):

- *Anterior cerebral artery* infarction damages the anterior and medial aspects of the frontal lobe. It typically

---

BOX 11.4	**Common Manifestations of Strokes**

Carotid artery
  Anterior cerebral
    Contralateral lower-extremity paresis
    Mutism, apathy, pseudobulbar palsy*
  Middle cerebral
    Contralateral hemiparesis
    Hemisensory loss
    Aphasia
    Hemi-inattention
  Posterior cerebral
    Contralateral homonymous hemianopia
    Alexia without agraphia (dominant hemisphere only)
Vertebrobasilar system
  Basilar artery
    Total occlusion
      Coma
      Locked-in syndrome^
    Occlusion of branch
      Cranial nerve palsy with contralateral hemiparesis^$
      Internuclear ophthalmoplegia^#
  Vertebral artery
    Lateral medullary (Wallenberg) syndrome^

*With bilateral infarctions
^No cognitive impairment
$See Chapter 4
#See Chapter 15

causes paresis and apraxia of the contralateral leg. With bilateral anterior cerebral artery infarctions, the resulting frontal lobe damage, which is extensive, typically causes pseudobulbar palsy, apathy, mutism, personality changes, and urinary incontinence (see Chapter 7), along with paresis and apraxia in both legs.

- *Middle cerebral artery* infarction, which is the most common stroke syndrome, usually results in contralateral hemiparesis, hemisensory loss, and either aphasia with dominant hemisphere lesions or neglect with nondominant hemisphere strokes.

Infarctions in the Basilar Artery Distribution

Infarctions in the basilar artery distribution cause brainstem, cerebellar, and posterior cerebral injuries. Small brainstem infarctions usually cause constellations of cranial nerve palsies and hemiparesis, while large ones can cause coma, if not immediate death. In contrast to cerebral hemisphere infarctions, brainstem infarctions generally spare language and other cognitive function and do not lead to seizures (see Box 11.4).

The posterior cerebral arteries, as previously noted, are actually terminal branches of the basilar artery. Infarction of a posterior cerebral artery causes a contralateral homonymous hemianopia and occasionally, if in the dominant hemisphere, alexia without agraphia (see Chapter 8). Bilateral posterior cerebral artery strokes can cause cortical blindness, which sometimes leads to Anton syndrome (see Chapter 12).

Continuing a tradition dating back to the nineteenth century, neurologists love to localize small brainstem infarctions for both clinical and academic reasons. Lesions of the midbrain may cause ipsilateral oculomotor nerve palsy and contralateral paresis (see Fig. 4.9). Those in the pons may cause ipsilateral abducens nerve palsy and contralateral paresis (see Fig. 4.11). Infarctions involving the midline of the midbrain or pons can affect the medial longitudinal fasciculus (MLF) and cause internuclear ophthalmoplegia (see Chapters 12 and 15). Finally, lateral medullary infarctions, which are the most common brainstem stroke syndrome, cause Wallenberg syndrome, a complex, apparently disparate, combination including ipsilateral limb ataxia, palatal paresis, Horner's syndrome, and crossed hypalgesia (diminished pain and temperature sensation in the ipsilateral face and contralateral body). The posterior inferior cerebellar artery (PICA) is the vessel that perfuses the lateral medulla, and is usually occluded due to thrombosis or embolism in its parent vessel, the vertebral artery (see Fig. 2.10).

The clinical implication of such precise localization indicates that if the lesion is situated in the brainstem, the patient's cognitive functions will remain intact. For example, a patient with right hemiparesis and a left sixth cranial nerve palsy is unlikely to have aphasia or dementia. Even brainstem lesions that extensively damage motor pathways can spare intellectual function and preserve cognition – as in the locked-in syndrome (see later).

Hemorrhages

Cerebral or cerebellar hemorrhages typically occur abruptly and, because of increased intracranial pressure, produce the triad of headache, nausea, and vomiting. Patients are likely to lose consciousness and have profound neurologic deficits determined by the hemorrhage's location. One special example is the *cerebellar hemorrhage* because it potentially leads to rapidly fatal compression of the fourth ventricle and the underlying medulla. Compression of the fourth ventricle blocks the flow of cerebrospinal fluid (CSF), which causes obstructive hydrocephalus. Pressure on the medulla depresses respiratory drive and causes coma. Physicians can diagnose cerebellar hemorrhage by its clinical manifestations: occipital headache, gait ataxia, dysarthria, and lethargy. Once imaging studies confirm a diagnosis of cerebellar hemorrhage with hydrocephalus, neurosurgeons often immediately evacuate the hemorrhage and/or insert a ventricular shunt to relieve the pressure on the fourth ventricle and brainstem.

Hemorrhages, which are most often the result of hypertension, usually erupt in the basal ganglia, thalamus, pons, or cerebellum (see Figs. 20.13 and 20.14). Trauma and use of cocaine or anticoagulant medication also cause hemorrhages, but their location is not as predictable as with hypertension-induced hemorrhage. In a classic scenario, patients who take a monamine oxidase (MAO) inhibitor antidepressant and then, inadvertently or in a suicide attempt, consume certain foods rich in tyramine (notoriously, aged cheese or red wine) or receive meperidine (Demerol) develop cerebral hemorrhages. These combinations cause sympathomimetic effects that lead to a surge in blood pressure sufficient to cause the hemorrhage. (Notably, MAO-A inhibitors may cause this interaction, but selective MAO-B inhibitors, such as those used to treat Parkinson disease, generally do not [see Chapter 9].)

Subarachnoid hemorrhage (*SAH*) may result from a ruptured berry aneurysm or from head trauma. SAH most often produces a prostrating headache that patients classically describe as the "worst headache" of their life. SAH also produces nuchal rigidity and lethargy, but usually no lateralized signs. Exercising, straining to pass stool, and other usually benign activities can rupture an aneurysm and precipitate an SAH. A diagnostic dilemma occurs when a sudden, profound headache interrupts sex. In most cases preorgasmic or orgasmic headache is responsible (see Chapter 9), but it is imperative to consider and rule out SAH. Thus, TGA, SAH, and a migraine variant are hazards of sexual activity.

When an aneurysm ruptures, CT and MRI usually reveal blood in the subarachnoid space at the base of the brain and/or within the ventricles. A lumbar puncture (LP) yields CSF colored blood-red or, if the hemorrhage is less acute, yellow (xanthochromic). Depending on the particular case, neurologists may order CT angiography, MRA, or conventional angiography to detect an aneurysm.

The traditional treatment of a ruptured aneurysm consisted of a craniotomy to insert a clip over the neck of the aneurysm. Even for aneurysms located in accessible positions, surgical complications included vascular spasm, rupture of the aneurysm that had only been leaking, and inadvertent occlusion of the parent vessel. Current treatment options, which represent a major medical advance, include minimally invasive procedures, such as intravascular insertion of coils, epoxies, and other substances that fill the aneurysm. However, for aneurysms inaccessible by an intravascular approach, surgery remains the only option.

NEUROPSYCHOLOGIC SEQUELAE

Several large or many small (lacunar) strokes cause *vascular cognitive impairment (VCI)*, previously labeled *vascular dementia* and before that *multi-infarct dementia*. The DSM-5 labels it, depending on the severity, Major or Mild Neurocognitive Disorder Due to Vascular Disease. Despite the implication of these terms, the dementia stems not only from disruption of the cerebral circulation, which deprives neurons of oxygen and other nutrients, but also from the neuropathologic changes of Alzheimer disease that accompany those of cerebral vascular disease (see Chapter 7).

Occlusion of a cerebral artery typically destroys a discrete area of the cerebral cortex. Commonly occurring strokes produce well-known neuropsychologic syndromes, such as aphasia, Gerstmann syndrome, and hemi-inattention (see Chapter 8). Strokes in both frontal lobes, which may occur either simultaneously or in succession, cause pseudobulbar palsy and executive dysfunction (see Chapters 4 and 8).

In another mechanism, hypoxia, hypotension, decreased cardiac output, carbon monoxide poisoning, or similar catastrophes cause generalized cerebral anoxia. This insult may lead to dementia, cortical blindness, a persistent vegetative state (see later), and postanoxic myoclonus (see Chapter 18). A less severe syndrome occurs when cerebral hypoperfusion – decreased blood flow – affects only the *watershed* or *border zone areas* of the cerebral cortex that lie at the boundary of two adjacent arterial territories. An episode of cerebral hypoperfusion that reduces the oxygen supply below a critical point in the watershed area produces a *watershed infarction*. These infarctions often leave patients with weakness, visual loss, and transcortical aphasia (see Fig. 8.3D).

Poststroke Depression

Depending on many variables – stroke severity, time since the stroke, and whether the patient remains in a rehabilitation facility or has returned home – the prevalence of depression in stroke victims ranges from 20% to 50% within the first year and peaks within the first 6 months of the stroke. Mood disturbances of all varieties follow stroke more frequently than they follow either a medical illness or orthopedic injury that produces similar disabilities. The majority of patients with poststroke depression enjoy a remission within the first year after the stroke, but 20% remain depressed at 3 years.

Risk factors for poststroke depression begin with the generally recognized risk factors for depression, such as a history of depression, close family member with depression, and ill health. Disease-specific risk factors reflect the severity of the stroke, such as physical dependence,

functional impairments, degree and extent of paresis, curtailed activities of daily living (ADLs), and cognitive impairment, including aphasia. By way of comparison, depression complicates vascular dementia more often than Alzheimer disease dementia.

When it occurs, poststroke depression impairs patients' recovery and lengthens their hospitalization. Depressed patients do not fully participate in their rehabilitation program or optimize their remaining cognitive function. They recover fewer ADLs. As a corollary of this fact, physicians might investigate stroke patients for depression when they fail to meet expectations for recovery.

In addition to inducing morbidity, post-stroke depression portends increased mortality. Mortality rates are significantly higher at 1 and 10 years for post-stroke depression patients. Moreover, even though the physical incapacity of many stroke victims prevents their acting upon suicide ideation, their suicide rate is two times that of age-matched controls. To place that figure in context, relative to the general population, suicide prevalence is increased up to ten-fold in Huntington disease patients, seven-fold in multiple sclerosis patients, and four-fold in epilepsy patients. Risk factors for suicide in stroke patients include prior stroke, impaired ADLs, and depressive symptoms.

In some, but not all studies, remission of poststroke depression has correlated with improved rates of recovery of ADLs and other physical measures. Remission also has correlated with improved cognitive function.

Before leaping to the diagnosis of post-stroke depression, physicians should keep in mind that some stroke symptoms may mimic depression. Failing to appreciate them may lead to misdiagnosis and unwarranted prescriptions. For example, patients with a nondominant hemisphere stroke may deny having a hemiparesis, not because of depression, but because of anosognosia. Also, their conversations may lose their emotional tone because of aprosody (see Chapter 8). In another situation, strokes – individually or in succession – that damage both frontal lobes frequently result in apathy, pseudobulbar palsy with unprovoked crying and emotional incontinence (see Chapter 4), or a paucity of verbal output because of abulia (see Chapter 7). Finally, following several strokes, patients often develop sleep disturbances and vegetative symptoms.

To compound the diagnostic difficulty, medical care itself may produce complications that mimic depression. For example, some medications – such as beta-blockers and antiepileptic drugs – frequently administered to stroke patients may induce or exacerbate depressive symptoms and cognitive impairment. Also, sleep deprivation, uncomfortable or painful procedures, and psychologic factors, such as disorientation, fear, and isolation, may express themselves as withdrawal and expressions of hopelessness.

Several studies have challenged the classic notion that strokes in the left frontal lobe most often cause poststroke depression. These studies have reported equally strong correlations between depression and lesions in the right as well as the left cerebral hemisphere, and occasionally depression secondary to strokes in the basal ganglia, thalamus, and other subcortical structures.

Several trials of treatment of poststroke depression have reported success with tricyclic antidepressants, selective serotonin reuptake inhibitors (SSRIs), and, in the elderly, psychostimulants. However, most trials found that antidepressants did not prevent depression or improve functional outcome. Moreover, no consensus emerged as to the best antidepressant, much less showed that any had a major impact. Psychological treatments in several studies improved patients' mood, but they did not help other parameters. Although electroconvulsive therapy may cause more confusion than usual in stroke patients, overall it is safe and effective.

Other Psychiatric Complications

Following a stroke, approximately 10% to 25% of patients, particularly women and younger patients, have anxiety. When it occurs, poststroke anxiety typically leads to unpleasant physical manifestations, including insomnia and decreased energy. It also impairs function and rehabilitation. In the majority of these patients, depression is comorbid. As with poststroke depression, poststroke anxiety has no consistent anatomic correlation. No specific therapy is approved for pure poststroke anxiety, but when it is comorbid with depression, antidepressants may help.

In contrast to the frequent occurrence of poststroke depression, mania follows a stroke only rarely. Moreover, studies have not determined its characteristics, underlying pathology, or treatment.

Delusions, hallucinations, and other symptoms of psychosis also rarely develop after a stroke. When these symptoms occur, they typically reflect preexisting dementia. Unlike other poststroke psychiatric problems, poststroke psychosis should prompt physicians to consider the possibility of seizures.

ALTERED LEVELS OF CONSCIOUSNESS

Depending on their etiology, multiplicity, and location, strokes may induce cognitive impairment, altered level of consciousness, or specific neuropsychologic deficits. These disturbances often affect patient's decisional capacity. Families, medical colleagues, and lawyers often ask psychiatrists and neurologists to determine if a patient's stroke has deprived them of their decisional capacity.

Neurologists usually describe the levels of consciousness with adjectives such as, in descending order, *alert, lethargic, stuporous,* or *comatose.* Not to belabor the obvious, but alert patients are characteristically awake and have their eyes open. Being alert is a prerequisite – but certainly not a guarantee – for the essential human qualities of awareness, cognitive functioning, and emotional capability. Being alert reflects a functioning cerebral cortex, brainstem, and reticular activating system. However, patients who appear alert have not necessarily retained consciousness or decisional capacity. For example, patients with advanced Alzheimer disease and those who have survived profound cerebral anoxia may seem alert because they have open eyes and look at physicians and family members, but they typically have incapacitating cognitive impairment. In the opposite situation, some patients with no motor function, such as those with the

locked-in syndrome (see later), retain their cognition, personality, and decisional capacity.

In contrast, lethargic patients remain with their eyes closed and appear asleep, but with sufficient stimulation they may open their eyes and temporarily assume an awake state. Nevertheless, even when awake they are typically inattentive, disoriented, and cognitively impaired.

Although lethargy is normal in certain circumstances, such as sleep-deprivation, it may represent dysfunction of the entire cerebral cortex or the brainstem, particularly its reticular activating system. Greater depression in the level of consciousness – stupor and coma – reflects even more profound impairment of these structures. Common disorders that cause lethargy and more depressed levels of consciousness include toxic-metabolic aberrations, multiple or large structural lesions, traumatic brain injury (TBI), and increased intracranial pressure. Lethargy is also the most common symptom of delirium, which neurologists call "toxic-metabolic encephalopathy"; however, patients in delirium often have hallucinations, physical agitation, and hypervigilance rather than lethargy.

Compared to lethargy, stupor is a more depressed level of consciousness. Stuporous patients remain unarousable and their eyes remain closed. Verbal or tactile stimuli elicit only rudimentary motor or verbal responses. Structural lesions, metabolic aberrations, and increased intracranial pressure may all cause stupor. In addition, structural lesions usually also produce lateralized signs, such as hemiparesis, and indications of increased intracranial pressure, such as papilledema.

Coma, which neurologists often grade using the Glasgow Coma Scale (see Chapter 22), is the most profound depression of consciousness. Comatose patients have closed eyes, make little or no verbal response, and move their limbs only as a reflex. They have no meaningful interaction with their environment.

In practice, these states of depressed levels of consciousness typically last several hours to weeks. Even patients with widespread neurologic injuries usually evolve into the locked-in syndrome, persistent vegetative state, or minimally conscious state.

Locked-in Syndrome

Among their innumerable patients who have sustained strokes, TBI, or other structural lesions and appear completely incapacitated, neurologists search for the rare patient with *locked-in syndrome*. These patients remain mute, quadriplegic, bedridden, and totally dependent on caregivers; however, they actually are alert, have *intact decisional capacity*, and can communicate by moving their eyes. In other words, their completely disabled body encases ("locks in") an intact mind.

The locked-in syndrome usually results from a stroke that damages the base (ventral portion) of the pons (*basis pontis,* see Fig. 2.9) and medulla. The cause is usually a thrombosis or embolus that occludes the basilar artery (see Fig. 11.2). The stroke causes bulbar palsy and interruption of the bilateral corticospinal tracts. It renders patients mute, quadriplegic, apneic, and dysphagic. Patients almost always require tracheostomy, ventilator support, and feeding tubes. Although locked-in patients have lost almost all their motor ability, their higher functions, like language comprehension and cognitive ability, remain intact.

The locked-in syndrome results not only from brainstem stroke. Several peripheral nervous system (PNS) diseases, such as myasthenia gravis, ALS, and Guillain–Barré syndrome (see Chapters 5 and 6), may weaken cranial and limb muscles sufficiently to abolish movement.

Despite the devastating damage in the locked-in syndrome, the upper brainstem, reticular activating system, and cerebral cortex remain intact. Moreover, the physiologic circuits between the cerebral cortex and upper brainstem, including the thalamus, remain intact (Fig. 11.3). Thus, locked-in patients retain cognition, affective capacity, and, given sufficient cues, a sleep–wake cycle. Patients who are otherwise completely paralyzed can still purposefully move their eyes and eyelids. By closing their eyelids in a "yes" or "no" pattern, they can communicate by answering questions.

Patients with locked-in syndrome retain cognizance and decisional capacity. They comprehend people talking and reading to them, and can convey their wishes, including decisions regarding their medical care. In fact, locked-in syndrome patients may direct the removal of their own artificial life-sustaining equipment. Patients in a locked-in syndrome from a brainstem stroke may partially recover, but their overall prognosis is poor. In contrast, patients debilitated from a PNS illness often fully recover.

Physicians might examine stroke victims (and those with severe, extensive PNS disease) for the locked-in syndrome if they are unable to speak or move their limbs, but have their eyelids open and voluntarily look from side to side. The physician should ask these patients to blink a certain number of times. If they correctly respond, the patient, physician, and family can establish a system of communication. If patients can blink meaningfully, the physician should test their ability to see and calculate. Afterward, physicians can undertake detailed mental status testing. A recent device allows locked-in patients to communicate by looking at a monitor and directing their gaze to a desired target among a variety of choices, including letters, objects, or common requests.

In a classic case, a Navy veteran with locked-in syndrome due to stroke communicated in Morse code using eyelid blinks. In another example, a motor vehicle crash left an editor of the Paris fashion magazine *Elle*, Jean-Dominique Bauby, in the locked-in syndrome. By blinking to an assistant, he dictated a short autobiography that was made into the film with the same title, *The Diving Bell and the Butterfly*.

Persistent Vegetative State

Extensive cerebral cortex damage sparing the brainstem may cause the *persistent vegetative state* (PVS). Like locked-in patients, PVS patients remain bedridden with quadriparesis and incontinence, but their eyelids open and their eyes move about. However, in contrast to locked-in patients, PVS patients lack awareness of themselves and their surroundings, have no cognitive function, and cannot communicate in any manner because of the damage to their cortex. Neurologists sometimes describe this state as "wakefulness without awareness" (Figs. 11.4 and 11.5). Nevertheless, the undamaged brainstem

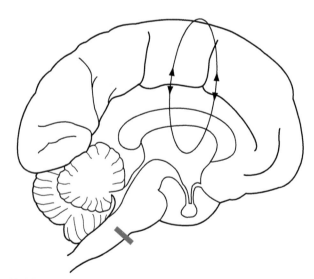

FIGURE 11.3 ■ The locked-in syndrome usually results from an infarction of the ventral or basilar portion of the lower brainstem, typically at the basis pontis (see Fig. 2.9). A lesion in this area (indicated by the bar) would sever the corticospinal tracts and directly injure cranial nerves IX through XII. However, it would not damage several vital systems: (1) the reticular activating system of the brainstem; (2) the cerebral hemispheres, particularly the cerebral cortex; and (3) the cerebral and brainstem system that governs ocular movement (see Fig. 12.11). This lesion, which is nowhere near the cortex, would not affect the brain's cognitive, language, or visual centers. The EEG is relatively normal because the lesion also spares the circuits reverberating between the thalamus and the cerebral cortex (indicated by the loop), which generate the organized, relatively regular background EEG activity.

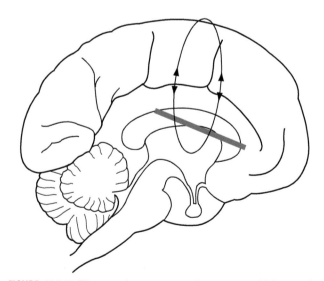

FIGURE 11.4 ■ The persistent vegetative state, which can be caused by cerebral anoxia or numerous other conditions, results from extensive damage to the cerebral cortex or the tissue immediately underlying it (indicated by the bar). These injuries impair all cerebral functions, including cognitive ability, purposeful motor activity, vision, and speech.

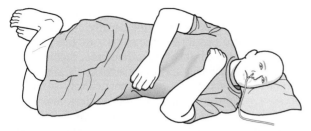

FIGURE 11.5 ■ Patients in the persistent vegetative state tend to assume a decorticate (flexed or fetal) posture because of extensive cerebral damage. Appearing to be awake, they remain mute, unable to respond to visitors or examiners, and motionless except for breathing and roving eye movements. Patients almost always require combinations of nasogastric tubes, intravenous lines, urinary catheters, and tracheostomies. Being immobile and requiring mechanical devices, they are vulnerable to aspiration pneumonia, urinary tract infections, and decubitus ulcers.

continues to regulate the body's vegetative functions, such as metabolism, breathing, temperature regulation, and digestion. Also, unlike comatose patients, PVS patients continue their sleep–wake cycle.

Damage to the cortex and cortical–brainstem connections in the PVS renders the EEG abnormal. The damage also causes positron emission tomography (PET) and functional MRI (fMRI) to show generalized, markedly reduced cerebral glucose metabolism and blood flow.

In what might constitute a misleading appearance of consciousness, PVS patients lie in bed with open eyelids, retain sleep–wake periods, and move their limbs as a reflex or in response to noxious stimulation. In addition, their eyes, moving spontaneously and randomly, may momentarily fix on a face or reflexively turn toward voices or other sounds. Yet PVS patients perform none of these actions consciously or deliberately. Unfortunately, relatives may misinterpret patients' appearance, eye movements, and other activities as appreciating their presence or understanding their words. Relatives often not only overestimate the patient's cognition and awareness, they may treat the patients as if they were suffering, in a state of suspended animation, or only partially unconscious.

Extensive cerebral insults, including TBI, anoxia, profound hypoglycemia, multiple or massive strokes, and progression of neurodegenerative illnesses – particularly Alzheimer disease and childhood-onset metabolic disorders – often lead to PVS. After an acute insult, some patients remain comatose for weeks before entering a vegetative state and after 1 month in that condition, patients fall into the category of *persistent* vegetative state. Patients with neurodegenerative illnesses usually slip into the PVS without first entering coma. Once patients have been in TBI-induced PVS for 1 year or from neurodegenerative illness for 3 months, they have no realistic chance of recovery.

Beyond its heart-wrenching aspects, PVS raises important ethical and legal considerations. Acting on patients' living wills or other directions that they "not live like a vegetable," health-care proxies have sought to discontinue nutrition and artificial support. Other proxies with different values have sought to maintain artificial support despite its futility. Several well-known legal cases have explored the limits of maintaining PVS patients in accordance with their own or their proxy's wishes in the absence of any known advanced directives. When documentation is lacking, courts generally have allowed the health-care proxy to make decisions, including removing food and nutrition.

Minimally Conscious State

Patients in the *minimally conscious state* have a reduced level of conscious and impaired awareness of themselves and their environment due to stroke or other cerebral insult, but not to the degree seen in either coma or vegetative state. Patients in this state display discernible behavioral evidence of consciousness. Their behavior must appear on a reproducible and sustained basis, and not merely constitute a reflex. As examples, patients must follow one or more simple commands; gesture or say "yes" and "no" (regardless of accuracy); speak intelligibly; smile or cry appropriately (not reflexively); respond to questions by speech or gesture; or use their hands to reach or manipulate objects. These patients may consciously perceive pain. Although the etiologies are similar, patients in the minimally conscious state generally have a more favorable outcome than those in the PVS.

In contrast to the EEG and PET in the persistent vegetative state, which fail to show meaningful cerebral cortical activity, these studies in the minimally conscious state may show some organized cerebral cortical activity.

MANAGING STROKE

Laboratory Tests

In most cases of stroke, CT or MRI confirms the diagnosis or reveals an alternative diagnosis such as brain tumor, abscess, or subdural hematoma (see Chapter 20). CT indicates the presence and location of most strokes, except those that are very acute, small, or located in the brainstem or elsewhere in the posterior fossa (where bone artifacts may obscure them). Compared to CT, MRI provides better resolution of small strokes, visualizes those in areas of the brain surrounded by bone, and, by using special imaging sequences, shows acute infarctions. MRA can visualize extra- and intracranial cerebral arteries and most regions of stenosis and occlusion (see Chapter 20).

Examination of the CSF through an LP is unnecessary for a routine stroke. However, if imaging does not show a stroke, LP is valuable for seeking evidence of SAH, meningitis, or encephalitis, all of which may mimic an ischemic stroke. Physicians must remember to avoid performing the procedure in the presence of an intracranial mass lesion (see Transtentorial Herniation, Chapter 19).

Therapy

For acute ischemic strokes, neurologists may administer thrombolytic agents, such as tissue plasminogen activator (tPA), which ideally will dissolve cerebral arterial occlusions and restore distal blood flow. As could be anticipated, tPA carries the potential for cerebral hemorrhage and other complications. Because of its dangers, neurologists must administer tPA according to a rigorous set of guidelines, including giving it within 3 hours in most patients and 4.5 hours in selected patients after the onset of a stroke, and withholding it if the patient has undergone major surgery within the previous 14 days, the blood pressure exceeds 185/110, bleeding parameters fall outside a narrow range, or a CT shows signs of intracranial hemorrhage. In recent years, interventional radiologists have developed potentially helpful techniques, such as administering thrombolytic agents intraarterially through an angiography catheter directly to a thrombus and retrieving clots by a mechanical device. Multiple trials of neuroprotective agents (medications intended to preserve ischemic brain tissue) have been disappointing. Steroids and vasoactive medicines have no proven benefit.

Medical and nursing care aims to prevent stroke complications, such as aspiration pneumonia, decubitus ulcers, deep vein thromboses (DVTs), and urinary tract infections. Treatment of fever and hyperglycemia may improve outcomes. If the patient is not alert or has a depressed gag reflex, neurologists administer medications and nutrition intravenously or through a nasogastric tube. To prevent decubiti, which are unsightly, malodorous, and liable to lead to sepsis, neurologists usually order air mattresses, sweat-absorbent bed surfaces (e.g., artificial sheepskins), and elbow and heel cushions for paretic limbs. Because urinary incontinence adds to the likelihood of developing decubitus ulcers, leaves patients cold and wet, and creates repugnant odors, neurologists generally order catheters or diapers. Prophylaxis against deep vein thrombosis is standard.

Poststroke medical care also aims to prepare the patient for rehabilitation. Staff should position patients in a way that allows them to interact optimally with their environment while accounting for deficits such as hemianopia or neglect.

In the initial phase, relatives of stroke patients can be helpful by orienting the patient and bringing a luminous dial clock, a calendar, and pictures; repositioning the patient; moving paretic limbs to avoid contractures; and locating appropriate rehabilitation facilities. Eventually many relatives have difficulty in coping with the patient's disabilities and develop caregiver stress. They have depression at about three times the usual rate.

Physical therapy will often maintain the patient's muscle tone, forestall decubitus ulcers, and prevent contractures. It will usually help patients with simple hemiparesis to regain the ability to walk, circumvent some impediments, and avoid expeditious but maladaptive physical compensations. Moreover, physical therapy necessarily entails the "laying-on of hands," which conveys emotional as well as physical support.

Speech therapy may help with dysarthria and dysphagia and offer patients encouragement; however, it probably does not restore language function in aphasia. "Cognitive and perceptual skill training" for impaired mentation, sensory impairment, and visual loss remains without proven value.

Hemi-inattention and anosognosia usually resolve spontaneously within the first month, and aphasia usually improves to almost its fullest extent by 4 to 6 weeks. Deficits persisting after that time usually do not resolve. Poor prognostic factors for recovery – as any physician might sense – are advanced age, dementia, incontinence, bilateral brain damage, and prior strokes. If asked for a consultation, psychiatrists might particularly search for depressive symptoms with or without anxiety, maladaptation, denial, and other defense mechanisms.

One influential trial found that fluoxetine imitated early after an ischemic stroke, when coupled with physical therapy, resulted in improved motor outcomes at 3 months. A 2012 meta-analysis concluded that SSRIs favorably impacted both dependence and disability in stroke patients. Although neurologists do not universally prescribe SSRIs following stroke, they certainly consider doing so if any suggestion of depression or anxiety is present.

REFERENCES

Ayerbe, L., Ayis, S., Crichton, S. L., et al. (2014). Explanatory factors for the increased mortality of stroke patients with depression. *Neurology*, *83*, 2007–2012.

Barnes, D. E., Haight, T. J., Mehta, K. M., et al. (2010). Second hand smoke, vascular disease, and dementia incidence: Findings from the cardiovascular health cognition study. *American Journal of Epidemiology*, *171*, 292–302.

Brott, T. G., Hobson, R. W., Howard, G., et al. (2010). Stenting versus endarterectomy for treatment of carotid-artery stenosis. *The New England Journal of Medicine*, *363*, 11–23.

Chimowitz, M. I., Lynn, M. J., Derdeyn, C. O., et al. (2011). Stenting versus aggressive medical therapy for intracranial arterial stenosis. *The New England Journal of Medicine*, *365*, 993–1003.

Chollet, F., Tardy, J., Albucher, J., et al. (2011). Fluoxetine for motor recovery after acute ischemic stroke (FLAME): a randomized placebo-controlled trial. *The Lancet. Neurology*, *10*, 123–130.

Cruse, D., Chennu, S., Chatelle, C., et al. (2011). Bedside detection of awareness in the vegetative state. *Lancet*, *378*, 2088–2094.

Dong, J. Y., Zang, Y. H., Tong, J., et al. (2012). Depression and risk of stroke: A meta-analysis of prospective studies. *Stroke; a Journal of Cerebral Circulation*, *42*(1), 32–37.

Easton, J. D., Saver, J. L., Albers, G. W., et al. (2009). Definition and evaluation of transient ischemic attack: A scientific statement for healthcare professionals from the American Heart Association/American Stroke Association Stroke Council; Council on Cardiovascular Surgery and Anesthesia; Council on Cardiovascular Radiology and Intervention; Council on Cardiovascular Nursing; and the Interdisciplinary Council on Peripheral Vascular Disease. *Stroke; a Journal of Cerebral Circulation*, *40*, 2276–2293.

Giacino, J. T., Ashwal, A., Childs, N., et al. (2002). The minimally conscious state: Definition and diagnostic criteria. *Neurology*, *58*, 349–353.

Henderson, K. J., Clark, C. J., Lewis, T. T., et al. (2013). Psychosocial distress and stroke risk in older adults. *Stroke; a Journal of Cerebral Circulation*, *44*, 367–372.

Jackson, C., & Mishra, G. D. (2013). Depression and risk of stroke in midaged women: a prospective longitudinal study. *Stroke; a Journal of Cerebral Circulation*, *44*, 1555–1560.

Johnston, S., Gress, D., Browner, W., et al. (2000). Short-term prognosis after emergency department diagnosis of TIA. *JAMA: The Journal of the American Medical Association*, *284*, 2901–2906.

Karaiskos, D., Tzavellas, E., Spengos, K., et al. (2012). Duloxetine versus citalopram and sertraline in the treatment of poststroke depression, anxiety, and fatigue. *The Journal of Neuropsychiatry and Clinical Neurosciences*, *24*, 349–353.

Kernan, W. N., Ovbiagele, B., Black, H. R., et al. (2014). Guidelines for the prevention of stroke in patients with stroke and transient ischemic attack: a guideline for healthcare professionals from the American Heart Association/American Stroke Association. *Stroke; a Journal of Cerebral Circulation*, *45*, 2160–2236.

Lovett, J., Dennis, M., Sandercock, P., et al. (2003). Very early risk of stroke after a first transient ischemic attack. *Stroke; a Journal of Cerebral Circulation*, *34*, e138–e140.

O'Donnell, M. J., Xavier, D., Liu, L., et al. (2010). Risk factors for ischaemic and intracerebral haemorrhagic stroke in 22 countries. *Lancet, 376,* 112–123.

Pan, A., Sun, Q., Okereke, O. I., et al. (2011). Depression and risk of stroke morbidity and mortality: A meta-analysis and systemic review. *JAMA: The Journal of the American Medical Association, 306,* 1241–1249.

Schmid, A. A., Kroenke, K., Hendrie, H. C., et al. (2011). Poststroke depression and treatment effects on functional outcomes. *Neurology, 76,* 1000–1005.

Solfrizzi, V., Scafato, E., Capurso, C., et al. (2010). Metabolic syndrome and the risk of vascular dementia: The Italian Longitudinal Study on Ageing. *Journal of Neurology, Neurosurgery, and Psychiatry, 81,* 433–440.

Surtees, P. G., Wainwright, N. W. J., Luben, R. N., et al. (2008). Psychological distress, major depressive disorder, and risk of stroke. *Neurology, 70,* 788–794.

Wechsler, L. R. (2011). Intravenous thrombolytic therapy for acute ischemic stroke. *The New England Journal of Medicine, 364,* 2138–2146.

Willey, J. Z., Disla, N., Moon, Y. P., et al. (2010). Early depressed mood after stroke predicts long-term disability. *Stroke; a Journal of Cerebral Circulation, 41,* 1896–1900.

QUESTIONS AND ANSWERS

1–10. Match the neurologic deficit (1–10) with the most likely artery or arteries responsible for the infarction (a–k).

Deficit

1. Left hemiparesis with relative sparing of the leg
2. Left lower-extremity monoparesis
3. Monocular blindness from optic nerve ischemia
4. Left homonymous hemianopia
5. Left palate paresis, left limb ataxia
6. Right third cranial nerve palsy with left hemiparesis
7. Right hemiparesis with aphasia
8. Quadriplegia and mutism with intact mentation
9. Left sixth and seventh cranial nerve palsy with right hemiparesis
10. Coma, quadriparesis

Artery

a. Right posterior cerebral
b. Left posterior cerebral
c. Right anterior cerebral
d. Right middle cerebral
e. Left anterior cerebral
f. Left middle cerebral
g. Ophthalmic
h. Vertebral or posterior inferior cerebellar
i. Perforating branch of basilar
j. Anterior spinal
k. Basilar

Answers: 1–d, 2–c, 3–g, 4–a, 5–h, 6–i, 7–f, 8–i and k, 9–i, 10–k.

11–20. Match the type of neurologic deficit (11–20) with the artery or arteries usually responsible for such a transient ischemic attack (TIA) or stroke (a–d):

Deficit

11. Hemianopia
12. Monocular amaurosis fugax
13. Paresthesias of right arm and aphasia
14. Vertigo, nausea, nystagmus, and ataxia
15. Right foot drop and areflexia
16. Locked-in syndrome
17. Diplopia
18. Cortical blindness
19. Transient hemiparesis
20. Paraparesis and anesthesia below the chest, but preserved position and vibration sensation

Artery

a. Carotid artery and its branches
b. Basilar artery and its branches
c. Both
d. Neither

Answers: 11–b, 12–a (ophthalmic artery), 13–a, 14–b, 15–d, 16–b, 17–b, 18–b, 19–c, 20–d.

21–30. After experiencing 1 week of a steadily worsening left-sided headache, a 74-year-old man seeks a neurologic evaluation. The examination reveals a nonfluent aphasia and right-sided homonymous hemianopia, hemiparesis, hyperreflexia, and Babinski sign. Which of the following should be considered as likely diagnoses (Yes/No)?

21. Cerebral hemorrhage
22. Subarachnoid hemorrhage
23. Brain tumor
24. Subdural hematoma
25. Basilar artery occlusion
26. Carotid artery occlusion
27. Brain abscess
28. Toxoplasmosis
29. Cerebral embolus
30. Multiple sclerosis (MS)

Answers:
21. No. Cerebral hemorrhages are usually catastrophic acute processes, heralded by a severe headache, that develop between several minutes and a few hours.
22. No. The headaches of a subarachnoid hemorrhage are usually cataclysmic and incapacitating. An examination of a patient with a subarachnoid hemorrhage likely would show nuchal rigidity and a depressed level of consciousness. Also, because subarachnoid hemorrhage occurs outside of the brain substance, patients usually do not have lateralized signs, such as aphasia and homonymous hemianopia. An exception would be a posterior communicating artery aneurysm rupture, which compresses the adjacent third cranial nerve.
23. Yes. A brain tumor is a valid diagnostic choice in this case. Tumors, such as a glioblastoma, produce symptoms over a period of weeks. Also, they may cause multiple signs because they infiltrate or, as in the case of metastases, are multicentric.
24. Unlikely. Although the headache and hemiparesis are consistent, subdural hematomas and other masses outside the brain substance (i.e., extra-axial lesions) rarely cause aphasia or hemianopia.

25. No. A basilar artery occlusion would interrupt the reticular activating system. It would cause coma, apnea, and quadriplegia.

26. Yes. Over the course of a week, progressive carotid artery stenosis can lead to complete occlusion and infarction of an entire cerebral hemisphere. Carotid artery stenosis may also cause ipsilateral headache.

27. Yes. As with a brain tumor, an abscess and its surrounding edema can expand rapidly enough to impair an entire cerebral hemisphere. Surprisingly, traditional signs of infection, such as fever and leukocytosis, are often minimal or entirely absent in cases of brain abscess.

28. No. Cerebral toxoplasmosis develops almost exclusively as a complication of immunosuppression. Moreover, because toxoplasmosis typically produces multiple sites of infection, it produces multifocal symptoms and signs.

29. No. Although the findings are compatible, the time course is inconsistent. Emboli occur acutely.

30. No. The single focus and older age are inconsistent with MS. Moreover, it usually does not cause a headache.

31–36. After a stroke, a 75-year-old man is alert, but mute and unable to move his palate, arms, or legs. He has bilateral hyperreflexia and Babinski signs. He responds appropriately by blinking his eyelids to verbal and written questions.

31. Does this man have aphasia, and if so is it fluent, nonfluent, or global? (Yes/No)
32. Is his vision impaired? (Yes/No)
33. Has he sustained cerebral damage? (Yes/No)
34. How would the EEG appear?
35. What is this syndrome called?
36. Where is the lesion?

Answers:

31. No. He does not have aphasia in any form because he can understand spoken language and respond appropriately. He cannot speak or write because of motor impairment.

32. No. His vision is not impaired because he can read written questions.

33. No. He has no indication of cerebral cortex damage. His ability to communicate indicates that cortical functions remain intact. Instead, the weakness of the palate and limbs reflects brainstem damage.

34. The EEG should appear normal because his cortical functions are intact.

35. His being fully alert, cognizant, and communicative, but almost completely paralyzed, indicate that he suffers from the locked-in syndrome.

36. The lesion is in the ventral surface of the lower brainstem, i.e., the base of the pons (basis pontis).

37–41. A 71-year-old woman sustained a right cerebral infarction the previous year. She has residual left-sided hemiparesis. Her family has just brought her to the emergency room after she developed the sudden, painless onset of mutism and right hemiparesis. On examination, she has bilateral paresis and no verbal output. Although her eyes are frequently open, she fails to establish eye contact or respond to either voice or gesture. She has no papilledema. She seems to have normal sleep–wake cycles.

37. Where is the probable site of the recent injury?
38. What is the probable cause?
39. Would the EEG be normal?
40. If she were not paralyzed, would she be able to write?
41. Would she have bulbar or pseudobulbar palsy?

Answers:

37. The new lesion is in the left (dominant) hemisphere. With the history of a prior right cerebral infarction, she now has bilateral cerebral infarctions.

38. The sudden, painless onset suggests a thrombotic or embolic stroke. The rapid onset and absence of signs of increased intracranial pressure exclude a mass lesion, such as a tumor or abscess.

39. The EEG will be abnormal because of extensive cerebral damage.

40. No. She has global aphasia with impairment of all avenues of communication. Moreover, as the result of extensive cerebral cortex strokes, she probably has vascular cognitive impairment (VCI), previously labeled "vascular dementia," which DSM-5 designates Major or Mild Neurocognitive Disorder Due to Vascular Disease.

41. Although proper clinical assessment requires more time, she probably will have pseudobulbar palsy due to bilateral cerebral infarctions.

42–52. A 20-year-old woman awakens from sleep and finds that she has a mild left hemiparesis. Which are the possible causes of her deficit (Yes/No)?

42. Cerebral thrombosis associated with high-dose estrogen oral contraceptives
43. Cerebral vasculitis from lupus or drug abuse
44. Cerebral embolus from mitral stenosis
45. Antiphospholipid syndrome
46. Septic cerebral embolus from bacterial endocarditis
47. Cerebral embolus from an atrial myxoma
48. Cocaine-induced stroke
49. Stroke from sickle cell disease
50. Migraine-induced transient paresis, i.e., hemiplegic migraine
51. A prolonged postictal (Todd's) paresis
52. Multiple sclerosis

Answers: All Yes. Approximately 12% of stroke victims are younger than 45 years. Causes vary somewhat by age group, but generally stroke results from diseases of the heart, blood, or blood vessels (42–49). The other processes (50–52), although not strictly strokes, may mimic them.

53–56. The family of a 25-year-old woman brings her to the emergency room because she suddenly stopped speaking and moving her right arm and leg. The patient looks directly forward and does not follow verbal or gestured requests. On inspection of her fundi, her eyes constantly evert. She seems to respond to visual images in all fields. The right arm and leg are flaccid and immobile, but her face is symmetric. The neurologist finds symmetric deep tendon reflexes (DTRs) and no Babinski sign. She does not react to noxious stimuli on the right side of her face or body.

53. Based upon the first sentence of this description, where does the lesion appear to be located?
54. (a) What abnormalities usually found with such a lesion are not present in the patient? (b) What non-neurologic features are present?
55. What is the most likely origin?
56. What readily available laboratory tests would lend great support to the diagnosis?

Answers:
53. A patient who seems to have global aphasia and a right hemiparesis would usually have a left cerebral hemisphere lesion.
54. (a) She lacks the expected right homonymous hemianopia, paresis of the right lower right face, asymmetrical DTRs, and Babinski sign. (b) Everting eyes during examination is almost always voluntary. Inability to perceive noxious stimuli is rare in cerebral lesions. Although individuals with cerebral strokes may have difficulty localizing pain, they feel it and respond. Likewise, a sharply demarcated vertical sensory loss – "splitting the midline" – is not neurologic.
55. A psychogenic disturbance is the most likely cause.
56. A normal computed tomography (CT), magnetic resonance imaging (MRI), and electroencephalogram (EEG) would support the diagnosis of a psychogenic disturbance.

57–60. A 50-year-old man experiences sudden onset of a severe occipital headache, nausea, vomiting, and an inability to walk. He has no paresis but a downward drift of the right arm and symmetrically hyperactive DTRs with equivocal plantar responses. He has dysmetria on right finger–nose and heel–shin movements. His gait is so unsteady that the medical staff must support him when he attempts to walk.

57. Where is the lesion?
58. Which side?
59. What is its origin?
60. What is the consequence of increased size of the lesion?

Answers:
57. Because he has ataxia and dysmetria the lesion is in the cerebellum.
58. When unilateral, cerebellar damage causes dysfunction on the ipsilateral side of the body, which, in this case, is his right side.
59. In view of the sudden onset of the cerebellar deficits, a stroke is the most likely cause. Because

he has a severe headache, physicians must first consider cerebellar hemorrhage. Hypertension, including cocaine-induced hypertension, is the most common cause of cerebellar hemorrhage. Occasionally, hemorrhage into a tumor results in a cerebellar hematoma.
60. If the hemorrhage were to expand, it would compress the fourth ventricle and cause obstructive hydrocephalus. With further expansion, the hemorrhage would compress the brainstem. At that point, a neurosurgeon should evacuate the cerebellar hematoma, lest it lead to coma and death.

61. Which one of the following is a typical finding in a 65-year-old man with transient global amnesia (TGA)?
    a. Retaining ability to recall his name and address
    b. Increased likelihood of a subsequent stroke
    c. A 50% chance of a TGA recurrence in the next year
    d. Retrograde amnesia much more pronounced than anterograde amnesia

Answer: a. Patients with TGA, despite amnesia, can typically state their personal identifying facts. The signature deficit is inability to recall information acquired after the onset of the attack, i.e., anterograde amnesia. TGA episodes recur in only about 10% of cases and do not represent a risk factor for stroke – factors weighing against considering TGA as a form of TIA. Preservation of patients' identity and the limited duration of the episode set TGA apart from dissociative amnesia.

62. Elevated serum concentration of homocysteine is a risk factor for stroke and myocardial infarction. Which is the best method to reduce an elevated serum homocysteine concentration?
    a. High-protein diet
    b. Statin medication
    c. Folic acid
    d. None of the above

Answer: c. Folic acid (folate) will reduce homocysteine concentration. However, that strategy, although innocuous and inexpensive, does not appear to reduce the risk of stroke or myocardial infarction. Lowering serum cholesterol, reducing blood pressure, and use of an anti-platelet medication will reduce the risk of stroke.

63. In B_{12} deficiency, which *two* serum constituents rise?
    a. Homocysteine
    b. Methylmalonic acid
    c. Folate
    d. Cystathionine

Answer: a, b: In the absence of B_{12}, which acts as a coenzyme, homocysteine and methylmalonic acid will accumulate. Administration of folate, which also acts as a coenzyme, will alleviate some features of B_{12} deficiency, such as the megaloblastic anemia. However, without concomitant administration of B_{12}, folate will not prevent subacute combined degeneration (see Fig. 5.9).

64. A 35-year-old woman sought chiropractic treatment of neck muscle spasms. In the middle of vigorous manipulation, she suddenly developed vertigo, nausea, and vomiting. On examination, a neurologist found dysarthria, nystagmus, right-sided ptosis and miosis, numbness of the left arm and leg, and ataxia on right finger-to-nose movement. What is the most likely etiology of her condition?
    a. Basilar artery occlusion
    b. Drug-induced brainstem injury
    c. Food poisoning
    d. A traumatic dissection of the right vertebral artery

Answer: d. Forceful, twisting neck movements (torsion), such as occurs in wrestling, whiplash neck injuries, and chiropractic manipulation, occasionally cause vertebral artery dissection. The dissection leads to a vertebral artery occlusion, which may lead to a stroke in the brainstem or cerebellum. In this case, a vertebral artery dissection caused the patient to have a right-sided lateral medullary syndrome.

65. Of the following, which medication category will reduce the incidence of neurocognitive disorder due to vascular disease?
    a. Estrogen replacement therapy
    b. Antioxidants, such as selegiline and alpha-tocopherol
    c. Antihypertensive medications
    d. Nonsteroidal anti-inflammatory drugs

Answer: c. Because antihypertensive medications unequivocally reduce the incidence of stroke, their use is associated with a lower incidence of stroke and its consequences, including neurocognitive disorder due to vascular disease.

66. Which of the following statements regarding post-stroke anxiety is *true*?
    a. Approximately 50% of patients with anxiety have comorbid depression.
    b. When anxiety complicates depression in stroke patients, depression has a longer duration.
    c. When it occurs without comorbid depression, poststroke anxiety does not impair function or rehabilitation.
    d. Poststroke anxiety correlates with strokes in the limbic system.

Answer: b. Almost all patients with poststroke anxiety have comorbid depression. When anxiety and depression complicate stroke recovery, depression outlasts anxiety. Even without comorbid depression, poststroke anxiety impairs function and rehabilitation. Neither poststroke depression nor poststroke anxiety has a consistent anatomic correlation.

67. An internist asked a psychiatry consultant to evaluate a 60-year-old stroke patient who, for no apparent reason, began to scream at the nurses, complained loudly about the food, and demanded that the physical therapists leave his room. The patient had woken up the previous day with left hemiplegia. Although the patient had obviously sustained a stroke, he was not eligible for tissue plasminogen activator (tPA) because more than 3 hours had elapsed since its onset. A CT and MRI showed an acute infarction in the distribution of the right middle cerebral artery. After a cardiac evaluation disclosed atrial fibrillation, the cardiologist planned to institute anticoagulation. The psychiatrist found the patient to be fully alert, attentive, and lucid, and learned that he had been functioning very well both at work and at home. He had no preceding psychiatric history and had been using no psychotropics, illicit drugs, or excessive alcohol. The patient insisted that he did not know why he was in the hospital or that he had any cardiac disease. He also said that he was "fine" and accused the admitting physician of confusing him with the other patient in the room, and giving him a "preposterous" diagnosis of stroke. He added that he wanted to leave the hospital that evening, but the nurses and the "idiot doctor" refused to discharge him. Which is the most likely explanation for the patient's irrational and potentially self-injurious behavior?
    a. Poststroke depression
    b. Poststroke psychosis
    c. Drug-seeking behavior
    d. Catastrophic reaction
    e. Toxic-metabolic encephalopathy

Answer: d. The internist most likely precipitated a catastrophic reaction in a patient with anosognosia for his left hemiplegia. The first three explanations – depression, psychosis, and drug-seeking – are tenable, but patients with those diagnoses usually are aware, perhaps overly so, of their physical deficits, and their denial is not limited to stroke-related deficits. This patient does not have toxic-metabolic encephalopathy (delirium) because he maintains a normal level of consciousness and attention.

Patients with anosognosia tend to employ classic defense mechanisms. Informing them about their deficits requires a great deal of skill. If possible, the discussion should be carried out over the course of several days. The physician might have to show patients that they have impediments rather than frankly stating the severity and extent of their paresis or other deficit. By continuing to deny their deficits, patients with anosognosia may not make realistic plans or participate in rehabilitation programs.

68. Following her third miscarriage, a 29-year-old woman sought psychiatric consultation for depression. In reviewing her history, the psychiatrists found that her migraines had flared-up and, because of a persistent recent calf cramp, she was no longer able to exercise. Which of the following tests should her physician order?
    a. Anticardiolipin antibodies
    b. Urine toxicology
    c. Lyme titer
    d. Thyroid function

Answer: a. The combination of repeated miscarriages, migraines, and deep vein thromboses indicates that she has the antiphospholipid syndrome. In this condition, anticardiolipin antibodies usually are present in the serum. Although the antiphospholipid syndrome does not directly cause depression, it causes a hypercoagulable state that leads to repeated miscarriages, migraines, and deep vein thromboses, and places her at risk of stroke and myocardial infarction.

69. A 10-year-old boy, according to his parents, has episodes of being unresponsive and having weakness on one side or the other of his body. The episodes began about 1 year before the visit, occur approximately once a month, and last several hours. He agrees with his parents' description and adds that during the episodes, his head hurts and he is nauseated. Between episodes, he is normal in every respect. Of the following, which is the most likely diagnosis?
    a. TIA
    b. Stroke
    c. Migraine
    d. Focal seizures

Answer: c. He probably has migraine with "alternating hemiplegia." Another possibility, although rarely occurring, is a mitochondrial encephalopathy with stroke-like episodes. Focal seizures are also a potential explanation, but they usually do not cause headache, paresis, or variable symptomatology.

70. Of the following, which is the most powerful stroke risk factor?
    a. "Type A" personality
    b. High-cholesterol diet
    c. Obesity
    d. Cigarette smoking
    e. Hypertension
    f. Lack of exercise

Answer: e. Hypertension is the statistically most powerful modifiable risk factor. All the others are powerful risk factors for myocardial infarction but carry relatively lower risk for stroke.

71. Which of the following is the standard therapy for vertebrobasilar artery TIAs?
    a. Endarterectomy
    b. Stenting
    c. Coumadin
    d. Aspirin

Answer: d. Aspirin or another antiplatelet agent is the usual treatment for vertebrobasilar artery TIAs. However, if the cause is a cardiac arrhythmia or cardioembolism, other treatments may be indicated.

72. Which of the following is the most important cause of neurocognitive disorder due to vascular disease?
    a. Carotid bifurcation atherosclerosis
    b. Cerebral emboli
    c. Generalized atherosclerosis
    d. Hypertension with small-vessel disease

Answer: d. Small lacunar strokes are the most important cause of neurocognitive disorder due to vascular disease; however, histologic examination generally shows Alzheimer disease pathology as well as infarctions in patients who had neurocognitive disorder due to vascular disease.

73. Which feature occurs more frequently in neurocognitive disorder due to vascular disease than in Alzheimer dementia?
    a. Depression
    b. Memory impairment
    c. Impaired judgment
    d. Delusions and hallucinations

Answer: a. Depression occurs much more frequently in vascular than Alzheimer dementia. Memory impairment is generally more pronounced in Alzheimer disease than neurocognitive disorder due to vascular disease.

74. A 28-year-old man with mild generalized headache has had a 3-day history of increasing left arm weakness and clumsiness. Examination reveals only mild left arm weakness and hyperactive DTRs. Routine medical evaluation reveals no abnormalities. Both CTs and MRIs show five large ring-enhancing cerebral lesions. Of the following, which is the most likely cause of his neurologic difficulties?
    a. Cerebral infarction
    b. Cerebral hemorrhage
    c. Toxoplasmosis
    d. Glioblastoma
    e. Meningioma

Answer: c. The most common cause of multiple ring-enhancing cerebral lesions in young adults is toxoplasmosis, which is a typical manifestation of AIDS. Cerebral lymphoma is another AIDS complication, but it usually causes only a single lesion. Cerebral infarctions in a 28-year-old man are rare; however, cocaine use, sickle cell disease, arterial dissections, antiphospholipid syndrome, and cardiac diseases that lead to emboli can cause them. Embolic strokes are usually wedge-shaped on CT or MRI. Cerebral hemorrhage is typically a sudden event, associated with blood-density on scans. A glioblastoma would also be rare in a 28-year-old individual, and the scans would have indicated an infiltrating tumor. A meningioma is likewise rare in young adults. When it does occur, a meningioma is extra-axial and slowly growing.

75–86. Match the sign (75–86) with (a) the locked-in syndrome, (b) the persistent vegetative state, (c) both, or (d) neither.

75. Mutism
76. Quadriparesis
77. Voluntary eye movement
78. Reflexive movement to light and sound
79. Sleep–wake cycles may be preserved
80. Capacity to suffer conscious pain

81. Intact cognition
82. Absence of cognition
83. Due to lesion in base of pons that spares reticular activating system
84. Due to lesions that damage virtually all of the cerebral cortex
85. Guillain–Barré syndrome or myasthenia gravis may be responsible
86. Severe cerebral anoxia or hypoglycemia may be responsible

Answers: 75–c, 76–c, 77–a, 78–c, 79–c, 80–a, 81–a, 82–b, 83–a, 84–b, 85–a, 86–b.

87. Which of the following characteristics most reliably distinguishes neurocognitive disorder due to vascular disease from Alzheimer dementia?
    a. Stepwise development
    b. Brain atrophy on MRI
    c. Aphasia
    d. Focal physical findings
    e. Greatest cognitive deficit is loss of memory
    f. Absence of plaques and tangles

Answer: d. Focal physical findings, such as hemiparesis, hemianopia, and pseudobulbar palsy, which are manifestations of infarctions in the cerebrum or brainstem, characterize neurocognitive disorder due to vascular disease. A stepwise progression of neurocognitive disorder due to vascular disease is classic, but that course is not diagnostically reliable and is not required for the diagnosis. Atrophy is seen in both conditions. Although aphasia is often comorbid with neurocognitive disorder due to vascular disease, anomic aphasia frequently occurs in Alzheimer disease. Loss of memory is a common feature and a diagnostic criterion for both conditions. Ironically, histologic examination discloses Alzheimer disease pathology, such as plaques and tangles, in the majority of cases of neurocognitive disorder due to vascular disease.

88. In patients with asymptomatic carotid stenosis, what degree of stenosis should prompt a carotid endarterectomy?
    a. 50%
    b. 70%
    c. 90%
    d. 100%
    e. Optimal medical management may be as effective as endarterectomy in preventing stroke in patients with asymptomatic carotid stenosis.

Answer: e. In the past, carotid stenosis of 70% or greater in an asymptomatic individual was felt to justify carotid endarterectomy, provided that it could be performed with little risk, i.e., morbidity of 3% or less. More recent data (e.g., the SAMMPRIS trial) suggest that optimal medical management with modern therapies (including aspirin and a statin) may be as effective as endarterectomy. Studies are underway that may help guide selection of appropriate management – medical therapy, carotid endarterectomy, or carotid artery stenting – for individual patients.

89. Which pattern is most likely found on positron emission tomography (PET) and single photon emission computed tomography (SPECT) in an individual with neurocognitive disorder due to vascular disease?
    a. Multiple, scattered hypometabolic regions
    b. Hypometabolism in the temporal and parietal association cortex
    c. Hypometabolism in the frontal lobes
    d. None of the above

Answer: a. In neurocognitive disorder due to vascular disease, multiple discrete areas of hypometabolism reflect underlying strokes. In patients with Alzheimer disease, scans initially show hypometabolism in the temporal and parietal association cortex and eventually in the frontal cortex.

90. For patients in a persistent vegetative state, who determines the health-care plans, goals of care, and whether artificial life-sustaining devices are to remain in place?
    a. Closest family member
    b. Health-care proxy
    c. Attending physician
    d. Patient

Answer: b. Patients in a persistent vegetative have lost cognitive capacity. Based on input from their physicians, their health-care proxy has the right to determine the nature and duration of medical care, even to terminate life-saving care.

91. A 73-year-old woman arises from a vigorous hair washing at her local beauty parlor and finds that she is vertiginous and nauseous. A physician finds nystagmus and truncal ataxia. Her symptoms and signs resolve over 1 hour. Which is the most likely cause of her disturbance?
    a. Carotid artery TIA
    b. Vertebrobasilar artery TIA
    c. A chemical in the hair wash
    d. Benign paroxysmal positional vertigo

Answer: b. She probably has had hyperextension (excessive backward bending) of her head and neck that compressed her vertebral arteries and caused a vertebrobasilar artery TIA. This scenario is most common in elderly people who have the combination of narrowed, atherosclerotic vertebral arteries and spinal osteophytes that press against the vertebral arteries as they pass upward through the cervical spine. This disorder is sometimes called the *vanity syndrome* because it was first described in patrons of beauty parlors who had their hair washed in basins (vanities). This case represents a variation of the cervical torsion injury that caused the vertebral artery dissection that led to the lateral medullary syndrome (Question 64).

92. Which condition involving neuronal death is characterized by cellular infiltrates but does *not* require cellular energy?
    a. Stroke
    b. Amyotrophic lateral sclerosis (ALS)

c. Huntington disease
d. Parkinson disease

Answer: a. Cellular infiltrates characterize necrosis, which is the histology of stroke, trauma, and most infections. In contrast, degenerative illnesses and normal age-related changes lead to cell death by apoptosis, which is programmed, energy-requiring, and free of cellular infiltrates.

93. Three months after surviving a drug overdose, a 30-year-old man lies in his hospital bed, quadriparetic and almost mute. However, he has regained enough strength to reach for his food and, with some assistance, feed himself with a spoon. He looks directly at examiners and appears to watch televised sports events. He usually says, "no, no" when someone begins to change the channel. His EEG when he is alert shows slow background activity and PET shows markedly decreased cerebral cortical metabolism. Which of the following diagnoses most accurately describes his condition?
    a. Malingering
    b. Locked-in syndrome
    c. Persistent vegetative state
    d. Minimal conscious state

Answer: d. His behavior fulfills the basic criteria for the minimal conscious state. His behavior is inconsistent and rudimentary. However, as he is aware of visitors and sports events, the patient shows partial preservation of conscious awareness. He reaches for at least one object (the spoon) and uses it appropriately. Thus, his mental and physical functions are much greater than those of persistent vegetative state patients. His abnormal EEG and PET results set him apart from malingering patients.

94. Studies consistently correlate poststroke depression with infarcts in the left frontal lobe. *True or false?*

Answer: False. Although classic studies reported an association of poststroke depression with strokes in the left frontal lobe, more recent studies have implicated the right cerebral hemisphere, other lobes, and subcortical structures, such as the basal ganglia and thalamus. Similarly, older studies reported as association of poststroke mania with right frontal lesions, but newer studies do not substantiate that association.

95. Which of the following would be the least statistically significant risk factor for stroke?
    a. Periodontal disease
    b. Marijuana use
    c. Cocaine use
    d. Elevated C-reactive protein (CRP)
    e. Elevated homocysteine levels

Answer: b. Although cocaine and other sympathomimetic stimulants lead to stroke by causing hypertension and vasoconstriction, marijuana has little or no relationship to stroke. Inflammation (as suggested by an elevated CRP), infections such as periodontal disease, and elevated homocysteine levels are less well known but powerful stroke risk factors.

96. The parents of a 4-year-old boy bring him to the emergency room after he suddenly developed aphasia and right-sided hemiparesis. There is no indication of trauma. CT confirms the clinical impression of a left middle cerebral artery stroke. Blood tests reveal marked lactic acidosis. Results of sickle cell testing and homocysteine levels are normal. Which of the following would be the most appropriate diagnostic test?
    a. Cerebral arteriography
    b. Temporal artery biopsy
    c. Genetic testing
    d. Echocardiogram

Answer: c. Lactic acidosis in a child who has suffered a stroke indicates a mitochondrial myopathy, such as MELAS (*m*itochondrial *e*ncephalomyopathy, *l*actic *a*cidosis, and *s*troke-like episodes). In many patients, genetic testing of blood or (more sensitively) skeletal muscle reveals a causative mutation in mitochondrial DNA. Histologic examination of a muscle biopsy also can be useful in diagnosing MELAS and would reveal ragged red fibers and abnormal mitochondria.

97. Which of the following statements most closely describes the course of poststroke depression in the majority of cases?
    a. The incidence of major depression peaks 3–6 months after a stroke and has a mean duration of 6–9 months.
    b. The incidence of major depression peaks within the first month after a stroke and has a mean duration of 1–2 months.
    c. Major depression begins almost immediately after a stroke and its incidence progresses steadily upward during the following 1–2 years.
    d. Major depression begins soon after the onset of the stroke, but its symptoms change during the next 6 months to a year.

Answer: a. Depression often begins soon after a stroke, but usually subsides by the end of the first year. Although the majority of depressed patients experience a remission within the year, 20% remain depressed at 3 years.

98. Which of the following characteristics is *least* closely associated with poststroke depression?
    a. History of depression or poor physical health before the stroke
    b. Severity of the physical deficits
    c. Curtailed activities of daily living
    d. Poststroke psychosis

Answer: d. Psychosis rarely develops after a stroke. It is much more closely associated with preexisting dementia than poststroke depression.

99. Which of the following statements concerning patients with poststroke depression is *untrue*?
   a. They tend to perform poorly in physical rehabilitation programs.
   b. They fail to optimize their remaining motor, cognitive, and language abilities.
   c. If ECT is indicated, it can be given with impunity.
   d. According to some studies, successful treatment of depression improves patients' outcome.

Answer: c. Although it is effective, ECT in stroke patients may cause more confusion than usual.

100–101. When asked to evaluate a 79-year-old man 6 months after two strokes and a cardiac arrest, a psychiatrist finds that the patient remains alert throughout a long evaluation but confined to bed, quadriplegic, mute, and completely dependent on health-care workers. The patient can establish eye contact with the psychiatrist and begins to follow several simple requests, such as "Please, show me your hand," but not more complicated ones, such as "Please, close your eyes and raise your thumb." The patient can also indicate when a stimulus is painful and if he is thirsty. He seems to take no pleasure in food, television, or family members' visits.

100. Which of the following terms best describes the patient's condition?
   a. Locked-in syndrome
   b. Persistent vegetative state
   c. Minimally conscious state
   d. Delirium
   e. Coma

Answer: c. Because the patient remains alert and attentive, he is neither in coma or delirium. His attentiveness, responses to requests, and appreciation of pain and thirst exclude the persistent vegetative state. In view of his having only those rudimentary neurologic functions and inability to appreciate any pleasure, his condition would best be described as the minimally conscious state.

101. In this patient, what would an EEG most likely show?
   a. Alpha activity over the occipital lobes
   b. Slow and disorganized background activity
   c. Triphasic waves
   d. Electrocerebral silence

Answer: b. The patient probably has extensive, severe cerebral injury, which would cause slow and disorganized background EEG activity. Alpha activity over the occipital lobes is the normal pattern of alert individuals with their eyes closed who are neither concentrating nor anxious. Triphasic waves are associated with hepatic encephalopathy and other metabolic disorders. In the locked-in syndrome, the EEG usually would show relatively normal activity. Electrocerebral silence ("flat wave") is an indication of brain death.

102. A 40-year-old man reported sudden development of weakness in his left arm and leg after slipping on ice and striking his neck and back. X-rays of his head, neck, and lower back showed no abnormalities. When the neurologist asked him to lie supine and raise his right leg, he pushed down with his left. His strength was so great in left leg extension that, using it as a level, she raised his lower trunk from the bed. What is the best description of his left leg movements?
   a. His weakness is psychogenic.
   b. His weakness is due to organic pathology.
   c. The patient demonstrated left-sided hemi-inattention.
   d. He has anosognosia.

Answer: b. The neurologist has looked for the Hoover sign, i.e., absence of extension of the contralateral leg with attempted flexion of the affected leg. If present, the Hoover sign is an indication of psychogenic hemiparesis, but in this case it was absent, suggesting an organic cause for weakness. Another sign of psychogenic hemiparesis is the abductor sign (see Chapter 3).

103. In the recovery room following coronary artery bypass surgery, an 85-year-old man complained that he was unable to move his legs. The neurologist found that he had a clear sensorium, good memory and judgment, intact cranial nerves, and normal strength and DTRs in his arms and hands. She also found that he had flaccid areflexic paraplegia, hypalgesia to pin below the umbilicus, and urinary retention that he did not appreciate. In contrast, position and vibration sensation were preserved in his legs and feet. Where is the lesion?
   a. Bilateral anterior cerebral arteries
   b. Cervical spinal cord
   c. Thoracic spinal cord
   d. Peripheral nervous system
   e. Cauda equina

Answer: c. The patient sustained an infarction of the anterior spinal artery where it perfuses the thoracic spinal cord, i.e., a stroke of the spinal cord. The anterior spinal artery is thin, delicate, and vulnerable to atheromatous debris dislodged during any surgery involving the aorta. The anterior spinal artery supplies the anterior two-thirds of the spinal cord (see Chapter 2). Infarctions in the territory of this artery cause paraplegia and anesthesia caudal to the lesion because of damage to the corticospinal and spinothalamic tracts. Immediately after acute spinal cord injuries, DTRs and muscle tone decrease because of "spinal shock," but days to weeks later patients develop hyperactive DTRs, Babinski signs, and spasticity. Because multiple small segmental arteries supply the posterior portion of the spinal cord, infarction of the anterior spinal artery spares the posterior columns. In this infarction, position and vibration sensations are spared (see Figure 11QA.1).

Bilateral anterior cerebral artery infarctions can cause paraplegia, but cognitive and personality changes are more prominent. Also, DTRs become hyperactive and Babinski signs are often present.

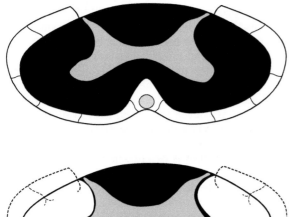

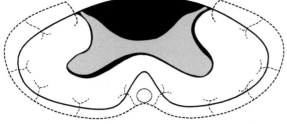

FIGURE 110A.1 ■ *Top,* A cross-section of the normal thoracic spinal cord shows that the anterior spinal artery perfuses the anterior two-thirds of the cord. This region contains the corticospinal and lateral spinothalamic tracts (see Fig. 2.15). *Bottom,* If the anterior spinal artery is occluded, this region of the spinal cord will undergo infarction. The patient would lose strength in the legs and sensation below the site of the infarction. However, because this lesion spares the posterior columns, the patient would still perceive position and vibration sensation.

104–105. A 75-year-old man came to the emergency room because he suddenly developed right hemiparesis. One year earlier he had sustained a right middle cerebral artery occlusion that resulted in a left hemiparesis. Neurologists had diagnosed him many years before with Alzheimer disease. CT showed an acute left middle cerebral artery distribution infarction and the old right middle cerebral artery infarction. Although the patient was breathing satisfactorily, he was unresponsive to verbal and tactile stimulation. He was quadriplegic. His eyes were closed and he moaned, but did not speak.

104. If he survives the acute stroke superimposed on his preexisting stroke and Alzheimer disease, which will most likely be his status?
a. He will remain permanently comatose.
b. Within several weeks, his eyes will open and he will resume periods of sleep and wakefulness, but he will never regain cognition or emotional capacity.
c. Within the year, he will eventually regain his cognition and emotional capacity, but remain quadriplegic and mute.
d. The strokes will have devastating psychologic effects and he will go into deep depression.

Answer: b. Each of the two strokes and the Alzheimer disease irreparably damage the cerebral cortex. Although his brainstem will continue to function and govern eating (chewing and swallowing), sleeping, and reflex activity, he will not regain cognitive and emotional capacity.

105. Which of the following terms will *least* likely describe his condition at the end of one year?
a. Locked-in syndrome
b. Persistent vegetative state
c. Minimally conscious state

Answer: a. The locked-in syndrome describes patients who retain cerebral function and their cognition and emotional capacity, but have quadriplegia and anarthria. This patient has had devastating cerebral insults and undoubtedly has lost all or almost all cerebral function.

106. When an immediate diagnosis is essential, as in the emergency room, which of the following is the best test to diagnose a cerebral hemorrhage?
a. MRI
b. CT
c. Lumbar puncture (LP)
d. Fundoscopic examination

Answer: b. CT requires only a few minutes and detects even small hemorrhages. Neurologists rely upon head CT to rule out intracranial hemorrhage rapidly and reliably before administering tPA for ischemic stroke within the limited time frame. MRI requires 20–40 minutes and precludes patients with metal devices and requires sedation for those with claustrophobia, which confuses the clinical situation. Patients with metal devices, including pacemakers, and those with claustrophobia can safely undergo CT. An LP will not provide useful information in cases of intracerebral hemorrhage. Moreover, in the case of a large cerebral hemorrhage, the procedure could lead to transtentorial herniation (see Fig. 19.3).

VISUAL DISTURBANCES

This chapter describes several common visual disturbances that frequently occur in psychiatric patients, including decreased visual acuity, glaucoma, visual field loss, and visual hallucinations (Box 12.1). In addition, it reviews the causes of visual impairments that may have psychiatric effects in individuals older than 65 years (Box 12.2).

EVALUATING VISUAL DISTURBANCES

After determining the patient's specific visual symptom, the physician's initial examination typically includes inspecting the globe or "eyeball" (Fig. 12.1) and eyelids; assessing visual acuity, visual fields, and optic fundi; and testing pupil reflexes and ocular movements. When appropriate, physicians also perform additional examinations for psychogenic blindness, visual agnosia, and other perceptual disturbances.

Examiners routinely measure visual acuity by having the patient read from either a Snellen wall chart, a hand-held card, or smartphone application. A person with "normal" visual acuity can read 3/8-inch letters at a distance of 20 feet. This acuity, the conventional reference point, is designated 20/20. People with 20/40 acuity must be as close as 20 feet to see what a person with normal acuity can see at a distance of 40 feet.

Optical Disturbances

People with *myopia* have poorer visual acuity at increasingly greater distances. Myopia often becomes troublesome during adolescence when it causes difficulty with seeing blackboards, watching movies, and driving. Because reading and other close-up activities that require "near vision" remain unimpaired, common parlance labels people with myopia as "nearsighted."

The usual causes of myopia are optical rather than neurologic, such as a lens that is too "thick" or a globe that is too "long" (Fig. 12.2). Occasionally medicines cause myopia. For example, topiramate (Topamax), a widely prescribed antimigraine and antiepileptic drug (AED), may produce an acutely occurring but transient myopia. (Topiramate can also lead to angle-closure glaucoma [see later].)

In contrast to myopia, people with *hyperopia* or *hypermetropia* have poorer visual acuity at increasingly shorter distances. The lay public commonly labels them "farsighted" because they can see distant objects, such as street signs, more clearly than closely held ones, such as newspapers. In hyperopia, the lens is usually too "thin," rendering its refractive strength insufficient. Occasionally the globe is too "short."

In *presbyopia*, older individuals cannot focus on closely held objects because their relatively inelastic and dehydrated lenses are unable to change shape. With their impaired near vision, people with presbyopia, as well as those with hyperopia, tend to hold newspapers and sew with needles at arms' length. Reading glasses usually can compensate for the refractory error by bringing the focal point into the proper working distance.

Disruption of the *accommodation reflex* is another common cause of visual disturbance. Normally, when a person looks at a nearby object, this reflex causes the ciliary body muscles to contract, thereby thickening the lens so that the image falls on the retina. This response also constricts the pupils and converges the eyes. In other words, the accommodation reflex focuses the image of closely held objects on the retina.

Because the parasympathetic nervous system mediates the accommodation reflex, many medications with anticholinergic side effects impair visual acuity for closely held objects by disrupting this reflex (Fig. 12.3). These medicines include selective serotonin reuptake inhibitors (SSRIs), selective norepinephrine reuptake inhibitors (SNRIs), tricyclic antidepressants, and clozapine. For example, duloxetine (Cymbalta) causes blurred vision in approximately 3% of patients; sertraline (Zoloft) and paroxetine (Paxil) in 4%; and venlafaxine (Effexor) at a dose of 75 mg in 9%. This side effect may be unsuspected because these medicines can impair accommodation without producing other anticholinergic effects, such as dry mouth, constipation, and urinary hesitancy.

Abnormalities of the Lens, Retina, and Optic Nerve

Cataracts (loss of lens transparency) may result from advanced age (senile cataract), trauma, diabetes, myotonic dystrophy (see Chapter 6), and chronic use of certain medicines, such as steroids. In prolonged high doses, phenothiazines and some second-generation neuroleptics may produce minute lens opacities, but these rarely are dense enough to impair vision.

Pigmentary changes in the retina can be a manifestation of injury, degenerative diseases, diabetes, infection, or the use of high doses of phenothiazines (Fig. 12.4). Among infants and children, *nonaccidental head injury* (child abuse), particularly violent head shaking or direct trauma, creates retinal hemorrhages. Other stigmata of repeated trauma – spiral fractures of the long bones, multiple skull fractures, and burns (see Chapter 22) – frequently accompany these retinal hemorrhages.

In 25% or more of Americans older than 65 years, the cells of the retina's pigment epithelium, mostly in the macula, degenerate through a variety of mechanisms, including proliferation of the underlying blood vessels. When degeneration involves cells in the macula, a condition known as *macular degeneration* disrupts central vision, which is critical for tasks such as reading. Patients use their remaining peripheral vision to negotiate around their living areas, but progressive deterioration ultimately may deprive them of all their eyesight. As with individuals who develop blindness from any cause, those beset by

macular degeneration are at risk of losing their independence, appearing to have cognitive dysfunction, and experiencing visual hallucinations (especially if they also have hearing or cognitive impairments [see Box 12.1]).

Among acquired immune deficiency syndrome (AIDS) patients, opportunistic organisms such as cytomegalovirus

BOX 12.1	Common Neurologic Causes of Visual Hallucinations

Blindness/sensory deprivation – Charles Bonnet syndrome
Palinopsia
Dementia-producing diseases
  Alzheimer
  Dementia with Lewy bodies*
  Parkinson^
Intoxications
  Alcoholic hallucinosis
    Delirium tremens (DTs)
  Hallucinogens
    Amphetamines
    Cocaine
    Lysergic acid diethylamide (LSD)
    Phencyclidine (PCP)
  Medicines
    Atropine, scopolamine
    Levodopa and dopamine agonists
    Steroids
Migraine with aura (classic migraine)
Narcolepsy: Hypnopompic (awakening) and hypnagogic (falling asleep) hallucinations (see Chapter 17)
Seizures
Peduncular hallucinations

---

*Although visual hallucinations are likely to complicate almost any form of dementia, they are characteristic of dementia with Lewy bodies disease.
^Dopaminergic medications such as levodopa-carbidopa (Sinemet) are more likely than Parkinson disease itself to produce hallucinations.

BOX 12.2	Common/Important Causes of Visual Impairments in Individuals Older Than 65 Years

Cataracts
Diabetic retinopathy
Macular degeneration
Glaucoma
Presbyopia and other accommodation problems
Temporal (giant cell) arteritis
Visual agnosia and cortical blindness from multiple strokes or Alzheimer disease

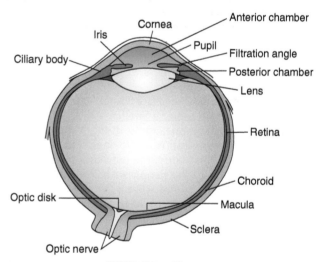

FIGURE 12.1 ■ The eye.

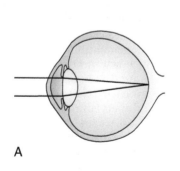

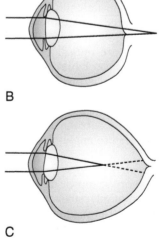

FIGURE 12.2 ■ Image focusing in hyperopic (farsighted) and myopic (nearsighted) eyes: *A,* In normal eyes, the lens focuses the image onto the retina. *B,* In hyperopic eyes, the shorter globe or improperly focusing lens causes the image to fall behind the retina. *C,* In myopic eyes, the longer globe or improperly focusing lens causes the image to fall in front of the retina. Corrective lenses (i.e., glasses or contact lenses) can compensate for the refractive errors of hyperopia and myopia. Alternatively, laser or surgical "flattening" of the lens can correct myopia.

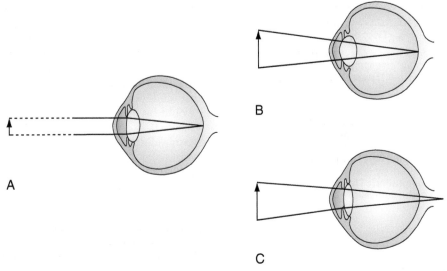

FIGURE 12.3 ■ Accommodation and accommodation paresis. *A*, When someone looks at a distant object, parallel light rays are refracted little by a relatively flat lens onto the retina. *B*, Accommodation: when someone looks at a closely held object, a normal ciliary muscle contracts, thereby increasing the curvature of the lens and greatly refracting the light rays. *C*, Accommodation paresis: If the ciliary muscles are paretic, the lens cannot form a rounded shape. Its weakened refractive power focuses light rays from closely held objects behind the retina; however, parallel light rays from distant objects still focus on the retina. Therefore accommodation paralysis blurs closely held objects but leaves distant ones distinct.

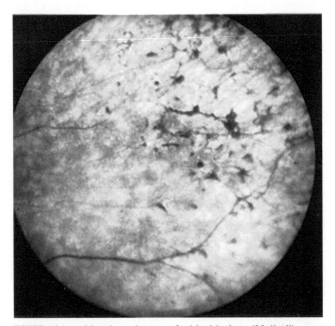

FIGURE 12.4 ■ Massive doses of thioridazine (Mellaril) may induce retinal hyperpigmentation – described as "black bone spicules" or "salt and pepper." Before these retinal pigmentary changes are visible on fundoscopic examination, patients may complain of blurred vision or impaired nighttime vision.

infect the retina. Current antiretroviral regimens have greatly reduced visual complications. In a more benign situation, several medicines lead to visual discoloration. For example, digoxin at toxic concentrations casts a yellow hue (*xanthopsia* [Greek, xanthos yellow + opsis sight]), and sildenafil (Viagra), a blue or yellow hue. On the other hand, a few, such as the AED vigabatrin (Sabril), sometimes cause permanent retinopathy.

Optic Nerve

Damage to the optic nerves, which are projections of the central nervous system (CNS), results in visual loss that may be limited to a scotoma (an area of blindness [see Fig. 15.2]), but may encompass the entire visual field. In addition, because the optic nerves serve as the afferent limb of the pupillary light reflex, unilateral (or asymmetric) optic nerve injury also causes an *afferent pupillary defect*: when the examiner shines a light into an eye with optic nerve dysfunction, both pupils fail to constrict; however, when the same light shines into the unaffected eye, both pupils normally constrict (see Fig. 4.2). With time, optic nerve injuries usually lead to atrophy of the optic disk (the most anterior segment of the optic nerve), visible as disk pallor on fundoscopic examination.

Optic nerve injuries may occur as isolated conditions or in conjunction with disorders of the cerebrum or other parts of the CNS. One of the most common is *optic neuritis*, inflammation of one or both optic nerves, which causes sudden visual loss (often affecting central vision), pain with eye movements, and an afferent pupillary defect (Fig. 12.5). In addition, color vision becomes "desaturated." For example, patients cannot appreciate the difference between fire engine red and brick red. In severe cases, they cannot distinguish red from green.

When optic neuritis affects the optic disk, physicians can see inflammation of the disk (*papillitis*) on fundoscopic examination. If the inflammation affects only the segment of the optic nerve posterior to the disk (*retrobulbar neuritis*), the optic disk will appear normal on fundoscopic examination. With recurrent attacks of optic neuritis, the optic nerve becomes atrophic, the disk white, the pupil unreactive, and the eye blind.

Of the many conditions that cause optic neuritis, demyelinating illnesses, particularly *multiple sclerosis (MS)*

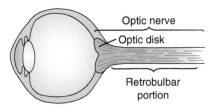

FIGURE 12.5 ◼ Neurologists consider the optic disk, which is visible on fundoscopic examination, to be the *bulbar portion* of the optic nerve. The long segment of the optic nerve behind the eye constitutes its *retrobulbar* portion. Multiple sclerosis usually attacks the posterior portion of the nerve and causes *retrobulbar neuritis*, which is characterized by visual loss, pain on eye movement, and color desaturation. These symptoms occur regardless of the location of the demyelination along the course of the nerve.

and its close relative *neuromyelitis optica* (*NMO*), are the most common (see Chapter 15). Importantly, optic neuritis frequently precedes other manifestations of MS or NMO. If an otherwise asymptomatic patient develops optic neuritis and the MRI shows two or more hyperintense lesions in the brain, that patient has greater than a 70% risk of developing MS. On the other hand, an otherwise asymptomatic optic neuritis patient who has no MRI lesions in the brain has only a 25% risk of developing MS.

Treatment of optic neuritis often includes a course of high-dose intravenous steroids; this may shorten an attack but probably does not alter the outcome. Physicians cautiously use steroids because of their potential side effects that include euphoria, agitation, and, in the extreme, psychosis.

Toxins, including some medications, can also damage the optic nerves. For example, alcoholics may inadvertently drink methanol (CH_3OH), a solvent component of antifreeze and cooking fuels, such as Sterno, and an illicit adulterant of everyday ethanol (C_2H_5OH). Drinking methanol causes a combination of gastroenteritis, delirium, and visual problems, particularly blurry vision and a scotoma. With severe methanol intoxication or merely its chronic intermittent consumption, optic nerves atrophy and victims become blind.

Temporal arteritis or *giant cell* arteritis, a form of vasculitis (an inflammatory condition of the blood vessels), typically begins in the temporal arteries, but often involves the arteries that supply the optic nerve, brain, or both (see Chapter 9). When it involves the arteries that supply the optic nerve, this disorder may cause blindness. Characteristically affecting only people older than 60 years, temporal arteritis usually begins with headache, malaise, and joint pains lasting weeks to months. These initial nonspecific symptoms understandably may lend the appearance of depression or a somatoform disorder. However, physicians should avoid missing this diagnosis because, if untreated, it can result in blindness and strokes. Finding giant cells and other signs of inflammation in a temporal artery biopsy will confirm the diagnosis. High-dose steroids usually reverse the illness and prevent blindness and strokes.

Leber hereditary optic atrophy, an illness attributable to a mitochondrial DNA mutation, also involves the optic nerves, but no other part of the CNS or the musculature (see Chapter 6). Most commonly affecting young males, it causes painless progressive visual loss culminating in blindness in one and then, within months, the other eye.

Several conditions simultaneously affect the cerebrum and the optic nerves. These conditions produce cognitive decline and personality changes as well as blindness. MS would be one example. Another is *Tay-Sachs disease*, a lysosomal storage disease due to a deficiency in hexosaminidase A, which is almost always fatal by age 5 years.

Another classic example of simultaneous injury of both the optic nerve and cerebrum is an olfactory groove or sphenoid wing *meningioma*. This tumor may compress the optic nerve (see Chapters 19 and 20) and the overlying frontal or temporal lobe. The cerebral damage can trigger complex partial seizures and cause cognitive decline and personality changes. At the same time, optic nerve damage causes optic atrophy and blindness in one eye.

Similarly, tumors of the pituitary region, such as *adenomas* or *craniopharyngiomas*, may also produce visual loss accompanied by psychologic changes. Unless detected and removed early, these tumors grow slowly upward to compress the optic chiasm and hypothalamus and downward to infiltrate the pituitary gland (see Fig. 19.4). Compression of the optic chiasm causes bitemporal hemianopia. Compression of the hypothalamus and pituitary gland causes headache and panhypopituitarism that result in decreased libido, diabetes insipidus, and loss of secondary sexual characteristics.

GLAUCOMA

In most cases, glaucoma consists of elevated intraocular pressure resulting from obstructed outflow of aqueous humor through the *filtration angle* of the anterior chamber of the eye (Fig. 12.6) – not from increased production of aqueous humor. If glaucoma remains untreated, it damages the optic nerve, causing visual field impairments and potentially leading to blindness. There are two common types of glaucoma – open-angle and angle-closure – but familiarity with the angle-closure type is especially important for psychiatrists, as it can be a side effect of certain psychotropic medications.

Open-Angle Glaucoma

Open-angle or *wide-angle glaucoma* occurs seven times more frequently than closed-angle glaucoma. People at greatest risk are those older than 65 years, those with diabetes or myopia, and relatives of glaucoma patients. Because symptoms are usually absent at the onset, this variety of glaucoma might be diagnosed only when an ophthalmologist detects elevated intraocular pressure, certain visual field losses, or changes in the optic nerve. Later, when central vision or acuity is impaired, the optic cup is abnormally deep and permanently damaged. Lack of symptoms in the initial phase of open-angle glaucoma is one of the most compelling reasons for annual ophthalmologic examinations.

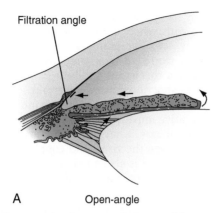
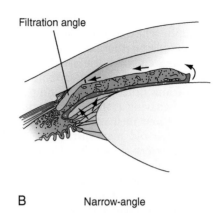

A Open-angle   B Narrow-angle

FIGURE 12.6 ■ *A,* Open-angle glaucoma: drainage of the aqueous humor becomes obstructed, and impaired flow from the eye leads to gradually increased intraocular pressure. *B,* Narrow-angle glaucoma: when the iris moves forward, as may occur during pupil dilation, the angle is narrowed or even closed. Obstruction of aqueous humor flow leads to angle-closure glaucoma.

Open-angle glaucoma usually responds to topical medications (eye drops) or laser treatment. Psychotropic medications do not precipitate open-angle glaucoma. In general, patients with open-angle glaucoma may take antidepressants and other psychotropic medications, provided that they continue their glaucoma treatment.

Angle-Closure Glaucoma

In *angle-closure glaucoma,* which is also called *closed-angle* or *narrow-angle glaucoma,* intraocular pressure is usually elevated due to impaired outflow of aqueous humor at the filtration angle, trapping the fluid behind the iris (see Fig. 12.6A). Patients with narrow-angle glaucoma are usually older than 40 years and often have a family history of the disorder, but they also frequently have a history of hyperopia and longstanding narrow angles. Few have had the classic symptoms, such as seeing halos around lights, preceding an attack of angle-closure glaucoma. In contrast to the relatively normal appearance of the eye in open-angle glaucoma, in acute angle-closure glaucoma the eye is red, the pupil dilated and unreactive, and the cornea hazy. Moreover, the eye and forehead are painful, and vision is impaired.

Angle-closure glaucoma is sometimes iatrogenic. For example, when pupils are dilated for ocular examinations, the "bunched-up" iris can block the angle (see Fig. 12.6B). Likewise, medicines with anticholinergic properties can precipitate angle-closure glaucoma, probably because they dilate the pupil.

The actual risk of glaucoma with tricyclic antidepressant use is low, and with SSRIs, it is almost nonexistent. However, as neurologists and other physicians prescribe tricyclics for numerous conditions – including chronic pain, headache, and diabetic neuropathy – many patients become vulnerable. In addition, other medications for neurologic diseases, particularly topiramate, can cause angle-closure glaucoma.

Whatever the cause of angle-closure glaucoma, prompt treatment can preserve vision. Topical and systemic medications open the angle (by constricting the pupil) and reduce aqueous humor production. Laser iridotomy immediately and painlessly creates a passage directly through the iris that drains aqueous humor.

Because glaucoma poses such a threat, individuals older than 40 years should have intraocular pressure measured every 2 years and those older than 65 years, every year. Most patients who are under treatment for either form of glaucoma may safely receive psychotropic medications. Glaucoma medications, such as pilocarpine (a cholinergic medicine that constricts the pupils), and ophthalmic beta-blockers, such as timolol (Timoptic), may seep into the systemic circulation and create psychologic and cardiovascular side effects, including orthostatic lightheadedness, bradycardia, and even heart block. Not surprisingly, elderly patients who use beta-blocker eye drops sometimes experience brief periods of confusion.

Children are also susceptible to systemic absorption. For example, when children receive scopolamine or other atropine-like eye drops for ocular examination, they often become agitated.

CORTICAL BLINDNESS

Bilateral damage of the occipital lobes, which house the visual cortex, can produce severe visual impairment, called *cortical blindness.* Bilateral posterior cerebral artery occlusions or trauma may produce damage restricted to the occipital lobes that will cause only cortical blindness. Alternatively, extensive brain injury from anoxia, multiple strokes, or MS may cause cortical blindness along with cognitive, other neuropsychological, and physical impairments. Reflecting occipital lobe damage, electroencephalograms (EEGs) characteristically lose their normal posterior 8–12-Hz (alpha) rhythm. Whether cortical blindness results from limited or generalized cortex injury, the pupils remain normal in size and reactivity to light because all elements of the pupillary light reflex – the optic nerves, midbrain, and oculomotor nerves (see Fig. 4.2) – remain intact.

Anton Syndrome

The dramatic neuropsychologic phenomenon of *Anton syndrome* – in which patients with cortical blindness explicitly or implicitly deny that they have lost all vision – characteristically complicates the sudden onset of blindness. Some patients demonstrate anosognosia (see Chapter 8); some simply refuse to admit that they have lost vision, while others blame external factors, like dim light, for their problem. Some may, if pressed, acknowledge visual loss but confabulate by "describing" their room, clothing, and various other objects. Blind patients with Anton syndrome, behaving as though they still have normal vision, stumble about their room.

For example, a 76-year-old man sustained a right-sided posterior cerebral artery stroke that was superimposed on a prior left-sided posterior cerebral artery stroke. He first blamed his inability to see the examiner's blouse on poor lighting and having misplaced his glasses. He then claimed to be uninterested in the exercise. When urged, still implicitly denying his blindness, he calmly described the blouse as "lovely" and "becoming," at one time elaborating that it was "obviously finely sewn and made from expensive material."

VISUAL PERCEPTUAL DISTURBANCES

Visual perceptual disturbances usually consist of impaired processing of visual information or inability to integrate visual input with other information. Although these fascinating conditions seem to be neatly defined, patients usually have incomplete or overlapping forms. Moreover, visual perceptual disturbances often coexist with other neuropsychologic disorders, such as dementia, aphasia, and apraxia.

Palinopsia

Palinopsia (Greek, *palin*, again; *opsis*, vision), which may be likened to visual perseveration or a visual echo, consists of recurrent or persistent images following removal of the visual stimulus. Technically a form of hallucinations, the visions usually appear to the patient within an area of visual loss, such as within a left homonymous hemianopia. Patients with palinopsia often have recurrent images of objects, scenes, or family members in rapid succession. Because palinopsia consists of duplicate images of common objects, it usually does not elicit an emotional response.

Both the left-sided visual impairment and the superimposed hallucinations stem from right-sided occipital and parietal lobe lesions, such as a stroke or tumor. Other causes of palinopsia include migraine and side effects of psychoactive medications, including mirtazapine, trazodone, and risperidone.

Palinopsia may represent a failure of the cortex to capture only a single image, but it rarely results from seizure activity. In palinopsia, compared to seizure activity, the visions are well formed, appearing as reproductions of objects in the environment, and unaccompanied by changes in emotion or level of consciousness. In cases where isolated repetitive visual hallucinations result from seizures, EEG should readily detect discharges originating in the occipital lobe.

Agnosia

Another visual perceptual disturbance, *visual agnosia*, consists of the inability to appreciate the meaning of an object by its appearance, despite an intact visual system. Patients with visual agnosia simply cannot comprehend what they see. For example, a man would be able to describe a stop sign by saying that it is octagonal, red, and displays the letters "S-T-O-P," but not be able to explain what action drivers must take.

Neurologists detect visual agnosia most often in patients with cognitive impairment from multiple small strokes or Alzheimer disease. They sometimes explain it as a disconnection between the visual and cognitive centers.

Visual agnosia is also a major component of the infamous, although uncommon, *Klüver–Bucy syndrome*. Neurosurgeons have produced this behavioral disorder in monkeys by resection of both anterior temporal lobes, which contain the amygdalae and other components of the limbic system. The resulting damage produces visual agnosia so severe that the monkeys not only touch all objects, but they compulsively seek to identify objects by putting them into their mouth ("psychic blindness"). Their behavior can be repetitive, compulsive, and indiscriminate. When the Klüver–Bucy syndrome occurs in humans (see Chapter 16), they display a muted variation of psychic blindness, *hyperorality*, which consists of their placing inedible objects in their mouth, although only briefly, partly, and absent-mindedly.

Color agnosia is an inability to identify colors by sight. The affected individual's problem is neither aphasia nor color blindness (which is a sex-linked inherited retinal abnormality), but rather a cognitive impairment due to a lesion in the ventral occipital cortex. Patients with color agnosia cannot specify (by speech or writing) the names of colors. When shown colored cards, for example, they cannot say or write the name of the colors. Despite those deficits, patients can match pairs of cards of the same color, read Ishihara plates (pseudoisochromatic numbered cards), and recite the colors of well-known objects, such as the American flag.

In a related impairment, *prosopagnosia*, patients cannot recognize familiar faces (Greek, *prosopon*, face, person; *agnosia*, lack of knowledge). An inability to identify objects out of their usual (visual) context, such as a shirt pocket cut from a shirt often accompanies prosopagnosia. Nevertheless, patients can continue to identify individuals by their voice, dress, and mannerisms. Neurologists usually attribute prosopagnosia to occipitotemporal dysfunction related to a structural lesion or neurodegenerative illness, such as Alzheimer disease or frontotemporal dementia.

In a variation of prosopagnosia, patients with right cerebral lesions cannot match pairs of pictures of *unfamiliar* faces. This condition represents a visual perceptual impairment possibly induced by a nondominant parietal lobe lesion.

Balint Syndrome

Balint syndrome, which neurologists attribute to bilateral parietal-occipital damage from strokes or Alzheimer disease, consists of three related elements concerned with visual attention: *ocular apraxia*, *optic ataxia*, and *simultanagnosia*. Ocular apraxia, which neurologists sometimes call "*psychic paralysis of fixation*," is the neuropsychologic inability of a patient to shift attention by looking away from an object to one located in the periphery of vision. Patients behave as though they were mesmerized by the original object or as a military radar system that has locked onto an approaching hostile aircraft. By briefly closing their eyes, which momentarily interrupts attention, patients can shift their gaze.

Optic ataxia, the second element of Balint syndrome, is the inability to use visual information to guide the hands accurately for reaching and other activities.

The third element, simultanagnosia, consists of inability to attend simultaneously to multiple objects in the field of vision. Patients will often focus on objects in the center of vision and ignore those in the periphery even though they might be more important or attractive. Because of simultanagnosia, patients cannot comprehend complicated scenes or intricate objects. For example, they would be unable to follow a baseball game, despite being able to see the individual players, the ball, and the bases.

Psychogenic Blindness

The medical literature has stated that *nonorganic visual loss*, also termed *psychogenic blindness*, accounts for the symptom of visual loss in as many as 5% of children and adults. However, cases of psychogenic blindness that convincingly mimic true blindness are rare. Because most people lack an intuitive knowledge of visual pathways, neurologists can readily detect nonanatomic patterns of psychogenic blindness. Even bedside testing can easily reveal its spurious nature.

Psychogenic blindness occurs in malingering and particularly in what the *Diagnostic and Statistical Manual of Mental Disorders, 5th Edition* (DSM-5) classifies as Conversion Disorder (Functional Neurological Symptom Disorder) with Special Sensory Symptom. One of the most common presentations of psychogenic blindness is monocular visual loss and ipsilateral hemiparesis. This combination defies the facts of neuroanatomy because the division of optic pathways at the optic chiasm dictates that a cerebral lesion causing hemiparesis will cause hemianopia – not monocular blindness. (Brainstem lesions may cause hemiparesis and diplopia, but not hemianopia or monocular blindness.) In another presentation, individuals with psychogenic blindness often needlessly wear sunglasses. This ploy seems to serve several purposes: it signals that they are blind, reduces visual distractions, and prevents observers from seeing when they establish eye contact.

Similarly, *tubular* or *tunnel vision* defies the laws of optics that dictate that the visual area expands with increasing distance (Fig. 12.7). Important exceptions to this general rule may occur when patients with migraine with aura have constriction of their peripheral vision, and also in some patients taking vigabatrin.

To unmask psychogenic blindness, an uninhibited examiner simply might make childlike facial contortions or ask the patient to read profane words. The patient's reaction to these provocations might reveal the ability to see. When only one eye is affected by psychogenic blindness, fogged, colored, or polarized lenses in front of the unaffected eye will often confuse (or fatigue) a patient into revealing that vision is present.

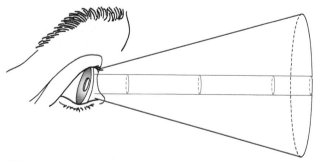

FIGURE 12.7 ■ The area seen by a person normally increases conically in proportion to the distance from the object. In *tubular* or *tunnel vision*, which defies the laws of optics, the "visible" area remains constant despite increasing distance.

Another technique that exposes intact vision is to draw a striped cloth or spin a striped cylinder (drum) in front of a person. The moving striped surface will elicit *optokinetic nystagmus* unless true blindness is present. Likewise, having patients stare at a large, moving mirror irresistibly compels them to follow their own image.

In a different approach, neurologists offer patients eyeglasses with lenses having negligible optical strength. Wearing these glasses allows patients to extract themselves from psychogenic blindness without embarrassment.

If clinical tests are inconclusive, EEG and other electrophysiologic testing may help. Alpha rhythm overlying the occipital lobes of patients at rest with their eyes closed, and loss of that rhythm when they open their eyes, indicates an intact visual system. However, because patients' anxiety or concentration suppresses alpha activity, its absence is not as meaningful as its presence. In visual evoked response (VER) testing, another noninvasive electrophysiologic test, visual system damage delays or abolishes the normal potentials (see Chapter 15).

VISUAL HALLUCINATIONS

Unlike auditory hallucinations, which typically result from psychiatric disorders, visual hallucinations in adults typically result from neurologic disorders. (In children, they may be a symptom of schizophrenia.) Specific qualities of visual hallucinations that should prompt a neurologic evaluation include stereotyped visions, alteration in the patient's level of consciousness, and concurrent behavioral abnormalities. Problems as diverse as toxic-metabolic encephalopathy, dementia-producing diseases, medication side effects, and structural lesions can produce visual hallucinations (see Box 12.1). Patients usually require an imaging study, routine blood tests, urinary toxicology analysis, and an EEG.

Seizures

Seizures originating from dysfunction of the frontal, temporal, or occipital cortex (see Chapter 10) can produce visual hallucinations. Seizure-induced visual hallucinations tend to be stereotyped and brief, can be "seen" in both eyes, and may even appear in a hemianopic area. They range from simple geometric forms (typical of occipital lobe seizures) to detailed visions accompanied by sounds, smells, thoughts, emotions, and, characteristically, impairment of consciousness (more characteristic of temporal or frontal lobe seizures).

Migraine Aura

The "aura" in migraine with aura (previous termed "classic migraine") consists of sensory disturbances – olfactory, sensory, or visual. In almost all cases, auras include stereotyped visual hallucinations (see Fig. 9.2). The majority consist of distinctive crescent scotomata or scintillating, patterned zigzag lines (fortification spectra) that move slowly across the visual field for 1 to 20 minutes before yielding to a hemicranial headache. In a potentially confusing situation, visual auras sometimes represent the sole manifestation of migraine. In rare individuals, migraine aura consists of elaborate visual distortions, such as *metamorphopsia*, in which individuals and objects appear to the patient to change size or shape, as in the celebrated Alice in Wonderland syndrome.

Narcolepsy

As an element of narcolepsy (see Chapter 17), visual hallucinations intrude into patients' partial consciousness while they are falling asleep (hypnagogic hallucinations) or waking up (hypnopompic hallucinations). Narcolepsy induced visual hallucinations are essentially dreams composed of variable, unpredictable – not stereotyped – intricate visions accompanied by rich thoughts and strong emotions. As with normal dreams, these hallucinations are associated with flaccid, areflexic paresis and rapid eye movements (REMs).

Neurodegenerative Illnesses

Visual hallucinations are also a hallmark of neurodegenerative diseases that cause dementia, particularly Alzheimer, Lewy bodies, and Parkinson diseases or their treatment (see Chapters 7 and 18). When manifestations of these disorders, hallucinations tend to be visually complex, have a paranoid aspect, and occur predominantly at night. As a clue to dementia with Lewy bodies disease, visual hallucinations occur frequently and begin early in its course. In contrast, when visual hallucinations complicate Alzheimer disease, they occur in its late stages. Hallucinations in Parkinson disease are usually medication-induced, at least in part.

Toxins

Many classes of medicines, in addition to anticholinergics or dopamine enhancers, may cause hallucinations as a side effect. In addition, many illicit drugs, by design, are hallucinogens (see Chapter 21). Even withdrawal from certain substances causes visual hallucinations. The best-known example is alcohol withdrawal causing *delirium tremens* (*DTs*). In this case, most patients have varied, sometimes frightening visions that stem from the environment. Agitation, confusion, fluctuating consciousness, sweating, and tachycardia accompany or overwhelm the

hallucinations. In some DT patients, however, the hallucinations seem to petrify the patients who then become hypervigilant, reticent, and immobile.

Sensory Deprivation

Visual loss from any cause results in sensory deprivation or "deafferentation" of the visual cortex. Without visual input, unregulated visual cortex activity emerges as hallucinations. When this phenomenon occurs, neurologists label it the *Charles Bonnet syndrome* or *release hallucinations*. Visual hallucinations occur in patients with visual loss in the absence of dementia, delirium, or psychiatric disorders.

For example, soldiers sustaining extensive eye wounds have periods of "seeing" brightly colored forms and even entire scenes. Patients with hemianopia may have hallucinations exclusively in their blind visual field. Individuals with sudden visual loss or even slowly progressive loss from cataracts or, more frequently, macular degeneration often present with the Charles Bonnet syndrome.

Release hallucinations are often complex and patients may "see" long-dead relatives, friends, or household pets. Despite vivid elaborate imagery, affected individuals typically experience the hallucinations quietly and harmlessly. The hallucinations usually elicit little or no emotional response. They are usually aware that their visions are merely hallucinations, and they may only reluctantly disclose them to their family and physicians.

Peduncular Hallucinosis

In *peduncular hallucinations*, patients with damage to the ventral midbrain (usually from a stroke) experience vivid images, often of people or animals. The cause may be disinhibition of the reticular activating system secondary to damage to structures that normally inhibit it. Comorbid findings include third cranial nerve palsy and ataxia (see later and Chapter 4).

With seizures, migraine, or narcolepsy, appropriate treatment of the underlying condition will usually eliminate visual hallucinations. Antipsychotics and occasionally AEDs may suppress hallucinations that complicate neurodegenerative illnesses, intoxications, and acute visual loss; however, physicians should avoid administering dopamine-blocking agents to patients with dementia with Lewy bodies (see Chapter 7).

VISUAL FIELD LOSS

As in so much of neurology where anatomy determines destiny, the pattern of a patient's visual loss is invaluable in localizing neurologic lesions (Fig. 12.8). Routine examination at the bedside can detect large visual field defects, but more subtle abnormalities may require formal visual field evaluation. Computerized techniques permit reproducible and objective assessment of visual fields.

Optic nerve lesions, such as optic neuritis or trauma, lead to a scotoma – loss of an area of the visual field – in the ipsilateral eye. This area is usually oval or kidney-shaped and, unlike most other visual field defects, crosses the midline. If a lesion transects the entire optic nerve,

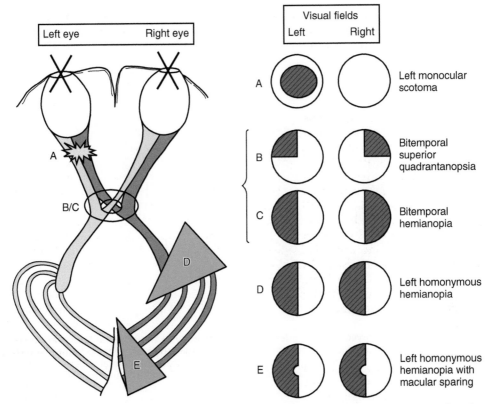

FIGURE 12.8 ■ The visual pathway (also see Fig. 4.1), which extends from the eyes to the occipital cortex, is vulnerable throughout its entire course. Lesions at specific sites produce characteristic visual field defects. The defects, in turn, indicate the lesion's location and give hints to its etiology and expected associated findings. *A,* Optic nerve lesions typically produce an ipsilateral scotoma. *B,* Optic chiasm lesions from below, when small (smaller ring), cause a superior bitemporal quadrantanopsia. *C,* When large (larger ring), optic chiasm lesions result in a bitemporal hemianopia. *D,* Cerebral lesions that disrupt the optic tract produce a contralateral homonymous hemianopia. *E,* Lesions that interfere with the occipital cortex also yield a contralateral homonymous hemianopia, sometimes with macular sparing. Although the determination of visual fields serves as a highly reliable sign of localized neurologic disease, their graphical representation is one of clinical neurology's most confusing exercises. In the standard manner, these sketches portray visual field defects as solid or crosshatched areas from the *patient's perspective.* For example, the sketch of the left homonymous hemianopia (*D*) portrays the abnormal areas on the left side of each circle – as when the patient looks at the paper. The sketch of cerebral optic tract pathways portrays the tracts as though a picture had been taken of the patient's brain from above (see Fig. 8.4). In contrast, CTs and MRIs traditionally show the brain in right-to-left reversal – for example, showing a left cerebral lesion on the right side of the image. Medical illustrations should include a notation to orient the reader.

that eye will lose all vision and the patient will have monocular blindness.

Pituitary adenomas often expand upward and compress the optic chiasm, disrupting the inferior nasal crossing fibers. The damage to these fibers causes *bitemporal superior quadrantanopsia.* If the adenoma continues to extend and grow upward, it can disrupt the superior as well as the inferior crossing fibers, and the visual field deficit will become a *bitemporal hemianopia.*

Injuries posterior to the optic chiasm – anywhere in the optic tract, lateral geniculate bodies, optic radiations, or occipital cortex – cause contralateral visual field deficits which are homonymous (approximately the same in both eyes) and may affect a superior or inferior quadrant (quadrantanopsia), a hemifield (hemianopia), or other portion of the visual field. One common example is a stroke in the distribution of the left posterior cerebral artery, which would cause infarction of the left occipital cortex and produce a right homonymous hemianopia. Similarly, strokes in the distribution of the left middle

cerebral artery cause a right homonymous hemianopia by damaging the optic radiations.

While posterior brain regions are associated most closely with hemianopia, large strokes affecting frontal or parietal lobes along with the occipital cortex usually cause physical abnormalities – such as gaze deviation, hemiparesis, hemisensory loss – and certain neuropsychological deficits along with homonymous hemianopia. For example, right-sided homonymous hemianopia is often associated with conjugate ocular deviation to the left, right-sided hemiparesis and hemisensory loss, and nonfluent aphasia. Likewise, left-sided homonymous hemianopia is often associated with conjugate ocular deviation to the right, left-sided hemiparesis and hemisensory loss, and left-sided anosognosia and hemi-inattention (see Chapter 8).

Unlike scotomas from optic nerve lesions and many cases of psychogenic visual loss, homonymous and bitemporal hemianopias respect the vertical midline. Although occipital lesions sometimes do not involve the center of

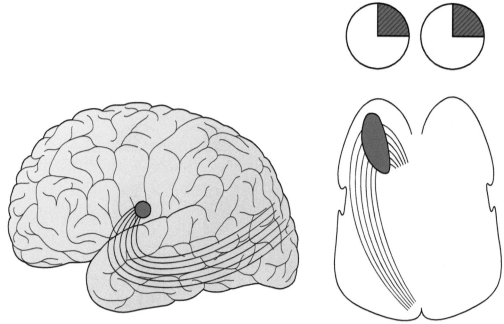

FIGURE 12.9 ■ *Left,* The optic radiations sweep from the lateral geniculate body to the occipital lobe's visual cortex. Some of the fibers sweep anteriorly from the lateral geniculate body through the temporal lobe's anterior tip before heading posteriorly; this detour is known as Meyer's loop. These fibers convey visual information from the contralateral superior quadrant. *Right,* If a large lesion or a surgical resection of the left temporal lobe damages Meyer's loop it produces a contralateral (right) homonymous superior quadrantanopsia.

vision (see later), hemianopias never drift over the center vertical meridian to affect the other visual field.

A rare but important situation is the *homonymous superior quadrantanopsia* (Fig. 12.9). This visual field deficit may be the only physical manifestation of a contralateral temporal lobe lesion. Thus, it may represent the only interictal physical finding in patients who have seizures arising from the temporal lobe or the residua of a temporal lobectomy for trauma or intractable epilepsy.

Hemianopia due to lesions restricted to the contralateral occipital lobe are unique in several respects. Unlike with damage of the anterior portion of the optic system, precise mapping of the visual fields in occipital lobe lesions may demonstrate that central vision is preserved within the hemianopia, a phenomenon known as macular sparing. This preservation of central vision may relate to representation of central vision in both hemispheres of the cerebral cortex or to dual blood supply perfusing the occipital pole, where central vision is housed. Another distinguishing feature of a homonymous hemianopia due to an occipital lesion is that no cognitive or other physical defects accompany the field cut.

CONJUGATE EYE MOVEMENT

In the normal, awake state, *(supranuclear)* gaze centers in the cerebral cortex (Fig. 12.10) innervate pontine gaze centers, which in turn innervate the nearby oculomotor, trochlear, and abducens cranial nerve nuclei (Fig. 12.11). Both eyes thus normally move together in a coordinated, paired (*conjugate*) manner. This system allows individuals

to slowly follow (*pursue*) moving objects, or rapidly shift their gaze from one location in space to another (perform a *saccade*).

When people are conscious and looking about, their cortical supranuclear gaze centers control gaze through conjugate movements of the eyes. When they are unconscious, tested in various ways, or beset by a variety of conditions that injure their cerebral cortex, their pontine nuclear gaze centers assume control of their conjugate eye movements. In particular, when people dream, pontine centers generate rapid eye movements (see REM sleep, Chapter 17). Also, during both *oculocephalic testing,* in which an examiner turns the patient's head to the side, and *cold caloric (oculovestibular) testing,* in which the examiner irrigates an ear canal with cold water, labyrinthine stimulation of the pontine centers overrides any supranuclear innervation, and the nuclear stimulation drives the eye movement. In *brain death,* of course, neither cortical nor brainstem stimulation produces any eye movement.

A disorder that classically causes eye movement abnormalities is *progressive supranuclear palsy* (PSP, see Chapter 7). This condition shares some features with Parkinson's disease (gait impairment, dementia); however, it is characterized by a patient's inability initially to voluntarily move the eyes upward or downward, and then, late in the disease course, the inability to move the eyes horizontally. The description of the condition as "supranuclear" connotes that the problem lies not in the extraocular muscles, cranial nerves, or cranial nerve nuclei in the brainstem, but rather in the innervation of those nuclei from higher centers in the cerebrum. For this reason, directly exciting the brainstem nuclei with oculocephalic (doll's eyes) or

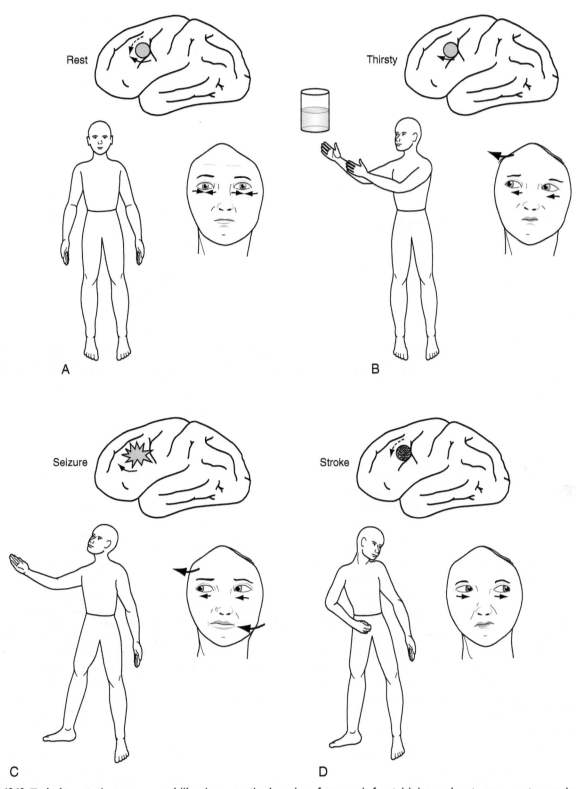

FIGURE 12.10 ■ *A,* At rest, the eyes are midline because the impulses from each frontal lobe conjugate gaze center are balanced, each "pushing" the eyes to the contralateral side. Maintaining eyes in one position is an active process. *B,* Voluntarily increased activity of the left cerebral gaze center (due to activation from other cortical areas) drives the eyes to the right (contralaterally). *C,* Similarly, involuntary activity originating in the left cerebrum, as occurs during a seizure, drives the eyes contralaterally. Seizure activity may also involve the nearby motor cortex, causing right arm and leg tonic-clonic movement. *D,* A stroke that destroys the left cerebral gaze center will permit the cortex on the right to push the eyes toward the left, the side of the lesion. It also disrupts the left cerebral motor strip, causing contralateral paresis. Thus, the eyes "look away" from the hemiparetic side of the body in this common stroke syndrome.

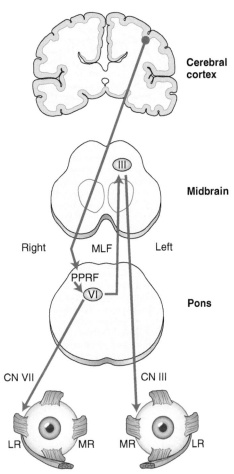

FIGURE 12.11 ■ To produce a saccadic eye movement to the right, the left frontal conjugate gaze center stimulates the right (contralateral) pontine gaze center, which neurologists also call the *pontine paramedian reticular formation (PPRF)*. The pontine gaze center, in turn, stimulates the adjacent right abducens nucleus, which sends motor axons to the right lateral rectus (LR) muscle and other axons upwards through the left medial longitudinal fasciculus (MLF) to the left (contralateral) oculomotor nerve nucleus in the midbrain, which then sends motor axons to the left medial rectus (MR). (Also see Fig. 15.3.)

oculovestibular (caloric) stimulation results in normal eye movements.

Conjugate Eye Deviation From Cerebral Lesions

In an alert person, each cerebral gaze center continuously emits impulses that go through a complicated pathway to "push" the eyes conjugately contralaterally. With the counterbalancing activity of each cerebral gaze center, the eyes remain midline. When a person wants to look to one side, the contralateral cerebral gaze center increases activity. For example, when someone wants to look toward a water glass on the right, the left cerebral gaze center activity increases and both eyes turn to the right. If this person wished to reach for the glass, the left cerebral motor strip, which is situated posterior to the gaze center, would mobilize the right arm.

Focal seizures can increase activity of the cerebral conjugate gaze center. They push the eyes contralaterally and, because the seizures usually encompass the adjacent motor cortex, they also push the head and neck contralaterally and produce tonic-clonic activity of the contralateral arm and leg (see Fig. 10.7).

In contrast, when patients have unilateral destructive cerebral injuries, such as large strokes, the activity of the gaze center on that side is abolished. The activity in the contralateral center, being unopposed, pushes the eyes toward the injured side of the brain. For example, with a left cerebral stroke, the eyes deviate toward the left. In addition, because the stroke would also damage the corticospinal tract, the right side of the body would be paralyzed. Thus, in a cerebral stroke, the eyes look *away from* the paralyzed side of the body.

Conjugate Eye Deviation From Brainstem Lesions

Each cerebral gaze center normally produces conjugate eye movements by stimulating a contralateral *pontine gaze center*, which neurologists also call the *pontine paramedian reticular formation (PPRF)*. In contrast to the movement generated by the cerebral center, each pontine center *pulls* the eyes toward its own side (Fig. 12.11). A lesion on one side of the pons thus allows the eyes to be pulled toward the opposite side. For example, if a stroke damages the right pontine gaze center, the eyes would deviate to the left. Also, because this stroke would damage the corticospinal tract in the right pons, the left arm and leg would be paralyzed. With a pontine lesion, the eyes look *toward* the paralyzed side of the body.

When the pontine gaze center receives impulses from the contralateral cerebral conjugate gaze center, it activates neurons in the adjacent abducens nucleus. Some of these neurons innervate the ipsilateral lateral rectus muscles and cause the ipsilateral eye to abduct, while others ascend through the contralateral *medial longitudinal fasciculus (MLF)* to the oculomotor nucleus, which causes the medial rectus muscle to contract and adduct the eye contralateral to the active PPRF. In this way, stimulation of the pontine gaze center results in conjugate lateral eye movement toward the stimulated side (see also Figs. 15.3 and 15.4).

MLF injury, as often occurs in MS and brainstem strokes, produces an *internuclear ophthalmoplegia (INO)*. This condition, which spares the cranial nuclei and nerves but severs the connection between them, causes a classic pattern of ocular movement impairment identifiable primarily by inability of the eye ipsilateral to the lesion to adduct past the midline, along with coarse nystagmus in the other, abducting eye (see Chapter 15).

Nystagmus, another important ocular movement abnormality, usually consists of rhythmic horizontal, vertical, or rotatory oscillations of both eyes. Many CNS injuries cause nystagmus, including strokes or MS lesions in the brainstem or cerebellum. In addition, it may be the most prominent physical finding from alcohol or drug intoxication. Physicians should particularly consider Wernicke–Korsakoff syndrome and phencyclidine

(PCP) intoxication in delirious patients with nystagmus. On the other hand, neurologists routinely detect nystagmus in epilepsy patients taking therapeutic doses of phenytoin or phenobarbital. In fact, its absence in patients who should be taking phenytoin may suggest noncompliance.

Although usually a sign of CNS dysfunction, nystagmus may be a normal variant. For example, many normal individuals have a few beats of horizontal nystagmus when looking far laterally (*end-point nystagmus*). Some have *congenital nystagmus*, which may seem disconcerting to people speaking with them, but it does not interfere with their vision. Congenital nystagmus is usually pendular (no alternation of fast and slow phases), direction-changing, and absent when the individual looks toward a particular point off to one side (the null point).

Sometimes nystagmus from the peripheral vestibular system (such as labyrinthitis) mimics nystagmus from brainstem dysfunction. However, patients with labyrinthitis have prominent vertigo, nausea, and vomiting, and signs of viral infection like sore throat, runny nose, cough, and fever are common.

Saccades and Pursuit Movement

Under ordinary circumstances, when an object of interest enters the periphery of the visual field, one's eyes dart toward it to redirect the line of sight and refocus gaze. The eyes rotate conjugately, smoothly, and rapidly. Their movement does not disturb the eyelids or move the head. These ocular movements, *saccades*, are characterized by their rapidity, which may exceed 700 degrees-per-second.

Neurologists examine saccades by asking a patient to stare at an object 45 degrees to one side and then suddenly look at another one 45 degrees to the other side. At the bedside, the primary abnormality is slowness. Other abnormalities are overshooting or undershooting (hypermetria and hypometria), irregular or jerky movements, and initiating the saccade by blinking or a head jerk.

Unlike saccades, which are responsible for rapid shift of gaze from one object to another, *pursuit* or *smooth pursuit* is the slow continual ocular tracking of a moving object, such as a bird in flight. In other words, unlike saccades, pursuits follow and maintain gaze on an object remaining in the field of vision. Bedside testing consists of asking the patient to follow the examiner's finger as it moves horizontally at about 30 degrees-per-second. The eyes should remain on the target and smoothly track the finger. The primary abnormality would be a jerky path rather than a smooth one. Numerous lesions and illnesses – even fatigue and inattention – impair smooth pursuit (Box 12.3).

Many conditions, including strokes, MS, tumors, neurodegenerative illnesses, and schizophrenia, can damage the intricate mechanisms that generate these movements. The responsible lesions may be located in the cerebral cortex, cerebellum, pons, or occasionally elsewhere in the CNS. Abnormal saccades are a signature of Huntington disease (see Chapter 18). For example, when an examiner asks a patient with Huntington disease to shift his gaze from the examiner's nose to an object to the left, the patient's eyes may move conjugately to the left, jerk momentarily to the right, and then resume their leftward

BOX 12.3	**Common Causes of Smooth Pursuit Abnormalities**

Medications
  Antiepileptic drugs
  Barbiturates and benzodiazepines
  Neuroleptics
Neurodegenerative diseases
  Alzheimer
  Huntington
  Parkinson
Psychiatric illnesses
  Affective disorders
  Attention deficit hyperactivity disorder
  Borderline personality disorder
  Obsessive-compulsive disorder
  Schizophrenia
Strokes, multiple

movement but overshoot the target. Abnormalities in smooth pursuit and, to a lesser degree, saccades characterize eye movements of schizophrenic patients and even some of their asymptomatic first-degree relatives. The abnormalities occur independent of medications. Similar abnormalities are also present, although less frequently, in individuals with depression, borderline personality disorder, and other psychiatric disturbances. Notably, in depression, they improve with successful treatment.

DIPLOPIA

Monocular diplopia is usually the result of either ocular abnormalities, such as a dislocated lens, or psychogenic factors. In either case, it persists in all directions of gaze and covering the affected eye should abolish it.

The form of diplopia most characteristic of a neurologic disorder – binocular diplopia – results from misalignment of the two eyes. Unlike monocular diplopia, it is usually present (or magnified) in certain directions of gaze and covering *either* eye will abolish it.

The neurologic causes of diplopia are almost always lesions in the brainstem or lower in the neuroanatomic hierarchy: internuclear ophthalmoplegia (INO) and other brainstem syndromes; oculomotor, trochlear, or abducens cranial nerve injury; neuromuscular junction disorders; or extraocular muscle paresis. In contrast, lesions above the brainstem, such as cerebral and other supranuclear lesions, characteristically cause conjugate gaze palsies but not diplopia.

Oculomotor (third cranial) nerve injury results in diplopia that is greatest when the patient looks laterally, away from the affected eye, due to weakness of the medial rectus muscle. The three findings that neurologists rely on when attributing diplopia on lateral gaze to a third nerve injury are ptosis, lateral deviation of the eye, and a dilated pupil (Fig. 12.12). With a third nerve palsy, diplopia will be most pronounced when the patient attempts to adduct the eye, i.e., bring it medially. For example, a patient with damage to the left oculomotor nerve will have difficulty adducting the left eye, and diplopia will be greatest upon looking to the right.

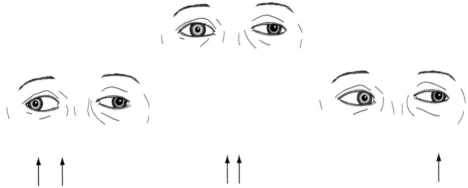

FIGURE 12.12 ■ In the center picture, a patient with a left oculomotor (third cranial) nerve palsy looks straight ahead. The left upper lid is lower (ptosis), the pupil larger, and the eye deviated slightly laterally. Because the eyes are disconjugate, the patient sees two arrows (diplopia) side-by-side when looking ahead. In the picture on the left, the patient looks to the right. Because the paretic left eye fails to adduct, the eyes are more disconjugate and there is greater diplopia. In the picture on the right, the patient looks to the left. The eyes are almost conjugate and there is little or no diplopia.

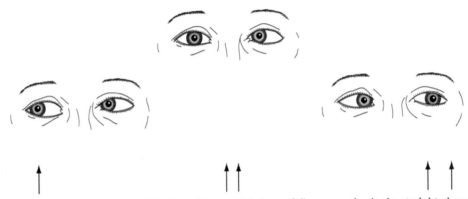

FIGURE 12.13 ■ In the center picture, a patient with a left abducens (sixth cranial) nerve palsy looks straight ahead. The patient's left eye is deviated medially. The eyes are disconjugate, and the patient sees two arrows when looking ahead. In the picture on the left, the patient looks to the right. The eyes are conjugate, and the patient sees only a single arrow. In the picture on the right, the patient looks to the left. The paretic left eye fails to abduct. The exaggeration of the disconjugate gaze increases the diplopia.

The full triad raises the concern of an extrinsic lesion compressing the third nerve, particularly an aneurysm arising from the posterior communicating artery. On the other hand, a third nerve infarction from diabetes is likely to cause ptosis and impaired adduction, but characteristically "spares the pupil," i.e., the pupil remains reactive to light and the same size as its counterpart. Diabetic infarctions of the third nerve are also often painful.

Abducens (sixth cranial) nerve injury also causes diplopia on looking laterally. In contrast to a third nerve palsy, the examination shows medial deviation of the affected eye at rest and inability of that eye to abduct. Also in contrast to a third nerve palsy, the examination shows neither ptosis nor pupil dilation (Fig. 12.13).

When diplopia results from *myasthenia gravis*, the classic neuromuscular junction disorder, patients have fluctuating, variable, and asymmetric combinations of ptosis and paresis of various ocular muscles. However, no matter how severe the diplopia and ptosis, patients' pupils are characteristically round, equal, and reactive to light (see Chapter 6).

Although congenital ocular muscle weakness, *strabismus*, causes dysconjugate gaze, children and adults with strabismus do not have diplopia because the brain suppresses the image from the weaker eye. With continuous suppression of vision from one eye, that eye will lose vision and become blind, i.e., *amblyopic*. Thus, ophthalmologists patch the "good" eye of babies and children with strabismus for several hours each day. The patching forces them to use the weakened eye, which strengthens its vision and muscular control. Alternatively, ophthalmologists perform muscle surgery or administer intramuscular botulinum toxin injections to reestablish conjugate gaze and thereby bring the affected eye into play.

Mitochondrial myopathies may cause *progressive external ophthalmoplegia* due to the delicate nature and high metabolic demands of the extraocular muscles (see Chapter 6). These disorders cause extraocular muscle paresis, including prominent ptosis, and sometimes diplopia. Although the paresis may mimic myasthenia gravis, mitochondrial myopathies progress insidiously, do not fluctuate, symmetrically weaken muscles, and usually spare facial, vocal, and limb muscles.

Psychogenic factors may also be responsible for symptoms of diplopia. Psychogenic diplopia is usually intermittent, inconsistent, and present in all directions of gaze. As previously mentioned, sometimes the diplopia is monocular. Recall that the symptoms of myasthenia gravis tend to fluctuate, and should not be interpreted as the inconsistency of a psychogenic condition!

In a related psychogenic disturbance, *convergence spasm*, patients (often children or young adults) fix their eyes in a downward and inward position as if looking at the tip of their nose, which superficially resembles bilateral sixth nerve palsies.

HORNER'S SYNDROME AND ARGYLL–ROBERTSON PUPILS

The sympathetic pathway from the brain to the eye follows a long and circuitous route (Fig. 12.14A). Injury to these fibers leads to *Horner's syndrome*: ptosis, miosis (a small pupil), and anhidrosis (lack of sweating) (Fig. 12.14B). Given the vulnerability of injury during its long route, sympathetic tract damage leading to a Horner's syndrome can result from injury to any of several widely separate locations, including lateral medullary infarction (see Wallenberg syndrome; Fig. 2.10); cervical spinal cord injury; apical lung (Pancoast) tumor; and internal carotid artery dissection.

A novice might confuse Horner's syndrome with a third nerve palsy because ptosis is a manifestation common to both conditions. However, the ptosis in Horner's syndrome is always mild, while in a third nerve palsy it may be quite severe. Also, the pupil in Horner's syndrome is small, while third nerve injury causes a dilated, unreactive pupil. Anhidrosis in Horner's syndrome is another clue, but one that is difficult to detect.

In a different situation, the astute physician confronting a small pupil must also bear in mind that the real problem may be that the contralateral one is abnormally large. Causes of a dilated pupil include lesions that damage the parasympathetic supply of the pupil sphincter muscles, including oculomotor nerve injury, because lack of parasympathetic innervation leaves the sympathetic innervation unopposed. An acquired benign variation, *Adie pupil*, exemplifies the pupil-dilating effect of depriving a pupil of its normal parasympathetic innervation (Fig. 12.15).

In yet another example, accidentally rubbing atropine-like substances into the affected eye can cause a dilated pupil. In a notorious variant, medical personnel surreptitiously instill eye drops with anticholinergic properties. The unilateral dilated pupil typically triggers hospitalization and a series of investigations.

Argyll–Robertson pupils are irregular, asymmetric, and small (1–2 mm). They characteristically constrict normally when patients look at closely held objects (i.e., during accommodation), but fail to react to light. The intact accommodation, but impaired light reflex, especially with the historic association with syphilis, has been memorialized in the simile, "Argyll–Robertson pupils are like prostitutes – they accommodate but do not react." Today's statistics belie that mnemonic: diabetic autonomic neuropathy and cataract surgery currently cause almost all of cases of Argyll–Robertson pupils.

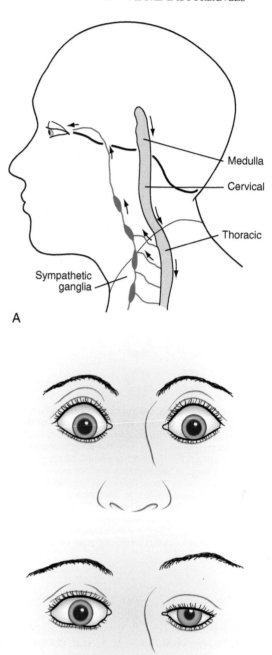

A

B

FIGURE 12.14 ■ *A*, Sympathetic nervous system fibers originate in the hypothalamus and descend through the brainstem into the lower cervical and uppermost thoracic spinal cord. Some sympathetic fibers leave the spinal cord and, after passing over the apex of the lung, ascend to form ganglia adjacent to the cervical vertebrae. Axons from these ganglia then travel superiorly wrapped around the common carotid and then internal carotid arteries until they enter the orbit with the ophthalmic division of the trigeminal nerve (V_1). Through these postsynaptic neurons, the sympathetic nervous system innervates the pupil dilator muscles, eyelid muscles, and facial sweat glands. *B, Top*, Sympathetic nervous system activity retracts the eyelid, dilates the pupil, and causes sweating. States of excitement, including amphetamine use, may induce these cardinal signs of the flight-or-fight response. *Bottom*, Interruption of the left sympathetic tract in this patient has caused *Horner's syndrome* – ptosis, miosis, and anhidrosis – on the left side. A subtle clue to Horner's syndrome ptosis is the eyebrow elevation, which is an unconscious contraction forehead (frontalis) muscles to uncover the pupil.

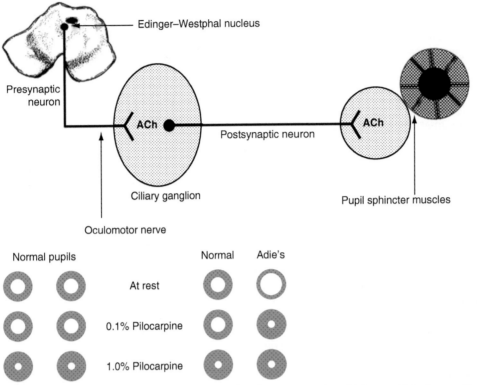

FIGURE 12.15 ■ *Top,* The parasympathetic innervation of the pupil sphincter muscle, which constricts the pupil, originates in the Edinger–Westphal nucleus (also see Fig. 4.2), part of the third cranial (oculomotor) nerve nucleus. Parasympathetic fibers from that nucleus travel along with the oculomotor nerve, then separate and synapse in the ciliary ganglion. From there, postsynaptic fibers form a neuromuscular junction with the sphincter muscles. Acetylcholine (ACh) is the neurotransmitter in both synapses. Through this pathway, light and various other stimuli cause pupil constriction. *Bottom,* In the Adie pupil, which is typically a unilateral condition, the ciliary ganglion degenerates and the pupil, deprived of parasympathetic innervation, dilates. The loss of the ciliary ganglion also subjects the pupil to denervation hypersensitivity. In this patient, the left (Adie) pupil is dilated at rest in room light due to loss of parasympathetic innervation. In response to bright light, it constricts weakly, incompletely, and slowly. Diluted cholinergic eye drops (0.1% pilocarpine), which have no effect on normal pupils including this patient's unaffected right eye, produce a brisk and long-lasting constriction of the Adie pupil. The reaction is exaggerated in the Adie pupil because its denervated postsynaptic neurons are overly sensitive due to denervation hypersensitivity. Normal pupils as well as the Adie pupil will constrict when physicians apply a more concentrated solution of pilocarpine (1%). The combination of Adie pupil with loss of deep tendon reflexes is known as *Holmes–Adie syndrome.*

REFERENCES

Bengtzen, R., Woodward, M., Lynn, M. J., et al. (2008). The "sunglasses sign" predicts nonorganic visual loss in neuroophthalmologic practice. *Neurology, 70,* 218–221.

Chen, J. J., Chang, H. F., Hsu, Y. C., et al. (2015). Anton-Babinski syndrome in an old patient: A case report and literature review. *Psychogeriatrics, 15,* 58–61.

Giussani, C., Roux, F. E., Bello, L., et al. (2009). Who is who: Areas of the brain associated with recognizing and naming famous faces. *Journal of Neurosurgery, 110,* 289–299.

Gersztenkorn, D., & Lee, A. G. (2015). Palinopsia revamped: A systemic review of the literature. *Survey of Ophthalmology, 60,* 1–35.

Holbrook, J. T., Jabs, D. A., Weinberg, D. V., et al. (2003). Visual loss in patients with cytomegalovirus retinitis and acquired immunodeficiency syndrome before widespread availability of highly active antiretroviral therapy. *Archives of Ophthalmology, 121,* 99–107.

Kang, S. S., Dionisio, D. P., & Sponheim, S. R. (2011). Abnormal mechanisms of antisaccade generation in schizophrenia patients and unaffected biological relatives of schizophrenia patients. *Psychophysiology, 48,* 350–361.

Liu, G. T., Volpe, N. J., & Galetta, S. L. (2010). *Neuro-Ophthalmology: Diagnosis and Management* (2nd ed.). Philadelphia: Saunders.

Schadlu, A. P., Schadlu, R., & Shepherd, J. B. (2009). Charles Bonnet syndrome: A review. *Current Opinion in Ophthalmology, 20,* 219–222.

QUESTIONS AND ANSWERS

1. Which *three* findings characterize Argyll–Robertson pupils?
   a. Miosis (small pupil)
   b. Ptosis
   c. Irregular shape
   d. Unresponsiveness to light
   e. Unresponsiveness to accommodation
   f. Failure to dilate with atropine drops

Answer: a, c, d. Small, irregular, and unreactive pupils – Argyll–Robertson pupils – classically characterize tertiary neurosyphilis. For example, neurologists find this constellation of abnormalities in 90% of tabes dorsalis cases. With neurosyphilis cases occurring so rarely, neurologists now find these changes most often as a result of diabetic ocular changes.

2. Which medication often produces transient visual impairment because of accommodation paresis?
   a. Haloperidol
   b. Amitriptyline
   c. Carbamazepine
   d. Phenobarbital

Answer: b. The anticholinergic side effects of tricyclic antidepressants lead to visual impairment.

3. Which one of the following does not cause cataracts that impair vision?
   a. Myotonic dystrophy
   b. Diabetes mellitus
   c. Ocular trauma
   d. Chlorpromazine

Answer: d. Myotonic dystrophy, diabetes, and ocular trauma may cause cataracts dense enough to impair vision. Phenothiazines, some atypical neuroleptics, and amiodarone cause lens opacities that do not reach the density of cataracts.

4. A 20-year-old soldier develops loss of vision in the right eye accompanied by retro-orbital pain, especially when looking from side to side. An ophthalmologist finds no ocular or neurologic abnormalities except for a decreased reaction to light shone into the right pupil. However, both pupils constrict to light shone into the left eye. After 1 week, vision returns except for a small central scotoma. Which is the most likely diagnosis?
   a. Charles Bonnet syndrome
   b. Optic neuritis
   c. Left cerebral infarction
   d. Pituitary adenoma
   e. Glaucoma

Answer: b. The loss of vision accompanied by an impaired direct light reflex but preserved consensual response in the right pupil indicates that the problem is in the right optic nerve. This cranial nerve forms the afferent limb of the pupillary light reflex. The pain indicates nerve inflammation, i.e., neuritis. In retrobulbar optic neuritis, the "patient sees nothing and the ophthalmologist sees nothing." Optic neuritis as an isolated condition or a manifestation of multiple sclerosis (MS) occurs relatively commonly among young adults.

5. Which cells produce the myelin covering of the optic nerve?
   a. Schwann cells
   b. Oligodendroglia
   c. Neurons
   d. Microglia

Answer: b. The optic nerve is actually an extension of the central nervous system (CNS). Oligodendroglia produce the myelin that covers the white matter of the CNS, which includes the optic nerve and a small proximal portion of the acoustic nerve. In contrast, Schwann cells produce the myelin that covers the peripheral nerves and the other cranial nerves. Microglia are supporting cells of the CNS.

6. As individuals age beyond 50 years they typically require reading glasses to discern closely held objects, such as newspapers and sewing. Without their glasses, they must hold such objects at arm's length. What accounts for this visual problem?
   a. Cataract formation impairs accommodation.
   b. Retinal degeneration prevents accommodation.
   c. Their lenses lose elasticity and dehydrate.
   d. They develop visual agnosia.

Answer: c. As people age, their lenses lose elasticity and fluid content. Aged lenses are unable to widen rapidly or fully, and thus cannot accommodate to focus on closely held objects.

7. A 79-year-old woman who has been blind since cataract surgery 5 years earlier discloses that she has been "seeing" her children as babies, her long deceased parents, and picturesque scenes. The visions last several minutes to an hour and occur at any time of the day. She is not frightened or inclined to act on them. She recognizes that the visions are hallucinations. An examination discloses no cognitive impairment or physical neurologic signs. What should be the next step?
   a. Perform an EEG
   b. Obtain an MRI

c. Administer an antipsychotic
d. Administer an antidepressant
e. Do none of the above

Answer: e. She has Charles Bonnet syndrome in which visually impaired individuals experience visual hallucinations in the absence of dementia, delirium, or a psychiatric disturbance. Because the hallucinations result from sensory deprivation ("deafferentation"), neurologists label them "release visual hallucinations" or more simply "release phenomena" and construct an analogy to phantom limb pain. Visual hallucinations, presumably also on the basis of sensory deprivation, may occur in the blind field of individuals with homonymous hemianopia. For example, in a patient with a left homonymous hemianopia from a right posterior cerebral artery stroke, visual hallucinations might arise in the left visual field. Being elderly and having other sensory impairments, particularly deafness, predispose blind individuals to experiencing visual hallucinations. If reassurance and providing alternative sensory input suppress the hallucinations, physicians do not have to proceed with administering medicines. Second-generation antipsychotics, on either an "as-needed" or nightly basis, may suppress the hallucinations.

8. Which of the following is a *true* statement regarding electroencephalogram (EEG) alpha activity in patients with ocular blindness?
   a. Alpha activity is located over the occipital lobes both at rest and when the eyes are open.
   b. Alpha activity is absent both at rest and when the eyes are open.
   c. Alpha activity is present when the eyes are open but not at rest.
   d. None of the above.

Answer: a. Sighted individuals at rest with their eyes closed have alpha activity, but when they open their eyes, alpha activity disappears as visual information is transmitted to the occipital lobe. In individuals blinded by ocular injury, the alpha activity persists because no visual information is transmitted to the occipital lobe. In contrast, if someone has psychogenic blindness, opening the eyes will abolish alpha activity. Of course, if individuals have a widespread occipital cortex injury, they will not be able to generate alpha activity with their eyes open or shut.

9. Which one of the following statements is *false* regarding glaucoma?
   a. Serotonin reuptake inhibitors are less likely than tricyclic antidepressants to precipitate glaucoma.
   b. Most cases of glaucoma in the United States are the angle-closure type.
   c. Beta-blocker topical medications (eyedrops) often enter the systemic circulation in concentrations great enough to cause transient mental changes.
   d. Patients being treated for glaucoma may safely be given tricyclic antidepressants.

Answer: b. Among glaucoma patients in the United States, about 90% have the open-angle variety. On the other hand, angle-closure glaucoma is more common in

Asian people, probably because their angles tend to be narrower.

10–15. Match the clinical presentation (10–15) with the accompanying visual field loss (a–f). Answers may be used more than once. These drawings follow the conventional practice of showing visual fields from the patient's perspective, i.e., "right is right," and colored areas represent regions that the patient cannot see. Also, the right eye appears on the right, and the left eye on the left.

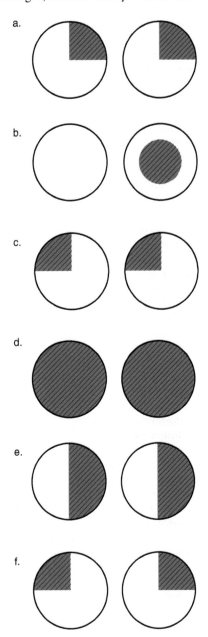

10. A 25-year-old woman has paraparesis and ataxia.
11. A 35-year-old woman has insidious onset of loss of peripheral daytime vision and all nighttime vision. Her mother has a similar illness.
12. A 30-year-old man has episodes of seeing the American flag and hearing the first five bars of "America the Beautiful."

13. A 21-year-old man has loss of bodily hair, gynecomastia, and diabetes insipidus.

14. A 70-year-old man has global aphasia, right hemiplegia, and right hemisensory loss.

15. A 75-year-old man has fluent aphasia.

Answers:

10–b. The patient has spinal cord, cerebellar, and right optic nerve injury, probably as the result of MS.

11–d. The patient and her mother have preservation only of central vision during daytime. If examination of her fundi showed clumping of retinal pigment, the diagnosis of retinitis pigmentosa would be certain. These visual fields might also be obtained from someone having tunnel vision.

12–a or c. The patient may have a lesion in one temporal lobe, giving rise to focal seizures and a contralateral homonymous superior quadrantanopsia.

13–f. The patient has a large pituitary tumor causing panhypopituitarism and bitemporal superior quadrantanopsia.

14–e. The patient probably has a large left hemisphere lesion, such as a stroke or tumor, giving a right homonymous hemianopia.

15–a. A lesion in the left temporal lobe is producing receptive aphasia and a right superior homonymous quadrantanopsia.

16–26. Match the characteristics of the visual hallucination or other symptom (16–26) with its most likely source(s) (a–c). More than one choice may be correct.

16. Co-occurrence of both visual and musical hallucinations

17. Co-occurrence of both visual and olfactory hallucinations

18. Flashes of bright lights in one visual hemifield

19. Rotating blotches of color

20. Formed hallucinations with impaired consciousness

21. Postictal aphasia

22. Throbbing unilateral headache

23. Nausea and vomiting

24. Simple blocks and stars of color

25. Twisting, complicated multicolored lights

26. Faces with distorted features or coloring
  a. Seizures that originate in the occipital lobe
  b. Seizures that originate in the temporal lobe
  c. Migraine with aura (classical migraine)

Answers: 16–b; 17–b, rarely c; 18–a, c; 19–a; 20–b; 21–b, rarely c; 22–c; 23–c; 24–a, c; 25–c, less likely b; 26–c, less likely b.

27–28. Match the symptom (27–28) with the possible cause(s) (a–d).

27. Diplopia when looking to the right

28. Diplopia when looking to the left
  a. Left third nerve palsy
  b. Left sixth nerve palsy
  c. Right third nerve palsy
  d. Right sixth nerve palsy

Answers: 27–a, d; 28–b, c.

29–30. Match the actions that cause blindness (29–30) with the mechanism (a–c).

29. Staring directly into the sun

30. Drinking adulterated alcohols
  a. Methanol-induced optic nerve injury
  b. Pigmentary retinal degeneration
  c. Retinal burns

Answers: 29–c; 30–a.

31. Which *four* conditions are common causes of ptosis?
  a. Third nerve palsy
  b. Sixth nerve palsy
  c. Pancoast tumor
  d. MS
  e. Myasthenia gravis
  f. Psychogenic disturbances
  g. Botulinum treatment of blepharospasm

Answer: a, c, e, g. Third nerve palsy, Horner syndrome, and myasthenia gravis are classic causes of ptosis. When neurologists inject botulinum toxin into the orbicularis oculi to treat blepharospasm, it may enter the levator palpebrae (either by inadvertent injection directly into this muscle or by diffusion) and cause ptosis. In addition, laxity of ligaments, muscles, and other soft tissues commonly occurs with normal aging, often causing older individuals' eyelids to sag and giving the appearance of ptosis. A rare cause of ptosis along with paresis of all ocular movement is progressive external ophthalmoplegia, due to mutation in mitochondrial DNA.

32. Which *three* conditions may cause internuclear ophthalmoplegia (INO)?
  a. MS
  b. Midbrain strokes
  c. Pons strokes
  d. Occlusion of the posterior inferior cerebellar artery (PICA)
  e. Dominant hemisphere strokes
  f. Psychogenic disturbances

Answer: a, b, c. MS plaques or strokes affecting the medial longitudinal fasciculus (MLF) in the pons or the midbrain may cause INO. Occlusions of PICA lead to the lateral medullary syndrome, which includes nystagmus and Horner syndrome, but do not involve the MLF, which is located in the medial, not lateral, brainstem. Cerebral lesions cannot damage the MLF. Individuals cannot feign an INO.

33. Which ocular motility abnormality is most closely associated with schizophrenia?
  a. Internuclear ophthalmoplegia
  b. Nystagmus
  c. Convergence spasm

d. Conjugate gaze paresis
e. Pursuit abnormalities

Answer: e. Schizophrenic patients often have slow, irregular pursuit movements and saccade abnormalities. However, those ocular motility abnormalities are not unique to schizophrenia. Even bedside examination will detect them in Huntington disease as well as in mood disorders. These ocular motility abnormalities appear independent of dopamine-blocking antipsychotic medications and are detectable in asymptomatic first-degree relatives of schizophrenic patients. Convergence spasm usually represents a psychogenic disturbance.

34. A 70-year-old man awakens with a right hemiparesis, vertigo, and his eyes deviated to the right. Which condition will also be found?
    a. Aphasia
    b. Right homonymous hemianopia
    c. Dementia
    d. Nystagmus

Answer: d. The right hemiparesis and eyes deviated to the right indicate that he has sustained an infarction in his left pons. He likely would have nystagmus because of damage to the vestibular nuclei, which are located in the pons. Neurologists would also predict left upper and lower facial paresis because of injury to the left facial nerve nucleus, which is also situated in the pons. He would not have hemianopia, aphasia, or other cognitive impairment because those are signs of cerebral injury.

35. Which condition indicates that the dopamine system is involved in conjugate eye movement?
    a. Internuclear ophthalmoplegia
    b. Nystagmus
    c. Progressive supranuclear palsy
    d. Oculogyric crisis

Answer: d. Phenothiazines, including those used for nonpsychotic conditions such as nausea and vomiting, precipitate oculogyric crises.

36. Which conditions have a predilection for people older than 65 years?
    a. Myopia
    b. Presbyopia
    c. Macular degeneration
    d. Classic migraines
    e. Temporal or giant cell arteritis
    f. Glaucoma
    g. Cataracts
    h. Optic neuritis

Answer: b, c, e, f, g. Moreover, combinations of these conditions may occur together in the same older patient. Whatever the cause of a visual impairment, it is a major threat to the wellbeing of patients, especially those with cognitive deficits or loss of other special senses.

37. A 70-year-old man suddenly developed right-sided homonymous hemianopia, hemisensory loss, and mild hemiparesis. In addition, although he can both say and write the names of objects that he feels, he is unable to name objects that he only sees, even when they are presented to his left visual field. What is the name of this condition?
    a. Aphasia
    b. Hemi-inattention
    c. Visual agnosia
    d. Gerstmann syndrome
    e. Balint syndrome
    f. Dementia
    g. Alexia

Answer: c. The patient has visual agnosia, a condition in which patients cannot process visually acquired information. Additional testing might reveal Gerstmann syndrome or alexia without agraphia (see Chapter 8) – conditions also resulting from posterior dominant hemisphere lesions. His problem is not aphasia: Once the examiner circumvents vision, by testing the patient's writing and speaking and allowing the patient to touch objects, language function is shown to be normal. The lesion causing visual agnosia is usually in the left parietal and occipital region.

38. With the onset of menopause, a 59-year-old woman experiences an increase in the frequency of her migraines from once a month to twice weekly. Her neurologist initiates preventative treatment with topiramate. Several weeks later, the woman reports bilateral visual impairment and eye pain. A consulting ophthalmologist finds that she has redness of the eyes, large pupils, and shallow anterior chambers. Which of the following conditions has most likely developed?
    a. Open-angle glaucoma
    b. Angle-closure glaucoma
    c. Optic neuritis
    d. Self-inflicted eye injury

Answer: b. She likely has developed angle-closure glaucoma with elevated intraocular pressure. Although the glaucoma may have developed spontaneously, the topiramate treatment probably precipitated it.

39–46. Match the patient's deficit (39–46) with the neuropsychologic disorder (a–j).

39. Cannot recognize familiar faces
40. Despite visual loss, willfully but erroneously describes hospital room and physician
41. After cardiac arrest, blindness with intact pupil light reflex
42. Cannot identify a red card, although able to match it to another red card and read a red-colored number on the Ishihara plates
43. Despite only a right homonymous hemianopia, inability to read. Writing ability is intact.
44. Congenital inability to read Ishihara plates
45. Inability to name common objects under any circumstances
46. Cannot name objects when seen, but can name them when described or grasped
    a. Cortical blindness

b. Visual agnosia
c. Color agnosia
d. Color blindness
e. Prosopagnosia
f. Anton syndrome
g. Psychogenic blindness
h. Alexia without agraphia
i. Congenital cerebral injury
j. Anomia

Answer: 39–e, 40–f, 41–a, 42–c, 43–h, 44–d, 45–j, 46–b.

47. Which *three* conditions cause stereotyped visual hallucinations?
    a. Temporal lobe seizures
    b. Occipital lobe seizures
    c. Tonic-clonic seizures
    d. Hypnagogic hallucinations
    e. Migraine with aura
    f. Migraine without aura
    g. D-lysergic acid diethylamide (LSD) ingestion
    h. Alcohol withdrawal

Answer: a, b, e. Focal seizures that originate in the temporal lobe or visual cortex and migraine with aura cause the patient to experience the same – stereotyped – visual hallucination with each attack. In contrast, primary generalized seizures (absences and tonic-clonic) seizures do not cause an aura or visual symptoms. Intoxications and withdrawal cause varied hallucinations – often tactile as well as visual – among other symptoms of delirium. Hypnagogic and hypnopompic hallucinations, which are essentially dreams that intrude into wakefulness (see Chapter 17), are variable.

48. Which *three* varieties of hallucinations appear predominantly or exclusively in hemianopic areas?
    a. Palinopsia
    b. Partial seizures
    c. Migraines
    d. REM-associated dreams
    e. Charles Bonnet syndrome

Answer: a, b, e. In palinopsia and focal seizures, visual hallucinations often appear exclusively within a hemianopic region. Benign visual hallucinations in an area of visual loss in the context of a clear sensorium – the Charles Bonnet syndrome – may appear in a hemianopic area as well as in complete blindness. Hallucinations related to migraines, dreams, and intoxications occur randomly and do not respect visual fields.

49. A 35-year-old woman seeks neurologic consultation because she has developed "droopy eyelids" and inability to look in any direction. Her symptoms persist evenly throughout the day. She explains that her sister, younger by 5 years, has begun to have the same facial appearance and paralysis of gaze. The patient has bilateral, symmetric ptosis and inability to move her eyes in any direction, but her pupils are round, equal, and reactive to light. She shows normal mentation, lower cranial nerves, muscle, and reflexes. Which is the most likely disorder?
    a. Myasthenia gravis
    b. Botulism
    c. Lambert–Eaton syndrome
    d. Progressive external ophthalmoplegia

Answer: d. Progressive external ophthalmoplegia, a mitochondrial myopathy, causes paresis of all the extraocular muscles, which produces ptosis and immobility of eye movement. As in myasthenia gravis, ptosis is prominent and pupillary reaction to light is preserved; however, progressive external ophthalmoplegia worsens insidiously and does not fluctuate, affects muscles symmetrically, and usually spares facial, vocal, and limb muscles. In progressive external ophthalmoplegia, genetic tests of mitochondrial DNA will show mutations, and tests for myasthenia, such as acetylcholine receptor antibodies, EMGs, and a Tensilon test, will be negative. Leber hereditary optic atrophy, which causes blindness, is another disorder attributable to a mitochondrial DNA mutation (see Chapter 6).

50. Which *two* of the following statements are *true* regarding saccades?
    a. Saccades are the smooth, steady tracking movements used to follow moving objects.
    b. They are the quick, conjugate movements that bring images from the periphery to the center of vision.
    c. They are governed by supranuclear centers.
    d. Unlike pursuit movements, they are resistant to structural lesions and degenerative illnesses.

Answer: b, c. Cerebral conjugate gaze centers generate saccades, which are high-velocity conjugate gaze movements.

51. A 68-year-old retired well-known actor sought neurologic consultation because he has frequently fallen while descending stairs or walking off a curb. His friends and ex-wife thought that he was showing the effects of alcoholism. The neurologist found a paucity of facial and limb movements, rigidity of limbs, and loss of postural reflexes, but no tremor. He was unable to look upward or downward in response to requests, but when the neurologist flexed and extended his head and neck (rocked his head up and down), his eyes moved in both vertical directions. Which is the most likely diagnosis?
    a. Parkinson disease
    b. Progressive supranuclear palsy (PSP)
    c. Psychogenic disturbance
    d. Wernicke–Korsakoff syndrome

Answer: b. PSP, a disorder related to Parkinson disease, characteristically causes loss of voluntary vertical eye movement and Parkinson-like rigidity, bradykinesia, and progressive cognitive impairment. The loss of vertical eye movements explains why patients fall or trip while descending stairs or a curb. The signature of PSP is preserved ocular movement in response to flexing and extending the head and neck, i.e., PSP patients have preserved oculocephalic reflexes.

52. Which of the following is *not* a characteristic of an Adie pupil?
   a. Loss of parasympathetic innervation
   b. Denervation hypersensitivity to noradrenergic stimulation
   c. Denervation hypersensitivity to cholinergic stimulation
   d. Constriction to 0.1% pilocarpine

Answer: b. The ciliary ganglion supplies parasympathetic innervation to the pupillary constrictor muscles. If it is damaged, as in an Adie pupil, unopposed sympathetic innervation dilates the pupil. The unaffected pupil remains normal in size and reactivity. Room light is insufficient to constrict an Adie pupil. Although bright light constricts it, the movement is slow and incomplete. The distinguishing feature of an Adie pupil is that, because of parasympathetic denervation, the pupillary constrictor muscles have denervation hypersensitivity to cholinergic stimulation. Thus, a dilute pilocarpine solution (0.1%) constricts an Adie pupil but not its unaffected counterpart. A more concentrated pilocarpine solution (1%), which can be used to treat glaucoma, will constrict normal as well as denervated pupils. In the Holmes–Adie syndrome, an Adie pupil is associated with absence of deep tendon reflexes.

53. In which *four* conditions is Horner syndrome commonly found?
   a. Migraine without aura
   b. Migraine with aura
   c. Cluster headache
   d. Trigeminal neuralgia
   e. Cervical spinal cord injury
   f. Apical lung tumor
   g. Lateral medullary infarction

Answer: c, e, f, g. Horner syndrome may result from lesions in the brainstem, cervical (or uppermost thoracic) portion of the spinal cord, apex of the lung, or the carotid artery – anywhere along the circuitous route of the sympathetic innervation of the pupil (see Fig. 12.14). Horner syndrome in cluster headache is thought to originate in the cavernous sinus, which transmits the internal carotid artery with associated sympathetic fibers, as well as trigeminal and parasympathetic fibers.

54. Which cerebral artery supplies the occipital lobes?
   a. Anterior cerebral
   b. Middle cerebral
   c. Posterior cerebral
   d. None of the above

Answer: c. The posterior cerebral arteries, which are the terminal branches of the basilar artery, perfuse the occipital lobes. Because the occipital lobes contain the primary visual cortex, occlusion of both posterior cerebral arteries causes cortical blindness. An occlusion of the left posterior cerebral artery that causes an infarction of the left occipital lobe and posterior corpus callosum (the splenium) may cause alexia without agraphia as well as a right homonymous hemianopia (see Chapter 8).

55. A 33-year-old man claims to have double vision in his right eye after a motor vehicle crash. When he covers the right eye, the diplopia disappears, but when he covers the left eye, he has persistent diplopia. The visual acuity in the left eye is 20/20 and in the right eye 20/400. Visual fields are normal in the left eye but cannot be determined in the right eye because of the diplopia. Which *three* statements regarding his situation are *true*?
   a. His symptom is monocular diplopia.
   b. With the available information, conclusions cannot be drawn concerning the presence of CNS injury causing the diplopia.
   c. Monocular diplopia may result from an ocular injury, such as a dislocated lens or retinal tear.
   d. The first step in determining the cause of diplopia is to establish whether it arises from a single eye. In other words, determine if covering one eye abolishes the diplopia.

Answer: a, c, d. When the brainstem or cranial nerves III, IV, and/or VI are injured, patients have diplopia only if both eyes are open. As a general rule, cerebral lesions do not cause diplopia. When diplopia originates from one eye, neurologists say that the patient has monocular diplopia. Its causes are usually an ocular injury or a psychogenic disorder.

56. In which structure is the nucleus of the third cranial nerve located?
   a. Midbrain
   b. Pons
   c. Medulla
   d. Cerebrum

Answer: a.

57. In which structure is the nucleus of the fourth cranial nerve located?
   a. Midbrain
   b. Pons
   c. Medulla
   d. Cerebrum

Answer: a.

58. In which structure is the nucleus of the sixth cranial nerve located?
   a. Midbrain
   b. Pons
   c. Medulla
   d. Cerebrum

Answer: b.

59. During an evaluation for possible dementia, a neurologist showed a 75-year-old man a picture of his anniversary party that had been held when he was 50 years old.

He recognized most friends and family members but could not identify the relationships between them. He could not recall the reason for the party despite a "Happy 25th Anniversary" banner in the background. He looked from one person to another, but he failed to survey the scene and was unable to direct his gaze. He was oriented and had satisfactory memory and judgment. His visual acuity and visual fields were within normal limits. Which is the best term describing his inability to comprehend the picture?
a. Dementia
b. Cortical blindness
c. Bilateral hemi-inattention
d. Gerstmann syndrome
e. Balint syndrome
f. Depression

Answer: e. Balint syndrome consists of ocular apraxia (psychic paralysis of fixation), optic ataxia, and simultanagnosia. Simultanagnosia prevents one from simultaneously perceiving objects in the periphery and in the center of vision. Ocular apraxia refers to inability to shift one's gaze from one object to another, as though the first object were overwhelmingly captivating. The simultanagnosia and ocular apraxia inhibit patients from exploring space. Optic ataxia refers to the inability to reach accurately with visual guidance.

60. In a stuporous 1-year-old infant, what further testing does the presence of retinal hemorrhages indicate?
a. Blood glucose for diabetes mellitus
b. HIV testing for AIDS-related retinal disease
c. X-rays of the long bones
d. Sickle cell determination

Answer: c. Retinal hemorrhages suggest the "shaken baby" syndrome, which physicians consider a nonaccidental head injury. Clinicians should seek other signs of child abuse, such as skin lesions and spiral fractures of the long bones. Of course, the physicians should also order a head CT in a stuporous infant with signs of trauma.

61. During her recovery from a lumbar laminectomy, a 35-year-old nurse complains of the sudden onset of poor vision in her right eye. That pupil is dilated and does not respond to light shone into either eye. Pilocarpine eyedrops (1%) also fail to constrict the pupil. Her extraocular movements are full and the fundoscopic examination reveals no abnormalities. The remainder of the neurologic examination is normal. A CT, MRI, and LP all produce normal results. The intraocular pressure is normal. A similar problem followed her hysterectomy the previous year. What is the most likely cause of her visual impairment?
a. Myasthenia gravis
b. A left-sided Horner syndrome
c. Adie pupil
d. None of the above

Answer: d. The failure of pilocarpine, a strong miotic agent, to constrict the pupil indicates that someone put a substance onto her eye. Cocaine, atropine, and hydroxyamphetamine eye drops dilate the normal pupil. In addition, several nonophthalmologic medicines, including Preparation H, which contains a sympathomimetic, dilate a normal pupil. Myasthenia gravis does not affect the pupils. An Adie pupil, unlike a normal pupil, constricts with even a dilute (0.1%) pilocarpine solution and slowly reacts to a bright light.

62. A 27-year-old woman has suddenly lost vision in her left eye. In room light her pupils are equal in size. When a light is shone into the left eye, neither pupil constricts; however, when light is shone into the right eye, both pupils constrict. Which portion of the light reflex is impaired?
a. Afferent limb from left eye
b. Afferent limb from right eye
c. Efferent limb to left eye
d. Efferent limb to right eye

Answer: a. Something has injured her left optic nerve, which constitutes the afferent arc of the light reflex.

63. In evaluating another patient with an impaired light reflex, the physician finds that when a light is shone into the left eye, only the right pupil constricts. When light is shone into the right eye, only the right pupil constricts. Which portion of the light reflex is impaired?
a. Afferent limb from left eye
b. Afferent limb from right eye
c. Efferent limb to left eye
d. Efferent limb to right eye

Answer: c. Something has injured her left oculomotor nerve, which constitutes the efferent arc of the light reflex. Alternatives include ocular trauma and instillation of eye drops.

64. A 72-year-old retired psychiatrist reported that suddenly and painlessly a gray curtain obscured vision in her left eye for 3 minutes. During the episode she assured herself that the vision in her right eye was normal by performing a visual field examination and reading newsprint. Which term most appropriately describes her symptom?
a. Amaurosis fugax
b. Left homonymous hemianopia
c. Acute angle-closure glaucoma
d. Palinopsia

Answer: a. She experienced transient (fugax) loss of vision (amaurosis). The intact vision in the right eye excludes a homonymous visual field cut. Amaurosis fugax is often caused by emboli that originate in the carotid artery and pass into the ophthalmic artery. When patients have this symptom, neurologists usually evaluate them for carotid stenosis and prescribe antiplatelet agents such as aspirin. Sometimes carotid artery surgery or stenting is warranted.

65. A 68-year-old man, a well-respected successful lawyer, remains personable, humorous, and a good ballroom dancer. Years ago he began to forget the

names of acquaintances and some colleagues. He consulted an ophthalmologist because he has begun to fail to recognize the faces of friends, acquaintances, and historic figures, such as George Washington. However, his visual acuity is 20/20 with glasses. Which is the most likely condition?
a. Mild cognitive impairment
b. Dementia, probably from Alzheimer disease
c. Visual acuity impairment
d. Prosopagnosia superimposed on mild cognitive impairment
e. Normal age-related cognitive changes

Answer: d. He has developed prosopagnosia, which is a visual perceptual problem consisting of an inability to recognize faces, superimposed on mild cognitive impairment. Prosopagnosia is usually attributable to a neurodegenerative illness, such as frontotemporal dementia or Alzheimer disease. Although the patient may have mild cognitive impairment, he does not have dementia because he still functions.

66. A 43-year-old man, who was well-known to the emergency room staff as a chronic alcoholic and "down on his luck," seemed to say that he was seeing "snow" in both his eyes. His symptom was difficult to understand because of confusion, disorientation, and dysarthria, but, as best as the staff could determine, his vision was 20/200 even with his glasses. His visual fields were full to confrontation. His pupils were slow to react to light. He had nystagmus with no paresis of extraocular muscles. His gait was ataxic. Blood tests detected an anion gap with profound metabolic acidosis. The staff administered intravenous thiamine. Which treatment(s) should they administer in addition to the thiamine?
a. Bicarbonate, ethanol, and hemodialysis
b. Fosphenytoin
c. A long-acting benzodiazepine
d. Pyridoxine and cobalamin

Answer: a. Because of the "snowy" vision, poor visual acuity, and slow pupillary light reaction, the emergency room staff correctly concluded that this alcoholic probably drank ethanol adulterated with methanol. To prevent cardiovascular collapse and toxic damage, they administered bicarbonate to counteract the acidosis; ethanol to divert the metabolism of methanol, which yields toxic metabolites (formaldehyde and formic acid); and hemodialysis to clear the methanol and its metabolites. In methanol poisonings, fomepizole may be more effective than ethanol in reducing formaldehyde and formic acid levels.

67. Which is a common permanent sequela of methanol poisoning?
a. Optic atrophy and blindness
b. Peripheral neuropathy
c. Stroke
d. Ataxia

Answer: a. Methanol preferentially damages the optic nerves. It also damages the putamen and may lead to parkinsonism.

68–71. Match the visual disturbance (68–71) with the etiology (a–e).

68. Psychic blindness
69. Night blindness
70. Cortical blindness
71. Transient monocular blindness
    a. Carotid stenosis
    b. Bilateral occipital damage
    c. Conversion reaction
    d. Bilateral temporal lobe damage
    e. Vitamin A deficiency

Answers: 68–d (Klüver–Bucy syndrome), 69–e, 70–b, 71–a (amaurosis fugax). In addition, night blindness is also a symptom of retinitis pigmentosa.

CONGENITAL CEREBRAL IMPAIRMENTS

Many perinatal cerebral injuries, brain malformations, and genetic mutations create distinctive and life-long neurologic, neuropsychologic, and physical impairments. Although usually apparent in infancy, some of these disorders do not become evident until childhood or adolescence. One explanation for the delay is that the time course of cerebral myelination, which begins in the third trimester of gestation and extends from the brainstem to the cortex, is not complete until the second year of life. Another explanation is that infants and young children, despite mild brain injury, may reach their early milestones, but eventually they cannot meet the progressively greater challenges first of learning to walk, then speaking and drawing, and eventually caring for themselves. Regardless of the age when neurologists detect children's congenital impairments, they know that these children will grow up to be adults with the same impairments.

From the viewpoint of the *Diagnostic and Statistical Manual of Mental Disorder, 5th Edition* (DSM-5), many of these disorders serve as a specifier – an underlying medical or genetic condition – for neurodevelopmental disorders and, in particular, autism spectrum disorder (ASD). For example, a psychiatrist would say that a child has ASD associated with Rett syndrome (Box 13.1). In contrast, neurologists look at the nomenclature from the perspective of the primary illness. They would say, for example, that a child has Rett syndrome with symptoms of social and language regression, epilepsy, and hand-washing stereotypies. Similarly, the current *10th International Statistical Classification of Diseases and Related Health Problems* (ICD-10) usually places the code for the primary underlying illness before its manifestations.

CEREBRAL PALSY

Cerebral palsy (CP) is a nonscientific but generally accepted term that describes the permanent, nonprogressive neurologic *motor system* impairments that result from injuries or genetic abnormalities of the immature brain during fetal development (*in utero*), delivery, infancy, or early childhood. Some textbooks and articles have begun to use the term "static encephalopathy" rather than "CP," but since "CP" remains ingrained in the medical and lay public's vocabulary, this book will continue to use it.

Several nonmotor problems routinely accompany but fall outside of the operational definition of CP. They include, most importantly, epilepsy and *intellectual disability*. As a general rule, the incidence of epilepsy roughly corresponds to the severity of physical impairments and intellectual disability (Fig. 13.1). Other common problems that accompany CP include deficits in vision and hearing, strabismus, dysarthria, poor school performance, and impaired social skills. The DSM-5 does not define CP but allows for several of its comorbidities, including Intellectual Disability, Language Disorder, and Developmental Coordination Disorder.

Neurologists attribute most cases of CP to prematurity and low birth weight, particularly weights less than 1.5 kg. Among premature infants, *periventricular leukomalacia* (damage of the white matter around the lateral ventricles) is the predominant pathology. Other risk factors include hypoxia before or during labor, prolonged bradycardia, 10 or 15 minute Apgar score of less than 4, in utero intracerebral hemorrhage, perinatal ischemia, and postpartum multisystem organ failure. Modern prenatal, obstetric, and postpartum care has reduced the incidence of CP to about 2% of births. However, intensive neonatal care, a counterbalancing factor, has allowed very premature infants to survive with persistent motor and other neurologic impairments.

Preventable obstetric injuries, such as anoxia, account for less than 10% of cases. In contrast, unalterable antepartum factors account for more than 70%. For example, CP is often a manifestation of congenital malformations, such as microgyria (small cerebral gyri), pachygyria (thickened gyri), hydrocephalus, and porencephaly (see Fig. 20.4). Also, because 5% of CP children have a first-degree relative with a similar condition, genetic factors undoubtedly determine or at least contribute in many cases.

Neurologists often divide CP into four varieties. Each one has a characteristic motor impairment, such as *spastic paresis* or *choreoathetosis* (Fig. 13.2), and incidence of its two major comorbidities, epilepsy and intellectual disability. Unlike the motor impairments, these comorbidities may not appear before age 5 years.

Neurologists usually do not diagnose CP until infants are at least 4 months old and, in some cases, not until they are 4 years old. Moreover, once children have an established motor deficit, it must not progress as they mature. In fact, impairments may seem to recede as children learn compensatory strategies and benefit from various therapies.

Once assured that a child has a stable, congenital neurologic impairment rather than a childhood-onset neurodegenerative illness, such as a leukodystrophy (see Chapter 15) or Rett syndrome (see later), which will follow a downhill course, neurologists concentrate on the problem at hand by evaluating the child's disabilities and abilities in intellect, learning, speech, and hearing as well as motor function. Because approximately 50% of children with CP have normal intelligence despite major motor deficits, neurologists have them undergo individualized evaluations that, as much as possible, bypass motor impairments, dysarthria, hearing impairments, and other disabilities.

As a related issue, caregiver stress is a major problem for parents and siblings of a child with CP. Moreover, unlike care for an adult with a neurodegenerative illness, such as Alzheimer disease, care for a CP child is endless.

Spastic CP

In spastic CP, spasticity usually impairs mobility more than paresis. It causes slow, clumsy, and stiff movements that force affected children to walk with extended, unbending legs. The spasticity also precludes them from making normal isolated movements, such as tapping one foot while keeping the other immobile. The usual signs of upper motor neuron injury – hyperactive deep tendon reflexes (DTRs), clonus, and Babinski signs – accompany spasticity.

As a result of the cerebral injury occurring prior to physical maturation, arms or, already weak and stiff, fail to grow to their proper length and have less than normal muscle bulk. If the deficit is asymmetric, the thumb and

great-toe nail beds are smaller on the abnormal side. A short Achilles' tendon forces children to walk on their toes. Neurologists say that the foreshortened limbs have *growth arrest* and *growth asymmetry*.

Diplegic CP (spastic diplegia) consists of bilateral symmetric paraparesis (Fig. 13.3). It usually forces children to hold their legs straight, drawn together (adducted), and crossed over each other (scissored). It also forces them to keep their feet and toes pointed downward (plantarflexed). When babies with diplegic CP try to walk, this posture forces them to stand on their toes with their legs held closely together, i.e., adducted, which is an unstable stance.

Neurologists usually find the diplegic CP variety in children who have been born prematurely and have sustained periventricular leukomalacia. Because the cerebral cortex has escaped major damage, both epilepsy and intellectual disability occur in a relatively small proportion (about 25%) of these children.

Hemiplegic CP consists of spastic hemiparesis affecting the face and arm more than the leg (Fig. 13.4). Although the motor impairments of children and adults with hemiplegic CP resemble adults with strokes from middle cerebral artery occlusions, the impairments differ in three respects. While normal infants younger than 2 years old do not show hand preference, infants with hemiplegic CP show premature handedness. For example, unequivocal right-handedness in infants younger than 1 year old may mean that the left hand, if not the entire left arm, is

BOX 13.1	Neurologic Syndromes That Include ASD Symptoms*
Angelman	
Fragile X	
Klinefelter	
Landau–Kleffner	
Rett	
Neurofibromatosis type 1	
Tuberous sclerosis	

*Regression, loss of language skills, and hand flapping and other stereotypies

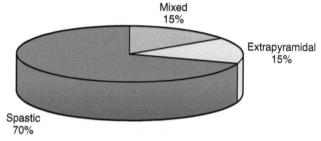

FIGURE 13.2 ■ Most cases of CP are varieties of spastic CP, but many are extrapyramidal or mixed. Because studies vary, the percentages are approximations.

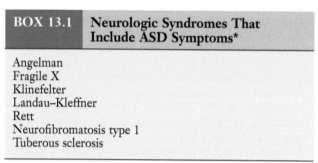
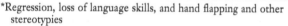
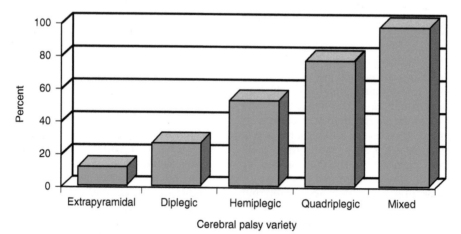

FIGURE 13.1 ■ The proportion of CP patients with intellectual disability and epilepsy increases from 10% in choreoathetosis or extrapyramidal CP to 95% in mixed CP.

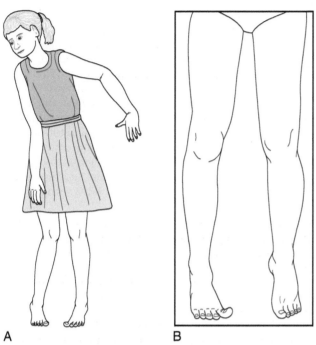

A   B

FIGURE 13.3 ■ *A*, Spastic diplegia in this 10-year-old girl with low-normal intelligence causes straightening, inturning, and adduction of her legs; a tiptoe stance; and scissor-like gait. Her uncoordinated, awkward arm movements (posturing) also reflect her CP. *B*, An 18-year-old college engineering student with spastic diplegia also shows adduction of his legs and toe-walking. He also has a spontaneous right-sided Babinski sign.

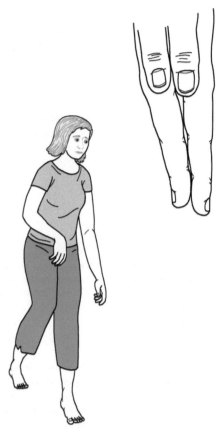

FIGURE 13.4 ■ Hemiparetic since birth, this 28-year-old woman with normal intelligence holds her spastic and weak arm, wrist, and fingers in a flexed posture. Her right hand has shortened fingers and a less broad thumb nail bed. Similarly, her right leg, especially the heel (Achilles) tendon, is short. The growth arrest causes her to walk on her right toes and circumduct that leg. Her posture and gait are similar to that of adults after a left middle cerebral artery infarction (see Figs. 2.3 to 2.5).

paretic. Another difference is that because left hemisphere injury during the perinatal period forces the right hemisphere to assume dominance, children and adults with congenital right hemiparesis usually have no language impairment (aphasia). Finally, older children and adults with hemiplegic CP show growth arrest of the affected limbs.

Quadriplegic CP consists of paresis of all four limbs usually accompanied by pseudobulbar palsy. Extensive cerebral damage, often from anoxia during delivery, usually underlies this CP variety. In contrast, cervical spinal cord birth injury causes quadriplegia without cerebral damage.

Physical and occupational therapy, bracing, and orthotics may help children with CP. Neurologists often recommend surgery that transposes or lengthens tendons to extend a joint's range of motion. To reduce spasticity, which will give the child greater mobility, they prescribe oral medications, such as baclofen, dantrolene, and tizanidine, and administer intramuscular injections of botulinum toxin to select muscle groups (see Chapter 18). However, epilepsy in these children resists treatment. Seizure control often requires two or more antiepileptic drugs (AEDs), which may produce undesirable side effects.

Extrapyramidal CP

Involuntary writhing movements (athetosis) of the face, tongue, hands, and feet punctuated by jerking movements (chorea) of the trunk, arms, and legs – embraced by the term *choreoathetosis* – define extrapyramidal or *dyskinetic CP* (Fig. 13.5). Although choreoathetosis may remain subtle throughout a patient's lifetime, it interferes with fine writing and other fine hand movements, walking, and even sitting. In addition, involuntary larynx, pharynx, and diaphragm movements lead to incomprehensible speech.

Physicians should distinguish choreoathetotic CP from *dopamine-responsive dystonia* (*DRD*), which produces similar involuntary movements in young children (see Chapter 18). In short, unlike CP, DRD is progressive (albeit slowly), fluctuating in a characteristic diurnal pattern at its onset, and, most important, responsive to small doses of levodopa (L-dopa). It mimics extrapyramidal CP so closely that many neurologists insist on a therapeutic trial of L-dopa in dystonic children before accepting a diagnosis of choreoathetotic CP.

Neurologists usually attribute choreoathetotic CP to combinations of low birth weight, anoxia, and neonatal hyperbilirubinemia damaging the basal ganglia (*kernicterus*). In addition, because these insults also damage the auditory pathways, hearing impairment frequently complicates the clinical picture.

Unlike spastic CP, choreoathetosis may not become clinically apparent until children are 2–4 years old. By

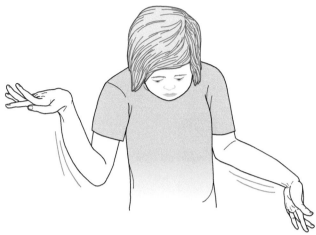

FIGURE 13.5 ■ Neurologists have diagnosed this 13-year-old girl with congenital choreoathetosis as having extrapyramidal or dyskinetic CP. Her wrists, hands, and fingers show slow sinuous movements (athetosis) and her trunk and limbs superimpose large-amplitude jerky movements (chorea). The athetosis forces her hands into flexion at the wrist and her fingers into extension with overlapping positions.

that time, when normal children should have acquired steady walking and some fine motor skills, these children's involuntary movements have usually delayed or prevented them from acquiring these and other milestones. Similarly, a hearing impairment may remain unnoticed until 1 year of age, when the rudiments of language should commence.

In contrast to the burden of these impairments, probably because kernicterus tends to spare the cerebral cortex, choreoathetotic CP is associated with a relatively low – 10% – incidence of epilepsy and intellectual disability. A superficial academic or medical evaluation may underrate children with choreoathetotic CP. Despite pronounced physical impediments, many CP patients are able to complete college. Thus, both choreoathetotic and diplegic CP qualify, along with polio, cervical spinal cord trauma, and DYT1 dystonia, as physically devastating pediatric neurology conditions that allow normal cognition.

Medications provide little relief from the choreoathetosis. Although deep brain stimulation reduces athetosis, the procedure is not yet optimized for this situation.

Finally, *mixed-form CP* – combinations of spastic paraparesis and choreoathetosis – account for about 15% of cases. This variety reflects the most extensive central nervous system (CNS) injury, which is naturally associated with the highest incidence of epilepsy and intellectual disability – 95%.

NEURAL TUBE CLOSURE DEFECTS

During the third and fourth weeks of gestation, dorsal ectoderm normally invaginates to form a closed, midline *neural tube*. The tube goes on to seal itself at both ends and form the brain and spinal cord (Fig. 13.6, top). While ectoderm thus gives rise to the CNS, mesoderm gives rise to its coverings – the meninges, vertebrae, and skull.

The neural tube sometimes does not follow the choreography and fails to fuse at one or both ends. In other words, the neural tube may not close at the prospective site of the brain or lower end of the spinal cord. These defects expand during embryogenesis and lead to malformations of the brain, lower spinal cord, or both. In addition, defects in the surrounding meninges and either lumbosacral vertebrae or skull fail to cover neural tube defects. Beyond the neurologic issues, neural tube defects create some of the most heart-wrenching controversies in medicine, such as the question of whether to continue treatment of severely malformed infants and the burden of tremendous health care costs for infants with a dismal prognosis.

Upper Neural Tube Closure Defects

In an extreme example of a neural tube defect, the entire upper end of the neural tube fails to form. In this case, *anencephaly*, the fetus lacks a brain or has one consumed by a major, often cavitary malformation.

In an *encephalocele*, a malformed brain, covered only by its skin and meninges, but bathed in its cerebrospinal fluid (CSF), protrudes through an occipital skull defect. In a similar malformation, the *Dandy–Walker syndrome*, the posterior portion of the upper neural tube fails to mature. Posterior brain structures, particularly the cerebellar vermis, remain at a small, embryonic stage. Expanding into the vacancy, the fourth ventricle forms a large cystic structure.

A group of malformations, collectively termed the *Arnold–Chiari malformation*, constitute a variety of upper neural tube closure defects. Not obvious by external appearances, the Arnold–Chiari malformation consists of downward displacement of the lower portion of the medulla and cerebellum through the foramen magnum (see Figs. 13.6 and 20.22). In older children and adults, who may previously have escaped detection, this malformation often produces head and neck pain (especially when bending) and, in severe cases, bulbar palsy. Patients with compression of the medulla or cerebellum require surgical "unroofing" of the upper cervical spine and occipital portion of the skull.

Lower Neural Tube Closure Defects

Upper neural tube defects are associated with comparable lower neural tube defects. In the most benign variety of lower neural tube defects, *spina bifida occulta*, lumbar vertebrae simply fail to fuse. With both the underlying spinal cord and cauda equina remaining intact, this disorder usually remains asymptomatic. In *meningocele*, a more serious variety, the meninges protrude through a lumbosacral spine and skin defect to form a large, CSF-filled bulge.

Meningomyelocele (*myelomeningocele*) consists of a tangle of a rudimentary lower spinal cord, lumbar and sacral nerve roots, and meninges that protrude into a sac-like structure overlying the lumbosacral spine (Fig. 13.7). The disrupted nerve tissue causes paraparesis, areflexia, incontinence, and hydronephrosis. In addition, hydrocephalus and other brain abnormalities are comorbid in about 25% of cases.

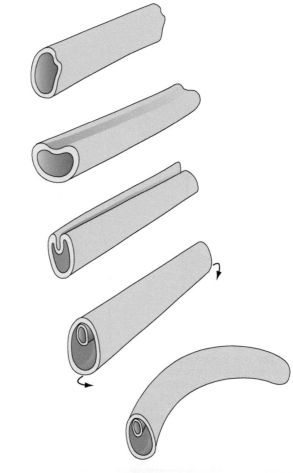

FIGURE 13.6 ■ *Top*, During the normal third and fourth weeks of gestation, the embryo's ectoderm invaginates to shape a distinct, midline neural tube that eventually closes at both ends. Once closed, the embryo assumes a curved shape with the tube on the outer surface. *Bottom left*, The MRI shows the normal relationship of several of the structures contained in the posterior fossa: the pons (P), medulla (M), cerebellum (C), and the fourth ventricle (the unmarked black, CSF-filled, triangular area between the pons and middle of the cerebellum). Note that the medulla and lower portion of the cerebellum remain above the foramen magnum. *Bottom right*, This MRI shows an Arnold–Chiari malformation. The lower portion of the cerebellum (C), which includes the tonsils, and the medulla (M), crowded together, protrude down through the foramen magnum.

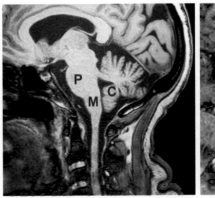

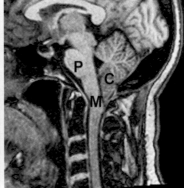

Meningoceles and meningomyeloceles also deprive the lower CNS of the multiple normal coverings – skin, vertebrae, and meninges – that shield it from the environment. To prevent bacteria from entering the CSF through defective meninges and causing meningitis, neonates with meningoceles must undergo neurosurgery within 3 days of birth not to correct the paraplegia, which is uncorrectable, but to prevent meningitis. Many neonates with a meningomyelocele eventually require permanent ventricular shunting to treat hydrocephalus. In addition, as affected children mature, they often require urinary- and fecal-diversion procedures, revision of ventricular shunts, and further spine surgery. Some recent publications have described in utero or "prenatal"

meningomyelocele surgery that reduces the risk of death and need for shunting, and may improve mental and motor function.

Causes

In the United States the incidence of neural tube defects is 1 in 2000 births. Studies have implicated genetic factors. For example, the risk of a neural tube defect occurring in a sibling of an affected child is 5%. With two affected children, the risk for a third increases to 10%. Similarly, the concordance rates for dizygotic twins is 4% and for monozygotic twins, almost 8%. Another indicator of a genetic basis of neural tube defects

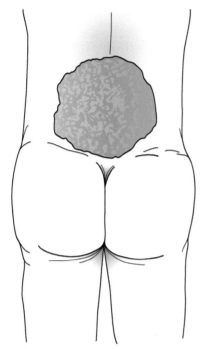

FIGURE 13.7 ■ The meningomyelocele of this newborn has a typical broad-based, loose, translucent sac of thin, friable skin arising from the lumbar area. It contains rudiments of the lumbosacral spinal cord and nerves of the cauda equina. Its surface weeps a mixture of serum and CSF. The infant's legs, lacking innervation, remain weak, flaccid, and areflexic. The bladder, also lacking innervation, distends and leads to hydronephrosis.

is its frequent occurrence in infants with trisomy 13 or trisomy 18.

Other studies have attributed neural tube defects to environmental factors: the AEDs carbamazepine and valproate, folic acid deficiency, autoantibodies to folate receptors, radiation, and toxins, including potato blight. There is no complete explanation for the link between AEDs and neural tube defects, but AEDs reduce serum folate levels and thus raise homocysteine levels. Whatever the explanation, neurologists avoid prescribing carbamazepine or valproate to women who are pregnant or planning to conceive. Offsetting the potential teratogenic effects of AEDs by folic acid supplements (see later) has not been shown to be safe or effective.

Prenatal testing may provide early warning of a neural tube defect. For example, excessive concentrations of α-fetoprotein in amniotic fluid and maternal serum indicate a neural tube defect. Fetal ultrasound examination, a complementary test, may show neural tube defects as well as other congenital malformations.

Reflecting that folic acid deficiency is a powerful risk factor for neural tube defects, studies have found that a folic acid intake of 5 mg daily before conception and during the first month of pregnancy reduces the incidence of neural tube defects by 85%. Even eating adequate amounts of fruits and vegetables, which contain folic acids and other nutrients, reduces the risk of neural tube defects by 70%. Based on these data, the United States Food and Drug Administration has mandated "folic acid fortification" of cereal grain products, such as breakfast cereals and corn meal.

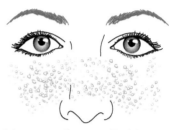

FIGURE 13.8 ■ Adenoma sebaceum (facial angiofibromas), the cutaneous component of tuberous sclerosis, consist of firm pale nodules several millimeters in diameter spread over the malar surface of the face. Although adenoma sebaceum may resemble acne, acne pimples have a liquid (pus) center surrounded by inflammation and accumulate on the trunk as well as the face.

NEUROCUTANEOUS DISORDERS

Embryologic defects in the ectoderm also give rise to neurocutaneous disorders that consist of paired abnormalities of the brain and skin. In addition, these disorders often include abnormalities of other organs. The neurocutaneous disorders, which neurologists sometimes call the *phakomatoses* (Greek *phakos*, lentil [bean-shaped]) allow for the quintessential diagnosis by inspection.

Neurocutaneous disorders usually develop either as spontaneous mutations or are inherited in an autosomal dominant pattern. Although patients' cutaneous component usually remains stable through adult life, they often have progressive neurologic deterioration. The symptoms and time course of some disorders mimic ASD.

Tuberous Sclerosis

The classic triad of tuberous sclerosis stigmata consists of epilepsy, intellectual disability, and conspicuous smooth and firm nodules, *facial angiofibromas* (adenoma sebaceum), on the malar surface of the face (Fig. 13.8). Although this illness-defining lesion often first appears only in adolescence, during infancy and childhood the skin shows several other characteristics: hypopigmented (hypomelanotic) macules and *ash-leaf spots*; *shagreen patches*, which are leathery, scaly areas on the lower trunk and buttocks; and ungual fibromas.

Almost any variety of seizure, which is the most common initial symptom of the illness, may be a manifestation of the epilepsy. Refractory epilepsy portends serious intellectual disability. The intellectual disability generally worsens as children mature. It frequently reaches the severity of dementia and forces them into institutions. On the other hand, some children with tuberous sclerosis have only minimal cognitive impairment and readily controlled epilepsy.

The CNS manifestation of the illness consists of subependymal tubers (Latin *tuber*, swelling), which are small, potato-like brain nodules, 1 to 3 cm in diameter that tend to line the ventricles. Another characteristic growth is subependymal giant cell astrocytomas (SEGAs) that frequently grow and compress and irritate the surrounding cerebral cortex, thus producing the epilepsy and progressive cognitive impairment. Growths blocking the foramen of Monro cause obstructive hydrocephalus.

As the tubers grow, children may display cognitive decline, attention-deficit/hyperactivity disorder (ADHD), or ASD symptoms. Thus, neurologists consider tuberous sclerosis as one of several neurologic causes of ASD symptoms (see Box 13.1).

Although an autosomal dominantly transmitted mutation causes tuberous sclerosis, the mutation has occurred *de novo* in about 70% of cases. Whether inherited or sporadic, the mutation involves either of two tumor suppressor genes: the tuberous sclerosis complex 1 (TSC 1) on chromosome 9, which codes for the protein hamartin, or the tuberous sclerosis complex 2 (TSC 2) on chromosome 16, which codes for the protein tuberin. Conventional genetic testing will uncover one or the other of these mutations in 80% to 90% of patients, leaving a few diagnosed by clinical, radiographic, and pathological criteria.

Especially because tubers tend to calcify, computed tomography (CT) and even plain skull X-rays may help to identify them by their telltale calcifications; however, magnetic resonance imaging (MRI) is the best diagnostic test. Removing the tubers may reduce intracranial pressure, relieve obstructive hydrocephalus, excise a malignancy, and reduce seizure frequency, but neurosurgery is usually not feasible when tubers are numerous and deeply situated. In a breakthrough, studies have shown that inhibitors of the *mammalian target of rapamycin (mTOR)*, such as everolimus and sirolimus, shrink subependymal giant cell astrocytomas. Topically applied mTOR inhibitors also reduce the facial angiofibromas.

Neurofibromatosis

Neurofibromatosis type 1 (NF1) – previously called von Recklinghausen disease or "peripheral type" neurofibromatosis – causes a clinical triad: multiple *café-au-lait spots, neurofibromas, and Lisch nodules. Café-au-lait* spots, the signature of neurofibromatosis, are areas of uniformly light-brown, oval, and flat skin (Fig. 13.9). Although individual *café-au-lait* spots are found in at least 10% of normal individuals, the presence of more than six, each larger than 5 mm in children and 1.5 cm in adults, is a reliable sign of NF1. Freckling in the axilla and groin – two skin surfaces sheltered from sun exposure – is a related sign of the disorder.

Neurofibromas consist of soft, palpable, subcutaneous growths, each a few millimeters to several centimeters in size that emerge along peripheral nerves (Figs. 13.10 and 13.11). They can also grow from nerve roots within the spinal canal and compress the spinal cord or cauda equina. They occasionally reach grotesque proportions or induce extraordinary growth of an affected limb. However, the famous 19th century "Elephant Man," Joseph Merrick, commonly cited as having neurofibromatosis, probably suffered from a different condition, Proteus syndrome.

Lisch nodules, the least obvious but most common manifestation, are multiple, asymptomatic, macroscopic, yellow-to-brown nodules (melanocytic hamartomas) situated on the iris (Fig. 13.12). Although ophthalmologists

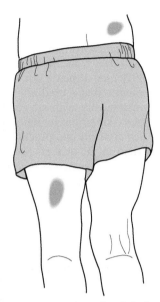

FIGURE 13.9 ■ *Café-au-lait* spots are flat, light-brown skin lesions.

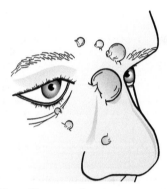

FIGURE 13.10 ■ Neurofibromas often grow to several centimeters of disfiguring protuberances on the face and elsewhere over the body.

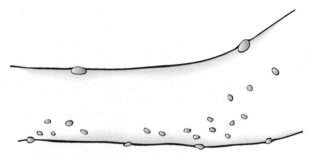

FIGURE 13.11 ■ Neurofibromas are often subtle, multiple, subcutaneous, soft, and typically less than 0.5 cm in size.

may need a slit-lamp examination to detect Lisch nodules and differentiate them from inconsequential pigment collections, Lisch nodules are almost pathognomonic of NF1.

Excision of neurofibromas, except for those compressing the spinal cord or other vital structures, is impractical because NF1 involves innumerable peripheral nerves. If necessary, laser therapy can blanch *café-au-lait* spots.

Far from being entirely peripheral, NF1 induces intracerebral tumors, particularly optic nerve gliomas, as well as intraspinal neurofibromas. It often induces ADHD, learning disabilities, social problems, and a decrease of about 5 to 10 IQ points; however, most NF1 children and adults do not greatly differ from the general population. Although 20% to 40% may display some ASD symptoms, most patients' problems consist predominantly of social-communication impairments without repetitive behaviors, eye contact failure, or language deficiency. Less than 10% show *intellectual disability* and psychosis occurs at no greater frequency than in the general population.

Approximately 50% of patients inherit NF1 in an autosomal dominant pattern. In the remainder, NF1 arises sporadically. The mutation consists of an abnormality in a tumor-suppressor gene on chromosome 17. (The mnemonic for recalling the abnormal chromosome is "von Recklinghausen contains 17 letters.") The incidence of spontaneous NF1, like the incidence of Down syndrome and achondroplasia, increases with advanced paternal age.

Neurofibromatosis type 2 (*NF2*), which occurs only 10% as frequently as NF1, is a completely different disorder.

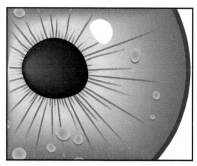

FIGURE 13.12 ■ Lisch nodules, nearly pathognomonic of NF1, are pigmented aggregations on the iris that are often visible with the unaided eye.

NF2, also called *familial acoustic neuroma* with good reason, is characterized by bilateral acoustic neuromas (vestibular schwannomas) that steadily impair hearing until deafness ensues (see Fig. 20.27). In fact, NF2 is usually unrecognized until acoustic neuromas are discovered. Gadolinium enhanced MRIs can readily show the acoustic neuromas. Gamma radiation or laser surgery may burn away the tumor while sparing the acoustic nerve.

Unlike NF1, NF2 does not cause behavioral, learning, or other cognitive impairments. Also, the NF2 mutation is carried on chromosome 22 and, in the majority of cases, transmitted in an autosomal dominant pattern. (The mnemonic for its inheritance is "Chromosome 22 carries the NF2 mutation.")

Sturge–Weber Syndrome

Sturge–Weber syndrome, more formally known as *encephalo-trigeminal angiomatosis*, consists simply of angioma of both the face and underlying cerebral hemisphere. Unlike the etiology of other neurocutaneous disorders, an embryonal developmental disorder rather than a genetic mutation causes Sturge–Weber syndrome. Thus, this disorder appears sporadically, does not strike multiple family members, and cannot be passed on by an affected individual.

The facial angioma consists of a deep red discoloration ("port-wine stain") in the distribution of one or more divisions of the trigeminal nerve (Fig. 13.13). Clinicians must distinguish this angioma from more common benign skin abnormalities, such as small forehead angiomas ("strawberry nevi"). The angioma's size does not correlate with the cerebral abnormality, but its location does. Overall, angiomas are associated with Sturge–Weber syndrome in only 8% of cases, but in about 33%

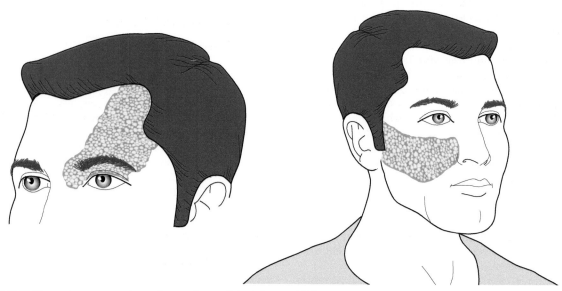

FIGURE 13.13 ■ The cutaneous angioma (port wine stain) of Sturge–Weber syndrome encompasses one or more divisions of the trigeminal nerve (see Fig. 4.12). The commonest sites are the anterior scalp, forehead, and upper eyelid, i.e., the first division. One-third of patients have bilateral involvement.

of cases where the nerve's first division is involved. Whether or not facial angiomas are a component of Sturge–Weber syndrome, laser therapy can bleach them.

The CNS component of Sturge–Weber syndrome consists of atrophic, calcified layers of cerebral cortex in the hemisphere underlying the facial vascular malformation. Although CT and even plain X-rays may reveal calcified cerebral abnormalities, neurologists usually require MRI with contrast to show the presence and extent of the lesion.

Sturge–Weber children almost always have seizures that begin in infancy and are often refractory to AEDs. Children with refractory seizures may need to undergo cerebral lobectomy, transection of the corpus callosum, or even hemispherectomy (see Chapter 10). Seizures in the first year of life portend intellectual disability. Especially if they have seizures, the majority of Sturge–Weber children have slowed acquisition of milestones and learning disabilities. Approximately one-third will have pronounced *intellectual disability*.

Depending on the underlying cerebral lesion, patients have contralateral neurologic deficits, such as homonymous hemianopia and spastic hemiparesis. Their physical and cognitive deficits often worsen as children age, probably because of increasing sclerosis surrounding the cerebral lesions. Another common manifestation of the disorder is glaucoma or enlargement of the eye (buphthalmos), particularly when the angioma affects the adjacent eyelids.

Ataxia-Telangiectasia

At one time called Madame Louis-Barr disease, making it one of the few conditions named after a woman physician, ataxia-telangiectasia's cutaneous component consists of telangiectasia – aggregations of small, dilated vessels – on the conjunctiva, bridge of the nose, and cheeks. The neurologic component, which precedes the appearance of the telangiectasia, appears in children aged 3 to 5 years as progressively severe gait ataxia, followed by other motor impairments. Eventually cognitive and language functions also deteriorate, but not to the extent of the motor deficits. As with Rett syndrome, ataxia-telangiectasia also causes deceleration of head growth that leads to a small head circumference (acquired microcephaly) as the child ages.

Unlike most other neurocutaneous disorders, ataxia-telangiectasia is inherited in an autosomal recessive pattern. It results from a mutation on chromosome 11 that interferes with DNA repair.

An almost unique feature of ataxia-telangiectasia is its consistent association with immunodeficiency. Children with ataxia-telangiectasia have both cellular immunity impairment and complete or nearly complete deficiency of immunoglobulin IgA or IgE. The immunodeficiency leads to severe sinus and respiratory tract infections. It also places these children at risk for lymphomas, leukemia, and other neoplasms. (The same association of immunodeficiency with lymphoma occurs in human immunodeficiency virus [HIV] infection and antirejection drug treatment for organ transplantation.)

OTHER GENETIC NEUROLOGIC DISORDERS

Often combinations of cognitive impairments that sometimes reach profound levels, distinctive physical signs, and peculiar behavior – including ASD symptoms – allow neurologists to diagnose one of the following genetically based neurologic syndromes.

Autosomal Chromosomal Disorders

Phenylketonuria (PKU) (Chromosome 12)

An autosomal recessive inherited deficiency in the catabolic enzyme, hepatic phenylalanine hydroxylase, produces PKU. A triumph of medicine – near universal neonatal testing and treatment with dietary restrictions for PKU – has either eliminated this disorder or markedly reduced its consequences.

In PKU, a deficiency of phenylalanine hydroxylase, which normally converts plasma phenylalanine to tyrosine, produces a triad of major biochemical ramifications:

1. The enzyme deficiency prevents most of the normal metabolism of phenylalanine to tyrosine. Affected untreated individuals thus have elevated concentrations of phenylalanine and reduced concentrations of tyrosine in their blood.
2. The deficiency prevents the normal synthesis of "downstream" neurotransmitters, including dopamine, melatonin, and norepinephrine (noradrenaline) (see Chapter 21).

$$\text{Phenylalanine} \xrightarrow{\textit{phenylalanine hydroxylase}}$$
$$\text{Tyrosine} \xrightarrow{\textit{tyrosine hydroxylase}} \text{DOPA} \xrightarrow{\textit{DOPA decarboxylase}}$$
$$\text{Dopamine} \xrightarrow{\textit{dopamine }\beta\textit{-hydroxylase}} \text{Norepinephrine}$$

3. It also diverts phenylalanine metabolism to secondary metabolic pathways that yield phenylpyruvic acid and phenylketones, which are excreted in the urine. Simple tests in the nursery readily detect excessive phenylalanine levels in the blood and phenylketones in the urine, i.e., phenylketonuria.

Normal Phenylalanine Metabolism

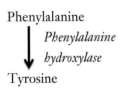

Diversion of Phenylalanine Metabolism in PKU

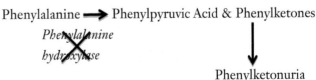

Before the introduction of effective treatment, PKU infants would appear normal from birth until as old as 1 year of age when they would then begin to fall behind in all areas of growth and development. Almost all of them were eventually left with intellectual disability, two-thirds of them with profound disability. In addition, because of reduced synthesis of melatonin, most of these infants lacked pigment. Without it, PKU children develop blond hair, blue eyes, a fair complexion, and eczema. Phenylketones in their urine turned it malodorous.

A mutation on chromosome 12 transmits PKU in a classic autosomal recessive pattern. The incidence of PKU varies widely between countries, being highest in Turkey and lowest in Japan. Most United States hospitals screen newborns for PKU among 40 or more other illnesses, including amino acid disorders, endocrine disorders, fatty acid disorders, hemoglobin disorders, lysosomal disorders, cystic fibrosis, hearing loss, and HIV infection. One note of caution: these tests may be invalid immediately after birth if residual maternal enzyme continues to metabolize phenylalanine or other substrate.

A phenylalanine-free diet usually prevents the development of intellectual disability. Noncompliance with the diet, as particularly occurs with PKU adolescents, produces a wide variety of psychiatric disturbances and cognitive impairment. Elevated phenylalanine blood levels correlate with the presence and severity of these symptoms. In another period of concern, if pregnant women with PKU do not strictly adhere to their diet, they accumulate toxic levels of phenylalanine and its metabolic products that pass through the placenta. In this case, even though the fetus is likely to be only heterozygous, its brain is vulnerable to the toxins.

Physicians should be aware that subsisting on phenylalanine-free foods is arduous, expensive, and apt to lead to short stature and anemia. The diet prohibits foods and beverages with artificial sweeteners because most, including Diet Coke and Diet Pepsi, contain phenylalanine. A phenylalanine-free diet also eliminates foods that contain large amounts of protein. Another therapeutic strategy rests on dietary manipulations that reduce the amount of phenylalanine entering the brain by consuming proteins with minimal phenylalanine. In a complementary strategy, physicians prescribe sapropterin (Kuvan), a synthetic tetrahydrobiopterin (a cofactor of phenylalanine hydroxylase), because it enhances the metabolism of phenylalanine.

Homocystinuria (Chromosome 21)

Cystathionine β-synthase, along with vitamin B_6, converts homocysteine to cystathionine (see Fig. 5.9). A deficiency of this enzyme leads to accumulation of homocysteine and its precursor, methionine. Chromosome 21 carries the mutation, which is so rare that physicians encountering a child with the illness might suspect consanguinity in the patents. Other conditions that produce an accumulation of homocysteine include vitamin B_{12} deficiency, exposure to nitrous oxide, and use of certain AEDs (such as carbamazepine and phenytoin).

Homocystinuria leads to intellectual disability in almost all cases, behavioral disturbances, obsessive-compulsive symptoms, and personality disorders. It also leads to strokes in young and middle-aged adults (see Chapter 11). Other features of homocystinuria consist of readily identifiable malformations of multiple organs, including dislocation of the ocular lens, pectus excavatum (a "sunken-in chest"), and a tall, thin and long-limbed, Marfan-like stature.

Treatment in the presymptomatic stage reduces the likelihood of children developing intellectual disability. Administering vitamin B_6, usually in the form of pyridoxine, increases the metabolism of homocysteine and reduces levels of methionine as well as homocysteine in approximately 50% of patients. However, administering folate and B_6 does not reduce the stroke risk in adults with elevated homocysteine levels.

Prader–Willi and Angelman Syndromes (Chromosome 15)

In addition to being commonly occurring examples of genetically determined intellectual disability, Prader–Willi and Angelman syndromes consist of different abnormal behaviors and serve as a prime example of *genomic imprinting*: the mutation is a microdeletion on chromosome 15 that when transmitted by the mother tends to produce Angelman syndrome, while the same mutation transmitted by the father tends to produce Prader–Willi syndrome. Neurologists diagnose Prader–Willi and Angelman syndromes in both boys and girls, without gender preference.

Of Prader–Willi syndrome cases, approximately 75% are paternally inherited – the rest arise sporadically. Children with Prader–Willi syndrome have intellectual disability and behavior problems, but their identifying symptom consists of hyperphagia with resultant morbid obesity. Of all the genetic causes of obesity, the Prader–Willi mutation is the most frequently occurring. More importantly, to say that children with Prader–Willi syndrome have obesity from hyperphagia understates the symptom. These children eat relentlessly and aggressively. They eat barely edible food, such as uncooked meat. They grab meals from family members' plates, break refrigerator locks, and rummage through garbage cans. Although these children, who later become adults with the same symptoms, show consistent abnormal behavior, the DSM-5 does not define Prader–Willi syndrome as a mental disorder.

Beyond their striking obesity and other physical anomalies (Fig. 13.14), Prader–Willi children have low-normal to below-normal intelligence. They comprise about 1% of children with intellectual disability. They also tend toward mood disorders that may, after adolescence, be accompanied by psychotic symptoms. Most commonly they have oppositional defiant disorder that often results in temper tantrums related and unrelated to food. Notably, the severity of the obesity does not correlate with either the presence or severity of the neuropsychiatric disturbances. Prader–Willi, like obesity in general, leads to hypoventilation, hypersomnia, hypertension, diabetes, stroke, and osteoporosis.

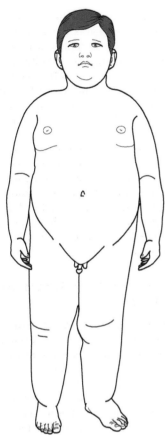

FIGURE 13.14 ■ An 8-year-old boy with Prader–Willi syndrome shows the typical obesity, which can reach grotesque proportions, small penis and testicles, short stature, short arms and legs, and small hands and feet.

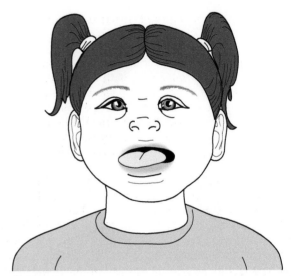

FIGURE 13.15 ■ Children with Down syndrome are short with low-set ears and a thickened neck. Their epicanthal folds are widened, the bridge of their nose depressed, and their face generally flat. The tongue, characteristically large, tends to protrude over a slack jaw. Their palms are broad, often with a single midline ("simian") crease, and their fingers are short and stubby.

Recombinant human growth hormone injections increase height and muscle mass and may provide cognitive benefits. Bariatric surgical procedures have produced equivocal benefits. Noninvasive ventilation assistance reduces hypoventilation and hypersomnia.

Carrying essentially the same mutation, Angelman syndrome children typically show profound intellectual disability with prominent deficiency of language skills; epilepsy; microcephaly; *stereotypies* (involuntary repetitive, patterned, and purposeless movements); spontaneous jerky and flapping movements; unsteady or frankly ataxic walking; a smiling face; and paroxysms of unprovoked laughter. Their jerky movements and superficially happy appearance have given rise to the term "happy puppet syndrome." Adults with Angelman syndrome generally continue to display the same laughter, require assistance with their daily activities, and suffer from refractory epilepsy.

Angelman syndrome in girls mimics Rett syndrome because both syndromes share intellectual disability, language impairment, microcephaly, and involuntary movements. Angelman syndrome in both boys and girls is associated with autism due to the presence of stereotypies, jerky and flapping movements, and poor language skills.

Down Syndrome (Trisomy 21)

Down syndrome children have distinctive physical features (Fig. 13.15) and mild to moderate intellectual disability, with a median IQ of 40 to 50. They are also plagued by hearing loss, congenital cardiac anomalies, and obstructive sleep apnea (see Chapter 17). As adults, they tend to develop hypothyroidism and leukemia. The cause of Down syndrome in 90% of cases is nondisjunction of chromosome 21 during gametogenesis; in 5% or less, a translocation is responsible.

An almost uniform complication by age 50 years, Down syndrome leads to an Alzheimer-like dementia with cerebral plaques, tangles, and accumulation of amyloid (see Chapter 7). One theory holds that because Down syndrome individuals have three copies of the gene for the amyloid precursor protein, which is situated on chromosome 21, they overproduce amyloid.

Down syndrome children retain social skills that partly compensate for their intellectual disability. In fact, Down syndrome has a negative statistical correlation with ASD. However, Down syndrome children occasionally have behavior that fulfills criteria for ADHD and, beginning when they are young adults, they often have depressive symptoms. Curiously, severely affected children with no neuroleptic exposure may have orofacial dyskinesias.

The incidence of Down syndrome correlates with increasing maternal age (especially after 40 years). Its incidence also increases, but not to the same degree, with increasing paternal age. Physicians may diagnose Down syndrome in utero by analysis of cell-free fetal DNA (cfDNA) in a pregnant woman's blood, ultrasound of fetal nuchal thickness, or amniocentesis. Even though it is obviously genetic, neurologists do not classify Down syndrome as an *inherited* cause of intellectual disability because it is not transmitted from generation to generation. This distinction allows neurologists to state that fragile X syndrome is the most common form of inherited intellectual disability.

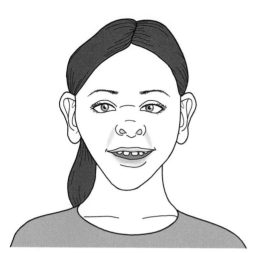

FIGURE 13.16 ■ This 10-year-old girl shows the characteristic elfin (elf-like) appearance of Williams syndrome. She is short. Her forehead is broad and her cheeks are prominent. Her nose has a flat bridge, and its nostrils are full and turned slightly upward. Her teeth are hypoplastic and widely spaced.

Williams Syndrome (Chromosome 7)

Life-long neuropsychologic oddities and a distinctive, "elfin" facial appearance (Fig. 13.16) characterize Williams syndrome. The disorder leads to defects in the elastic qualities of the skin and congenital abnormalities at the root of the aorta, which cause supravalvular aortic stenosis, but they have no gross physical neurologic abnormalities, such as microcephaly, stereotypies, or epilepsy.

Williams syndrome children are slow to acquire motor milestones, have a strikingly poor sense of visual–spatial relationships, and cannot perform construction or copying tasks. The majority has ADHD, phobias, or both. In general, they perform in the mild-to-moderate disability range on testing with an average IQ of approximately 65 points. As adults, Williams syndrome individuals rarely find steady employment and develop memory impairment at a greater rate than controls.

Most striking, the disorder paradoxically seems to enhance certain neuropsychologic functions. For example, remarkably and so far inexplicably, Williams individuals frequently possess unusual musical talent, many possessing perfect pitch. Their conversations, although lacking substance and often one-sided, are garrulous, bubbly, and engaging. They are extroverts with no fear of strangers. Neurologists often call their interactions "hypersocial" and describe their "cocktail-party personality."

Although some Williams syndrome cases have followed an autosomal dominant inheritance pattern, *de novo* mutations have led to most cases. The genetic abnormality consists of a microdeletion in chromosome 7.

Velocardiofacial (VCF) Syndrome (Chromosome 22)

Neurologists and psychiatrists have come to recognize VCF, along with Prader–Willi, Williams, and Lesch–Nyhan, as genetic disorders with distinctive neuropsychiatric manifestations. As its name implies, VCF consists primarily of abnormalities, in various combinations and degrees of severity, of the soft palate (*velum palatinum* [Latin, *velum*, veil]), *c*ardiac system, and *f*ace. Neurologists and other specialists have also called this constellation of disorders DiGeorge sequence, DiGeorge syndrome, 22q11 deletion syndrome, and Shprintzen syndrome. VCF, which occurs in 1/3000 children, is an autosomal dominant genetic disorder that stems from a microdeletion in chromosome 22q11.2. However, with 75% or more cases occurring sporadically, VCF is an inherited disease in only a minority of cases. Interestingly, the size of the deletion does not correlate with the disease's phenotype.

Palatal or velopharyngeal dysfunction, the most obvious symptom, gives the VCF child's voice a nasal tone. Hearing the nasality, physicians may further suspect the diagnosis by inspection of the palate at rest and during voluntary retraction. In addition, VCF children may have external ear malformations that cause hearing impairment and worsen the speech impediment. The facial appearance of children with VCF has several characteristic, if not pathognomonic, features (Fig. 13.17). Finally, VCF children typically have congenital cardiac anomalies, usually ventricular septal defects, that often necessitate surgery.

Although VCF's primary components are physical, its neuropsychiatric manifestations generally determine the child's life course. VCF children's IQ scores typically fall into the borderline range. Moreover, beginning in young adulthood, major depression occurs in up to 40% and psychotic symptoms, which are usually indistinguishable from schizophrenia, occur in up to 30% of VCF patients.

VCF offers a clue to the basis of schizophrenia. The VCF 22q 11.2 microdeletion and several other mutations associated with schizophrenia localize to the same region on chromosome 22. Of all of them, the VCF mutation carries the most statistically powerful genetic risk factor for schizophrenia not confined to an ethnic group.

Sex-Linked Chromosomal Disorders

Fragile X Syndrome

The *fragile X syndrome*, like many other genetic disorders, consists of intellectual disability, behavioral disturbances, and distinctive nonneurologic physical stigmata (Fig. 13.18). About 70% of boys who inherit the entire or "full" mutation have moderate-to-severe intellectual disability. In contrast, most females carrying the mutation on one chromosome – typically the mother and sisters of affected boys – show none of the syndrome's physical stigmata. However, about one-third of them have borderline or lower IQs, and many have a mood disorder, executive impairment, or social anxiety.

Fragile X syndrome boys display strikingly abnormal behavior, including stereotypies, particularly flapping or wringing of their hands. Many bite their fingers and engage in other self-injurious behavior. Fragile X syndrome is the quintessential, most common monogenetic cause of ASD symptoms.

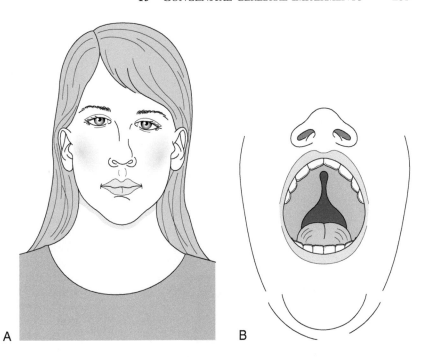

FIGURE 13.17 ■ *A*, The face of children with VCF typically appears long, tapering to a small lower jaw (micrognathia). A tubular nose with a broad tip and small nasal alae, and deformed ears are also typical. Many VCF children have microcephaly. *B*, The cleft may be difficult to appreciate because most are submucosal.

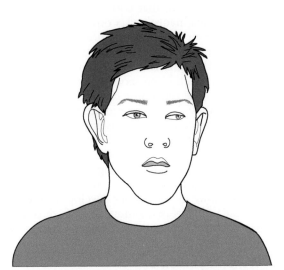

FIGURE 13.18 ■ This boy with the full fragile X syndrome mutation has an IQ of 65 and shows the syndrome's typical prominent forehead and jaw; long, thin face; and large, low-set, "seashell-shaped" ears. Although his penis will remain normal in size for his age, his testicles will grow during puberty to a remarkably large size – two- to three-fold greater in volume than normal. This *macro-orchidism* occurs in almost all fragile X syndrome boys and represents the single most consistent physical anomaly.

The mutation (FMR1) consists of excessive repetitions of the CGG trinucleotide on the X chromosome.* Occurring in about 1 in 1200 males and half as frequently in females, and responsible for as many as 10% of all cases of intellectual disability, fragile X syndrome ranks as the most common cause of inherited intellectual disability as well as the single most common monogenetic cause of

ASD. Unlike inheritance in Down syndrome, fragile X syndrome parents regularly and predictably transmit the mutation to one or more of their children. Thus, neurologists often find that the child presenting for fragile X evaluation has a male relative with mild if not overt intellectual disability. Some neurologists have stated that of children with ASD, boys should undergo testing for fragile X and girls for the Rett mutation.

Compared to the normal complement of 5 to 44 CGG repeats, the full fragile X mutation typically has 200 or more CGG repeats. Individuals with only 55 to 200 repeats have the *premutation*, which leads to no major intellectual impairment or physical stigmata. Nevertheless, the premutation has several ramifications. In successive generations, as with other excessive trinucleotide repeat disorders, the fragile X mutation tends to increase in size, its symptoms emerge at an earlier age (anticipation), and its symptoms seem more pronounced. As an example of anticipation, the number of repeats in germ cells may expand from premutation levels to ones greater than 200. Thus, an asymptomatic mother who carries the premutation may have boys with the full syndrome and girls with a muted version of it. Even the premutation induces developmental problems, including ADHD, depression, and ASD symptoms. Sometimes the premutation may produce manifestations only after an individual has reached 40 years of age. For example, women with the premutation undergo premature ovarian failure and menopause, and men with it may develop a tremor-ataxia syndrome, cognitive impairment, and mood disorders.

Rett Syndrome

Generally restricted to girls, *Rett syndrome* symptoms emerge at 6 to 18 months of age after an initial normal birth and development. Over the next several years, Rett syndrome girls lose their language skills, ability to walk, and other learned motor activities. They typically regress

---

*Excessive trinucleotide repeats in other mutations produce Friedreich ataxia and other spinocerebellar degenerations, myotonic dystrophy, and Huntington disease (see Chapters 2, 6, and 18, respectively, and Appendix 3C). Neurologists refer to illnesses caused by excessive trinucleotide DNA repeats as polyglutamine illnesses

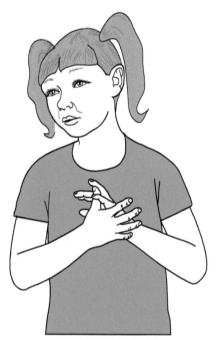

FIGURE 13.19 ■ A 6-year-old girl with Rett syndrome, displaying stereotypies, incessantly moves her hands as though she were washing or clapping, and pulls her hair. In another hallmark of the disease, her head circumference is only 48 cm, which is two standard deviations below the mean for her age (51 cm). Because her head circumference had been normal during her first 2 years, neurologists determined that she had developed *acquired microcephaly*. She has also progressively lost her language ability and now cannot speak in a meaningful manner. When her symptoms first appeared, her pediatrician understandably suggested the diagnosis of autism.

in all phases of psychomotor function to a state of profound intellectual disability. Moreover, 60–90% of them develop epilepsy beginning at the age of 3 years.

Rett syndrome girls display two striking neurologic abnormalities: stereotypies and acquired microcephaly (Fig. 13.19). Their stereotypies, which first appear at about 18 months of age, consist of incessant hand movements, particularly hand wringing and hand washing, hair pulling, clapping, or flapping. As these stereotypies progress, Rett children often lose hand function. Most of them also develop stereotypies beyond hand movements, such as bruxism, mouthing, and body twisting.

Head growth follows a normal trajectory from birth to about 6 months, but then its growth decelerates while relatively normal body growth continues. When the head's size becomes relatively small for the body, neurologists diagnose *acquired microcephaly*. By way of contrast, in *congenital microcephaly* – for example, as the result of congenital rubella infection, the recently emergent Zika virus, and other prenatal insults – the head is small from birth.

Rett syndrome is attributable in about 85% of cases to a mutation in a gene – methyl-CpG-binding protein 2 (MECP2) – on the X chromosome. The mutation is presumably lethal to a male fetus, but occasionally a male fetus will inherit the mutation and survive with a *forme fruste* of the disorder.

Rett syndrome symptoms of regression, loss of language, prevalence of epilepsy, and stereotypies mimic

those of an ASD. In fact, preceding versions of the DSM included Rett syndrome as a category of Autism or ASD. Rett syndrome children, for practical purposes, are only girls, have microcephaly, and regress in their motor and language skills. Also, in contrast to children with the common storage diseases, Rett syndrome children have neither organomegaly nor retinal abnormalities.

Landau–Kleffner Syndrome

In a condition similar to Rett syndrome, but not transmitted in a sex-linked pattern or by any single mutation, *Landau–Kleffner syndrome* (*LKS*) or *acquired epileptic aphasia*, both boys and girls who have had a normal development begin to regress between ages 2 and 8 years. With boys outnumbering girls by 2 : 1, these children lose their comprehension of words then phrases and then their ability to express themselves, i.e., they develop aphasia. They also show behavioral regression and other ASD symptoms, but most retain some personal interaction. The majority has focal seizures, generalized seizures, or both (see Chapter 10). The electroencephalogram (EEG) shows epileptiform abnormalities, especially during slow-wave sleep, that correlate with the clinical deterioration. Thus, neurologists order a 24-hour EEG when attempting to make the diagnosis of LKS. AEDs often suppress seizures and normalize the EEG, but they do not improve the aphasia or ASD symptoms. Approximately one-third of children spontaneously recover their language ability. The remaining children have persistent disabilities, but they do not deteriorate further.

Although LKS occurs rarely, it is important for several reasons. LKS may present with ASD symptoms or simply aphasia. In girls, it mimics Rett syndrome. It exemplifies the need to check children's hearing not only routinely, but also particularly if they regress, lose communication skills, have learning difficulties, or develop ADHD. LKS also shows the utility of performing an EEG during sleep to capture nocturnal epileptic events (see Chapter 10).

Lesch–Nyhan Syndrome

The Lesch–Nyhan syndrome – the quintessential example of genetically determined abnormal behavior – consists of intellectual disability, dystonia, and, its hallmark, self-mutilation. This illness is transmitted in a recessive sex-linked pattern and therefore appears, with rare exceptions, only in boys. Because the dystonia is its most consistent feature, this book includes Lesch–Nyhan syndrome among the involuntary movement disorders (see Chapter 18).

Turner Syndrome (X0)

Individuals with Turner syndrome have a mutation in or, more usually, absence of one of their sex chromosomes. With a complement of only 45 fully functioning chromosomes, physicians usually say that these individuals have an "XO" chromosome pattern. They are outwardly phenotypically female; however, they are dysmorphic (Fig. 13.20) and, because of their gonadal dysgenesis, they do not undergo puberty.

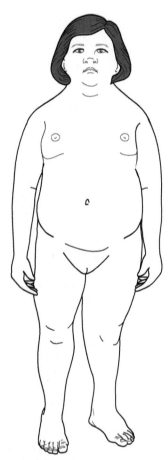

FIGURE 13.20 ■ This 16-year-old girl with Turner syndrome (XO) has intellectual disability and the distinctive short stature and webbed neck. As with several other genetic disorders, her ears are low-set (but hidden by a low hairline), her nose is flat, and its bridge spreads into broad epicanthal folds. Because she characteristically failed to undergo puberty, she lacks breast development and other secondary sexual characteristics. Also, her elbows' carrying angles are relatively straight, which is the male pattern.

A minority (10% to 20%) of Turner syndrome girls has mild-to-moderate intellectual disability; however, the majority – up to 70% – has learning difficulties. As with Williams syndrome children, Turner syndrome girls have greater impairment on performance than verbal IQ testing.

Klinefelter Syndrome (XXY)

With an additional X chromosome, Klinefelter syndrome boys are tall and eunuchoid (Fig. 13.21). As young men, their unusual height and lack of secondary sexual characteristics may draw medical attention, but physicians often diagnose Klinefelter syndrome only after the boys fail to go through puberty. Sometimes physicians first diagnose the disorder when an infertility evaluation reveals small testes and a lack or near lack of sperm. Testosterone treatment improves their sexuality and sperm counts.

Klinefelter syndrome boys usually have an IQ between 80 and 90 and tend to have dysarthria, dyslexia, and other learning disabilities. According to some reports, they have a passive personality.

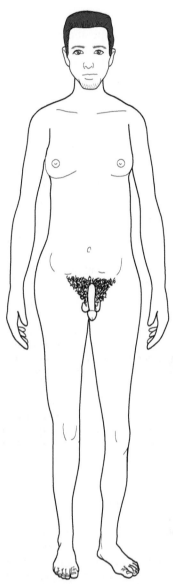

FIGURE 13.21 ■ After a delayed and then incomplete puberty, this 30-year-old man with Klinefelter syndrome (XXY) has grown taller than 6.5 feet, largely due to his disproportionately long legs. He has grown into a eunuchoid habitus with gynecomastia, sparse facial hair, and small testicles. Conditions characterized by excessive height include the XYY and Marfan syndromes and homocystinuria as well as the Klinefelter syndrome.

XYY Syndrome

Males who carry an extra Y chromosome are also tall, averaging 6'3". However, unlike those with Klinefelter syndrome (XXY), those with XYY syndrome often have macrocephaly and macro-orchidism (a large head and large testes), but otherwise normal secondary male sexual characteristics, and prominent acne in adolescence. Moreover, they are able to father children, and those children usually have a normal chromosome complement.

The original studies of the XYY syndrome, which were performed in prisons, suggested that the disorder expressed itself as deviant, violent, and aggressive behavior. With their size and behavior, affected men were labeled "super-males." In retrospect, the population base for those studies had tainted the results.

Modern studies have rejected a causal relationship between an XYY karyotype and aggression. They found that XYY men often, but not necessarily, have delays in acquiring speech and other neurodevelopmental milestones. They frequently show learning disabilities, and their IQ is 10 to 20 points lower than their sibs. If they commit a crime, it is typically nonviolent; however, because of their developmental delays, they are likely to be apprehended and incarcerated.

ENVIRONMENTAL TOXINS

Heavy Metals

The gastrointestinal tract absorbs the organic form of mercury (methylmercury [CH_3Hg^+]). In pregnant women, it readily crosses the placenta and tends to accumulate in fetal brain tissue. Mercury intoxication in fetuses, children, and adults causes cognitive impairment and other signs of brain damage. Exposure to debris from industrial accidents (such as occurred in Japan's Minamata Bay) and inhaling environmental gases has caused mercury intoxication. However, eating certain fish causes most mercury toxicity in neonates and infants. Large sea fish, such as swordfish, shark, king mackerel, and tuna, and certain fresh-water fish, such as pike and bass, have relatively high mercury concentrations. Pregnant women should avoid eating all of them.

On the other hand, the mercury in old-style dental fillings dissolves, if at all, at such a slow rate that it carries no significant risk. Even dentists who prepared the fillings on a daily basis had no mercury-related illnesses. Removing mercury-containing dental fillings offers no benefits.

Several researchers and many parents proposed an ominous association between autism and an old form of the measles, mumps, and rubella (MMR) vaccination because it contained an ethylmercury ($C_2H_5Hg^+$) preservative, thimerosal. Because the vaccination may have led to a brief but significant mercury exposure in infants, several studies – now discredited – suggested that it caused autism and other disorders. Even though vaccine manufacturers stopped adding mercury preservatives during the 1990s, the reported incidence of autism continued to climb. Those epidemiologic data and many other studies have exonerated both the current and older MMR vaccinations as a cause of autism and other neuropsychologic impairments.

Lead intoxication in infants and children, depending on its intensity, causes intellectual disability, learning disabilities, and other signs of cerebral impairment. This intoxication has usually originated in infants and children ingesting lead-based paint chips and environmental pollution. Acute intoxication causes seizures. The more common low-level exposure leads to subtle cognitive impairment.

Alcohol

A pregnant mother's drinking of alcoholic beverages, in certain quantities, and for a long enough duration, leads

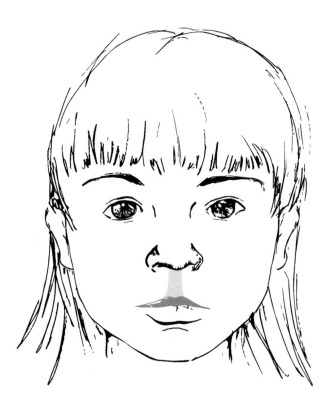

FIGURE 13.22 ■ The three most prominent and consistent facial abnormalities of the fetal alcohol syndrome occur in the mid-face and give this 6-year-old girl the distinctive appearance: 1. short palpebral fissures that hide the medial and lateral portions of her eyes, 2. smooth philtrum (the normally indented vertical groove between the bottom of the nose and the upper lip), and 3. thin upper lip.

to the *fetal alcohol syndrome*. In addition, adverse socioeconomic circumstances and certain genes constitute risk factors. This syndrome consists of developmental delays, three abnormalities of the face (Fig. 13.22), and life-long cognitive and behavioral impairments. Severely affected children have microcephaly, dysarthria, epilepsy, and intellectual disability. The fetal alcohol syndrome is probably the most common nongenetic cause of intellectual disability.

Not only does *in utero* alcohol exposure lead to learning and attention impairments and the resultant aversion to school, it is associated with antisocial and criminal behaviors, including substance abuse. Unlike most other young men with intellectual disability, except perhaps for XYY syndrome men, those with fetal alcohol syndrome are apt to be incarcerated.

REFERENCES

Adzick, N. S., Thom, E. A., Spong, C. Y., et al. (2011). A randomized trial of prenatal versus postnatal repair of myelomeningocele. *The New England Journal of Medicine, 364*, 993–1004.

Bardsley, M. Z., Kowal, K., Levy, C., et al. (2013). 47 XYY syndrome. *The Journal of Pediatrics, 162*, 1085–1094.

Bilder, D. A., Burton, B. K., Coon, H., et al. (2013). Psychiatric symptoms in adults with phenylketonuria. *Molecular Genetics and Metabolism, 108*, 155–160.

Caraballo, R. N., Cejas, N., Chamorro, N., et al. (2014). Landau-Kleffner syndrome: A study of 29 patients. *Seizure: The Journal of the British Epilepsy Association, 23*, 98–104.

Cianfaglione, R., Clarke, A., Kerr, M., et al. (2015). A national survey of Rett syndrome: Age, clinical characteristics, current abilities, and health. *American Journal of Medical Genetics. Part A, 167,* 1493–1500.

Cope, H., McMahon, K., Heise, E., et al. (2013). Outcome and life satisfaction of adults with myelomeningocele. *Disability and Health Journal, 6,* 236–243.

Curatolo, P., Moavero, R., & de Vires, P. J. (2015). Neurological and neuropsychiatric aspects of tuberous sclerosis complex. *The Lancet. Neurology, 14,* 733–745.

Deonna, T., & Toulet-Perez, E. (2010). Early-onset acquired epileptic aphasia (Landau-Kleffner syndrome, LKS) and regressive autistic disorders with epileptic EEG abnormalities. *Brain and Development, 32,* 746–752.

El Bashir, H., Dekair, L., Mahmoud, Y., et al. (2015). Neurodevelopmental and cognitive outcomes of classical homocystinuria: Experience from Qatar. *JIMD Reports, 21,* 89–95.

Elison, S., Stinton, C., & Howlin, P. (2010). Health and social outcomes in adults with Williams syndrome. *Research in Developmental Disabilities, 31,* 587–599.

Garg, S., Plasschaert, E., Descheemaeker, M. J., et al. (2015). Autism spectrum disorder profile in neurofibromatosis type 1. *Journal of Autism and Developmental Disorders, 45,* 1649–1657.

Green, T., Gothelf, D., Glaser, B., et al. (2009). Psychiatric disorders and intellectual functioning throughout development in velocardiofacial (22q11.2 deletion) syndrome. *Journal of the American Academy of Child and Adolescent Psychiatry, 48,* 1060–1068.

Grieco, J., Pulsifer, M., Seligsohn, K., et al. (2015). Down syndrome: Cognitive and behavioral functioning across the lifespan. *American Journal of Medical Genetics. Part C, Seminars in Medical Genetics, 169,* 135–149.

Hadders-Algra, M. (2010). *The Neurological Examination of the Child with Minor Neurological Dysfunction* (3rd ed.). London: MacKeith Press.

Jagtap, S., Srinivas, G., Harsha, K. J., et al. (2013). Sturge-Weber syndrome: Clinical spectrum, disease course, and outcome of 30 patients. *Journal of Child Neurology, 28,* 725–731.

Jarvien, A., Korenberg, J. R., & Bellugi, U. (2013). The social phenotype of Williams syndrome. *Current Opinion in Neurobiology, 23,* 414–422.

Jones, K. L., & Jones, M. C. (2013). *Smith's Recognizable Patterns of Human Malformation* (7th ed.). Philadelphia: Elsevier.

Keen, J. R., Przekop, A., Olaya, J. E., et al. (2014). Deep brain stimulation for the treatment of childhood dystonic cerebral palsy. *Journal of Neurosurgery. Pediatrics, 14,* 585–593.

Klein-Tasman, B. P., Lira, E. N., Li-Barber, K. T., et al. (2015). Parent and teacher perspectives about problem behavior in children with Williams syndrome. *American Journal on Intellectual and Developmental Disabilities, 120,* 72–86.

Kraan, C. M., Hocking, D. R., Bradshaw, J. L., et al. (2013). Neurobehavioral evidence for the involvement of the FMR1 gene in female carriers of fragile X syndrome. *Neuroscience and Biobehavioral Reviews, 37,* 522–547.

Lo, S. T., Collin, P. J., & Hokken-Koelega, A. C. (2015). Psychiatric disorders in children with Prader-Willi syndrome. *American Journal of Medical Genetics, 167A,* 983–991.

May, P. A., Baete, A., Russo, J., et al. (2014). Prevalence and characteristics of fetal alcohol spectrum disorders. *Pediatrics, 134,* 855–866.

Moss, J., & Howlin, P. (2009). Autism spectrum disorders in genetic syndromes: Implications for diagnosis, intervention and understanding the wider autism spectrum disorder population. *Journal of Intellectual Disability Research, 53,* 852–873.

Nelson, K. B., & Blair, E. (2015). Prenatal factors in singletons with cerebral palsy born at or near term. *The New England Journal of Medicine, 373,* 946–953.

Neul, J. L., Kaufman, W. E., Glaze, D. G., et al. (2010). Rett syndrome: Revised diagnostic criteria and nomenclature. *Annals of Neurology, 68,* 944–950.

Northrup, H., & Krueger, D. A. (2013). Tuberous sclerosis complex diagnostic criteria update. *Pediatric Neurology, 49,* 243–254.

Philip, N., & Bassett, A. (2011). Cognitive, behavioral and psychiatric phenotypes in 22q11.2 deletion syndrome. *Behavior Genetics, 41,* 403–412.

Plasschaert, E., Descheemaeker, M. J., Van Eylen, L., et al. (2015). Prevalence of autism spectrum disorder symptoms in children with neurofibromatosis type 1. *American Journal of Medical Genetics, 168B,* 72–80.

Siegel, M. S., & Smith, W. E. (2010). Psychiatric features in children with genetic syndromes: Toward functional phenotypes. *Child and Adolescent Psychiatric Clinics of North America, 19,* 229–261.

Stinton, C., Elison, S., & Howlin, P. (2010). Mental health problems in adults with Williams syndrome. *American Journal on Intellectual and Developmental Disabilities, 115,* 3–18.

Swaiman, K. F., Ashwal, S., Ferriero, D. M., et al. (2012). *Swaiman's Pediatric Neurology: Principles and Practice* (5th ed.). London: Elsevier.

Urv, T. K., Zigman, W. B., & Silverman, W. (2010). Psychiatric symptoms in adults with Down syndrome and Alzheimer's disease. *American Journal on Intellectual and Developmental Disabilities, 115,* 265–276.

Vinck, A., Verhagen, M. M., Gerven, M., et al. (2011). Cognitive and speech-language performance in children with ataxia telangiectasia. *Developmental Neurorehabilitation, 14,* 315–322.

Wallingford, K. B., Niswander, L. A., Shaw, G. M., et al. (2013). The continuing challenge of understanding, preventing, and treating neural tube defects. *Science, 339,* 1047–1054.

Walker, A., Kaufman, D. M., Solomon, G., et al. (2008). *Child and Adolescent Neurology for Psychiatrists.* Philadelphia: Lippincott Williams & Wilkins.

Williams, C. A. (2010). The behavioral phenotypes of the Angelman syndrome. *American Journal of Medical Genetics. Part C, Seminars in Medical Genetics, 154C,* 432–437.

CHAPTER 13

QUESTIONS AND ANSWERS

1–11. Match the neurocutaneous disorder (a–d) with its manifestation (Q1–11).
a. Tuberous sclerosis
b. Neurofibromatosis type 1 (NF1)
c. Sturge–Weber syndrome
d. Neurofibromatosis type 2 (NF2)

1. Acoustic neuroma
2. Facial lesions vaguely resemble rhinophyma
3. Progressive dementia
4. Neurofibromas
5. Angiofibromas (adenoma sebaceum)
6. Hypopigmented macules (ash leaf spots)
7. Intractable epilepsy
8. *Café-au-lait* spots
9. Facial angioma
10. Optic glioma
11. Shagreen patches

Answers: 1–d, 2–a, 3–a, 4–b, 5–a, 6–a, 7–a, 8–b, 9–c, 10–b, 11–a.

12–17. For each of the following disorders, state whether it frequently causes episodic inattention or changes in mood in children (Yes/No):

12. Migraine
13. Focal seizures
14. Antihistamines
15. Cerebral palsy
16. Sedative medications
17. Mitochondrial disorders

Answers: 12–yes, 13–yes, 14–yes, 15–no, 16–yes, 17–yes.

18. Which genetic illness causes short stature?
a. XXY
b. XYY
c. XO
d. Marfan syndrome

Answer: c. Turner (XO), trisomy 21, XXX, and numerous metabolic syndromes cause short stature. Klinefelter (XXY), "supermale" (XYY), homocystinuria, and Marfan syndromes all cause tall stature.

19. A son of college professors, an 8-year-old boy has slowly and incompletely acquired milestones. Unlike his parents and sibs, he has suffered childhood obesity. His pediatrician recently found that he developed diabetes. He eats incessantly and disregards any limits that his parents place on his calorie consumption. He stole food from the rabbit cage at

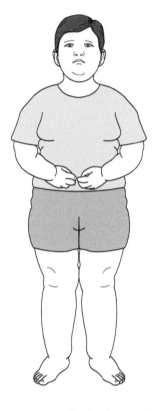

the children's zoo. Which abnormality explains his appearance and behavior?
a. Attention deficit hyperactivity
b. Fragile X syndrome
c. Valproate use
d. A DNA deletion
e. A hypothalamic tumor

Answer: d. He has Prader–Willi syndrome which results from a deletion in a chromosome 15. This disorder accounts for small but significant segments of the childhood obesity and intellectual disability populations. It may hold clues to the mechanism of satiety because children with this disorder lack negative feedback (to stop eating) when either their blood sugar rises or their stomach is distended. Bariatric surgical procedures so far have failed to alleviate the obesity. Although obesity and intellectual disability characterize Prader–Willi syndrome, the presence and severity of these two manifestations do not correlate in individual cases. Valproate leads to weight gain but not of this magnitude and not with the compulsive eating. Hypothalamic tumors may cause obesity classically accompanied by headache, visual impairment, and sleep disorders.

20. A woman reports to her doctor that her 40-year-old brother with Down syndrome has had a decline in

his functional ability, the development of apathy, and loss of his social skills. Which of the following conditions should the physician consider?

a. Depression
b. Neurocognitive disorder (dementia)
c. Leukemia
d. Hypothyroidism
e. All of the above

Answer: e. During and after their teenage years, Down syndrome individuals are vulnerable to depression, hypothyroidism, acute leukemia, obstructive sleep apnea, and hearing loss. Because Down syndrome individuals harbor three copies of the chromosome 21, which carries the amyloid precursor protein, they tend to develop Alzheimer disease routinely and at a young age.

21. In the DSM-5, which of the following conditions is *not* defined as a Neurodevelopmental Disorder?

a. Tourette's disorder
b. Language disorder
c. Nightmare disorder
d. Intellectual developmental disorder

Answer: c. Nightmare disorder is a Parasomnia, which is a category of Sleep–Wake Disorders.

22. The mother of a 5-year-old daughter who has received a diagnosis of ASD but has no physical stigmata of neurologic illness asks a consulting psychiatrist if her daughter should be referred for a neurologic examination, genetic analysis, and other testing. What would constitute the ideal response?

a. Yes
b. No
c. Maybe
d. Because the ASD patient is a girl, she should undergo further testing.

Answer: a. Pediatricians and psychiatrists sometimes ask when they should send a child with ASD, even with no physical abnormalities, for a neurologic examination, genetic analysis, and other testing. Answering that question is more than an academic exercise. With the maximum available knowledge, parents can more easily accept that some illnesses, such as fragile X, do not respond to treatment and others, such as Rett syndrome, follow a relentlessly downhill course. However, some aspects of some illnesses respond to treatment. For example, mTOR inhibitors may shrink tuberous sclerosis-induced SEGAs and metabolic interventions may reduce renal damage in Lesch–Nyhan syndrome. For illnesses that result from a single gene mutation, parents can learn that future children or grandchildren will have a certain chance of expressing or merely carrying the illness or that children of only one gender are at risk. Many pediatric neurologists recommend that girls with ASD symptoms undergo testing for the MECP2 and other Rett syndrome mutations, and boys with ASD symptoms undergo testing for fragile X. Of course, children who show regression, focal seizures, neurocutaneous disorders, or macrocephaly should undergo an MRI. However,

physicians should avoid sending children for CT (see Chapter 19). Children with ASD symptoms should undergo an EEG not only if they have seizures but also if they have Rett or Landau–Kleffner syndrome, where seizures complicate the majority of cases.

23. Which syndrome carries the lowest incidence of intellectual disability?

a. Klinefelter
b. Trisomy 21
c. Angelman syndrome
d. Down syndrome
e. Fragile X
f. Prader-Willi

Answer: a. Except for Klinefelter syndrome (XXY), intellectual disability is an integral part of all these conditions. Only about 30% of Klinefelter syndrome individuals have intellectual disability and, when present, it is usually mild. In fact, Klinefelter syndrome often remains undiagnosed until men undergo an evaluation for infertility.

24. Because he has sickle-cell disease, a 1-year-old boy sustained an occlusion of his left middle cerebral artery. Which of the following consequences will probably *not* appear?

a. Aphasia
b. Right-sided spasticity
c. Stunted growth (growth arrest) of right arm and leg
d. Right-sided hemiparesis

Answer: a. He will probably not develop aphasia because his right hemisphere will emerge as dominant for language and fine motor function. However, he will develop right-sided spastic hemiparesis with a foreshortened arm and leg. Strokes in infancy, childhood, and adolescence most often result from congenital heart disease, homocystinuria, mitochondrial disorders, migraine, drug abuse, and sickle-cell disease.

25–30. Match the neurologic deficit (Q25–30) with its cause.

25. Choreoathetosis
26. Spastic quadriplegia
27. Spastic hemiparesis
28. Deafness
29. Seizure disorder
30. Progressive areflexic, atrophic paresis

a. Cervical spinal cord injury
b. Kernicterus
c. Werdnig–Hoffmann disease
d. Stroke in utero

Answers: 25–b, 26–a, 27–d, 28–b, 29–d, 30–c.

31. Which chromosome carries the mutation that determines VCF?

a. Chromosome 22
b. Chromosome 7
c. Chromosome 15
d. Chromosome 12

Answer: a. A microdeletion on chromosome 22 determines VCF. Because the disorder appears as a sporadic mutation in 75% of cases, neither parent usually has the disorder; however, when VCF passes from parent to child, it follows an autosomal dominant pattern. This mutation is a major risk factor that cuts across ethnic lines for schizophrenia. Mutations in chromosome 7 determine Williams syndrome; 15, Prader–Willi and Angelman syndromes; and 12, PKU.

32. Regarding PKU, which one of the following statements is *false*?
    a. The disease is transmitted in an autosomal recessive pattern.
    b. The blood phenylalanine is high and tyrosine is low in affected individuals.
    c. If a woman with PKU were to conceive, the fetus would most likely be heterozygous for the PKU gene, and would therefore be unaffected by the mother's diet.
    d. Diet sweeteners and many other "foods" contain phenylalanine, which individuals with PKU should avoid.

Answer: c. Women with PKU, who are necessarily homozygous for the disorder, bear children who, with rare exception, are heterozygote. If the father were heterozygote, 50% of their offspring will be homozygous. If the father had PKU and was therefore homozygote for the disorder, 100% of their offspring will be homozygous. Assuming that a pregnant woman with PKU strays from her diet and consumes foods with phenylalanine, such as diet soda, she will accumulate excessive concentrations of phenylalanine. The phenylalanine and metabolic products readily cross the placenta and overwhelm the fetus' immature enzyme system and damage its brain. Pregnant women with PKU must adhere strictly to their phenylalanine-free diet. A synthetic tetrahydrobiopterin, sapropterin (Kuvan), offers some protection.

33. When asked to assess a 9-year-old girl, a psychiatrist learns that she had late acquisition of her developmental milestones, her IQ is 88, and she has poor arithmetic and visual-spatial skills. However, she is friendly, articulate, and verbal. In an entirely one-sided conversation, she explained that she has learned two foreign languages and plays two musical instruments. She has an upturned nose and her teeth hypoplastic and wide-spaced. Which is the most likely disorder?
    a. Rett syndrome
    b. Turner syndrome
    c. Williams syndrome
    d. Angelman syndrome

Answer: c. She has Williams syndrome, which the psychiatrist immediately identified by her elflike face and small and wide-spaced teeth. She also has the characteristic mild-to-moderate intellectual disability with poor visual-spatial relationships resulting in constructional apraxia juxtaposed to remarkable verbal and musical abilities.

34. Which other manifestation is likely to be present in the girl in Question 33?
    a. Supravalvular aortic stenosis
    b. Microcephaly
    c. Stereotypies
    d. Hepatosplenomegaly

Answer: a. Williams syndrome involves impaired formation of tissue elastin, which leads to supravalvular aortic stenosis. Microcephaly is a manifestation of Rett syndrome, ataxia-telangiectasia, Angelman syndrome, congenital rubella infection, and congenital Zika virus infection, but not Williams syndrome. In Rett syndrome and ataxia-telangiectasia, microcephaly is "acquired." Stereotypies – repetitive, involuntary, meaningless movements, usually of the hands – are characteristic of Rett, Angelman, and fragile X syndromes.

35. Which one of the following statements concerning individuals with the XYY karyotype is *true*?
    a. They live up to their appellation, "super-males."
    b. They are usually taller than 6' and they tend to have acne.
    c. They frequently have aggressive behavior and commit violent crimes.
    d. Their karyotype is a valid defense against criminal prosecution.

Answer: b. Individuals with the XYY karyotype are phenotypic men and they can father children. They average 6'3" and have acne, but they do not have pronounced muscle bulk, great strength, or athletic abilities. Their intellectual growth is slow and often falls short of average. They probably do not commit crimes more frequently or more violently than other individuals with comparable intellect or socioeconomic status. However, they are less able to evade arrest than criminals with normal intellectual capacity. They remain cognizant of their activities.

36. Which condition is characterized by macrocephaly?
    a. Rett syndrome
    b. Congenital rubella
    c. Angelman syndrome
    d. Ataxia-telangiectasia
    e. Tay–Sachs disease
    f. Fetal alcohol syndrome

Answer: e. Tay–Sachs and other storage diseases, XYY syndrome, and hydrocephalus cause macrocephaly. In contrast, Rett and Angelman syndromes, ataxia-telangiectasia, congenital rubella or Zika infection, cerebral anoxia at birth, and fetal alcohol syndrome cause microcephaly. For Rett and Angelman syndromes and ataxia-telangiectasia, two distinguishing features are that their microcephaly has a genetic basis and it develops many months to several years after birth, i.e., they have acquired microcephaly.

37. Meningomyeloceles are *not* associated with which one of the following conditions?
    a. Spastic paraparesis
    b. Intellectual disability

c. Incontinence

d. Flaccid quadriparesis

Answer: a. A meningomyelocele is a congenital neural tube closure defect. It causes flaccid, not spastic, paraparesis because of malformation of the junction of the lowest portion of the spinal cord and its emerging nerve roots. In addition, meningomyeloceles are often associated with comparable defects in the upper neural tube that lead to hydrocephalus and intellectual disability.

38. Which neurologic condition is associated with immunodeficiency?
    a. Neurofibromatosis
    b. Meningomyelocele
    c. Sturge–Weber syndrome
    d. Ataxia-telangiectasia

Answer: d. Ataxia-telangiectasia is associated with IgA and IgE immunoglobulin deficiency, cellular immunity impairment, and lymphomas. Of the common neurocutaneous disorders, it is the only one inherited in an autosomal recessive pattern.

39. During the past year, a previously healthy 5-year-old girl has slowly begun to ignore her parents and older siblings conversations and then to lose her ability to express herself – at least with words. She had a seizure while asleep. A pediatrician concluded that she had regressed in her psychomotor skills and developed aphasia. Her head circumference was normal and she had no abnormal movements or physical findings. An MRI was normal. An EEG showed epileptic discharges during slow-wave sleep. Which is the most likely diagnosis?
    a. Autism spectrum disorder (ASD)
    b. Deafness
    c. Landau–Kleffner syndrome (LKS)
    d. Rett syndrome

Answer: c. LKS, also known as acquired epileptic aphasia, is a rare childhood-onset illness characterized by the development of aphasia and, in most cases, epilepsy. It is one of many identifiable causes of ASD symptoms (Box 13.1). Although deafness is not the primary problem in this girl, physicians should test the hearing of neonates, all children during routine appointments, and children with intellectual disability, learning disabilities, hyperactivity, aphasia, and other neuropsychologic disorders. Physicians should consider Rett syndrome in girls who show ASD symptoms, but this girl probably does not have it because of her normal head circumference and lack of stereotypies.

40. Which of the following statements regarding Sturge–Weber syndrome is *false*?
    a. Of all port-wine stains involving the face, less than 10% are associated with cerebral abnormalities.
    b. Of port-wine stains involving the first division of the trigeminal nerve, only about 33% are associated with cerebral abnormalities, i.e., represent the Sturge–Weber syndrome.

c. Whether or not facial angiomas are a manifestation of Sturge–Weber syndrome, laser therapy can bleach them.

d. Like most other neurocutaneous disorders, Sturge–Weber is inherited in an autosomal dominant pattern.

Answer: d. Sturge–Weber is the result of an embryonal developmental disorder rather than a genetic mutation. Ataxia-telangiectasia is inherited in an autosomal recessive pattern, but neurofibromatosis and tuberous sclerosis are inherited in an autosomal dominant pattern.

41. Which pair of disorders exemplifies genomic imprinting?
    a. Neurofibromatosis 1 and 2 (NF1 and NF2)
    b. Prader–Willi and Angelman syndromes
    c. XXY and XYY
    d. Tuberous sclerosis 1 and 2 (TSC1 and TSC2)

Answer: b. Essentially the same mutation, a microdeletion on chromosome 15, usually produces Prader–Willi syndrome if the father has transmitted it to an offspring, but Angelman syndrome if the mother has transmitted it. This pattern of transmission is an example of genomic imprinting, i.e., the parent-of-origin determines the phenotype. Chromosome 17 carries the mutation causing NF1 and chromosome 22 carries the one causing NF2. Chromosome 9 carries the mutation causing TSC1 and chromosome 16 carries the one causing TSC 2.

42. Which of the following supplements reduces the incidence of meningomyelocele?
    a. Thiamine
    b. Vitamin A
    c. Folic acid
    d. Omega 3

Answer: c. Studies have found that 5 mg a day of folic acid before conception and during the first month of pregnancy reduces the incidence of neural tube defects by 85%. As a public health measure, food producers fortify breakfast cereals and breads with folic acid.

43. Soon after his school year began, 8-year-old Johnny, shorter than average with mild dysarthria, punched and bit several classmates. After he attacked several children during a game, the teacher sent him for an evaluation. As best as his mother recalled, he reached language and motor milestones later than his cousins. She seemed unaware that her son lacked the ability to sustain his concentration and socialize with neighborhood children or classmates. What is the child most likely to look like?
    a. Micrognathia, tubular nose with a broad tip and small nasal alae, and deformed ears
    b. Prominent forehead, long face, and large, low-set, "seashell-shaped" ears
    c. Webbed neck, low-set ears, flat nose, and broad epicanthal folds

d. Short palpebral fissures, smooth philtrum, and thin upper lip

Answer: d. Short palpebral fissures, smooth philtrum, and thin upper lip indicate the fetal alcohol syndrome (Fig. 13.22). While his delay in reaching milestones, dysarthria, inattention, and learning disabilities also indicate the fetal alcohol syndrome, the strongest indication is his aggression and lack of socialization. The physician might see if the mother has been an alcoholic. In contrast to this scenario, children with most other congenital neurodevelopmental disorders do not exhibit aggression. Micrognathia, tubular nose with a broad tip and small nasal alae, and deformed ears characterize VCF (Fig. 13.17). Of course, defects in the palate have greater diagnostic importance. A prominent forehead, long face, and large "seashell-shaped" ears characterize fragile X syndrome (Fig. 13.18). A webbed neck, low-set ears, flat nose, and broad epicanthal folds characterize Turner (XO) syndrome (Fig. 13.20).

44. In which condition is CT generally indicated in children?
    a. Dyslexia
    b. Regression in developmental milestones
    c. Three or more ASD symptoms
    d. Intermittent migraine
    e. Acute penetrating head trauma

Answer: e. Acute penetrating head trauma is an emergency that requires a rapidly obtained picture of the bones, foreign bodies, and acute blood as well as brain damage. These structures may be indistinct on MRI, which requires much more time and greater sedation to perform than a head CT. Although CT involves exposure to ionizing radiation and thus carries a small but measurable risk of an increase in a child's lifetime cancer risk, the benefits justify its use in acute penetrating trauma. CT is not indicated in the other conditions, but MRI is sometimes indicated.

45. Which is the most common pathology among premature infants who develop CP?
    a. Periventricular leukomalacia
    b. Kernicterus
    c. Microgyria
    d. Porencephaly

Answer: a. In premature infants, the destruction of the white matter surrounding the lateral ventricles – periventricular leukomalacia – is closely associated with the subsequent development of CP. Kernicterus, bilirubin staining of basal ganglia associated with the development of athetosis, is uncommon because of the prevention of hemolysis from Rh factor incompatibility and effective treatments of hyperbilirubinemia with exchange transfusion and phototherapy. Microgyria is small gyri of unknown cause throughout the entire cerebrum or in a limited area. Neurologists or pathologists sometimes find this condition in children with intellectual disability. Porencephaly is essentially a hole in the brain that might

have resulted from an in utero arterial occlusion or simply maldevelopment (see Fig. 20.4).

46. Which one of the following statements is *true* regarding fragile X syndrome?
    a. Its symptoms occur exclusively in boys.
    b. When trinucleotide repeats are abnormally long, but still within the 55–200 range, affected boys and girls may remain completely or almost completely asymptomatic.
    c. Fragile X syndrome is a rare cause of intellectual disability.
    d. When it causes intellectual disability, the cognitive impairment is unaccompanied by behavioral changes.

Answer: b. Boys with 55 to 200 trinucleotide repeats – the premutation – on their X chromosome have few if any symptoms. Girls with the premutation are generally asymptomatic, but detailed neuropsychologic testing may reveal impairments.

47. Which of the following syndromes is least likely to include ASD symptoms?
    a. Fragile X
    b. Rett
    c. Klinefelter
    d. Angelman
    e. Tuberous sclerosis
    f. Landau–Kleffner

Answer: c. Physicians often diagnose ASD children as having underlying fragile X, Rett, Angelman, tuberous sclerosis, or Landau–Kleffner syndrome. In DSM-5 terminology, these syndromes are *specifiers for ASD*. Fragile X syndrome is the most common diagnosable cause of ASD.

48. A 78-year-old man sought consultation for the onset of ataxia and tremor of his arms. One of his grandsons has ASD. After routine tests do not reveal a diagnosis, which one of the following tests should be ordered?
    a. Ataxia-telangiectasia
    b. CAG trinucleotide length on chromosome 4
    c. CGG trinucleotide length on the X chromosome
    d. TSC 1 and TSC 2
    e. A microdeletion on chromosome 15

Answer: c. More than 200 CGG trinucleotides on the X chromosome cause fragile X syndrome. Some men with a mild form of this mutation remain asymptomatic or unrecognized until their 7th decade or later, but then they develop ataxia and tremor of their limbs. Meanwhile, they have transmitted the mutation, which naturally expands in succeeding generations, to their children and grandchildren. In this case, the grandson has ASD associated with fragile X syndrome. Ataxia-telangiectasia presents in childhood. Excessive CAG trinucleotides on chromosome 4 cause Huntington disease. TSC 1 and TSC 2 mutations cause tuberous sclerosis. A microdeletion on chromosome 15 causes Prader–Willi or Angelman syndromes.

49. Which of the following might expose a fetus to high levels of mercury?
   a. Maternal dental fillings
   b. The mother eating canned tuna every day
   c. The mother eating fresh salmon every day
   d. The mother eating trout every day

Answer: b. Large, predatory fish – shark, tuna, king mackerel, and swordfish – have relatively high concentrations of methylmercury, which readily crosses the placenta and enters the fetal circulation. Old-style mercury-containing dental amalgams cause an insignificant mercury exposure.

50. In the mid-1990s vaccine manufacturers stopped using ethylmercury (thimerosal), as a preservative in measles, mumps, and rubella (MMR) vaccinations. What effect did this change in policy have on the incidence of ASD?
   a. The incidence continued to rise with no change in rate
   b. The incidence continued to rise but at a slower rate
   c. The incidence began to fall
   d. The incidence immediately fell to zero

Answer: a. Following the elimination of thimerosal from MMR vaccinations, the increasing rate of ASD diagnosis persisted.

51. Asked to see a 19-year-old woman who is recovering from ventricular septal defect surgery, a psychiatrist learns from her parents that she has had depressive episodes at least since she was 16 years old and a cleft palate that required surgical repair in infancy. The psychiatrist finds that the woman has nasal speech, external ear deformities, and mild-to-moderate intellectual disability. Which of the following disorders or syndromes is most likely to underlie the woman's defects?
   a. Prader–Willi
   b. Turner
   c. Velocardiofacial (VCF)
   d. Williams

Answer: c. With anomalies of her heart, palate, and ears, and intellectual disability, this patient has the VCF syndrome. An important aspect of VCF is the prevalence of mood disorder and schizophrenia in adults with this syndrome. Congenital cardiac disease may complicate Turner and Williams syndromes as well as VCF.

52. A 6-year-old girl, born after a normal gestation and delivery to neurologically normal, unrelated parents, began to lose her developmental milestones at 3 years of age. Her language suffered the most, but then she stopped playing and simply clapped her hands for hours at a time. Looking back at her head circumference determinations, her pediatricians calculated that she had acquired microcephaly. Which

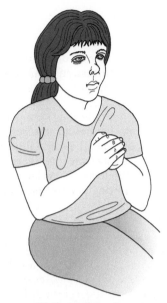

mutation most likely explains her appearance, behavior, and development?
   a. MECP2 mutation
   b. Excessive trinucleotide repeats on the X chromosome
   c. Microdeletion on chromosome 15
   d. Excessive trinucleotide repeats on the short arm of chromosome 4

Answer: a. She has Rett syndrome, which is caused by a mutation in the gene MECP2 (methyl CpG binding protein 2) in about 85% of cases. That gene governs the synthesis of methyl CpG binding protein, which is critical to cell function because, in large part, it silences other genes.

53. In which trimester of pregnancy does cerebral myelination begin?
   a. First
   b. Second
   c. Third
   d. None of the above

Answer: c. Cerebral myelination begins only in the third trimester of pregnancy and is not complete until the second year of life.

54. What is the common underlying cause of the following illnesses: Williams syndrome, Prader–Willi, and Angelman syndrome?
   a. They result from excessive trinucleotide repeats.
   b. They result from microdeletions.
   c. They result from mitochondrial DNA mutations.
   d. They are sex-linked disorders.

Answer: b. These disorders each result from minute DNA deletions – microdeletions – in chromosomal DNA.

55. What is the incidence of epilepsy in Rett syndrome?
   a. 10–20%
   b. 33%

c. 50%
d. ≥60%

Answer: d. The incidence of seizures in Rett syndrome is 60–90%. In contrast, in ASD of all causes, the incidence is approximately 33%.

56. A 7-year-old boy with life-long slow development has an IQ score of 60. He has no seizures, physical neurologic deficits, or general medical illness. His parents and two sisters have average intelligence. His X chromosomes tend to break in certain culture media. Which of the following is most likely to occur?

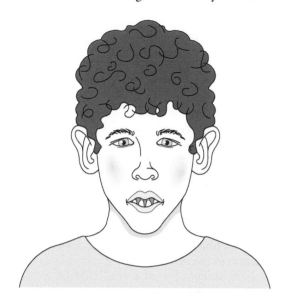

    a. He is apt to suffer further decline in his IQ.
    b. Some of his sisters' sons will have low IQ scores.
    c. Some of his brothers' sons will have low IQ scores.
    d. All his progeny will be unaffected.

Answer: b. His intellectual disability and low-set ears indicate that this boy has fragile X syndrome. Once he reaches puberty, examination will reveal *macro-orchidism* (large testicles). Fragile X syndrome boys show symptoms of ASD in 15% to 30% of cases. In fact, the fragile X mutation is the single most common monogenetic cause of ASD. Because the mutation consists of a mutation on the X chromosome containing excessive trinucleotide repeats, it tends to expand in successive generations. This expansion makes symptoms appear earlier and more profoundly (anticipation) in children and grandchildren. Fragile X syndrome causes mild to profound intellectual disability.

57. Which is the most common cause of intellectual disability in the United States?
    a. Trisomy 21
    b. Fragile X
    c. Fetal alcohol syndrome
    d. Obstetrical injuries
    e. Unknown or idiopathic

Answer: e. Trisomy 21 is often cited as the most common genetic cause; fragile X the most common

inherited cause; fetal alcohol syndrome the most common acquired cause; and obstetrical injuries the most common cause in legal proceedings. However, neurologists simply cannot determine the cause in most cases of intellectual disability.

58. A 17-year-old high school student who was diagnosed at birth with PKU has recently begun to do poorly academically and has had depressive symptoms. He has denied using drugs and alcohol, and claims to have adhered to his phenylalanine-free diet. Which is the best test to check that he has adhered to the diet?
    a. Urine phenylketones
    b. Serum phenylalanine
    c. Serum tyrosine
    d. Serum ceruloplasmin

Answer: b. Determining the serum phenylalanine levels is the best test for the status of PKU treatment. Elevated phenylalanine levels correlate with cognitive impairment and other neuropsychologic symptoms of PKU. Although serum tyrosine levels will be low in PKU, the correlation with neuropsychologic symptoms is not clear. Serum ceruloplasmin concentrations will be low in Wilson disease. Of course, as a general rule, physicians should perform urine toxicology studies on depressed high school students.

59. A child psychiatrist notices that an unusually tall 6-year-old boy with mild intellectual disability has thin and long arms and legs, sunken-in chest, and a dislocated ocular lens. Which of the following conditions is the most likely cause of the intellectual disability?
    a. Klinefelter syndrome
    b. Marfan syndrome
    c. Homocystinuria
    d. Fragile X syndrome

Answer: c. When inspection recognizes a lanky boy with mild-to-severe-mild intellectual disability has pectus excavatum and a dislocated ocular lens, the diagnosis is probably homocystinuria. Klinefelter syndrome (XXY) and Marfan syndromes also consist of tall, thin and longed-limbed statures, but neither causes chest deformity, lens dislocation, or, for the most part, significant intellectual disability. The XYY syndrome also consists of an abnormally tall frame and below-average intelligence, but normal muscle bulk and neither chest deformity nor lens dislocation.

60. In the previous case, absence of which of the following enzymes is the most likely cause of his disease?
    a. Tyrosine hydroxylase
    b. Cystathionine β-synthase
    c. Phenylalanine hydroxylase
    d. Dopamine β-hydroxylase

Answer: b. Cystathionine β-synthase along with vitamin B_6 metabolizes homocysteine to cystathionine. Its absence characterizes homocystinuria. A deficiency of tyrosine hydroxylase characterizes Parkinson disease. A deficiency of phenylalanine hydroxylase characterizes

PKU. A deficiency of dopamine β-hydroxylase leads to norepinephrine deficiency disorders.

61. In cases of homocystinuria, which is the best treatment?
    a. Inhibitors of the mammalian target of rapamycin (mTOR)
    b. Phenylalanine-free diet
    c. Tetrahydrobiopterin
    d. Pyridoxine

Answer: d. Vitamin B$_6$, usually in the form of pyridoxine, helps metabolize and reduce blood concentrations of homocysteine and its metabolite, methionine. Inhibitors of the *mammalian target of rapamycin (mTOR)* suppress the growth of subependymal giant cell astrocytomas (SEGAs), which are a characteristic of tuberous sclerosis. Tetrahydrobiopterin enhances phenylalanine metabolism.

62. Which of the following statements concerning tuberous sclerosis is *false*?
    a. A mutation in either of two genes, tuberous sclerosis complex 1 (TSC 1) on chromosome 9 or TSC 2 on chromosome 16, may cause the tuberous sclerosis complex.
    b. The majority of cases have been transmitted in an autosomal dominant pattern.
    c. Inhibitors of mTOR reduce the size of SEGAs.
    d. Tuberous sclerosis complex is one of several neurologic illnesses that cause ASD symptoms (see Box 13.1).

Answer: b. The majority (70%) of tuberous sclerosis cases occur *de novo*. The rest are transmitted in an autosomal dominant pattern by mutations in either TSC 1 or TSC 2. In a recent medical breakthrough, administering mTOR inhibitors, such as everolimus and sirolimus, has been shown to reduce the size of SEGAs. Tuberous sclerosis complex is one of several neurologic illnesses that cause ASD symptoms (see Box 13.1).

63. Mitochondrial disorders typically present in childhood with neurologic symptoms. Which of the following statements is *true* regarding normal mitochondria?

    a. They primarily perform anaerobic metabolism.
    b. During mitosis, they segregate equally.
    c. They perform oxidative phosphorylation to produce the energy source, adenosine triphosphate (ATP).
    d. They are invulnerable to cyanide poisoning.

Answer: c. Normal mitochondria perform aerobic metabolism that drives the "respiratory chain" that creates the energy source, ATP. Unlike segregation of chromosomes during mitosis, mitochondria segregate unequally even within the same organ, i.e., they show heteroplasmy. They are particularly vulnerable to cyanide poisoning.

64. Which of the following statements is *false* regarding abnormal mitochondria?
    a. Disorders resulting from genetically defective or otherwise abnormal mitochondria characteristically produce elevated blood levels of lactic acid and pyruvate.
    b. These disorders produce symptoms at all times rather than intermittently.
    c. The genes in mitochondria usually operate independently of those in the chromosomes.
    d. The proportion of mutant mitochondrial DNA (mtDNA) in an organ determines the symptoms.

Answer: b. Mitochondria rendered ineffective either by mtDNA mutations or certain poisons, such as many rodenticides or herbicides, cannot perform aerobic metabolism. Cells forced to rely on anaerobic metabolism produce elevated blood levels of lactic acid and pyruvate. The threshold proportion of mutant mitochondrial DNA (mtDNA) in an organ determines its functional capacity. Symptoms emerge when energy demand peaks, but at other times patients may remain asymptomatic. In many conditions, mutations in chromosomal DNA affect mitochondria function, and in some conditions, mutations in mitochondria DNA (mtDNA) affect chromosomal function.

NEUROLOGIC ASPECTS OF CHRONIC PAIN

More than just a persistent symptom, chronic pain is a complex endless condition with unique qualities, impaired activities of daily living, and psychiatric comorbidities. Traditional medical approaches to chronic pain emphasized diagnosis, distinguished between its psychologic and physiologic components, and sought its eradication. Currently, multidisciplinary pain teams focus on symptomatic management, reducing pain's affective component (suffering), and restoring function. These teams describe their role as pain *management* specialists without holding out the expectation that they will eliminate the pain.

As a member of a team or an individual treating physician, psychiatrists should be aware of common chronic pain syndromes and their underlying neuroanatomy, psychiatric comorbidity, and treatments involving long-term use of opioids (narcotics) and adjuvant medications (primarily nonanalgesic drugs, such as antidepressants and antiepileptics [AEDs]).

TYPES OF PAIN

Nociceptive pain results from acute, ongoing tissue damage, such as trauma, metastasis to bone, dental infection, or disease of the viscera. It usually consists of dull aching pain at the site of the tissue damage. Diseased viscera, however, may also refer pain to another region, such as when gallbladder stones seem to produce pain in the scapula. Wherever the location, tissue damage triggers specific receptors (*nociceptors*) in the peripheral nervous system (PNS) and certain cranial nerves. Either peripheral or cranial nerves transmit the noxious stimuli to the central nervous system (CNS). Removing diseased tissue and other direct treatments may reduce or eliminate nociceptive pain. Until the injury responds to treatment or heals, analgesics reduce the pain.

Neuropathic pain, in contrast, results from pain signals transmitted by the nervous system, often without actual tissue injury. It is a symptom of a wide variety of CNS and PNS disorders, such as cranial neuropathies, mononeuropathy or polyneuropathy, brachial or lumbar plexus injury, lumbar spine disorders, complex regional pain syndrome, and thalamic injury.

Unlike the dull ache of nociceptive pain, neuropathic pain consists of electric, sharp, lancinating, or burning sensations. Also, not confined to the site of an injury, neuropathic pain and spontaneously occurring painful paresthesias radiate throughout the distribution of an injured nerve and often well beyond it. Other features are that painful or even neutral stimuli elicit an intense, distorted, or exaggerated response – *hyperalgesia* or *allodynia* (see Chapter 5).

Especially because physicians cannot remove or repair the injured nerves, they can rarely abolish neuropathic pain. Another reason is that nerve injury may eventually reorganize CNS pain perception through *plasticity*, the capacity of the CNS to reorganize its functions. Although plasticity is usually beneficial, in this case it amplifies, distorts, and perpetuates pain. Whatever its source, neuropathic pain is common, disabling, and usually unrelenting. Moreover, it carries great psychiatric comorbidity.

The *Diagnostic and Statistical Manual of Mental Disorders, 5th Edition* (DSM-5) categorizes pain somewhat differently. The former DSM diagnosis of Pain Disorder has now been subsumed into Somatic Symptom Disorder. In this diagnosis, pain represents the major focus of the clinical presentation and causes distress or functional impairment. It allows psychological factors to have an important role in the pain's onset, severity, or maintenance. The diagnosis excludes pain better explained by a mood disorder, anxiety, or psychosis. The symptomatic state must last at least 6 months. It considers pain resulting from a neurologic or medical condition, such as headaches, peripheral neuropathy, or low back injury to be a component of those conditions.

The DSM-5 labels individuals as malingering who knowingly falsely claim severe and prolonged pain. In addition to financial expectations, incentives to malinger include freedom from work assignments, receiving attention, and seeking retribution. Even though the proportion of malingering individuals may be less than 1% of all pain cases, the number of such individuals is quite large.

Although neurologic disorders generally have a psychiatric component, probably none has a greater psychiatric component than chronic pain. Pain management centers report that as many as 50% of patients with chronic pain have dual diagnoses – particularly depression, but also somatoform and personality disorders, substance abuse, and posttraumatic stress disorders. Moreover, chronic pain is linked to drug and alcohol dependency, dysfunctional family relationships, and exaggeration of physical deficits.

The closest association remains between depression and chronic pain, which is almost invariably neuropathic. When present, depression lowers the threshold for pain, makes it refractory to treatment, and increases disability. In many patients the causal relationship between pain and depression is unclear. For example, painful injuries lead to depression, but certainly preexisting depression leads to chronic pain following injuries. With respect to chronic pain, major depression is more closely associated with the *number* of painful sites or painful conditions than the severity or duration of pain.

PSYCHIATRIC CONSULTATIONS

Physicians often refer patients with chronic pain for evaluation of depression and anxiety, posttraumatic stress disorder, or drug or alcohol abuse. Instead of waiting to be consulted as a last resort, psychiatrists might urge their colleagues to solicit consultations for patients (1) who have vegetative symptoms, regardless of the apparent connection to the pain, (2) whose pain or disability is refractory to medical treatment, (3) who seem to require excessive medication, (4) for psychopharmacology consultation, (5) for whom inpatient treatment or surgical procedures have been unsuccessful, or (6) who may have psychopathology that complicates their management.

When possible, psychiatrists should examine the physical location of a patient's pain. An examination involving physical touch of the painful area, where appropriate, probably has therapeutic benefit, albeit the primitive one of "laying on of hands." Also, in evaluating pain-related functional disability, psychiatrists should watch the patient sit, walk, and, if possible, use the affected part of the body.

PAIN PATHWAYS

Ascending pathways rapidly bring information from the periphery to the brain. They identify a pain's nature and location, arouse central mechanisms, and activate the limbic system. Analgesic pathways originating in the brain and descending in the spinal cord modulate pain perception. This neuroanatomy for pain and analgesia serves as the basis of many treatment strategies.

Peripheral Pathways

Painful conditions, such as contusions and menstrual cramps, liberate inflammatory mediators including prostaglandins, arachidonic acid, and bradykinin that stimulate nociceptors. These mediators initiate pain transmission by triggering voltage-gated sodium channels in the PNS and CNS. Aspirin and nonsteroidal anti-inflammatory agents (NSAIDs) block cyclooxygenase (COX), an enzyme crucial in the synthesis of prostaglandins, thereby reducing tissue inflammation and alleviating pain. Lidocaine, several AEDs, and tricyclic antidepressants (TCAs) block these channels and reduce pain.

Central Pathways

The PNS fibers enter the CNS at the spinal cord's dorsal horn and, either immediately or after ascending a few segments, synapse in its *substantia gelatinosa* (Fig. 14.1). At many of these synapses, the fibers release an 11-amino-acid polypeptide, *substance P*, which constitutes the major neurotransmitter for pain at the spinal cord level.

After the synapse, pain sensation ascends predominantly within the *lateral spinothalamic tract* to the brain

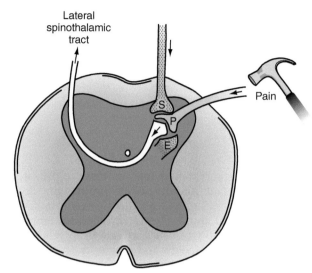

FIGURE 14.1 ■ Pain sensation travels along the *A-delta* and *C* fibers of peripheral nerves. These fibers enter the dorsal horn of the spinal cord where, using *substance P* (P), they synapse onto second-order neurons. The second-order neurons cross to the contralateral side of the spinal cord and, forming the *lateral spinothalamic tract*, ascend to the thalamus. Two powerful pain-dampening or pain-modulating analgesic systems (*stippled*) play upon the dorsal horn synapse. One tract descends from the brain and releases *serotonin* (S). The other system is composed of spinal interneurons that release enkephalins (E).

(see Figs. 2.6 and 2.15). This crucial tract crosses from the substantia gelatinosa to the spinal cord's other side and ascends contralateral to the injury to terminate in specific nuclei of the thalamus. Additional synapses relay the stimuli to the somatosensory cerebral cortex, enabling the individual to locate the pain.

In the *spinohypothalamic tract*, another ascending pain pathway, ipsilateral and contralateral fibers travel up the spinal cord and terminate directly in the hypothalamus. This pathway may explain pain-induced disturbances in temperature regulation, sleep, and other autonomic functions. The spinal cord also transmits pain in other, less well-defined ipsilateral and contralateral tracts.

In addition to relaying pain to the thalamus and hypothalamus, these tracts convey pain to the limbic system, reticular activating system, and other brainstem regions. These connections partially explain why individuals awaken when given a painful stimulus during sleep. It also accounts for chronic pain patients' sleeplessness, loss of appetite, and a tendency to develop anxiety and mood disturbances. On the other hand, loss of this connection – from trauma, anoxia, or other insult – explains why patients who are unconscious cannot experience pain or suffer.

ANALGESIC PATHWAYS

Many analgesic pathways interfere with pain transmission within the brain or spinal cord. Several pathways that originate in the frontal lobe and hypothalamus terminate in the gray matter surrounding the third ventricle and aqueduct of Sylvius (*periaqueductal gray matter*). They contain large amounts of *endogenous opioids*, which are

BOX 14.1 Glossary

β-endorphin: An endogenous opioid concentrated in the pituitary gland and secreted with ACTH. It consists of amino acid numbers 61–91 of β-lipotropin and gives rise to the enkephalins (see Fig. 14.2).

β-lipotropin: A 91-amino-acid polypeptide, which may be an ACTH fragment. It gives rise to β-endorphin but has no opioid activity itself (that is, β-lipotropin is not an endogenous opioid).

Dynorphin: An endogenous peptide opioid that binds to kappa opioid receptors.

Endogenous opioids: Polypeptides (amino acid chains) found within the CNS that create effects similar to those of morphine and other opioids. The effects of both endogenous and exogenous opioids are characteristically reversed by naloxone.

Endorphins: Endogenous morphine-like substances or opioid peptides. This term is virtually synonymous with endogenous opioids.

Enkephalins: Short (5-amino-acid) polypeptide endogenous opioids that include met-enkephalin and leu-enkephalin. They are found primarily in the amygdala, brainstem, and dorsal horn of the spinal cord.

Naloxone (Narcan): A pure opioid antagonist that reverses the effects of endogenous and exogenous opioids.

Substance P: An 11-amino-acid polypeptide that is probably the primary pain neurotransmitter at the first synapse of the primary afferent neuron in the spinal cord.

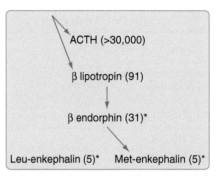

FIGURE 14.2 ■ Endogenous opioids are synthesized and secreted, along with adrenocorticotropin (ACTH), from the pituitary gland in times of stress or acute pain. A large precursor molecule (not pictured) gives rise to ACTH and β-lipotropin, which are often released together. β-Lipotropin gives rise to β-endorphin and met-enkephalin, but another precursor gives rise to leu-enkephalin. (The asterisks denote the important endogenous opioids, and the numbers within parentheses denote the number of amino acids in the polypeptide chains.)

powerful analgesics (Box 14.1). Implanted electrodes that stimulate the periaqueductal gray matter area may provoke the release of endogenous opioids and thereby induce profound analgesia.

Similarly, short neurons located entirely within the spinal cord, *interneurons*, inhibit incoming PNS stimuli. These neurons release endogenous opioids and other neurotransmitters that reduce pain transmission.

Analgesic pathways also originate in the brainstem and descend in the spinal cord's *dorsolateral funiculus*. They provide "descending analgesia" relief of pain by inhibiting both spinal cord synapses and their ascending pathways. Unlike most other analgesic pathways, they release *serotonin*.

ENDOGENOUS OPIOIDS

Often called *endorphins* (*end*ogenous m*orphin*e-like substances), endogenous opioids – endorphins, enkephalins, and dynorphins – are amino acid chains (polypeptides) synthesized in the CNS with powerful analgesic properties (Fig. 14.2). Endogenous opioids bind to receptors in the limbic system, periaqueductal gray matter, dorsal horn of the spinal cord, and other CNS sites. The "runner's high" and the initial painlessness reported by wounded soldiers serve as examples of endorphins' analgesic effects.

Synthetic (exogenous) opioids, particularly morphine and other medicines, are virtually identical to endogenous opioids. They bind to the same CNS receptors and produce the same effects – analgesia, mood elevation

(euphoria), sedation, and respiratory depression. *Naloxone* (Narcan), an antagonist that competitively binds to the opiate receptor, reverses the effects of endogenous, as well as exogenous, opioids. Indeed, naloxone's opioid antagonist effect is so characteristic that *naloxone-reversibility* serves as a criterion for ascertaining that opioid pathways mediate an analgesic's effect.

TREATMENTS

Physicians prescribe numerous medications for pain and administer them through various routes. Some alleviate pain by reducing tissue damage, interrupting pain transmission through peripheral or central pathways, or blunting its impact on cerebral structures. The addition of psychologic treatment and physical therapy may further reduce pain and, as part of a complete care plan, decrease suffering, restore activities of daily living, and return control to patients. Because chronic pain remains notoriously refractory to conventional treatment, neurologists aim for pain management, not pain cure.

Nonopioid Analgesics

As previously mentioned, aspirin, other salicylates, NSAIDs, steroids, and acetaminophen – nonopioid analgesics – inhibit prostaglandin synthesis at the injury (Box 14.2). Through this mechanism, these medicines relieve acute and chronic pain of mild-to-moderate severity.

Nonopioid analgesics generally provide steady analgesia for weeks to months and avoid several potential problems. In particular, after completing a course of treatment, patients do not experience withdrawal symptoms. Also, except for the potential for high-dose steroids to cause steroid psychosis (see Chapter 15), these analgesics do not induce mood, cognitive, or thought disorders.

On the other hand, large doses of NSAIDs and aspirin cause gastric irritation or hemorrhage, and prolonged use increases the risk of cardiovascular disease. In addition,

BOX 14.2	Examples of Analgesics

Acetaminophen (Tylenol and others)
Aspirin
   Choline magnesium trisalicylate (Trilisate)
   Diflunisal (Dolobid)
Nonsteroidal anti-inflammatory agents
   Ibuprofen (Motrin, Advil)
   Indometacin (Indocin)
   Ketorolac (Toradol)
   Naproxen (Naprosyn)
Opioids
   Fentanyl (Duragesic)*
   Hydromorphone (Dilaudid)
   Levorphanol (Levo-Dromoran)
   Methadone^
   Morphine$
   Oxycodone (Percocet)

*Available for transcutaneous (skin patch) and transmucosal (lollipop) administration
^Long-acting
$Available in long-acting forms (MS Contin, Oramorph SR)

although nonopioid analgesics provide dose-dependent pain relief, they do so only up to a point. Once these medicines provide their maximum pain relief, greater doses do not increase their benefit (the "ceiling effect").

Nonopioid analgesics are more effective if patients take them on a prophylactic basis. For example, taking nonopioid analgesics prior to dental procedures or menses will avert much of the pain. They are also more effective if taken in a generous initial "loading" dose.

Although nonopioid analgesics alone offer minimal benefit in cases of neuropathic pain, they act synergistically when taken in combination with opioids. In other words, peripherally acting nonopioid analgesics enhance centrally acting opioid analgesics. For example, adding NSAIDs to morphine helps alleviate the pain of metastases to bone. Because nonopioid analgesics allow a smaller dose of opioids to be effective, they have an "opioid-sparing effect."

With routine use, acetaminophen by itself or as an enhancement to opioids provides effective, reasonably safe analgesia. Stern warnings about acetaminophen compounds, such as oxycodone-acetaminophen (Percocet) and hydrocodone-acetaminophen (Vicodin), as well as acetaminophen itself, causing permanent liver damage are justifiable, but usually when looking at the aftermath of an overdose or their use by alcoholic individuals or patients with pre-existing hepatic disease.

Opioids

When chronic pain results from cancer, neurologists categorize it as "cancer" or "malignant" pain, but when it results from other conditions, as "noncancer" pain. Opioids are unquestionably indicated for cancer pain (see Box 14.2). In addition, a number of studies suggest that they are also useful for chronic noncancer pain syndromes.

Opioids have no ceiling effect. Greater doses or more potent preparations increase their analgesic effect. Adding NSAIDs or other nonopioid analgesics enhances opioids' effect without risking their side effects. On the other hand, when treating patients with noncancer pain who do not find relief with opioid treatment, physicians should slowly discontinue opioids rather than increase the dosage.

Chronic pain patients may obtain opioid treatment from pills, transdermal patches, intranasal sprays, rectal suppositories, and epidural injections. A particularly innovative technique, *patient-controlled analgesia (PCA)*, allows patients to regulate continual or intermittent intravenous opioid infusions. Through controls in the system, patients regulate the depth of analgesia without causing respiratory depression. Even 6-year-old children can safely and effectively administer PCA.

Compared to older opioids, newer ones provide more rapid onset and longer duration of action. Some are long-acting because they are embedded in a matrix that slowly releases its medication.

Administering opioids by PCA, patches, or long-acting oral preparations on a *regular prophylactic* or *time-dependent* basis, such as every 2 to 4 hours, is more effective than administering them only at the onset of pain. Administering opioids only after pain has developed makes it more difficult to control, creates a pattern of "hills and valleys" (undertreatment alternating with overtreatment), prevents restful sleep, and increases side effects. Moreover, because patients, fearful about pain recurrence, develop anxiety and preoccupation with obtaining their medicines, they may even seem to behave like addicts (see later).

Physicians who prescribe narcotics should select long-acting preparations, such as methadone or a transdermal opioid. Also, because various opioids affect different regions of the mu (μ) and related opioid receptors, physicians should vary the opioid for patients with intractable pain. However, because of the potential of large accumulated doses, transdermal and extended-release oral opioid formulations carry a disproportionately greater risk of morbidity and mortality.

Physicians should also avoid changing from an oral to parenteral form of opioid at a given dose because the substitution will likely lead to an overdose. In the reverse situation, changing the same dose from an intramuscular or intravenous injection to pills is likely to produce undertreatment, which can cause withdrawal symptoms and recurrence of pain.

In an attempt to control indiscriminate prescription of opioids, the Food and Drug Administration (FDA) launched Risk Evaluation and Mitigation Strategies (REMS) in 2012 for physicians who prescribe opioids. REMS will hopefully reduce inappropriate prescriptions, abuse, overdose, and other untoward effects. Additionally, physicians are accountable in many states with a requirement to check an electronic database of a patient's controlled substance prescription history prior to writing a new prescription.

"Addiction"

In a situation akin to drug addiction, within weeks of beginning opioid treatment, patients require increasingly greater quantities to produce the same level of anesthesia (*tolerance*) as the opioids desensitize receptors. Similarly, abruptly stopping opioid treatment produces unpleasant symptoms (*withdrawal*). However, because the two situations differ in several important respects, physicians certainly do not label a terminal cancer patient who requires opioids a drug addict.

Although tolerance and withdrawal characterize physical dependence, pain management physicians as well as neurologists define addiction primarily in behavioral terms, such as harmful drug-seeking activity and overwhelming involvement with use of a drug. They consider tolerance and dependence, which often occur together but can occur independently, as physiologic responses, an expectable aspect of medical treatment, and not peculiar to opioids. They also note that inadequate treatment and development of tolerance drives pain patients to be overly concerned about their opioid schedule and to seek larger doses. Physicians unfamiliar with pain management may interpret this behavior as "drug-seeking" and an indication of addiction, but many pain-management physicians consider it iatrogenic *pseudoaddiction*. On the other hand, some pain management physicians remain skeptical and consider pseudoaddiction to be true addiction.

Some pain management specialists contend that physicians' fear of creating addiction has led to the most common side effect of opioid treatment – undertreatment. In fact, addiction rarely develops in previously opioid-naive individuals who develop an acute painful illness that requires opioids for several weeks. Pain management physicians have been advocating continual opioid treatment of moderate-to-severe noncancer as well as cancer pain, though the American Academy of Neurology noted in a position paper that strong evidence supporting this treatment modality is limited.

Other Opioid Side Effects

For the psychiatric consultant, a dilemma is the similarity of opioid-induced mental status changes to those induced by head trauma, metabolic aberrations, and cerebral metastases. It is because opioids may cause delirium and depress the level of consciousness, which obscure the clinical picture, that neurologists and neurosurgeons avoid treating head trauma patients with opioids when possible.

Hypoventilation – slow and shallow breathing – represents the primary life-threatening side effect of opioids. However, in practical terms, administering opioids to patients with pulmonary disease, rather than an overdose in an otherwise healthy patient, is the usual cause of hypoventilation. Also, patients develop tolerance to hypoventilation along with their other side effects.

Although depression of sensorium and hypoventilation loom large to physicians as major iatrogenic problems, constipation remains the most troublesome side effect for patients. Rather than trying to reverse this inevitable complication, physicians can prevent it by ordering a combination of laxatives, such as senna (Senokot), and stool softeners, such as docusate sodium (Colace). They can also prescribe an oral selective μ (mu)-opioid receptor antagonist that does not cross the blood–brain barrier, such as alvimopan (Entereg), lubiprostone (Amitiza), or naloxegol (Movantik).

To prevent or alleviate opioid-related nausea, physicians should prescribe antiemetics, but they should cautiously prescribe antiemetics containing phenothiazine or another dopamine receptor-blocking agent because they can cause dystonic reactions or parkinsonism (see Chapter 18). In another caveat, pharmacologic marijuana, such as dronabinol (Marinol) and nabilone (Cesamet), generally reduces nausea, pain, and anxiety; however, robust formal studies have not established that it is the most effective treatment when cancer or chemotherapy has been responsible these symptoms. Moreover, it may cause transient mood and thought disorders.

The use of specific opioids is fraught with difficulties. For example, phenytoin and carbamazepine – whether prescribed for their antiepileptic activity, mood modulation, or pain control – accelerate methadone metabolism. Therefore giving either of these AEDs to patients on methadone maintenance may precipitate withdrawal symptoms. To avoid that problem physicians should increase the methadone dose when they add those medications (see Chapter 10).

Heroin, a problematic opioid, is no more effective in relieving pain or improving mood than morphine, but its potential for abuse is much greater. Regardless of several medical and nonmedical groups' assertions, heroin has no legitimate use that cannot be better fulfilled by the current array of medicines.

As with other medicines, physicians should discontinue opioids when unnecessary. Rather than abruptly stopping opioids, which would probably lead to withdrawal, physicians might use an exit strategy of tapering opioids by reducing their dose by 50% every 3 days. Alternatively, physicians might briefly replace a short-acting opioid, such as morphine, with a long-acting one, such as methadone, and then prescribe a nonopioid analgesic. If withdrawal still complicates the process, benzodiazepines may alleviate the physical or mental discomfort, and clonidine (Catapres) may blunt autonomic nervous system hyperactivity (see Chapter 21).

Chronic Opioid Therapy Debate

Over the past decade, neurologists, pain management specialists, and other physicians began to prescribe long-term opioid treatment for many noncancer conditions, including osteoarthritis, headache, postoperative low back pain, and fibromyalgia. These physicians offer several arguments that have gained increased acceptance. They claim that when used to control otherwise intractable pain, opioids are not addictive; opioids are effective, safe, and allow patients to work, use machinery, and drive; and, more than other medicines, opioids increase function, reduce suffering, and restore sleep.

Physicians prescribing chronic opioid therapy expect patients to agree, often with a written contract, to use the opioid in preset amounts and only from a single physician. Patients must also give permission for random urine testing for illicit substances, particularly drugs of abuse. Physicians monitor the patient's social and occupational functioning as well as their pain and urine tests.

Physicians who have opposed expanding opioid prescriptions offer several counterarguments. Opioids reduce pain less than 2 to 3 points on a 0 to 10 scale. Chronic opioid therapy may be counterproductive in several conditions. It portends worse long-term outcomes for headache and low back pain, and tends to convert episodic migraines or tension-type headache to persistent daily headache (see Chapter 9). Patients demand opioids when less potent or alternative measures, even nonpharmacologic ones, would suffice. In addition, patients may subvert medical treatment. They may seek opioids for their euphoric effect rather than for pain relief. Falsely reporting the persistence and severity of pain to obtain opioids prolongs disability. Some patients, claiming intractable pain, demand excessive quantities, but sell or pass along their opioids. To avoid this "diversion" of opioids, some physicians go so far as to ask a patient who has been prescribed fentanyl patches to return the used ones, which should have the patient's hair stuck to the patch's adhesive. Some patients use opioids to tide them over an addiction to illicit drugs. For many patients, obtaining opioids takes over their day-to-day concerns.

Some neurologists feel that chronic opioid therapy is rife with misuse. Examples include using alcohol and illicit substances in addition to the opioids, selling or trading the opioids, and surreptitiously obtaining additional quantities of opioids. Risk factors for misuse are a family as well as a personal history of substance abuse; age 16 to 45 years; presence of a "psychiatric condition," including schizophrenic disorders, affective psychosis, neurotic disorders, and personality disorders; and, in women, preadolescent sexual abuse. Rates of misuse of opioids among chronic opioid therapy patients range from 3% to 30%.

Long-term opioid treatment, especially at high dosage or following a dose increase, generally produces sedation, impairs cognition, and interferes with psychosocial function. In addition to leading to these neuropsychologic effects, it also leads to the usual opioid side effects, particularly chronic constipation and hypogonadism.

Finally, physicians prescribing opioids are subject to administrative oversight that may be stringent and punitive. Both state and federal investigators pursue possible irregularities. That being said, the number of opiate prescriptions in the US increased 700% from 1997 to 2007 and in 2010 alone there were more than 27,000 admissions to health-care facilities for opiate-related problems (including unintended pediatric ingestion). Consequently, physicians prescribing opiates must insist upon their own close patient monitoring to ensure safe administration.

Adjuvants

Antidepressants

Adjuvants enhance the effect of opioid and nonopioid analgesics and modulate the affective component of chronic pain. For example, TCAs help alleviate neuropathic conditions, particularly painful diabetic neuropathy. In addition, TCAs help restore patients' normal sleep–wake schedule and improve their mood.

In general, TCAs are helpful for chronic pain patients with or without comorbid depression. They are suitable for chronic pain in children. When used to treat pain, TCAs are effective at low doses and have a rapid onset of action. However, even at the low doses, TCAs may cause side effects, such as dry mouth, urinary retention, and in elderly patients, confusion. Also, unlike opioid treatment, substituting one TCA for another will probably not improve analgesia.

Selective serotonin reuptake inhibitors (SSRIs), compared to TCAs, have little analgesic effect – surprising given serotonin's crucial analgesic role. However, SSRIs may offer some pain relief in patients with comorbid depression. There have been several case reports of serotonin syndrome (see Chapter 6) precipitated by the concomitant use of SSRIs and fentanyl, both in the IV form (perioperative) and in the patch form (chronic pain management). Thus, a full medication history is crucial when combination therapy is being considered. Selective norepinephrine reuptake inhibitors (SNRIs), such as duloxetine (Cymbalta), have greater analgesic potential in neuropathic conditions, especially if patients have comorbid depression.

In general, antidepressants are more effective than AEDs as adjunctive pain medicines. Without considering their potential side effects, the most potent antidepressant adjuvants in pain management in *descending* order are TCAs, SNRIs, and SSRIs.

Antiepileptic Drugs

Like antidepressants, several AEDs – carbamazepine, clonazepam, gabapentin and pregabalin, phenytoin, and valproate – are effective alone or in combination with opioids for many neuropathic conditions. For example, carbamazepine and oxcarbazepine relieve trigeminal neuralgia so effectively that a positive response confirms the diagnosis. Not all of their analgesic effects are attributable to their anticonvulsant properties, but to their tendency to improve mood. In fact, carbamazepine is structurally similar to TCAs.

Other Adjuvants

Neurologists prescribe other adjuvants to ameliorate comorbid symptoms. If anxiety complicates the picture, benzodiazepines may produce calm, permit sleep, and counteract muscle spasms. By treating those symptoms, they indirectly reduce pain and suffering. On the other hand, benzodiazepines may interact with opioids or other medicines to depress the sensorium or create mental status changes. Similarly, antipsychotic agents alleviate severe anxiety and thus reduce pain and suffering. In addition, antipsychotic agents with dopamine-blocking action contribute a valuable antiemetic effect.

Finally, diverse medicines unexpectedly serve as adjuvants. For example, clonidine, an alpha-2 adrenergic agonist, purportedly reduces pain in various chronic neuropathic conditions. In an apparent paradox, adrenergic alpha-receptor blockers, such as phentolamine, that do not cross the blood–brain barrier also have been beneficial for some patients. Even cardiac antiarrhythmics, such as mexiletine, have reduced pain.

Other Treatments Directed at the Peripheral or Central Pathways

When the skin is affected by postherpetic neuralgia (see later) or other painful conditions, applying patches of a long-acting anesthetic agent such as lidocaine gel (Lidoderm) directly over the lesion interrupts the transmission of pain stimuli. Alternatively, for a region of occipital scalp, chronic chest, or abdominal pain, physicians may perform a *nerve block* by injecting anesthetic agents near a superficial nerve, such as the greater occipital nerve in the patient with occipital neuralgia (see Chapter 9), or one of the cervical, thoracic, and lumbar nerve roots, which are readily accessible as they emerge from the spine.

Long-acting local preparations provide pain relief for days or, with an alcohol, months. However, nerve blocks are impractical for chronically painful limbs because the blocks may cause paresis as well as analgesia. Nor are they useful for facial pain within the first division of the trigeminal nerve (V_1), because analgesia involving the eye leads to corneal ulceration.

Sometimes a sympathetic plexus or ganglion block reduces pain. For patients with pancreatic carcinoma, physicians can deaden the celiac plexus with alcohol injections. Similarly, for patients with the shoulder-hand syndrome, physicians can inactivate the stellate ganglion (the sympathetic ganglion adjacent to the upper cervical vertebrae) with alcohol injections. Nevertheless, their benefit in complex regional pain syndrome (see later) remains controversial.

To interrupt pain transmission in the spinal cord, physicians have introduced several different treatments. Capsaicin cream, applied to a painful area, is absorbed through the skin and drawn up along sensory nerves. When it reaches the spinal cord synapse, capsaicin depletes substance P, the crucial neurotransmitter, and thereby impairs pain transmission (Fig. 14.1). This treatment, which complements systemic medicines, helps alleviate pain from arthritis, diabetic neuropathy, and postherpetic neuralgia. Its usefulness is limited by its own tendency to cause painful local burning and tingling.

Anesthetics administered intrathecally, the basis of spinal anesthesia, completely block transmission of all sensory and motor nerve impulses. Although suitable for surgical procedures, spinal anesthesia is not selective enough for treatment of chronic pain. Preliminary studies suggest that certain intrathecally administered nonopioid voltage-gated calcium channel blockers, such as ziconotide, create anesthesia without producing paresis or incontinence. Another approach to interrupting spinal cord pain transmission, dorsal column stimulation, applies a low-intensity current to the spinal cord (see later).

Stimulation-Induced Analgesia

The idea that stimulation of a neurologic pathway inhibits a complementary one has given rise to stimulation-induced analgesia. The *gate control theory*, which embodies this idea, supposedly found practical application in *transcutaneous electrical nerve stimulation* (*TENS*). TENS devices, which stimulate the skin proximal to the painful area, generate low-intensity impulses that theoretically dampen adjacent pain-transmitting ones. Despite their widespread use, with many pain patients reporting substantial relief without side effects, studies have shown no benefit for their most popular application, chronic low back pain, but some relief for painful diabetic neuropathy.

A similar but invasive technique (*dorsal column*) *spinal cord stimulation*, involves insertion of electrodes into the epidural space overlying the spinal cord. A stimulator, which the patient controls, generates an electric current that presumably interferes with nerve transmission. The device alleviates pain and improves the quality of life for patients with complex regional pain syndrome or chronic low back pain.

Another noninvasive procedure is repetitive transcranial magnetic stimulation (*rTMS*, or *TMS*), which has been used for patients with fibromyalgia, chronic regional pain syndrome, debilitating neuropathic pain and even chronic migraine. Studies describe increased pain threshold and activation of distant pain processing areas of the brain as possible mechanisms of action.

Some studies found that acupuncture provides analgesia in people with mild-to-moderate pain. Placing the needles in dermatomes (see Fig. 16.2) creates more analgesia than placing them in the traditional regions (meridians). When acupuncture includes electrostimulation, the procedure doubles in effectiveness. Because traditional acupuncture induces a rise in brainstem, limbic system, and cerebrospinal fluid (CSF) endorphins and its benefit is naloxone-reversible, acupuncture may work in part through the endogenous opioid system (Box 14.3).

In another CNS stimulation technique, neurosurgeons implant electrodes into the periventricular and periaqueductal gray matter and adjacent brainstem regions. As noted earlier, stimulation of these sites, which releases stored endogenous opioids, may induce profound analgesia. Despite the strong rationale, the procedure remains investigational.

For patients with intractable pain confined to a single limb, neurosurgeons have experimented with severing the lateral spinothalamic tract in the spinal cord contralateral to the pain. This procedure, a *cordotomy*, based on the neuroanatomy of the spinothalamic tract, provides profound and almost immediate analgesia. However, because the improvement lasts for only a few months,

---

BOX 14.3	Analgesics Mediated by the Endogenous Opioid System*

Acupuncture
Opioids
Placebo
Stimulation^
   TENS (transcutaneous electrical nerve stimulation)
   Dorsal column stimulation
   rTMS (repetitive transcranial magnetic stimulation)
   Periaqueductal gray matter stimulation

*Because naloxone partially or entirely reverses these analgesics, the endogenous opioid system presumably mediates their actions. In contrast, naloxone does not reverse analgesia induced by tricyclic antidepressants or hypnosis
^See text regarding efficacy

physicians have abandoned the procedure. Neurologists attributed the brevity of its effect to plasticity of central pain pathways. Bilateral cordotomies for extensive pain were also unacceptable because they were complicated by respiratory drive impairment (Ondine's curse) and urinary incontinence.

Epidural Analgesia

Anesthesiologists administer epidural analgesia, an *epidural*, for vaginal birth, caesarean section, or other pelvic surgical procedures. Epidurals anesthetize lower thoracic, lumbar, and sacral nerve roots, including T10 through L1, which innervate the uterus and cervix, and S2–S4, which, through the pudendal nerves, innervate the vaginal canal and perineum (see Fig. 16.1). They create analgesia throughout the pelvis, but do not cause respiratory depression in the woman or affect the fetus.

The procedure typically consists of the anesthesiologist's introducing a catheter into the lumbar epidural space and injecting a local anesthetic, such as lidocaine, along with an opioid anesthetic, such as morphine. The anesthetics permeate the lumbosacral epidural space, but, to a limited extent, they also diffuse into the underlying subarachnoid space. Depending on the duration of the procedure, required depth of analgesia, and other factors, the anesthesiologist continually administers anesthetics through the catheter. When the anesthetic bathes only the lowermost nerves, as for delivery and other obstetric procedures, patients retain strength in their legs and remain able to walk.

A related procedure, spinal anesthesia, a *spinal*, may supplement an epidural (Fig. 14.3). In this procedure, the anesthesiologist injects anesthetic directly into the lumbar subarachnoid space. This technique, which is similar to a lumbar puncture, provides rapid-onset anesthesia. It also causes paraparesis, which resolves as the medication

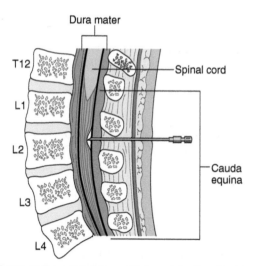

FIGURE 14.3 ■ To administer spinal anesthesia, the physician advances a needle through the subcutaneous tissue into the lumbar subarachnoid space and sometimes then passes an indwelling catheter over or through the needle. The lumbar and sacral nerve roots run through this space, where the medicines bathe them. This injection, at the L2 level, is comfortably below the spinal cord, which terminates at T12–L1.

wears off. However, the anesthetic may diffuse upward in the subarachnoid space to compromise the spinal cord. If the anesthetic rises to the cervical region, it may cause quadriplegia and respiratory arrest.

Placebos, Hypnosis, and Psychologic Therapies

Placebos produce a brief period of analgesia for at least 30% of patients. They suppress severe acute pain, especially when anxiety is comorbid, but have little effect on mild continual pain. Contrary to popular belief, a positive response to placebo does not mean that pain is psychogenic. Because the analgesic effect of placebos is partially naloxone-reversible, placebos probably stimulate the endogenous opioid system.

Hypnosis also reduces pain for a limited period in a wide variety of chronic conditions, including cancer. Because patients' susceptibility to hypnosis does not correlate with their response to placebos, neurologists do not equate hypnosis with treatment by placebo. In another difference from placebos, naloxone does not reverse hypnosis-induced analgesia.

When pharmacologic treatment provides insufficient relief or the pain exceeds the severity or chronicity warranted by the injury, patients may respond to various psychologic therapies, such as relaxation techniques, cognitive-behavioral therapy, operant conditioning, biofeedback, or group therapy. These techniques are also useful in some cases of abnormal behavior, opioid abuse, or when family members reinforce maladaptive activities.

CANCER PAIN

Cancer can cause neuropathic and nociceptive pain that, if improperly treated, may be excruciating and unrelenting. Such pain may originate in a variety of sources, particularly from metastases in bones, which are richly innervated, and nerves. The medical and surgical treatments themselves may also cause pain. Moreover, disease-induced and iatrogenic pain superimposed on the underlying illness routinely engenders depression and anxiety.

Physicians should generally accept patients' accounts of their pain without reservation and monitor their pain as regularly as they check the temperature and pulse (Fig. 14.4). In fact, pain has come to be regarded as the *fifth vital sign*. Patients should have access to nonpharmacologic treatments as well as the full arsenal of medicines. Physicians should prescribe medicines from the three categories – nonopioid, opioid, and adjuvant – early if not preemptively, and then frequently and generously. As opioid tolerance develops, physicians should readily increase the doses. In addition, they should suppress "breakthrough pain" with supplements to regularly scheduled opioids.

NONCANCER PAIN SYNDROMES

Although agonizing pain is generally associated with malignancies, several noncancer syndromes cause comparable

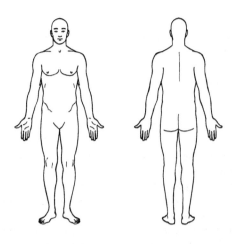

0–10 NUMERIC PAIN INTENSITY SCALE

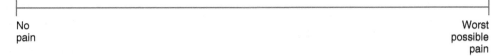

| 0 | 1 | 2 | 3 | 4 | 5 | 6 | 7 | 8 | 9 | 10 |

No
pain

Moderate or
distressing pain

Worst
possible pain

VISUAL ANALOG SCALE

No
pain

Worst
possible
pain

Wong–Baker FACES® Pain Rating Scale

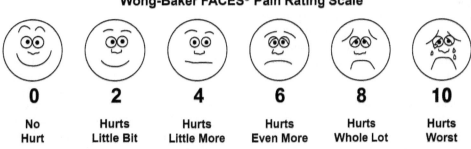

| 0 | 2 | 4 | 6 | 8 | 10 |

No
Hurt

Hurts
Little Bit

Hurts
Little More

Hurts
Even More

Hurts
Whole Lot

Hurts
Worst

FIGURE 14.4 ■ Graphics are replacing verbal reports of the site and severity of pain. Patients describe their pain by circling the most painful area on the sketch. Then they circle the single number on the Numeric Pain Scale or mark the Visual Analog Scale at the point that describes the intensity of their pain. Most children 8 years or older can use the analog scale. For children as young as 3 years, physicians may substitute the Wong–Baker smiling–crying faces icons. Although useful for assessing acute pain intensity, these scales are literally one-dimensional and fail to capture suffering, functional impairment, insomnia, or changes in mood. Moreover, they do not allow the patient to describe symptoms of neuropathic pain, such as allodynia. (Adapted from Agency for Health Care Policy and Research (AHCPR) [now the Agency for Healthcare Research and Quality (US); Rockville, MD]. AHCPR Quick Reference Guides. Rockville (MD): Agency for Health Care Policy and Research (US); 1992–1996. 9, Management of Cancer Pain: Adults: Quick Reference Guide Number 9. 1994 Mar. Available from: http://www.ncbi.nlm.nih.gov/books/NBK52131/; Wong-Baker FACES Foundation (2016). Wong-Baker FACES® Pain Rating Scale. Retrieved 10/14/16 with permission from http://www.WongBakerFACES.org.)

pain, suffering, and disability. In addition, insomnia, drug-seeking behavior, depression, and other psychiatric comorbidities complicate these syndromes.

Neurologists often successfully apply guidelines for management of cancer-related pain to noncancer pain syndromes. Nevertheless, some differences exist. Patients and physicians should acknowledge that while most of these conditions are chronic and incurable, they are not fatal. The goals in these treatment strategies – different from the single-minded one of complete pain relief – should be to reduce suffering, restore ability to work, and allow a return to social roles. The goals should be clear, acceptable to the patient and caregivers, and attainable within several months.

Physicians should strive to control if not alleviate pain. The treatment plan, which usually requires patient and family cooperation, should aim to minimize suffering, medication side effects, and preoccupation with pain and obtaining medications. Medications should maintain patients' mental clarity and function.

This book has already reviewed several common non-cancer pain syndromes, including diabetic neuropathy (see Chapter 5) and trigeminal neuralgia (see Chapter 9). This chapter continues by discussing six others. Their pharmacologic management typically begins with analgesics, which often include chronic opioids. TCAs, SNRIs, gabapentin, and pregabalin are more effective in treatment of neuropathic than nociceptive pain. Patients may still require opioids. Physical and occupational therapy, psychotherapy, hypnosis, behavioral therapies, and social service intervention may further reduce suffering, improve mobility, and increase function.

Postmastectomy Axillary Pain

During a mastectomy, as surgeons explore the axilla and remove lymph nodes, they occasionally damage or sever the cutaneous branch of the first thoracic nerve root, the *intercostobrachial nerve*. Several weeks after the surgery, some women develop searing axillary pain that extends to the inner aspect of the upper arm, well beyond the incision. (In contrast, common incision pain is only mildly to moderately intense, has an itching quality, and is confined to the scar.) Postmastectomy pain, like many painful conditions, worsens at night. Because shoulder movement provokes postmastectomy pain, pain-induced immobility may lead to a "frozen shoulder."

Approximately 50% of women undergoing mastectomy will suffer postoperative pain and 10% will describe it as "moderate to severe." Neurologists attribute postmastectomy pain to intercostobrachial neuralgia, phantom breast pain, pain related to implants, other surgical reconstruction, and other types of neuropathy. Some unfortunate women may develop similar pain if they have a cancer recurrence with metastatic invasion of the brachial plexus. Risk factors for postmastectomy pain include preoperative chronic pain, repeated surgery, outstanding litigation, surgery that involved axillary node dissection, breast-conserving procedures, and insertion of implants.

Opioid or nonopioid analgesics and adjuvants usually help women with routine postmastectomy pain. Local treatments, such as lidocaine gel or nerve blocks, provide topical anesthesia that complements systemic treatment. In addition, physical measures such as massage, shoulder exercises, and vapor-coolants, e.g., ethyl chloride spray, may reduce the pain.

Even though postmastectomy pain carries little prognostic significance, it intensifies the surgery's psychological impact. Moreover, it tempts psychologically oriented physicians and nonphysicians to suggest that postmastectomy pain stems from emotional factors.

Postherpetic Neuralgia

An acute herpes zoster infection, from reactivated varicella virus that has lain dormant in dorsal (sensory) nerve root ganglia, changes one or two adjacent dermatomes into a field of vesicular eruptions, known as *shingles*. The infection causes an unrelenting and moderately severe burning sensation that may precede eruption of the vesicles by several days. This pain typically lasts several weeks. Although the infection may strike any dermatome, it most commonly affects the thoracic dermatomes and the first branch of the trigeminal nerve, which includes the cornea. It causes pain not only during several weeks of the acute infection but then, in many cases, a recurrence involving chronic severe pain, i.e., the pain often has a bimodal course.

Herpes zoster commonly afflicts individuals older than 65, even those in good health, and patients with immunosuppressive illnesses, such as lymphoproliferative disorders and acquired immune deficiency syndrome (AIDS). A vaccine against herpes zoster may prevent, reduce the incidence of, or at least decrease the severity of the infection and all of its painful sequelae. Because one-third of all people may experience a herpes zoster infection during their lifetime, this vaccine has the capacity to produce a public health improvement.

The pain of acute herpes zoster infection usually merits a prescription of an opioid. Antiviral agents, such as acyclovir (Zovirax) and famciclovir (Famvir), may speed healing of vesicles, shorten duration of the pain, and prevent spread of infection to the eye.

For 3 to 6 months after the initial infection has resolved, patients are at risk of developing an even more painful secondary phase, *postherpetic neuralgia*. In an age-related risk pattern, postherpetic neuralgia develops in few individuals younger than 50 years, but in 50% of those older than 60 years and in 75% of those older than 70 years.

The neuralgia has a continual quality of excruciating severity with superimposed lancinating paresthesias. The agony it causes leads to anorexia, insomnia, and mood changes. Although postherpetic neuralgia eventually resolves spontaneously, it may torture patients for years and leave them with a band of anesthetic (numb) scarred skin and, if a major motor nerve is involved, muscle weakness and atrophy. Physicians should prescribe adjuvants, particularly gabapentin and pregabalin, as well as generous doses of long-acting opioids. If the affected area does not include the eye, patients might also benefit from long-acting topical anesthetics, such as lidocaine gel. As a general rule, the earlier the diagnosis and treatment of postherpetic neuralgia, the more likely treatment is to be effective.

Complex Regional Pain Syndrome

Reflex sympathetic dystrophy (RSD), and sympathetically maintained pain (SMP) fall under the rubric of *complex regional pain syndrome* (CRPS). By definition, CRPS type 1 (*causalgia*) stems from no definable nerve injury, but CRPS type 2 has underlying associated nerve damage. Terms suggesting that the sympathetic nervous system is at fault are misleading because studies have demonstrated no consistent abnormalities in it.

The severity, chronicity, and disability of patients' pain are typically much greater than expected for the injury. In addition, the pain often extends far beyond the injury to include the entire limb, although predominantly in its distal portions, and in many cases into adjacent limbs. For example, after several months of left arm pain, a patient may describe similar symptoms in the left leg and then in the right leg.

Patients typically describe the pain as relentless burning or lancinating sensations superimposed on irritating numbness. Sometimes their descriptions of the pain seem extravagant. Neurologists find allodynia and hyperalgesia in CRPS patients more often than in any of the other noncancer pain syndromes. Because even touching or moving an affected limb increases the pain, patients tend to be preoccupied with the affected limb and go to great lengths to guard it. For example, they assiduously shield an afflicted hand by wearing a sling and glove, or they protect a foot by using crutches. The combination of the injury, sensitivity, and protective maneuvers incapacitate the affected limb.

Fingernails remain uncut and grow thick, long, and brittle. Although the skin may sweat excessively (*hyperhidrosis*), it is usually smooth, shiny, scaly, and dry. Similarly, the skin of affected regions usually turns pale, sometimes changing to a dusky color with superimposed livedo reticularis. Severe cases include peripheral edema, bone reabsorption, and muscle wasting (dystrophy), which gave rise to the term RSD. Tremor, dystonia, and other involuntary movement disorders complicate some cases.

CRPS follows minor as well as major injuries of a limb. The injuries may not necessarily have involved overt nerve damage, as with a penetrating wound. Compressive or traction injuries may have preceded its development. Common causes are knife and gunshot wounds, fractures, myocardial infarctions, and peripheral vascular disease.

In addition to prescribing the standard treatments for neuropathic pain, physicians order intensive physical therapy to mobilize the affected limb, including pain-exposure therapy. Other nonpharmacologic therapies include mirror therapy and guided motor imagery.

Pain management specialists also prescribe blockade of regional sympathetic ganglia in selected cases. For example, patients with causalgia of the hand may benefit from blocking the stellate ganglion with an anesthetic agent. Intravenous infusions of bretylium or guanethidine, which block the region's α- and β-adrenergic sympathetic ganglion receptors, occasionally produce dramatic pain relief. Response to such blocks, even though brief, has diagnostic as well as therapeutic value.

In intractable cases, physicians attempt to block the pain pathways in the spinal cord by implanting spinal stimulators, but the procedures are invasive, dangerous, and remain experimental. Similarly, ziconotide, the calcium channel blocker, holds promise as a potential treatment (see earlier).

Phantom Limb Pain

Phantom limb pain occurs in areas that had belonged to a limb before it was amputated. For example, a man with this disorder who lost his left leg at the thigh when it was severed in an automobile accident still felt pain in his left ankle for many months. In addition, nonpainful sensations often accompany painful ones. For example, patients with an amputation will often feel that their limb remains an integral part of their body and sense it making purposeful movements. The phenomena are not restricted to limb injuries but may follow amputation of a breast, ear, or other body part.

Neurologists often classify the pain from phantom limb, brachial plexus avulsion, and thalamic infarction (see later) as *deafferentation pain* because sensory deprivation underlies all of these conditions. Whatever their origin, abnormal sensations or misperceptions reach the level of somatic hallucinations. They resemble the visual hallucinations that stem from blindness (see Chapter 12).

Pain at the site of a surgical incision, stump pain, differs from phantom limb pain because it is confined to the injury and attributable to nerve scars (neuromas). Nevertheless, phantom and stump pain may occur together.

Even in its most typical settings, phantom limb pain varies in quality, severity, and accompanying psychological symptoms. It usually begins soon after a traumatic amputation and has a self-limited duration of several weeks. The pain is even more likely to develop and persist if the affected body part were chronically painful before the amputation (as with osteomyelitis). Because most cases result from war wounds, victims are usually young or middle-aged veterans. Many patients also have sustained other injuries, including facial disfigurement, loss of several limbs, and castration.

In addition to prescribing the usual treatments for noncancer pain syndromes, some physicians have claimed to help patients by using hypnosis which induces the imagery that the phantom limb is shrinking to the point of disappearing. Another nonpharmacologic approach is "mirror therapy," which induces changes in the primary sensorimotor and supplementary motor cortex.

Thalamic Pain

Thalamic infarctions initially cause contralateral hemianesthesia, but no pain. Depending on the location of the damage, hemiparesis, hemiataxia, or a visual field cut may accompany the hemianesthesia. Subsequently, many patients develop spontaneous painful sensations on the hemianesthetic side of the body (*Déjérine–Roussy syndrome*). This condition most often causes face and hand pain. As with complex regional pain syndrome, patients are beset with allodynia and hyperalgesia, and they try to ward off pain by wearing hats, long sleeves, and gloves. Fortunately, this pain usually subsides after 6 to 12 months.

Low Back Pain

As opposed to acute low back pain from a herniated intervertebral disk (see Chapter 5), chronic low back pain seems to stem from ill-defined or nonspecific injury of the lumbar vertebrae, intervertebral disks, or the supporting ligaments. Affecting over 2 million individuals, chronic low back pain is one of the most prevalent disabling conditions in the United States.

As much as in any neurologic condition, nonmedical factors contribute to persistent pain and prolonged disability. In fact, disability bears little relationship to structural abnormalities visible on magnetic resonance imaging (MRI). Work-related injuries, job dissatisfaction, psychological distress, outstanding litigation, and other painful conditions are risk factors for a poor prognosis. Although depression, distress, somatization, and substance abuse also play a major role, their effects are often hidden. Psychological screening tests, including the Minnesota Multiphasic Personality Inventory-2 (MMPI-2), cannot reliably predict which chronic low back pain patients will have a satisfactory surgical outcome.

Most patients with chronic low back pain should be advised to accept it as a chronic condition that medical care might ameliorate but not cure. Physicians might shift their goal from abolishing pain to improving function. For example, goals, which should be kept modest, might include completing a 6-hour workday or walking one mile.

Although the usual treatments for noncancer pain help, severe cases defy treatment. For example, despite even obvious MRI abnormalities, surgery on herniated disks, spinal stenosis, and other orthopedic conditions fails in the majority of cases to eliminate pain and enable patients to return to work. In fact, surgery may even worsen the pain and disability. Also, many popular techniques – acupuncture, back-strengthening exercises, massage, spinal manipulation, and sleeping on a firm mattress – produce mild, short-lived, or no improvement.

Neurologists often refer to patients who remain incapacitated despite surgery and other treatment as having the "failed back surgery syndrome" (FBSS). Studies of these patients have postulated multiple causes of FBSS, such as neural fibrosis and recurrent or retained herniated disks, but show no explanation in a significant proportion of cases.

Finally, both physicians and patients should acknowledge, when relevant, that litigation often promises large amounts of money for *permanent* pain, suffering, and disability. This incentive discourages improvement, effective treatment, a return to work, and even accurate reporting. Some neurologists recommend concluding litigation before expecting successful treatment.

REFERENCES

Abramowicz, M. (Ed.). (2010). Medical marijuana. *The Medical Letter*, *52*, 5–6.

Backonja, M. M., & Krause, S. J. (2003). Neuropathic pain questionnaire – short form. *The Clinical Journal of Pain*, *19*, 315–316.

Benarroch, E. E. (2007). Sodium channels and pain. *Neurology*, *68*, 233–236.

Benarroch, E. E. (2012). Endogenous opioid systems: current concepts and clinical correlations. *Neurology*, *79*, 807–814.

Berman, B. M., Langevin, H. H., Witt, C. M., et al. (2010). Acupuncture for chronic low back pain. *The New England Journal of Medicine*, *363*, 454–461.

Birklein, F., O'Neill, D., & Schlereth, T. (2014). Complex regional pain syndrome: an optimistic perspective. *Neurology*, *84*, 89–96.

Boyer, E. W. (2012). Management of opioid analgesic overdose. *The New England Journal of Medicine*, *367*, 146–155.

Carragee, E. J. (2005). Persistent low back pain. *The New England Journal of Medicine*, *352*, 1891–1898.

Carragee, E. J., Alamin, T. F., Miller, J. L., et al. (2005). Discographic, MRI, and psychosocial determinants of low back pain disability and

remission: A prospective study in subjects with benign persistent back pain. *The Spine Journal*, *5*, 24–35.

Carroll, L. J., Cassidy, J. D., & Cote, P. (2004). Depression as a risk factor for onset of an episode of troublesome neck and low back pain. *Pain*, *107*, 134–139.

Cherkin, D. C., Sherman, K. J., Deyo, R., et al. (2003). A review of the evidence for the effectiveness, safety and cost of acupuncture, massage therapy, and spinal manipulation for low back pain. *Annals of Internal Medicine*, *138*, 898–906.

Chey, W. D., Webster, L., Sostek, M., et al. (2014). Naloxegol for opioid-induced constipation in patients with noncancer pain. *The New England Journal of Medicine*, *370*, 2387–2396.

Diers, M., Christmann, C., Koeppe, C., et al. (2010). Mirrored, imagined and executed movements differentially activate sensorimotor cortex in amputees with and without phantom limb pain. *Pain*, *149*, 296–304.

Dubinsky, R. M., Kabbani, H., El-Chami, Z., et al. (2010). Assessment: Efficacy of transcutaneous electric nerve stimulation in the treatment of pain in neurologic disorders (an evidence-based review). *Neurology*, *74*, 173–176.

Dworkin, R. H., O'Connor, A. B., Audette, J., et al. (2010). Recommendations for the pharmacological management of neuropathic pain: an overview and literature update. *Mayo Clinic Proceedings. Mayo Clinic*, *85*(3 Suppl.), S3–S14.

Foley, K. M. (2003). Opioids and chronic neuropathic pain. *The New England Journal of Medicine*, *348*, 1279–1281.

Franklin, G. M. (2014). Opioids for chronic noncancer pain: a position paper of the American Academy of Neurology. *Neurology*, *83*, 1277–1284.

Galhardoni, R., Correia, G., Araujo, H., et al. (2015). Repetitive transcranial magnetic stimulation in chronic pain: a review of the literature. *Archives of Physical Medicine and Rehabilitation*, *96*, S156–S172.

Hawkins, J. L. (2010). Epidural analgesia for labor and delivery. *The New England Journal of Medicine*, *362*, 1503–1510.

Hayden, J. A., van Tulder, M. W., Malmivaara, A. V., et al. (2005). Meta-analysis: Exercise therapy for nonspecific low back pain. *Annals of Internal Medicine*, *142*, 765–775.

Jamison, R. N., & Mao, J. (2015). Opioid analgesics. *Mayo Clinic Proceedings. Mayo Clinic*, *90*, 957–968.

Jung, B. F., Ahrendt, G. M., Oaklander, S., et al. (2003). Neuropathic pain following breast cancer surgery. *Pain*, *104*, 1–13.

Nasreddine, Z. S., & Saver, J. L. (1997). Pain after thalamic stroke: Right diencephalic predominance and clinical features in 180 patients. *Neurology*, *48*, 1196–1199.

Pincus, T., Burton, A. K., Vogel, S., et al. (2002). A systemic review of psychological factors as predictors of chronicity/disability in prospective cohorts of low back pain. *Spine*, *27*, 109–120.

Rang, S. T., Field, J., & Irving, C. (2008). Serotonin toxicity caused by an interaction between fentanyl and paroxetine. *Canadian Journal of Anaesthesia*, *55*, 521–555.

Rastogi, R., Swarm, R. A., & Patel, T. A. (2011). Case scenario: opioid association with serotonin syndrome: implications to the practitioners. *Anesthesiology*, *115*, 1291–1298.

Rowbotham, M. C., Twilling, L., Davies, P. S., et al. (2003). Oral opioid therapy for chronic peripheral and central neuropathic pain. *The New England Journal of Medicine*, *348*, 1223–1232.

Sampathkumar, P., Drage, L., & Martin, D. (2009). Herpes zoster (shingles) and postherpetic neuralgia. *Mayo Clinic Proceedings. Mayo Clinic*, *84*(3), 274–280.

Slipman, C. W., Shin, C. H., Patel, R. K., et al. (2002). Etiologies of failed back surgery syndrome. *Pain Medicine (Malden, Mass.)*, *3*(3), 200–214.

Webster, L. R., & Webster, R. M. (2005). Predicting aberrant behaviors in opioid-treated patients. *Pain Medicine (Malden, Mass.)*, *6*, 432–442.

Williams, L. S., Jones, W. J., Shen, J., et al. (2004). Outcomes of newly referred neurology outpatients with depression and pain. *Neurology*, *63*, 674–677.

QUESTIONS AND ANSWERS

1–7. Match the substance (1–7) with its effect on the pain pathways (a–e). More than one answer may be correct.

1. Morphine
2. Endogenous opioids
3. Serotonin
4. Substance P
5. Enkephalin
6. β-endorphin
7. Nonsteroidal anti-inflammatory drugs (NSAIDs)
    a. Reduces tissue inflammation
    b. Interferes with prostaglandin synthesis
    c. Provides analgesia by acting within the CNS
    d. Acts as a neurotransmitter of pain in the spinal cord
    e. Is liberated in a spinal cord descending analgesic tract

Answers: 1–c, 2–c, 3–c and e, 4–d, 5–c, 6–c, 7–a and b.

8. Which action of morphine is *not* shared with endogenous opioids?
    a. Causes tolerance
    b. Affects deep brainstem structures and spinal cord
    c. Causes mood changes as well as analgesia
    d. Naloxone reverses effects
    e. Causes pulmonary edema

Answer: e. Excessive morphine, usually from an overdose, causes pulmonary edema, but endogenous opioids do not.

9–17. Match the substance (9–17) with its composition (a–h).

9. Leu-enkephalin
10. ACTH
11. Morphine
12. β-endorphin
13. Heroin
14. β-lipotropin
15. Met-enkephalin
16. Serotonin
17. Substance P
    a. 11-amino-acid polypeptide
    b. 5-amino-acid polypeptide
    c. Diacetyl morphine
    d. Greater than 30,000 amino-acid polypeptide
    e. Indole
    f. Alkaloid of opium
    g. 91-amino-acid polypeptide
    h. 31-amino-acid polypeptide

Answers: 9–b, 10–d, 11–f, 12–h, 13–c and f, 14–g, 15–b, 16–e, 17–a.

18. A young soldier who recently lost his left arm in a firefight still "feels" his entire limb. On at least a conscious level, he is aware of the amputation and its implications. At night he has pain in an area that extends from his fingers to shoulder. Which is the most likely diagnosis?
    a. Stump pain
    b. Complex regional pain syndrome
    c. Phantom limb pain
    d. Post-traumatic stress disorder (PTSD)

Answer: c. All of these conditions may befall wounded soldiers. Many are comorbid. Because this soldier's sensory disturbances have developed in the distribution of his amputated limb, he most likely has phantom limb pain. As part of a multimodal approach, nonpharmacologic interventions, such as mirror therapy and cognitive-behavioral therapy, may reduce phantom limb pain and complement treatment of PTSD.

19. In which spinal cord tract does most pain sensation ascend?
    a. Fasciculus gracilis
    b. Fasciculus cuneatus
    c. Lateral corticospinal tract
    d. Lateral spinothalamic tract

Answer: d.

20. In which tract do serotonin-based analgesic fibers descend within the spinal cord?
    a. Lateral spinothalamic tract
    b. Dorsolateral funiculus
    c. Fasciculus gracilis
    d. Dentatorubral tract

Answer: b.

21. Which *two* forms of analgesia are *not* naloxone-reversible?
    a. Acupuncture
    b. Opioid
    c. Transcutaneous electrical nerve stimulation (TENS)
    d. Aspirin
    e. Hypnosis
    f. Placebo
    g. Stimulation of periventricular gray matter
    h. Intrathecal morphine injections

Answer: d, e.

22. Why would the addition of aspirin or an NSAID increase the effectiveness of opioids?
    a. They are also opioids.
    b. They actually do not increase analgesia.

c. They stimulate endogenous opioid release.
d. They interfere with prostaglandin synthesis.
e. They inhibit serotonin reuptake.

Answer: d.

23. Which of the following statements regarding tricyclic antidepressants (TCAs) is *incorrect*?
   a. TCAs treat comorbid depression.
   b. TCAs help restore restful sleep.
   c. TCAs are more effective than antiepileptics as adjunctive pain medicines.
   d. TCAs are less effective than selective serotonin reuptake inhibitors (SSRIs).

Answer: d. Although TCAs help suppress pain, treat comorbid depression, and restore restful sleep, their adverse effects on the autonomic nervous system often limit their analgesic usefulness. Blocking re-uptake of norepinephrine and increasing serotonin levels are both analgesic, but enhancing norepinephrine activity is much more effective. Although SSRIs have usually been disappointing, SNRIs show promise in certain painful conditions, such as diabetic neuropathy. As a general rule, antidepressants are less effective than antiepileptic drugs (AEDs) as adjunctive pain medicines.

24. Which of the following is *not* a complication of mixed agonist-antagonist opioids, such as pentazocine (Talwin)?
   a. Normeperidine accumulation
   b. Addiction
   c. Delirium
   d. Respiratory depression
   e. Precipitating withdrawal symptoms in patients using meperidine (Demerol)
   f. Skin and subcutaneous scarring (sclerosis)
   g. All of the above

Answer: a.

25. Which of the following is *true* about postmastectomy pain?
   a. Emotional factors surrounding the loss of a breast play a large role in the development of postmastectomy pain.
   b. Very few women will experience postmastectomy pain.
   c. Postmastectomy pain may lead to a "frozen shoulder."
   d. Topical anesthetics such as lidocaine are not useful in the treatment of postmastectomy pain.

Answer: c. Because shoulder movement can exacerbate postmastectomy pain, guarding and immobility may lead to a frozen shoulder. Up to 50% of women may experience postmastectomy pain. Although postmastectomy pain may intensify the psychologic impact of the surgery, there is no evidence that "emotional factors" play a role in its development. Topical anesthetics, along with opioid and nonopioid analgesics, may act as an effective adjuvant therapy.

26. Which of the following is *not* characteristic of complex regional pain syndrome?
   a. The skin often takes on a shiny and scaly appearance.
   b. The pain is often relieved with blockade of the sympathetic ganglia.
   c. The trunk and abdomen are typically involved.
   d. The pain spreads beyond the injured nerve.

Answer: c. Complex regional pain syndrome usually involves a limb, but almost never the face, head, or trunk. The pain rarely spreads beyond an affected limb. Changes in skin temperature, turgor, color, and moisture characterize the disorder. An examination may also detect long, brittle nails. Prolonged observation usually reveals that the patient fails to use an affected limb and usually protects it with a sling, sock, or glove.

27. A 39-year-old headache patient who has had migraine since childhood has been taking an aspirin-butalbital-caffeine compound (Fiorinal) daily for at least 10 years. When the patient attempts to stop the medication, unbearable generalized dull headaches develop. What is the best descriptive term for this phenomenon?
   a. Chronic migraine headache
   b. Medication overuse headache
   c. Status migrainosus
   d. Addiction

Answer: b. Headaches following withdrawal of analgesics, especially if they are combined with vasoconstrictive medications, represent a major problem in headache management. "Medication overuse headache" is a form of withdrawal (see Chapter 9).

28. Which of the following is *not* a complication of infarction of the thalamus and its surrounding structures?
   a. Hemianesthesia
   b. Allodynia
   c. Hyperpathia
   d. Abnormal sweating

Answer: d. The thalamus is the brain's major sensory relay station. Infarctions in this structure prevent the transmission of pain and other sensations to the cerebral cortex, which leads not only to hemianesthesia but deafferentation. Manifestations of deafferentation include the neuropathic pain symptoms: spontaneously occurring pain (painful paresthesias), perception of pain in response to an ordinarily nonpainful stimulation (allodynia), and perception of great pain in response to a mildly painful stimulation (hyperpathia or hyperalgesia).

29. Which of the following statements regarding the periaqueductal gray matter is *incorrect*?
   a. Stimulation of the periaqueductal gray matter produces analgesia.
   b. Thiamine deprivation causes hemorrhage into the periaqueductal gray matter.
   c. The periaqueductal gray matter surrounds the aqueduct of Sylvius.

d. The aqueduct of Sylvius is the conduit for cerebrospinal fluid (CSF) between the lateral and third ventricles.

e. The aqueduct of Sylvius is the conduit for CSF between the third and fourth ventricles.

Answer: d. In experimental procedures in humans as well as animals, deep brain stimulation of the periaqueductal gray matter produces analgesia. The aqueduct of Sylvius is the conduit for CSF between the third and fourth ventricles. The foramina of Monro provides the communication from the lateral ventricles to the third ventricle.

30. Which of the following statements regarding enkephalins is *true*?
    a. They are tricyclic.
    b. They are secondary messengers.
    c. Naloxone inhibits them.
    d. They are part of the serotonin system.

Answer: c. The enkephalins are peptide neurotransmitters that have a powerful inhibitory effect on spinal cord interneurons. Their effects mimic those of morphine because they are part of the endogenous opioid system.

31. Which of the following statements regarding serotonin's role in pain and analgesia is *false*?
    a. Serotonin often reduces pain before affecting mood.
    b. Descending serotonin-based spinal cord tracts induce analgesia.
    c. In its analgesic role, serotonin is an inhibitory neurotransmitter.
    d. Serotonin is an endogenous opioid.

Answer: d.

32. Which factor is *not* associated with misuse of opioid therapy of noncancer pain?
    a. Faith-based spirituality
    b. Age between 16 and 45 years
    c. Personal history of alcohol or drug abuse
    d. Family history of alcohol or drug abuse
    e. Neurotic disorders

Answer: a. A wide range of psychiatric disturbances, as well as young age and a family or personal history of drug or alcohol abuse, are risk factors for misuse of opioid therapy of noncancer pain. Up to 30% of patients receiving chronic opioid therapy for noncancer pain, in some studies, have misused the opioids. Careful selection and monitoring of patients will reduce abuse to approximately 2%.

33. Which *three* statements describe NSAIDs?
    a. When used in excess, they cause gastrointestinal bleeding.
    b. Additional medication produces greater analgesia, i.e., they have no "ceiling."
    c. Patients develop a tolerance to the analgesia.

d. They are as effective as some opioids.
e. They can be combined with opioids to produce additional analgesia.

Answer: a, d, e.

34. For a given dose, which route of administration of an opioid provides the lowest blood concentrations?
    a. Intramuscular
    b. Oral release
    c. Intravenous

Answer: b. About 50% of an orally administered opioid is metabolized on its first pass through the liver. Parenteral and transcutaneous administration is generally more effective than oral administration.

35. Which of the following is *not* an advantage of patient-controlled analgesia (PCA) over analgesia administered on a "by-the-clock" or an "as-needed" basis?
    a. Lower cost
    b. Steadier levels of analgesia that avoid under- and over-treatment
    c. More regular sleep schedules
    d. Earlier hospital discharge

Answer: a. Despite the expense of training, close monitoring, and equipment, PCA is a widely accepted and successful innovation that empowers patients in the management of their postoperative and chronic cancer pain. However, unless patients have the dexterity and cognitive capacity to adjust the system, PCA may be ineffective or dangerous. Also, in patients with pulmonary disease, respiratory depression may complicate PCA as well as conventional administration of opioids.

36. Where do pain-carrying peripheral nerves synapse with the lateral spinothalamic tract?
    a. Dorsal columns
    b. Substantia gelatinosa
    c. Limbic system
    d. Thalamus

Answer: b. These peripheral nerves synapse with the lateral spinothalamic tract in the spinal cord's substantia gelatinosa. That tract then ascends a short distance, crosses, and continues to ascend contralateral to the painful site to synapse in the thalamus.

37. Which *two* of the following painful conditions are considered examples of deafferentation pain?
    a. Brachial plexus avulsion
    b. Insect stings
    c. Trigeminal neuralgia
    d. Carcinoma metastatic to bones
    e. Thalamic infarction
    f. Migraine
    g. Postherpetic neuralgia

Answer: a, e. When an injury deprives the brain of normal continual sensory input, the deafferentation produces a variety of spontaneously occurring neuropathic pain that neurologists call deafferentation pain. When conditions, such as trigeminal neuralgia or postherpetic neuralgia, injure nerves, patients may develop other varieties of neuropathic pain.

38. A passing automobile catches the shirtsleeve of a 40-year-old man. The force drags him by the arm and dislocates his shoulder. Even after the shoulder has apparently healed, the entire arm develops an intense burning sensation that increases on movement or touching. The patient avoids using the arm and often wears a glove. The skin of the hand becomes smooth, dry, and edematous. He cannot cut his fingernails because the pain is too intense. Which *three* of the following statements are *true* concerning this condition?
    a. Studies of the hand would likely show bone reabsorption.
    b. The skin changes are an integral part of the condition.
    c. TENS is usually effective in such cases.
    d. Sympathetic blockage may provide partial temporary relief in such cases.
    e. Shoulder dislocations are painful injuries, but they do not cause nerve damage.

Answer: a, b, d. He has developed complex regional pain syndrome from a traction injury of the brachial plexus. It has caused changes of the skin, nails, and soft tissue and provoked protective maneuvers. Nuclear bone scans and even routine X-rays will probably reveal bone reabsorption.

39. What is the effect of acupuncture on CNS endorphin levels?
    a. It induces an increase in brainstem, limbic system, and CSF endorphin levels.
    b. It induces an overall, nonspecific increase in CNS endorphin levels.
    c. It induces an increase in spinal cord endorphin levels at the meridian of the needle insertion.
    d. It has no effect on CNS endorphin levels.

Answer: a. Acupuncture increases brainstem, limbic system, and CSF endorphin levels. The increased endorphin levels correlate with the analgesia. As would be expected in opioid-based system, naloxone reverses the analgesia.

40. Which of the following descriptions of withdrawal is *incorrect*?
    a. Withdrawal symptoms suggest dependence.
    b. Abruptly discontinuing regular use of caffeine, tobacco, or alcohol causes withdrawal symptoms.
    c. Requiring additional doses of a substance to avoid symptoms is termed withdrawal.
    d. Abruptly discontinuing many medications causes withdrawal symptoms.
    e. The most common symptom of discontinuing opioids is a flulike syndrome and anxiety.

Answer: c. Requiring additional doses of a substance is termed *tolerance*.

41. Match the term (a–d) with the closest description (1–5). More than one answer may be appropriate.
    a. Allodynia
    b. Deafferentation pain
    c. Physical dependence
    d. Hyperpathia
    1. Testing for pain perception with a safety pin evokes reports of severe pain
    2. Spontaneous pain apparently originating from denervated areas
    3. Increasing opioid requirement with disease progression
    4. Flu-like symptoms that follow discontinuing opioids
    5. Nonpainful stimuli, such as touch with a feather, provoke pain

Answer: a–5, b–2, c–4, d–1.

42. Which of the following is *least* likely to occur in patients prescribed opioids for noncancer pain?
    a. Potentially harmful drug-seeking behavior
    b. Need for increasing doses of the narcotic
    c. Physical dependence
    d. Tolerance

Answer: a. Patients prescribed opioids for noncancer pain rarely engage in criminal or other activities potentially harmful to themselves or others. Although patients typically develop tolerance and experience symptoms if the opioid is withdrawn, they rarely meet criteria for addiction.

43. Which of the following is an example of nociceptive pain?
    a. Postherpetic neuralgia
    b. Diabetic neuropathy
    c. Painful HIV-associated neuropathy
    d. Complex regional pain syndrome
    e. Fractured tooth pain

Answer: e. Although quite painful, a fractured tooth causes pain that will subside after it is repaired. Until then, NSAIDs, opioids, and other analgesics will suppress the pain. The other conditions are examples of neuropathic pain that typically persists despite apparent healing of nerve injury. For them, although analgesics, including opioids, and local treatments will help, adjuvants like AEDs and antidepressants are usually necessary.

44. Which of the following is known as the "fifth vital sign"?
    a. Pulse
    b. Blood pressure
    c. Respiration
    d. Temperature
    e. Pain

Answer: e.

45. When under treatment with opioids, to which effect is a patient unlikely to develop tolerance?
    a. Respiratory depression
    b. CNS depression
    c. Analgesia
    d. None of the above

Answer: d. With opioids, tolerance to their side effects parallels tolerance to their analgesic effects.

46. Which receptor subtype mediates most of the analgesic effect of opioids?
    a. α
    b. β
    c. κ
    d. μ

Answer: d. Opioids characteristically bind to the μ (mu) receptor and sometimes also to related receptors, such as the κ.

47. After incessant low back pain ended the successful career of a screen actor at the age of 65 years, he went through a series of surgical procedures on his lumbar spine for herniated disks and degenerative changes. Physical therapy and psychotherapy provided little relief. By prescribing opioids, adjuvant medications, and physical therapy, his pain management physicians controlled his pain and returned him to part-time work making radio commercials. Several months later, his physicians found that he was requiring increasing doses of opioids to maintain his improvement. Suspecting drug abuse, they sent him for a psychiatric consultation. Which of the following conditions is *least* likely to explain his increased demand for opioids?
    a. Addiction
    b. Pseudoaddiction
    c. Onset of depression
    d. Use of another medication that reduces the opioid's effectiveness

Answer: b. Pseudoaddiction refers to a patient's concern to the point of obsession with securing a pain-relieving medication, hoarding it, and other addiction-like behavior. Provided that the patient receives adequate medication at the appropriate dose and time, patients' behavior should be normal. On the other hand, the patient may have developed addiction once he began opioid treatment or even before. Alternatively, he may be self-medicating for depression, anxiety, personality disorder, or other psychiatric disorder. Several medications, particularly phenytoin, may interfere with opioids. Finally, physicians dispensing opioids must guard against their patients engaging in "criminal diversion," i.e., selling their narcotic medications.

48. A Gulf War veteran who had lost both legs and his genitalia was in a methadone maintenance program partly as pain control and partly to prevent his returning to street narcotics. His psychiatrist was prescribing an SSRI as well as providing supportive psychotherapy. One night he was left in the emergency room where physicians found him comatose, almost apneic, and with miotic pupils. He was in pulmonary edema. Which would be the best immediate treatment?
    a. Naloxone
    b. Oxygen
    c. Atropine
    d. Scopolamine

Answer: a. Deliberately or not, he has taken an overdose of his methadone, heroin, or other street narcotic drug. Opioid overdoses classically cause apnea, miosis, and pulmonary edema. Naloxone will counteract the opioid and save his life.

49. Which is the youngest age at which most children may reliably use the Visual Analog Scale to indicate the intensity of their pain?
    a. 3 years
    b. 5 years
    c. 8 years
    d. 12 years

Answer: c.

50. Which is the youngest age at which children may reliably use the Wong–Baker smiling–crying faces icons to indicate the intensity of their pain?
    a. 3 years
    b. 5 years
    c. 8 years
    d. 12 years

Answer: a.

51. In which condition does TENS provide analgesia?
    a. Painful diabetic neuropathy
    b. Chronic low back pain
    c. Complex regional pain syndrome

Answer: a. Although popular and supported by many anecdotes, TENS is helpful in painful diabetic neuropathy but not in chronic low back pain, complex regional pain syndrome, and a variety of other disorders.

52. Which nerve roots innervate the uterus and cervix?
    a. T10–L1
    b. L2–L4
    c. L4–S1
    d. S2–S4

Answer: a.

53. Which nerve roots innervate the perineum?
    a. T10–L1
    b. L2–L4
    c. L4–S1
    d. S2–S4

Answer: d. S2–S4, which form the pudendal nerves, innervate the vaginal birth canal and perineum.

54. An 80-year-old man sustains a cerebral infarction that initially causes loss of almost all sensation on the left face, trunk, and limbs. Several weeks later, the sensory loss recedes but is replaced by continual burning pain in the left face and arm. Also, the slightest stimulation, including people brushing against his hand or physicians examining it, causes intolerable pain. He carefully shields the hand and arm under a glove and covers his arm with a blanket. What is the name of this condition?
    a. Trigeminal neuralgia
    b. Thalamic pain
    c. Temporal arteritis
    d. Postinfarction neoplasm
    e. Psychogenic pain

Answer: b. The initial sensory loss indicates that the underlying lesion was a thalamic infarction. The subsequent condition, the thalamic pain syndrome, is its frequently occurring complication. The extraordinary sensitivity, allodynia is a feature of neuropathic pain.

55. Which of the following is *not* used in the treatment of chronic pain?
    a. Acupuncture
    b. Transcutaneous electrical nerve stimulation (TENS)
    c. Repetitive transcranial magnetic stimulation (rTMS)
    d. Corticospinal tract stimulation

Answer: d. Spinal cord stimulation is used as a treatment of chronic pain, but neurosurgeons insert epidural electrodes to generate interfering current in the dorsal columns, not the corticospinal tracts. All of the other therapies are used in the treatment of chronic pain.

56. A 47-year-old woman with major depressive disorder is admitted to the hospital for profound vaginal bleeding and is found to have multiple large uterine fibroids, requiring emergent total abdominal hysterectomy and bilateral salpingo-oophorectomy. Postoperatively, she is given cefazolin to prevent perioperative infection. Because of relative hemorrhagic shock, she is unable to be immediately extubated. She is started on a fentanyl infusion at 50 mcg/h to provide mild sedation and pain control. Over the next 24 hours, she develops a low-grade fever, agitation, rigidity, vital sign instability, and myoclonus. What is the best intervention at this time?
    a. Increase the fentanyl
    b. Decrease the fentanyl
    c. Initiate bromocriptine and dantrolene therapy
    d. Change the antibiotic

Answer: b. This clinical scenario likely represents a medication–medication interaction. Given the patient's history of major depressive disorder, she is probably taking an SSRI, which has been known to cause serotonin syndrome (see Chapter 6) when co-administered with fentanyl. Decreasing or stopping the fentanyl in favor of another mild sedative agent will likely lead to resolution of the patient's symptoms. While serotonin syndrome resembles neuroleptic malignant syndrome, bromocriptine and dantrolene are not used therapeutically in this condition.

MULTIPLE SCLEROSIS

Multiple sclerosis (MS) is the most common disabling neurologic illness of North American and European young and middle-aged adults. It is also the primary example of a central nervous system (CNS) autoimmune illness.

Neurologists base a diagnosis of MS on repeated neurologic symptoms and signs disseminated in both space and time. The current diagnostic criteria, named for the senior member of an international panel, Dr. W. Ian McDonald, rely on the number of clinical episodes or "attacks" and the number and location of magnetic resonance imaging (MRI) lesions. Neurologists also use certain cerebrospinal fluid (CSF) findings and evoked potentials (see later) to support a diagnosis.

Still maintaining a high sensitivity and specificity, neurologists may now diagnose MS during its first attack. They can institute therapy and attenuate, although not halt, the illness early in its course. Monitoring clinical findings and MRI changes allows neurologists to follow the disease's subclinical as well as clinical progression and judge patients' response to treatment.

ETIOLOGY

MS – usually a chronic recurring illness – typically begins with 1-mm to 3-cm patches of inflammation developing in the oligodendrocyte-generated myelin sheaths of CNS axons. T cell-mediated inflammation strips myelin from (demyelinates) axons and eventually leaves sclerotic (Greek *sklerosis*, hard) *plaques* scattered throughout the CNS. Plaques disseminated throughout the myelin or "white matter" of the cerebrum, cerebellum, spinal cord, ocular motility system, and optic nerves constitute the signature of MS.

When deprived of their myelin insulation, axons transmit nerve impulses slowly or not at all. Some deficits resolve as myelin inflammation spontaneously subsides or anti-inflammatory medications, such as steroids, suppress it. As plaques recur, develop in new areas, and accumulate, MS evolves from an acute inflammatory to a chronic degenerative condition. Sooner or later the plaques leave permanent neurologic deficits.

Although MS acts primarily as a CNS demyelinating disorder, its pathology includes prominent axon degeneration. In contrast to demyelination associated with plaques, axon degeneration regularly produces permanent mental and physical disabilities.

The mean age of onset of MS is 33 years, with 70% of cases developing between 21 and 40 years. Some studies have reported that many patients suffered their first or a subsequent MS attack after a medical insult, such as infection, childbirth, head or spine trauma, intervertebral disk surgery, or electrical injury. Other studies have reported that psychologic stress preceded the first MS or subsequent attacks. However, most carefully controlled prospective studies have shown that these factors do not play a major role in either causing or exacerbating MS.

The specific cause remains unknown, but studies suggest that genetic susceptibility and environmental factors – or, more likely, their interaction – allow MS to develop. Epidemiologic studies that indicate the importance of genetic factors have found that MS occurs in individuals in proportion to their relatives with MS. For example, compared to its incidence in the general population, MS occurs 20 to 40 times more frequently in first-degree relatives of MS patients. It occurs in 5% of dizygotic twins of MS patients, and in 25% of monozygotic twins of MS patients. It also occurs three to four times as frequently in women than men. Although some studies link several different chromosome mutations to the development of MS, none appears to be necessary or sufficient.

Although genetic factors clearly confer susceptibility, they do not constitute the entire explanation. The concordance rates in twins, while striking, are far smaller than if the illness resulted from conventional genetic inheritance. Moreover, affected twins tend to display different symptomatology and follow different disease courses.

Epidemiologic studies have shown the powerful effect of environmental factors. In general, the prevalence of MS increases with the distance from the equator. A compelling group of studies consistently found a relatively high incidence of MS among people born and raised in cool climates. For example, the incidence of MS is higher in residents of Boston than New Orleans, is high in states north of the 37th parallel north in the United States, and is higher in Scandinavian countries compared to Italy and Spain. The reverse pattern naturally applies in the Southern Hemisphere. For example, the incidence is relatively high in Australia's cool, southern regions. Similarly, the incidence is low in the tropical areas of Asia, Latin America, and sub-Saharan Africa.

Other studies have linked a lack of sun exposure in late childhood to risk of subsequently developing MS. Similar studies have correlated MS with lack of ultraviolet exposure. Vitamin D has also entered the spotlight, with studies showing that vitamin D deficiency is a risk factor for MS development and increased disease severity. With its relationship to the northern latitudes, vitamin D deficiency may account for some of the geographical distribution of MS.

Related epidemiologic findings suggest that an individual's "geographic risk" of developing MS is fixed by the age of 15 years. These studies correlate the development of MS with the location where individuals spend their childhood. Studies have found a higher incidence of MS in individuals who spent their childhood in Northern Europe and immigrated to Israel as adults than those who emigrated from Northern Europe to Israel as infants. In other words, those who left Europe during childhood, before they were exposed to an environmental factor – as-yet unknown, but perhaps an infectious agent or relative lack of sunlight or UV radiation – were unlikely to develop MS. Because spouses are not particularly vulnerable, environmental factors that adults encounter are probably not the cause.

CLINICAL MANIFESTATIONS

Course

The initial episode of MS may range from a single trivial impairment lasting several days to a group of debilitating deficits that remain for several weeks and never fully recede. Subsequent episodes vary considerably in their manifestations, severity, and permanence. Relapse rates are highly variable among individuals, but most untreated patients will have a clinical relapse approximately every 1 to 2 years. During exacerbations, the initial symptoms, accompanied by additional ones, generally reappear.

Almost all MS patients follow one of four reasonably distinct courses, *disease categories*, characterized by multiple attacks, steady deterioration, or several attacks followed by steady deterioration (Fig. 15.1, top). The categories reflect the clinical status as it relates to time. They do not take into account the severity or results of MRIs.

Relapsing-remitting MS, the category that initially includes about 80% of cases, consists of discrete attacks followed by partial or complete recovery. Although deficits may accumulate following each attack, patients remain stable between them. Unfortunately, at an annual rate of about 3% per year, most patients in the relapsing-remitting category evolve into *secondary progressive* MS, which consists of further, steady deterioration.

Primary progressive MS, characterized by unremitting, steady deterioration from onset of the illness, accounts for only about 10–15% of cases. Unlike the other disease categories, primary progressive MS typically develops in individuals who are in their fifth or sixth decade, rather than their third or fourth, and predominantly or exclusively affects the spinal cord. *Progressive-relapsing* MS, the least frequently occurring presentation, consists of a steady deterioration with superimposed acute attacks. Although many neurologists consider progressive-relapsing MS to be a distinct category, it likely represents a subset of primary progressive MS.

In addition to being descriptive, MS categories indicate a patient's prognosis and likely response to immuno-modulating treatments. Of the various categories, relapsing-remitting MS is the most amenable to treatment; progressive MS, the least (see later).

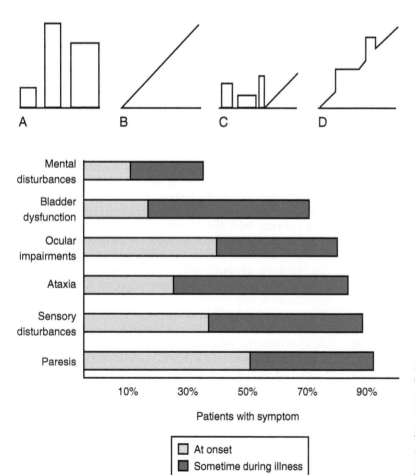

FIGURE 15.1 ■ *Top*, Graphs of different clinical courses – with severity of MS attacks (vertical axis) plotted against time (horizontal axis) – reveals four patterns or disease categories: *A*, Relapsing-remitting; *B*, primary progressive, *C*, secondary progressive; *D*, progressive-relapsing. *Bottom*, This chart of initial and cumulative manifestations of MS indicates that mental disturbances develop infrequently at the onset and ultimately less often than physical impairments.

Frequent Symptoms

Lesions in the white matter tracts of the CNS cause various symptoms during the course of a patient's illness (see Fig. 15.1, bottom). Moreover, simultaneous involvement of two separate CNS areas often produces combinations of disparate symptoms. For example, plaques may simultaneously develop in the cerebellum and thoracic spinal cord, which would cause ataxia and paraparesis.

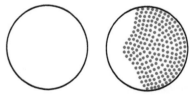

FIGURE 15.2 ■ Optic or retrobulbar neuritis impairs vision in a large, irregular area (*scotoma*) of the affected eye.

Cerebellar Signs

As some of their earliest manifestations, MS patients often develop ataxia, intention tremor, and other signs of cerebellar and cerebellar outflow tract injury. When the cerebellum is involved, patients typically develop an ataxic gait (see Fig. 2.13); however, with minimal cerebellar involvement, the gait impairment may consist only of difficulty walking in a heel-to-toe (*tandem gait*) pattern. Cerebellar involvement also may cause *scanning speech*, analogous to "ataxia of speech," characterized by irregular cadence and uneven emphasis on words. For example, when asked to repeat a pair of short syllables, such as "ba…ga…ba…ga…," a patient might place unequal stress on different syllables, blur them together, or pause excessively. Other manifestations of cerebellar involvement include intention tremor (see Fig. 2.11), dysdiadochokinesia, and an irregular, conspicuous, head tremor (*titubation*).

Sensory Disturbances

Both lack of sensation and abnormal sensations occur frequently and prominently. Patients often describe hypesthesia, paresthesias, or dysesthesias in their limbs or trunk, or below a particular spinal cord level. They typically lose ability to appreciate vibration and position sensation more than other modalities. At their onset, sensory symptoms may not conform to expected neurologic patterns or be unaccompanied by objective findings. Physicians may understandably mistake this situation as a psychogenic disturbance.

Ocular Impairments

Impaired visual acuity and disordered ocular motility occur frequently not only at the onset of MS but also throughout its course. In fact, the absence of eye signs in patients believed to have MS often prompts neurologists to reconsider the diagnosis (see later).

Decreased Visual Acuity

The optic nerve is involved in MS because its covering consists entirely of CNS myelin (i.e., myelin produced by oligodendrocytes, as opposed to peripheral nervous system myelin, which comes from Schwann cells). The acoustic nerve (cranial nerve VIII) is only partially covered by CNS myelin and is rarely if ever involved in MS. No other cranial nerves are covered by CNS myelin.

Neurologists usually attribute visual acuity impairment in MS to inflammation in the optic nerve, known as *optic neuritis*. When inflammation is restricted to the portion of the nerve behind the optic disk, neurologists apply the more specific term, *retrobulbar neuritis* (see Fig. 12.5). Optic neuritis typically causes an irregular area of visual loss in one eye, a *scotoma*, which classically includes the center of vision (Fig. 15.2). Optic neuritis also leads to *color desaturation*, in which colors, especially red, lose their intensity.

In addition to reducing vision, optic neuritis characteristically causes pain in the affected eye. Probably because ocular movement puts traction on an inflamed optic nerve, eye pain increases when patients look from side to side.

Optic neuritis, as well as other lesions of the optic nerve, causes a readily identifiable, surprising pupillary light reaction (see Fig. 4.2). In the "swinging flashing test," shining a flashlight first into the normal eye and then into the eye with optic neuritis will lead to dilation, rather than continued constriction, of both pupils. This dilation results from less light entering the defective optic nerve compared to when the light was shone into the normal eye. Because the abnormality lies in the afferent limb of the light reflex pathway, neurologists call this response a "relative afferent pupillary defect" or "Marcus Gunn pupil," and recognize it as a sign of optic nerve pathology.

Unless the optic disk is swollen, routine ophthalmoscopic examination usually reveals no abnormality. This discrepancy between visual loss and the normal appearance of the disk has given rise to the saying, "The patient sees nothing and the physician sees nothing." As an optic neuritis attack subsides, most vision returns and pain subsides. However, with repeated attacks, progressive visual loss ensues and the disk becomes pale and atrophic.

Statistics vary on the relationship of optic neuritis to MS. They indicate that approximately 25% of MS patients present with optic neuritis as their initial symptom and 50% of MS patients suffer an optic neuritis attack during their illness. A single attack of optic neuritis with no other neurologic symptoms and an MRI showing no lesions means that the individual has only about a 25% likelihood of developing MS in the following 10 years; however, when one or more MRI lesions accompany optic neuritis, the individual's likelihood increases to about 70% during the same period. Therefore neurologists closely monitor any patient with a single attack or *clinically isolated syndrome*. Depending on the presentation and evaluation, neurologists consider initiating "disease-modifying therapy" in hopes of reducing the probability of another attack.

Ocular Motility Abnormalities

MS also causes ocular motility abnormalities, including *nystagmus* and the characteristic *internuclear ophthalmoplegia* (*INO*), which is also known as the *medial longitudinal fasciculus (MLF) syndrome*. Either brainstem or cerebellar involvement can cause nystagmus. Although it is clinically indistinguishable from nystagmus induced by other conditions (see Chapter 12), MS-induced nystagmus classically occurs in combination with dysarthria and tremor (Charcot's triad).

In MS-induced INO, MLF demyelination interrupts nerve impulse transmission from the pontine conjugate gaze centers to the oculomotor nuclei (Figs. 12.11, 15.3, and 15.4). The primary symptom of INO is diplopia on lateral gaze because of paresis of the adducting eye. INO is strong evidence of MS; however, systemic lupus erythematosus (SLE [see later]) and small basilar artery strokes may also cause it. In addition, Wernicke–Korsakoff syndrome, myasthenia gravis, and botulism can produce patterns of ocular muscle weakness that mimic INO. From a physiologic viewpoint, INO is analogous to a disconnection syndrome, such as conduction aphasia, in which communicating links are severed but each neurologic center remains intact (see Chapter 8).

Spinal Cord Symptoms and Signs

Patients with spinal cord involvement, typically the primary and sometimes the only source of disability in primary progressive MS, have paraparesis with hyperactive DTRs and Babinski signs. They usually have three troublesome, common symptoms (the 3 "*Is*") – incontinence, impotence, and impairment of gait. Another frequent, often incapacitating feature of spinal cord involvement consists of spasticity of the legs. Even in the absence of paraparesis, spasticity impairs patients' gait and causes painful leg spasms. Patients with cervical spinal cord involvement often describe electrical

sensations elicited by neck flexion that radiate from the neck down the spine (*Lhermitte's sign*).

Spinal cord involvement also typically leads to *urinary incontinence* from a combination of spasticity, paresis, and incoordination (*dyssynergia*) of the bladder sphincter muscles (Fig. 15.5). MS patients initially often have incontinence during sleep and sexual intercourse. As the disease progresses, patients develop intermittent urinary retention and then complete loss of control. They often require intermittent or continuous catheterization, which leads to frequent, chronic, or recurrent urinary tract infections.

Erectile dysfunction, decreased libido, and other forms of sexual impairment plague the majority of MS patients (see Chapter 16). About 40% of women with MS do not engage in sexual intercourse. Even before developing erectile dysfunction, men often experience premature or retrograde ejaculation. Sexual dysfunction, with or without urinary incontinence, is attributable to MS involving the spinal cord. With spinal cord damage severe enough to cause paraplegia, men have abnormal sperm production, but women can conceive and bear children.

Fatigue and Other Important Symptoms

An inexplicable, constant sense of fatigue, which neurologists sometimes call "lassitude" (weariness of body or

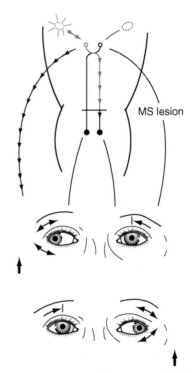

INTERNUCLEAR
OPHTHALMOPLEGIA

MS lesion

FIGURE 15.4 ■ In *internuclear ophthalmoplegia* (*INO*), also known as the *MLF syndrome*, an interruption of the MLF prevents impulses from reaching the oculomotor (third) nuclei. Because those nuclei themselves remain intact, the pupils and eyelids are normal in both eyes. However, when looking to the right, because the left oculomotor nucleus is not stimulated, the left eye fails to adduct. The right eye abducts, but nystagmus develops. With bilateral INO, which is characteristic of MS, neither eye adducts and abducting eyes have nystagmus.

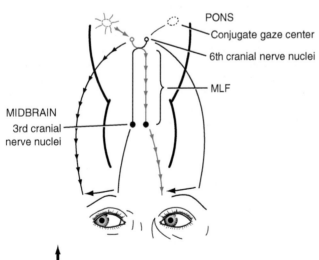

MEDIAL LONGITUDINAL
FASCICULUS (MLF)

PONS
Conjugate gaze center
6th cranial nerve nuclei
MLF

MIDBRAIN
3rd cranial
nerve nuclei

FIGURE 15.3 ■ Under normal conditions, when looking laterally, the pontine conjugate gaze center stimulates the adjacent abducens (sixth) nerve nucleus and, through the *medial longitudinal fasciculus* (*MLF*), the contralateral oculomotor (third) nerve nucleus. For example, when looking to the right, as in this illustration, the right pontine gaze center stimulates the right abducens and the left oculomotor nuclei (also see Fig. 12.11).

BLADDER

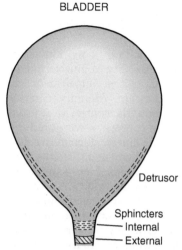

Detrusor

Sphincters
— Internal
— External

FIGURE 15.5 ■ The urinary outflow of the bladder has two sphincters: an internal sphincter controlled by the autonomic nervous system (ANS), and an external one under voluntary control. Normal urinary bladder emptying (urination) occurs when the detrusor (wall) muscle contracts and *both* sphincter muscles relax. Purposefully urinating requires voluntary action (to relax the external sphincter) and reflex parasympathetic (ANS) activity (to contract the detrusor and relax the internal sphincter). Urinary retention occurs with either anticholinergic medication or excessive sympathetic activity because both inhibit detrusor contraction and internal sphincter muscle relaxation. Urinary retention also occurs with spinal cord injury because the external sphincter is unable to relax because it is spastic and paretic (dyssynergic).

mind), affects up to 80% of MS patients. This symptom, which is entirely subjective, does not correlate with patients' age or degree of paresis. It reduces MS patients' quality of life, ability to work, and compliance with medical regimens. In addition, it intensifies other MS symptoms, including depression and cognitive impairment. MS-induced fatigue represents a physiologic cause of the chronic fatigue syndrome (see Chapter 6). Although many studies found that depression is comorbid with MS-induced fatigue, antidepressants do not alleviate it.

Various pain syndromes also commonly occur in MS. For example, approximately 2% of MS patients suffer from trigeminal neuralgia (see Chapter 9) and 10% exhibit Lhermitte's sign. Many MS patients have pain in their limbs or trunk. These pains probably arise from MS plaques that irritate pain-transmitting fibers in, respectively, the brainstem and cervical spinal cord. As with other forms of neuropathic pain (see Chapter 14), antiepileptic drugs, particularly gabapentin and carbamazepine, provide some relief.

Because MS attacks, in general, spare CNS structures that contain little or no myelin, symptoms that originate in gray matter injury rarely complicate the early stages of illness. For example, MS patients seldom develop signs of focal cerebral cortical dysfunction, such as seizures or aphasia, as an initial symptom. Similarly, because the basal ganglia, like the cerebral cortex, are devoid of myelin, MS patients almost never develop parkinsonism or related movement disorders (see Chapter 18). Using newly introduced imaging techniques, however, neurologists are able to see gray matter injury in chronic MS patients. Gray

matter involvement helps explain the global cerebral atrophy and progression of cognitive symptoms that cannot be attributed solely to white matter involvement.

Pregnancy

Women with MS remain fertile. Oral contraceptives do not influence MS. If women conceive, they do not have an increased rate of miscarriages, obstetric complications, or fetal malformations. Throughout pregnancy, the rates of both first MS attacks and MS exacerbations significantly fall. In fact, during the third trimester, the exacerbation rate falls to 70% of its baseline. If MS exacerbations occur, they do not affect the pregnancy. After delivery, women who breastfeed extend the protection associated with pregnancy.

As for delivery, MS patients require cesarean sections for only the usual indications. Epidural anesthesia also has no effect on the course of MS.

Although the pregnancy and delivery pose little or no threat, during the first 3 postpartum months, 20% to 30% of mothers with MS have an exacerbation. Postpartum exacerbations are more incapacitating than those that strike before conception. In the long run, neither pregnancy nor parity worsens the course of MS.

PSYCHIATRIC COMORBIDITY IN MS

Depression

Depression is the most common psychiatric comorbidity of MS. The *Diagnostic and Statistical Manual of Mental Disorders, 5th Edition* (DSM-5) includes it in the category of Depressive Disorder due to another medical condition. Depression develops more frequently in patients with MS than in patients with most other chronic, equally debilitating nonneurologic illnesses, such as rheumatoid arthritis. Depressive symptoms arise frequently at the onset of the illness, during exacerbations, and late in its course. They also correlate with cognitive and physical impairment, loss of bodily function, inability to work, and lack of family and social support. A history of depression and "trait anxiety" predisposes MS patients to depression. Depressive symptoms occur more when MS involves the cerebrum rather than only the spinal cord, and when MRIs show cerebral atrophy and a great total MS lesion area or volume (*lesion load* or *burden*).

Unlike depressive illness that occurs in families without MS, genetic influence in MS-induced depression is negligible. For example, the rate of depression in first-degree relatives of depressed MS patients is considerably lower than the rate of depression in first-degree relatives of depressed individuals who do not have MS. Also, MS-induced depression equally affects men and women.

Even when depressive symptoms do not reach the severity and duration of a major depression, which occurs in 25% to 50% of MS patients during their lifetime, they interfere with MS patients' adherence with their arduous regimen of self-injecting medicines, self-catheterization, and participating in rigorous physical therapy programs.

Largely reflecting the high incidence of depression, the suicide rate of patients in MS clinics is up to seven times greater than that of comparably aged individuals. Compared to all MS patients, those who have attempted or completed suicide have been younger than 30 years and symptomatic for less than 1 year. In addition, their history includes depression in themselves or their family, alcohol abuse, and limited psychosocial support. However, MS-induced cognitive impairment is not a risk factor for suicide.

Well-controlled studies failed to prove that antidepressants improve MS patients' mood. Moreover, antidepressants with anticholinergic side effects may precipitate urinary retention and SSRIs may increase spasticity. Nevertheless, neurologists prescribe antidepressants for patients with MS in the same regimen as for patients with other neurologic illnesses. Electroconvulsive therapy (ECT) may be effective and can be administered with only the usual precautions. In other words, MS cerebral lesions are not a contraindication to ECT. Whichever treatment physicians and their patients choose, adding psychotherapy, social services, occupational counseling, or physical therapy would benefit them.

Although bipolar disorder occurs at twice the rate in MS patients than in the general population, mania rarely develops. If it occurs, consultants must consider the possibility of a side effect from treatment with steroids.

Consultants may also encounter "MS-induced euphoria" – an elevation of mood clearly inappropriate to these patients' disability. This euphoria is associated with physical deterioration, chronicity of the illness, and at least subtle intellectual impairment, as well as steroid treatment. Some euphoric patients are masking depression or protecting themselves with denial. Others simply sense relief as an MS attack subsides. Whether or not psychologic factors seem to explain the euphoria, extensive cerebral involvement usually underlies it. In particular, pseudobulbar palsy may explain pathological laughter (see Chapter 4).

Psychosis

The prevalence of psychosis, unlike the prevalence of depression, is not significantly greater in MS patients than unaffected individuals. In fact, the prevalence of psychosis in MS is less than in most other neurologic illnesses, including Alzheimer disease, Parkinson disease, head trauma, and epilepsy. Except for cases in scattered reports, MS does not present with psychosis.

Nevertheless, severely disordered thinking occurs in MS patients. On a practical level, psychiatrists should begin by assuming that it reflects adverse effects of medications or concomitant physical illness, such as a urinary tract infection, i.e., delirium superimposed on cognitive impairment.

Cognitive Impairment

Almost all MS patients in the initial phase of their illness have normal cognitive capacity. They satisfactorily complete their day-to-day functions, routine mental status evaluation, and Mini-Mental State Examination (MMSE) (see Fig. 7.1). However, more demanding measures, such as the Wechsler Adult Intelligence Scale (WAIS),

Selective Reminding Test, and Halstead Category Test, reveal at least clinically silent deficits in 45% to 65% of MS patients.

With greater duration of the illness and, to a lesser extent, physical disability, cognitive function unequivocally declines. Cognitive impairment correlates with fatigue and depression. Memory deterioration occurs first and, throughout the course, most prominently. Language function, in contrast, is comparatively spared. Late in the course of the illness, all cognitive domains deteriorate to the point of dementia. Patients would then fulfill DSM-5 criteria for Major Neurocognitive Disorder due to another medical condition.

MS-induced cognitive impairment can hamper activities of daily living, prevent full compliance with medical regimens, and burden care-givers (see later). Moreover, it can precipitate thought and mood disorders.

Cognitive impairment in MS differs from that in Alzheimer disease in several respects. MS produces a subcortical dementia and any cortical symptoms from gray matter injury (see earlier) come late in disease, if at all. Also, cognitive impairment typically appears late in the course of MS and long after physical disability has developed, but in Alzheimer disease, cognitive impairment long precedes the onset of physical disability. Also by way of contrast, in vascular dementia, intellectual and physical deficits appear and worsen together.

Physicians attempting to reduce cognitive deficits in MS might institute cognitive rehabilitation, enhanced structure, occupational therapy, and psychotherapy. Immunomodulators possibly delay the onset or slow the progression of cognitive as well as physical disabilities (see later), but donepezil (Aricept) does not help.

Pediatric MS

Approximately 4% of cases develop in children and adolescents. Pediatric MS patients present with the same neurologic symptoms and signs and are subject to similar neuropsychiatric comorbidities as their adult counterparts. However, their course is almost always relapsing-remitting at its onset and evolves into a secondary progressive pattern only after decades.

Cognitive impairments, which typically interfere with their schoolwork, develop in 30% of pediatric MS patients. Only about 6% of pediatric MS patients develop major depression, but up to 75% develop fatigue. Despite widespread cerebral disease, they are not prone to develop attention deficit hyperactivity disorder, autism symptoms, or specific learning disabilities. While the disease pathology is likely the same in children and adults, pediatric MS patients are less equipped to compensate for attacks because their brains have not had the opportunity to complete full developmental myelination prior to onset of disease.

Caregiver Stress

Distress and reduced quality of life can overwhelm caregivers of MS patients. Characteristics of both the patients and their caregivers determine the stress' nature and severity. Patient characteristics associated with high stress levels include not only their physical disabilities, but also their overall poor quality of life, presence of depression and anxiety, and degree of cognitive impairment. Caregiver characteristics associated with high stress levels include a change in their life role and the onset or exacerbation of a preexisting, subclinical depression. To reduce the stress, the patient and caregiver require assistance from family, friends, and perhaps a support group; social and financial services; and current, valid information about all aspects of the illness.

LABORATORY TESTS

When patients' clinical evaluation is equivocal, several tests are required to diagnose MS and exclude other illnesses. None is diagnostic and all yield false-negative and false-positive results.

Imaging Studies

Computed tomography (CT) can show atrophy, reveal large areas of demyelination, and exclude large mass lesions that can masquerade as MS. However, it is too insensitive and too nonspecific to be useful in diagnosing MS.

MRI – certainly the most valuable test – can readily reveal demyelinated areas indicative of MS plaques. The revised McDonald criteria call for combinations of one gadolinium-enhanced lesion or nine T2-weighted hyperintense MRI lesions located in various regions of the brain, particularly in the periventricular area (Figs. 15.6 and 20.25), or spinal cord (Fig. 15.7). Although not pathognomonic, these hyperintensities are detectable in more than 90% of MS patients.

MRI readily detects lesions in large, heavily myelinated tracts of the CNS, such as the corpus callosum, periventricular area, MLF and other brainstem tracts, cerebellum, optic nerves, and spinal cord. It can show asymptomatic as well as symptomatic lesions.

Because gadolinium enhances MS lesions during the first month after they arise, gadolinium-enhanced MRI can distinguish between new and old lesions. Neurologists accept the appearance of new MRI lesions, even in the absence of acute symptoms, as a marker of active disease.

In addition to showing lesions, the MRI may reveal atrophy of the corpus callosum and cerebrum. Communicating hydrocephalus or hydrocephalus ex vacuo, which occurs commonly, reflects cerebral atrophy and compensatory enlarged ventricles. The cerebral and corpus callosum atrophy correlates with chronicity and cognitive impairment; however, overall lesion load and, more so, periventricular white matter demyelination correlate more closely with cognitive impairment.

Despite its reliability, MRI may be misleading. Small T2-weighted hyperintensities, "unidentified bright objects" (UBOs), appear in numerous conditions besides MS, including migraine, hypertensive cerebrovascular disease, and benign age-related changes. When accompanied by neurologic symptoms, MRI UBOs may lead to a misdiagnosis. As another pitfall, the MRI reveals demyelination – although usually not multiple, large, periventricular plaques – in neurologic diseases other than MS, such as the leukodystrophies (see later).

Cerebrospinal Fluid

Routine CSF analysis during an MS attack will usually contain protein concentrations that are either normal (40 mg/100 ml or less) or only slightly elevated, and a mild, nonspecific gamma globulin elevation (9% or greater), but no increase in white blood cells (WBCs).

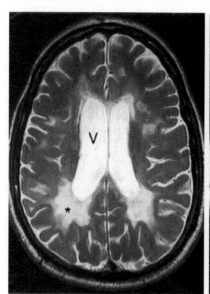 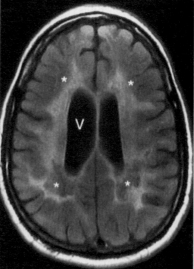 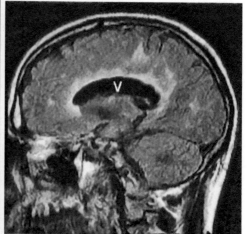

FIGURE 15.6 ■ *Left*, This axial T2-weighted MRI through the cerebrum of an MS patient shows multiple plaques (*) concentrated around the ventricles (V), particularly in the posterior regions. The MS plaques are characteristically white (hyperintense), sharply demarcated, and located in the periventricular region. *Center*, This axial T2-weighted, fluid-attenuated inversion recovery (FLAIR) image of the same study also shows hyperintense lesions (*) surrounding the ventricles (V). FLAIR images, in which CSF remains black, highlight demyelinated areas. *Right*, The sagittal T2 FLAIR image of the same study shows the periventricular hyperintensities surrounding the lateral ventricle (V).

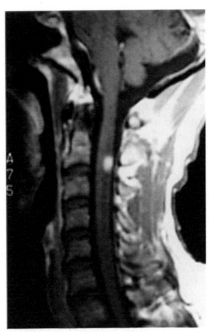

FIGURE 15.7 ■ This MRI of an MS patient reveals a plaque – the hyperintense lesion – in the high cervical spinal cord.

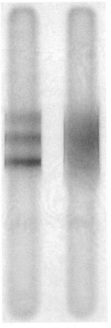

FIGURE 15.8 ■ Electrophoresis of CSF of a patient with MS (left), compared to the CSF of one with no CNS inflammatory disease (right), shows three distinct, horizontal oligoclonal bands.

One suggestive feature is that the CSF of 90% of MS patients contains CSF *oligoclonal bands* that consist of discrete IgG antibodies (see Fig. 15.8). However, oligoclonal bands are also present in other inflammatory diseases involving the CNS, such as lupus, chronic meningitis, sarcoidosis, neurosyphilis, Lyme disease, acquired immune deficiency syndrome (AIDS), and paraneoplastic limbic encephalitis.

Myelin basic protein, another protein not normally present in CSF, is essentially a myelin breakdown product. As with oligoclonal bands, myelin basic protein occurs in many inflammatory CNS diseases. In diagnosing MS, CSF myelin basic protein carries even less weight than CSF oligoclonal bands.

Evoked Responses

Although routine electroencephalograms (EEGs) do not help in the diagnosis, another electrophysiologic test, *evoked response* or *evoked potential testing*, can reveal characteristic interruptions in the visual, auditory, or sensory pathways. Evoked potential testing is based on repetitive stimulation of these pathways, which are heavily myelinated, and then detecting the responses with scalp electrodes similar to those used for EEGs. The responses are so small that they are lost in normal cerebral electrical activity and background "noise." In evoked testing, hundreds of responses are computer-averaged to cancel out unrelated electrical activity, thereby revealing an otherwise undetectable composite wave pattern. MS injury slows and distorts electrophysiologic conduction. Any injury lengthens the interval between the stimulus and composite response, which is reflected in an abnormally increased latency and distortion of the final composite wave pattern.

Evoked response tests are particularly useful in demonstrating lesions that are undetectable on neurologic examination. For example, if a patient has deficits referable only to the spinal cord, but evoked response tests reveal a subclinical optic nerve injury, the physician would know that at least two CNS areas were injured and that the illness was disseminated in space.

Visual evoked responses (*VERs*) reveal visual pathway lesions. The patient stares at a rapidly flashing pattern on a television screen and a computer averages responses detected over the occipital cortex. Optic neuritis increases the latency or distorts the waveform. Because VERs can indicate the site of an interruption in the visual pathway, they are helpful in distinguishing ocular, cortical, and psychogenic blindness (see Chapter 12).

Brainstem auditory evoked responses (*BAERs*) reveal auditory pathway lesions. By measuring responses to a series of clicks in each ear, BAERs may indicate MS brainstem involvement. They are also useful in characterizing hearing impairments, diagnosing acoustic neuromas, and evaluating hearing in people unable to cooperate, such as infants and those with autism.

Somatosensory evoked responses reveal lesions anywhere along the sensory pathways from the limbs to the cerebral cortex. This test involves stimulating the limbs with electrical impulses and detecting the resulting cerebral potentials. MS and other disorders of the spinal cord and even nerve injuries in the limbs interfere with neurophysiologic transmission and produce evoked response abnormalities.

THERAPY

For attacks of MS or optic neuritis, with or without other signs of MS, neurologists generally administer high doses

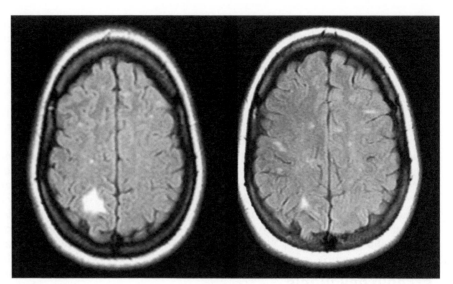

FIGURE 15.9 ■ *Left,* A 38-year-old woman who had MS for 9 years developed left-sided paresthesias and left homonymous hemianopia. Her MRI showed a large region of high signal (hyperintensity) in the white matter of her right parietal-occipital cerebrum. *Right,* After a 6 months' course of steroids for the exacerbation, her deficits remitted and the MRI lesion almost completely resolved, but new, small lesions appeared.

of intravenous steroids, such as methylprednisolone, which shorten attacks and possibly reduce residual disability. Recent data suggest that oral steroids may be no less effective, but intravenous steroids remain the standard at this time. Physicians must cautiously administer steroid treatment because it potentially leads to steroid psychosis (see later) or other serious complications (Fig. 15.9).

Acknowledging that no cure is available, neurologists prescribe "disease-modifying therapies." This strategy, which relies on immunomodulation, attempts to reduce the frequency, severity, and residual disability of relapses. It reduces the lesion load and disease activity as determined by the MRI.

Immunomodulatory treatment, in general, aims to reduce the number of T-cell lymphocytes or impair their ability to penetrate the blood–brain barrier. Some treatments require that patients inject themselves with recombinant human interferon preparations, such as intramuscular beta-interferon-1a (Avonex), subcutaneous beta-interferon-1a (Rebif), beta-interferon-1b (Betaseron), or a preparation of four amino acids similar to myelin basic protein (glatiramer acetate [Copaxone]).

Natalizumab (Tysabri), a unique immunomodulator that neurologists administer intravenously, consists of humanized monoclonal antibodies directed against molecules on the cell surface of leukocytes. It reduces entry of inflammatory cells into the CNS, and thereby reduces their destructive potential. When withdrawn, even if started on alternative therapy, half of patients previously on natalizumab show new MRI activity. Thus, neurologists continue natalizumab as long as possible.

Most recently, several oral immunomodulators have been approved for use in MS. They are an appealing option to patients frustrated with years of injections and those who resist injectable therapy because of needle phobia. Fingolimod (Gilenya), the first oral medicine approved for MS, sequesters lymphocytes within lymph nodes. Teriflunomide (Aubagio) inhibits immune cell proliferation. Dimethyl fumarate (Tecfidera) activates a cellular neuroprotective and anti-inflammatory pathway. Despite these options, most neurologists do not transition an MS patient from an

injectable medication to an oral medication if they have been free of attacks and have no evidence of new activity on surveillance MRI scans.

Immunomodulators are expensive (see Appendix 2). For example, one population-based study that examined their cost-effectiveness showed that each quality-adjusted year cost $800,000.

Immunomodulators are contraindicated in pregnant women. Neoplasms, especially leukemias and lymphomas, on rare occasions complicate long-term immunosuppression in MS patients.

While natalizumab blunts lymphocytes' destructive effects in the CNS, it similarly impairs lymphocytes' protective effects. Probably as a result of natalizumab-induced immunosuppression, 1 person for every 1000 MS patients treated for 1.5 years with natalizumab for MS initially developed progressive multifocal leukoencephalopathy (PML) (see later). Subsequent studies found that the MS patients who developed PML had anti-JC virus* antibodies before their natalizumab treatment, suggesting that they harbored a quiescent infection which the medication reactivated. Neurologists now exclude patients with those antibodies from natalizumab treatment or limit their treatment to less than 2 years, when the risk of PML emergence still appears to be low. Surveillance for PML has become an even more important issue as some of the new oral disease-modifying agents, specifically fingolimod and dimethyl fumarate, have also been associated with PML.

Although ultimately unsubstantiated, initial reports indicated that interferons caused or exacerbated preexisting depression in MS patients. Nevertheless, many neurologists still avoid prescribing interferons to patients with a history of depression. (Alpha-interferon, when used as a treatment for hepatitis, may lead to depression.)

Popular, "natural treatments," such as snake venom, bee extracts, and megadoses of vitamins, have been ineffective when scientifically tested.

---

*Not to be confused with Jakob–Creutzfeldt, in this context *JC* stands for John Cunningham, a patient infected with the virus.

In addition to seeking to modify the underlying disease course, neurologists also treat many individual symptoms of MS. For example, depending on the nature of a patient's bladder dysfunction, either cholinergic medications such as bethanechol (Urecholine) or anticholinergic ones such as oxybutynin (Ditropan) might reduce incontinence; however, patients with advanced disease may require self-catheterization or sphincter bypass. Although paresis cannot be improved, the accompanying spasticity, which may be just as much of an impediment, usually responds to baclofen, diazepam, muscle relaxants, or injections of botulinum toxin (see Chapter 18). Formal exercise programs reduce disability and promote social contacts. Although inhaled cannabis purportedly reduces bladder dysfunction, spasticity, and pain, it impairs stamina and cognition.

STEROID PSYCHOSIS

Steroid treatment of MS – as with steroid treatment of lupus, organ transplant rejection, and acute asthma – can induce anxiety, euphoria, mania, depressive symptoms, and psychosis. Likewise, Cushing's syndrome, other medical conditions that generate excessive steroid production, and even surreptitious use of steroids for bodybuilding can lead to personality and behavioral changes. In addition to inducing mental changes, steroids often produce insomnia, ravenous appetite, and tremor (see Chapter 18), any of which may constitute the first sign of steroid toxicity.

Glucocorticoid steroids such as prednisone and dexamethasone are more apt than mineralocorticoid steroids such as fludrocortisone to induce psychosis. The incidence of steroid psychosis, which usually begins 1 to 4 days after starting treatment, is 4% in patients receiving less than 40 mg of prednisone daily and increases to 20% in patients receiving more than 80 mg daily. When physicians discontinue steroid treatment, its adverse symptoms recede within 6 weeks in 90% of patients. As brain damage from MS or other illness increases patients' vulnerability, high-dose steroid treatment can readily cause mental changes that would fulfill DSM-5 criteria for Delirium, Medication-induced Psychotic Disorder, or Occasionally Medication-induced Depressive Disorder.

Psychosis in a patient with lupus or other systemic inflammatory disease receiving high-dose steroids poses a clinical dilemma. Because these diseases can directly affect the CNS, abruptly decreasing the steroids might intensify the illness' cerebral involvement. In addition, at a time when the body is under stress and consequently requires an increased dose of steroids, suddenly stopping them may precipitate adrenal insufficiency. As a general rule, in patients with a systemic inflammatory disease, physicians should maintain or increase the steroid dose at least until the evaluation is complete. On the other hand, because steroids are not life-saving in MS and chronic use may increase the risk of suicidal behavior, physicians should reduce or discontinue them as soon as possible. In the interim, first- or second-generation antipsychotics may suppress psychosis, but antidepressants may exacerbate it. According to a few reports, if the situation requires continued steroid treatment, prophylactic use of lithium may prevent steroid psychosis.

CONDITIONS THAT MIMIC MS

Physicians may reasonably confuse MS with conversion disorder or other psychiatric illness when patients present with nonspecific symptoms like clumsiness, sexual impairments, vague sensory loss, or fatigue. Perhaps some young paraplegic patients described in the original psychoanalytic literature, who improved during psychoanalysis, may actually have enjoyed the spontaneous resolution of an MS episode.

Common symptoms and signs that should point to a disease other than MS – "red flags" – include the onset of symptoms before the age of 20 years or after the age of 50 years, multiple family members with the same symptoms, lack of eye signs, a single manifestation, systemic symptoms, and normal results on MRI, evoked potential, and CSF testing.

Demyelinating Diseases That May Mimic MS

Guillain–Barré Syndrome

Most neurologic disorders that mimic MS are demyelinating illnesses of the CNS. Even though it is a demyelinating disease of the peripheral nervous system (PNS) rather than of the CNS, Guillain–Barré syndrome may resemble MS because it generally strikes young adults and causes paraparesis or quadriparesis (see Chapter 5). In contrast to MS, Guillain–Barré syndrome is characterized by a single, monophasic attack, lasting several weeks to months, of symmetric, flaccid, areflexic paresis. Additionally, Guillain–Barré syndrome usually progresses over several days, whereas an MS attack usually progresses over hours.

Neuromyelitis Optica

In contrast to individuals with MS, those with *neuromyelitis optica (NMO)* characteristically suffer nearly exclusively from the combination of visual loss in one or both eyes and paraparesis, a combination due to demyelinating lesions in one or both optic nerves and the spinal cord (i.e., unilateral or bilateral optic neuritis and myelitis). Compared to MS attacks, NMO attacks cause greater clinical deficits with more severe demyelination, but they are less likely to cause cognitive impairment or fatigue.

Also in contrast to MS patients, NMO patients' serum contains an NMO antibody that is directed against aquaporin-4 on astrocytes. Their CSF may contain a moderate number of WBCs and their MRIs show a longitudinal plaque of demyelination in the spinal cord, more extensive than typical MS spinal cord plaques (Fig. 15.10), but the brain remains relatively free of demyelination. Also, NMO patients tend to have other comorbid autoimmune illnesses, particularly lupus. Interferon treatment is ineffective or even deleterious in NMO. Neurologists treat acute NMO attacks with steroids, but, if

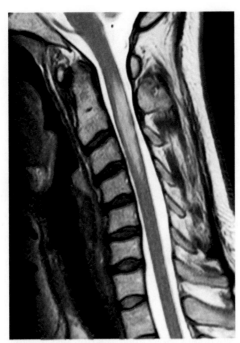

FIGURE 15.10 ■ An MRI of the cervical spinal cord in a patient with NMO shows the longitudinally extensive demyelinating plaque, which appears white. NMO spinal cord lesions, such as this, are characteristically longer than those in MS (see Fig. 15.7).

there is no significant improvement, move quickly to other immunosuppressants or plasmapheresis.

Leukodystrophies

Destruction of CNS myelin, alone or in combination with PNS myelin, is the hallmark of an uncommon group of genetically transmitted illnesses, *leukodystrophies*. As with MS, leukodystrophies cause optic nerve, cerebellum, and spinal cord myelin degeneration that leads to progressively severe visual impairment, ataxia, and spastic paraparesis. In contrast to MS, the leukodystrophies are entirely genetically determined and cause unremitting physical and mental deterioration. Their symptoms usually first appear in infants or children, but occasionally not until the teen or young adult years. In those older victims, the leukodystrophies may present with behavioral problems, emotional changes, and cognitive impairment. Whether the leukodystrophies appear in infants or young adults, they cause dementia within several years.

Two well-known leukodystrophies are *adrenoleukodystrophy* (*ALD*) and *metachromatic leukodystrophy* (*MLD*; see Chapter 5). ALD, which is transmitted in an X-linked pattern, typically first produces neurologic symptoms and adrenal insufficiency in boys between 5 and 15 years old. However, sometimes symptoms emerge only when men carrying the defective gene reach 20 to 30 years. When ALD develops at these later ages, CNS demyelination may cause mania, gait impairment, and eventually dementia. In addition to CNS demyelination, which often has an inflammatory component, MLD causes peripheral neuropathy.

An oxidation enzyme defect in *peroxisomes*, which are intracellular organelles, causes ALD. The defect results

in accumulation of saturated unbranched very long chain fatty acids (VLCFAs) in the brain, adrenal glands, other organs, and serum. Lorenzo's oil, a widely publicized therapy developed by two self-trained biochemists whose son inherited the illness, reduces VLCFA concentrations; however, it fails to alter the course of the disease. Similarly, treatment by adrenal hormone replacement does not arrest the demyelination. Preliminary studies indicate that bone marrow or hematopoietic stem cell transplants before symptoms develop may prevent both brain and adrenal damage.

Infections

Several organisms, which are usually viruses, produce demyelination not by an actual infection of the CNS but by provoking an immunologic response that invades the CNS and attacks its myelin. For example, *postinfectious encephalomyelitis*, which is probably identical to *acute disseminated encephalomyelitis* (*ADEM*), occurs 1 to 4 weeks after an exanthematous or other infectious illness and consists of an extensive and destructive immune attack on cerebral and spinal cord myelin. ADEM affects children more frequently than adults, presumably because of their propensity to contract exanthematous illnesses. Unlike MS, ADEM consists of a single episode, i.e., it is a single, monophasic illness. Neurologists also treat ADEM with intravenous steroids, which produce a full recovery in the majority of patients.

Progressive multifocal leukoencephalopathy (PML), due to infection with the JC virus (a polyomavirus), produces one or more large areas of CNS demyelination (Fig. 15.11) and multiple neurologic deficits. PML is usually a late complication of AIDS and other illnesses characterized by immunologic impairment (see Chapter 7). It also complicates medication-induced immunosuppression for organ transplantation and cancer chemotherapy as well as several newer MS therapies. The presence of JC virus antibodies in CSF detected with polymerase chain reaction (PCR) testing confirms the diagnosis of PML and frequently obviates the need for a brain biopsy.

Several other CNS infections – directly or through antibodies – indirectly attack CNS myelin and mimic MS. In particular, infection with the *human T-lymphotropic virus type 1* (*HTLV-1*) causes a demyelinating *myelitis* that particularly affects the corticospinal tracts in the spinal cord (see Fig. 2.15), i.e., HTLV-1 myelitis. Thus, its clinical manifestations resemble MS involving only the spinal cord. HTLV-1, a retrovirus related to the *human immunodeficiency virus* (*HIV*), is endemic in the Caribbean islands, where MS is uncommon, and some areas of Japan. Sexual intercourse, pregnancy, and contaminated blood transmit HTLV-1, just like HIV; however, fewer than 5% of individuals infected with HTLV-1 develop symptoms. When it occurs, HTLV-1 myelitis typically produces a slowly evolving, painless, MS-like spastic paraparesis. However, HTLV-1 infection rarely causes cognitive impairment or personality change. In infected individuals, antibodies to HTLV-1 are detectable in both serum and CSF, which typically shows an atypical lymphocytic pleocytosis.

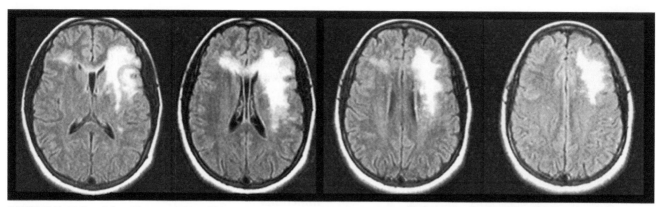

FIGURE 15.11 ■ Surviving 20 years with a kidney transplant and enduring a decade of aggressive immunosuppression, a 40-year-old man insidiously developed right-sided hemiparesis and pseudobulbar speech and affect. His MRI showed an extensive area of hyperintensity in his left frontal lobe that extended through his anterior corpus callosum and involved a small area of his right frontal lobe. However, unlike the MRI in MS, his MRI showed lesions that were patchy and extensive and not periventricular. The MRI appearance in this setting is indicative of PML. He had the right hemiparesis from damage to the corticospinal tract in his left frontal lobe, and pseudobulbar palsy from the bilateral frontal lobe damage. Because the PML spared his cerebral cortex, he did not have aphasia.

Toxins

CNS myelin is particularly vulnerable to numerous toxins. For example, a contaminant of certain homemade Italian red wines probably causes degeneration of the heavily myelinated corpus callosum, the *Marchiafava–Bignami syndrome*. Theoretically at least, Marchiafava–Bignami syndrome can damage the corpus callosum severely enough to produce the split brain syndrome (see Chapter 8).

Chronic toluene exposure, whether from inadequate industrial ventilation or recreational volatile substance use ("huffing"), damages CNS myelin (see Chapter 5). Although appropriate industrial toluene levels should not produce problems, when individuals regularly inhale high concentrations, they develop cognitive disabilities, personality changes, and MS-like physical findings, including ataxia, corticospinal tract signs, nystagmus, and even optic nerve impairment. MRI changes from toluene-induced demyelination, which may be more pronounced than those from MS, correlate with cognitive and physical impairment.

A small group of lawyers and physicians, but not neurologists, had claimed that silicone breast implants caused MS, "multiple sclerosis-like symptoms," chronic fatigue syndrome, cognitive impairment, chronic inflammatory demyelinating polyneuropathy, and other neurologic disorders. However, several major studies concluded that silicone breast implants did not cause any of these problems. Women who reported neurologic disorders after receiving the implants had no consistent pattern of symptoms, virtually no objective signs, and no significant laboratory abnormalities – except in the normal number of women who would be expected to have coincidentally contracted various neurologic illnesses. Also, women with unruptured implants reported the same incidence of postoperative neurologic problems as women with ruptured implants. Women in Sweden and Denmark who received the implants reported essentially the same incidence of neurologic symptoms as those who underwent breast reduction. In other settings, such as its use as cardiac pacemaker coverings, silicone has not been associated with neurologic disease. In many cases, physicians established more plausible alternative diagnoses – most often, depression and anxiety, carpal tunnel syndrome, neuropathies, and MS.

Systemic Lupus Erythematosus

Like MS, lupus and other systemic vascular inflammatory and autoimmune diseases produce various neurologic symptoms that follow a chronic course punctuated by exacerbations. Of all of these diseases, lupus most often causes neurologic, especially neuropsychiatric, symptoms. Moreover, it may cause neuropsychiatric disturbances in the absence of either systemic physical or neurologic manifestations of the disease.

Also like MS, lupus predominantly strikes women more frequently than men (nine times more frequently) and it affects children as well as adults. Lupus affects the CNS as the initial organ of involvement in only about 5% of cases, but it eventually produces neurologic complications in 25% to 75% of all cases. The wide range reflects different age groups and diagnostic criteria in various studies. One explanation of the high prevalence of neurologic complications in some studies had been that the American College of Rheumatology had considered tension and migraine headaches and mild cognitive impairment as "neuropsychiatric syndromes associated with SLE." Another is the complex, seemingly ever-changing serologic criteria for lupus.

When lupus affects the CNS, neurologists usually find that major neuropsychiatric symptoms are cognitive impairment and thought disturbances to the point of dementia and psychosis, respectively. Mood disorders are also common. These symptoms occur with or without other neurologic or systemic manifestations. Physical signs of CNS lupus, particularly seizures and strokes, frequently occur alone or accompany these neuropsychiatric complications. Uncommonly occurring neurologic complications include chorea and INO.

Lupus neurologic complications are associated with various serologic abnormalities: antiphospholipid antibodies, low albumin, and antibodies to double-stranded DNA. CNS complications also induce CSF oligoclonal bands. MRIs may reveal white matter signal abnormalities and cerebral infarctions. However, no laboratory test abnormality is necessary or sufficient to assure clinicians of the diagnosis.

Lupus affects the CNS in up to 85% of children hospitalized with the illness. Of children with CNS lupus, approximately 50% develop depression, inattention, memory impairment, psychosis, or other mental status abnormalities. They are also frequently beset by headache and delirium. Of lupus patients older than 50 years, by contrast, less than 20% have CNS involvement. Moreover, their manifestations are relatively mild and responsive to treatment.

Manifestations of lupus-induced PNS involvement, which occur alone or in conjunction with CNS involvement, include polyneuropathy and mononeuritis multiplex (see Chapter 5). Studies have attributed both the CNS and PNS neurologic complications to autoantibodies, immune complexes, arteritis or vasculitis, and intrathecal production of cytokines. Many complications clearly reflect cardiac valvular disease, a tendency to develop thromboses, opportunistic infections, hypertension, renal failure, or possibly the elaboration of false neurotransmitters. Sometimes, because steroids remain a mainstay of lupus treatment, steroid psychosis rather than the underlying disease explains the eruption of a thought disorder, change in mood, or abnormal behavior. As with mental status changes in MS, those that develop in lupus may fall into the category of delirium, psychotic disorder due to another medical condition, medication-induced psychotic disorder, or medication-induced depressive disorder.

Smallpox Vaccinations

A serious inflammatory demyelinating reaction, *postvaccinal encephalomyelitis* (*PVEM*), has complicated smallpox vaccination in a small proportion of individuals. Affected individuals develop paraparesis and other MS-like symptoms 1 to 2 weeks after receiving their primary vaccination; however, sometimes PVEM only complicates revaccination. Compared to the demyelination in MS, the demyelination in PVEM is more extensive, the course more fulminant, and the mortality rate (10%) much greater. Postimmunization encephalomyelitis, although rare and unpredictable, imposes a tremendous liability risk on the pharmaceutical industry and a burden on public health officials who seek to vaccinate the population against common infectious illnesses, including measles, polio, and rubella.

PVEM and the almost complete worldwide eradication of smallpox have halted routine vaccinations. Nevertheless, physicians still vaccinate individuals at risk of smallpox exposure, such as soldiers and some medical personnel. Although no reliable data exist, neurologists hesitate to allow their MS patients to undergo vaccination against smallpox.

On the other hand, studies support routinely vaccinating MS patients against influenza, hepatitis B, varicella,

BOX 15.1	Frequently Occurring Causes of Painless Paraparesis

Inflammatory CNS diseases
   Multiple sclerosis (MS)
   Neuromyelitis optica (NMO)
Genetic disorders
   Spinal cerebellar ataxias (SCAs)
   Hereditary spastic paraparesis (HSP)
Infectious illnesses
   Human T-lymphotropic virus type 1 (HTLV-1) myelopathy
Compressive lesions*
   Cervical spondylosis
   Spinal meningiomas
   Metastatic tumors
Neurodegenerative illnesses
   Amyotrophic lateral sclerosis (ALS)
Nutritional deficiencies
   Copper deficiency
   Vitamin B_{12} deficiency (combined system disease)

*May be associated with spine pain

and tetanus. While carrying a risk, these vaccinations protect MS patients against infectious illnesses that might seriously debilitate them.

Spinal Cord Disorders

Insidiously developing, painless paraparesis is a relatively common, important clinical problem (see Chapter 2). Numerous categories of neurologic illnesses in addition to MS that primarily or exclusively affect the spinal cord may cause it (Box 15.1)

REFERENCES

Multiple Sclerosis

Amato, M., Goretti, B., Ghezzi, A., et al. (2008). Cognitive and psychosocial features of childhood and juvenile MS. *Neurology, 70,* 1891–1897.

Chanson, J. B., Zephir, H., Collongues, N., et al. (2011). Evaluation of health-related quality of life, fatigue and depression in neuromyelitis optica. *European Journal of Neurology, 18,* 836–841.

Fardet, L., Petersen, I., & Nazareth, I. (2012). Suicidal behavior and severe neuropsychiatric disorders following glucocorticoid therapy in primary care. *The American Journal of Psychiatry, 169,* 491–497.

Feinstein, A. (2004). The neuropsychiatry of multiple sclerosis. *Canadian Journal of Psychiatry. Revue Canadienne de Psychiatrie, 49,* 157–163.

Figved, N., Myhr, K. M., Larsen, J. P., et al. (2007). Caregiver burden in multiple sclerosis: The impact of neuropsychiatric symptoms. *Journal of Neurology, Neurosurgery, and Psychiatry, 78,* 1097–1102.

Fox, R. J., Cree, B. A. C., Seze, J. D., et al. (2014). MS disease activity in RESTORE: a randomized 24-week natalizumab treatment interruption study. *Neurology, 82,* 1491–1498.

Gay, M. C., Vrignaud, P., Garitte, C., et al. (2010). Predictors of depression in multiple sclerosis patients. *Acta Neurologica Scandinavica, 121,* 161–171.

Ghaffar, O., Reis, M., Pennell, N., et al. (2010). APOE e4 and the cognitive genetics of multiple sclerosis. *Neurology, 74,* 1611–1618.

Goodin, D. S., Cohen, B. A., O'Connor, P., et al. (2008). Assessment: The use of natalizumab (Tysabri) for the treatment of multiple sclerosis (an evidence-based review): Report of the Therapeutics and Technology Assessment Subcommittee of the American Academy of Neurology. *Neurology, 71,* 766–773.

Kale, N., Agaoglu, J., & Tanik, O. (2010). Neuropsychiatric manifestations in multiple sclerosis: Correlation of fatigue and depression with disease progression. *Neurological Research, 32*, 221–223.

Koch, M., Glazenborg, A., & Uyttenboogaart, M. (2011). at al. Pharmacologic treatment of depression in multiple sclerosis. *The Cochrane Database of Systematic Reviews*, (2), CD007295.

Koopman, W. J., Benbow, C. L., & Vandervoort, M. (2007). Top 10 needs of people with multiple sclerosis and their significant others. *The Journal of Neuroscience Nursing: Journal of the American Association of Neuroscience Nurses, 38*, 369–373.

Krupp, L. B. (2004). *Fatigue in Multiple Sclerosis: A Guide to Diagnosis and Management*. New York: Demos.

Langer-Gould, A., Huang, S. M., Gupta, R., et al. (2009). Exclusive breastfeeding and the risk of postpartum relapses in women with multiple sclerosis. *Archives of Neurology, 66*, 958–963.

Le Page, E., Veillard, D., Laplaud, D. A., et al. (2015). Oral versus intravenous high-dose methylprednisolone for treatment of relapses in patients with multiple sclerosis (COPOUSEP): a randomized, controlled, double-blind, non-inferiority trial. *Lancet, 386*, 974–981.

Lee, M., & O'Brien, P. (2008). Pregnancy and multiple sclerosis. *Journal of Neurology, Neurosurgery, and Psychiatry, 79*, 1308–1311.

Li, J., Johansen, C., Bronnum-Hansen, H., et al. (2004). The risk of multiple sclerosis in bereaved parents: A nationwide cohort study in Denmark. *Neurology, 62*, 726–729.

Lublin, F. D., Reingold, S. C., Cohen, J. A., et al. (2014). Defining the clinical course of multiple sclerosis: the 2013 revisions. *Neurology, 83*, 278–286.

Major, E. O. (2009). Reemergence of PML in natalizumab-treated patients. *The New England Journal of Medicine, 361*, 1041–1043.

Noye, K., Bajorska, A., Chappel, A., et al. (2011). Cost-effectiveness of disease-modifying therapy for multiple sclerosis. *Neurology, 77*, 355–363.

Palmer, A. M. (2014). New and emerging immune-targeted drugs for the treatment of multiple sclerosis. *British Journal of Clinical Pharmacology, 78*, 33–43.

Patten, S. B., Francis, G., Metz, L. M., et al. (2005). The relationship between depression and interferon beta-1a therapy in patients with multiple sclerosis. *Multiple Sclerosis, 11*, 175–181.

Polman, C. H., Reingold, S. C., Banwell, B., et al. (2011). Diagnostic criteria for multiple sclerosis: 2010 revisions to the McDonald Criteria. *Annals of Neurology, 69*, 292–302.

Renoux, C., Vukusic, S., Mikaeloff, Y., et al. (2007). Natural history of multiple sclerosis with childhood onset. *Neurology, 356*, 2603–2613.

Riise, T., Mohr, D. C., Munger, K. L., et al. (2011). Stress and the risk of multiple sclerosis. *Neurology, 76*, 1866–1871.

Sirois, F. (2003). Steroid psychosis: a review. *General Hospital Psychiatry, 25*, 27–33.

Smith, P. (2007). Symptomatic treatment of multiple sclerosis using cannabinoids: recent advances. *Expert Review of Reurotherapeutics, 7*, 1157–1164.

Solomon, A. J., & Whithan, R. H. (2010). Multiple sclerosis and vitamin D: a review and recommendations. *Current Neurology and Neuroscience Reports, 10*, 389–396.

The Optic Neuritis Study Group. (2008). Multiple sclerosis risk after optic neuritis. *Archives of Neurology, 65*, 727–732.

Therapeutics and Technology Assessment Subcommittee of the American Academy of Neurology. (1999). The relationship of MS to physical trauma and psychologic stress. *Neurology, 52*, 1737–1745.

Van Munster, C. E., Jonkman, L. E., Weinstein, H. C., et al. (2015). Gray matter damage in multiple sclerosis: Impact on clinical symptoms. *Neuroscience, 303*, 446–461.

Zabad, R. K., Patten, S. B., & Metz, L. M. (2005). The association of depression with disease course in multiple sclerosis. *Neurology, 64*, 359–360.

Other Illnesses

Abrahams, B. C., & Kaufman, D. M. (2004). Anticipating smallpox and monkeypox outbreaks: Complications of the smallpox vaccine. *The Neurologist, 10*, 265–274.

Angell, M. (1996). Shattuck Lecture – Evaluating the health risks of breast implants: The interplay of medical science, the law, and public opinion. *The New England Journal of Medicine, 334*, 1513–1518.

Argyriou, A. A., & Makris, N. (2008). Neuromyelitis optica: A distinct demyelinating disease of the central nervous system. *Acta Neurologica Scandinavica, 118*, 209–217.

Ferguson, J. H. (1997). Silicone breast implants and neurologic disorders: Report of the Practice Committee of the American Academy of Neurology. *Neurology, 48*, 1504–1507.

Joseph, F. G., Lammie, G. A., & Scolding, N. J. (2007). CNS lupus. *Neurology, 69*, 644–654.

Muscal, E., & Brey, R. L. (2010). Neurologic manifestations of systemic lupus erythematosus in children and adults. *Neurologic Clinics, 28*, 61–73.

Novak, J. C., Lovett-Racke, A. E., & Tacke, M. K. (2008). Monoclonal antibody therapies and neurologic disorders. *Archives of Neurology, 65*, 1162–1165.

Ramos-Rios, R., Berdullas, J., Arauxo, A., et al. (2009). Schizophrenic psychosis at onset of adrenoleukodystrophy. *CNS Spectrums, 14*, 711–712.

Trebst, C., Jarius, S., Berthele, A., et al. (2014). Update on the diagnosis and treatment of neuromyelitis optica: recommendations of the Neuromyelitis Optica Study Group. *Journal of Neurology, 261*, 1–16.

QUESTIONS AND ANSWERS

1–4. Over 4 days, a 25-year-old salesman became unable to walk because his legs would not support him. He also says that his left eye has become painful and blind. On examination, his left pupil reacts slowly to light and actually dilates when a light is shone first into his right eye and then switched to his left eye. Its visual acuity is 20/200. His legs have moderate weakness, hyperactive deep tendon reflexes (DTRs), and bilateral Babinski signs. He has irregularity on finger–nose testing and clumsiness and breakdown of rapid alternating movements of his hands. Which of the following disorders is the most likely cause of his neurologic deficits?
a. Spinal cord tumor
b. Psychogenic disturbances
c. Multiple sclerosis (MS)
d. Acute disseminated encephalomyelitis (ADEM)
e. HTLV-1 myelitis
f. Neuromyelitis optica (NMO)

Answer: c. Because the patient has lesions in his left optic nerve, cerebellum, and spinal cord, and even though they are not disseminated in time, he probably has developed MS. Alternative explanations include illnesses that cause widespread CNS lesions: other demyelinating conditions, such as ADEM and lupus, metastatic tumors, abscesses, and exposure to toxins. ADEM usually occurs in young patients immediately following a viral illness. Although NMO causes paraparesis and visual impairment with an afferent pupillary defect from optic neuritis (see Chapter 12), it would not be as likely to cause his cerebellar signs (dysmetria and dysdiadochokinesia). Spinal cord tumors would create spastic paraparesis but, of course, not visual or cerebellar impairment. Psychogenic disturbances might lead to many of the findings including feigned Babinski signs; however, patients cannot mimic an afferent pupillary defect. HTLV-1 myelitis typically causes spastic paraparesis but not cerebellar dysfunction or abnormal pupil reactions.

2. His physicians perform laboratory tests. Which one of the following results would be most likely?
a. Oligoclonal bands in the cerebrospinal fluid (CSF)
b. Serum antibodies to aquaporin-4
c. Abundant leukocytes in the CSF
d. Serum antiphospholipid antibodies

Answer: a. Although they may be present in other inflammatory conditions, oligoclonal bands in the CSF are indicative of MS (see Fig. 15.8). The NMO antibody consists of serum antibodies to aquaporin-4 on astrocytes. Numerous conditions provoke abundant leukocytes in the CSF. In this case that finding might have suggested NMO or ADEM. Serum antiphospholipid antibodies and double-stranded DNA antibodies suggest lupus.

3. After a 2-month course of rehabilitation, the patient became ambulatory and had recovered his vision and coordination. He even returned to work and resumed his social life. Nevertheless, 1 year later, he reported persistent erectile dysfunction and urinary incontinence. Where do those symptoms originate?
a. Frontal lobes
b. Cerebellum
c. Brainstem
d. Spinal cord
e. Lumbosacral plexus

Answer: d. Erectile dysfunction and incontinence are referable to lesions interrupting the delicate circuits in the spinal cord. Large bilateral frontal lobe lesions, which would create numerous other signs, are the only other possible cause for such symptoms. Despite the importance of these symptoms, MS patients may not discuss them. In the midst of a first attack or relapse, MS patients' visual loss, paraparesis, sensory loss, and incoordination usually overwhelm less incapacitating symptoms. Subsequently, patients may be reluctant to reveal them.

4. At the 1-year visit, what will the magnetic resonance imaging (MRI) of the brain probably show?
a. Multiple ring-enhancing lesions
b. Areas of demyelination in the periventricular region, cerebellum, and brainstem
c. Wallerian degeneration
d. None of the above

Answer: b. The MRI will probably show demyelination in the periventricular white matter and clinically affected areas. Eventually, the corpus callosum and other white matter regions areas undergo atrophy.

5. Of the various MRI abnormalities in MS, which one correlates most closely with cognitive impairment?
a. Enlarged cerebral ventricles
b. Corpus callosum atrophy
c. Lesions seen with gadolinium enhancement
d. Total lesion area or volume

Answer: d. MS-associated cognitive impairment most closely correlates with total MRI lesion area or volume ("the lesion load"), particularly in the periventricular region.

6. Which *two* of the following substances produce optic neuropathy?
a. Tobacco
b. Oral contraceptives

c. Heroin
d. Methanol
e. Penicillin

Answer: a, d.

7. Which *four* of these illnesses are associated with optic neuritis?
   a. Rubella
   b. Gonorrhea
   c. MS
   d. AIDS
   e. Sarcoidosis
   f. Syphilis
   g. Neuromyelitis optica (NMO)

Answer: c, e, f, g. Although MS is not the only cause of optic neuritis, it has the most common association. For individuals who are otherwise asymptomatic and have no MRI lesions, the risk of developing MS in the next 15 years is about 25%. If the MRI shows three or more cerebral lesions, at the time of an optic neuritis attack, those individuals have almost an 80% risk of developing MS in the next 15 years. By definition, NMO includes optic nerve involvement. Because NMO is an inflammatory condition, the CSF typically contains WBCs. Neurologists often require CSF and serum tests, MRI, and other studies to distinguish all the conditions that potentially cause optic neuritis.

8. Which *three* of the following conditions may lead to internuclear ophthalmoplegia (INO)?
   a. MS
   b. Subdural hematoma
   c. Conversion reaction
   d. Lupus
   e. Brainstem infarctions

Answer: a, d, e. INO, more so than optic neuritis, is indicative but not pathognomonic of MS. Normal conjugate gaze requires an intact medial longitudinal fasciculus (MLF), which is a long, delicate, heavily myelinated brainstem tract. It is vulnerable to infarctions and demyelinating lesions. A damaged MLF causes INO.

9–11. A 60-year-old man has a broad-based gait with excessive lifting of his knees. Although the strength in his legs is normal, his DTRs are absent. Also, he has lost position sense, but not pain or touch sense, in his feet. He has small pupils that are unreactive to light.

9. Which one of the following is the most likely cause of his gait disturbance?
   a. Cerebellar damage
   b. Spinal cord compression
   c. MS
   d. Posterior column dysfunction

Answer: d. The loss of proprioception in his legs causes him to have ataxia and a "steppage gait" (see Fig. 2.20). Neurologists might say that he has "sensory ataxia."

10. Although his pupils are small and unreactive to light, they constrict when he looks at a closely held object. What is the pupillary disturbance called?
    a. Argyll–Robertson pupils
    b. Optic neuritis
    c. Internuclear ophthalmoplegia (INO)
    d. Miosis

Answer: a. He has small pupils with lack of light reaction but preserved accommodation. Neurologists label this pattern *Argyll–Robertson pupils*. His gait impairment and sensory deficit indicate tabes dorsalis. Argyll–Robertson pupils are present in about 90% of cases of tabes dorsalis.

11. Which laboratory finding would be most reliable in confirming a diagnosis of CNS syphilis?
    a. A positive CSF microhemagglutination assay (MHA)
    b. Periventricular white matter changes on an MRI
    c. A positive CSF VDRL
    d. Detecting oligoclonal bands in the CSF

Answer: c. Because serum test results are often false-negative, the most reliable test for confirming CNS syphilis is a positive CSF VDRL. The CSF MHA is unreliable. Periventricular white matter changes on the MRI indicate MS. CSF oligoclonal bands are found in a variety of infectious or inflammatory CNS illnesses, including MS.

12. Paresis of the oculomotor cranial nerve (CN III) shares many clinical features with internuclear ophthalmoplegia (INO). Which of the following distinguishes INO from CN III palsy?
    a. Patients with INO have no ptosis or dilation of the pupil.
    b. In those with INO, the affected eye fails to adduct on attempted lateral gaze.
    c. The adducting eye has nystagmus in INO.
    d. Ptosis, miosis, and anhidrosis characterize CN III palsy.

Answer: a. Ptosis and dilation of the pupil characterize CN III palsy. In both INO and CN III palsy, the affected eye cannot adduct. In INO, the abducting eye has nystagmus. Horner's syndrome consists of ptosis, miosis, and anhidrosis.

13. During which obstetrical period is MS most likely to relapse?
    a. First trimester
    b. Second trimester
    c. Third trimester
    d. First 3 postpartum months

Answer: d. MS usually goes into remission throughout pregnancy, especially during the third trimester. However, the first 3 postpartum months are associated with MS relapses.

14. Which of the following tests should be performed to diagnose neuromyelitis optica (NMO)?
    a. Serum NMO antibody
    b. CSF oligoclonal bands

c. CSF myelin basic protein
d. CSF 14-3-3 protein

Answer: a. Serum NMO antibody determination is the best test for NMO. CSF oligoclonal bands and myelin basic protein, although supportive of a diagnosis of MS in the appropriate clinical setting, are nonspecific findings. MRI is helpful in diagnosing NMO when it shows lesions only in the optic nerves and in a longitudinal region of the spinal cord. Multiple cerebral and cerebellar lesions, for practical purposes, almost exclude the diagnosis. In cases of NMO, tests of the CSF also reveal NMO antibody. In many cases of Jakob–Creutzfeldt disease, tests of the CSF reveal the 14-3-3 protein.

15. Which statement regarding pregnancy and MS is *true*?
    a. MS causes a high rate of miscarriages.
    b. MS frequently causes complications during delivery.
    c. Fetal malformations in MS patients are common.
    d. Cesarean sections are frequently indicated when MS women deliver.
    e. Offspring have a greater risk than the general population of developing MS.

Answer: e. Children of MS patients have an increased incidence of the illness. MS does not cause miscarriages, obstetric complications, fetal malformations, or problems that require cesarean sections.

16. Which MS features are correlated with cognitive impairment?
    a. Physical impairments
    b. Duration of the illness
    c. Enlarged cerebral ventricles
    d. Corpus callosum atrophy
    e. Periventricular demyelination
    f. Total lesion area
    g. Cerebral hypometabolism
    h. All of the above

Answer: h. All of these features are risk factors for cognitive impairment in MS, but total lesion area is the most statistically powerful one.

17. What is the approximate concordance rate of MS among monozygotic twins?
    a. 25%
    b. 50%
    c. 75%
    d. 100%
    e. 200%

Answer: a. Most studies describe an MS concordance rate of 25% to 30% for monozygotic twins and 5% for dizygotic twins. When both twins have MS, their phenotypes (symptoms and signs) differ.

18–24. Match the ocular motility disorder (18–24) with its most likely cause (a–g).
    a. Wernicke's encephalopathy
    b. Labyrinthitis
    c. Psychogenic disorders
    d. Myasthenia gravis
    e. MS
    f. Midbrain infarction
    g. None of the above

18. Pupillary dilation, ptosis, and paresis of adduction
19. Bilateral ptosis
20. Bilateral horizontal nystagmus
21. Bilateral horizontal nystagmus, unilateral paresis of abduction, and absent DTRs
22. Nystagmus in abducting eye and incomplete adduction of the other eye when looking horizontally
23. Ptosis bilaterally, paresis of adduction of one eye, and normal pupils
24. Nystagmus in adducting eye and paresis of abduction of the other eye

Answers:
18–f (oculomotor nerve palsy)
19–d, f (myasthenia gravis, oculomotor nucleus damage)
20–a, b, e (Wernicke's encephalopathy, labyrinthitis, MS)
21–a (Wernicke's encephalopathy)
22–e (MS-induced INO)
23–d (Myasthenia gravis)
24–g (None of the above)

25. The partner of a 58-year-old man with longstanding MS brings him to the emergency department for urinary incontinence. He has a distended bladder, paraparesis, and decreased sensation in his lower trunk and legs, but no back pain. Which should be the first step in alleviating his distress?
    a. Administer cholinergic medications
    b. Do an MRI of the spinal cord
    c. Stop any anticholinergic medications
    d. Administer analgesics that have no anticholinergic side effects
    e. None of the above

Answer: e. He has overflow incontinence and should have a catheter inserted into his bladder to drain the urine. To avoid precipitating a hypotensive episode, the drainage should be interrupted after removing each liter. Not all cases of bladder distention and overflow incontinence in MS are due to the illness. Instead, the cause may be prostatic hypertrophy, other obstructions, anticholinergic medications, or detrusor muscle weakness.

26. A 9-year-old boy has developed social and academic difficulties. He has hyperactive DTRs, clumsiness, and an awkward gait. His older brother had similar symptoms and signs before succumbing to adrenal failure. The patient's MRI shows extensive demyelination in the brain. Which of the following statements is *correct*?
    a. Lorenzo's oil will arrest the disease.
    b. The illness is transmitted in an autosomal recessive pattern.
    c. The illness results from defective mitochondria.
    d. The disease is characterized by the accumulation of unbranched saturated very long chain fatty acids (VLCFAs).

Answer: d. The patient, like his brother, probably has adrenoleukodystrophy (ALD), a leukoencephalopathy in which defective peroxisomes lead to the accumulation of VLCFAs. It is an X-linked disorder that usually presents in boys and runs its course over 5 years. Neither Lorenzo's oil nor adrenal replacement therapy compensates for the defective peroxisomes.

27. Which one of the following descriptions best characterizes MS-induced MRI changes?
    a. Multiple, white areas scattered in the cerebrum
    b. Conversion of the cerebral hemisphere white matter to gray
    c. Loss of the myelin signal throughout the corpus callosum
    d. Periventricular high-intensity abnormalities
    e. Periventricular low-intensity abnormalities

Answer: d. MS is characterized by multiple relatively large patches (plaques) in the cerebral periventricular white matter. MS plaques are also often routinely detected in other areas of the cerebrum, especially the corpus callosum, and the cerebellum. High-resolution MRI can show these plaques in the optic nerves and spinal cord. MS plaques on MRIs show high intensity on T2 images and low intensity on T1 images. However, scattered, small white matter hyperintense lesions – unidentified bright objects (UBOs) – are a nonspecific finding often confused with MS plaques.

28. Natives of which of the following cities have the highest MS incidence?
    a. New Orleans
    b. Boston
    c. Philadelphia
    d. Seattle

Answer: b. Boston. Higher latitudes are usually associated with a greater incidence of MS.

29. Which of the following regions has the lowest MS incidence?
    a. New England
    b. Colorado
    c. Scotland
    d. Caribbean islands

Answer: d. Caribbean residents have a very low incidence of MS, but they are subject to HTLV-1 infection that mimics spinal cord MS.

30. Of the following Israeli groups, which would have the highest incidence of MS?
    a. Native Israelis (Sabras)
    b. Adult European immigrants to Israel
    c. Israeli immigrants raised to age 18 years in sub-Saharan Africa

Answer: b. Classic studies have shown that adult European immigrants, like other individuals who grow up in cool climates, have a relatively high risk of developing MS. The period of vulnerability includes the years

from birth to about 16 years. In other words, adults emigrating from one climate to another carry the incidence of their homeland. Sabras and sub-Saharan Africans have a low incidence no matter to where they immigrate.

31. In which four conditions do visual evoked responses (VERs) typically show prolonged latencies or other abnormal pattern?
    a. Asymptomatic optic neuritis
    b. Retrobulbar neuritis
    c. Long-standing MS
    d. "Blindness" from a conversion reaction
    e. Optic nerve gliomas
    f. Deafness

Answer: a, b, c, e. Almost any lesion in the visual pathway slows the nerve action potential, which prolongs the latency and distorts its waveform.

32. In MS patients, which three findings are most often associated with urinary incontinence?
    a. Leg spasticity
    b. Ataxia
    c. Spasticity of the external sphincter of the bladder
    d. Sexual impairment
    e. Medial longitudinal fasciculus (MLF) syndrome

Answer: a, c, d. Urinary incontinence, sexual impairment, and spastic paraparesis all result from spinal cord involvement. In MS, the spinal cord is often the sole or primary site of involvement. Its pathways are exquisitely sensitive.

33. Which is the most common psychiatric comorbidity of MS?
    a. Anxiety
    b. Dementia
    c. Depression
    d. Psychosis

Answer: c. Depression complicates the course of MS from its onset and affects a large proportion of patients. If psychosis and dementia occur, they are late-developing comorbidities. Depression is also the most common comorbidity of epilepsy and stroke.

34. After two decades of enduring relapsing-remitting MS unresponsive to interferon therapy, a 45-year-old former Broadway actress switched to immunosuppressant treatment with a humanized monoclonal antibody. One year later she developed the rapid development of pseudobulbar speech, cognitive impairment, and left-sided hemiparesis. Her MRI showed new large, demyelinated patches in several subcortical regions. Which is the most likely explanation for her deterioration?
    a. She has had a relapse of MS.
    b. Her MS has entered a secondary progressive phase.
    c. Progressive multifocal leukoencephalopathy (PML) has complicated her new immunosuppressant treatment.
    d. She has developed a cerebral lymphoma.

Answer: c. Humanized monoclonal antibody treatments, such as natalizumab, are used for rheumatoid arthritis and inflammatory bowel disease as well as MS. PML has complicated their use in MS. Cerebral lymphomas, which may develop simultaneously in several areas, may also complicate immunosuppressive therapy. However, like other brain tumors, cerebral lymphomas exert a mass effect that would be evident on clinical examination and MRI. Although neurologists might reasonably attribute this woman's new symptoms to a relapse of MS, the MRI shows subcortical rather than periventricular areas of demyelination.

35. Regarding the previous question, which of the following would best confirm a clinical diagnosis of progressive multifocal leukoencephalopathy (PML)?
    a. A brain biopsy
    b. CSF analysis for JC virus
    c. Repeat MRI in 3 months
    d. VERs

Answer: b. Unsuppressed cerebral JC virus infection leads to PML. Finding it in the CSF would confirm the diagnosis of PML and obviate a biopsy.

36. A 32-year-old actress, who had been entirely well all of her life, presented to a neurologist with the sudden loss of vision in her left eye and weakness in both legs. Her examination revealed inability to count fingers in her left eye and 20/100 vision in her right eye. She had paraparesis with hyperactive DTRs and bilateral Babinski signs. The MRI of her brain showed signs of demyelination in both optic nerves. MRI of her cervical spine shows a longitudinal segment of demyelination. Which is the most likely diagnosis?
    a. MS
    b. Neuromyelitis optica (NMO)
    c. Drug abuse
    d. Progressive multifocal leukoencephalopathy (PML)

Answer: b. Clinical and MRI demyelinating abnormalities confined to her optic nerves and a longitudinal segment of the spinal cord indicate NMO rather than MS. PML and drug abuse, except for methanol, do not attack the optic nerves, and neither attacks the spinal cord.

37. Which of the following cells produces CNS myelin?
    a. Astrocytes
    b. Neurons
    c. Schwann cells
    d. Oligodendroglia

Answer: d. Oligodendroglia produce CNS myelin. Schwann cells produce peripheral nervous system myelin.

38. In regard to the allegation that silicone breast implants cause MS, which of the following statements is *true*?
    a. The incidence of symptoms is greater in women with ruptured than unruptured implants.
    b. The incidence of symptoms is greater in women who have had breast implants than in women who have undergone breast reduction surgery.
    c. Silicone-covered pacemakers produce similar neurologic problems.
    d. Neurologic symptoms associated with silicone breast implants are consistent from patient to patient.
    e. None of the above

Answer: e. There is no credible evidence that silicone breast implants cause neurologic disease.

39. A 22-year-old woman is admitted to a hospital because she has nystagmus, scanning speech, hyperactive DTRs in all limbs, Babinski signs, and a spastic-ataxic gait. She has inappropriate euphoria, impaired recent and remote memory, and impaired judgment. The MRI of her brain shows diffuse loss of myelin in her entire brain and spinal cord. Her HIV test was negative. She smokes two packs of cigarettes each day and admits to daily "huffing" (deliberately inhaling volatile substances for their euphoric effect). Which is the most likely diagnosis?
    a. HTLV-1 infection
    b. MS
    c. Chronic solvent abuse
    d. Progressive multifocal leukoencephalopathy (PML)

Answer: c. She probably has been inhaling toluene or other hydrocarbon solvent, which are frequent volatile drugs of abuse. Toluene, a solvent used in furniture, shoe, and heavy machinery manufacturing, acts as a CNS demyelinating agent. When used for recreation, it produces a mild but immediate euphoria. HTLV-1 affects the spinal cord primarily or exclusively and it usually does not produce cognitive changes. PML would have been possible if she had AIDS or another immunodeficiency condition.

40. Which of the following statements is *true* regarding depression in MS?
    a. Patients typically have several family members with depressive illness.
    b. Among MS patients, depression affects women two to five times more frequently than men.
    c. Fatigue is a risk factor.
    d. Although depression is common in MS patients, it does not lead to suicide.

Answer: c. Risk factors for depression in MS include cognitive impairment, physical impairment, and fatigue. Unlike patients with major depressive disorder, MS patients with depression do not have a family history of depression. Although the incidence of MS is twice as great in women as in men, men and women with MS are equally likely to be affected. Depression in MS patients leads to suicide with a seven-fold incidence compared to the general population. Suicidal MS patients often have a personal or family history of depression, history of alcohol abuse, and limited psychosocial support.

41. Following exposure to a prairie dog infected with monkeypox, public health officials administered smallpox vaccinations to a 19-year-old waitress and a dozen other young adults. Several days later she developed a high fever, stupor, INO, and spastic paraparesis. From which condition does she probably suffer?
    a. Monkeypox
    b. Smallpox
    c. MS
    d. Postvaccinial encephalomyelitis

Answer: d. She most likely developed an adverse reaction, postvaccinal encephalomyelitis, to the smallpox vaccination. This reaction causes acute MS-like demyelination throughout the CNS. The reaction is explosive, severe, extensive, and associated with 10% mortality, but it is a monophasic condition. It was one of the main reasons that public health officials halted routine smallpox vaccinations. However, smallpox vaccinations are still administered to individuals exposed to cowpox and monkeypox, which are caused by species of the DNA virus *Orthopoxvirus*.

42. Why do evoked responses show an increased latency when an MS plaque has damaged the pathway?
    a. The plaque reduces the amplitude of the action potentials.
    b. Demyelinated pathways, deprived of their insulation, conduct impulses slowly or unreliably.
    c. Axon damage speeds nerve conduction.
    d. None of the above

Answer: b. In MS, impaired conduction by axons that have lost their myelin or have been directly injured causes increased latency and waveform distortion on evoked potential testing.

43. Which of the following statements is *true* regarding MS in the pediatric age range (18 years or younger)?
    a. Autism symptoms are comorbid with pediatric MS.
    b. Attention-deficit hyperactivity is comorbid with pediatric MS.
    c. The majority of such cases develop cognitive impairment, depression, or both.
    d. The majority of them develop fatigue.

Answer: d. Fatigue develops in about 75% of pediatric MS cases, but cognitive impairment in 30% and depression in 6%. Neither autism symptoms nor attention-deficit hyperactivity is comorbid with pediatric MS.

44. Which one of the following cranial nerves is covered by CNS-type myelin?
    a. CN II
    b. CN III
    c. CN VI
    d. CN VII

Answer: a. Unlike the other cranial nerves, the optic nerve (CN II) is an outgrowth of the CNS. CNS myelin covers only the optic nerve and a small portion of the acoustic nerve (CN VIII). PNS-type myelin covers the others. In practical terms, CNS demyelinating illnesses classically attack the optic nerve as well as the spinal cord and brain, but not the other cranial nerves. For example, patients with MS or ALD do not develop deafness, loss of taste, or isolated CN III or CN VI palsies.

45. Which statement is *false* regarding caregiver stress in MS?
    a. MS patients' depression, anxiety, and cognitive impairment add to caregiver burden.
    b. The caregiver is at risk for depression or reemergence of preexisting depression.
    c. Social and financial counseling may reduce the stress.
    d. Caregiver stress is greater in MS than in other neurologic disorders.

Answer: d. The loss of productivity, inability to care for the family, unpredictability of relapses, psychiatric comorbidity, and sexual impairments, as well as the physical disability, lead to depression and other sequelae of stress in the patient and caregiver. However, neurodegenerative illnesses (Parkinson, Alzheimer, and Huntington diseases), stroke, and many congenital illnesses (autism, Rett syndrome) produce comparable or greater lifelong, heart-wrenching situations.

46. A 33-year-old woman, who has just returned from a camping trip, awoke with decreased vision in her right eye. She also had pain in and around that eye when she looked from side to side. An ophthalmologist found that she had a dense central scotoma and visual acuity of 20/400 in her right eye. The patient's pupils were both 4 mm in room light and, when the ophthalmologist aimed a flashlight in her left eye, both pupils constricted to 2 mm; however, when the ophthalmologist swung the light to the right eye, both pupils dilated back to 4 mm. What is the term for this pupillary reaction to light?
    a. Afferent pupillary defect
    b. Efferent pupillary defect
    c. Adie's pupil
    d. Argyll–Robertson pupil

Answer: a. Her pupils both dilated when the flashlight was switched in the "swinging flashlight test" from the normal to the affected eye. This response reflects decreased light input to the entire light reflex arc (see Fig. 4.2). Inflammation of the right optic nerve – optic neuritis – impaired the direct and consensual light reflex when light was shone into the right eye. Neurologists often refer to this afferent pupillary defect as a "Marcus Gunn pupil."

47. Which one of the following statements concerning CNS lupus is *true*?
    a. Physical neurologic complications always accompany neuropsychiatric complications.
    b. Chorea and internuclear ophthalmoplegia (INO) are common complications.
    c. Seizures, strokes, and psychosis are frequently occurring manifestations.

d. The presence of CSF oligoclonal bands mandates a diagnosis of MS rather than lupus.

Answer: c. Seizures, strokes, and psychosis, along with cognitive impairment and depression, are frequently occurring complications of CNS lupus. Neurologists sometimes quip, "The most common neurologic manifestations of lupus are the "3 'S's: seizures, strokes, and psychosis." In about 5% of lupus cases, neurologic complications, including purely neuropsychiatric ones, are the presenting feature. Even subsequently, physical neurologic complications do not necessarily accompany neuropsychiatric ones. Chorea and INO occur in only about 1% of lupus cases, but neurologists usually include lupus in the differential diagnosis of these conditions. CSF oligoclonal bands and serum antiphospholipid antibodies and double-stranded DNA are often detectable when lupus neurologic complications occur.

48. Which of the following disease-modifying therapies for MS has *not* been associated with the development of progressive multifocal leukoencephalopathy (PML)?
    a. Glatiramer acetate (Copaxone)
    b. Dimethyl fumarate (Tecfidera)
    c. Fingolimod (Gilenya)
    d. Natalizumab (Tysabri)

Answer: a. Of all the choices, only glatiramer acetate has not been associated with an increased risk of PML during treatment. This often devastating infection, while still rare, has complicated the success of many of the new MS therapies. One newer therapy, teriflunomide, has not had any reported cases of PML. Similarly, the oldest therapy still in use, interferon-beta, has not had any associated cases of PML.

NEUROLOGIC ASPECTS OF SEXUAL FUNCTION

Whatever its underlying psychology, sexual function depends on two complex and delicate neurologic pathways: (1) a connection between the brain and the genitals, and (2) a reflex loop between the genitals and spinal cord. Both involve the central nervous system (CNS), peripheral nervous system (PNS), and autonomic nervous system (ANS).

In the first pathway, the brain converts various stimuli, including sleep-related events, into neurologic impulses that are usually excitatory, although occasionally inhibitory. These impulses travel down the spinal cord. Some impulses descend all the way down to the cord's sacral region (S2–S4) where they exit through the sacral nerve roots to travel through the *pudendal nerve*. Upon exiting the spinal cord, they leave the CNS to join the PNS (Fig. 16.1). Other impulses travel through the same nerve roots, but travel through the *parasympathetic* division of the ANS. Meanwhile, as if diverted to a parallel route, some impulses leave the spinal cord at its low thoracic and upper lumbar regions (T11-L2) to travel through the sympathetic division of the ANS.

Excitatory descending stimuli increase parasympathetic ANS activity, which reduces (relaxes) tone in the wall muscles of genital arteries. As the relaxed arteries dilate, they allow increased blood flow. In men, increased blood flow inflates the penis and produces an erection. In women, it produces clitoral engorgement.

With continued excitatory stimulation, a complex series of predominantly sympathetic ANS-mediated events produce an orgasm. Afterward, a return to normal, relatively constricted arterial wall muscle tone reduces blood flow. The resultant reduced vascular engorgement results in detumescence.

Although the sympathetic and parasympathetic components of the ANS are complementary, they depend on different neurotransmitters – acetylcholine in the parasympathetic and monoamines in the sympathetic. Moreover, the ANS components have different roles. An admittedly crude mnemonic describes the *p*arasympathetic and *s*ympathetic ANS roles in sexual response: "*point* and *shoot*." (The mnemonic also reflects that current knowledge of sexual function rests primarily on male physiology, evaluation, and treatment.)

The second pathway – the genital–spinal cord reflex – is shorter and simpler. In it, erotic impulses from genital stimulation pass through the pudendal nerve to the spinal cord. Most impulses synapse in the sacral region of the spinal cord and return, via the ANS, to the genitals.

NEUROLOGIC IMPAIRMENT

Without accepting a complete distinction between neurologic and psychologic sexual impairment, certain elements of the patient's history (Box 16.1) and neurologic examination (Box 16.2) reliably indicate a neurologic origin. For example, either spinal cord or peripheral nerve injury might lead to a pattern of weakness and sensory loss below the waist or only around the genitals, anus, and buttocks – the "saddle area" (Fig. 16.2). Plantar and deep tendon reflex (DTR) testing will indicate which system is responsible: spinal cord injury causes hyperactive DTRs and Babinski signs, whereas peripheral nerve injury causes hypoactive DTRs and no Babinski signs. Both CNS and PNS impairment lead to loss of the relevant "superficial reflexes": scrotal, cremasteric, and anal (Fig. 16.3).

Signs of ANS impairment, although often subtle, carry great weight. For example, *orthostatic hypotension*, usually defined as a fall of 20 mmHg in systolic blood pressure upon standing, reliably indicates ANS impairment, as might result from diabetes, medications, or idiopathic systemic conditions. Similarly, *anhidrosis*, lack of sweating, indicates ANS impairment. In this condition, *urinary incontinence* and hairless and sallow skin usually accompany dry axillae, groins, and legs. Finally, if microscopic examination of urine obtained after orgasm reveals sperm, the man probably has *retrograde ejaculation*, which usually reflects a disorder of the finely tuned, ANS-based mechanism.

In many conditions, such as spinal cord injury or severe ANS damage, urinary and fecal incontinence accompany neurologic-induced sexual impairment because the bladder, bowel, and genitals share many elements of innervation. The anus, like the bladder, has two sphincters (see Fig. 15.5). Its internal sphincter, more powerful than the external one, constricts in response to increased sympathetic activity and relaxes to parasympathetic activity. The external sphincter of the anus is under voluntary control through the pudendal nerves and other branches of the S3 and S4 peripheral nerve roots. Thus, to produce a bowel movement, individuals must deliberately relax their external sphincter while the internal sphincter, under involuntary parasympathetic control, simultaneously relaxes.

As could be anticipated, excess sympathetic ANS activity, as in the "fight or flight" response, inhibits both urinating and defecating by constricting the sphincters.

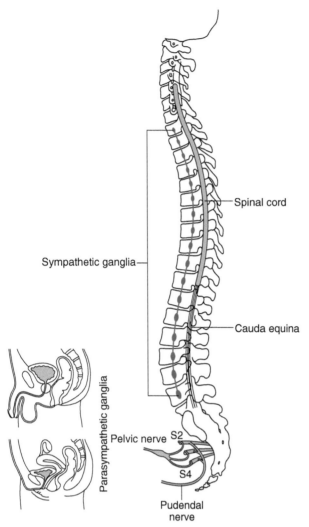

FIGURE 16.1 ■ The sacral spinal cord segments (S2–S4) give rise to the pudendal nerves, which supply the genital muscles and skin. Those segments also supply the vaginal canal. They convey sensations for pleasure during sex and pain during vaginal delivery. The sympathetic and parasympathetic components of the ANS also innervate the genitals, and the reproductive organs, bladder, sweat glands, and arterial wall muscles.

BOX 16.1	Symptoms Suggesting Neurologic Sexual Impairment

Continual erectile dysfunction
    Absence of morning erections
        No erection or orgasm during masturbation or sex with
            different partners
Related somatic complaints
Sensory loss in genitals, pelvis, or legs
Urinary incontinence
Certain neurologic conditions
    Spinal cord injury
    Diabetic neuropathy
    Multiple sclerosis
    Herniated intervertebral disk
Use of many medications

BOX 16.2	Signs of Neurologic Sexual Impairment

Signs of spinal cord injury
    Paraparesis or quadriparesis
    Leg spasticity
    Urinary incontinence
Signs of autonomic nervous system injury
    Orthostatic hypotension or lightheadedness
    Anhidrosis in groin and legs
    Urinary incontinence
    Retrograde ejaculation
Signs of peripheral nervous system injury
    Loss of sensation in the genitals, "saddle area," and legs
    Paresis and areflexia in legs
    Scrotal, cremasteric, and anal reflex loss

Moreover, excess ANS activity, typically caused by anxiety, often impairs sexual arousal, inhibits an erection, and precipitates premature ejaculation.

Laboratory Tests

Sleep-Related Studies

From infancy to old age, normal men have erections and other signs of ANS activity during their rapid eye movement (REM) periods of sleep. The erections develop during dreams, regardless of their overt content. Thus, normal men have three to five erections per night, each lasting about 20 minutes. In a *nocturnal penile tumescence* (*NPT*) study, a device monitors a man's erections and correlates them with REM periods over 1 to 3 nights.

Because NPT studies take place in a secluded setting, the testing frees men with erectile dysfunction from most social and psychologic influences. During NPT studies, some men casually diagnosed as having erectile dysfunction actually develop erections. Those who develop no erections usually have a physiologic disturbance; however, some of them suffer from depression, a sleep disorder, or a test-induced artifact.

Other Tests

Depending on the circumstances – peripheral vascular disease, atherosclerosis, diabetes, or pelvic injuries – physicians may assess men with erectile dysfunction and other sexual impairments by measuring the blood pressure and blood flow in the dorsal artery of the penis using a small blood pressure cuff, Doppler ultrasound apparatus, and other devices. Barring vascular disease, an injection of a vasodilator into the penis (i.e., an intracorporeal vasodilator injection) produces an erection. In fact, such injections provide a treatment option.

If physicians suspect polyneuropathy, pudendal nerve damage, or spinal cord injury, neurologists may perform electrophysiologic studies, such as peripheral nerve conduction velocity, penile nerve conduction velocity, and somatosensory evoked potentials for women as well as men. These tests help in the diagnosis of patients with diabetic neuropathy, prostate cancer, pelvic or spine trauma, or multiple sclerosis (MS) (see later).

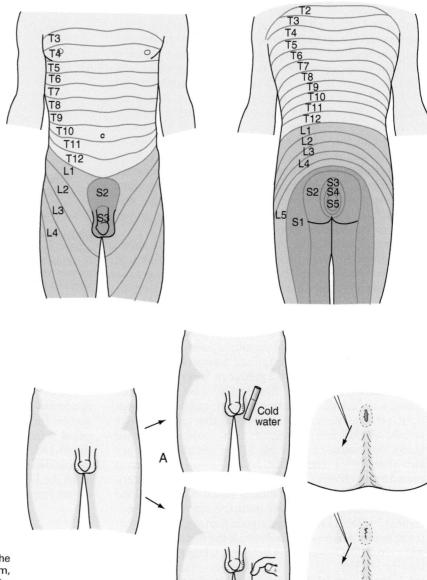

FIGURE 16.2 ■ The sacral dermatomes (S2–S5) innervate the skin overlying the genitals and anus, but the lumbar dermatomes innervate the legs.

FIGURE 16.3 ■ *A*, The *scrotal reflex*: When the examiner applies a cold surface to the scrotum, the ipsilateral skin contracts and testicle retracts. *B*, The *cremasteric reflex*: Stroking the inner thigh elicits the same response. *C*, The *anal reflex*: When the examiner scratches the skin surrounding the anus, it tightens.

Individuals with an endocrinologic basis of their sexual dysfunction usually have other signs of hormone imbalance. Relevant screening tests usually measure blood glucose, prolactin, testosterone, estrogen, and gonadotropic hormone concentrations. Other tests may reveal hypogonadism, hypothyroidism, diabetes, or a disruption of the hypothalamic–pituitary–gonadal axis. In performing an endocrinologic evaluation, physicians should note that although an elevated prolactin concentration usually indicates a pituitary adenoma, antipsychotics and other medicines also might elevate it.

Medical Treatment of Erectile Dysfunction

Several medications can produce erections adequate for sexual intercourse despite neurologic injury or vascular insufficiency. They can also restore erections in men experiencing psychogenic erectile dysfunction and in those taking psychotropic medication.

Many physicians prescribe yohimbine, a centrally acting α_2-adrenergic antagonist (see Chapter 21). This medicine may slightly increase sympathetic vasomotor activity, provide mild psychologic stimulation, and create an aphrodisiac sensation. Although yohimbine may alleviate psychogenic erectile dysfunction, it does not help in cases of sexual function due to medical or neurologic illness. Moreover, it often causes anxiety.

Testosterone injections are popular mostly because they may increase muscle mass, especially in body builders, and provide psychologic stimulation. However, except in cases of hypogonadism, testosterone injections have no effect on sexual function and, in high doses for long periods, they may induce prostate cancer.

In contrast, intracorporeal injections of vasoactive medicines – although briefly painful – are effective. They induce erections in men with spinal cord damage, peripheral neuropathy, or vascular disease. The most effective medicines are papaverine, a nonspecific smooth muscle relaxant; phentolamine, an α-adrenergic antagonist; and alprostadil, a synthetic prostaglandin E1. A man with erectile dysfunction can inject these medicines – individually or as a mixture – into the base of his corpus cavernosum (the vascular erectile tissue of the penis).

Phentolamine-induced erections illustrate an important physiologic distinction. In contrast to α-adrenergic *antagonists* such as phentolamine which produce erections by increasing blood flow into the penis, adrenergic *agonists* such as epinephrine (adrenaline) (see later) soften erections by reducing blood flow.

Using an alternative treatment, men insert a short, thin alprostadil suppository into the urethra. Although initially uncomfortable, it leads to an erection by greatly promoting blood flow into the penis. This method, unlike sildenafil (Viagra) treatment, does not require physical stimulation to achieve an erection.

Sildenafil and related medicines – tadalafil (Cialis), vardenafil (Levitra), and avanafil (Stendra) – have simplified the treatment of erectile dysfunction and dispensed with expensive and lengthy testing. To a greater or lesser degree they assist men with erectile dysfunction from age-related changes, diabetes, MS, spinal cord injury, and nerve damage from prostate surgery. Furthermore, they often correct erectile dysfunction associated with anxiety, decreased libido, depression, or other psychiatric disturbances. They also partially or completely reverse sexual dysfunction caused by psychotropic medications in both sexes (see later).

Sildenafil and related medicines have a well-established mechanism of action. Under normal circumstances, psychologic or tactile sexual stimulation provokes parasympathetic neurons to produce and release the neurotransmitter nitric oxide (NO) within the penis. NO, in turn, promotes the production of cyclic guanosine monophosphate (cGMP). In turn, cGMP dilates the arteries that promote blood flow and creates an erection. When the enzyme cGMP-phosphodiesterase metabolizes cGMP, the erection subsides.

As their primary mechanism of action, these medicines – *phosphodiesterase inhibitors* – inhibit cGMP-phosphodiesterase. The resulting increased cGMP concentration promotes blood flow in the penis (Fig. 16.4).

Hardly a panacea, phosphodiesterase inhibitors help only about 60% of men with erectile dysfunction. In particular, they are often ineffective in men older than 70 years, with diabetes (especially when it is uncontrolled), undergoing cancer chemotherapy, or who smoke. In addition, they carry some risk; men taking nitroglycerin, other nitrates, doxazosin, or most α_1-adrenergic antagonists should not take phosphodiesterase inhibitors because excess vasodilation may lead to orthostatic hypotension.

Invasive treatments are rarely satisfactory. Delicate and tedious arterial reconstructive procedures are usually disappointing except in men with localized vascular injuries. Surgically implanted devices, such as rigid or semirigid silicone rods or a balloon-like apparatus, can mimic an erection. Unfortunately, implants are costly, unaesthetic,

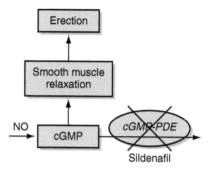

NO = Nitrous oxide
cGMP = Cyclic guanosine monophosphate
PDE = phosphodiesterase, which metabolizes cGMP
but is inhibited by sildenafil

FIGURE 16.4 ■ As its mechanism of action, sildenafil inhibits cGMP-phosphodiesterase (cGMP-PDE). The resulting increase in cyclic guanosine monophosphate (cGMP) leads to smooth muscle relaxation that promotes vascular congestion in the penis and thus an erection.

and prone to infections and mechanical failures. In contrast, silicone penile implants have never been accused, like silicone breast implants, of causing rheumatologic or MS-like symptoms (see Chapter 15).

Curiously, although NO and cGMP mediate clitoral blood flow and engorgement in women, use of phosphodiesterase inhibitors in women has not shown great success for female sexual dysfunction. A new multifunctional serotonin agonist-antagonist medication, flibanserin (Addyi) was approved in 2015 for the treatment of hypoactive sexual desire disorder (HSDD) in women. Of note, the DSM-5 now classifies HSDD as part of Female Sexual Interest/Arousal Disorder.

UNDERLYING CONDITIONS

Age-Related Changes

In men aged 50 years and older, although their libido generally remains intact, erections decrease in rigidity and duration. Their penis, like other bodily areas, begins to lose sensitivity to touch and vibration. Also, these men's refractory period between orgasms, which was 20 minutes when they were in their sexual prime, at age 18 years, lengthens to days and then to weeks. Their serum testosterone concentration decreases, but changes correlate poorly with erectile function. For example, although restoring testosterone concentrations reverses a diminished libido, it does not improve erectile dysfunction.

One credible explanation for their erectile dysfunction implicates the normal age-related increased smooth muscle tone throughout the body. Not only does increased arterial wall smooth muscle tone cause or contribute to essential hypertension, it also leads to reduced blood flow into the penis.

In addition to hypertension, other factors common among middle-aged and older men that may cause or at least predispose them to erectile dysfunction include atherosclerotic disease, smoking, alcohol abuse, and television viewing time. Whether in isolation or as a group, these factors also blunt the response to phosphodiesterase inhibitors.

Spinal Cord Injury

Spinal cord injury produces a triad of symptoms that varies according to the injury's level and whether it partially or completely transects the spinal cord:

- Paraparesis or quadriparesis with spasticity, hyperactive reflexes, and Babinski signs
- Sensory loss up to a certain spinal level (see Fig. 16.2)
- Bladder, bowel, and sexual difficulties.

In addition, upper cervical cord injuries compromise respiration. They also release the sympathetic nervous system from CNS control.

Cervical and Thoracic Spinal Cord Injury

When injuries sever the cervical spinal cord, patients develop quadriparesis. When injuries sever the thoracic portion, they develop paraparesis. In both of these situations, the injury interrupts ascending sensory impulses, and patients cannot sense genital stimulation. Nevertheless, because the genital–spinal cord loop remains intact, patients retain the capacity for reflex genital arousal. They can achieve an orgasm even though they are unable to perceive it.

In these cases, erections are usually too weak for intercourse. If orgasms occur, they may produce an excessive, almost violent ANS response, called *autonomic hyperreflexia*. This response often causes hypertension, bradycardia, nausea, and lightheadedness. Occasionally the hypertension is so severe that it leads to an intracerebral hemorrhage.

Most spinal cord injury patients also suffer from urinary incontinence and constipation, requiring catheters and enemas. Infections of the urinary tract and decubitus ulcers constantly threaten them. Furthermore, men lose fertility because of inadequate and abnormal sperm production. However, women continue to ovulate and menstruate. They retain their capacity to conceive and bear children.

Incomplete spinal cord damage, as typically occurs in MS and nonpenetrating trauma, causes less pronounced neurologic deficits. Still, because of the delicate nature of the sexual neurologic pathways, even incomplete injuries impair genital arousal and inhibit orgasm.

Lumbosacral Spinal Cord Injury

As with patients who sustain thoracic spinal cord transection, those with lumbosacral spinal cord transection (at approximately the level of the T10–L1 vertebrae; recall that the spinal cord ends at the L1 level in adults) also have paraparesis and incontinence. In addition, because this lower lesion interrupts both the genital–spinal cord reflex and ascending and descending spinal cord tracts, neither genital nor mental stimulation produces erection or orgasm.

Nevertheless, the ANS, which travels in a parallel pathway, may remain undamaged and able to innervate the genitals. This innervation preserves fertility in men and women. Also in contrast to higher spinal cord injuries, sensation of the breasts and their erotic capacity is preserved – and relatively enhanced – because upper chest sensation remains unaffected.

Poliomyelitis and Other Exceptions

Several neurologic illnesses can be so devastating that the untrained physician might assume that their victims have lost their sexual capacity. However, careful evaluations may reveal that many patients with these illnesses have retained sexual desire and function.

For example, two relatively common motor neuron diseases, poliomyelitis (polio) and amyotrophic lateral sclerosis (ALS) (see Chapter 5), devastate the voluntary motor system. Polio often left survivors confined to wheelchairs and braces, but with stable deficits. ALS, in contrast, causes progressively greater disability that usually results in death after several years. Nevertheless, both these illnesses relatively spare victims' intellect (see Chapter 5), sensation, involuntary muscle strength, and ANS functions. Thus, they allow patients to have normal sexual desire and function, genital sensation, bladder and bowel control, and fertility.

Similarly, most extrapyramidal illnesses (see Chapter 18), despite causing difficulties with mobility, do not impair sexual desire, sexual function, or fertility. For example, adolescents with athetotic cerebral palsy and other varieties of congenital birth injury – even those with marked physical impairments – often have intact libido and sexual function. Among older patients, those with Parkinson disease have preserved sexual drive; however, it may remain unexpressed until dopaminergic medications, such as levodopa and ropinirole, allow it to reemerge. Moreover, neurologic conditions, such as frontal lobe trauma, frontotemporal dementia, Parkinson-related impulse control disorder, and Alzheimer disease, may cause loss of inhibition that sometimes leads to sexual aggressiveness.

Diabetes Mellitus

Retrograde ejaculation and erectile dysfunction eventually affect almost 50% of diabetic men. These sexual impairments result predominantly from ANS injury, but there are contributions from PNS injury and also from atherosclerosis of the genital arteries (see later). Erectile dysfunction is associated with age greater than 65 years, duration of diabetes longer than 10 years, obesity, and the frequently occurring complications of diabetes, such as retinopathy, neuropathy, and peripheral vascular disease. Although phosphodiesterase inhibitors alleviate erectile dysfunction in many men with various illnesses or conditions, they provide uncertain benefits to diabetic men (see later).

The data conflict regarding sexual impairment in diabetic women, though most show some degree of dysfunction in comparison to women without diabetes. Some investigators found that diabetic women had anorgasmia, decreased arousal, reduced vaginal lubrication, or dyspareunia, and that sexual impairment was related to neuropathy; however, others found that diabetic women were not especially prone to sexual impairment and that even those with profound neuropathy experienced full sexual function. All agree, though, that diabetic women are prone to vaginal infections and that, while they remain fertile, miscarriages and fetal malformations often complicate their pregnancies. Given the presumed ANS and PNS injury, it is not clear that the new medication flibanserin (see above) would be effective in treating these women.

Urinary incontinence often accompanies sexual dysfunction in both diabetic men and women because the bladder and genitals share a common ANS innervation. Lack of innervation allows the bladder to dilate excessively and lose its tone. In addition, patients with diabetes-induced sexual dysfunction typically experience other complications of ANS impairment, such as anhidrosis and orthostatic hypotension. However, they do not necessarily have other complications of diabetes, such as retinopathy, nephropathy, or peripheral vascular disease.

Multiple Sclerosis

Sexual impairment can be the most bothersome and sometimes even the sole symptom of MS (see Chapter 15). Patients in an early stage of the disease may have few persistent neurologic deficits, but as attacks recur, the incidence of sexual impairment rises. When sexual impairment occurs, urinary bladder dysfunction accompanies it in 90% of cases. MS-induced sexual impairment is also often associated with paresis and spasticity of the legs. Although spinal cord involvement probably underlies most cases of MS-induced sexual impairment, psychiatric comorbidity contributes. Whatever the precise mechanism, sexual dysfunction greatly reduces quality of life in MS patients and their partners.

Between 70% and 90% of male MS patients experience sexual impairment, particularly erectile dysfunction. Less frequently the illness also causes premature ejaculation, retrograde ejaculation, and anorgasmia. Decreased sperm production, another complication, impairs fertility. Phosphodiesterase inhibitors help correct erectile dysfunction and improve quality of life in most affected men.

Among female MS patients, a somewhat smaller proportion – between 50% and 75% – have sexual dysfunction. Women with MS remain fertile, but have decreased sexual desire, inadequate vaginal lubrication, and anorgasmia.

Medication-Induced Impairment

More than 100 medications impair one or another aspect of sexual function. Several categories are consistently responsible. Antidepressants, antipsychotics, and antiepileptics constitute a major category. Another is the standard antihypertensive medicines, such as clonidine, thiazide diuretics, and β-blockers. However, newer antihypertensive agents, including angiotensin-converting enzyme (ACE) inhibitors and the calcium-channel blockers, cause little or no sexual impairment.

Although many psychiatric patients are prone to sexual dysfunction because of their disorder, psychotropic medications may precipitate or exacerbate it. In both men and women, such medication-induced sexual dysfunction is primarily dose-related. Medication-induced sexual dysfunction also correlates with medications' suppression of

dopamine activity and its correlate, elevated serum prolactin concentration; increase in serotonin activity; and inhibition of NO synthetase.

In general, the sexual side effects of antidopaminergic antipsychotic medications are consistent with the hypothesis that decreased dopamine activity, usually accompanied by increased prolactin concentration, leads to sexual dysfunction. For example, typical antipsychotics routinely decrease libido, impair erectile function, and cause other sexual problems in both men and women. In contrast, clozapine, olanzapine, quetiapine, and several other atypical antipsychotics carry a relatively low risk of sexual side effects. Interestingly, almost all typical and atypical antipsychotic agents on rare occasion cause priapism (see later).

Even though dopamine plays little role in their mechanism of action, tricyclic, heterocyclic, monoamine oxidase inhibitor, and selective serotonin reuptake inhibitor (SSRI) antidepressants also routinely lead to sexual dysfunction. This side effect often so troubles patients that they fail to comply with their medication regimen.

SSRIs more so than tricyclic antidepressants delay or prevent orgasm. Furthermore, approximately one-third of men taking SSRIs experience erectile dysfunction. These medicines also interfere with vaginal lubrication. For any particular SSRI, the rate of adverse sexual side effects greatly varies among different studies.

When an antidepressant causes sexual side effects, physicians may prescribe a phosphodiesterase inhibitor such as sildenafil, which frequently alleviates the problem. Sometimes switching from one to another antidepressant is helpful. Several reports show that bupropion and trazodone have a lower association with sexual side effects than conventional antidepressants.

Anticholinergic medications, which psychiatrists often prescribe to counteract neuroleptic-induced parkinsonism, also cause sexual impairment. In addition, these medicines cause other bothersome symptoms that reflect ANS dysfunction: dry mouth, orthostatic hypotension, urinary hesitancy, and accommodation paresis (see Chapter 12). According to some studies, many antiepileptic drugs depress serum testosterone levels in men, which might impair their sexual function.

On the other hand, physicians treating men with premature ejaculation may capitalize on certain psychotropic medications' propensity to delay orgasm. For example, use of clomipramine (Anafranil) or sertraline (Zoloft) may be desirable to prolong arousal and delay orgasm.

Priapism

Phosphodiesterase inhibitor or trazodone treatment may inadvertently produce an uncomfortable and embarrassing persistent erection (priapism) in men who have an unexpected sensitivity, take too large a dose, or have an underlying structural abnormality. Priapism may also complicate spinal cord injury.

Other conditions that lead to priapism include sickle cell crises, leukemia, vascular abnormalities, and venous thrombosis from self-injection of narcotics. These insults block the venous drainage of the penis and thereby engorge it with blood. In addition, although typical and atypical antipsychotic medications usually dampen sexual function, they occasionally produce priapism because, to a certain extent, they block α-adrenergic activity.

Besides inducing pain, priapism can cause ischemia or, in severe cases, necrosis of the penis. Furthermore, repeated bouts lead to fibrosis. Urologists consider priapism an emergency. To stop blood flow into the penis, they inject it with epinephrine to produce arterial vasoconstriction (see Chapter 21). Cases that do not respond to epinephrine may require surgical drainage.

THE LIMBIC SYSTEM AND THE LIBIDO

From a neurologic viewpoint, the *limbic system* provides libido. This system consists of a large horseshoe-shaped reverberating subcortical circuit that connects several structures: the hippocampal formation and the adjacent amygdala in the temporal lobe, thalamic and hypothalamic regions, including the mamillary bodies, midbrain nuclei, and frontal lobe (Fig. 16.5). Among its many functions, the limbic system generates, conveys, and stores memory, emotion, programs for "flight or fight," eating and drinking behavior, and sexual and reproductive urges.

Structural lesions and neurodegenerative illnesses that strike the frontal or temporal lobes often damage the limbic system. For example, head trauma, strokes, or frontotemporal dementia (see Chapter 7) regularly reduce patients' psychic energy, including their sexual appetite. Although most frontal lobe injuries cause apathy and hyposexuality, they occasionally lead to aggressive, sexually charged behavior.

The Klüver–Bucy Syndrome

In the classic laboratory model that produced the *Klüver–Bucy syndrome*, neurosurgeons performed bilateral anterior temporal lobectomies, which included removing both amygdalae (Greek, almond [the shape of the amygdala]) in rhesus monkeys. Postoperatively, the animals displayed aggression and rampant, indiscriminate heterosexual and homosexual activity. In addition, as if they had lost their vision, the monkeys continually grasped objects and placed inedible as well as edible materials in their mouth. The investigators labeled this behavior *psychic blindness* or *oral exploration* (terms related to *visual agnosia*, see Chapter 12).

When even fractions of the Klüver–Bucy syndrome occur in human children or adults, they constitute a dramatic example of limbic system injury. Although the human Klüver–Bucy syndrome also results from bilateral temporal lobe injury, the usual causes consist of herpes simplex encephalitis, frontotemporal dementia including Pick disease, bilateral posterior cerebral artery infarctions, and paraneoplastic limbic encephalitis – conditions that have a predilection for striking the temporal lobes. Conditions that affect the brain diffusely or nonspecifically, such as anoxia, trauma, and Alzheimer disease, sometimes predominantly injure the temporal lobes and also may cause elements of this syndrome.

The manifestations of the human version differ considerably from those that occur in monkeys. Only about one-half of humans show any increase in heterosexual activity or masturbation. Most only speak or gesture in an

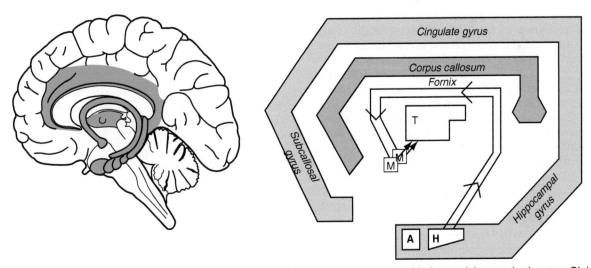

FIGURE 16.5 ■ *Left,* The *limbic system* (shaded) is a circuit deep in the brain that connects with the overlying cerebral cortex. *Right,* This schematic portrayal of the limbic system shows its main features:

Hippocampus (H) with the adjacent amygdala (A)
↓
Fornix (Latin, *fornix*, arch)
↓
Mammillary bodies (M) that send off a mammillothalamic tract
↓
Anterior nucleus of the thalamus (T)
↓
Cingulate gyrus that connects to the overlying cerebral cortex and back to the hippocampus
↑
Cerebral cortex and subcallosal and hippocampal gyri

aggressive or sexually suggestive manner. Showing a variety of oral exploration, humans with the Klüver–Bucy syndrome tend to eat excessively and smoke or drink compulsively; however, they rarely become obese. Whatever their behavior, other manifestations of temporal lobe injury, such as amnesia, aphasia, and dementia, cause more of a handicap. In particular, children with the Klüver–Bucy syndrome, which usually results from hypoxic cerebral damage, are most impaired by the amnesia.

Other Conditions

Certain medications and drugs of abuse, including hallucinogens, amyl nitrate, "ecstasy," dopamine agonists, and levodopa, may increase sexual interest and activity. Although numerous other substances are purported to have aphrodisiac qualities, their effect is minimal or nil, and many may be dangerous. For example, sildenafil, despite its ability to enhance erectile function, is not an aphrodisiac because it requires stimulation to be effective and does not affect the libido.

Another neurologic cause of heightened sexuality is damage to the inhibitory centers of the frontal lobes. Loss of inhibition may unleash suppressed sexual interest in patients with Alzheimer disease, frontotemporal dementia, vascular dementia, Parkinson-related impulse control disorder, and traumatic brain injury. However, other neuropsychologic manifestations of these illnesses – impaired cognitive function, reduced executive ability, and apraxia – often leave patients' actions rudimentary and clumsy.

Although epilepsy is usually associated with hyposexuality (see Chapter 10), seizures occasionally induce activity with sexual overtones. For example, during a seizure, patients may tug at their clothing, partially undress, or even engage in rudimentary masturbation. However, the seizures do not cause interactive, purposeful sexual activity.

Disturbances in the hypothalamic–pituitary axis occasionally lead to decreased sexual activity. Hypothalamic tumors, for example, may induce a ravenous appetite, but without accompanying increased sexual activity. Also, the Kleine–Levin syndrome (see Chapter 17) includes increased rudimentary sexual activity, which is almost always masturbation, along with hypersomnia.

In contrast to those few examples of neurologic illnesses increasing sexuality, most decrease it. Lesions of the pituitary, hypothalamus, and diencephalon usually cause hyposexuality. For example, in Sheehan's syndrome (see Chapter 19) women experience weight loss, amenorrhea, lack of sexual interest, and other symptoms of hypothalamic–pituitary insufficiency. Strokes with or without comorbid depression usually reduce both sexual interest and physical ability.

Although the libido resists mild fatigue, hunger, and fear, pain almost always dampens it. Patients with chronic pain not only have comorbid depression, they also take potent analgesics, such as opioids, that reduce sexual interest or function.

Neurologic Sequelae of Sexual Activity

Despite its pleasures, sexual activity occasionally produces several untoward neurologic consequences. In the simplest scenario, vigorous activity may precipitate a stroke because of exercise-induced hypertension or herniate a lumbar intervertebral disk because of low back strain. A migraine-like headache during sex (coital cephalgia, see Chapter 9) occasionally occurs. In a rare but more worrisome scenario, a powerful, "thunderclap" headache during sex sometimes signals the onset of a subarachnoid hemorrhage. Thus, when sexual activity precipitates a unique headache, neurologists generally recommend further evaluation, including magnetic resonance imaging (MRI) and angiography (MRA), as the first step in identifying an aneurysm. If sexual activity produces a cardiac arrhythmia, hypertension or, because of a Valsalva maneuver, hypotension, it may cause an episode of transient global amnesia (TGA, see Chapter 7).

REFERENCES

Baum, N., & Essell, A. (2008). Treating erectile dysfunction in nonresponders to PDE5 inhibitors. *Res and Staff Phys, 54*, 20–25.

Corona, G., Giorda, C. B., Cucinotta, D., et al. (2014). Sexual dysfunction at the onset of type 2 diabetes: The interplay of depression, hormonal and cardiovascular factors. *The Journal of Sexual Medicine, 11*, 2065–2073.

Fowler, C. J., Miller, J. R., Sarief, M. K., et al. (2005). A double blind, randomized study of sildenafil citrate for erectile dysfunction in men with multiple sclerosis. *Journal of Neurology, Neurosurgery, and Psychiatry, 76*, 700–705.

Frohman, E. M. (2002). Sexual dysfunction in neurologic disease. *Clin Neuropharm, 25*, 126–132.

Harden, C. (2006). Sexuality in men and women with epilepsy. *CNS Spectrums, 11*(Suppl. 9), 13–28.

Hellstrom, W. J., Kaminetsky, J., Belkoff, L. H., et al. (2015). Efficacy of avanafil 15 minutes after dosing in men with erectile dysfunction. *The Journal of Urology, 194*, 485–492.

Herzog, A. G., Drislane, F. W., Schomer, D. L., et al. (2006). Differential effects of antiepileptic drugs on neuroactive steroids in men with epilepsy. *Epilepsia, 47*, 1945–1948.

Rudkin, L., Taylor, M. J., & Hawton, K. (2004). Strategies for managing sexual dysfunction induced by antidepressant medication. *The Cochrane Database of Systematic Reviews*, (4), CD003382.

Simon, J. A., Kingsberg, S. A., Shumel, B., et al. (2014). Efficacy and safety of flibanserin in postmenopausal women with hypoactive sexual desire. *Menopause, 21*, 633–640.

Smith, S. M., O'Keane, V., & Murray, R. (2002). Sexual dysfunction in patients taking conventional antipsychotic medication. *The British Journal of Psychiatry: The Journal of Mental Science, 181*, 49–55.

Stahl, S. M. (2015). Mechanism of action of flibabserin, a multifunctional serotonin agonist and antagonist (MSAA) in hyposexual sexual desire disorder. *CNS Spectrums, 20*, 1–6.

Virseda-Chamorro, M., Salinas-Casado, J., Lopez-Garcia-Moreno, A. M., et al. (2013). Sexual dysfunction in men with spinal cord injury. *International Journal of Impotence Research, 25*, 133–137.

QUESTIONS AND ANSWERS

1. A 40-year-old man, wheelchair-bound since he survived childhood poliomyelitis, reports developing erectile dysfunction. He has a history of low back pain, hypertension, and diabetes. Which of the following is the *least* likely cause of his sexual dysfunction?
   a. Herniated lumbar intervertebral disk
   b. Antihypertensive medications
   c. Diabetic neuropathy
   d. Poliomyelitis

Answer: d. Poliomyelitis and several other neurologic illnesses may cause debilitating deficits, but typically spare sexual function. Factors a–c routinely cause erectile dysfunction. Sexual function requires a complex, delicate system that is vulnerable at any of its components: the central nervous system (CNS), peripheral nervous system (PNS), and autonomic nervous system (ANS).

2. A 24-year-old man who complains of premature ejaculation also has experienced several month-long episodes of unsteady gait, diplopia, and paraparesis. Which of the following might a neurologic examination reveal?
   a. Internuclear ophthalmoplegia
   b. Absent abdominal reflexes
   c. Ataxia of gait
   d. Babinski signs
   e. Hyperactive deep tendon reflexes (DTRs)
   f. All of the above

Answer: f. The patient probably has multiple sclerosis (MS) with cerebellar, brainstem, and spinal cord involvement. Between episodes, he is likely to retain neurologic impairments (a–e), particularly sexual dysfunction. Premature ejaculation and erectile dysfunction are frequent symptoms – and sometimes the only ones – of MS in remission.

3. Which of the following conditions often causes retrograde ejaculation?
   a. Depression
   b. Diabetic autonomic neuropathy
   c. Psychogenic influence
   d. Sexual inexperience

Answer: b. In retrograde ejaculation, semen is propelled by involuntary mechanisms into the bladder instead of the urethra. It is always the result of neurologic, muscular, or other organic impairment – particularly of the ANS or spinal cord – that diverts the flow of semen.

4. In which illnesses should a physician assume that sexual dysfunction has a neurologic basis?
   a. XYY syndrome
   b. Mild mental retardation
   c. Parkinson disease
   d. Poliomyelitis
   e. Amyotrophic lateral sclerosis
   f. None of the above

Answer: f. Although each of these illnesses may cause neurologic dysfunction, the patient's sexual drive, genital sensation, and orgasmic reactions are preserved. Physicians should not assume that a patient's physical immobility impairs libido.

5. Immediately after sexual intercourse with his wife of almost 40 years, a retired baseball player seemed to forget his whereabouts and the events of the previous several hours, which included his 65th birthday party. When his wife brought him to the emergency room, he could not recall the name of the physician, despite three introductions, or a list of three objects; however, he recalled his age, telephone and Social Security numbers, and the names and birthdays of all his family members. He became frustrated, anxious, and distressed. A neurologist found no physical deficits. Which is the most likely diagnosis?
   a. Conversion disorder
   b. Alcohol intoxication
   c. Transient global amnesia
   d. Substance abuse

Answer: c. The development of acute amnesia in an elderly man after sexual intercourse or other strenuous activity, especially when antegrade amnesia predominates and personal information is preserved, indicates transient global amnesia (TGA).

6. During sleep, when do erections and seminal emissions ("wet dreams") occur?
   a. NREM
   b. REM
   c. Both REM and NREM, equally

Answer: b. Erections and emissions occur during REM sleep. Erections characteristically remain present on awakening, when the final REM period is waning.

7. In which situation is fertility lost?
   a. Women with cervical spinal cord transection
   b. Men with cervical spinal cord transection
   c. Men with diabetes mellitus and neuropathy
   d. Women with diabetes mellitus and neuropathy

Answer: b. Men with upper spinal cord injury tend to have reduced sperm concentration and abnormalities in the sperm that are present. Women are able to conceive and bear children despite spinal cord injury. Both men and women with diabetes remain fertile.

8. A 43-year-old man describes 2 days of erectile dysfunction each time he completes a 3-hour bicycle ride. He has no diabetes and takes no medications. Which is the most likely cause of his sexual difficulty?
   a. Compression of the pudendal nerve
   b. Excessive sympathetic autonomic nervous system activity
   c. A muscle disorder
   d. Excessive parasympathetic autonomic nervous system activity
   e. Psychologic factors

Answer: a. When he rides his bicycle, pressure between the seat and his symphysis pubis compresses his pudendal nerve. Bicycle riders also sometimes compress the adjacent blood vessels, which causes erectile dysfunction.

9. In which *two* conditions would cremasteric reflexes be lost?
   a. Diabetic autonomic neuropathy
   b. Anxiety
   c. Sacral spinal cord injury
   d. Frontal meningioma

Answer: a, c. Cremasteric reflexes, which are superficial reflexes rather than DTRs, require intact pudendal nerves, ANS, and spinal cord.

10. One month after falling down a flight of stairs, a 35-year-old man complains of low back pain and erectile dysfunction. Examination reveals loss of pinprick sensation below the waist, but intact position, vibratory, and warm–cold sensation. Deep tendon and cremasteric reflexes are intact, and plantar reflexes are flexion. Which is the most likely cause of the erectile dysfunction?
    a. Spinal cord injury
    b. Autonomic nervous system dysfunction
    c. Peripheral neuropathy
    d. Multiple sclerosis (MS)
    e. Alcoholism
    f. None of the above

Answer: f. The lack of objective neurologic deficit indicates that no neurologic injury has occurred. In fact, a structural lesion cannot cause the dissociation of pinprick and warm–cold sensation because both sensations travel in the same nerve pathways. Alcoholism may blunt the libido and cause a neuropathy. In alcoholic peripheral neuropathy, DTRs and sensation are lost.

11. Which is *not* an aspect of the Klüver–Bucy syndrome in monkeys?
    a. Psychic blindness
    b. Apathy
    c. Dementia
    d. Visual agnosia
    e. Increased homosexual, heterosexual, and autosexual activity

Answer: c. After temporal lobectomy, which includes removal of the amygdalae, monkeys demonstrate oral exploratory behavior. When the monkeys do not identify objects by their appearance even though their vision is intact, researchers label their behavior as visual agnosia or psychic blindness. In another characteristic behavior, the monkeys lose extreme emotion. For example, while they may appear fearless, the monkeys are actually apathetic. Most striking, they display intermittent aggressive behavior and increased, indiscriminate sexual activity.

12. In humans, which *two* of the following are frequent manifestations of bilateral temporal lobe damage?
    a. Memory impairment
    b. Placing food and inedible objects in their mouths
    c. Hypersexuality
    d. Rage attacks
    e. Obesity

Answer: a, b. In humans bilateral temporal lobe damage causes a modified version of the Klüver–Bucy syndrome consisting of impaired memory, a tendency to eat excessively, and, as in monkeys, an inclination to place inedible objects in the mouth. Contrary to the behavior in monkeys, affected humans control their sexual appetite and show no violent outbursts.

13. In humans, which one of the following conditions does *not* usually preferentially damage the limbic system?
    a. Herpes simplex virus
    b. Alcoholism
    c. TIAs of the posterior cerebral arteries
    d. Varicella zoster virus
    e. Frontotemporal dementia
    f. Paraneoplastic encephalitis

Answer: d. Because the amygdala and hippocampus are situated in the temporal lobes, these components of the limbic system are vulnerable to conditions that damage the temporal lobes. Herpes zoster due to varicella zoster virus often causes painful neuralgia in the trigeminal nerve distribution and other dermatomes, but it rarely infects the CNS. In contrast, herpes simplex virus, which has a predilection for the frontal and temporal lobes, frequently causes encephalitis characterized by memory impairment and partial complex seizures. Posterior cerebral TIAs lead to ischemia of the temporal lobes that causes confusion and memory impairment. Chronic alcohol abuse can cause Wernicke–Korsakoff syndrome, which is associated with hemorrhage into the mammillary bodies and other parts of the limbic system. Frontotemporal dementia, which includes Pick disease, causes early and severe atrophy of the frontal and temporal lobes. Paraneoplastic limbic encephalitis, a remote effect of carcinoma, causes memory impairment, seizures, and behavioral disturbances.

14. Which *two* of the following conditions are *not* consequences of a pituitary microadenoma?
a. Headaches
b. Hyperprolactinemia
c. Optic atrophy
d. Homonymous superior quadrantanopia
e. Irregular menses

Answer: c, d. Optic atrophy and homonymous superior quadrantanopia are manifestations of macroscopic but not microscopic pituitary adenomas. Physicians often diagnose microadenomas when patients present with headaches or infertility. Hyperprolactinemia or magnetic resonance imaging (MRI) changes in the pituitary may lead to the diagnosis of microadenoma. Whether the result of medications or microadenomas, hyperprolactinemia may cause sexual impairment.

15. In normal males, which of the following is *not* associated with REM-induced erections?
a. Dreams with or without overt sexual content
b. Most dreams, even with frightful or anxiety-producing content
c. Increased pulse and blood pressure
d. Increased testosterone level
e. An EEG that appears, aside from eye movement artifact, as though the patient were awake

Answer: d. Testosterone levels are not associated with erections. Treatment with testosterone usually increases muscle mass, but it not only fails to correct erectile dysfunction, it increases the risk of prostate cancer. During REM sleep, individuals have increased ANS activity and an EEG that has ocular movement artifact superimposed on an "awake" background pattern.

16. Which substance will usually reverse medication-induced (iatrogenic) priapism?
a. Epinephrine
b. Phentolamine
c. Papaverine
d. Prostaglandins

Answer: a. Injections into the dorsum of the penis (intracorporeal injections) of phentolamine, papaverine, or prostaglandins, which are vasodilators, will produce an erection in many men who have erectile dysfunction because of diabetes, multiple sclerosis (MS), spinal cord injury, adverse effects of medications, or psychogenic factors. However, men with vascular disease must use these injections with caution. Should priapism occur, an injection of epinephrine, a vasoconstrictor that reduces blood flow into the penis, can usually bring it to an end.

17. What is the origin of the sexual organs' sympathetic innervation?
a. Lower cranial nerves
b. Cervical and upper thoracic spinal cord
c. Lower thoracic and upper lumbar spinal cord
d. Sacral spinal cord

Answer: c.

18. What is the origin of the sexual organs' parasympathetic innervation?
a. Lower cranial nerves
b. Cervical and upper thoracic spinal cord
c. Lower thoracic and upper lumbar spinal cord
d. Sacral spinal cord

Answer: d.

19. What proportion of men with erectile dysfunction are helped by phosphodiesterase inhibitors, such as sildenafil?
a. 100%
b. 80%
c. 60%
d. 30%

Answer: c. Phosphodiesterase inhibitors help about 60% of men with erectile dysfunction. They are least effective in men who are older than 70 years, have poorly controlled diabetes, or smoke. However, they are helpful in men with erectile dysfunction from minor age-related changes, decreased libido, depression, and SSRIs.

20. What is the mechanism of action of phosphodiesterase inhibitors, such as sildenafil?
a. They provoke the release of nitric oxide (NO).
b. They promote the production of cyclic guanosine monophosphate (cGMP).
c. They enhance cGMP-phosphodiesterase, which metabolizes cGMP.
d. By inhibiting cGMP-phosphodiesterase, they increase or prolong cGMP activity.

Answer: d. Phosphodiesterase inhibitors inhibit the enzyme cGMP-phosphodiesterase. Increased or prolonged cGMP activity promotes genital blood flow.

21. Which president survived poliomyelitis (polio)?
a. J. Carter
b. T. Roosevelt
c. F. D. Roosevelt
d. J. F. Kennedy

Answer: c. As a young man, President Roosevelt contracted polio. He eventually required heavy braces for his legs and later was confined to a wheelchair. His case illustrates that polio may cause marked physical disability but typically spares intellectual abilities. (According to some authors, FDR's illness may have been Guillain–Barré syndrome and not polio, but this is a minority opinion.)

22. Which of the following sequences describes the path of the limbic system?
a. Fornix, mammillothalamic tract, amygdala, anterior nucleus of the thalamus, cingulate gyrus

b. Cingulate gyrus, mammillary bodies, mammillo-thalamic tract, anterior nucleus of the thalamus, hippocampus and adjacent amygdala

c. Hippocampus and adjacent amygdala, fornix, mammillary bodies, mammillothalamic tract, anterior nucleus of the thalamus, cingulate gyrus

d. Hippocampus and adjacent amygdala, mammil-lothalamic tract, fornix, hippocampus and adjacent amygdala, mammillary bodies, anterior nucleus of the thalamus, cingulate gyrus

Answer: c.

23. Which of the following acts as the neurotransmitter for *sympathetic* nervous system activity during sexual function?
    a. Acetylcholine
    b. Monoamines
    c. Serotonin
    d. Nitric oxide

Answer: b. Norepinephrine, a monoamine, acts as the neurotransmitter in the sympathetic nervous systems urging sexual function.

24. Which of the following acts as the neurotransmitter for *parasympathetic* nervous system activity during sexual function?
    a. Acetylcholine
    b. Monoamines
    c. Serotonin
    d. Dopamine

Answer: a. Acetylcholine acts as the neurotransmitter in the parasympathetic nervous system. The actual genital engorgement is mediated by nitric oxide (NO).

25. Which autonomic nervous system effect produces an erection?
    a. Increase in parasympathetic tone
    b. Decrease in parasympathetic tone
    c. Increase in sympathetic tone
    d. Decrease in sympathetic tone

Answer: a.

26. Which autonomic nervous system activity produces ejaculation?
    a. Increased parasympathetic tone
    b. Decreased parasympathetic tone
    c. Increased sympathetic tone
    d. Decreased sympathetic tone

Answer: c. Under normal circumstances, a switch from predominately parasympathetic to sympathetic tone advances the sexual response from arousal to orgasm. In highly anxious individuals, excessive sympathetic activity may suppress an erection or, if one occurs, precipitate a premature ejaculation.

27. At which age do men have the shortest orgasm latency (interval between orgasms)?

a. 8 years
b. 18 years
c. 28 years
d. 58 years

Answer: b. Men at age 18, who are in their sexual prime, have a latency as short as 20 minutes. As men age, their latency increases to days to weeks.

28. Which of the following is *not* a normal age-related sexual change in men older than 50 years?
    a. Erections decrease in rigidity.
    b. The penis loses its sensitivity to touch and vibration.
    c. Because of end-organ damage, serum testosterone concentrations rise.
    d. Erections decrease in duration.

Answer: c. In men over 50 years, erections decrease in rigidity and duration, and nerves in their penis, like their other peripheral nerves, lose sensitivity to touch and vibration. Although their serum testosterone concentrations are also frequently low, the decrease correlates poorly with erectile dysfunction. Testosterone injections will not restore erectile function, but they may restore a diminished libido.

29. Which of the following statements concerning α-adrenergic agonists and antagonists is *false*?
    a. α-Adrenergic antagonists, such as phentolamine, induce erections.
    b. Typical and atypical antipsychotic medications, which have α-adrenergic antagonist properties, occasionally produce priapism.
    c. Because epinephrine, an α-adrenergic agonist, reduces blood flow into the penis, it can abort priapism.
    d. Men taking phosphodiesterase inhibitors should not simultaneously take α_1-adrenergic antagonists because the combination may lead to generalized vasodilation and profound orthostatic hypotension.
    e. All of the above are true.

Answer: e. The general rule is that α-adrenergic agonists, such as epinephrine, lead to smooth muscle constriction of the arteries in the systemic circulation and the penis. When urologists inject epinephrine into the penis for treatment of priapism, it constricts the arteries and reduces blood flow into the penis. Blood drains out through the veins. In the opposite situation, α-adrenergic antagonists relax smooth muscle, allowing greater blood flow into the penis. Phosphodiesterase inhibitors, such as sildenafil, promote the accumulation of potentially dangerous concentrations of vasodilators, such as nitroglycerin.

30. A 48-year-old man, under treatment with an SSRI for depression, complains that he has developed erectile dysfunction. On the other hand, he reports that he is pleased that it has greatly improved his mood and energy level, and he has returned to work and resumed a social life. What would be the best treatment for the erectile dysfunction?

a. Stop the SSRI.
b. Reduce the dose of the SSRI.
c. Switch to a different class of antidepressant.
d. Add a phosphodiesterase inhibitor.

Answer: d. Although each of the options might be reasonable, the best initial step would be to try a phosphodiesterase inhibitor.

31. A 49-year-old man with diabetes, hypertension, and coronary artery disease described having erectile dysfunction. His primary care physician had prescribed a phosphodiesterase inhibitor. Although the medicine produced satisfactory erections, he developed postcoital severe throbbing headaches and on several occasions postcoital fainting. He returned very discouraged. Which of the following medicines would be best next step?
    a. A triptan for medication-induced migraine
    b. Tadalafil
    c. Vardenafil
    d. None of the above

Answer: d. The patient is probably taking an antihypertensive medicine or coronary vasodilator containing a nitrate in addition to the phosphodiesterase inhibitor. The interaction causes a vasodilatory effect that leads to migraine-like headaches and orthostatic hypotension. To correct this interaction, the physicians should change the antihypertensive or coronary vasodilator medicine.

32. A 34-year-old woman experiences throbbing hemicranial or generalized headaches at the moment of orgasm. Her neurologic examination is normal. Which is the most likely explanation?
    a. She has psychogenic headaches.
    b. The partner's sildenafil seeps into her circulation.
    c. She has repeated subarachnoid hemorrhages.
    d. She has a variety of migraine.

Answer: d. She is experiencing orgasmic cephalgia, which is a variety of migraine. Sildenafil may cause mild bilateral headaches, but only in the individual who takes it. Subarachnoid hemorrhage is usually a cataclysmic event and victims have nuchal rigidity, photophobia, and prostration. Moreover, it is not an event that recurs.

33. What is the role of nitric oxide (NO) in production of erections?
    a. NO acts as a neurotransmitter that promotes the production of cyclic guanosine monophosphate (cGMP).
    b. NO reduces cGMP production.
    c. NO promotes the production of cGMP-phosphodiesterase.
    d. NO reduces the production of cGMP-phosphodiesterase.

Answer: a. NO promotes the production of cGMP. An enzyme, cGMP-phosphodiesterase, metabolizes and thus inactivates cGMP.

34. Is the following statement *true* or *false*? Because clitoral blood flow and engorgement is controlled by nitric oxide (NO) and cyclic guanosine monophosphate (cGMP), phosphodiesterase inhibitors such as sildenafil are equally effective in treating female sexual dysfunction.
    a. True
    b. False

Answer: b. Despite the similar physiologic control systems, phosphodiesterase inhibitors have shown disappointing results in the treatment of female sexual dysfunction. A new medication, flibanserin, has been approved, however, for the treatment of hypoactive sexual desire disorder (HSDD), part of Female Sexual Desire/Arousal Disorder in DSM-5.

SLEEP DISORDERS

Neurologists describe sleep and its components, variations, abnormalities, and response to treatment through the lens of the *polysomnogram* (*PSG*). Although the clinical manifestations of a condition remain paramount, the PSG provides a unique physiologic correlate for most Sleep–Wake Disorders in the *Diagnostic and Statistical Manual of Mental Disorder, 5th Edition* (DSM-5). In sleeping individuals, the full PSG simultaneously records:

- Cerebral activity through several electroencephalogram (EEG) channels
- Ocular movements through right and left ocular channels (ROC and LOC)
- Chin, limb, or other muscle movement and tone through electromyography (EMG)
- Oxygen saturation and other vital signs
- Video of body movements, vocalizations, and other activity.

PSG studies readily distinguish the two phases of sleep. A *rapid eye movement* (*REM*) phase consists of dream-filled sleep accompanied by predominantly horizontal rapid eye movements and flaccid limb paralysis. A *nonrapid eye movement* (*NREM*) phase consists of relatively long stretches of essentially dreamless sleep accompanied, approximately every 15 minutes, by repositioning movements of the body (Table 17.1).

NORMAL SLEEP

REM Sleep

Because most people awakened during REM sleep report that they were dreaming, physicians equate this phase with dreaming. Dreams that occur during REM sleep possess emotional or intellectual complexity, at least on a superficial level, and rich visual imagery.

Except for the eye movements and normal breathing, people in REM sleep remain immobile with paretic, flaccid, and areflexic muscles. EMGs recorded from chin and limb muscles, which are a standard placement, show little or no electric activity (Fig. 17.1). This paralysis is fortuitous because it prevents people from acting out their dreams.

In marked contrast to the flaccid muscle paralysis during REM sleep, autonomic nervous system (ANS) activity increases and produces an increased pulse rate, elevated blood pressure, raised intracranial pressure, increased cerebral blood flow, greater muscle metabolism, and, in boys as well as men, erections. As though defying psychoanalytic interpretation, erections develop regardless of the content of the dreams. Investigators have implicated ANS overactivity associated with REM sleep as a factor contributing to the increased incidence of myocardial infarctions and strokes that strike sleeping individuals in the early morning.

Aside from eye-movement artifact, the EEG during REM sleep appears similar to the EEG during wakefulness. Overall, REM sleep – with its ANS activity and EEG patterns – resembles wakefulness far more than NREM sleep.

Dopamine, serotonin, histamine, and acetylcholine activity is associated with wakefulness. Activity of hypocretin (also known as orexin) is associated with wakefulness and lack of its activity is strongly associated with sleep. Despite its association with wakefulness, hypocretin maintains wakefulness rather than causes it. As far as sleep is concerned, decreased dopamine and serotonin activity, but increased gamma-aminobutyric acid (GABA) activity, characterize both NREM and REM phases. Curiously, increased acetylcholine activity is associated with REM sleep as well as wakefulness, but not NREM sleep. In general, medicines with anticholinergic side effects, including tricyclic antidepressants (TCAs) and many serotonergic antidepressants, suppress or delay the onset of REM sleep. As commonly seen in patients treated for allergies, antihistamines induce sleep. Lack of

---

TABLE 17.1 REM and the Three Stages of NREM in Normal Sleep

Stage		Bodily Movements	Ocular Movements	EMG	EEG
NREM					
N1	Light	Persistent face and limb tone with repositioning every 15–20 minutes	Slow, rolling	Continual activity	Attenuation or slowing of alpha (8–12 Hz) activity
N2	Intermediate	Same	Slow, rolling or none	Further reduction	Sleep spindles and/or K complexes. Low amplitude
N3	Slow-wave, deep, delta	Same	Absent	Further reduction	Slow (0.5–2 Hz) wave/delta activity
REM	Activated, paradoxical	Flaccid, areflexic conjugate paresis, except for brief face and limb movements	Rapid, ocular movement	Silent with artifact	Low amplitude, mixed frequency

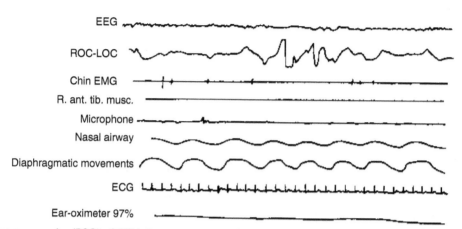

FIGURE 17.1 ■ Polysomnography (PSG) of REM sleep uses many channels to monitor physiologic functions. The EEG shows low-voltage, fast activity similar to the EEG activity of awake individuals. The electro-oculogram (EOG) channel – ROC-LOC – reflects several rapid eye movements (REM) by large-scale, quick fluctuations. Electromyograms (EMGs) of the chin and right anterior tibialis muscles show virtually no activity, which indicates an absence of muscle movement and tone (flaccid paresis). The microphone detects a snore. The regular, undulating airway and diaphragm recordings indicate normal breathing and air movement.

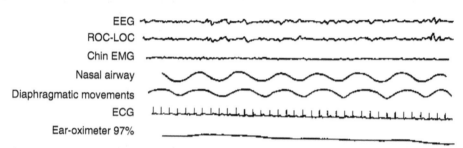

FIGURE 17.2 ■ The polysomnogram (PSG) of N1 stage sleep, which neurologists previously called stage I NREM sleep, shows low-voltage, 7-Hz activity. The ROC-LOC channel shows occasional slow ocular movement (i.e., no REM activity). The chin EMG shows continual low-voltage activity that reflects persistent muscle tone.

hypocretin causes episodic loss of wakefulness (narcolepsy with cataplexy, see later).

On an anatomic level, the perilocus ceruleus nuclei, situated in the pons immediately adjacent to the locus ceruleus nuclei (see Chapters 18 and 21), drive the eye movements, diminish muscle tone, and trigger dreaming during REM sleep.

NREM Sleep

NREM sleep, in contrast to REM sleep, has three stages (N1, N2, and N3) distinguishable primarily by progressively greater depths of unconsciousness and slower, higher-voltage EEG patterns. During early NREM sleep, eyes roll slowly and cognitive activity consists only of brief, rudimentary, and readily forgotten thoughts or notions. Unlike their ability to recall dreams that occur during their REM sleep, individuals have little or no recall of any thought content that might occur in NREM sleep.

Also unlike sleepers in an REM stage, those in an NREM stage have conspicuous repositioning movements, relatively normal muscle tone, and preserved DTRs. Their chin and limb muscles display readily detectable EMG activity (Fig. 17.2). In addition, NREM sleepers have a generalized decrease in ANS activity that may lead to hypotension and bradycardia. Similarly, their cerebral blood flow and oxygen metabolism fall to about

75% of the awake state, which is equivalent to the level induced by light anesthesia.

Nevertheless, important hypothalamic–pituitary (neuroendocrine) activity occurs during NREM sleep. For example, the daily secretion of growth hormone occurs almost entirely during NREM sleep, about 30 to 60 minutes after sleep begins. In another endocrine surge, serum prolactin secretions rise to their highest level at about the same time. Cortisol concentration is also sleep-dependent, but its secretion occurs in five to seven discrete late nighttime episodes, which accumulate to yield the day's highest cortisol concentration within a half-hour after awakening.

Overall, N3 sleep, often called *slow-wave* sleep, probably provides most of the physical recuperation derived from a night's sleep. After sleep "squeezes" N3 into the beginning of the night, sleep depth lightens and it allows more dreams, i.e., sleep shifts to N1, N2, and REM sleep.

Patterns

After going to bed, people usually fall asleep within 10 to 20 minutes. The interval between going to bed and falling asleep, *sleep latency*, is inversely related to sleepiness: the greater the sleepiness, the quicker people fall asleep, i.e., the shorter the latency. During daytime, sleep latency shrinks to its shortest duration at approximately 3 pm to 4 pm. However, social and physiologic factors alter the duration of sleep latency and the time of day when it is shortest (Box 17.1).

Another variable – *sleep efficiency* – is the ratio of the total time asleep to the time in bed. Reduced sleep efficiency, with a ratio significantly less than 1.0, characterizes insomnia and other disorders.

Once asleep, normal individuals enter NREM sleep and pass in succession through its three stages. After 90 minutes to 120 minutes of NREM sleep, they enter the initial REM period. Abnormalities in the interval between falling asleep to the first REM period, *REM latency*, characterize several sleep disorders, particularly narcolepsy (Box 17.2).

The NREM–REM cycle repeats throughout the night with a periodicity of approximately 90 minutes. REM periods develop four or five times in total, but in the latter half of the night they lengthen and occur more frequently (Fig. 17.3). Also, in the latter half of sleep, when the tendency toward REM sleep peaks, body temperature falls to its lowest point (the nadir). The final REM period typically merges with awakening. Consequently, people can most easily recall their final dream, which may incorporate surrounding morning household activities. In addition, because of residual REM influence, men's erections often persist on awakening.

Without external clues, an "internal biological clock," centered in the *suprachiasmatic nucleus* of the hypothalamus, sets the daily (*circadian*) sleep–wake cycle at 24.5 to 25 hours (Fig. 17.4). This nucleus also sets the circadian hormone and metabolic rhythms. Individuals forced to rely exclusively on their internal biologic clock such as participants in experiments that isolate them from their environment and its cues, for example, living in caves for months – gradually lengthen their circadian cycle to almost 25 hours.

Melatonin

Light–dark cycles regulate the sleep–wake cycle in large part through their effect on the pineal gland's synthesis and release of *melatonin* (*N*-acetyl-5-methoxytryptamine). The pineal gland synthesizes melatonin, which is an indolamine, through the following pathway:

$$\text{Tryptophan} \rightarrow \text{Serotonin} \rightarrow N\text{-acetyl-serotonin} \rightarrow \text{Melatonin}$$

Darkness promotes melatonin synthesis and triggers its release into the plasma. Thus, melatonin concentrations rise during the night. Similarly, because both natural and artificial light suppress melatonin synthesis and release, its concentration falls during daylight. The sleep–wake cycles of adolescents and teenagers, however, show a variation of that pattern. Their melatonin levels rise and fall at later times than in adults' cycles. That shift is consistent with their tendency to remain awake into the early morning and stay asleep until the late morning. Several studies have suggested that adolescents may show greater alertness and improved mood following a delay in the start of their school day.

BOX 17.1	Sleep Latency* Changes

Shortened sleep latency
    Alcohol- and drug-induced sleep
    Narcolepsy
    Sleep apnea
    Sleep deprivation
Prolonged sleep latency
    Delayed sleep phase syndrome
    Poor sleep hygiene
    Psychiatric disorders
    Restless legs syndrome

*Normal sleep latency is usually 10 to 20 minutes

BOX 17.2	Shortened REM Latency* or Sleep-Onset REM

Depression
Narcolepsy
Sleep apnea
Sleep deprivation^
Withdrawal from alcohol, hypnotics, and TCAs

*Normal REM latency is approximately 90 to 120 minutes
^As part of REM rebound

Sleep Deprivation

Although various sleep disorders cause *excessive daytime sleepiness* (*EDS*), the most common cause is sleep deprivation from environmental demands: social life, family

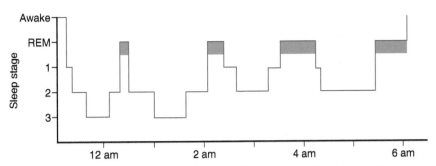

FIGURE 17.3 ■ In the conventional representation of a normal night's sleep pattern – its sleep *architecture* or *hypnogram* – the first REM period starts approximately 90 minutes after sleep begins and lasts about 10 minutes. Later in the night, REM periods recur more frequently and have longer duration. NREM sleep progresses through its three stages (N1–N3).

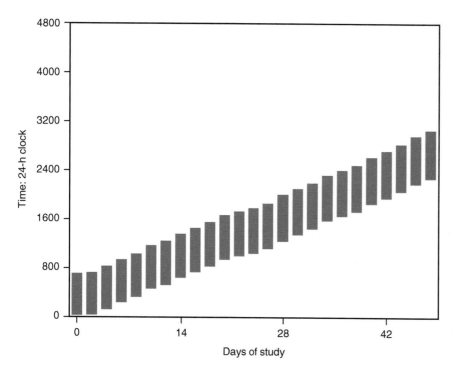

FIGURE 17.4 ■ When healthy young adults are allowed to sleep and arise at will in rooms protected from time cues, such as clocks, daylight, daytime sounds, and delivery of meals on a fixed schedule – "*free run*" – they typically go to sleep later each day (delay their sleep phase) and extend their sleep–wake (circadian) cycle to 24.5 to 25 hours.

obligations, and work. Physicians often use the Epworth Sleepiness Scale (Box 17.3) to quantifying sleepiness.

Sleep deprivation primarily impairs an individual's ability to concentrate. PSG studies following sleep deprivation show a short sleep latency, increased sleep time, a greater depth and duration of N3, and then REM rebound. REM rebound consists of three major components: the first REM period occurs within 15 minutes of falling asleep (*sleep onset-REM period* [*SOREMP*]); subsequent REM periods are longer than normal; and REM sleep occupies a greater proportion than normal of sleep time. Simply put, after missing sleep, people fall asleep early and deeply, dream plentifully, and remain asleep longer.

REM rebound commonly follows withdrawal from *REM-suppressing substances*, such as cocaine, amphetamines, opioids, alcohol, many hypnotics, and many antidepressants and hypnotics. People who suddenly stop chronic use of an REM-suppressing substance often undergo a period of frequent, vivid dreams that can reach the severity of nightmares. In a related example, during interrogations that include sleep deprivation, victims experience hallucinations, delusions, and cognitive disorganization.

Sleep deprivation, so commonplace that it is a public health problem, causes poor work performance and leads to increased appetite, weight gain, and a prediabetic state. Perhaps in a reciprocal situation, it aggravates chronic pain. Moreover, sleep deprivation is a major risk factor for motor vehicle crashes. It was implicated as a factor in the Chernobyl nuclear disaster, the near meltdown at the Three Mile Island nuclear reactor, and, along with alcohol, the Exon Valdez oil spill.

Studies have linked short sleep phase as well as frank sleep deprivation to coronary and cerebrovascular artery diseases, cancer, and "all-cause" mortality. They have not

---

BOX 17.3 | **The Epworth Sleepiness Scale**

How likely are you to doze off or fall asleep in the following situations, in contrast to just feeling tired? This refers to your usual way of life in recent times. Even if you have not done some of these things recently, try to work out how often they would have affected you. Use the following scale to choose the most appropriate number for each situation.

0 = would never doze
1 = slight chance of dozing
2 = moderate chance of dozing
3 = high chance of dozing

Situation	Chance of dozing
Sitting and reading	_____
Watching TV	_____
Sitting inactive in a public place, e.g., a theater or a meeting	_____
As a passenger in a car for 1 hour without a break	_____
Lying down to rest in the afternoon when circumstances permit	_____
Sitting and talking to someone	_____
Sitting quietly after a lunch without alcohol	_____
In a car, while stopped for a few minutes in traffic	_____
Total Score _____	

This widely used scale allows for a quantitative assessment of sleepiness and determination that an individual has excessive daytime sleepiness. A total score of <8 is normal; a total score of 9–12 indicates that the patient is possibly sleepy; a total score of >13 indicates that the patient is abnormally sleepy. Typical scores are 6 for normal individuals, 12 for patients with sleep apnea, and 18 for patients with narcolepsy.

From Johns MW. A new method for measuring daytime sleepiness: The Epworth Scale. Sleep 1991; 14:540–545.

only linked sleep deprivation to anxiety, depression, and psychosis, but also to more subtle disturbances, such as impaired recognition of human emotions.

EDS in children, whether from sleep deprivation, narcolepsy, or another disorder, leads to somewhat different symptoms than in adults. Instead of being merely sleepy, sleep-deprived children typically are inattentive, hyperactive, and appear to have learning disabilities.

Effects of Age

Infants and Children. Neonates sleep 16 to 20 hours a day, with about 50% of that time spent in REM sleep. Infants between 3 and 6 months begin to establish a circadian rhythm. Children aged 1 to 3 years spend 12 to 14 hours sleeping during the night and in afternoon naps, with about 30% of sleep in REM. Their NREM sleep, like adults' NREM sleep, predominates in the early night and increases following sleep deprivation and exhaustion.

As children grow, they sleep less and dream even less. By 3 to 4 years, they usually give up their afternoon nap by consolidating their entire sleep period into the night. As if by coincidence, growing out of their afternoon nap allows children to start a full day of school. The corollary of this development is that sleepiness in school children is abnormal. By the age of 5 years, the proportion of children's REM proportion falls to the adult level of 20% to 25% and their REM latency reaches the adult duration of 90 minutes.

Adolescents, Teenagers, and Adults. Adolescents and teenagers allow themselves too little time for sleep, despite their great need for it. They often remain chronically sleep-deprived. In these age groups, social behavior often leads to delayed or erratic sleep patterns.

Adults average 6 to 8 hours of total sleep time, but they require 7 to 9 hours. Consistently longer or shorter times are associated with poor health and reduced life expectancy. Compared to children and young adults' sleep, middle-age and older adults' sleep has a decreased proportion of deep NREM sleep and increased proportion of light REM sleep. REM continues to occupy the same proportion of sleep (20% to 25%).

Individuals Older Than 65 Years. Compared to young and middle-aged adults, those older than 65 years sleep less at night and have multiple brief awakenings, especially in the early morning. Although they spend more time in bed, they spend less time asleep, i.e., their sleep efficiency is low. However, they recoup some sleep during daytime naps, especially after meals and in the late afternoon. In another difference, they go to sleep in the earlier evening and awaken earlier in the early morning, i.e., they phase-advance their sleep. Thus, early morning awakening in the elderly does not necessarily constitute a sign of depression. PSG studies generally show that the proportion of N3 phases progressively declines with age.

In addition to these expected age-related changes, the elderly are vulnerable to several sleep–wake disorders, including restless legs syndrome, REM sleep behavior disorder, and breathing-related sleep disorders (such as sleep apnea). They are also vulnerable to other factors

BOX 17.4	DSM-5 Sleep–Wake Disorders: Major Categories and Some Subcategories

Insomnia disorder
Hypersomnolence disorders
Narcolepsy
    Narcolepsy without cataplexy
    Narcolepsy with cataplexy
Breathing-related sleep disorders
    Obstructive sleep apnea hypopnea
Circadian rhythm sleep–wake disorder
    Delayed sleep phase type
    Advanced sleep phase type
    Shift work type
Parasomnias
    Nonrapid eye movement sleep arousal disorders
        Sleepwalking type with or without sleep-related eating or sexual behavior (sexsomnia)
        Sleep terror type
    Nightmare disorder
    REM sleep behavior disorder
    Restless legs syndrome
    Substance/medication-induced sleep disorder

that disrupt sleep, including cardiovascular disturbances, medications, pain, and depression.

SLEEP DISORDERS

The DSM-5 defines Sleep–Wake Disorders on the basis of their PSG and other physiologic parameters as well as their clinical characteristics (Box 17.4). Its classification allows physicians, for the most part, to correlate abnormal sleep-related behavior with physiologic disturbances.

Insomnia Disorder

The DSM-5 diagnostic criteria for Insomnia Disorder require: (1) a dissatisfaction with sleep quantity or quality associated with difficulty initiating or maintaining sleep, and (2) that the sleep disturbance cause distress or functional impairment for at least 3 nights per week for 3 months. The criteria exclude sleeplessness from medicines or illicit drugs. Neurologists typically see insomnia as the most common sleep–wake disorder and difficulty maintaining sleep as its most common variety. They also encounter patients with insomnia as a distinct condition and as a manifestation of a medical or psychiatric illness. In an interesting twist, they sometimes find that despite certain individuals' reports of being sleepless, an accurate sleep–wake diary or a PSG will reveal that they sleep 6 or more uninterrupted hours almost every night. Neurologists term these underestimates *pseudoinsomnia* or *sleep state misperception*.

Nonpharmacologic Treatment of Insomnia

Studies generally have found that cognitive behavioral therapy (CBT), in one or another method, although sometimes supplemented by hypnotics, is the most effective, longest-lasting, and least hazardous therapy for insomnia disorder. CBT for insomnia consists first of practicing good *sleep hygiene*. Individuals with insomnia should adhere to a regular sleep schedule even on weekends; exercise on a regular basis, but only 4 to 6 hours before bedtime; avoid medicines that conceivably might interfere with sleep; stop evening coffee, alcohol, and large meals; dim the household lights, which should be amber-colored, for the hours before bedtime; restrict evening use of computers, which have bright screens, blue light, and exciting images; avoid daytime naps or allow themselves, at most, only a brief (<30 minute) early afternoon nap; and use the bed exclusively for sleeping.

In another nonpharmacologic CBT strategy, physicians institute *sleep restriction therapy* that essentially creates mild sleep deprivation to enhance sleep efficiency. Individuals using this strategy first reduce the time in bed to slightly less than the previous night's time asleep. They then postpone bedtime until they immediately fall asleep when getting into bed. Continuing to awaken at the customary time, they are deliberately sleep-deprived. Once sleeping almost the entire time while in bed and thus maintaining a high state of sleep efficiency, the individuals then expand the time in bed to increase sleep time.

Other CBT methods effective in insomnia include stimulus control, relaxation therapy, and cognitive therapy.

Pharmacologic Treatment of Insomnia

Almost all medicines that have secured a Food and Drug Administration (FDA) indication as a hypnotic fall into one of three categories (Box 17.5). Benzodiazepines, which activate $GABA_A$ receptors, decrease sleep latency by about 10 minutes, increase total sleep time by 30 to 60 minutes, and reduce the number of awakenings. On the other hand, they decrease REM and, more so, N3 sleep, which is sleep's most physically restorative phase. Moreover, depending on their dose, duration of action, and concomitant use of alcohol or other medicines, benzodiazepines tend to cause anterograde amnesia and confusion, unsteady gait and falls, hazardous driving, and EDS. With continued use, tolerance develops and patients require larger doses. Additionally, if patients abruptly stop long-term benzodiazepine treatment, they may suffer rebound insomnia and, in the extreme, withdrawal seizures.

BOX 17.5   **Major Groups of Hypnotic Agents**

Agents active at the benzodiazepine receptor
  Benzodiazepines
  Benzodiazepine receptor agonists ("Z drugs")
    Eszopiclone (Lunesta)
    Zaleplon (Sonata)
    Zolpidem (Ambien)
Melatonin receptor agonists
  Melatonin
  Ramelteon (Rozerem)
Orexin receptor agonists
  Suvorexant (Belsomra)

Benzodiazepine receptor agonists, which also activate $GABA_A$ receptors, not only offer similar benefits to benzodiazepines, they have minimal effect on sleep architecture and do not suppress REM or N3 sleep. Thus, when patients stop taking benzodiazepine receptor agonists, REM rebound and insomnia are less likely to occur. However, their adverse effects have been so daunting that the FDA has required a reduction in the recommended dose of at least one of them (zolpidem) for women and suggested a reduction for men. In addition to the benzodiazepines' adverse effects, benzodiazepine receptor agonists' adverse effects have been pronounced amnesia, hallucinations, violent outbursts, and complex, often dangerous behavior, including sleepwalking, driving while asleep, and nocturnal binge eating. The FDA classifies benzodiazepine receptor agonists, like benzodiazepines, as controlled substances.

Melatonin receptor agonists, such as ramelteon, naturally occurring melatonin, and pharmaceutically prepared melatonin, all bind to melatonin receptors in the suprachiasmatic nucleus. Like benzodiazepine receptor agonists, melatonin receptor agonists reduce sleep latency and, subjectively at least, improve sleep quality. They are not only effective in the treatment of insomnia, they help reverse jet lag, seasonal affective disorder, and delayed sleep phase (see later).

In contrast to benzodiazepine receptor agonists, melatonin receptor agonists do not impair cognition, cause imbalance, induce dangerous complex behavior, or fall into the category of controlled substances. Because fluvoxamine inhibits CYP1A2, which is the enzyme that metabolizes ramelteon, concurrent administration of fluvoxamine and ramelteon may lead to toxic concentrations of ramelteon.

The third category, which is new but will probably expand, consists of an orexin (hypocretin) receptor antagonist, suvorexant. Orexin, a peptide neurotransmitter, ordinarily maintains wakefulness. Its absence leads to sleepiness and sleep attacks, as in narcolepsy (see later). Presumably by blocking the orexin receptor, suvorexant reduces sleep latency, improves sleep efficiency, and lengthens sleep time. Like many other hypnotics, its tendency to produce sleepiness may extend into the following morning and may impair driving and other complex tasks. Withdrawal may cause rebound insomnia. Suvorexant is also a controlled substance.

Hypersomnolence Disorder

The core criteria of the DSM-5 category of Hypersomnolence Disorder are a main sleep period of at least 7 hours with one or more additional sleep periods during the same day, 9 hours or longer of unrefreshing ("nonrestorative") sleep periods, and difficulty on fully awakening from sleep. The DSM-5 also requires that the hypersomnia give rise to distress or functional impairment. However, it does not require PSG confirmation of a patient's report of the sleep schedule or any reaction to it. Neurologists see most cases of multiple or recurrent episodes of hypersomnia as a manifestation of drug or alcohol abuse, focal seizures, status migrainosus, tumors involving the hypothalamus, depression with atypical features, or the depressed phase of bipolar disorder. More rarely, they diagnose patients with recurrent, prolonged episodes of hypersomnia as having *Kleine–Levin syndrome*.

Kleine–Levin Syndrome

In this rare, idiopathic disorder, also called recurrent or periodic hypersomnia, patients – who are predominately adolescent or young adult males – sleep about 18 hours a day for periods of 1 to 4 weeks, one to four times a year until the episodes gradually disappear after about 14 years. As remarkable as the hypersomnia, Kleine–Levin patients remain in a trance for about one to several hours when seemingly awake during the episodes. In that twilight, they typically eat voluminous quantities of food (i.e., show hyperphagia or "morbid hunger"), display rudimentary sexuality (e.g., masturbate or expose themselves), and, when questioned, are confused, withdrawn, apathetic, or surly. If undisturbed, they return to bed to resume sleeping. After a hypersomnia episode resolves, Kleine–Levin patients show no overt neurologic deficits, resume a normal sleep–wake pattern, and have no psychiatric symptoms. Infections, drug or alcohol use, or traumatic brain injury (TBI) may precede a hypersomnia episode, but most arise spontaneously.

PSG, endocrine evaluation, and other physiologic studies have not discovered a consistent, significant abnormality. Neither antiepileptics (AEDs) nor antidepressants prevent or shorten episodes. Lithium may help. Modafinil may counteract the hypersomnia, but not the behavioral abnormalities.

Narcolepsy

A DSM-5 diagnosis of Narcolepsy requires primarily periods of irrepressible need to sleep that culminate in sleep and at least one of the following: cataplexy, hypocretin deficiency, or a confirming physiologic study (a nocturnal PSG showing sleep-onset REM periods or a *multiple sleep latency test* [*MSLT*] showing at least two sleep-onset REM periods with a sleep latency less than 8 minutes on average across all five naps). Neurologists, relying on the clinical presentation, look for the *narcoleptic tetrad*:

- Excessive daytime sleepiness with sleep attacks
- Cataplexy
- Sleep paralysis
- Sleep hallucinations.

Recent studies have discovered that narcolepsy is an adolescent- and young adult-onset illness. In 90% of patients, its symptoms first emerge between adolescence and age 30 years. However, its diagnosis is often not secured until patients reach their mid-30s. Young people with narcolepsy often remain undiagnosed or misdiagnosed as lazy, neurotic, or depressed.

The nearly universal clinical feature of narcolepsy, which affects males and females, is EDS. Not only do individuals with narcolepsy have perpetual sleepiness, they have irresistible naps (sleep attacks) that initially mimic normal daytime naps because they typically occur when patients are bored, comfortable, and engaged in monotonous activities. Each nap usually lasts less than 15 minutes

and can be easily interrupted by noise or movement. Narcolepsy-induced naps evolve into naps that have an unexpected, abrupt onset, occur many times each day, and, more strikingly, take place when patients are standing, during a lively interchange, or in the middle of activities that require constant attention, including driving.

Although a characteristic, sleep attacks are not found only in narcolepsy. They may also be a manifestation of sleep deprivation, sleep apnea, hypothalamic injury, Parkinson disease, or, ironically, dopamine agonist treatment for Parkinson disease.

Cataplexy accompanies narcolepsy in about 70% of narcolepsy cases, leading to the DSM-5 distinction of Narcolepsy With Cataplexy and Narcolepsy Without Cataplexy. When cataplexy develops, it appears in 50% of cases at 1 year and 70% of cases at 4 years into the illness. It consists of a sudden loss of muscle tone typically lasting between a few seconds and several minutes and occurring one to four times daily. During cataplexy, patients remain alert, but immediately afterwards they may have a sleep attack. Cataplexy-induced weakness tends to be symmetric and proximal. Most commonly, the neck muscles first weaken and the head falls forward. The legs or merely the knees frequently lose their tone. However, in cataplexy's most sensational form, which rarely occurs, patients' entire body musculature suddenly becomes limp and they collapse to the floor. When only the jaw, face, or neck muscles weaken, physicians might not recognize that the jaw dropping or head nodding represents cataplexy. The most common precipitant of cataplexy is hearing or telling a joke. In general, strong emotions – negative ones, such as anger, frustrations, and fear, as well as positive ones – provoke it.

Regardless of whether a group of muscles or the entire musculature weakens, affected muscles become flaccid and areflexic – as in REM sleep. Nevertheless, also as in REM sleep, patients breathe normally and retain full ocular movement.

Sleep paralysis and sleep hallucinations, which may each develop on awakening (hypnopompic) or falling asleep (hypnagogic), affect 25% to 50% of narcolepsy with cataplexy patients. Like cataplexy, they may appear several years after the onset of narcolepsy. In sleep paralysis, patients are unable to move or speak for as long as several minutes after awakening or when falling asleep, but they remain cognizant of their surroundings, breathe, and move their eyes. This situation may terrify the patients who vainly attempt to scream or move about. Sleep paralysis is a characteristic feature of narcolepsy, but it is not diagnostic because it may occur in sleep-deprived individuals and anyone else with REM deprivation.

During hypnopompic or hypnagogic hallucinations, patients essentially see vivid dreams while awake. Thus, narcolepsy qualifies as an organic cause of visual hallucinations (see Chapters 9 and 12). As with the other elements of narcolepsy, hypnopompic or hypnagogic hallucinations represent REM sleep intruding into people's wakefulness (Fig. 17.5).

In addition to this tetrad of symptoms, multiple, brief, spontaneous awakenings interrupt narcolepsy patients' nighttime sleep. These interruptions cause inadequate nighttime sleep that exacerbates the EDS.

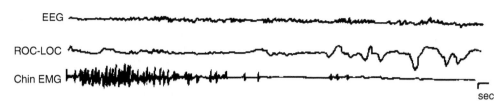

FIGURE 17.5 ■ During an event captured on a PSG, a narcoleptic attack begins when the EEG channel shows the low-voltage fast activity of REM sleep. The absence of chin EMG activity indicates that muscles are flaccid. After several seconds, rapid eye movements begin.

Testing

Neurologists use the MSLT to support a clinical diagnosis of narcolepsy. This test determines both sleep latency and REM latency during five "nap opportunities" offered at 2-hour intervals during the daytime. The DSM-5 criteria for Narcolepsy on the MSLT require a sleep latency of 8 minutes or less and two or more SOREMPs. A short REM latency (15 minutes or less) on the PSG the night before the MSLT supports the diagnosis or substitutes for one of the SOREMPs on the MSLT.

In a newly delineated aspect of narcolepsy, the most specific test finding for narcolepsy with cataplexy has been a low or absent concentration of hypocretin in the cerebrospinal fluid (CSF). Hypocretin is composed of a pair of polypeptide excitatory neurotransmitters, *hypocretin* 1 and 2, which are also known as *orexin* A and B. One research group named hypocretin for its location in the *hypo*thalamus, and another named the same molecule orexin (Greek, *orexis*, appetite).

Hypocretin normally maintains wakefulness and stimulates the appetite. Cells in the hypothalamus synthesize hypocretin and secrete some of it into the CSF. Hypocretin-producing cells project to several centers involved with sleep regulation, particularly the locus ceruleus and hypothalamic nuclei. Distinctive findings in narcolepsy with cataplexy are degeneration of hypocretin-synthesizing cells in the hypothalamus and the resulting near absence of CSF hypocretin (<110 pg/mL). Low levels of CSF hypocretin correlate much more closely with narcolepsy with cataplexy than narcolepsy without cataplexy. Curiously, in both conditions serum hypocretin concentrations remain normal, which suggests that cells outside the CNS also synthesize it.

Etiology

The most credible theory of the pathogenesis of narcolepsy is that an environmental factor, such as TBI or an infection, probably triggers an autoimmune process in genetically vulnerable individuals. Then the interaction destroys hypocretin-producing cells in the hypothalamus and thus causes narcolepsy or at least the variety accompanied by cataplexy. Evidence supporting this theory is that streptococcal antibody titers are often elevated in narcolepsy with cataplexy patients.

First-degree relatives have a 10- to 40-fold increased risk of developing the illness, but the concordance rate between monozygotic twins is only 25%. Narcolepsy with hypocretin deficiency also occurs in an autosomal recessive inheritance pattern in certain pony and dog families. Researchers use these animals as laboratory models of the disorder.

Almost 90% of narcolepsy with cataplexy patients carry a certain major histocompatibility complex, designated human leukocyte antigen (HLA) DQB1*0602, on chromosome 6. Despite the antigen's prevalence among narcolepsy patients, and its use as a screening test, the antigen is neither necessary nor sufficient for the diagnosis because approximately 25% of the asymptomatic general population carries it and most carriers show no signs of the illness.

Treatment

The primary goal in treatment of narcolepsy is for the patient to remain awake during critical times, particularly when driving, attending school, and working. In one approach, stimulants such as methylphenidate (Ritalin) and amphetamines, which enhance adrenergic and dopaminergic activity, reduce EDS and the naps. The major problem with this approach is its potential for abuse. For example, individuals may falsely but convincingly report symptoms of narcolepsy with cataplexy in order to secure these stimulants and then use them or sell them to others. Also, stimulants induce tolerance and, even at therapeutic doses, create psychiatric side effects.

In a newer approach to counter the EDS and tendency to napping, prescribing "wake-promoting agents" – the nonamphetamine medication modafinil (Provigil) or its long-acting, R-enantiomer version armodafinil (Nuvigil) – helps assure wakefulness without causing excitation or nighttime insomnia. Moreover, unlike stopping amphetamines and other stimulants, stopping these medicines does not lead to EDS or a rebound in NREM sleep. In other words, they do not merely keep people awake by postponing sleep. Modafinil increases the release of dopamine and serotonin, and elevates the levels of histamine. It also may interact with the dopamine transporter to inhibit dopamine reuptake and thus increase dopamine activity.

Despite these medicines' help in keeping patients awake, they have little effect on cataplexy. Instead, a rapid-acting hypnotic, oxybate (Xyrem), also known as gamma-hydroxybutyrate (GHB), reduces cataplexy. It provides for a more restful night of sleep, decreases EDS by reducing nighttime awakenings and increasing N3 sleep, and reduces hypnopompic hallucinations and sleep paralysis. A combination of GHB and modafinil is most effective. Imipramine and protriptyline also suppress cataplexy.

Although beneficial, illicitly prepared or illicitly used oxybate has caused many complications, including profound amnesia (which earned it the name "date-rape drug"), coma, seizures, and, with continued use, addiction (see Chapter 21). Even a pharmaceutical preparation in narcolepsy patients has led to sleepwalking, enuresis, confusion, and suicide ideation. It may also lead to depression in predisposed patients.

BREATHING-RELATED SLEEP DISORDERS

Obstructive Sleep Apnea-Hypopnea

Neurologists, other physicians, and this book use the term "sleep apnea" for the DSM-5 disorder Obstructive Sleep Apnea Hypopnea is the most clinically important type of Breathing-Related Sleep Disorders. Its DSM-5 diagnostic criteria require PSG evidence of five episodes per hour of obstructive apneas (absent airflow) or hypopneas (reduced or near absent airflow) and either: (1) clinical manifestations, such as snoring, snorting, gasping, or breathing pauses, or (2) EDS. Alternatively, the DSM-5 will accept as sufficient for the diagnosis a PSG demonstration of 15 or more episodes hourly of obstructive apneas or near-apneas, regardless of symptoms. In practice, loud nighttime snoring in individuals with daytime napping and sleepiness suggests sleep apnea.

Sleep apnea is one of the most common causes of EDS. The apneas produce at least partial awakenings ("microarousals"); however, patients remain unaware of them because they are so brief and incomplete. Nevertheless, the awakenings lead to restless sleep and EDS.

As breathing resumes at the end of an apneic episode, patients usually briefly snore or make other noises. During the daytime, because of their EDS, sleep apnea patients succumb to brief, unrefreshing naps. In a potentially misleading scenario, sleep apnea patients may describe their symptoms as chronic fatigue rather than chronic sleepiness.

In obstructive sleep apnea, fat-laden or weak soft tissues of the pharynx, congenital deformities, hypertrophied tonsils or adenoids, or other pharyngeal abnormalities block the airway. Neuromuscular disorders, such as bulbar poliomyelitis, can also narrow the airway by producing weakness of the pharynx.

Sleep apnea can produce arterial blood oxygen desaturation, cardiac arrhythmias, pulmonary hypertension, and systemic hypertension. Thus, sleep apnea constitutes a risk factor for stroke and myocardial infarction. It also causes or contributes to the metabolic syndrome, headache, and symptoms of depression. Like other causes of EDS, sleep apnea predisposes patients to motor vehicle crashes, impairs their cognitive function, and interferes with their social responsibilities. Some neurologists assert that sleep apnea is a cause of dementia and depressive symptoms. Moreover, given the effective therapies (see later), sleep apnea is a correctable cause of these problems.

In the classical conception, sleep apnea develops in obese middle-aged men. However, current studies have shown that it occurs frequently in other demographic groups. With the epidemic of obesity, teenagers have been developing sleep apnea. About 30% of all patients are not obese. Postmenopausal woman often develop sleep apnea that manifests as sleep-maintenance insomnia.

In addition, sleep apnea may develop in children. When it does, their symptoms, etiology, and treatment differ from those in adults. Instead of saying that they are sleepy, children with sleep apnea typically have attention deficits, hyperactivity, learning disabilities, and even aggression. They usually have airway obstruction from enlarged tonsils and adenoids. These children are not obese. Children with Down syndrome, because of the architecture of their neck, lax oropharyngeal muscles, and large tongue, are particularly susceptible. Tonsillectomy and adenoidectomy or reconstructive surgery generally alleviates sleep apnea in children.

In both children and adults, the PSG shows periods of apnea, hypoxia, and then arousals. It reveals episodes of loss of airflow despite chest and diaphragm respiratory movements (Fig. 17.6). Because of the sleep deprivation, sleep latency and REM latency both shorten and SOREMPs appear. During nighttime sleep, apnea episodes occur in either phase but more frequently during REM sleep because in that sleep phase, palatal and pharyngeal muscles are lax.

Treatment of sleep apnea should markedly reduce EDS, its systemic physiologic manifestations, particularly hypertension, and cognitive impairments. The initial management, in most cases, attempts to have patients lose weight, give up smoking, and stop using hypnotics and alcohol. If those strategies do not alleviate the

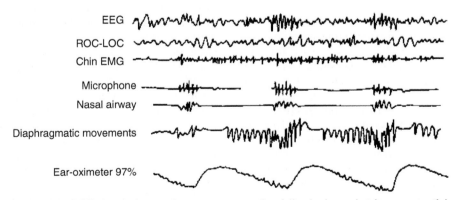

FIGURE 17.6 ■ In sleep apnea, the PSG shows that as the oxygen saturation falls, the hypoxia triggers a partial arousal, indicated by fast EEG activity. Diaphragmatic movements reach a crescendo and loud snoring begins. After strenuous diaphragm movements, air moves through the nasal passage and oxygen saturation improves.

problem, physicians prescribe ventilation by nasal continuous positive airway pressure (CPAP). Although the device is cumbersome, CPAP remains the mainstay of treatment. Other devices that might assure a patent airway include a tongue-retainer and mandibular advancement prosthesis. The addition of modafinil may further reduce EDS. Physicians should avoid prescribing benzodiazepines, other hypnotics, and opioid analgesics because they depress respirations. They should also avoid prescribing psychotropics that increase weight.

Central sleep apnea, which is less common than obstructive sleep apnea, results from reduced or inconsistent CNS ventilatory effort or congestive heart failure. For example, patients who have sustained lateral medullary infarctions and other injuries to the medulla (see Chapter 2), which houses the respiratory drive center, are susceptible to central sleep apnea.

Circadian Rhythm Sleep–Wake Disorders

In these disorders, individuals maintain an unconventional sleep–wake schedule. These disorders lead to insomnia, EDS, or both. Their variants include schedules in which sleep-time constantly begins later or earlier than usual and, most commonly, where the sleep-time varies week by week (shift-work). Even though the DSM-5 no longer includes them, neurologists would include in this category sleep–wake schedule disruptions because of travel across time zones, i.e., "jet lag."

Delayed Sleep Phase Type

In this variation, sleep starts at least 2 hours later than a conventional sleep-time, but thereafter has a normal quality and duration. Body temperature and melatonin concentration correlate with the sleep–wake cycle.

Although genetic predisposition may play a role, delayed sleep phase commonly develops in adolescents during a vacation when they remain active until the early morning. Although the pattern may seem benign during a vacation, it may persist after the vacation ends. With the unconventional timing, they cannot attend either to school or work without being tardy, and they are sleepy at school and work. In addition, because they cannot fall asleep at a conventional time, they appear to have sleep-onset insomnia. Uncorrected delayed sleep phase in university students portends daytime dysfunction after graduation.

The insomnia and EDS associated with delayed sleep phase separate it from sleep–wake schedules that conform to the lifestyle where individuals happily work and live, such as those in the entertainment industry. Depression and personality disorders are also associated with delayed sleep phase.

Delayed sleep phase resists the usual sleep-altering interventions, such as hypnotics and instruction to go to bed earlier. Fortunately, two complementary, predominantly nonpharmacologic therapies are able to restore a conventional schedule. Both require about 2 weeks and then sometimes supplementary melatonin once the desired schedule is reached.

Chronotherapy incrementally shifts the patient's sleep-wake schedule. One strategy is to phase-advance the schedule by advising the patient to go to sleep each night 15 minutes earlier and awaken each morning 15 minutes earlier until the desired schedule is reached. Another, complementary strategy is to phase-delay the schedule by advising the patient to delay sleep and the time of awakening by 1 to 3 hours each day. In these chronotherapy strategies, patients may need to resort to using coffee, sunlight, strong artificial light, or stimulating activities to awaken themselves in the morning and postpone sleep at night. Once at the desired sleep–wake schedule, melatonin may maintain it.

Light therapy (*phototherapy*) phase-advances patients' sleep–wake schedule. It probably relies in part on the melatonin release triggered by darkness. Patients use bright, artificial lights to awaken themselves in the morning and dim or amber lights to create a soporific mood in the evening.

Advanced Sleep Phase Type

In *advanced sleep phase*, the less frequently occurring counterpart of delayed sleep phase, patients fall asleep and awaken at substantially earlier times than the conventional schedule. As with delayed sleep phase patients, advanced sleep phase patients secure the full duration and restfulness of sleep. Also, PSGs show normal architecture, and body temperature and melatonin concentration fluctuations coincide with their sleep pattern. However, they are vulnerable to insomnia and EDS.

Individuals following this schedule go to sleep, for example, at 9 pm and awake at 5 am. Some accommodate their propensity to this schedule by seeking work in occupations that require full early morning activity, such as living in California and following the New York Stock Exchange. Many normal older individuals who awake early in the morning have Advanced Sleep Phase. In certain families, a genetic variation underlies Advanced Sleep Phase. Individuals with bipolar and depressive disorders sometimes follow an advanced sleep phase pattern.

Shift-Work Type

"Shift work" refers to a schedule of either rotating work or perpetual evening or nighttime work. Almost 20% of American workers have schedules that change on a weekly, monthly, or seasonal basis. Shift work tends to cause sleepiness, poor performance at work, and numerous problems when not working. Shift work problems plague medical house-staff, police officers, factory workers, and other individuals who must work daytime shifts and then rotate to evening or nighttime shifts. For example, medical house officers completing shifts longer than 16 hours report committing many more errors than those working fewer hours. Nurses also make fewer errors with less time on night shifts. Reports have implicated shift work in major public transportation accidents, such as recent New York City train crashes and interstate trucking accidents. Studies have found that shift work is associated with an increased incidence and increased severity of obesity, diabetes, hypertension, congestive heart failure, depression, and substance abuse.

Although most workers can transition to a new schedule after several days, some are unsuccessful because their internal schedule is deeply ingrained or, during weekends or holidays, they revert to their old schedule. While working a midnight shift, for example, their "daytime sleepiness" tends to occur at 4 am. Older workers are less resilient than younger workers.

Several strategies may help. Workers should remain on a given shift for as long as possible and maintain their work schedule through weekends and short holidays. Management should enhance the light at the workplace. If workers are sleepy on the job or driving home, they should drink coffee, seek bright light, and postpone potentially dangerous activities. Severely affected workers may benefit from taking modafinil, which has received an FDA indication for shift work sleep disorder. If insomnia is a problem, especially when beginning a new schedule, melatonin may help.

Jet Lag

Even though DSM-5 has omitted jet lag – perhaps because it is a brief, benign, and self-limited disorder – most physicians still recognize jet lag and attempt to prevent or treat it. Previously known as time zone change syndrome, jet lag consists of travelers across two or more time zones having several days of insomnia and EDS. Until they transition, their temperature fluctuations and hormone secretions, as well as their sleep–wake schedule, remain pegged to their home city.

East-to-west (westward) trips create fewer problems than west-to-east (eastward) ones because travelers can more easily postpone (delay) their night's sleep than fall asleep earlier (advance it). For example, travelers from New York to Los Angeles can, with a little effort, postpone their sleep-time by 3 hours, but those traveling in the opposite direction cannot so easily fall asleep 3 hours earlier.

When going in either direction, travelers can minimize jet lag by adopting the schedule of their destination several days to a week before their trip. For important events, travelers should arrive several days ahead of time. When going from New York to Los Angeles, for example, travelers should remain in sunlight as long as possible in the late afternoon on the West Coast to maintain their alertness. Those arriving in New York from the West Coast, the more taxing trip, should seek a sun-exposed location and drink a strong cup of coffee in the early morning. If they wish to go to sleep at a conventional East Coast time, they should avoid bright lights after sunset. In addition, once they reach their destination on long west-to-east flights, travelers can take a hypnotic to adopt the earlier local sleep time. On long east-to-west trips, travelers may adjust more easily if they nap.

PARASOMNIAS

Parasomnias (Latin, *para*, next to; *somnia*, sleep) are abnormal events that interrupt otherwise normal sleep. They usually last 1 to 10 minutes and arise during either the NREM or REM phase. They are prime examples of physiologic disturbances causing complex mental or behavioral aberrations. Focal seizures (see Chapter 10),

TABLE 17.2	**Sleep Terrors Compared to Nightmares**	
	Sleep Terrors	**Nightmares**
Trigger	Partial awakening from deep sleep	Anxiety, fear; withdrawal from medicines or drugs
Onset	Early in night	Anytime during night
Sleep stage	N3 (slow-wave sleep)	REM
Verbalization	Crying, screaming	Speaking words, conversing
Autonomic discharge	Marked	Little
Behavior after episode	Returns to deep sleep without recall	Awakens, recalls dream content, fearfulness

REM, rapid eye movement

nightmares (Table 17.2), panic attacks, and adverse reactions to medications or illicit drugs may mimic parasomnias. However, a PSG will distinguish a parasomnia from these other conditions.

NREM Sleep Arousal Disorders

The DSM-5 diagnostic criteria require recurrent episodes of incomplete awakening (partial arousal) from sleep for a diagnosis of Sleep Terrors, Sleepwalking, or both. Because NREM sleep arousal disorders usually arise out of N3 sleep, they usually occur within the first third of sleep – in the early night – when this stage predominates. Although sleep walking and sleep terrors generate a great deal of activity, individuals are not acting out a dream, which only takes place within REM sleep. Also, they will not recall the episode or thought content, if any were present, on awakening the next morning. In most cases, an outside event, such as a household noise, passing fire truck, or an internal sensation, such as thirst or a full bladder, arouses a susceptible person and triggers these parasomnias. Sleep deprivation makes children and adults susceptible because, when "overtired," they tend to fall rapidly into N3 sleep. Thus, these parasomnias frequently develop or increase in frequency when toddlers grow old enough to give up their afternoon nap. The parasomnias presumably occur when an immature, exhausted, or disordered physiology cannot make an orderly transition from deep sleep to wakefulness.

Children may have more than one variety of parasomnia and display complex behavior during each of them. For example, sleepwalking is comorbid with sleep terrors. However, in children, psychiatric disturbances are not comorbid with parasomnias.

During episodes of NREM sleep arousal disorders, the individuals' eyes are open and they are confused. In fact, neurologists continue to diagnose another NREM parasomnia, *confusional arousals*. In this variation, which the DSM-5 does not include, individuals display mental confusion or confusional behavior for several minutes to several hours following arousal from deep, N3 sleep. Immediately after the episode, they return to sleep.

Parents trying to prevent sleepwalking and sleep terrors should encourage predisposed children to increase sleep. They should minimize arousal by sleep disruptors, such as siblings' loud noise. Similarly, they should limit children to only a few sips of water at bedtime to avoid awakening to urinate. In the case of sleepwalking, parents should ensure the child's safety by installing night-lights, blocking windows and staircases, removing toys and other obstacles from the floor, and placing alarms in strategic locations. Medications to interrupt these parasomnias are not feasible because each episode is too brief. Preventative medications, especially in children, are rarely warranted.

Sleep Terrors

Sleep terrors, also called "night terrors," consist of episodes in which children suddenly, after a partial arousal from N3 sleep, behave as though they were in great danger. They stare, moan, and sometimes scream incessantly with their eyes fully open and their pupils dilated. They sweat, hyperventilate, and have tachycardia. Parents cannot fully wake them, put them back to bed, or comfort them. The children often leave their parents' arms to walk aimlessly, which constitutes simultaneous sleepwalking. Although the sleep terrors seem interminable to distraught parents, the episodes usually last 1 to 10 minutes and end abruptly with a return to deep sleep. Despite the episodes' vivid and awesome features, children characteristically do not recall them in the morning.

Sleepwalking

Sleepwalking (*somnambulism*) usually consists of sitting, standing, or walking, but occasionally more complex activities, including sleep talking, in the midst of sleep. Sleepwalking children rarely display any emotion. In a typical episode, a child walks slowly, with eyes open and a blank facial expression, along familiar pathways. While in the trance, sleepwalking children may urinate in a bathtub or closet. Although they appear partially awake, their parents cannot completely awaken them or capture their attention. When questioned during their trip, children cannot recall their whereabouts, remember recent events, or even converse sensibly; however, they will follow a lead back to bed. As with other NREM parasomnias, children will have no recall of the event.

Sleepwalking in adults, unlike sleepwalking in children, often arises during N1 or N2 sleep, rather than N3 sleep. Also in adults, various psychiatric disturbances, a history of violence, sleep apnea, and use of hypnotics, particularly zolpidem, are risk factors for sleepwalking. In some cases, sleepwalking and other NREM parasomnias have a genetic basis.

The DSM-5 recognizes two variants of sleepwalking. In one, Sleep-related Eating, individuals have episodes lasting 5 minutes or less that interrupt NREM or occasionally REM sleep, during which they consume high-calorie ("junk") food and barely edible foods, such as frozen pizza or raw meat. Although they most often eat food that they have left on their night table, they sometimes prepare an entire meal. These individuals may binge, but they do not purge. Probably because they remain asleep while preparing food, they tend to accidentally cut or burn themselves. As with other parasomnias, they have little or no recollection of the night's events in the morning, i.e., they have partial or complete amnesia. However, debris from the food or scattered kitchenware may prompt them to recognize their night's foraging. Depending on many factors, episodes may constitute manifestations of an eating disorder (night eating syndrome, nocturnal eating, or nighttime eating), Prader–Willi syndrome, or Kleine–Levin syndrome rather than a variation of sleepwalking.

The other variant is Sleep-Related Sexual Behavior. Better known among some as "*sexsomnia*" or "*sleepsex*," sleep-related sexual behavior consists of any variety of sexual activity during sleep. The partner may be a lover or merely an acquaintance in the same room, or anyone of either sex. Sometimes a bed partner is receptive, but often the partner is unwilling and shocked. After awakening, the sexual aggressor has little or no recollection of the sexual behavior.

Episodes usually occur during NREM sleep, where voluntary muscles are potentially fully mobile. Unlike other parasomnias, physical contact and alcohol consumption are frequent triggers. Also, unlike other parasomnias, sleep-related sexual behavior begins during adolescence and tapers off during the fifth decade. It occurs more frequently in men than women.

Nightmare Disorder

The DSM-5 defines Nightmare Disorder essentially as repeated nightmares that cause significant impairment. It excludes those attributable to either substance abuse or a medication. In contrast to sleep terrors, nightmares are essentially dreams with frightening content and complex imagery ("bad dreams"). Also they occur in the second half of sleep, which is heavily weighted with REM periods. Children and adults who experience nightmares typically recall them and re-orient themselves when awakened. Nightmares cause only a muted sympathetic response. Because they almost all arise in REM sleep, which causes quadriparesis, nightmares generally do not cause bodily movement. Also, the eyes are closed during a nightmare.

In adults as well as children, nightmares occur during REM periods. Adults also tend to have frequent and intense nightmares as a part of REM rebound. Therefore, an evaluation of nightmares in adults should explore not only the circumstances and content of the dreams, but the patient's use of alcohol, drugs, and medications and the possibility of sleep deprivation, especially from sleep apnea. Adults also have nightmares as a symptom of Posttraumatic Stress Disorder (PTSD). In PTSD, successful treatment of nightmares reduces its overall burden – if only by allowing a restful night's sleep. In addition to distinguishing nightmares from sleep terrors, physicians might consider *panic attacks*, which most often strike during the transition from drowsiness into light NREM rather than during deep NREM or REM sleep. Panic attacks usually contain no visual imagery, but they fully awaken the patient who is able to recall the fears. Another reasonable alternative to a diagnosis of nightmares is nocturnal focal seizures. One clinical difference is that nightmares differ in content, but seizures tend to create the same imagery. A PSG will readily capture seizures through its EEG leads.

REM Sleep Behavior Disorder

For the diagnosis of REM Sleep Behavior Disorder, which is one of the most dramatic neurologic conditions, the DSM-5 primarily requires repeated episodes of vocalization, complex movements related to dream content, or both during REM sleep. It also requires either PSG documentation that the patient was in REM sleep during episodes unless they arise in patients with a synucleinopathy, particularly Parkinson disease or dementia with Lewy bodies disease (see Chapters 7 and 18). The DSM-5 diagnostic criteria exclude situations where medications, illicit drugs, or medical conditions may be responsible for the episodes.

During normal REM sleep, even during nightmares, the perilocus ceruleus nuclei induce quadriparesis, atonia (flaccidity), and areflexia in limb and trunk muscles. This normal immobility, among other purposes, protects people from acting out their dreams. In comparison, REM Sleep Behavior Disorder releases individuals from the physical inhibitions of REM sleep. With the capability of moving and with normal muscle tone, patients show *dream enactment behavior* during an episode. They move their limbs and thrash, hit, or make running movements. They may also speak, shout, or scream. All this activity may injure a bed-partner.

Like other dreaming individuals, REM sleep behavior disorder patients' eyes are closed and, when awakened, they are alert and usually able to recall the dream. In their case, however, the dream typically has entailed defending themselves or avoiding an attack. Their recall contrasts with that of patients with sleep terrors, an NREM parasomnia, who typically remain amnestic for the episode.

Individuals with REM sleep behavior disorder are usually men older than 65 years. REM sleep behavior disorder develops before, during, or after the onset of Parkinson disease in 30% to 50% of cases and Lewy bodies dementia in 50% to 80% of cases. In these synucleinopathies, REM sleep behavior disorder correlates with cognitive impairment.

Although antidepressants and other medicines suppress REM sleep, they all may paradoxically create all the symptoms and signs of REM sleep behavior disorder. One possible explanation is that these medicines allow persistent muscle activity during REM sleep. The REM rebound that follows medication withdrawal may also precipitate attacks. The DSM-5 would probably not accept these situations as examples of REM sleep behavior disorder because they are secondary causes.

A PSG during an episode would show the signature of *REM sleep without atonia* and that the episodes arise in REM sleep. In addition, a PSG may diagnose other conditions that cause movement or vocalization during sleep, including seizures, sleepwalking, and other NREM parasomnias, sleep apnea, and willful violence. When comorbid with a synucleinopathy, the DSM-5 does not require PSG confirmation of REM Sleep Behavior Disorder.

Clonazepam 1 mg taken at night reduces or abolishes episodes of REM sleep behavior disorder. In fact, clonazepam suppresses the episodes so consistently that successful treatment supports the diagnosis. Melatonin in high doses may help.

Restless Legs Syndrome

The DSM-5 criteria for Restless Legs Syndrome (RLS) require painful or uncomfortable paresthesias that generate an irresistible urge to move. In an absolute requirement for the diagnosis, the urge should arise primarily or exclusively during rest, inactivity, or, particularly, bedtime. Also, the movement must satisfy the urge. The criteria exclude cases in the presence of peripheral vascular disease or other local tissue damage, where patients use cocaine or other illicit drugs, or where patients use dopamine-blocking antipsychotics that cause akathisia (see Chapter 18).

Neurologists would add that the movements should occur predominantly when patients rest or try to sleep, but not when they are actually asleep. They find that RLS patients typically seek relief by arising from bed and walking around; moving their feet back and forth while sitting in a chair; or, while lying in bed, performing bicycling movements. Most patients are adults, but children may have the disorder.

Like patients with tics or akathisia, those with RLS have psychologic discomfort if they fail to respond to the urge and then a sense of relief after they comply. In addition, about 80% of RLS patients have comorbid *periodic limb movement disorder* or its limited form, *periodic leg movements* (see later). RLS not only interferes with falling asleep, it causes sleep-onset insomnia, and then it disrupts sleep. All the movement causes EDS in both the bed-partner and the patient.

Several other conditions cause an urge to move and actual movement of the legs, but the DSM-5 precludes psychiatrists from diagnosing RLS in their presence. For example, polyneuropathy – from ischemia, diabetes, or uremia, and iron-deficiency anemia, characterized by low concentrations of serum ferritin (an iron protein complex) – causes RLS symptoms. In their third trimester, pregnant women often develop RLS symptoms, presumably because their expanded uterus irritates the adjacent lumbosacral nerves, but not because of low ferritin concentrations. According to some studies, selective serotonin reuptake inhibitors and selective serotonin and norepinephrine inhibitors (SSRIs and SNRIs) cause RLS symptoms. Dopamine receptor-blocking antipsychotic agents cause akathisia. A benign condition characterized by involuntary nocturnal leg movements, but lacking a sensory component, comprises the familiar, benign, leg thrusts – *sleep starts* or *hypnic* or *hypnagogic jerks* – in which people feel as if they are falling.

An observation that many otherwise healthy individuals with RLS have close relatives with the same problem indicates a genetic basis or susceptibility. Indeed, studies reveal a genetic polymorphism on chromosome 6 in many patients.

For treatment of idiopathic RLS, dopaminergic medications – particularly dopamine agonists such as ropinirole, pramipexole, and rotigotine – reduce the urge to move, suppress the movements, and promote restful sleep. A nondopaminergic medicine, pregabalin, also helps. For patients with polyneuropathy-induced RLS symptoms, medicines that reduce paresthesias, such as gabapentin, reduce or alleviate symptoms and restore sleep. Correcting iron-deficiency anemia frequently reduces the paresthesias and movements.

Periodic Limb Movement Disorder

Undefined in DSM-5, periodic limb movement disorder consists of regular (periodic), episodic stereotyped movements of the legs or, less often, arms during sleep that interrupt sleep or cause daytime sleepiness. Most often individuals with this disorder repetitively jerk both feet upward (dorsiflex at the ankle) in brief (0.5- to 5.0-second) thrusts. When the movements are confined to the legs, neurologists call the disorder *periodic leg movements*. Movements take place at 20- to 40-second intervals, for episodes of 10 minutes to several hours primarily but not exclusively during stages of NREM sleep (Fig. 17.7).

The movements occur in close association with RLS, use of antidepressants, and the onset of certain medical illnesses, particularly anemia and uremia. Despite the frequent comorbidity of RLS and periodic leg movements, these conditions differ in many respects. Periodic limb movements occur at regular intervals, only during sleep, and do not arise as a response to either paresthesias or an urge. Although the movements do not interrupt the patient's sleep or cause EDS, they may disrupt the sleep of a bed partner who may then develop EDS.

Substance/Medication-Induced Sleep Disorder

Within the category of Substance/Medication-Induced Sleep Disorder, the DSM-5 includes the effects on sleep produced by intoxication, chronic use, or withdrawal from numerous medicines, illicit drugs, and foodstuffs.

The effects may consist of insomnia, EDS, parasomnias, or a combination of those disturbances. The DSM-5 criteria exclude from this category sleep disturbances that occur exclusively during delirium. Here are examples of common substances causing sleep–wake disorders. Later, the book discusses sleep–wake disorders attributable to illicit substances (see Chapter 21).

Alcohol

One of the most common sleep-altering substances is alcohol, especially because its consumption is widespread and its chronic overuse is often surreptitious. The first few hours of sleep after imbibing alcohol-containing drinks may be tranquil as alcohol often induces deep sleep. For the remainder of the night, after the body metabolizes the alcohol, sleep is light, fragmented, and filled with dreams. For the first portion, the PSG generally shows a short sleep latency and then N3 sleep. For the second portion, it shows N1 and N2, with fragmentation, and abundant REM sleep.

During withdrawal from alcohol, which replicates withdrawal from hypnotics, individuals suffer from insomnia and REM rebound. Hallucinations and agitation from the REM rebound may merge into delirium tremens and impair an alcoholic's ability to remain sober. Studies have shown that the severity of REM rebound and other sleep disturbances during alcohol withdrawal closely correlate with relapse.

Caffeine

Caffeine, the world's most common stimulant, is a major ingredient in coffee, tea, and soft drinks; chocolate and other foodstuffs; and over-the-counter medicines (Table 17.3). Individuals who deliberately or unknowingly ingest excessive caffeine (250 mg or more daily) frequently develop *caffeinism*, which consists of insomnia accompanied by combinations of restlessness, nervousness, and excitement with physical signs, such as diuresis, gastrointestinal disturbance, tachycardia, and cardiac arrhythmias. These symptoms form the basis of the DSM-5 disorder, Caffeine Intoxication, which is a variety of Substance-Related Disorders. Even with mild consumption, caffeine reduces N3 sleep and total sleep time.

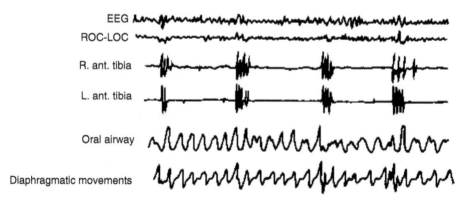

FIGURE 17.7 ■ A PSG in a patient with *periodic limb movement disorder* shows that at approximately 30-second intervals, synchronous anterior tibialis contractions cause the patient's ankles to dorsiflex.

TABLE 17.3 Caffeine Content (mg.) of Popular Beverages, Medicines, and Foods

Coffees*	
Brewed	
Generic	80–175
Decaffeineted	2–4
Dunkin' Donuts	143
Espresso^	100
General foods	
Café Vienna	90
Swiss mocha	55
Instant, generic	60
Starbucks	
Grande (16 oz)	330
Teas	
Lipton	
Brewed	40
Peppermint	0
Celestial Seasonings	
Ginseng	50
Herbal	0
Generic	
Black	45
Green	20
White	15
Green tea	30
Snapple	
Black	14
Lemon, peach	21
Sweet	8
Mistic Lemon	12
Nestea Lemon Sweet	11
Soft drinks	
7-UP	
Regular	0
Diet	0
AMP energy drink	71
Cocoa	2–20
Coca-Cola	
Classic 12 oz	35
Diet 12 oz	47
Dr. Pepper	28
Jolt	72
Mountain dew 12 oz	55
Pepsi-Cola	25
Sprite	
Regular	0
Diet	0
Medicines	
Anacin 2 tablets	64
Coryban-D Cold	30
Excedrin 2 tablets	130
NoDoz 1 tablet	200
Vivarin 1 tablet	200
Miscellaneous	
Ben & Jerry's Coffee	
Frozen Yogurt	85
Chocolate#	
Dark	20
Milk	6
Chocolate cake	20–30
Starbucks Coffee	
Ice Cream	40–60

*For coffees and teas, caffeine content varies by the type of bean or leaf, preparation, and duration of brewing as well as by the size of the serving
^1.5–2 oz
#One bar, approximately 1.5 oz

In the opposite situation, when habitual coffee drinkers abruptly stop taking caffeine, they experience headache, EDS, and various psychologic symptoms – fatigue or drowsiness, dysphoric mood, and inattentiveness – that the DSM-5 naturally labels Caffeine Withdrawal, another substance-related disorder.

Caffeine also alters the metabolism of several psychotropics. Probably because caffeine inhibits the cytochrome P-450 liver enzyme CYP1A2, caffeine consumption may potentiate many antidepressants (monoamine oxidase inhibitors [MAOIs], SSRIs, and duloxetine) and antipsychotics (clozapine, haloperidol, and olanzapine). In the opposite direction, some psychiatric medicines, such as fluvoxamine, a powerful CYP1A2 inhibitor, may increase caffeine levels. In another word of caution, caffeinated "energy drinks" are especially likely to raise plasma caffeine levels to levels that cause arrhythmias and other problems. These drinks contain high concentrations of caffeine and athletes who are dehydrated may gulp them thirstily.

Other Disorders

Depression

The effects of depression are pervasive. Depression disturbs sleep's onset, continuity, architecture, and duration. Depression can cause insomnia, EDS, and often both.

PSG changes in depression, which are more consistent than in any other psychiatric illness, consist of a characteristic triad of abnormalities:

- Short REM latency
- Increased REM duration and amount of eye movement per REM period (*REM density*)
- Decreased N3 (slow-wave or restorative) sleep.

Depression's most consistent feature is REM latency considerably shorter than the normal 90 minutes. It is often reduced to SOREMP. When they occur, REM periods are unusually long and occur in quick succession. The large number of REMs per minute (increased REM density) during the early nighttime leaves the latter portion of the night almost devoid of REM. Another typical abnormality consists of reduced and fragmented slow-wave, N3 sleep, which accounts for sleep's failure to refresh depressed patients and the subsequent onset of EDS. Finally, early morning awakening characterizes the sleep schedule of many depressed individuals; however, because the elderly also phase-advance their sleep schedule, early morning awakening is not always indicative of depression.

In addition, depressed individuals have neuroendocrine abnormalities related to their sleep alterations. Their body temperature nadir occurs several hours earlier than normal. Likewise, they have an earlier excretion of cortisol and the norepinephrine (noradrenaline) metabolite MHPG. Overall, the earlier onset of so many features of sleep – the first REM period, the bulk of REM sleep, the temperature nadir, and nocturnal hormone excretion – results from an advance of the normal circadian rhythm. When depressed people fall asleep, they seem to skip into the middle of a normal sleep and neuroendocrine cycle. Sleep disturbances are such an integral part of depression that when it remits spontaneously or responds to medication, sleep disturbances are one of the last symptoms to improve.

As a general rule, antidepressants decrease REM and delay remaining REM activity, i.e., restore normal REM latency. Curiously, fluoxetine induces prominent REM-like ocular movements during NREM sleep that may persist after it has been discontinued. In general, the following psychotropics decrease REM activity and delay its onset (prolong REM latency): TCAs, SSRIs and SNRIs, MAO inhibitors, lithium, benzodiazepines, and amphetamines. The opposite also applies. Withdrawal of these REM-suppressing psychotropics increases REM activity, advances its onset (decreased REM latency), and often provokes REM rebound.

Posttraumatic Stress Disorder

Sleep problems also constitute an integral part of PTSD. The DSM-5 cites "recurrent distressing dreams … related to the event" as one of several intrusion symptoms of PTSD. Other common PTSD symptoms include insomnia, nightmares, excessive awakenings, arousals, and EDS. In addition, several PTSD comorbidities cause sleep problems. For example, many PTSD patients have – alone or in various combinations – concussions and traumatic brain injury (TBI), painful conditions, obstructive sleep apnea, or substance use disorder, especially with opioids or cannabis. Early treatment of PTSD sleep symptoms may hasten recovery. Unless they respond to treatment, persistent PTSD-associated sleep symptoms constitute a risk for poor overall outcome.

Parkinson Disease

Parkinson disease's tremor and rigidity, as well as chorea and hemiballismus (see Chapter 18), characteristically disappear during sleep. On the other hand, Parkinson disease and medicines that treat it cause daytime sleepiness with unintentional napping and fragmented nighttime sleep. As with other synucleinopathies, REM sleep behavior disorder is comorbid with Parkinson disease. Also, Parkinson disease medicines, particularly dopamine agonists, may cause episodes of irresistible sleep (*sleep attacks*) that interrupt activities, preclude driving, and prompt vivid, frightening dreams.

In general, sleep disorders affect most Parkinson patients who have moderate to advanced disease. Of the many symptoms of the disease, sleep disturbances are the ones that most often force caregivers to place Parkinson disease patients in nursing homes. To alleviate some of the sleep problems, neurologists reduce the number and dosage of medications and administer the last doses early in the evening. Although antipsychotic agents may reduce nighttime hallucinations and agitation, they generally worsen rigidity and bradykinesia.

Other Movement Disorders

Stereotyped, forceful teeth grinding or clenching, *bruxism*, makes a loud, disconcerting sound and leads to the wearing away of teeth, headaches, and temporomandibular joint

dysfunction. Although it occurs in all sleep stages, bruxism generally develops in the transition from wakefulness to sleep and during light sleep. To some authors, bruxism falls within the category of NREM parasomnia. Individuals with major neurocognitive disorder, intellectual disability, or Parkinson disease often have bruxism while awake as well as when asleep. Use of SSRIs, cocaine, or other psychotropic substances may also cause transient bruxism. Nighttime dental devices help by cushioning the teeth.

In a similar condition, *rhythmic movement disorder*, infants, children, and occasionally adults have rocking of their head, trunk, or entire body while lying in bed during the transition from wake to sleep or during the initial stages of sleep at night. The condition usually begins in infancy and disappears by age 5 years. The movement usually consists merely of children's slowly rocking their head back and forth on a pillow; however, they sometimes increase the force and extent of the movement until it reaches the point of *head banging* or vigorous side-to-side rocking of the entire body.

Fatal Familial Insomnia

Fatal familial insomnia (*FFI*) consists of progressively severe insomnia, refractory to hypnotics, that appears on the average at 50 years of age. Like Creutzfeldt–Jakob disease (see Chapter 7), FFI is caused by a mutation of the prion protein gene (PRNP) that results in accumulation of abnormal prion protein (PrP^{Sc}). Cognitive impairments, including inattentiveness, amnesia, sequencing problems, and confusion, develop and worsen along with the insomnia. Later in their course, patients also develop hyperactive ANS activity (tachycardia, hyperhidrosis), endocrine abnormalities (elevated catecholamine and other hormone levels), and motor abnormalities (myoclonus, ataxia). FFI follows a relentless fatal course over 6 to 36 months.

Headaches

In some migraine patients, headaches arise only during sleep (nocturnal migraines, see Chapter 9). REM sleep coincides with the onset of migraine and, even more closely, with cluster headache. Migraines often begin during early-morning REM sleep. As a result, excessive sleep or other conditions that increase REM sleep may exacerbate migraines. The opposite is also true. Naturally occurring or medication-induced sleep often aborts migraines, and medications that suppress REM sleep, such as TCAs, reduce migraines.

Cardiovascular Disorders

Sleep may also trigger life-threatening cardiovascular disorders. Angina and myocardial infarctions take place much more often during REM sleep, when pulse and blood pressure fluctuate, than during NREM sleep. Strokes have a predilection for the REM periods in the hours just before awakening. Thus, a family often discovers that an elderly relative has sustained a stroke only when the individual fails to arise in the morning.

Exacerbations of asthma, chronic obstructive lung disease, gastroesophageal reflux, and peptic ulcer disease also tend to develop during sleep; however, they occur with equal frequency in both sleep phases. Whatever their cause, these nighttime disturbances interrupt sleep and lead to insomnia and EDS. In cases of "nocturnal asthma," physicians must not overlook the alternative of nocturnal panic attacks.

INDICATIONS FOR A POLYSOMNOGRAM

A PSG study is expensive and time-consuming, but it is indicated and probably cost-effective in diagnosing many sleep-related disorders. Most important, PSG can confirm a clinical diagnosis of sleep apnea, REM sleep behavior disorder, periodic limb movements, and parasomnias. It is particularly valuable in helping to diagnose sleep apnea in children who snore, especially if they have Down syndrome. PSG acts as a preliminary test for narcolepsy, but MSLT results, in the right clinical setting, can be diagnostic. In addition, PSG can also diagnose seizures that develop exclusively during sleep and those that mimic sleep-related disorders (see Chapter 10). Conversely, by demonstrating a normal sleep pattern, the PSG may indirectly assist in identifying nocturnal panic attacks, pseudoinsomnia, and factitious sleep–wake disorders. To be fair, PSG has a limited role in the evaluation of insomnia. However, PSG has some usefulness in evaluating sleep maintenance insomnia because it may detect an underlying sleep disorder, such as obstructive sleep apnea, that interrupts sleep.

REFERENCES

Abramowicz, M. E. (2015). Drugs for insomnia. *The Medical Letter on Drugs and Therapeutics, 57,* 95–98.

Ariño, H., Iranzo, A., Gaig, C., et al. (2014). Sexsomnia: Parasomnia associated with sexual behavior during sleep. *Neurologia (Barcelona, Spain), 29,* 146–152.

Arnulf, I. (2015). Kleine-Levin syndrome. *Sleep Medicine Clinics,* 151–161.

Asaoka, S., Komada, Y., Aritake, S., et al. (2014). Effect of delayed sleep phase during university life on the daytime functioning in work life after graduation. *Sleep Medicine, 15,* 1155–1158.

Barger, L. K., Cade, B. E., Ayas, N. T., et al. (2005). Extended work shifts and the risk of motor vehicle crashes among interns. *The New England Journal of Medicine, 352,* 125–134.

Buysse, D. J. (2013). Insomnia. *JAMA: The Journal of the American Medical Association, 309,* 706–716.

Capaldi, V. F., Guerrero, M. L., & Killgore, W. D. (2011). Sleep disruptions among returning combat veterans from Iraq and Afghanistan. *Military Medicine, 176,* 879–888.

Cooke, J. R., & Ancoli-Israel, S. (2011). Normal and abnormal sleep in the elderly. *Handbook of Clinical Neurology, 98,* 653–665.

Dolder, C. R., & Nelson, M. H. (2008). Hypnosedative-induced complex behaviors: Incidence mechanisms, and management. *CNS Drugs, 22,* 1021–1036.

Edwards, C., Mukherjee, S., Simpson, L., et al. (2015). Depressive symptoms before and after treatment of sleep apnea in men and women. *Journal of Clinical Sleep Medicine : JCSM : Official Publication of the American Academy of Sleep Medicine, 11,* 1029–1038.

Farrell-Carnahan, L., Franke, L., Graham, C., et al. (2013). Subjective sleep disturbance in veterans receiving care in the Veterans Affairs Polytrauma System following blast-related mild traumatic brain injury. *Military Medicine, 178,* 951–956.

Frauscher, B., Jennum, P., Ju, Y. E. S., et al. (2014). Comorbidity and medication in REM sleep behavior disorder. *Neurology, 82,* 1076–1079.

Hogl, B., Zucconi, M., & Provini, F. (2007). RLS, PLM, and their differential diagnosis – a video guide. *Movement Disorders: Official Journal of the Movement Disorder Society, 22*(Suppl. 18), S414–S419.

Howell, M. J., & Schenck, C. H. (2015). Rapid eye movement sleep behavior disorder and neurodegenerative disease. *Journal of the American Medical Association: Neurology, 72,* 707–712.

Howell, M. J., Schenck, C. H., & Crow, S. J. (2009). A review of nighttime eating disorders. *Sleep Medicine Reviews, 13,* 23–34.

Lam, S. P., Fong, S. Y., Yu, M. W., et al. (2009). Sleepwalking in psychiatric patients: Comparison of childhood and adult onset. *The Australian and New Zealand Journal of Psychiatry, 43,* 426–430.

Lavault, S., Golmard, J. L., Groos, E., et al. (2015). Kleine-Levin syndrome in 120 patients: Differential diagnosis and long episodes. *Annals of Neurology, 77,* 529–540.

Liira, J., Verbeek, J. H., Costa, G., et al. (2014). Pharmacological interventions for sleepiness and sleep disturbances caused by shift work. *The Cochrane Database of Systematic Reviews,* (8), CD009776.

Mahowald, M. W., Schenck, C. H., & Cramer-Bornemann, M. A. (2005). Sleep-related violence. *Current Neurology and Neuroscience Reports, 5,* 153–158.

Morrison, I., Rumbold, J. M., & Riha, R. L. (2014). Medicolegal aspects of complex behaviors arising from the sleep period. *Sleep Medicine Reviews, 18,* 249–260.

Neikrug, A. B., & Ancoli-Israel, S. (2010). Sleep disorders in the older adult. *Gerontology, 56,* 181–189.

Owens, J. A., Belon, K., & Moss, P. (2010). Impact of delaying school start time on adolescent sleep, mood, and behavior. *Archives of Pediatrics & Adolescent Medicine, 164,* 608–614.

Palagini, L., Baglioni, C., Ciapparelli, A., et al. (2013). REM sleep dysregulation in depression: State of the art. *Sleep Medicine Reviews, 17,* 377–390.

Pilon, M., Montplaisir, J., & Zadra, A. (2008). Precipitating factors of somnambulism: Impact of sleep deprivation and forced arousals. *Neurology, 70,* 2284–2290.

Ramadan, M. Z., & Al-Saleh, K. S. (2014). The association of sleep deprivation on the occurrence of errors by nurses who work the night shift. *Current Health Sciences Journal, 40,* 97–103.

Sack, R. L. (2010). Jet lag. *The New England Journal of Medicine, 362,* 440–447.

Scammell, T. E. (2015). Narcolepsy. *The New England Journal of Medicine, 373,* 2654–2662.

Serra, L., Montagna, P., Mignot, E., et al. (2008). Cataplexy features in childhood narcolepsy. *Move Disord, 23,* 858–865.

Sivertsen, B., Harvey, A. G., Pallesen, S., et al. (2015). Mental health problems in adolescents with delayed sleep phase. *Journal of Sleep Research, 24,* 11–18.

Thorpy, M. J., & Plazzi, G. (2010). *The Parasomnias and Other Sleep-Related Movement Disorders.* Cambridge: Cambridge University Press.

Trauer, J. M., Qian, M. Y., Doyle, J. S., et al. (2015). Cognitive behavioral therapy for chronic insomnia. *Annals of Internal Medicine, 163,* 191–204.

Viorritto, E. N., Kureshi, S. A., & Owens, J. A. (2012). Narcolepsy in the pediatric population. *Current Neurology and Neuroscience Reports, 12,* 175–181.

Winkelman, J. W. (2015). Insomnia disorder. *The New England Journal of Medicine, 373,* 1437–1444.

Also, see National Center on Sleep Disorders web site https://www.nhlbi.nih.gov/about/org/ncsdr/.

QUESTIONS AND ANSWERS

1–15. Are these statements, as they apply to normal adult sleep, *true* or *false*?

1. Normal sleep generally progresses through the three NREM stages before the first REM sleep period.
2. Because the first REM sleep period usually begins about 90 to 120 minutes after the onset of sleep, normal REM latency is 90 to 120 minutes.
3. The bulk of REM sleep occurs in the early night, whereas the bulk of NREM sleep occurs in the early morning.
4. The normal sequence of NREM–REM sleep recurs with a periodicity of about 90 minutes.
5. REM sleep is almost entirely devoid of physical and mental activity.
6. N3 sleep provides great physical restfulness.
7. When a sleep-related activity, such as falling asleep, shifts to later in the daily cycle, the change constitutes a phase delay.
8. Aside from eye movement artifact, REM sleep EEGs resemble those during wakefulness.
9. EEG slow-wave activity characterizes N3 sleep.
10. The proportion of REM sleep in normal adults is unchanged from birth.
11. Social and occupational factors override most individuals' intrinsic sleep–wake schedule.
12. The proportion of time spent in slow-wave sleep increases in the elderly.
13. Consistently sleeping shorter than 6 hours or longer than 10 hours is associated with increased mortality and morbidity.
14. When an activity, such as falling asleep, shifts to earlier in the daily cycle, the change constitutes a phase advance.
15. After they pass through adolescence, men no longer have penile erections during REM sleep.

Answers: 1–True, 2–True, 3–False, 4–True, 5–False, 6–True, 7–True, 8–True, 9–True, 10–False, 11–True, 12–False, 13–True, 14–True, 15–False.

16. In the night following sleep deprivation, which of the following characteristically occurs?
    a. REM and N3 sleep phases rebound.
    b. Epileptiform discharges may emanate from the temporal lobe of a patient with complex partial epilepsy.
    c. N1, N2, N3, and then REM will occur in quick succession.
    d. REM sleep will not appear until early morning.

Answer: a. Once allowed to sleep, sleep-deprived individuals will have deep sleep with many dreams. A polysomnogram (PSG) will show increased N3 (slow-wave sleep) and increased REM phases.

17–24. Which of the following are characteristic of sleep terrors (a), nightmares (b), both (c), or neither (d)?

17. Onset during N1 and N2 of NREM sleep
18. Onset during slow-wave sleep
19. Onset during REM sleep
20. A disturbing variety of common dreams
21. Amnesia for any content
22. Partial arousals during NREM often precipitate them
23. Parents cannot interrupt them
24. Are associated with somnambulism

Answers: 17–d, 18–a, 19–b, 20–b, 21–a, 22–a, 23–a, 24–a.

25–37. Which of the following phenomena typically occur during REM sleep (a), NREM sleep (b), either phase (c), or neither phase (d)?

25. Somnambulism
26. Areflexic DTRs
27. EEG delta waves
28. Enuresis
29. Vulnerability to primary generalized seizures
30. Cluster headache
31. REM sleep behavior disorder
32. Sleep spindles on PSG
33. Body repositioning
34. Low-voltage, mixed-frequency EEG activity
35. K complexes
36. Parkinson tremor
37. Hemiballismus

Answers: 25–b, 26–a, 27–b, 28–b, 29–b, 30–a, 31–a, 32–b, 33–b, 34–a, 35–b, 36–d, 37–d.

38. Where are the nuclei that generate the rapid eye movements that accompany dreams?
    a. Diencephalon
    b. Midbrain
    c. Pons
    d. Medulla

Answer: c. The pons contains conjugate gaze centers that, when stimulated, produce high-velocity conjugate ocular movements, i.e., rapid eye movements.

39. During combat, a soldier loses both eyes. Without external clues, which circadian rhythm will he most likely follow?

a. A conventional 24-hour sleep–wake cycle
b. A progressively shorter cycle
c. A steady 24.5- to 25-hour cycle
d. A random sleep–wake cycle

Answer: c. Without external clues, the soldier will most likely follow a 24.5- to 25-hour cycle (Fig. 17.4). This pattern is the same circadian rhythm that volunteers follow when they "free run" while isolated in caves during experiments.

40. In this synthetic pathway, what does X represent?
Tryptophan –> X –> N-acetyl-X –> melatonin
a. A catecholamine
b. An indolamine
c. An amino acid
d. A steroid

Answer: b. X is serotonin, which is an indolamine.

41. A 34-year-old woman reports having developed an uncomfortable sensation in her feet that she cannot describe. However, she says that the sensation is so severe at night that it forces her to rub her calves and feet and that it prevents her from sleeping. She is only able to relieve the discomfort by pacing for 1–2 hours. She has no ongoing medical illnesses and takes no medications. Her neurologic examination is normal. Even with the numerous causes of this condition, which of the following laboratory tests is *inappropriate*?
a. Serum ferritin
b. Pregnancy
c. BUN or creatinine
d. PSG

Answer: d. PSG is inappropriate because she remains awake during the movements. The other tests are standard. She has restless legs syndrome (RLS), which has *four* elements:
• Uncomfortable paresthesias occurring prior to sleep onset.
• An irresistible urge or a psychologic drive to move the legs.
• Relief of the paresthesias with leg movement.
• Return of paresthesias with stopping the movement.

42. For the patient in the previous question, assuming that all of the tests were negative or normal, which of the following medicines is a first-line treatment?
a. Serotonin reuptake inhibitors
b. Dopamine-receptor blocking neuroleptics
c. Dopamine agonists
d. Sedatives

Answer: c. Dopamine agonists will most likely reduce the uncomfortable sensations (dysesthesias), stop the movements, and enable sleep. In the absence of an underlying or comorbid condition, RLS presumably results from decreased D2 receptor binding in striatum. Although RLS mimics akathisia, neither typical nor atypical neuroleptics will ameliorate it.

43–47. Is each statement *true* or *false*?

43. Narcolepsy typically begins in middle age when normal afternoon fatigue becomes prominent.
44. Sleep apnea is a disorder only of adults.
45. Sleep apnea is associated with morning headaches, cardiovascular disorders, and obesity.
46. In children, sleep apnea may lead to learning disability and poor school performance.
47. Hypnopompic refers to phenomena that occur on awakening, and hypnagogic refers to phenomena that occur on falling asleep.

Answers:
43. False. About 90% of cases develop between adolescence and age 25 years.
44. False. Children, especially those with nasopharyngeal abnormalities, have sleep apnea.
45. True. However, about 30% of sleep apnea patients are not obese.
46. True.
47. True.

48. Which of the following statements concerning melatonin is *true*?
a. It is synthesized in the nucleus of Meynert.
b. Serotonin is a precursor in its synthesis.
c. Its maximum secretion coincides with the brightest time of the day.
d. SSRIs decrease melatonin plasma concentration.

Answer: b. Melatonin is synthesized in the pineal gland through the following pathway: tryptophan –> serotonin –> N-acetyl-serotonin –> melatonin. Melatonin, which is secreted in the dark, increases sleepiness and advances the sleep phase. SSRIs decrease melatonin plasma concentration. Acetylcholine is synthesized in the nucleus basalis of Meynert.

49. A 34-year-old woman reports that she "tosses and turns," worrying that she is not getting adequate sleep, every night when she goes to bed at 10:45 pm until she falls asleep at about midnight. She awakes, refreshed at 6:45 AM and usually has a productive day and pleasant evening. Which approach should a prudent physician take?
a. Prescribe a benzodiazepine receptor agonist.
b. Send her for a polysomnogram (PSG).
c. Prescribe an antidepressant.
d. Suggest CBT.

Answer: d. CBT would be to help her accept that she probably requires only 7 hours of sleep each night and explore why she is restless when she goes to bed. CBT has become a well-established first-line treatment for insomnia.

50. When falling asleep, a 5-year-old girl thrusts her head up and down on her pillow. Her parents can rouse her and interrupt the movements. She does not injure herself and, if left alone, falls asleep

within 5 minutes. She is otherwise well. Which is the *correct* statement concerning this activity?
a. It is a variety of epilepsy, which has a predilection to cause seizures in light sleep.
b. It is a stereotypy that is a criterion of autistic spectrum disorder.
c. She is trying to remain awake by willfully resisting sleep.
d. The movement is head banging, a variety of rhythmic movement disorder.

Answer: d. She has "head banging," which is a common childhood sleep-related condition that is innocuous and helps children fall asleep. Head rolling and body rocking are varieties of the disorder. These and other movements also occur in older children and adults with intellectual disability and autistic spectrum disorder. Although focal seizures have a predilection to arise in light (N1 and N2) sleep, the movements in this case are unlikely to be seizures because of their pattern and because her parents can interrupt them.

51. Which characteristic is common to the sleep patterns of both depression and sleep following sleep deprivation?
a. Increased sleep latency
b. Shortened REM latency
c. Sleep terrors
d. Interruptions in sleep

Answer: b.

52. Which effect will fluvoxamine have on the metabolism of caffeine?
a. Fluvoxamine will raise caffeine levels.
b. Fluvoxamine will lower caffeine levels.
c. Fluvoxamine will have no effect on caffeine levels.

Answer: a. Fluvoxamine inhibits cytochrome P450 (CYP-450) liver enzyme 1A2. Inhibition of this enzyme will increase serum caffeine concentration, possibly to the point of toxicity.

53. A psychiatrist prescribes a standard dose of olanzapine to an individual who, unbeknownst to the psychiatrist, drinks six cups of coffee each day. Which effect will the patient's coffee consumption have on the serum concentration of olanzapine?
a. The olanzapine concentration will be unexpectedly high.
b. The olanzapine concentration will be unexpectedly low
c. There will be no effect.
d. The olanzapine concentration will be expectable, but the caffeine concentration will rise to toxic levels.

Answer: a. Because caffeine also acts as an inhibitor of the metabolic enzyme CYP-450, it will lead to elevated levels of olanzapine. Similarly, caffeine inhibits the metabolism of haloperidol, clozapine, duloxetine, and tricyclic antidepressants.

54. Which physiologic change is associated with normal REM sleep?
a. Absent respirations
b. Lower pulse and blood pressure
c. High-voltage, slow EEG activity
d. Muscle atonia

Answer: d. Flaccid muscle tone (muscle atonia), reflected in absent limb and chin muscle EMG activity on the PSG, characterizes normal REM sleep.

55. In depressed patients, which one of the following is the most typical sleep-related change?
a. Delay in the nighttime body temperature nadir
b. Delayed cortisol secretion and first REM period
c. Increased cortisol secretion and advanced REM period
d. Delay in 3-methoxy-4-hydroxyphenylglycol (MHPG) secretion

Answer: c.

56. The parents of 7-year-old Tim bring him to a child psychiatrist because he has developed inattention and hyperactivity in school, especially in the early afternoon. Among their many observations, Tim's parents note that he has begun to snore loudly when he sleeps. The psychiatrist refers him to a pediatrician who finds enlarged tonsils and adenoids and diagnoses obstructive sleep apnea. A PSG confirms the diagnosis. What will be the probable outcome of a tonsillectomy and adenoidectomy?
a. The procedure will not benefit the boy as much as continuous positive airway pressure (CPAP).
b. It will improve his sleep and thus reduce his inattention and hyperactivity.
c. Unless the child also has trisomy 21, the procedure will not help.
d. It will probably improve his sleep but it will not improve his behavior.

Answer: b. The most important clinical feature of this case of childhood sleep apnea is that it leads not to excessive daytime sleepiness (EDS), but to hyperactivity, irritability, and inattention. Parents often describe their children as being "overtired." When the tonsils and adenoids are enlarged, which is often the case, their removal will probably improve sleep and reduce inattention and hyperactivity. If Tim were to have trisomy 21, the diagnosis would be more certain because of the lax oropharyngeal muscles and large tongue.

57. Joe, a recently retired salesman who appears in good physical and psychological health complains of inability to fall asleep until 1 AM. Moreover, Joe says that when he awakes, he has failed to obtain a

restful night's sleep. Of the following, which advice should he physician offer him?
a. Try one of the newer hypnotics.
b. Undergo a PSG.
c. Limit daytime naps, avoid alcohol, use the bed only for sleeping, exercise during the daytime, and practice other elements of good sleep hygiene.
d. Accept insomnia as an age-related impairment.

Answer: c. Practice good sleep hygiene before embarking on expensive testing or taking a hypnotic. The next step would be CBT rather than hypnotics.

58. Which is the following is a *Diagnostic and Statistical Manual of Mental Disorders, 5th Edition* (DSM-5) requirement for the diagnosis of Insomnia Disorder?
a. Inability to sleep more than 6 hours
b. Distress or impairment in social, occupational, or other important area of functioning
c. Sleeping at 2 AM and arising at 10 AM
d. Resulting excessive daytime sleepiness (EDS)

Answer: b. The DSM-5 diagnosis of Insomnia Disorder requires dissatisfaction with sleep quantity or quality, distress or impairment in function, certain time requirements, and the absence of an underlying physiologic disturbance or alternative mental illness. The diagnosis does not apply if the patient requires less than a normal duration of sleep or follows an unconventional sleep–wake schedule. Although insomnia may lead to EDS, the diagnosis does not require it.

59. Which of the following statements concerning suvorexant is *true*?
a. It promotes wakefulness.
b. It blocks the orexin receptor.
c. It induces narcolepsy-cataplexy
d. It stimulates the orexin receptor.

Answer: b. Suvorexant, a new hypnotic agent, blocks orexin receptors. It reduces sleep latency, improves sleep efficiency, and lengthens sleep time. Like most other hypnotics, it causes rebound insomnia on withdrawal.

60. Which is the most important factor in determining most individuals' sleep schedule?
a. Early learning
b. Social and occupational demands
c. Cerebral cortical "time clocks"
d. Melatonin secretion
e. Suprachiasmatic nucleus of the hypothalamus

Answer: b. The suprachiasmatic nucleus, located in the hypothalamus, serves as the biologic clock. However, social and occupational demands and exposure to light override the biologic clock.

61. Which light bulb color alerts people and tends to prevent sleep?
a. Green
b. Amber
c. Blue
d. Red

Answer: c. Blue lights and white lights, which necessarily contain some blue light, are the most stimulating. Computer screens and hand-held electronic devices are weighted toward blue light. The blue color intensifies the effect of the action and excitement of electronic devices.

62. Which light bulb color gives a relatively soporific effect?
a. Green
b. Amber
c. Blue
d. Red

Answer: b. Amber light, relative to other light, lends a calming effect and eases sleep. Amber light bulbs would be useful in the evenings in general and particularly during phototherapy when attempting to advance the sleep phase.

63. Charles, a 50-year-old man, struggles to stay awake during the day. He has restless nighttime sleep and, according to his girlfriend, snores loudly. His PSG shows decreases in the blood oxygen concentration followed by brief arousals. What is the best treatment for his excessive daytime sleepiness (EDS)?
a. CPAP
b. Tracheostomy
c. Uvula surgery
d. Stimulants

Answer: a. Charles has sleep apnea – the primary breathing-related sleep disorder. CPAP is the first-line treatment. Modafinil (Provigil) has an indication to promote daytime wakefulness in sleep-apnea patients. If possible, Charles should lose weight.

64. A college student accused his roommate of sexually attacking him on several occasions while he was asleep between 2 AM and 3 AM. He said that each time his roommate must have crossed their room, climbed into his bed, and fondled him. Although the accused student conceded that he awoke in or near his roommate's bed, he denied any sexual advances and could not recall any details. He admitted that he had been sleep-deprived and consumed excess alcohol before the event. After physicians conducted a full evaluation, which did not reveal alcoholism or paroxysmal EEG activity, they obtained a PSG that revealed masturbation during NREM sleep. Which is the most likely diagnosis?
a. Klein–Levin syndrome
b. Focal seizures
c. NREM sleep arousal disorder with sexual behavior (sexsomnia)
d. REM sleep behavior disorder

Answer: c. With the information available the accused roommate most likely experienced episodes of sexsomnia, formerly known as "sleep sex behavior," which DSM-5 categorizes as a Parasomnia, NREM Arousal Disorder. As with other parasomnias, sleep deprivation may precipitate a sexsomnia episode. Alcohol consumption and proximity to a sexual object also precipitate episodes. Focal seizures lead to only rudimentary sexual behavior, such as rubbing the genitals, and, if a seizure had occurred, the PSG would have shown paroxysmal EEG discharges. In REM sleep behavior disorder, the PSG would have shown that the episodes arose during REM sleep. Klein–Levin syndrome is excluded primarily because its sleep episodes last weeks and the sexual activity, which is only rudimentary, occurs when patients are awake.

65. Which sleep change represents a beneficial effect of benzodiazepines?
    a. Increase in total sleep time of 10%
    b. Increase in total sleep time of 30%
    c. Increase in total sleep time of 50% or more
    d. Increase in slow-wave NREM sleep

Answer: a. Benzodiazepines increase total sleep time by 10% and reduce sleep fragmentation. However, these are modest benefits. For long-term use, their potential adverse effects often overshadow their benefits.

66. When used as hypnotics for chronic insomnia, benzodiazepines have many potential adverse effects. Which one of the following is *not* an adverse effect of benzodiazepines?
    a. Hip fractures from an increased tendency to fall
    b. Anterograde amnesia
    c. With long-acting preparations, daytime sleepiness
    d. With short-acting preparations, insomnia in the early morning hours and daytime anxiety
    e. Lowered seizure threshold

Answer: e. Except for little or no increase of the seizure threshold, benzodiazepines have all these potential adverse effects when used for chronic insomnia. Benzodiazepines have an anticonvulsant effect, but abrupt withdrawal from chronic use may lead to status epilepticus.

67. During the summer after his freshman year in college, Lester slept incessantly for 10 days and would awaken only to use the toilet and eat large amounts of food – "like a hibernating bear," according to his mother. His father, who described Lester as a "zombie" when he was not completely asleep, found him masturbating several times. When his parents questioned him, Lester was reticent, unengaged, disoriented, and unable to recall recent events. He had a similar episode during the previous summer, but it lasted only 6 days. In addition, his parents heard that another occurred while he was away at college. Between these episodes, Lester was affable, bright, and industrious. During episodes, his medical examinations, routine blood tests, magnetic resonance imaging (MRI), lumbar puncture (LP), electroencephalogram (EEG), and toxicology studies all showed no significant abnormalities. Which disorder most likely has affected Lester?
    a. Hypersomnolence disorder
    b. Drug abuse
    c. Encephalitis
    d. Focal seizures

Answer: a. In view of the description of multiple events, his behavior, and all the negative laboratory tests, Lester probably has the Kleine–Levin syndrome, which DSM-5 includes as a Hypersomnolence Disorder. The DSM-4 had labeled this disorder Periodic Hypersomnia. Kleine–Levin syndrome, which is usually idiopathic, affects predominantly adolescent males and consists primarily of episodes of the "3 H's:" hypersomnia, hyperphagia, and hypersexuality. During sleep episodes, patients are confused, withdrawn, and apathetic. Between episodes, they usually have no identifiable psychiatric, neurologic, or internal medical illness.

68. In which direction is travel most likely to produce jet lag?
    a. East-to-west
    b. West-to-east
    c. North-to-south
    d. South-to-north
    e. None of the above

Answer: b. Jet lag, which is not included in the DSM-5, was known as *time zone change syndrome* in DSM-4, and is greater following eastward travel because individuals cannot advance their sleep schedule as easily as they can delay it. In other words, when flying from Los Angeles to New York, most travelers cannot easily go to sleep 3 hours earlier. When returning westward, most travelers can more easily delay going to sleep by the 3 hours. Travelers subject to jet lag should prepare for their trip by changing their sleep–wake schedule to conform to their destination's schedule several days before the trip. After arriving, they should expose themselves to sunlight in the morning and immediately follow the local time schedule. Eastward travelers can take melatonin or a hypnotic to facilitate their falling asleep earlier than normal, i.e., advance their sleep phase.

69. A 23-year-old aspiring actor requested evaluation for a sensation of falling coupled with a sudden contraction in his leg and back muscles upon falling asleep. He felt as if he were preventing the fall. This sequence occurs once or twice a month. It was most apt to occur after a particularly exhausting day. It not only frightens him, but then it prohibits him from sleeping for another 30 minutes. Which strategy should the physician recommend?
    a. Reassure him that he is experiencing a benign condition
    b. Send him for a PSG
    c. Prescribe him a mild hypnotic
    d. Prescribe a mild tranquilizer

Answer: a. The patient has described the near universal, benign phenomenon of hypnic jerks that consist of sudden contraction of antigravity muscles during the wake–sleep phase that occurs in response to a sensation of falling. Further investigation and treatment are not indicated. The physician should advise him that the condition is benign and to avoid sleep deprivation and physical exhaustion.

70. Which of the following hypnotics reduces slow-wave NREM sleep?
    a. Temazepam
    b. Eszopiclone
    c. Zaleplon
    d. Ramelteon
    e. Zolpidem

Answer: a. Benzodiazepines, such as temazepam (Restoril), reduce slow-wave NREM sleep, which is unfortunate because this stage is especially restorative. Melatonin and its agonists, such as ramelteon (Rozerem), and the "Z drugs" – eszopiclone (Lunesta), zaleplon (Sonata), and zolpidem (Ambien) – preserve sleep architecture.

71. Which statement concerning sleep maturation from infancy to older childhood is *true*?
    a. Children reach the normal REM latency (90 minutes) at the start of puberty.
    b. The proportion of REM falls to the adult level of 20% to 25% at puberty.
    c. Children establish a circadian rhythm between 5 and 6 years.
    d. As they mature, children sleep less and dream even less.

Answer: d. Children sleep less and dream even less as they mature. Children's REM latency reaches the adult duration of 90 minutes and the proportion of their REM falls to the adult level of 20% to 25% at age 5 years. They establish a circadian rhythm between 3 and 6 months.

72. Which of the following is a DSM-5 requirement for the diagnosis of Hypersomnolence Disorder?
    a. Polysomnogram (PSG) documentation of the main sleep period of 9 or more hours
    b. Self-reported excessive sleepiness despite sleeping 7 hours
    c. Sleep-onset REM periods (SOREMPs)
    d. Daytime sleep attacks

Answer: b. The DSM-5 requires a self-report, for which PSG documentation is not necessary, of excessive sleepiness despite sleeping 7 hours. In addition, the patient must have recurrent periods of sleep within the same day, a nonrestorative (unrefreshing) 9-hour sleep, or difficulty becoming fully awake after an abrupt awakening. Neither SOREMPs nor daytime sleep is required.

73. In which condition is a polysomnogram (PSG) most likely to show consistent abnormalities?
    a. Anxiety
    b. Mania
    c. Major depression
    d. Schizophrenia

Answer: c. PSG in major depression generally shows a short REM latency, increased REM duration, and increased frequency of eye movement in REM sleep (REM density), but decreased N3 (slow-wave or restorative) sleep. PSG results in the other illnesses are inconsistent.

74. A 25-year-old woman with anxiety disorder reports frequent episodes of various frightening thoughts that jar her awake from sleep. Once awake, she can recall her fears and is oriented and coherent. She then remains awake for an hour before returning to sleep. PSG shows that the episodes arise from NREM sleep and the EEG electrodes do not show paroxysmal discharges. Which is the most likely diagnosis?
    a. Nightmares
    b. Sleep terrors
    c. Nocturnal panic attacks
    d. Frontal lobe seizures

Answer: c. This woman, who has a history of anxiety disorder, has episodes of fear that arise from NREM sleep and awaken her – nocturnal panic attacks. Because they do not arise from REM sleep, they are not dreams, i.e., nightmares. They differ from sleep terrors in that they contain material that she recalls. The absence of stereotyped thinking, physical behavior during the episodes, and paroxysmal EEG activity exclude a diagnosis of frontal lobe seizures. Before the PSG, a physician would hopefully have obtained a thorough history including her mood, experiences, precipitants of the episodes, recall of any cognition during them, and possible use of alcohol, medicines, or illicit drugs.

75. After having worked the previous day, Dora, a medical intern, fell asleep at 3 AM. Her resident called her an hour later to ask her about the status of a patient, but Dora did not know that she was at work and could not speak coherently. Her resident recognized the situation, terminated the conversation, and advised her to return to sleep. In the morning Dora could not remember the call. Which is the best term for the episode?
    a. Transient global amnesia
    b. REM sleep behavior disorder
    c. Confusional arousal
    d. Nocturnal panic attack

Answer: c. The call undoubtedly interrupted Dora's deep sleep (probably slow-wave, N3 sleep), which she needed to make up for her sleep deprivation. She suffered a "confusional arousal," which neurologists classify as a variety of parasomnia, but the DSM-5 does not recognize. In her case, the call precipitated the confusional arousal, but many times confusional arousals occur with spontaneous, unprovoked awakening.

76. As individuals age, which of the following changes is most apt to occur?
    a. Increase in REM, slow-wave, and total sleep time

b. Decrease in total sleep time, but an increase in REM and slow-wave sleep
c. Decrease in slow-wave sleep and total sleep
d. None of the above

Answer: c. As individuals age, they have decreased slow-wave and total sleep. Moreover, their sleep is phase-advanced and frequent awakenings interrupt it. The early morning awakenings of older people are a manifestation of the normal phase advance. Therefore, early morning awakenings, by themselves, are not an indication of depression.

77. By what age do children consolidate their sleep into nighttime and give up their afternoon nap?
    a. 2 years
    b. 4 years
    c. 6 years
    d. 8 years

Answer: b. Children usually give up their afternoon nap by 3 to 4 years old. If loss of their afternoon naps leaves them sleep-deprived, children tend to be irritable or hyperactive rather than sleepy.

78. Buffy, an 18-year-old college freshman who works part-time as a waitress, described having excessive daytime sleepiness (EDS). For the last 2 years she has had irresistible urges to sleep about twice daily, weakness when laughing, and occasionally total paralysis when attempting to wake for morning classes. Which one of the following is the next best step?
    a. A therapeutic trial of methylphenidate or modafinil
    b. After 7 full nights of sleep, a PSG followed by a multiple sleep latency test (MSLT)
    c. MRI
    d. LP to determine cerebrospinal fluid (CSF) orexin concentration

Answer: b. Several of Buffy's symptoms – EDS, cataplexy, and sleep paralysis – suggest narcolepsy. However, she does not nap at inopportune or dangerous times. She may have EDS from its most common cause among young adults – sleep deprivation from social, academic, and occupational demands. However, she should still undergo urine toxicology testing, an evaluation for depression, and, after 7 nights of sleep, PSG and MSLT.

79. An elderly man flails his arms and strikes his wife while sleeping. He has minimal cognitive impairment. PSG shows REM without atonia. A consultant correctly labels his behavior, "dream enactment." Which of the following is the best treatment?
    a. Clonazepam
    b. Phenytoin
    c. Carbamazepine
    d. Tricyclic antidepressants

Answer: a. The combination of REM without atonia and dream enactment behavior is diagnostic of REM

sleep behavior disorder. Clonazepam treatment is highly effective in suppressing the disorder. In contrast, tricyclic antidepressants, monoamine oxidase inhibitors, and serotoninergic antidepressants are ineffective even though they may suppress or delay REM sleep. Moreover, these medicines may trigger dream enactment. DSM-5 criteria exclude episodes precipitated by medicines from the diagnosis of REM sleep behavior disorder.

80. Dr. Anna, a 32-year-old psychiatry resident in the third trimester of her first pregnancy, reports the development of unusual feelings in her legs to her training analyst. Beginning 2 weeks before, whenever she was "on the couch," she wanted to move her feet and walk around – as if to avoid further insights. Although characteristically reticent, the analyst remarked that it was more than a fantasy because he had leaned over and saw her feet moving. Dr. Anna had no other symptoms and was taking no medications. Which is the most likely Pregnancy-Related Disorder according to DSM-5 definitions?
    a. Tremor
    b. Eclampsia
    c. Restless leg syndrome (RLS)
    d. None of the above

Answer: d. Symptoms identical to RLS frequently complicate pregnancy. However, the presence of pregnancy or other medical conditions, such as edema or neuropathy, that cause the symptoms, preclude a DSM-5 diagnosis of RLS. Pregnancy also causes chorea gravidarum (see Chapter 18).

81. Jacob, a 50-year-old man is brought for psychiatric consultation by his wife because he has become "distant, inattentive, and confused" during the previous several months. Two months before those symptoms developed, he began to have progressively severe insomnia, which hypnotics, antidepressants, and other psychotropic medicines did not alleviate. Jacob's older sister recently died after 18 months of a similar illness. The psychiatrist found that the patient had personality changes, cognitive deficits, and subtle myoclonus. An internist found that he had tachycardia and labile hypertension. Of the following, which is the most likely illness?
    a. Creutzfeldt–Jakob disease
    b. Fatal familial insomnia
    c. Iatrogenic sleep disorder
    d. Lewy bodies disease

Answer: b. Because Jacob and his sister have had refractory insomnia, dementia, myoclonus, and autonomic nervous system (ANS) dysfunction, the most likely diagnosis is fatal familial insomnia. This illness, like Creutzfeldt–Jakob disease, is a prion disease characterized by accumulation of a prion protein (PrP^{Sc}).

82. Jacob undergoes further evaluation. Which of the following features is likely to be present?
    a. Lewy bodies in the cerebral cortex and the basal ganglia

b. Intracellular tau accumulations
c. Spongiform cerebral cortical changes
d. Elevated catecholamines and other endocrine abnormalities

Answer: c. Because this patient has a prion illness, fatal familial insomnia, his cerebral cortex would have a spongiform appearance. Lewy bodies in the cerebral cortex and the basal ganglia would indicate dementia with Lewy bodies disease and intracellular tau accumulations would indicate frontotemporal dementia. The DSM-5 labels these illnesses Major or Mild Neurocognitive Disorder due to Lewy bodies disease and Frontotemporal Lobar Degeneration.

83. Which of the following fulfills a diagnostic requirement for obstructive sleep apnea hypopnea?
    a. PSG evidence of at least five obstructive apneas or hypopneas per hour of sleep and either snoring or other breathing disturbance or EDS
    b. Regardless of symptoms, PSG evidence of at least 10 obstructive apneas or hypopneas per hour of sleep
    c. Loud snoring and EDS
    d. Hypercapnia during sleep

Answer: a. The presence of PSG evidence of at least five obstructive apneas or hypopneas per hour of sleep and either snoring or other breathing disturbance or EDS fulfills a diagnostic requirement for the diagnosis. Alternatively, the DSM-5 accepts PSG evidence of at least 15 obstructive apneas or hypopneas per hour of sleep regardless of the symptoms. Loud snoring, EDS, and hypercapnia are commonplace in the disorder, but DSM-5 does not require any of them.

84. When used to treat narcolepsy, which is the mechanism of action of methylphenidate and amphetamine?
    a. They enhance dopamine activity.
    b. They act as α_1-adrenergic agonists.
    c. They inhibit adrenergic reuptake.
    d. None of the above.

Answer: a.

85. Which of the following precludes a DSM-5 diagnosis of Substance/Medication-Induced Sleep Disorder?
    a. Insomnia
    b. Symptoms began only on withdrawal of a medicine
    c. Symptoms occur exclusively during delirium
    d. Symptoms develop during substance intoxication

Answer: c. The DSM-5 requires that symptoms develop during intoxication or withdrawal, but not exclusively during the course of delirium.

86. John-Philip, a 17-year-old student, has spent the summer starting a band. He went to sleep every night at 4 am. Anticipating the start of school on September 1, he requests that his physician prescribe an "upper" to help him remain awake during the transition. What would be the best method to change to a sleep schedule of 11 PM to 6:30 AM?
    a. Use an amphetamine during the transition.
    b. Suddenly switch to a new schedule, much like overcoming the change to a new time zone when traveling.
    c. Go to bed 1 hour earlier each night beginning August 16.
    d. Delay sleep by 1 hour each night beginning August 11.

Answer: d. John-Philip has a circadian rhythm sleep–wake disorder, delayed sleep phase type. The best way for him to reach a conventional schedule would be to delay sleep by 1–3 hours each night until sleep onset reaches the desired schedule. Simply going to bed early usually only increases sleep latency, but delaying sleep decreases the latency. An alternate therapy – phototherapy – is to shine bright light in the mornings, create a dim environment in the evening, and not allow any light after 11 PM.

87. Of the following, which is the most effective treatment of cataplexy?
    a. Modafinil
    b. Sodium oxybate
    c. Nortriptyline
    d. Amphetamine

Answer: b. Sodium oxybate (Xyrem), the same substance as gamma-hydroxybutyrate (GHB), the "date-rape drug," markedly reduces cataplexy. It is a rapidly acting hypnotic that increases slow-wave sleep, but does not affect REM sleep.

88. In the DSM-5, which of the following sleep disturbances may fulfill a diagnostic requirement for Posttraumatic Stress Disorder (PTSD)?
    a. Sleep terror
    b. Sleepwalking
    c. Recurrent distressing dreams in which the content of the dream is related to the traumatic event
    d. Insomnia

Answer: c. Dreams with affect or content related to the trauma constitute a DSM-5 intrusion symptom indicative of PTSD.

89. Charlie, a 35-year-old woman, sought psychiatric consultation for mild depression, insomnia, and obesity. When discussing her obesity, which seems refractory to her stringent diet, Charlie mentions that she cannot recall eating at night; however, she states that in the morning she occasionally finds open tuna cans and once an open cat food can on the kitchen floor. Which is the most likely explanation of the debris on the kitchen floor?
    a. Dream enactment
    b. Hypoglycemia
    c. Sleep-related eating
    d. Hunger

Answer: c. Charlie has sleep-related eating, a variation of sleepwalking, which consists of a partial arousal during which individuals eat for a few minutes. They often consume inedible as well as high-calorie or junk food, but they do not purge. Because this behavior occurs during NREM sleep, it falls into the category of a parasomnia. It sometimes causes individuals to burn or cut themselves while preparing food. Patients usually have amnesia for the episode the next morning. Zolpidem may cause or precipitate it, and may add to the amnesia. Alternatively, eating during the night may be a manifestation of an eating disorder (night eating syndrome), Prader–Willi syndrome, or Kleine–Levin syndrome.

90. What effect do tricyclic and serotoninergic antidepressants exert on REM sleep?
    a. Increase it
    b. Decrease it
    c. Have no effect
    d. Have an unpredictable effect

Answer: b. As a general rule, antidepressants decrease REM sleep and prolong REM latency. This effect counters one of depression's hallmarks – decreased REM latency.

91. Which is the most common situation or emotion that precipitates cataplexy in individuals with narcolepsy-cataplexy?
    a. Sexual arousal
    b. Anger
    c. Surprise
    d. Hearing or telling a joke

Answer: d. Strong emotions or surprises typically precipitate cataplexy in susceptible individuals. Even stronger than sexual arousal, hearing or telling a joke is the most powerful factor.

92. Which of the following hypnotics is free of the risk of complex sleep-related behavior?
    a. Ramelteon (Rozerem)
    b. Eszopiclone (Lunesta)
    c. Zolpidem (Ambien)
    d. Zaleplon (Sonata)
    e. None of the above

Answer: e. Treatment with either nonbenzodiazepine receptor agonists (eszopiclone, zolpidem, and zolpidem) or melatonin receptor agonists (ramelteon) may precipitate sleepwalking (a parasomnia), hallucinations, nocturnal binge eating, driving while asleep, or other complex sleep-related behavior.

93. A 58-year-old man has RLS. His wife reports that once he falls asleep, his legs jerk in flurries at approximately 30-second intervals. A polysomnogram (PSG) confirms the periodic bursts of muscle activity and leg movement. What is the name of these movements?
    a. Akathisia
    b. RLS
    c. Periodic limb movements
    d. Hypnic jerks

Answer: c. He has periodic limb movements superimposed on RLS. These movements complicate about 80% of RLS cases. Even if this patient were taking dopamine-blocking medications, he does not have akathisia because his movements occur predominantly in bed and do not occur in response to an inner urge. Hypnic jerks occur on falling asleep.

94. In which sleep stage do sleep spindles and K complexes appear?
    a. N1 of NREM
    b. N2 of NREM
    c. N3 of REM
    d. Sleep-induced seizures

Answer: b. Spindles and K complexes emerge in N2 NREM sleep and define this stage.

95. Of the following parasomnias, which one arises in REM sleep?
    a. REM sleep behavior disorder
    b. Sexsomnia
    c. Somnambulism
    d. Sleep terrors

Answer: a. Most parasomnias arise in slow-wave NREM (N3) sleep, but REM sleep behavior disorder episodes (by definition) arises during REM sleep. Unlike the other disorders, REM sleep behavior disorder occurs predominantly in older adults. Also notable is that the eyes are closed during episodes of REM sleep behavior disorder, but open in somnambulism.

96. Which ratio determines sleep efficiency?
    a. Total sleep time to time in bed
    b. Time in bed to total sleep time
    c. NREM to REM sleep time
    d. REM to NREM sleep time

Answer: a. Sleep efficiency equals the ratio of total sleep time to time in bed, when the bed is used only for sleeping.

97. Which of the following statements is *true* regarding sleep and schizophrenia?
    a. The hallucinations of individuals with schizophrenia represent intrusions of REM sleep into their daytime wakefulness.
    b. PSGs in chronic schizophrenia show consistent, specific abnormalities.
    c. Individuals with schizophrenia usually remain able to distinguish their dreams from hallucinations.
    d. PSG studies are helpful in the diagnosis and management of schizophrenia.

Answer: c. Not only can chronic schizophrenia patients usually distinguish their dreams from hallucinations, but also PSG studies show that hallucinations do not reflect REM activity, i.e., hallucinations are not dreams.

98. Which of the following statements is *false* concerning somnambulism persisting or developing in adults?
a. Zolpidem may precipitate it.
b. It occurs in N1 of NREM sleep.
c. PSGs supplemented by EEG leads reveal paroxysms of spike-and-wave activity.
d. Various psychiatric conditions are often comorbid.

Answer: c. EEGs during somnambulism, as during other parasomnias, do not reveal paroxysms of spike-and-wave activity or any other epileptiform activity. Physicians should distinguish parasomnias from nocturnal seizures on clinical grounds, but PSGs are indicated if the episodes remain refractory to prevention, occur frequently, or endanger the patient. Sleep deprivation and partial arousals typically precipitate somnambulism in children. In adults, psychologic stress and certain medicines, such as zolpidem, may precipitate somnambulism. In addition, unlike parasomnias in children, somnambulism in adults occurs in early NREM sleep and during the late portion of the night. Various neurologic and psychiatric disorders are comorbid with parasomnias that persist or develop in adults. Somnambulism has been raised, occasionally successfully, as a criminal defense.

99. At what daily dose does caffeine consumption lead to caffeine toxicity?
a. 100 mg
b. 150 mg
c. 200 mg
d. 250 mg

Answer: d. Daily consumption of 250 mg of caffeine typically leads to caffeine toxicity, caffeine intoxication, or simply caffeinism. This disorder, a hazard of modern culture, consists of insomnia along with restlessness, nervousness, and excitement in combination with diuresis, gastrointestinal disturbance, tachycardia, and cardiac arrhythmia. It is easy for people to consume excessive quantities of caffeine, either knowingly or unknowingly.

100. A 40-year-old secretary reports inability to fall asleep, frequent awakenings, and arising hours before necessary. She has excessive daytime sleepiness (EDS) that she attributes to her insomnia. Her PSG shows prolonged sleep latency, frequent arousals interrupting sleep, reduced slow-wave and REM sleep, and advanced awakening. Which is the most likely diagnosis?
a. Sleep apnea
b. Insomnia
c. Advanced sleep phase type, circadian rhythm sleep–wake disorder
d. Alcoholism

Answer: b. She has the symptoms and PSG results of typical, nonspecific insomnia. Depression, misuse of medicines, or medical illnesses may be responsible.

101. Which of the following is *true* concerning zolpidem and zaleplon?
a. These medicines are hypnotic agents probably because they increase $GABA_A$ activity.
b. They suppress REM and slow-wave sleep.
c. In general, benzodiazepine receptor agonists have a longer half-life than benzodiazepines.
d. Reports have discounted amnesia, hallucinations, nocturnal binge eating, and driving while asleep as adverse effects.

Answer: a. These hypnotics are benzodiazepine agonists and, therefore, increase $GABA_A$ activity. They have a relatively short half-life. With judicious use, patients have no morning grogginess. They preserve sleep architecture and maintain the restorative phases of sleep – slow-wave (N3) and REM. However, reports have linked their use to amnesia, hallucinations, nocturnal binge eating, and driving while asleep.

102. Ms. Brooks, a 45-year-old schoolteacher reports having insomnia when attempting to fall asleep at 11 PM. She remains awake – reading, using her computer, and doing household tasks. Once in bed between 1 am and 2 am she immediately falls asleep. She sleeps without interruption until the alarm clock awakens her at 6:30 am. Then she has trouble awakening and during the school day has constant excessive daytime sleepiness (EDS). On weekends and holidays, Ms. Brooks goes to bed and immediately falls asleep between 1 am and 2 am. She then sleeps until about 10 am. On those days she awakes refreshed and has no EDS. On all days, she has only a single cup of coffee in the morning, and does not use other caffeine-containing beverage or food. She takes no alcohol or medications that would affect her sleep. She has no symptoms of a mood disorder or other psychiatric disturbance. Which would be the best treatment?
a. An antidepressant
b. Phototherapy or chronotherapy
c. Sleep restriction
d. An amphetamine

Answer: b. Ms. Brooks' sleep-onset insomnia is a manifestation of the delayed sleep-phase type of circadian rhythm sleep–wake disorder. Unlike many employees in entertainment, nursing, and others fields who perform nighttime work, this schoolteacher's sleep–wake schedule is out of sync with her occupational demands. If she wishes to remain healthy and continue her current job, she must allow herself about 8 hours of restful sleep. Assuming she does not want to switch to teaching night-school, she might advance her sleep–wake schedule to a conventional sleep-time, e.g., 11 PM by using phototherapy (bright lights in the morning) or a hypnotic in the evening. Alternatively, using chronotherapy, she might delay her sleep-time by successively postponing it 1–3 hours each night until she would fall asleep at 11 PM.

Sleep restriction is useful if patients have insomnia from prolonged sleep latency. It creates more efficient sleep by initially causing sleep deprivation. Ms. Brooks already has sleep deprivation and has no lengthening of her sleep latency. Antidepressants do not help nondepressed patients overcome insomnia. Amphetamines are inappropriate treatment of EDS from insomnia because they often eventually lead to dependence, greater insomnia, and other adverse effects.

Once she has achieved an acceptable schedule, she must maintain it throughout the entire week. She should not even allow herself to sleep late on weekends and holidays.

103. Which neurodegenerative illness is frequently comorbid with REM sleep behavior disorder?
    a. Dementia with Lewy bodies
    b. Huntington disease
    c. Alzheimer disease
    d. Frontotemporal dementia

Answer: a. Synucleinopathies – including dementia with Lewy bodies, and Parkinson disease, develop in as many as 50% of REM sleep behavior disorder patients within 3–10 years.

104. Into which category does the DSM-5 place Sleep-Related Sexual Behavior Disorder (Sexsomnia)?
    a. REM parasomnia
    b. Hypersomnolence disorder
    c. REM sleep behavior disorder
    d. NREM parasomnia

Answer: d. The DSM-5 classifies Sexsomnia as a NREM Sleep Arousal Disorder. Neurologists similarly categorize sleep-related eating in the sleepwalking type.

105. In episodes of which disorder are the individual's eyes typically open?
    a. REM sleep behavior disorder
    b. Nightmare disorder
    c. NREM sleep arousal disorders
    d. NREM sleep

Answer: c. In sleepwalking and sleep terrors – NREM sleep arousal disorders – individuals maintain open eyes. Fortuitously, having open eyes is protective in sleepwalking.

106. Which condition is *not* associated with sleep-onset REM periods (SOREMPs)?
    a. RLS
    b. Sleep deprivation
    c. Depression
    d. Narcolepsy

Answer: a. RLS affects individuals attempting to sleep or merely rest. They are awake when RLS movements occur. SOREMPs characterize the sleep architecture of the other conditions, all of which may result in EDS; however, depression commonly results in insomnia as well as EDS.

107. A 45-year-old diabetic man undergoing evaluation for erectile dysfunction fails to have erections during nocturnal penile tumescence (NPT) studies. Which of the following is the *least* likely explanation?
    a. Profound depression
    b. A sleep disorder
    c. Use of medications or alcohol
    d. Anxiety

Answer: d. Men with anxiety-induced or other psychologic erectile dysfunction, as well as normal men, typically develop erections during REM sleep. Absence of erections during NPT studies, however, does not necessarily indicate a serious neurologic or vascular disease. Depression, a sleep disorder (especially ones that abolish REM sleep), and long-term use of certain medicines or alcohol may also inhibit erections during the test.

INVOLUNTARY MOVEMENT DISORDERS

Involuntary movement disorders occur frequently and cause serious physical disabilities. In some of these disorders, dementia and depression routinely precede or overshadow the movements, but others show neither psychiatric nor cognitive impairment despite profound physical disability.

Abnormalities of the basal ganglia underlie the classic movement disorders: Parkinson disease, athetosis, chorea, hemiballismus, Wilson disease, and generalized dystonia. In contrast, for several other disorders – including myoclonus, focal dystonias, essential tremor, and tics and Tourette disorder – the neuroanatomic basis is not understood but the basal ganglia are at least grossly normal. In some cases, adventitious movements, such as tremor or dystonia, can stem from psychiatric disorders or malingering.

Neuroimaging or laboratory tests may confirm the clinical diagnosis of many movement disorders; however, for all of them, the initial diagnosis rests on clinical grounds. Even more than other neurologic conditions, the diagnosis of a movement disorder relies upon careful observation and examination.

THE BASAL GANGLIA

The basal ganglia comprise five subcortical gray matter macroscopic nuclei (Figs. 18.1 and 18.2):

- The *caudate nucleus* and *putamen*, which together constitute the *striatum*
- The *globus pallidus*, which, together with the putamen, constitute the *lenticular nuclei*
- The *subthalamic nucleus* (*of Luys*)
- The *substantia nigra*.

The basal ganglia are linked to each other, to the thalamus, to the cerebral cortex, and to other structures via interconnections of dizzying complexity. Projections from the basal ganglia, along with tracts originating in the cerebellum, constitute the *extrapyramidal* motor system, in contrast with the *pyramidal* (corticospinal) tract. The extrapyramidal system modulates the corticospinal tract. It promotes, inhibits, and sequences movement. In addition, it maintains appropriate muscle tone and adjusts posture. Unlike the cerebellum and the pyramidal tract, the basal ganglia do not directly receive input from – or send output to – the spinal cord; rather, they project within the brain and act upon thalamocortical connections to inhibit or disinhibit the corticospinal tract.

The striatum is the main input nucleus of the basal ganglia and receives projections from numerous and widespread areas of the brain. The clinically most important input comes via the *nigrostriatal tract*, which, as its name suggests, extends from the substantia nigra to the striatum (Fig. 18.3). These projections use dopamine as their neurotransmitter, which interacts with medium spiny neurons in the striatum expressing either D1 or D2 dopamine receptors. Dopamine binding to D1 receptors stimulates adenylate cyclase activity, but dopamine binding to D2 receptors inhibits adenylate cyclase activity (see Table 21.1). Output from the striatum travels through two pathways: a *direct pathway* projecting (from striatal neurons expressing D1 receptors) to the globus pallidus internal segment (GPi), and an *indirect pathway* (from neurons expressing D2 receptors) which synapses in the globus pallidus external segment (GPe) and then the subthalamic nucleus en route to the GPi. The GPi uses gamma-aminobutyric acid (GABA) to send inhibitory output to the thalamus and thereby regulate thalamocortical pathways.

Damage to the basal ganglia (due to stroke, toxins, neurodegeneration, etc.), which produces excessive inhibitory output from the GPi, typically causes *hypokinesia* (too little movement) and, when patients move, *bradykinesia* or *akinesia* (slow or near-absent movement), rigidity, and impaired postural reflexes. Alternatively, insults that reduce the inhibition on the thalamus lead to *hyperkinesia* (increased movement), which takes the form of tremor, athetosis, chorea, hemiballismus, or dystonia. For most clinical purposes, Parkinson disease and parkinsonism (see below) constitute the sole hypokinetic movement disorder. However, sometimes hypokinesia and hyperkinesia may occur in combination; for example, Parkinson disease causes both bradykinesia and tremor.

As with other lesions of the brain – excluding those in the cerebellum – unilateral injuries of the basal ganglia induce clinical abnormalities in the contralateral side of the body. When illnesses exclusively affect the extrapyramidal tracts, patients show no evidence of pyramidal (corticospinal) tract damage, such as paresis, spasticity (though they do have rigidity – see below), hyperactive reflexes, or Babinski signs. Similarly, they have no signs of cerebral cortex damage, such as dementia and seizures.

GENERAL CONSIDERATIONS

Involuntary movement disorders share several clinical features. Anxiety, exertion, fatigue, and stimulants (including caffeine) increase the movements, but willful concentration and sometimes biofeedback may suppress them, at least

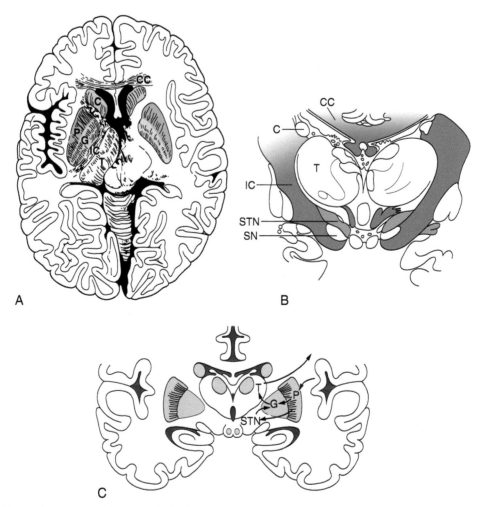

FIGURE 18.1 ■ *A*, This axial view of the brain shows the basal ganglia in relation to other brain structures, as displayed in CT and MRI studies. The heads of the caudate nuclei (C) indent the lateral undersurface of the anterior horns of the lateral ventricles. The caudate and putamen (P) constitute the *striatum*. The globus pallidus (G), which has internal and external segments, and the putamen form the *lenticular nucleus*, named for its resemblance to an old-fashioned lens (also see Fig. 18.1C). The posterior limb of the internal capsule (IC) separates the lenticular nucleus from the thalamus (T), which is not a component of the basal ganglia. *B*, This coronal view of the diencephalon demonstrates the substantia nigra (SN) and the subthalamic nuclei (ST) below the thalamus. The substantia nigra, because of its characteristic shape and pigmentation, serves as a landmark. The lateral ventricles are bounded laterally by the heads of the caudate nuclei (C) and superiorly by the corpus callosum (CC). *C*, A coronal view shows extrapyramidal circuits. The putamen sends input to the internal segment of the globus pallidus (GPi) via a direct pathway and an indirect pathway. Dopaminergic neurons in the substantia nigra project to the putamen, where neurons with D1 receptors project directly to the GPi (the direct pathway). Putaminal neurons with D2 receptors project through the globus pallidus external segment (GPe) and subthalamic nucleus and thence to the GPi (the indirect pathway). The GPi projects to the ventrolateral nucleus of the thalamus, which projects to the motor cortex. The cortex, completing a circuit, innervates the putamen.

transiently. Most involuntary movements disappear during sleep. The exceptions – hemifacial spasm, myoclonus, palatal tremor, and certain sleep-related disorders – persist in sleep (see Chapter 17).

Neurologists find it useful to classify involuntary movements along several dimensions. One axis is their anatomic distribution: whether they are focal (involving one body part), multifocal (involving more than one discrete body part), or generalized (involving the entire body). Another is whether they occur continuously or intermittently.

The diagnosis of patients with involuntary movement disorders is fraught with at least two potential errors.

Although possibly debilitated by uncontrollable movements and inarticulate speech, patients may remain fully alert, intelligent, and, possibly by resorting to unconventional techniques, able to communicate. Unless physicians are astute, they may misdiagnose these individuals as having cognitive impairment. On the other hand, dementia is characteristic of some movement disorders and its presence should not be overlooked.

Another error may occur when patients, at first glance, appear to have a psychogenic movement disorder (see later and Chapter 3). In many situations, the lack of a definitive confirmatory laboratory test forces neurologists to rely exclusively on their clinical judgment.

PARKINSON DISEASE

Essential tremor and restless legs syndrome (RLS) (see Chapter 17) are more prevalent than Parkinson disease (PD), but PD remains the quintessential movement disorder. It has three cardinal features:

- Tremor
- Rigidity
- Bradykinesia.

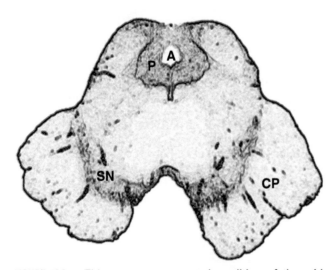

FIGURE 18.2 ■ This computer-generated rendition of the midbrain should be compared to a photograph (see Fig. 2.9), functional drawings (see Figs. 4.5 and 4.9), and an idealized sketch (see Fig. 21.1). The lower third of the midbrain, which lies just caudal to the diencephalon, contains the pair of horizontal but gently curved, elongated, pigmented nuclei – the substantia nigra (SN). In Parkinson disease, the substantia nigra and other pigmented nuclei lose their pigment and, compared to normal, thus appear blanched. The midbrain also houses the dorsally located aqueduct of Sylvius (A) surrounded by the periaqueductal gray matter (P), and cerebral peduncles (PD), which contain the descending corticospinal tract.

The initial and ultimately most disabling physical feature of PD is usually bradykinesia or, in the extreme, akinesia. Slow or absent movement produces the classic *masked face* (Fig. 18.4), paucity of trunk and limb movement (Figs. 18.5 and 18.6), and impairment of activities of daily living. Patients sometimes liken their slow movements to slogging through hip-deep mud, wearing lead clothing, or driving a car with an engaged emergency brake.

Rigidity typically accompanies bradykinesia (Fig. 18.7). Although rigidity is one of the cardinal features of PD, it often appears as a manifestation of other extrapyramidal disorders. No matter the context, physicians

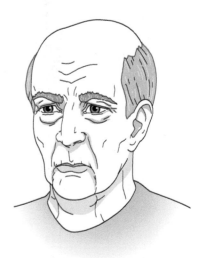

FIGURE 18.4 ■ Compared to normal individuals of the same age, Parkinson disease patients blink less frequently, show less facial expression, and move their head less often. Neurologists have called patients' facial appearance a "stare" or "masked facies" (Latin, face or countenance). Even when subtle, the masked face gives the appearance of apathy or depression.

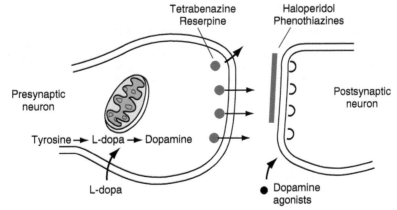

FIGURE 18.3 ■ A succession of enzymes normally converts tyrosine to dopamine in the presynaptic nigrostriatal neuron. In Parkinson disease the nigrostriatal tract degenerates, but the postsynaptic dopamine receptors remain intact. As a result of the degeneration, an absence of tyrosine hydroxylase leads to insufficient L-dopa and consequently markedly reduced synthesis of dopamine. Levodopa, the standard oral medication for Parkinson disease, penetrates the blood–brain barrier and substitutes for the deficient endogenous L-dopa in dopamine synthesis. (D-dopa, the dextro-isomer, does not cross the blood–brain barrier and cannot enter the synthetic pathway. It is therefore useless as a treatment for Parkinson disease.) Dopamine agonists, such as rotigotine (Neupro), pramipexole (Mirapex), and ropinirole (Requip), act directly on the D2 receptor and, to a lesser extent, other postsynaptic dopamine receptors. Although dopamine agonists treat Parkinson disease, they produce a less powerful effect than levodopa. Because reserpine and tetrabenazine deplete dopamine from its presynaptic sites, each reduces hyperkinesia in chorea, tardive dyskinesia, and Tourette disorder. However, presumably because these drugs create a dopamine-deficiency state, they produce lethargy, parkinsonism, and depression.

should not confuse rigidity with spasticity, which signals corticospinal tract disease (see Chapter 2).

Tremor is often the most conspicuous feature of Parkinson disease; however, it is the least specific sign, least debilitating symptom, and least associated with dementia and depression. In Parkinson disease, the affected body part usually oscillates in a single plane with a regular rate, although with a variable amplitude. It primarily involves the upper extremities asymmetrically. Even more characteristically, the tremor appears when patients rest quietly with their arms supported. This *resting tremor* (Fig. 18.8) distinguishes it from the *action tremor* of cerebellar tremor and essential tremor. When patients have tremor as their primary symptom, neurologists describe them as having "tremor-predominant" PD.

These cardinal features, in contrast to signs of most other movement disorders, typically first develop in an asymmetric or unilateral pattern. Even as PD progresses to involve both sides of the body, its manifestations continue to predominate on the side initially involved.

Another important feature of PD is its response in almost 80% of cases to levodopa (L-dopa) treatment. In the absence of a definitive laboratory test for the illness, a positive response to levodopa confirms the diagnosis for most neurologists. Likewise, failure to respond prompts them to consider alternative diagnoses, such as medication-induced parkinsonism, progressive supranuclear palsy, spinocerebellar ataxia, and Wilson disease (see below).

Additional symptoms and signs may emerge, despite treatment, as PD advances. Posture may become stooped. Patients lose their *postural reflexes*, which are neurologic compensatory mechanisms that adjust muscle tone in response to change in position. Loss of these reflexes, in

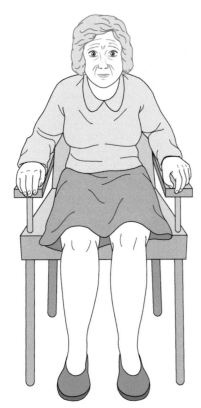

FIGURE 18.5 ■ Parkinson disease patients typically sit motionless with their legs uncrossed and their feet flat. Their arms remain on the chair or in their lap and rarely participate in normal gestures or repositioning movements. In contrast to normal individuals and especially those with chorea, Parkinson disease patients do not shift their weight from one hip to another or make any unnecessary movements.

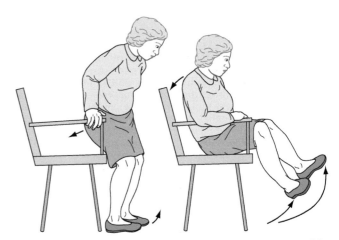

FIGURE 18.6 ■ Patients with akinesia and rigidity cannot rapidly flex their spine, hips, or knees. When sitting, they tend to fall slowly and solidly backward into a chair. Unable to bend rapidly, their feet rise several inches off the floor. Sitting and turning en bloc signal early parkinsonism.

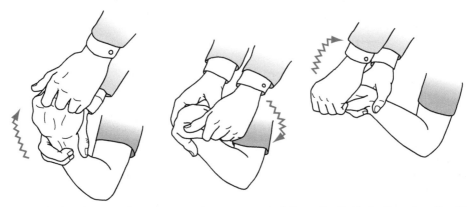

FIGURE 18.7 ■ When neurologists detect resistance to passive movement of the patient's limbs they describe this as rigidity. When present, rigidity causes an increased tone in all directions of movement. A superimposed tremor creates ratchet-like *cogwheel rigidity*.

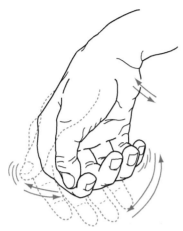

FIGURE 18.8 ■ *Resting tremor* – a cardinal feature of Parkinson disease – consists of a relatively slow (4 to 6 Hz) to-and-fro flexion movement of the wrist, hand, thumb, and fingers most apparent when patients sit comfortably. Its similarity to rolling a pill or a coin between the thumb and index finger gave rise to the description "pill-rolling" tremor. The tremor is exaggerated or sometimes apparent only when patients are anxious. However, voluntary movement or intense concentration may momentarily reduce the tremor, and sleep abolishes it. Rigidity and akinesia almost always accompany Parkinson disease's resting tremor.

combination with akinesia and rigidity, results in a characteristic gait impairment, *marche à petit pas* or *festinating gait*, which consists of patients' tendency to take short shuffling steps and accelerate their pace (Fig. 18.9A). In a test of postural reflexes, the *pull test*, the examiner stands behind the patient and quickly pulls the shoulders backward (Fig. 18.9B). Normal individuals merely sway. Patients who have mild impairment of their postural reflexes take a few steps back, exhibiting *retropulsion*. More severely affected patients rock stiffly backwards without flexion or other compensatory movement and topple en bloc into the examiner's arms.

PD patients' gait abnormality and impaired postural reflexes prevent them from walking safely. Many fall and fracture a hip. These disabilities eventually confine them to bed and contribute to morbidity and mortality.

Even at the onset of the illness, patients' handwriting deteriorates to a small and tremulous script, *micrographia* (Fig. 18.10). In parallel, their voice loses both volume and normal fluctuations in pitch and cadence, i.e., their speech becomes *hypophonic* and *monotonous*. Also, because of their illness or the medications used to treat it, PD patients develop sleep disturbances, characteristically REM sleep behavior disorder (see Chapter 17).

After several years of disease, patients usually develop fluctuating symptoms, termed "on–off phenomena." This problem likely results from inadequate buffering, storage, release, and reuptake of dopamine – whether from endogenous or exogenous sources. During "on" periods, patients remain well treated and asymptomatic, but during "off" periods, which may last hours, they are impaired by rigidity and bradykinesia. Even if patients reach a state of complete rigidity resembling catatonia in their off-periods, they have no change in their level of consciousness or electroencephalogram (EEG).

Nonmotor physical problems also emerge. For example, PD patients characteristically lose their sense of smell. The anosmia, which also occurs in Alzheimer disease, reflects the neurodegenerative nature of these illnesses (see Chapters 4 and 7). PD patients also routinely develop problems with their autonomic nervous system, including dysphagia, constipation, urinary incontinence, and abnormal sweating.

Parkinsonism

Tremor, rigidity, and bradykinesia constitute the clinical syndrome of *parkinsonism*. "Parkinson disease" connotes the neurodegenerative disease, which is the most common cause of parkinsonism but not the only one. The most important example of parkinsonism occurs when dopamine receptor-blocking antipsychotics produce tremor, rigidity, and bradykinesia; neurologists say that such patients have parkinsonism, not Parkinson disease. Parkinsonism characterizes many neurologic illnesses, including dementia with Lewy bodies disease (see later), chronic traumatic encephalopathy (CTE) (previously known as dementia pugilistica, see Chapter 22), and Parkinson-plus diseases, as well as Parkinson disease.

Psychiatric Conditions Comorbid with Parkinson Disease

Depression

For the first several years after onset of PD, patients' mood may reflect their failing health, isolation from coworkers and friends, reduced income, and loss of independence. A second phase of depression emerges after several years as the disease, despite optimal treatment, begins to incapacitate patients. Reports of prevalence of depression in PD patients vary widely because of variability in definitions and criteria among studies. Testing patients at different stages of the illness, including or excluding psychiatric comorbidities, and failing to weigh manifestations of the illness that may reflect either mood disorder or motor impairment (such as hypophonia, facial immobility, and sleep disturbances) all affect the reported prevalence of depression. By any measure, however, the prevalence of depression is substantial. Studies typically report that at least 30% of all PD patients manifest depression. The *Diagnostic and Statistical Manual of Mental Disorders, 5th Edition* (DSM-5) diagnosis of Depressive Disorder Due to Another Medical Condition would be appropriate in these cases.

The most powerful risk factors for depression include a history of depression, cognitive impairment, and akinesia, but not tremor. In addition, a young age at onset and longer duration of illness constitute powerful risk factors.

When it occurs, depression accelerates cognitive decline, interferes with sleep, and accentuates physical disabilities. Of the nonmotor PD symptoms, this one correlates most closely with a poor quality of life. The depression provokes anxiety, which may occur as another comorbidity. PD with or without comorbid depression generally does not increase the suicide rate.

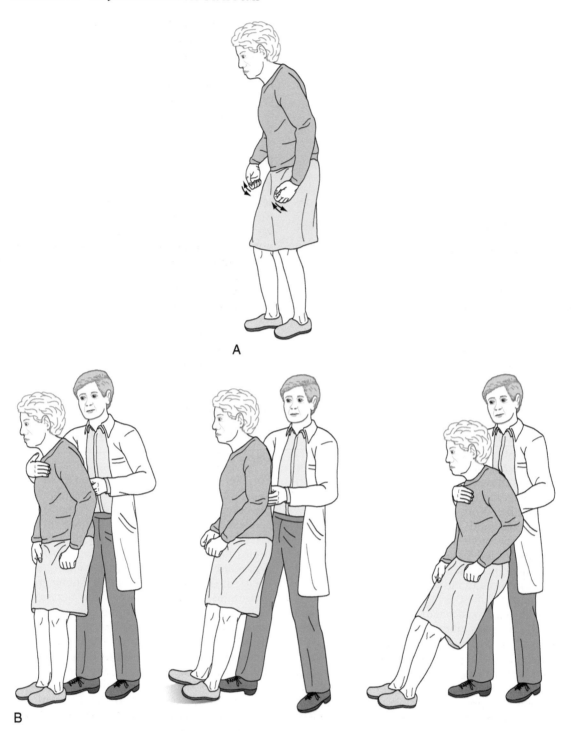

A

B

FIGURE 18.9 ■ *A*, Parkinson disease often produces a characteristic gait, in which patients take short, shuffling steps. Their neck and lower spine are typically flexed. When walking, they fail to swing their arms, look about, or have other normal accessory movements. They may have *festination*, i.e., acceleration with trouble stopping. Likewise, while turning they simultaneously move their head, trunk, and legs en bloc. *B*, The *pull test* consists of the physician's gently but rapidly pulling the patient's shoulders backward. Unaffected individuals will compensate by taking one or two steps backward. Parkinson patients, who generally have impaired postural reflexes, will take many steps backward (exhibiting *retropulsion*) because they are unable to stop through reflexive weight-shifting compensatory maneuvers. In pronounced cases, as the one pictured here, patients unable to alter their posture will tilt backwards en bloc and fall into the physician's arms. (PSP patients have similar bradykinesia, lack of accessory movements, and a positive pull test, but their posture is extended or erect rather than flexed.)

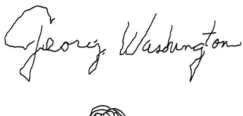

FIGURE 18.10 ■ The handwriting in this sample from a Parkinson disease patient shows progressive decrease in height (*micrographia*) and a superimposed tremor. Abnormalities in signatures, such as those on checks, can often date the onset of Parkinson disease. Although essential tremor may also cause tremor in handwriting samples, micrographia indicates that parkinsonism is the underlying condition.

Physicians should keep in mind the well-being of the patient's caregivers. Studies show that affective disorders and reduced quality of life are commonplace among caregivers and anxiety scores are high among women caregivers. As the illness progresses, caregivers shoulder an ever-increasing burden that may overwhelm them. Caregivers are especially susceptible to depression if the patient is depressed or has had a lengthy illness.

Treatment of Comorbid Depression

Psychological support, social services, and rehabilitation often help during the first several years of PD. However, as the disease progresses, optimum treatment almost always requires antidepressants. Neurologists should optimize the patient's antiparkinson medication regimen before anyone prescribes antidepressants because PD medicines can improve mood as well as motor symptoms.

However it is done, treatment of depression improves PD patients' quality of life and reduces their disability. Antidepressants may be just as effective in treating depression comorbid with PD as they are in treating depression unassociated with PD.

Several considerations should guide the choice of an antidepressant. Antidepressants and other psychotropics should be anxiolytic. Earlier studies found tricyclic antidepressants (TCAs) to be more effective than selective serotonin reuptake inhibitors (SSRIs). However, Parkinson disease patients, who are generally elderly, are susceptible to the anticholinergic side effects of TCAs, and more recent research has demonstrated efficacy of SSRIs in this population.

Although SSRIs carry fewer side effects than TCAs, they may cause a unique problem in PD patients. Prescribing an SSRI in conjunction with a monoamine oxidase (MAO) inhibitor (such as selegiline or rasagiline) can theoretically cause the serotonin syndrome because SSRIs prevent serotonin reuptake while MAO inhibitors prevent its breakdown (see Chapter 6). The actual incidence of serotonin syndrome is very low because at the doses used for treating PD selegiline selectively inhibits only MAO-B, which metabolizes dopamine, whereas the serotonin syndrome is mostly a complication of inhibition of MAO-A, which metabolizes serotonin. Similarly, when physicians

prescribe the selegiline patch (Emsam) for depression, as long as the dose remains below 12 mg/day, which is standard, it selectively inhibits MAO-B; however, selegiline patch doses greater than 12 mg/day inhibit MAO-A as well as MAO-B, and leave patients at risk of tyramine-induced hypertension or serotonin syndrome.

Electroconvulsive therapy (ECT) is effective and safe for depression in PD. In addition, it temporarily improves the rigidity and bradykinesia.

Dementia

During the first 5 years after onset of PD, patients typically continue to work, manage a household, participate in leisure activities, and remain free of cognitive impairment. Even when physically incapacitated, patients may retain sufficient cognitive capacity for routine intellectual activities.

However, as PD progresses and patients age, dementia commonly complicates the illness. In these cases, the DSM-5 would apply the diagnosis of Major Neurocognitive Disorder Due to Parkinson's disease. Dementia affects 24% to 50% of patients with PD. Its prevalence increases in proportion to the patient's age, duration of the illness, and physical impairments. Dementia is more frequent when akinesia and rigidity rather than tremor predominate. When dementia and depression both complicate Parkinson disease, dementia is usually more severe than when it occurs without depression.

PD dementia, which differs clinically from that of Alzheimer disease dementia, is distinguished by inattention, poor memory, difficulty shifting mental sets, and *bradyphrenia* (slowed thinking, the cognitive counterpart of bradykinesia). With its almost invariable gait impairment and preserved language function, the dementia of PD serves as a prime example of "subcortical dementia" (see Chapter 7). The Mini-Mental State Examination (MMSE) and the Montreal Cognitive Assessment (MoCA) are both valid screening tests for cognitive impairment in Parkinson disease; however, the MoCA is more sensitive. PD patients typically lose 2.3 points annually on the MMSE.

Of the potential causes of dementia in PD, studies have not implicated dopamine deficiency. The simplest evidence is that dopaminergic medicines do not prevent or alleviate the dementia. One possible cause or contributor is an acetylcholine deficiency. PET studies have shown a cerebral cortex cholinergic deficit in PD patients with dementia that is more pronounced than in Alzheimer disease.

A special diagnostic hazard when evaluating a patient with parkinsonism and dementia is failing to recognize *Lewy bodies disease*. This illness shares important features with PD including rigidity and bradykinesia, delusions and hallucinations, and sleep disturbances as well as cognitive impairment. One major clinical difference is that in Lewy bodies disease, dementia constitutes an early manifestation (see Chapter 7), but when dementia occurs in PD, it is a relatively late development. On a histologic level, Lewy bodies disease features Lewy bodies in the cerebral cortex, not just in the substantia nigra.

As with comorbid depression, treatments that reduce PD motor symptoms do not ameliorate comorbid dementia. For example, dopaminergic medicines alleviate tremor and rigidity, but they fail to improve cognitive function. Likewise, deep brain stimulation (DBS), which greatly reduces Parkinson disease motor symptoms (see later), does not reverse dementia. On the other hand, cholinesterase inhibitors may slow cognitive decline and reduce visual hallucinations.

Psychosis

PD patients commonly experience visual hallucinations, such as complex visions of people and animals that fluctuate throughout daytime and worsen at night. During hallucinations, PD patients initially maintain a clear sensorium and retain some insight. As the disease progresses, the majority of patients develop vivid hallucinations, disordered thinking, and often paranoid ideation that may center on physicians and family members.

Psychosis in PD correlates most closely with dementia and the duration and severity of the illness. It also correlates with the number and dosage of dopaminergic medications and signs of excessive medication, particularly dyskinesias. Notably, although PD medications often precipitate psychosis, they cause neither comorbid depression nor dementia. Other risk factors for psychosis include advanced age, sleep disturbances, and visual impairment. Finally, intercurrent illnesses, such as pneumonia or a urinary tract infection, readily precipitate psychosis or delirium; such reversible causes should always be sought, especially when symptoms begin abruptly in the absence of another identifiable trigger (such as an increase in medication). Thus, depending on the circumstances and clinical features of an individual case, appropriate DSM-5 diagnoses may be Delirium, Substance/Medication-Induced Psychotic Disorder, or Psychotic Disorder Due to Another Medical Condition.

In any case, once psychosis develops, it predisposes patients to dementia (which may have already developed), nursing home placement, and death within 2 years. Compared to the physical disabilities and cognitive impairment, psychosis imposes the greatest stress on caregivers.

Treatment of Comorbid Psychosis

Because of antiparkinson medications' role in causing or exacerbating psychosis, neurologists usually attempt to taper them or adjust their schedule before adding antipsychotics. They generally reduce medicines in order of likelihood of their causing mental aberrations: anticholinergics, then dopamine agonists, and lastly levodopa. Of course, patients can tolerate medication withdrawal only up to a point, after which disabling motor impairments return. In general, patients, physicians, and caregivers prefer mild rigidity and some immobility to psychosis.

Because administration of antiparkinson medication before bedtime tends to cause nightmares and hallucinations, neurologists advance the last daily dose to the early evening. Also, they avoid suddenly stopping these medicines because their abrupt withdrawal may lead to irreversible motor deterioration, complications of immobility, or even the neuroleptic malignant syndrome (NMS) (see Chapter 6).

Despite the "black box" warnings and other caveats, when psychosis is severe physicians eventually may have no alternative than to prescribe an antipsychotic. They should avoid agents that block dopamine receptors because they exacerbate parkinsonism. Clozapine and quetiapine, which target serotonin receptors, are the safest; clozapine is more effective but requires monitoring due to risk of agranulocytosis. Another approach involves use of an anticholinesterase – rivastigmine, donepezil, or galantamine – in hopes of reducing visual hallucinations and improving cognitive impairments.

Other Psychiatric Conditions

In contrast to the frequency of comorbid depression, bipolar disorder and schizophrenia rarely complicate PD. In fact, the rare coexistence of schizophrenia and PD contradicts the "dopamine hypothesis" of schizophrenia, which would predict that these two conditions, one from decreased dopamine activity and the other from increased dopamine activity, would be mutually exclusive. (Neurologists primarily should consider the diagnoses of Lewy bodies disease and drug-induced parkinsonism when PD and schizophrenia appear to co-occur.)

Impulse control disorders, a group of dramatic PD psychiatric complications, afflicts about 14% of Parkinson disease patients with one or more of the following aberrant behaviors: compulsive or pathological gambling, sexual behavior, shopping, or eating. Treatment with a dopamine agonist is the most powerful risk factor. Others include being unmarried, cigarette smoking, and a personal or family history of gambling. Reducing dopamine agonists or, when appropriate, performing DBS usually eliminates them. Cognitive-behavioral therapy may reduce the severity of impulse control behaviors in PD.

Another medication-induced behavioral complication of Parkinson disease consists of mindless, repetitive, purposeless behavior – *punding*. Common examples include patients' incessantly arranging peas on their plate into small piles, dismantling small constructions and then rebuilding them, opening and shutting a door, and folding and unfolding a newspaper without reading it. Not only does punding capture the patient's entire attention, it displaces normal daily activities and prohibits caregivers' assisting the patient. Punding does not seem to yield any pleasure or excitement. Similar behavior occurs in children with autism and adults with amphetamine intoxication. Other impulse control behaviors that beset PD patients include "hobbyism" (repetitive activities but at a higher level than punding) and hoarding. Reducing dopaminergic medicines or adding an antipsychotic medicine should decrease these behaviors but at the risk of exacerbating parkinsonism.

In a related disorder, *dopamine dysregulation syndrome* (formerly known as *hedonistic homeostatic dysregulation*), some PD patients curiously tend to overmedicate themselves. They express much greater concern for their medication (usually levodopa) than their symptoms warrant, and describe their medication requirements in terms associated with an obsession or addiction. At the other extreme, rapidly tapering or abruptly stopping dopaminergic medicines may send PD patients into a state of withdrawal – with cravings, anxiety, and drug-seeking behavior – akin to when amphetamine abusers are deprived of their stimulants.

Fatigue may be severe and may not readily respond to standard treatments. Apathy and anxiety are also common in PD and may have significant impact on patients' quality of life.

Pathology of Parkinson Disease

A well-established synthetic pathway in presynaptic nigrostriatal tract neurons normally converts phenylalanine to dopamine:

$$\text{Phenylalanine} \xrightarrow{\text{phenylalanine hydroxylase}} \text{Tyrosine}$$
$$\xrightarrow{\text{tyrosine hydroxylase}} \text{L-DOPA}$$
$$\xrightarrow{\text{DOPA decarboxylase}} \text{Dopamine}$$

(L- = L-3, 4-dihydroxyphenylalanine)

In PD, the nigrostriatal neurons slowly degenerate and lose their tyrosine hydroxylase. This degeneration of neurons places PD in the category of "neurodegenerative diseases." Amyotrophic lateral sclerosis (ALS), Alzheimer disease, Huntington disease, and several other chronic progressive illnesses also fall into this category.

The loss of tyrosine hydroxylase represents the critical failure in the pathogenesis of PD because this enzyme is the rate-limiting enzyme in dopamine synthesis (see Fig. 18.3). With the tyrosine hydroxylase deficit, the ever-shrinking pool of remaining nigrostriatal tract neurons cannot sustain the essential synthetic pathway. Once approximately 60% of these neurons degenerate, the nigrostriatal tract cannot synthesize adequate dopamine and PD symptoms appear. The illness also impairs synthesis of other neurotransmitters. For example, it leads to reduced concentrations of serotonin in the brain and cerebrospinal fluid (CSF).

The characteristic neuropathology of PD, which is immediately evident on gross examination of the brain, consists of loss of normal pigment (depigmentation) in certain brainstem nuclei: the substantia nigra (black), locus ceruleus (Latin, cerulean, blue), and vagus (Latin, wandering) motor nuclei (black).

On a microscopic level, neurons in these locations characteristically accumulate *Lewy bodies*, which contain a core of *α-synuclein* (see Chapter 7). In contrast, Lewy bodies located in the cerebral cortex, as well as the basal ganglia, constitute the histologic hallmark of Lewy body disease. With their abundance of Lewy bodies, both Parkinson disease and Lewy bodies fall under the rubric of *synucleinopathies*.

Positron emission tomography (PET) using radiolabeled fluorodeoxyglucose or fluorodopa usually shows asymmetrically decreased dopamine activity in the basal ganglia in presymptomatic individuals as well as in those with overt PD. Imaging presynaptic dopamine transporters with ioflupane (123-iodine) and single-photon emission computed tomography (SPECT) may distinguish PD from nonparkinsonian conditions, including essential tremor and drug-induced parkinsonism (see later). Other tests, such as magnetic resonance imaging (MRI), computed tomography (CT), transcranial ultrasound examination of the substantia nigra, and routine serum and CSF analyses, fail to reveal consistent abnormalities. Given the lack of specificity or sensitivity and expense of these tests, the diagnosis of PD continues to rely upon the patient's clinical features and response to levodopa treatment. As with Alzheimer disease research (see Chapter 7), much current research into PD focuses on efforts to identify useful biomarkers for the disease.

Possible Causes of Parkinson Disease

Parkinson disease ranks second to Alzheimer disease as the most common neurodegenerative illness. In contrast to the absence of responsible toxins in Alzheimer disease, studies have implicated various environmental and industrial toxins as causes of or even potential protectors against Parkinson disease. As with Alzheimer disease, genetic studies have discovered several mutations as risk factors and causes of Parkinson disease in a minority of patients.

Toxins

Parkinson disease has an increased incidence in people who drink well water, particularly farmers and other workers exposed to herbicides, insecticides, and pesticides. For example, exposure to the commercial insecticides rotenone and paraquat, which share a chemical structure with 1-methyl-4-phenyl-1,2,3,6-tetrahydropyridine (*MPTP*, see later), at least doubles the risk of Parkinson disease. Exposure to solvents is also a risk factor. The relationship between welding or other manganese exposure and risk of developing PD is controversial; while these previously were considered to be significant risk factors for PD, more recent epidemiologic studies have not indicated increased risk. Nevertheless, high levels of manganese (manganism) lead to parkinsonism (see below).

The most infamous PD-producing toxin is MPTP. This substance, a by-product of the illicit manufacture of meperidine (Demerol) and other narcotics, caused fulminant and often fatal PD in dozens of drug abusers who unknowingly administered it to themselves. Researchers have shown that MPTP selectively poisons nigrostriatal tract neurons and now use it in the laboratory to produce the standard animal model of PD.

In the opposite situation, some otherwise toxic substances fail to produce Parkinson disease. For example, contrary to initial reports, 3,4-methylenedioxy-methamphetamine (*MDMA*), commonly known as *ecstasy*, which depletes serotonin, probably does not cause PD. Although several young adults developed parkinsonism after using ecstasy, they may have used MPTP or other illicit drugs or possibly carried a genetic mutation (see below). Moreover, the small number of cases compared to the large number of probable ecstasy users suggests that ecstasy is benign in this particular regard.

Cigarette smoking varies inversely with the incidence of PD: based on statistics, cigarette smokers develop PD at lower rates. Coffee drinkers, those with elevated uric acid levels, and those who take ibuprofen regularly also have a reduced incidence of Parkinson disease. These associations do not necessarily denote a protective effect of these behaviors, though such an effect has been hypothesized.

In addition to the potential for dopamine receptor-blocking agents to cause reversible parkinsonism (see below), recent publications have raised the possibility that exposure to neuroleptics may increase the risk of eventually developing PD. More research is needed for confirmation of such a relationship and elucidation of the possible mechanisms behind it.

Oxidative Stress

Research stemming from the neurotoxicity of MPTP led to the *oxidative stress theory*, which proposes that defective mitochondria in Parkinson disease patients cannot detoxify potentially lethal endogenous or environmental oxidants, particularly *free radicals*, such as superoxides and nitric oxide. Free radicals are atoms or molecules that are unstable because they contain a single, unpaired electron. To complete their electron pairs, free radicals snatch electrons from neighboring atoms or molecules. Loss of electrons oxidizes cells and causes fatal injury.

When endogenous MAO oxidizes MPTP, the product, methylphenylpyridinium (MPP^+), generates intracellular free radicals that inhibit complex I of the mitochondrial respiratory chain. In laboratory animals, pretreatment with MAO inhibitors blocks this reaction. It thereby prevents MPP^+ formation, subsequent tissue oxidation, and development of parkinsonism.

Accepting the theory, neurologists have blamed oxidative stress and free radicals for numerous neurologic illnesses. However, the theory remains unproven. Moreover, antioxidants do not prevent or alter any of the illnesses.

Head Trauma

Even head trauma severe enough to cause loss of consciousness and posttraumatic amnesia only slightly increases the subsequent risk of a patient's developing PD. However, if the patient who sustains comparable head trauma carries one or more alpha-synuclein genes, the subsequent risk of PD rises approximately 3 to 11 times.

Repeated head injuries may cause a Parkinson-like syndrome, *dementia pugilistica* or, in current parlance, *chronic traumatic encephalopathy* (*CTE*). This condition consists of the insidious development of intellectual deterioration, dysarthria, stiffness, clumsiness, spasticity, and striking bradykinesia. Boxers who have been lightweight, alcoholic, and lost many matches have been most susceptible. The impairments, which often end their career, typically progress after retirement.

CT and MRI show white matter changes, focal contusions, and cerebral atrophy in proportion to the number of boxing matches. Autopsy studies reveal hydrocephalus and atrophy of the corpus callosum and cerebrum. Histologic examination shows Alzheimer-like neurofibrillary tangles and, with special stains, amyloid plaques, but no Lewy bodies.

Genetic Factors

Genetic factors play a significant role when the onset of PD symptoms occurs before 50 years of age and, obviously, when multiple family members have the illness. Overall, only 10% to 15% of PD patients have a first-degree relative with the same illness and only about 5% of all patients have a genetic cause. Even among PD patients younger than 50 years, only about 17% carry a mutation and many of those mutations show low penetrance.

When they cause the illness, mutations characteristically lead to early-onset illness, but follow either an autosomal dominant or recessive pattern. Symptoms of hereditary forms of PD appear on average as young as 45 years, and occasionally in adolescence or childhood. Genetically determined varieties also differ from the sporadically occurring illness in that their histology usually lacks Lewy bodies.

Several different mutations, including ones in the *parkin, leucine-rich repeat kinase-2* (*LRRK2*), and *α-synuclein* genes, either cause or allow Parkinson disease in some families. In fact, 30% or more of North African Arab and Ashkenazi (Eastern European) Jewish PD patients who have a family history of the illness carry a *LRRK2* mutation.

Recent studies have also linked a mutation in the GBA gene encoding glucocerebrosidase to PD. Deficiency in this enzyme, which ordinarily leads to Gaucher disease, occurs in approximately 15% of Ashkenazi Jewish and 3% of non-Jewish PD patients. Although the association is undoubtedly close and perhaps the most frequently occurring mutation among PD patients, it may confer susceptibility rather than act as a cause.

Prions

As discussed in Chapter 7, prion diseases result from misfolding of proteins that deposit in the brain and disrupt normal neuronal structure and activity. Recently, investigators have begun to consider the idea that α-synuclein might act as a prion-like protein. This hypothesis is based on observations that mutations in the gene coding for α-synuclein, which are known to cause familial PD, cause a conformational change in the protein that promotes aggregation in the brain. Using an animal model, researchers have even succeeded in documenting spread of Lewy bodies following inoculation of misfolded α-synuclein, as would be expected of an infectious agent. This concept could offer a novel avenue for therapeutic interventions in PD.

Parkinsonism

Parkinson disease is the most common cause of the clinical condition *parkinsonism*, but conditions other than PD per se can produce the same clinical manifestations. For example, when dopamine receptor-blocking neuroleptics produce tremor, rigidity, and bradykinesia, the patient has parkinsonism, not PD. Notably, in many illnesses characterized by parkinsonism – dementia pugilistica, Parkinson-plus diseases, and dementia with Lewy bodies disease (see later) – dementia may appear as the first or most prominent symptom.

Medication-Induced Parkinsonism

When medicines, as opposed to illicit drugs, induce parkinsonism, rigidity is the most prominent feature. In fact, all three cardinal features of parkinsonism occur in only about one-third of cases. As with PD, individuals older than 60 years are particularly susceptible to medication-induced parkinsonism. Typical and most atypical antipsychotic agents – because to a greater or lesser degree they block D2 receptors – routinely cause parkinsonism. Likewise, nonpsychiatric medicines that block D2 receptors – such as metoclopramide (Reglan), prochlorperazine (Compazine), and promethazine (Phenergan) – produce the same problem. Tetrabenazine (Xenazine) induces parkinsonism because it depletes dopamine (see later and Figs. 18.3 and 18.13). Case reports have also implicated valproate (Depakote), lithium, amiodarone, and calcium channel blockers – medicines with no direct connection to D2 receptors.

Medication-induced parkinsonism so closely resembles PD that clinical examination cannot reliably distinguish them. As one clue, medication-induced parkinsonism usually causes symmetric, bilateral signs from the onset, but PD tends to cause asymmetric signs at its onset and remain asymmetric throughout its course. Also, antipsychotic agents often induce akathisia and dyskinesias along with the parkinsonism.

Once physicians discontinue the offending drug, medication-induced parkinsonism usually resolves in a few weeks, but sometimes it lasts for 3 months and occasionally for 1 year. However, physicians must be careful with persistent parkinsonism patients because approximately 10% harbor PD or a Parkinson-plus syndrome that perhaps was unmasked by the medication. In children and young adults, persistent parkinsonism following antipsychotic treatment suggests several neurologic illnesses (see later).

If reducing or withdrawing the suspected medicine fails to reverse medication-induced parkinsonism, physicians may institute treatment while they reconsider the diagnosis. They should, however, resist the temptation to override an antipsychotic's block of the D2 receptors by administering dopaminergic medicines. That plan will not work and it may precipitate delirium or psychosis. Administering anticholinergics to counterbalance the lack of dopamine activity may help, but their side effects may outweigh their benefits. Administering amantadine, which mildly enhances dopamine activity, may also help (see later). If these medicines reduce the parkinsonism, physicians should taper them after 3 months to determine if they remain necessary.

Parkinson-Plus Diseases

A group of related neurodegenerative illnesses – loosely termed *Parkinson-plus diseases* – shares many physical signs with PD and its predominantly subcortical dementia. However, other features set them apart from PD and separate one from another. Overall, compared to PD, Parkinson-plus diseases follow a more rapid course and respond less well to dopaminergic medications.

Multisystem atrophy (*MSA*), a family of Parkinson-plus diseases, includes a cerebellar subtype (formerly *olivopontocerebellar degeneration*), which is notable for ataxia, and a subtype with pronounced autonomic dysfunction (formerly *Shy–Drager syndrome*). MSA, like PD, is a synucleinopathy; however, in contrast to PD, MSA does not respond to levodopa treatment.

Progressive Supranuclear Palsy

Patients with progressive supranuclear palsy (PSP) usually present with parkinsonism, except that they rarely have a tremor. Eventually they develop dementia, which the DSM-5 would label as Major Neurocognitive Disorder Due to Another Medical Condition.

PSP patients have predominantly axial rigidity that forces their head, neck, and entire spine to remain overly upright and unnaturally straight. Their posture contrasts with the flexed head and neck and kyphosis of the spine typical of patient with PD (see Fig. 18.9A). In addition, their postural instability occurs at the onset of PSP and accounts for their falling, which is sometimes incapacitating or even fatal. PSP patients show a slight male predominance and typically begin showing signs of their illness between 60 and 70 years. They inexorably deteriorate over approximately 7 years.

The pathognomonic feature of PSP, which may not appear until 3 years after the onset of parkinsonism, consists of patients losing their ability to look voluntarily in vertical directions. As the disease progresses, they eventually lose lateral eye movement, and finally their eyes stay fixed in a straight-ahead position. To circumvent the lack of supranuclear (cortical) input, neurologists can recruit the labyrinthine system and brainstem systems: they typically passively flex and extend the patient's neck to elicit "doll's eye" or oculocephalic vertical reflex movements. In PSP, despite the absence of supranuclear control, this maneuver directly stimulates the brainstem nuclei and causes the eyes to move up and down (Fig. 18.11). This constellation of eye movement abnormalities constitutes the best clinical diagnostic test for PSP.

PSP, like frontotemporal dementia, is considered a tauopathy (see Chapter 7) because tau-containing neurofibrillary tangles accumulate in neurons. As with frontotemporal dementia patients, PSP patients generally show apathy, aberrant behavior, disinhibition, executive disability, reduced verbal output, and pseudobulbar palsy. Both groups of patients also share cognitive decline to the point of dementia. Many patients with PSP have a variety of pathologic changes in the brain at autopsy, including evidence of concomitant Alzheimer disease, PD, dementia with Lewy bodies, and other abnormalities.

In PSP, the frontal cortex, basal ganglia, and upper brainstem undergo degeneration. MRI can be helpful by demonstrating the hummingbird sign: on sagittal views, due to atrophy of the rostral midbrain, the brainstem looks like a hummingbird. PET shows predominant frontal lobe hypometabolism, but not as distinctively as in frontotemporal dementia. Unfortunately, levodopa replacement does not significantly correct the parkinsonism of PSP, and cholinesterase inhibitors have little or no impact on the dementia.

Parkinsonism in Children and Young Adults

Although PD occasionally arises in individuals younger than 21 years, such early onset is rare and usually the expression of a gene mutation. Among patients in this age

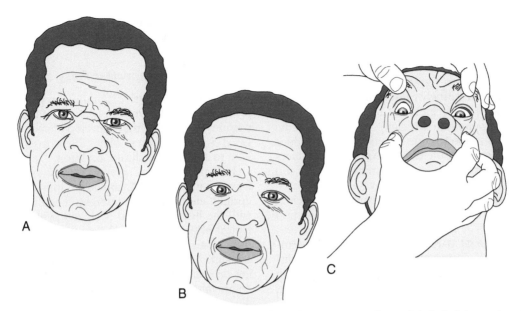

FIGURE 18.11 ■ *A*, PSP patients typically have a grimace because of continuous contractions of their facial muscles. *B*, Due to the loss of the ability to voluntarily move the eyes vertically, the hallmark of PSP, this patient cannot comply with the examiner's request to look downward. *C*, However, when the examiner rocks the patient's head back (performs an oculocephalic maneuver), his eyes dip well below the meridian.

group, parkinsonism more commonly arises secondary to another condition such as one of these:

- Dopa-responsive dystonia
- Early-onset generalized (DYT1) dystonia
- Juvenile Huntington disease
- Side effects of medications or illicit drugs
- Wilson disease.

In some of these disorders, dementia, psychosis, depression, a personality disorder, or another psychiatric abnormality regularly accompanies the parkinsonism.

Therapy of Parkinson Disease

Levodopa (L-DOPA)

Treatments for Parkinson disease alleviate motor symptoms for many years, but do not reverse – or even retard – the neurodegeneration. Medicines maintain normal dopamine activity by enhancing dopamine synthesis, inhibiting its metabolism, or acting as agonists at dopamine receptors. The most effective treatment consists of substituting orally administered levodopa to replace the deficiency of endogenous L-DOPA in the synthetic pathway for dopamine (see Fig. 18.3):

$$\text{Phenylalanine} \xrightarrow{\text{phenylalanine hydroxylase}} \text{Tyrosine}$$
$$\xrightarrow{\text{tyrosine hydroxylase}} \text{L-DOPA}$$
$$\xrightarrow{\text{DOPA decarboxylase}} \text{Dopamine}$$

To bypass the tyrosine hydroxylase deficiency, levodopa penetrates the blood–brain barrier and inserts itself into the synthetic chain where it substitutes for endogenous L-DOPA and undergoes decarboxylation to form dopamine. (Oral administration of dopamine itself is not useful because it does not cross the blood–brain barrier.) Levodopa remains

effective until almost all the nigrostriatal tract neurons degenerate and the remaining ones can no longer synthesize, store, and appropriately release dopamine.

In contrast to the degenerating presynaptic neurons, the postsynaptic nigrostriatal neurons, which express the dopamine receptors, remain intact in PD. They not only respond to dopamine but also can be stimulated by synthetic dopamine agonists; however, dopamine itself remains the most effective stimulus.

Prescribing levodopa as a "precursor replacement strategy" maintains most patients' functional status for approximately the first 5 years of the illness. During that time, enough nigrostriatal neurons remain intact to synthesize, store, and release the levodopa-derived dopamine. This strategy provides the most powerful, easiest to use, and least complicated symptomatic treatment. Neurologists typically prescribe levodopa as a therapeutic trial and then continue treatment until deterioration requires supplementation with another agent.

Dopa- and Dopamine-Preserving Medications

Several medications increase nigrostriatal L-DOPA by inhibiting two enzymes – *dopa decarboxylase* and *catechol-O-methyltransferase (COMT)* – that metabolize it in the systemic circulation (Fig. 18.12). With a relative increase in nigrostriatal L-DOPA, the dopamine concentration increases.

One enzyme-inhibiting medication, *carbidopa*, inactivates peripheral dopa decarboxylase, resulting in increased penetration of levodopa through the blood–brain barrier and higher concentrations in the brain. In turn, this strategy permits the dose of levodopa to be kept low to avoid systemic dopaminergic side effects – particularly nausea, vomiting, cardiac arrhythmias, and hypotension. The nausea and vomiting, which can be troublesome, result from high doses of dopamine stimulating the emesis

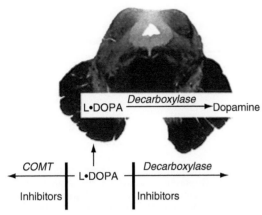

L•DOPA *Decarboxylase* → Dopamine

COMT ← | L•DOPA | → *Decarboxylase*

Inhibitors | | Inhibitors

FIGURE 18.12 ■ Medicines that inhibit catechol-*O*-methyltransferase (COMT), such as entacapone, and those that inhibit decarboxylase, such as carbidopa, slow the metabolism of L-dopa. Therapeutically, these enzymes can be coadministered with levodopa, permitting smaller levodopa doses and minimizing systemic side effects.

(vomiting) center in the medulla, which is one of the few areas of the brain not protected by the blood–brain barrier. Pharmaceutical firms have marketed fixed combinations of carbidopa and levodopa as Sinemet (Latin *sine* without, *emesis* vomiting) in recognition of the dramatic reduction of this side effect with the addition of carbidopa.

Another enzyme-inhibiting medication, entacapone (Comtan), inhibits COMT. A commercial preparation, Stalevo, combines both enzyme inhibitors – carbidopa and entacapone – with levodopa.

A complementary therapeutic strategy consists of blocking MAO-B, one of the main enzymes responsible for metabolizing and thus deactivating nigrostriatal dopamine. The MAO-B inhibitors selegiline (Eldepryl) and rasagiline (Azilect) preserve dopamine activity because they impair the oxidation of both endogenous and medically derived dopamine. As an added benefit of selegiline, its own metabolism produces minute amounts of methamphetamine and amphetamine, which provide a small but definite antidepressant effect. At least on a theoretical level, MAO-B inhibitors may also confer some neuroprotection by providing an antioxidant effect and reducing free radical formation.

On the other hand, although they ameliorate some symptoms and provide a modicum of antidepressant effect, MAO-B inhibitors carry a caveat. At high doses, they inhibit MAO-A as well as MAO-B. Because MAO-A is important in both serotonin and catecholamine metabolism, MAO-B inhibitors place patients in a position where they are vulnerable to the serotonin syndrome or a hypertensive crisis (see previously and Chapters 6, 9, and 21).

Dopamine Agonists

As an initial medication or when dopamine production eventually falls to inadequate levels, dopamine agonists provide stimulation of postsynaptic dopamine receptors (see Fig. 18.3). Bypassing dysfunctional presynaptic neurons, dopamine agonists act directly on D2 and to a lesser extent on other postsynaptic dopamine receptors.

Two oral dopamine agonists are currently on the market, pramipexole (Mirapex) and ropinirole (Requip). Another, rotigotine (Neupro), is available as a transdermal patch. One dopamine agonist – injectable apomorphine (Apokyn) – rescues Parkinson disease patients from a sudden loss of dopamine activity but has a short duration of action. Importantly, it also rapidly reverses dopamine activity deficiency in NMS.

Problems With Dopaminergic Medicines

Even though dopamine precursors and agonists effectively reverse rigidity and bradykinesia of PD, at least in its early stages, they often fail to alleviate these symptoms in its later stages and even from the outset have little effect on others. In particular, these dopaminergic medicines do not alleviate dysarthria, dysphagia, gait freezing, tendency to fall, dementia, hallucinations, depression, or other psychiatric comorbidities – symptoms that often reduce patients' quality of life.

In addition to failing to help certain symptoms, the dopaminergics may cause significant adverse effects, such as dyskinesias, sleep disturbances, visual hallucinations, thought disorders, and other mental status changes. The dyskinesias consist of oral-buccal-lingual movements, chorea, akathisia, dystonic postures, and rocking. Most of the dyskinesias are transient and do not inhibit patients' function; however, sometimes they cause gait impairment or resemble tardive dyskinesia (see later). Despite most patients' problems with dyskinesias, they prefer overactivity, which allows them to walk and care for themselves, to understimulation with its rigidity and immobility.

Other Medications

Alpha tocopherol (vitamin E), an antioxidant and free radical scavenger, should protect dopamine from destruction by free radicals and other toxins. Despite that solid rationale, a major study in Parkinson disease showed that tocopherol, either alone or in combination with selegiline, failed to slow progression of the illness. Coenzyme Q10 is another antioxidant. In a preliminary study, it appeared to slow progression in PD, but more rigorous research did not support a protective role.

Anticholinergic agents reduce tremor in PD and other forms of parkinsonism. By reducing cholinergic activity, these medicines seem to act by maintaining the balance with the diminished dopamine activity (Fig. 18.13). On the other hand, anticholinergics routinely produce mental and physical side effects, especially in the elderly.

Amantadine enhances dopamine activity by acting on presynaptic neurons to facilitate dopamine release and inhibit its reuptake. It also has anticholinergic properties. In early mild PD, amantadine provides a temporary, modest improvement in tremor, rigidity, and bradykinesia. Later in the disease it may also ameliorate levodopa-induced dyskinesias.

Deep-Brain Stimulation

Studies have not yet established the ideal location for the electrodes, the parameters of stimulation, or even its

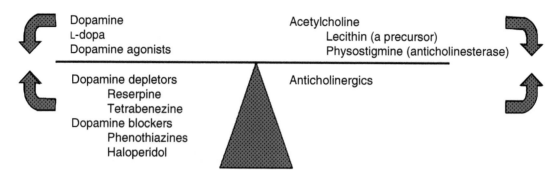

FIGURE 18.13 ■ In a classic but limited model, dopaminergic and cholinergic (acetylcholine) activity normally balance each other. When Parkinson disease reduces dopamine activity, the left side of the scale rises. Dopamine precursors, dopamine agonists, and anticholinergics – Parkinson disease treatments – restore the balance. Conditions characterized by excessive dopamine activity, such as chorea, push the left side downward. Substances that either antagonize or deplete dopamine, or enhance cholinergic activity, restore the balance.

mechanism of action, but DBS has unequivocally improved the quality of life of patients with Parkinson disease, dystonia, and essential tremor. It also has helped in many cases of Tourette disorder, spasmodic torticollis, tardive dyskinesias, chronic pain, and certain psychiatric conditions, including treatment-resistant depression and obsessive-compulsive disorder.

In DBS surgery for PD patients, neurosurgeons insert tiny electrodes into the subthalamic nucleus or GPi. They then connect the electrodes to a pacemaker-like device inserted into the subcutaneous tissues of the chest. Potential surgical complications include cerebral hemorrhage, infection, and electrode fracture. Unlike the first devices, current ones allow patients to undergo MRI.

DBS often allows PD patients to reduce their medication regimen and maintain their mobility with a great reduction in dyskinesias. It also helps reduce on–off episodes. However, DBS does not ameliorate gait impairment, postural instability, cognitive impairment, or depression. In one study, depending on the target, postoperative dopaminergic medication regimen, and other postoperative factors, some PD patients developed or had worsening of depression, approximately 0.5% to 1.0% had suicide ideation or attempts, and a larger proportion showed apathy. Of course, in many of these cases the symptoms were mild, transient, or amenable to treatment. Moreover, DBS does not hasten cognitive deterioration.

ATHETOSIS

Athetosis consists of involuntary slow, continually changing, twisting movements predominantly affecting the face, neck and distal limbs (Fig. 18.14). It sits at the beginning of a sequence – athetosis, choreoathetosis, chorea, and hemiballismus – of progressively larger and more irregular involuntary movements. Additional involuntary movements may coexist with athetosis. For example, rapid jerks of chorea or powerful twists of dystonia may punctuate or interrupt the slow movements of athetosis.

Athetosis is often encountered as a variety of *cerebral palsy* (see Chapter 13), and may not be apparent until early childhood. Most often athetosis results from combinations of perinatal hyperbilirubinemia (kernicterus), hypoxia, and prematurity. Genetic factors are unimportant.

Because athetosis originates in brain injuries that occur during the first 30 days after birth as well as *in utero*, seizures and mental retardation frequently accompany this movement disorder. However, with damage confined to the basal ganglia, as in many cases of athetosis, patients have normal intelligence despite disabling movements and garbled speech. Physicians, schoolteachers, family members, and friends should recognize that these patients retain cognitive and emotional capacities despite devastating physical neurologic disabilities.*

Dopamine antagonists may suppress athetosis, but their long-term use may lead to complications. Paradoxically, neurologists often offer an empiric trial of levodopa to children with athetosis for the possibility that the movements do not represent cerebral palsy but a different illness, dopa-responsive dystonia (see later). According to preliminary reports, DBS may also reduce athetosis. Injections of one of the formulations of *botulinum toxin* – onabotulinumtoxinA (Botox), abobotulinumtoxinA (Dysport), incobotulinumtoxinA (Xeomin), or rimabotulinumtoxinB (Myobloc) – may offer several months of reduced particularly troublesome movement or co-existent spasticity. (This book refers to all these medicines as "botulinum toxins.") When neurologists inject botulinum toxins for spasticity, dystonia, or other reason (see below), it may induce temporary weakness. Moreover, because the affected neurons reconstitute themselves, neurologists must repeat the injections – usually every 3 months.

CHOREA

Huntington Disease

Of the many causes of chorea (Box 18.1), Huntington disease, previously called "Huntington's chorea," remains preeminent. Chorea, dementia, and behavioral abnormalities characterize this disorder, which is inherited in

---

*Illnesses that produce incapacitating physical disability yet allow normal intelligence include athetotic and spastic diplegia varieties of cerebral palsy, primary dystonia, locked-in syndrome, spinal cord transection, amyotrophic lateral sclerosis (ALS), poliomyelitis, and some muscular dystrophies.

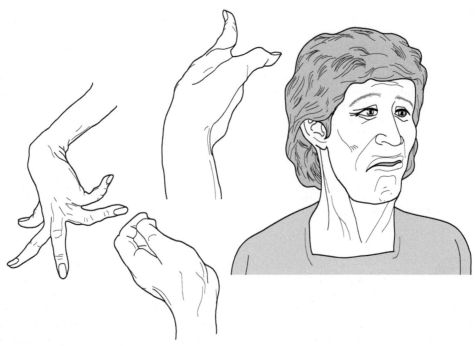

FIGURE 18.14 ■ Athetosis involving the face causes incessant grimacing. Fragments of smiles alternate with frowns. Pulling of one or the other side distorts the appearance of the face. In addition, neck muscles contract and rotate the head. Laryngeal contractions and irregular chest and diaphragm muscle movements cause an irregular speech cadence, nasal pitch, and dysarthria. The fingers writhe constantly and tend to assume hyperextension postures. At the same time, the wrists rotate, flex, and extend. Involuntary limb activity prevents writing, buttoning, and other fine tasks, but usually permits deliberate larger-scale shoulder, trunk, and hip movement.

BOX 18.1	Common Causes of Chorea

Basal ganglia lesions
  Perinatal injury, e.g., anoxia, kernicterus
  Stroke
  Tumor, abscess, toxoplasmosis*
Genetic disorders
  Huntington disease
  Wilson disease
Metabolic derangements
  Hyperglycemia
  Hyperthyroidism
Drugs
  Cocaine, amphetamine, methylphenidate
  Dopamine precursors and agonists
  Neuroleptics (see Box 18.2)
  Oral contraceptives[+]
Inflammatory conditions
  Sydenham chorea
  Systemic lupus erythematosus

*Acquired immunodeficiency syndrome (AIDS) indirectly causes chorea when toxoplasmosis involves the basal ganglia
[+]Estrogens from contraceptives or pregnancy (chorea gravidarum) cause chorea

autosomal dominant fashion. Symptoms first emerge when patients are, on average, approximately 37 years. However, approximately 10% of patients develop symptoms in childhood or adolescence and 25% when they are older than 50 years. Adults with the illness usually succumb to aspiration pneumonia and inanition from one to two decades after the diagnosis.

With a prevalence of 2 to 6 out of 100,000, Huntington disease represents a relatively frequent cause of dementia, which the DSM-5 would label Major Neurocognitive Disorder Due to Huntington Disease. Neurologists also consider it, along with frontotemporal dementia, human immunodeficiency virus (HIV)-associated dementia, and Wernicke–Korsakoff disease as a relatively common cause of dementia in middle-aged individuals. Although it affects individuals from all races and ethnic backgrounds, the majority of patients in the United States have descended from a small cohort of 17th century English immigrants.

Clinical Features

In contrast to the slow, writhing, continuous movements of athetosis, chorea consists of random, discrete, rapid movements that jerk the pelvis, trunk, and limbs (Fig. 18.15). Chorea also includes involuntary facial movements that produce brief, meaningless expressions (Fig. 18.16). When patients walk, the chorea characteristically interrupts their cadence and stability (Fig. 18.17). In fact, the gait abnormality gave rise to the term *chorea* (Greek, dance).

Movements in chorea occur with random timing and distribution. In other words, chorea consists of *nonstereotyped* movements. Also, chorea is associated with no psychic investment in the movements. In contrast, akathisia, RLS, and tics follow a premonitory urge to move, entail a compulsion to move, and bestow relief upon movement. In addition, in these disorders patients experience psychologic discomfort if they resist moving (see later).

Chorea in its earliest stage merely resembles nonspecific "fidgety" movements as seen with anxiety, restlessness, discomfort, or clumsiness. Later it may consist of excessive face or hand gestures, weight shifting, leg crossing, or finger twitching (Fig. 18.18). Chorea also impairs the ability to sustain a voluntary muscle contraction, which causes *motor impersistence*. Because of it, patients cannot either hold a firm grasp or extend their hands or tongue for more than 10 seconds. For example, when asked by the examiner to squeeze two fingers, patients exert irregular, variable pressure that neurologists call the "milkmaid's sign." Patients also show motor impersistence by intermittently, involuntarily withdrawing the tongue when neurologists ask them to protrude it for 30

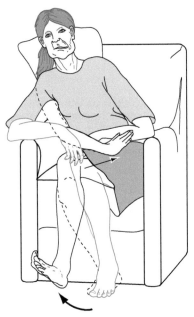

FIGURE 18.15 ■ As in this woman with Huntington disease, chorea consists of intermittent, random involuntary movements, such as brisk contractions in pelvic, trunk, and limb muscles. It also encompasses a mere flick of a finger or wrist, forward jutting of the leg, or shrugging of the shoulder.

seconds. Motor impersistence also prevents patients from sustaining postures. For example, when "standing at attention," patients' fingers twitch outward and their torso bends.

Huntington disease also disrupts normal eye movements. In particular, Huntington disease impairs *saccades*, which are the rapid conjugate eye movements that people normally use to glance from one object to another. In Huntington disease, patients cannot make a rapid, smooth, and accurate shift of their gaze toward an object that suddenly enters their visual field. They routinely first blink or jerk their head to initiate the saccade. Although characteristic, impaired saccades are not peculiar to Huntington disease. Patients with schizophrenia, for example, also have abnormal saccades.

In addition, Huntington disease impairs ocular *pursuit movements*, which are the normal, relatively slow conjugate eye movements that follow (track) moving objects, such as a baseball thrown into the air or ducks flying across the horizon. Huntington disease patients typically show irregular, inaccurate, and slow pursuit movements. As with abnormal saccades, abnormal pursuit movements are not peculiar to Huntington disease.

Even before dementia, which inevitably appears, patients display inattentiveness, erratic behavior, apathy, personality changes, and impaired judgment. Dementia typically begins within 1 year of the chorea. Poor memory, impaired planning ability, and faulty judgment, especially in financial matters, characterizes their dementia. In Huntington disease, as in Parkinson disease, the MoCA is more sensitive than the MMSE in detecting subtle cognitive impairment.

As almost an integral part of the disease, about 50% of patients have comorbid depressive symptoms that generally strike earlier rather than later in the illness. Most patients have agitation, anxiety, apathy, dysphoria, and irritability, and about 10% develop psychotic thinking. Sometimes these symptoms precede both the dementia and chorea.

At a higher rate than in other neurodegenerative illnesses, up to 10% of individuals who are carriers or have overt signs of Huntington disease commit suicide. They

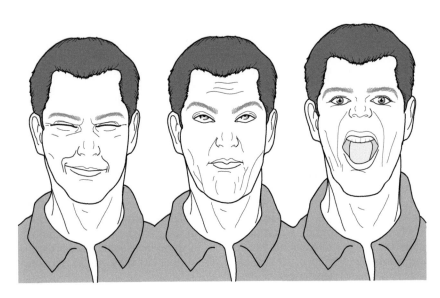

FIGURE 18.16 ■ Huntington disease patients characteristically make unexpected, inappropriate, and incomplete facial expressions. Without provocation, they frown, raise eyebrows, and smirk. Because their tongue frequently protrudes, this chorea occasionally mimics tardive dyskinesia.

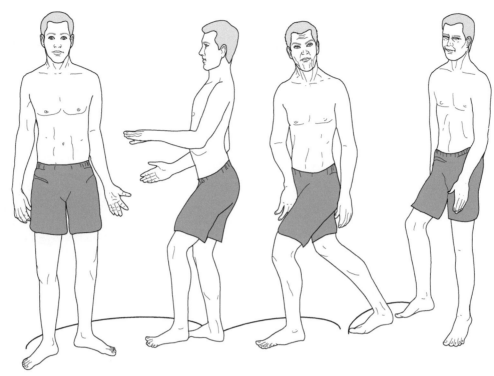

FIGURE 18.17 ■ The signature of Huntington disease is a jerky gait that results from intermittent, unexpected trunk and pelvic motions, spontaneous knee flexion and extension, lateral swaying, variable cadence, and unequal stride length.

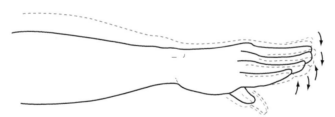

FIGURE 18.18 ■ With their arms and hands extended, Huntington disease patients fidget with their fingers and wrists. Neurologists label these movements "piano playing."

tend to have had depression or anxiety, aggression, impaired judgment, or impetuous behavior – alone or in combination. They commit suicide most often before learning the results of their genetic testing or later when beginning to lose their independence. Notably, the suicide rate immediately before undergoing a diagnostic test exceeds that after receiving a positive result.

The caregiver stress involved with Huntington disease exceeds that with Alzheimer disease, because Huntington patients almost always have behavioral as well as cognitive impairments. Moreover, if the spouse of the Huntington patient has the role of caregiver, that person is also often the parent of one or more children with overt or presymptomatic disease.

Physicians can base a preliminary diagnosis of Huntington disease on a patient's having chorea, dementia, and a relative with a similar disorder. Readily available DNA testing for patients and potential carriers, including a fetus, can confirm or exclude the diagnosis.

Neurologists seek to reduce chorea by prescribing either dopamine receptor-blocking antipsychotic agents or tetrabenazine, which depletes dopamine. However, these medicines neither improve other motor functions nor reverse dementia. Moreover, because tetrabenazine depletes stores of norepinephrine (noradrenaline) and serotonin as well as dopamine, it sometimes also leads to sedation, depression, suicidal ideation and parkinsonism. In mild cases of anxiety, benzodiazepines may suffice. Both TCAs and SSRIs may improve the depression.

Juvenile Huntington Disease

Sometimes symptoms appear in children and adolescents – individuals younger than 21 years of age. This variant, *juvenile Huntington disease* (also known as the Westphal variant of Huntington's disease), comprises 10% of all cases and exhibits different manifestations from the more common adult form. Patients' schoolwork declines and behavioral disturbances develop as the first signs. Also, rather than causing chorea as its initial physical symptom, juvenile Huntington disease presents with rigidity, dystonia, and akinesia (Fig. 18.19). Many affected children and adolescents look as though they have Parkinson disease. Another difference is that, unlike the adult variety, juvenile Huntington disease causes seizures. More importantly, juvenile Huntington disease progresses much more quickly and leads to death twice as rapidly as the adult form.

Genetics

As mentioned above, Huntington disease is transmitted in an autosomal dominant pattern. The DNA abnormality underlying juvenile and adult varieties of Huntington

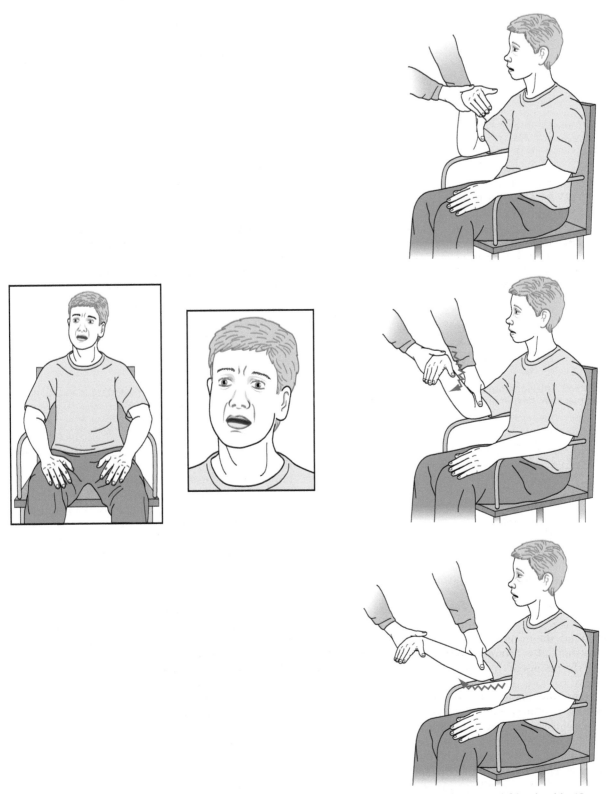

FIGURE 18.19 ■ Having had deteriorating grades and progressively greater isolation from his family and friends, this 18-year-old high-school student came for evaluation. During the interview, he sat motionlessly, had few facial or limb gestures, and moved slowly; however, he had no tremor. He was apathetic and lacked insight. He did not fully cooperate with routine mental status testing, but cognitive deficits appeared to be present. When the neurologist flexed and extended his right arm, she detected rigidity. After a routine evaluation, she ordered tests for conditions that cause parkinsonism accompanied by mental deterioration in teenagers – drug abuse, Wilson disease, and the juvenile variety of Huntington disease. The genetic testing showed 85 CAG trinucleotide repeats, confirming a diagnosis of Huntington disease. Examination of the patient's father disclosed subtle but definite chorea and cognitive impairment. His genetic testing revealed 50 CAG repeats.

disease – as with myotonic dystrophy, several spinocerebellar ataxias, fragile X syndrome, and other disorders – is a genetic mutation consisting of excessive *trinucleotide repeats* (see Chapter 6 and Appendix 3D). The *huntingtin* gene, located on the short arm of chromosome 4, normally consists of 11 to 35 repeats of the trinucleotide base cytosine-adenine-guanine (CAG). Individuals with 36–39 trinucleotide repeats, whom neurologists classify as "indeterminate," have no clinical signs of Huntington disease or merely a *forme fruste* of the disease; however, because of the gene's tendency to enlarge (see later), their children may have unequivocal disease. Individuals with 40 or more trinucleotide repeats invariably develop all manifestations of the illness and their age at onset of symptoms correlates inversely with the number of their repeats.

In general, with higher numbers of trinucleotide repeats, the disease shows itself at a younger age and pursues a more rapid course. When the mutation consists of 60 or more trinucleotide repeats, the juvenile variant develops.

As with other genes containing expanded trinucleotide sequences, the huntingtin gene is unstable and tends to increase further in length in successive generations. The progressive expansion of the gene (*amplification*) explains why carriers of the mutation show signs at progressively younger ages in successive generations (*anticipation*). In addition, the gene's trinucleotide sequences enlarge further in sperm than in eggs. Thus, there is a preponderance of affected fathers among children with the disease; moreover, paternal inheritance confers a greater likelihood of an earlier onset and greater severity of the disease.

Pathology

In Huntington disease, the excess of CAG repeats leads to an increased number of glutamine amino acids in the cytoplasmic protein *huntingtin*, which in turn causes neurodegeneration of neurons containing this protein. Thus, neurologists designate Huntington disease and other illnesses transmitted by excessive CAG repeats as *polyglutamine diseases*. At the molecular level, glutamate and other excitatory amino acids overstimulate N-methyl-D-aspartate (*NMDA*) receptors. This pathologic interaction, *excitotoxicity*, allows a fatal influx of calcium into neurons (see Chapter 21) that leads to cell death via apoptosis.

Apoptosis, the cell death that occurs in Huntington disease, ALS, and several other neurodegenerative illnesses, differs from *necrosis*, the more common cell death that occurs in strokes, trauma, and tumors. Apoptosis is programmed, sequential, and energy-requiring. It often occurs as a normal, vital process. For example, apoptosis characterizes the cell death that allows for closure of the patent ductus arteriosus and involution of the thymus. On a histologic level, apoptosis does not provoke inflammation. For example, macrophages and other mononuclear cells do not infiltrate the area of cells dying of apoptosis. Neurologists regard apoptosis as an expectable, clean, orderly, and dignified cell death, but necrosis as an unpredictable, bloody, and messy cell death.

Pathologists note that Huntington disease causes degeneration through apoptosis of the striatal medium spiny neurons that produce GABA. The caudate, which is part of the striatum, shows pronounced atrophy, and its GABA concentrations fall to less than 50% of normal.

Atrophy of the caudate nuclei, almost a pathognomonic macroscopic finding, correlates roughly with the severity of dementia. The atrophy of the caudate nuclei permits the lateral ventricles to balloon outward, i.e., develop a convex outline. They expand so much that neurologists call them "bat-wing ventricles." CT and MRI readily show the caudate atrophy and enlarged, convex ventricles (see Fig. 20.5). As Huntington disease progresses, the cerebral cortex also undergoes atrophy. PET studies demonstrate caudate hypometabolism even early in the illness.

By way of contrast, while normal aging and Alzheimer disease also cause cerebral atrophy, their atrophy does not preferentially affect the caudate nuclei. In these non-Huntington conditions, the caudate nuclei still bulge into the lateral ventricles. The ventricles enlarge, but they maintain a concave contour (see Figs. 20.2, 20.3, and 20.18).

Other Varieties of Chorea

Sydenham Chorea

Sydenham chorea, originally known as St. Vitus' dance, is one of the major diagnostic criteria for and complications of rheumatic fever. In fact, rheumatic fever accounts for almost all cases of acute chorea in childhood. Sydenham chorea predominantly affects children between the ages of 5 and 15 years and, in children older than 10 years, girls twice as frequently as boys.

In the most plausible explanation, group A β-hemolytic streptococcal infections, which cause rheumatic fever, inadvertently trigger an antibody-mediated attack on the basal ganglia. The chorea usually coincides with rheumatic fever, but it may begin as long as 2 to 6 months afterwards, when children have apparently recovered their health. It lasts for an average of 2 months, but often reappears during recurrences of rheumatic fever. With the decreasing incidence of rheumatic fever, Sydenham chorea seems restricted to small outbreaks – "mini-epidemics" – occurring mostly in neighborhoods with cramped living space and limited access to health care. Often siblings and friends develop the disorder simultaneously or in quick succession.

The chorea begins insidiously with grimaces and limb movements (Fig. 18.20). Sometimes the movements make the child seem willfully hyperactive. Sydenham chorea is one of the commonest neurologic causes of hyperactivity in children. A list of those causes would also include attention deficit hyperactivity disorder (ADHD), side effects from medications or illicit drugs, Tourette disorder and other tics, and withdrawal-emergent syndrome (see later).

The chorea's significance lies not only in its warning of an underlying life-threatening condition, but also because of its neuropsychiatric comorbidity. Obsessive compulsive behavior, obsessive compulsive disorder (OCD), and ADHD occur several-fold more frequently in children with Sydenham chorea compared to healthy controls. In addition, psychiatrists sometimes hold up

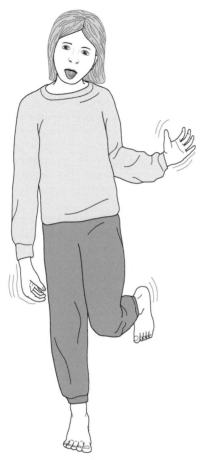

FIGURE 18.20 ■ Children with Sydenham chorea may appear to have coy smiles and brief grimaces, and walk with a playful sashay. However, the pathologic nature of their movements – chorea – can be made obvious if the children attempt to maintain a fixed position, such as standing at attention, standing on the ball of one foot, or protruding their tongue. The involuntary movements cause dysarthria that occasionally is so severe that children refuse to speak. Surprisingly, the chorea may be asymmetric or unilateral in at least 20% of cases. It usually lasts between several weeks and 2 months.

Sydenham chorea along with Tourette disorder as examples of PANDAS, but neurologists remain dubious about this concept (see later).

Some children reportedly also have learning disabilities following Sydenham chorea; however, in many cases their lower socioeconomic status may have already compromised their educational status. In any case, despite the serious nature of the illness, Sydenham chorea does not lead to frank cognitive impairment.

The chorea usually spontaneously resolves, but if it causes discomfort, functional impairment, sleeplessness, or exhaustion, neurologists prescribe a short course of either valproate or a dopamine receptor-blocking agent. In some cases, neurologists have sought to interrupt the inflammatory process and reduced the symptoms by administering steroids or immunoglobulins.

In adults, chorea of autoimmune etiology is rare but can occur as a paraneoplastic syndrome, mostly in association with small-cell carcinoma and adenocarcinoma. Male gender, concomitant peripheral neuropathy, and weight loss raise the likelihood of an underlying cancer.

Autoimmune chorea can also accompany other autoimmune conditions, such as systemic lupus erythematosus or antiphospholipid syndrome.

Estrogen-Related Chorea

Oral contraceptive-induced chorea occasionally complicates the use of oral estrogen-containing contraceptives. This variety of chorea, which is not associated with mental abnormalities, other than anxiety, develops in young women several months after starting these contraceptives and resolves after stopping them.

Chorea gravidarum, a related disorder, develops almost exclusively in young primigravidas in the first two trimesters of their pregnancy. Emotional lability, delirium, and rarely psychotic thinking are comorbid with the chorea. The chorea sometimes causes so much exhaustion that a woman spontaneously aborts. To relieve severe chorea, women must undergo a therapeutic abortion. Once the pregnancy is terminated, symptoms resolve.

Many women affected by oral contraceptive-induced chorea or chorea gravidarum have had previous episodes of either condition or Sydenham chorea. Also, their close relatives often have had one of these conditions. Nevertheless, if chorea develops in a woman who is pregnant or taking oral contraceptives, physicians must consider conditions in addition to the estrogen-related choreas, including Sydenham chorea, systemic lupus erythematosus, antiphospholipid syndrome (see Chapter 11), hyperthyroidism, and even Huntington disease.

HEMIBALLISMUS

Hemiballismus consists of intermittent, large-scale flinging movements of one side of the body. The movements resemble chorea, except that they are unilateral, less predictable, and more forceful (Fig. 18.21). Ballismus sits at the end of the sequence of progressively larger and more irregular involuntary movements.

Classic papers associated hemiballismus with lesions in the contralateral subthalamic nucleus, but contemporary studies have found lesions in that area in less than one-third of cases. Another piece of evidence exonerating the subthalamic nucleus is that when neurosurgeons deliberately implant DBS electrodes there, the damage rarely leads to postoperative hemiballismus or other movement disorders. Alternatively, lesions in the caudate nucleus or other basal ganglia may be responsible. In any case, because the responsible lesion is small and situated nowhere near the cerebral cortex, patients with hemiballismus do not have comorbid cognitive impairment, seizures, or paresis.

Whatever the location of the lesion, the most common etiology is an occlusion of one or more of the small perforating branches of the middle cerebral artery that perfuse the basal ganglia. Similarly, vasculitis can affect those arteries. In individuals infected with HIV, toxoplasmosis lesions have a tendency to develop in the basal ganglia and produce hemiballismus (see Fig. 20.11).

Most cases resolve spontaneously, which is fortunate because neurologists have few treatments to offer. In

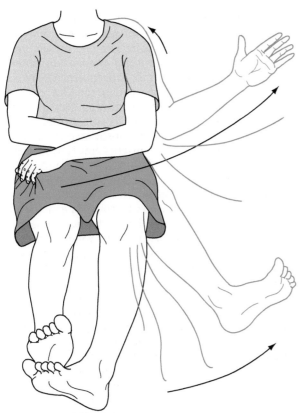

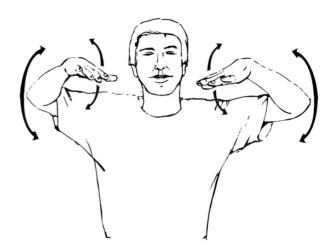

FIGURE 18.22 ■ Wilson disease characteristically induces parkinsonism, dystonia, dysarthria, and various tremors, including a *wing-beating tremor*. This particular tremor, which is a hallmark of the disease but occurs in only about one-third of cases, consists of rhythmic, coarse, up-and-down arm movements based at the shoulders. It gives patients the appearance of flapping their arms as though they were attempting to fly.

FIGURE 18.21 ■ Beset by hemiballismus, this woman has sudden large-scale movements of the limbs on the left side of her body. Even when hemiballismus has a more modest amplitude, patients use a variety of strategies to suppress it. In this case, the patient typically uses her left hand to grip her skirt in order to anchor her moving left arm. Sometimes patients press their body or unaffected limb against an involuntarily moving limb. They also attempt to camouflage the involuntary movements by converting them into apparently purposeful movements. For example, if her arm were to fly upward, she might incorporate the movement into a gesture such as waving to someone or smoothing her hair.

cases that persist, dopamine receptor-blocking agents or dopamine-depleting agents may suppress the movements. Neurosurgeons have implanted DBS or ablated basal ganglia nuclei in an attempt to relieve the movements, with varying degrees of success.

WILSON DISEASE

The insidious development of psychiatric disturbances, cognitive impairment, and a variety of involuntary movements in adolescents or young adults characterizes Wilson disease (*hepatolenticular degeneration*). Because early diagnosis and treatment can reverse its manifestations, neurologists consider Wilson disease as a cause of dementia or parkinsonism in children, adolescents, and young adults (see Box 7.3).

Wilson disease is transmitted via autosomal recessive inheritance. It results from a mutation in a gene carried on chromosome 13, which codes for a protein necessary for copper transport. The mutation leads to insufficient serum copper binding and hepatic excretion. The resulting

surplus of unbound serum copper, in turn, leads to destructive copper deposits in the brain, liver, cornea, and other organs. As its formal name implies, the illness primarily causes destruction of the liver and the lenticular nuclei of the basal ganglia (see Fig. 18.1A).

Symptoms usually first appear during the late teenage years. The psychiatric symptoms, which may emerge before the physical neurologic signs, initially consist of disturbances in personality, conduct, and mood. With further deterioration, patients develop thought disorder and then cognitive impairment, which culminate in dementia, which the DSM-5 would label Major Neurocognitive Disorder Due to Another Medical Condition. Wilson disease symptoms, especially in young adults, easily mislead physicians toward a diagnosis of schizophrenia.

The neurologic signs are dysarthria, dysphagia, gait impairment, anosmia, and those reflecting basal ganglia damage: rigidity, akinesia, dystonia, nonspecific tremor, and the characteristic *wing-beating tremor* (Fig. 18.22). These movements tend to occur in combination and may be accompanied by corticospinal or corticobulbar tract signs.

Especially in adolescents, nonneurologic manifestations often overshadow neurologic signs. For example, liver involvement leads to cirrhosis, which is sometimes so severe that it causes hepatic encephalopathy and then liver failure. Also, deposits of copper in the cornea produce the signature *Kayser–Fleischer ring* (Fig. 18.23).

Despite its infrequent occurrence (1 per 30,000 persons), neurologists routinely test for Wilson disease in adolescents and young adults who develop any of a wide variety of symptoms, including dysarthria, tremor, parkinsonism, dystonia, atypical psychosis, dementia, or cirrhosis. Because a Kayser–Fleischer corneal ring appears in almost all Wilson disease patients with neurologic manifestations, individuals suspected of having Wilson disease should undergo a slit lamp examination by an

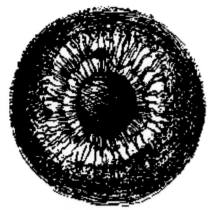

FIGURE 18.23 ■ The Kayser–Fleischer ring, which appears bilaterally, consists of green, brown, or orange copper pigment deposits in the periphery of the cornea. Most obvious at the superior and inferior margins of the cornea, the ring usually obscures the fine structure of the iris. Ophthalmologists must use a slit lamp to see the Kayser–Fleischer ring in its early stages. Although the ring develops in about 70% of cases when Wilson disease affects only the liver, it develops in almost 100% of patients when the disease affects the brain. In those cases, the ring's size and density correlate with the duration of the disease. However, because the Kayser–Fleischer ring also develops in primary biliary cirrhosis and several other liver diseases, it is not pathognomonic of Wilson disease. With successful treatment of Wilson disease, the ring dissolves.

ophthalmologist. They should also undergo determination of their serum ceruloplasmin (the serum copper-carrying protein) concentration, which in this illness is low to absent. Even when Wilson disease does not affect the brain, ceruloplasmin concentrations fall to very low levels. Another test, but a more cumbersome one, is measurement of the 24-hour urinary copper excretion: in Wilson disease, the absence of ceruloplasmin greatly increases urinary copper excretion. Genetic studies may confirm the diagnosis. MRI may help diagnose the illness, but characteristic changes often do not emerge until irreparable damage has occurred.

Assuming that physicians diagnose Wilson disease in a timely manner, medical intervention will usually prevent progression and reverse some or all of the mental deterioration, abnormal movements, and nonneurologic manifestations, including Kayser–Fleisher rings. Patients should avoid copper-containing foods, which includes many vegetables. Copper-chelating agents such as penicillamine and other medications, such as zinc, reduce the body's copper burden. When the disease is refractory to medical treatment, liver transplantation can rescue the patient. Case reports describe improvement in dystonia with DBS of bilateral GPi in patients with Wilson disease, but this approach requires further investigation.

DYSTONIA

Neurologists use the term *dystonia* to describe involuntary movements due to sustained muscle contractions. Unlike other movement disorders, which result from unopposed contractions of a muscle group (such as chorea) or alternating contractions of agonist and antagonist muscle groups (tremor), dystonia results from the simultaneous contractions of agonist and antagonist muscle groups. Dystonia can involve one muscle group (*focal dystonia*) or many (*generalized dystonia*). In generalized dystonia, patients' limb (appendicular) muscles and neck, trunk, and pelvis (axial) muscles contract, causing prolonged twisting or turning (torsion), and forcing patients into grotesque postures. Generalized dystonia often progresses over years to involve more and more regions until it encompasses the entire bodily musculature.

When dystonia is a manifestation of a known underlying condition, such as Wilson disease, neurologists refer to the movements as *secondary dystonia*. When the dystonic movements occur in isolation – without other neurologic abnormalities – neurologists refer to them as *primary dystonia*. Genetic traits play more of an important role in primary and several secondary generalized dystonias (see later) than in focal dystonias.

Primary dystonia, as previously noted, may cause physical incapacity but not dementia. On the other hand, depending on the variety of dystonia and degree of disability, depression may be comorbid.

Dystonia, whatever its cause or area of involvement, usually has several unusual features. For example, "tricks" will suppress the movements. Skipping, walking backward, or dancing (with or without music) overcomes the gait abnormality. Similarly, pressing lightly against a twisted body part (a *geste antagoniste*, see later) will straighten it temporarily. In another unusual feature, dystonia tends to trigger compensatory movements that give patients a bizarre appearance. Probably more frequently than with any other involuntary movement disorder, neurologists misdiagnose dystonia as a psychogenic disturbance because the movements are so unusual, idiosyncratic tricks override the movements, and compensatory movements force patients into strange postures. Conversely, psychogenic movements can mimic dystonia (see later).

Generalized Dystonias

Early-Onset Primary Dystonia (DYT1 Dystonia)

Early-onset primary dystonia or *idiopathic torsion dystonia* typically appears in 9- to 11-year-old children, but almost always by the age of 26 years. It is most prevalent among Ashkenazi Jews due to a founder effect. The dystonia usually begins with torsion of one hand or foot (Fig. 18.24) and subsequently spreads to the other limbs, pelvis (*tortipelvis*), trunk, and neck (*torticollis*). Untreated, it eventually incapacitates its victims (Fig. 18.25). A mutation in the *DYT1* gene, located on chromosome 9, carries the illness in an autosomal dominant pattern, but its penetrance is only 30%. DNA testing for the DYT1 gene nevertheless can establish the diagnosis. In contrast to genes characterized by excessive trinucleotide repeats, this mutation consists of deletion of the trinucleotide GAG. Several other genes also carry dystonia, but they vary as to whether they express the illness in a dominant or recessive pattern, which ethnic groups carry them, and their physical manifestations.

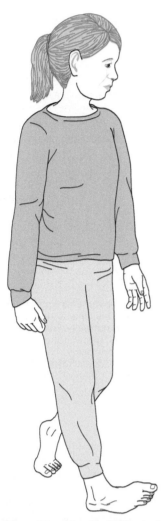

FIGURE 18.24 ■ When this girl with DYT1 dystonia walks, her right foot slowly inverts, causing her to limp. Because the dystonia is task-specific she can correct her limp by skipping, dancing, or walking backward.

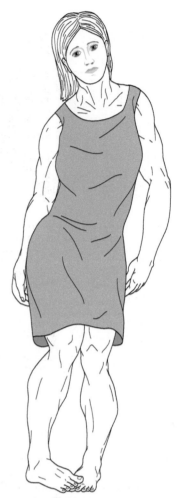

FIGURE 18.25 ■ As DYT1 dystonia spreads to involve the remaining limb and axial musculature, patients develop generalized dystonic postures. Because muscles continually contract, they hypertrophy. Patients lose their subcutaneous fat from the incessant exertion. When dystonia becomes generalized, these patients may resemble those with other forms of generalized dystonia, such as Wilson disease or tardive dystonia.

Routine tests – blood chemistry, MRI or CT, PET, and brain tissue analysis – reveal no consistent abnormality, and the mechanism through which the mutations produce the movements remains unknown. Several observations implicate a dopamine disturbance: dopamine alleviates dopamine-response dystonia and either prolonged or acute dopamine receptor blockade can cause dystonia (see later).

As for treatment, anticholinergics, baclofen (Lioresal), and benzodiazepines provide only modest and generally inconsistent benefit. However, DBS directed at the GPi greatly relieves dystonia, restores mobility, improves quality of life, and lifts mild-to-moderate depression. The benefit is often dramatic and lasts at least a decade. DBS usually permits reduction or elimination of oral medicines, often with improvement in mental status. Also, dystonia patients who undergo DBS, unlike PD patients, do not exhibit postoperative cognitive changes. Children as well as adults are candidates. DYT1 positivity and minor motor deficits preoperatively are predictors for a favorable outcome from DBS.

Dopa-Responsive Dystonia

In an illness first described by Segawa and his Japanese colleagues and often named after him, *dopa-responsive dystonia (DRD; DYT5)* appears in children and follows a distinctive diurnal pattern. The dystonia becomes evident in children, on the average, when they are 8 years old. The dystonia is typically absent in the morning but pronounced by the late afternoon and evening (Fig. 18.26). As with early-onset dystonia, DRD first affects children's legs, interfering with walking, and then progresses to become generalized. In a related sign, DRD sometimes superimposes parkinsonism on the dystonia.

The label "DRD" describes not only the diagnostic test for the illness, but also its treatment. Small levodopa doses, typically 300 mg per day or less, dramatically ameliorate DRD. Because of the success of levodopa in DRD, neurologists routinely give it as a therapeutic trial to children who have developed dystonia or almost any movement disorder resembling dystonia. If patients improve, the neurologist can order genetic testing to confirm the diagnosis.

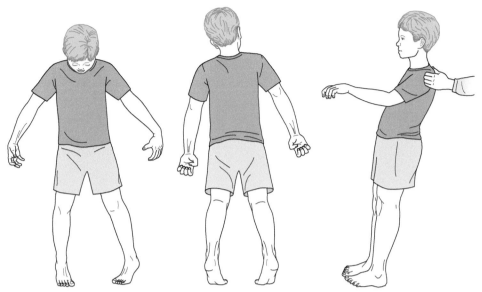

FIGURE 18.26 ■ During the previous year, this 8-year-old boy began to have leg and trunk movements upon returning home from school in the afternoon. In the evening, his arms and hands showed dystonic posturing and his legs assumed a straightened position that forced him to walk on his toes. When he awoke in the morning, he walked and ran normally. His parents initially thought that he had developed a psychologic disturbance. A pediatric neurologist detected dystonia, more in his legs than his arms, and elicited a positive response to the pull test (see Fig. 18.9B). Cognitive testing showed no abnormality. The physician administered a therapeutic trial of a daily low dose of levodopa. The boy immediately reverted to normal. Genetic tests later confirmed the diagnosis of dopa-responsive dystonia.

DRD exists in all ethnic groups. In affected families, cases usually appear in an autosomal dominant pattern with incomplete penetrance. Many different mutations of a gene carried on chromosome 14 impair the synthesis of tetrahydrobiopterin, which is a cofactor for both phenylalanine hydroxylase and tyrosine hydroxylase. The tetrahydrobiopterin deficiency, in turn, eventually leads to serotonin and dopamine deficiencies that become more pronounced over the course of a day as activities deplete their stores.

Secondary Generalized Dystonia

Several other neurologic illnesses – such as Wilson disease, juvenile Huntington disease, and many types of spinocerebellar degeneration – occasionally express themselves as generalized dystonia. Cerebral anoxia, stroke, encephalitis, brain tumors, and toxins also may be responsible. When an underlying condition causes the dystonia, neurologists designate it *secondary* or *symptomatic dystonia*.

One of these dystonia-producing illnesses, *Lesch–Nyhan syndrome*, an X-linked recessive genetic disorder, produces one of neurology's most bizarre symptoms: 2- to 13-year-old boys (or, extraordinarily rarely, girls) develop ferocious self-mutilation (Fig. 18.27). In this quintessential neuropsychiatric abnormal behavior, children exhibit a compulsion for biting their own lips and fingers. This self-injurious behavior begins abruptly and furiously. In addition to the self-mutilation, they have mental retardation, spasticity, and seizures, as well as dystonia. By way of contrast, in mental retardation accompanied by autism, self-injurious behavior usually consists of head banging and hitting that begins insidiously and remains relatively mild.

The basic abnormality in Lesch–Nyhan syndrome consists of a deficiency of a purine metabolism enzyme attributable to a mutation in the *hypoxanthine phosphoribosyl transferase (HPRT1)* gene. By late childhood, the mutation leads to an accumulation of uric acid in the blood (hyperuricemia) and renal insufficiency or failure. Although allopurinol corrects the hyperuricemia, it does not prevent the neurologic damage.

Focal Dystonias

In contrast to generalized dystonia, *focal dystonias* usually develop sporadically, occur 10 times more frequently than generalized dystonia, tend to arise in individuals in their fifth decade and older, and involve muscles in a single region of the body: most commonly the face or head (cranial dystonia), neck (cervical dystonia), or arm (brachial dystonia, or writer's cramp). Because focal dystonias recur in a particular pattern, neurologists refer to them as stereotyped. Certain actions may cause focal dystonias. For example, writing, but not drawing or typing, may precipitate writer's cramp (see later). Likewise, job-related motion may precipitate an *occupational dystonia*. Nevertheless, as with primary generalized dystonia, patients' cognitive capacity remains intact.

Rarely, focal dystonia relates to an identifiable cause, but more often, the etiology of focal dystonia remains unknown. Probably as an error in almost all cases, classic neurologists and psychoanalysts – who used to be one and

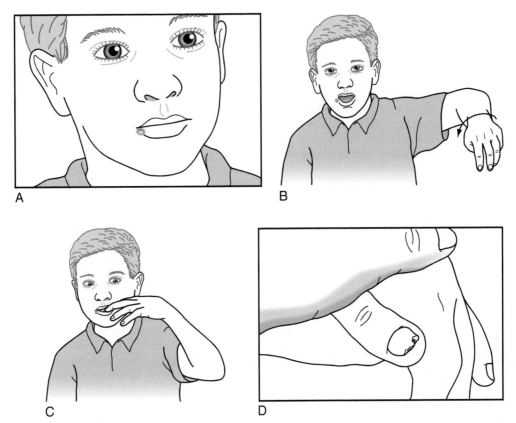

FIGURE 18.27 ■ This mentally retarded boy shows the self-mutilation and dystonia that characterize Lesch–Nyhan syndrome. *A*, His right lower lip has the scars of where he gnawed through it, even after his parents and physicians had his front teeth removed to prevent him from continuously biting himself. *B*, His limbs writhe and his thumb curls into his palm. *C*, In an apparent compulsion, he uncontrollably chews his fingers and already has amputated the tip of the smallest one. *D*, Prying away the boy's thumb shows that he has gnawed its nail and macerated its cuticle.

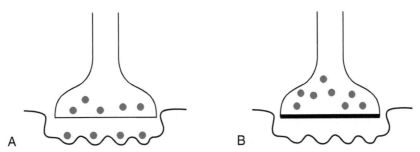

FIGURE 18.28 ■ *A*, At the normal neuromuscular junction, the presynaptic membrane releases packets of ACh (the pink dots) that cross the cleft and bind to postsynaptic membrane receptors, triggering muscle contractions. *B*, Botulinum toxin, injected directly into affected muscles, is taken up into the presynaptic motor nerve terminal and prevents the release of ACh, thereby weakening the injected muscle. The treatment reduces the abnormal contractions for about 3 months. To maintain the improvement, physicians must repeat the injections. Undesired weakness may occur if the dose is too high or the toxin diffuses into unintended muscles. Physicians can also inject botulinum toxins for cosmetic purposes to relax the facial muscles that cause undesirable furrows (rhythides) of the forehead, eyebrow ("frown lines"), lateral canthus ("crow's feet"), and other areas of the face and neck.

the same – attributed focal dystonias to subconscious conflicts. At another time, neurologists considered focal dystonias as a form of tardive dyskinesia because the movements sometimes followed administration of dopamine receptor-blocking medications. However, while neuroleptics can cause focal tardive dystonia, most patients with focal dystonia have had no exposure to such medications and, aside from disturbances that the movements induce, they usually have no psychiatric issues. In most cases dystonia relates to insults of the central nervous system, but some neurologists believe that dystonia can also result from peripheral nervous system damage, often from trauma.

Injections of botulinum toxin into affected muscles may effectively, but temporarily, eliminate focal dystonia (Fig. 18.28). Botulinum toxin may also treat particularly troublesome isolated muscle groups in DYT1 dystonia or tardive dystonia.

Cranial Dystonias

Blepharospasm, an easily recognizable and frequently occurring focal dystonia, consists of bilateral, simultaneous contractions of the orbicularis oculi (eyelid) and sometimes the frontalis (forehead) muscles (Fig. 18.29). The muscle spasms force the eyelids to close completely or partially, and also cause disfiguring facial expressions. Although neurologists cannot establish the cause in most cases, various eye diseases, including "dry eye," represent powerful risk factors.

To overcome the involuntary contractions, patients unconsciously learn tricks that temporarily suppress the contractions (Fig. 18.30). As with other focal dystonias, botulinum toxin injections usually reduce or abolish blepharospasm, at least on a temporary basis, with each set of injections.

Oromandibular dystonia consists of prominent contractions of the lower facial muscles and jaw muscles. Unlike the oral-buccal-lingual movements of tardive dyskinesia, the oral-buccal movements of oromandibular dystonia are symmetric and tongue protrusion is usually absent.

When the contractions involve both the upper and lower face, causing both blepharospasm and oromandibular dystonia, neurologists call the condition *Meige syndrome* (Fig. 18.31). This disorder mimics tardive dyskinesia except that, like oromandibular dystonia, it lacks tongue involvement. Neurosurgeons have performed DBS of the GPi to suppress the movements of Meige syndrome.

Cervical Dystonias

In *cervical dystonia*, the most frequent focal dystonia, one or more neck muscles involuntarily contract to rotate or tilt the head and neck (Figs. 18.32 and 18.33). The resultant posture may consist of turning of the head to one side (torticollis), tilting to one side (laterocollis), or flexion (anterocollis) or extension (retrocollis); most often these occur in complex combinations. The movements initially occur intermittently, but as the condition progresses, the abnormal postures become sustained and a superimposed "dystonic tremor" often complicates the picture. Unlike other forms of dystonia, cervical dystonia causes pain because the muscle contractions forcefully compress and rotate the cervical vertebra on each other and irritate the cervical nerve roots that emerge between them.

Cervical dystonia most commonly represents primary dystonia, though it can occur from structural lesions in the brain or cervical spine. Some cases are familial. In tardive dystonia due to long-term use of dopamine receptor-blocking agents, retrocollis often is prominent. Whatever the cause, intramuscular botulinum toxin injections reduce the movements as well as the pain. In severe cases, DBS has been helpful.

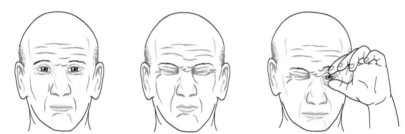

FIGURE 18.29 ■ This man with blepharospasm has repeated unprovoked closure of both eyelids lasting about 5 seconds at a time due to involuntary contractions of his orbicularis oculi muscles. Because the spasms block his vision, he often resorts to prying open his eyelids. In contrast to eyelid closure as a tic, the closures in blepharospasm are longer, more forceful, and not preceded by an urge to close the eyes.

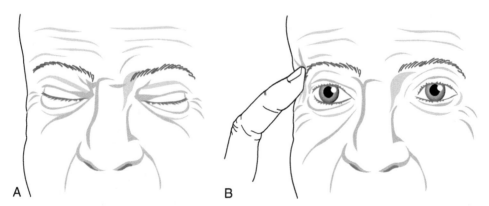

A   B

FIGURE 18.30 ■ *A,* During periods of blepharospasm, this man cannot open his eyelids. He attempts, perhaps unconsciously, to open them by contracting his frontalis muscle. *B,* He has instinctively learned that the sensory trick of lightly touching one eyebrow (a *geste antagoniste*) suppresses the spasms briefly.

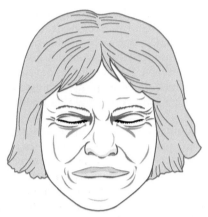

FIGURE 18.31 ■ This patient with Meige syndrome (cranial dystonia) has contractions of her entire facial musculature.

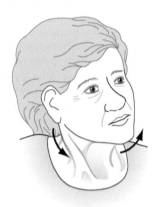

FIGURE 18.32 ■ Cervical dystonia consists of contraction of neck muscles that causes rotation (torticollis), tilting (laterocollis), flexion (*anterocollis*), or extension (*retrocollis*) – usually in combination – of the head and neck. Shoulder elevation often accompanies the other movements. Continuous contractions result in muscle hypertrophy and pain.

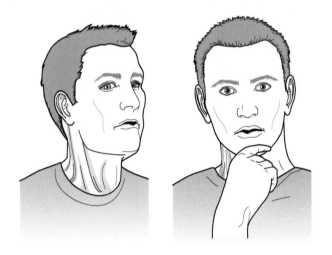

FIGURE 18.33 ■ As with blepharospasm and other focal dystonias, patients with cervical dystonia instinctively learn sensory tricks, such as lightly touching the chin, which is a classic *geste antagoniste*.

Spasmodic dysphonia consists of a distinctive speech abnormality caused by involuntary contraction of the laryngeal muscles when patients speak. In the most common type, the vocal cords adduct and lend the voice a strained tone – as if trying to speak while being strangled. Nevertheless, patients can shout, sing, and whisper. Likewise, patients can use the appropriate neighboring muscles normally to swallow and breathe.

Other cranial and cervical dystonias and head tremors often accompany spasmodic dysphonia. Clinical evaluation, often with laryngoscopy, can distinguish it from related conditions, such as essential tremor, vocal cord tumors, and pseudobulbar palsy (see Chapter 4). Electromyography-guided botulinum injections through the anterior of the throat directly into the laryngeal muscles reduce or eliminate involuntary contractions of the vocal folds and restore the voice.

Limb Dystonias

Limb dystonias usually involve arms more than legs. When hand muscles contract shortly after individuals engage in a repetitive action that forms the basis of their livelihood, neurologists term the disorder *occupational dystonia*. The disorder prevents workers from continuing their job. These dystonias are often task-specific, such that they emerge only with that particular action, while patients remain able to perform other functions with their affected hand.

In *writer's cramp*, a clear example of an occupational dystonia, shortly after authors begin to write, spasmodic contractions seize their finger and hand muscles. The contractions distort the hand and prevent it from properly grasping a pen or pencil (Fig. 18.34). However, writer's cramp does not prevent eating, buttoning clothing, or manipulating small objects – movements that require dexterity equal to handwriting.

Because affected individuals can still dictate or type material that they cannot write, writer's cramp differs from the psychologic phenomenon of *writer's block*. Fatigue-induced cramps also differ from writer's cramp in that they occur only after hours of performing the same task, cause considerable pain, and prohibit using the hand for any purpose.

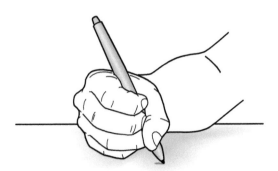

FIGURE 18.34 ■ This patient is an author with writer's cramp. She develops finger and hand muscle spasms several minutes after starting to write. The spasms force her hand into a fist and flex her wrist, preventing her from holding a pen. They also cause moderate pain. However, she does not develop the cramps when she uses the same hand to type, eat, or button clothing.

Other examples include *pianist's*, *guitarist's*, and *violinist's cramps*, in which repetitive, rapid, and intricate movements of these musicians' hands and fingers precipitate cramplike movements. Similarly, brass and woodwind players are vulnerable to *embouchure dystonia*, in which playing their instrument triggers debilitating lip, jaw, and tongue muscle contractions. Focal occupational dystonias strike professional musicians as frequently as 1/200, which is greater than in any other professional group, and signal the end of high-level performances. Although occupational dystonias that affect these individuals readily attract neurologists' attention, they also affect workers in less illustrious occupations, such as bricklaying and sewing.

ESSENTIAL TREMOR

Essential tremor consists of rhythmic oscillations (6 to 9 Hz) in one plane. It most often involves the upper and/or lower extremities, head and voice. When tremor involves the limbs, it is usually, but not always, symmetric. Performing particular actions or holding the arms in certain postures elicits or accentuates the limb tremor (Fig. 18.35). Tremors of the head usually conform to a "yes–yes" or "no–no" pattern.

Essential tremor usually develops in young and middle-aged adults. In the majority of cases, it follows autosomal dominant inheritance, but with variable penetrance. The pathophysiology underlying essential tremor is not clear. Some researchers have found reduced density of Purkinje cells in the cerebellum of patients with essential tremor, but not all studies have replicated this finding.

About 50% of affected individuals find that drinking alcohol-containing beverages suppresses their tremor. In almost all patients with tremor, as with many other neurologic conditions, anxiety precipitates or intensifies the movements. When anxiety does affect the tremor, it increases the tremor's amplitude but not its frequency.

Nonpharmacologic treatments may suffice for mild cases or they may supplement medication. Patients may benefit from wearing weights on their wrists, using capped mugs and a straw to drink fluids, and writing with thick rubber-covered pens. For the sake of safety, they should use electric shavers.

Of the pharmacologic treatments available, none is completely effective. However, β-adrenergic blockers, such as propranolol (Inderal), can help many cases of essential tremor and usually at doses that do not cause depression. The beneficial effect of these medicines supports the hypothesis that excessive β-adrenergic activity causes or

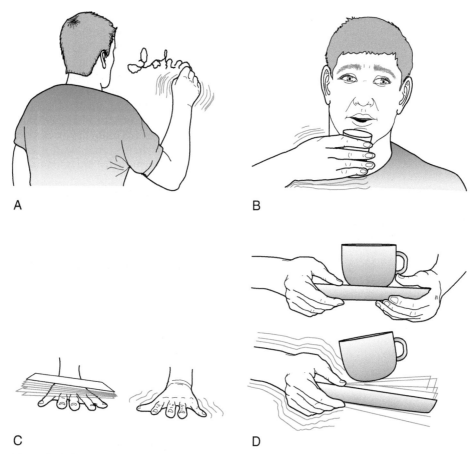

A   B

C   D

FIGURE 18.35 ■ Physicians elicit this 34-year-old gentleman's essential tremor by having him *A*, write his name, *B*, drink from a filled glass, *C*, support an envelope on his outstretched and pronated hand, or *D*, transfer a cup and saucer from one hand to the other. When his hands rest in his lap, the tremor completely subsides. Essential tremor is a prime example of an *action tremor*.

exacerbates essential tremor. Primidone (Mysoline), an anti-epileptic drug closely related to phenobarbital, alone or in combination with propranolol, also is effective in reducing the tremor. Medicines with less efficacy include benzodiazepines and other β-blockers.

For cases refractory to oral medications, DBS directed at the ventral intermediate (VIM) nucleus of the thalamus dramatically suppresses the tremor. To minimize risk, neurosurgeons can reduce operative time and likelihood of infection by implanting the electrodes unilaterally to improve the dominant hand. If successful, they can implant the electrodes contralaterally in a second procedure. While seemingly highly invasive for a relatively benign condition, DBS carries little risk. Neurosurgeons are currently investigating other methods for targeting the VIM nucleus, including focused ultrasound and gamma knife therapy.

Other Tremors

Other fine, rapid tremors, because they also respond to β-blockers, probably originate in excessive adrenergic system activity. These tremors often represent a physical manifestation of anxiety, as in stage fright (*performance anxiety*), or the DSM-5 diagnosis Social Anxiety Disorder (*social phobia*). They may also result from hyperthyroidism and other medical illnesses. Caffeine, the world's most popular drug, and other stimulants induce tremors (see Table 17.3, Caffeine Content of Popular Beverages, Medicines, and Foods). Also, tremors are often medication-induced – by steroids, the antiarrhythmic drug amiodarone, β-adrenergic agonists (such as those inhaled as bronchodilators), and psychotropics, including amitriptyline, lithium, valproate, SSRIs, and dopamine-blocking antipsychotics. Lithium and valproate may induce tremor even at therapeutic concentrations. From another perspective, tremor also can be a symptom of withdrawal from alcohol, benzodiazepines, opiates, or many other substances.

In contrast to the tremor of Parkinson disease, which characteristically occurs at rest, these tremor types are more prominent with action. The tremor of PD also differs from essential tremor by its "pill rolling" appearance (Fig. 18.8). Cerebellar dysfunction causes a coarse, irregular tremor elicited by movement (see Fig. 2.11). Except for the characteristic wing-beating pattern (Fig. 18.22), the tremors induced by Wilson disease remain difficult to categorize, especially because they can appear similar to those of PD, cerebellar disease, or essential tremor. Nevertheless, in young adults who develop a tremor, physicians should always consider Wilson disease. The fragile X tremor-ataxia syndrome, which appears in adults, includes tremor as well as mental retardation (see Chapter 13).

Palatal tremor, which neurologists until recently called *palatal myoclonus*, consists of uninterrupted symmetric, rhythmic contractions of the soft palate. The frequency – approximately 2 Hz – is consistent from patient to patient. It too persists during sleep or coma. Most cases are caused by small brainstem infarctions that involve the medulla's inferior olivary nucleus or its connections (see Fig. 2.9).

TICS

Tics consist of sudden, rapid, recurrent, and nonrhythmic movements. Neurologists classify them as *simple* or *complex*, and as *motor* or *vocal* (*phonic*) tics. *Simple motor tics* include the common head toss, prolonged eye blink, shoulder jerk, and asymmetric smile. *Simple vocal tics* consist of short, inarticulate sounds, such as throat clearing, grunting, and sniffing. The distinction between these two simple tics, however, is artificial because many vocal tics are simply the audible component of motor tics of the larynx, pharynx, or thoracic diaphragm. For example, tics of the diaphragm forcefully withdraw air through the nose, causing sniffles.

Complex motor tics consist of coordinated actions of several muscle groups, such as jumping, stomping, skipping, and mimicking movements (*echopraxia* or *echokinesis*). *Complex vocal tics* range from words to phrases and include repeated words (*echolalia*) and obscenities (*coprolalia*, see later).

Tics often occur in bursts that persist for several seconds, vary, and recur. Over periods of weeks, months, or years, tics develop and subside. Tics may occur during sleep. Except for anxiety, no factor consistently exacerbates them. Using intense concentration and learned strategies, individuals can temporarily suppress tics.

Another feature is that a premonitory sensation – commonly interpreted as a compulsion or irresistible urge – seems to provoke or at least precede tics in most patients. Patients gain relief if they allow tics to emerge, and suffer anxiety and an unpleasant intensification of the sensation if they do not. While characteristic of tics, a similar but less intense sensation precedes the movements in akathisia and RLS.

Simple motor tics develop at least briefly in as many as 30% of school-aged children, but, by the end of adolescence, almost all enjoy a spontaneous, complete remission. A disproportionate number of children with tics have a close relative with one or more tics. When their parents or siblings have tics, children are not only more apt to develop tics but also to develop them at a young age.

Tics in Adults

When adults display tics, they usually have either persistence of a childhood-onset disorder or, after a quiescent period, the reemergence of one. Compared to motor tics in children, which usually involve primarily the head, those in adults typically involve the neck and entire trunk. As individuals age, tics move from cephalad to caudal structures, i.e., move from head to toe. Also, tics in adults carry different comorbidities, including substance abuse, mood disorders, and anxiety and depression. Moreover, tics in adults may reflect use of cocaine or similar psychoactive substances.

Gilles de la Tourette Disorder

For a diagnosis of Tourette Disorder, the DSM-5 requires the presence of *both* vocal and multiple motor tics,

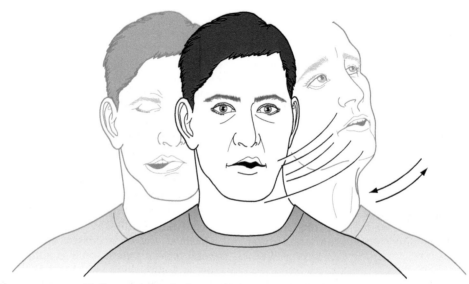

FIGURE 18.36 ■ This young man with Tourette disorder has multiple motor tics, including head jerking (head toss), grimacing of the right side of his mouth (half-smile), and depression of his forehead (frowning). Vocal tics of throat clearing and a short blowing sound accompany his motor tics. All of his tics continue throughout the day and briefly during sleep. Conversation, eating, and social situations have little influence, but with effort he can suppress his tics for several minutes.

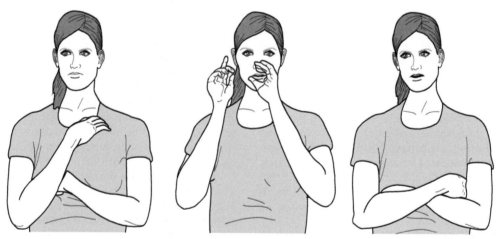

FIGURE 18.37 ■ This woman has compulsive obscene gestures – copropraxia. Similar to coprolalia, they have no affective or sexual content.

although not necessarily concurrently, for longer than 1 year, with onset before 18 years of age (Fig. 18.36). Neurologists, who use similar criteria, tend to use the term *Tourette syndrome*.

Tourette disorder affects boys more frequently than girls. This male preponderance also occurs in many other neurodevelopmental conditions, including dyslexia, stuttering, and autism. Tics appear on average at age 6 to 7 years, and in 90% of cases by age 13 years. They generally relapse at the beginning of the school year and remit during the summer months. By their adult years, about 30% of affected individuals enjoy a complete remission and another 30% a substantial improvement.

At the onset of Tourette disorder, tics usually involve only the face, eyes, and head, but in succeeding years different tics spread caudally to affect the neck and shoulders, then arms and hands, and finally the trunk and legs. Because each tic may recede or replace another, Tourette disorder varies from year to year in its repertoire, tempo, and intensity.

Vocal tics, an essential feature of Tourette disorder, consist of irresistible, repetitive, stereotyped utterances – sounds, words, or, in the extreme, coprolalia. Vocal tics usually arise several years after the onset of motor tics and remain simple. They typically consist of only inarticulate sounds, such as sniffing, throat clearing, or clicks. However, many vocal tics rise to loud and disconcerting noises, such as grunting, snorting, or honking. Complex vocal tics consist of formed words that can culminate in unprovoked outbursts of obscene words, *coprolalia*. Although most coprolalia consists of only fragments of scatological words, such as "shi" or "fu," some consist of strings of unequivocal obscenities. Equivalents of coprolalia, such as intrusions of obscene thoughts (*mental coprolalia*) or involuntary obscene movements or gestures (*copropraxia*, Fig. 18.37), may represent a form of coprolalia.

When coprolalia complicates Tourette disorder, it does not appear until about 6 years after the onset of motor tics. Usually coprolalia is merely socially reprehensible but occasionally it can be dangerous, such as when a young Chinese girl's vocal tic belittled Chairman Mao, a Bronx teenager endlessly and uncontrollably repeated two words disparaging the New York Yankees, or a devoutly Catholic adolescent girl incessantly damned a particular saint. Despite its dramatic and notorious aspects, physicians and the public have overemphasized coprolalia. It is not a diagnostic criterion for Tourette disorder and less than 25% of patients exhibit it.

Comorbid Psychiatric Conditions

Psychiatric disturbances complicate Tourette disorder in about 80% of cases. Those few patients who are unencumbered by psychiatric comorbidity enjoy relatively few behavioral disabilities and a better overall outcome. For the majority, one or more psychiatric comorbidities threatens to dominate the clinical picture. ADHD, the most frequently occurring comorbidity, affects about 60% of boys and one-half of girls with Tourette disorder. It precedes the development of tics by 1 to 2 years.

A dilemma regarding hyperactive children with Tourette disorder has centered on the concern that prescribing stimulants to control hyperactivity could worsen the tics. Studies have shown that, although stimulants such as methylphenidate may cause a transient flare-up in tics, in many cases the stimulants' benefits outweigh their risks.

Another common comorbidity of Tourette disorder consists of obsessive-compulsive symptoms, either alone or as part of OCD. This comorbidity occurs in about 30% of both males and females, and also emerges several years after the onset of tics. Obsessions and compulsions in Tourette disorder differ somewhat from those of pure OCD without comorbid Tourette disorder. For example, obsessions in Tourette disorder relate to sex, violence, and aggression, but those in pure OCD relate to dirt, germs, and illness. Similarly, compulsions in Tourette disorders typically consist of checking and ordering, but those in pure OCD consist of more elaborate activities, such as handwashing or housecleaning.

Anxieties, phobias, and related disturbances also complicate Tourette disorder in about 20% of patients of both genders. Their frequency and severity vary directly with the severity of the tics.

Children with Tourette disorder have normal intelligence and no propensity toward psychosis. Although many of them have learning disabilities, this problem may relate to the disorder only indirectly – for example, through ADHD and social factors that interfere with children's early education.

Other Associations

Many patients have soft neurologic signs and minor nonspecific EEG abnormalities. Their CT, MRI, functional MRI, PET, and diffusion imaging do not reveal consistent, specific abnormalities. However, some studies have found decreased volume of the caudate nucleus, and others have reported increased D2 receptor activity in the caudate.

Etiology

Genetic factors influence the risk of Tourette disorder. For example, penetrance reaches almost 90% in monozygotic twins, and, depending on the criteria, 10% to 15% of an affected individual's first-degree relatives will have the disorder. In some cases, Tourette disorder appears to be transmitted with autosomal dominant inheritance, but no single causative gene has been identified.

Environmental factors are also likely to play a part in the etiology of Tourette disorder. The theory of *pediatric autoimmune neuropsychiatric disorder associated with streptococcal infections* (*PANDAS*) proposes, at least for a subset of patients, that *group A β-hemolytic streptococcus* infections cause or trigger tics, Tourette disorder, and Sydenham chorea and, more important, induce obsessive-compulsive symptoms – all through antibody cross-reactivity or "molecular mimicry." Despite its popularity, this theory lost some traction after several clinical and basic science studies challenged it.

Some evidence suggests that dopamine supersensitivity leads to the tics. For example, agents that reduce dopamine activity suppress tics and dopamine-enhancing substances, such as cocaine, exacerbate them. Other authors have reported that severity of Tourette disorder is associated with maternal smoking during pregnancy or with low birth weight, but these observations remain unconfirmed and speculative.

Treatment

Behavioral therapy, including "habit-reversal training," may reduce tics or at least postpone them to more socially acceptable times. When tics require pharmacologic treatment, neurologists may try several approaches.

Clonidine and guanfacine, α-adrenergic agonists, suppress tics through unknown mechanisms of action. In addition, guanfacine may also help ADHD. A more potent treatment consists of reducing dopaminergic activity. For example, dopamine receptor antagonists, such as haloperidol, fluphenazine, and pimozide, suppress both vocal and most motor tics in about 80% of patients. Likewise, the dopamine depleter tetrabenazine lessens tics. The Food and Drug Administration (FDA) has given an indication to only haloperidol and fluphenazine for use in Tourette disorder. Putting aside withdrawal dyskinesias and other transient complications, dopamine receptor antagonist treatment of Tourette disorder rarely causes tardive dyskinesia. In fact, one paper reporting an extremely low complication rate quipped, "Does Tourette syndrome prevent tardive dyskinesia?"

Botulinum injections may temporarily eliminate particularly bothersome, relatively focal motor tics. Several studies have shown that DBS suppresses motor and vocal tics; however, they have not established if the best target for electrode placement is the GPi or thalamus or answered various technical questions. Even so, DBS directed at controlling tics will probably not improve the comorbid OCD.

Related Conditions

A *stereotypy* consists of a repetitive, patterned, rhythmic, and often complex involuntary movement. Examples include slapping, flapping of the hands; twisting and wringing of fingers; repetitive forceful closure of the jaw with grinding of the teeth (bruxism); and rocking, twirling, and weight shifting of the body.

Stereotypies may be manifestations of autism, Rett syndrome, or Sydenham chorea, as well as Tourette disorder. In blind or mentally retarded individuals, stereotypies such as continual rocking appear to compensate for sensory deprivation. Stereotypies also appear during focal motor seizures – sometimes as their only outward manifestation. Cocaine use can cause 2 to 6 days of various stereotypies as well as tics, akathisia-like leg movements ("crack-dancing"), and punding (see above). Despite their potential association with these disorders, stereotypies can also be perfectly benign, occurring in perhaps 7% of neurologically normal children.

MYOCLONUS

Myoclonus consists of generalized or focal, irregular, rapid jerks. It differs from most movement disorders in several respects. Myoclonus originates in abnormal discharges from motor neurons in the cerebral cortex, brainstem, or spinal cord rather than the basal ganglia. It may persist when patients are asleep or comatose. Also, unlike the spontaneous movements of chorea or Parkinson disease, myoclonic jerks can be triggered by voluntary movements or external stimuli such as noise, touch, or light. In other words, myoclonus is often *action-* or *stimulus-sensitive*.

A wide variety of disorders can produce myoclonus. Cerebral cortex dysfunction is most often the cause of generalized myoclonus. Survivors of cerebral anoxia often show *postanoxic myoclonus*. Myoclonus is a common side effect of many medications, including gabapentin, pregabalin, meperidine (Demerol) and other opiates, SSRIs and SNRIs, bismuth, and cyclosporine. For many of these agents, renal insufficiency increases the risk of drug-induced myoclonus. In fact, uremia itself can lead to myoclonus. In toxic-metabolic aberrations, myoclonus commonly co-occurs with delirium. Myoclonus is one of the most prominent physical manifestations of subacute sclerosing panencephalitis (SSPE) (see Chapter 7), Creutzfeldt–Jakob disease (see Chapter 7), certain mitochondrial disorders (see Chapter 6), and paraneoplastic limbic encephalitis (see Chapter 19).

When possible, remedying the underlying toxic-metabolic disturbance usually results in resolution of the myoclonus. Treatment with clonazepam, levetiracetam, or valproate may suppress myoclonus, but, of course, it does not affect the underlying disorder.

Psychiatrists may encounter myoclonus in their patients taking SSRIs, SNRIs, clozapine, or lithium. When myoclonus develops in patients taking an SSRI or SNRI, it suggests the serotonin syndrome (see Chapter 6). Physicians should avoid prescribing serotonergic agents in combination with medications that inhibit their metabolism, such as nonselective monoamine oxidase inhibitors.

Not all myoclonus reflects pathology. Benign forms include hiccups, which are merely physiologic shocklike contractions of the diaphragm, and hypnagogic and hypnopompic jerks, which are the sudden, generalized muscle contractions that accompany the transitions into or out of sleep.

Hemifacial Spasm

Hemifacial spasm, a type of focal myoclonus, consists of contractions of one or more muscles innervated by the facial nerve (the seventh cranial nerve) on one side (Fig. 18.38). In this disorder, spasms occur irregularly at 1 to 10 per minute, often in flurries or clusters. Depending on their severity and anatomic distribution, spasms may disfigure the face and close the eyelids. Like other types of myoclonus, hemifacial spasm routinely persists during sleep.

Hemifacial spasm often has an identifiable and correctable cause. In most cases, an aberrant vessel compresses and presumably irritates the facial nerve as it exits from the pons at the cerebellopontine angle. Sometimes, aberrant regeneration of the facial nerve after an injury, including Bell's palsy, leads to the disorder.

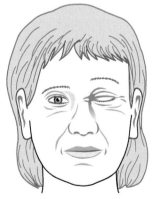 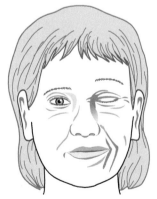 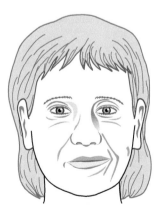

FIGURE 18.38 ■ This 53-year-old woman has hemifacial spasm manifesting as bursts of left-sided facial muscle contractions. The contractions repetitively squeeze shut her left eyelid and pull her mouth to her left side, but the upper and lower face muscles do not contract synchronously. As a compensatory mechanism to lift her left eyelid, she elevates the left eyebrow.

Neurosurgeons can alleviate hemifacial spasm resulting from an aberrant blood vessel by performing a *microvascular decompression* of the facial nerve. This procedure consists of inserting a cushion between the vessel and the facial nerve, which is a similar to microvascular decompression of the fifth cranial nerve for treatment of trigeminal neuralgia (see Chapter 9).

MOVEMENT DISORDERS DUE TO DOPAMINE-BLOCKING MEDICATIONS

As previously discussed, antipsychotic agents and other medicines that block dopamine potentially may cause NMS, lower the seizure threshold, alter the EEG (see Chapter 10), and produce retinal abnormalities (see Chapter 12). They may also cause dramatic involuntary movements as well as parkinsonism.

When considering movement disorders (dyskinesias) induced by dopamine receptor-blocking agents, neurologists find it helpful to classify them as acute or tardive (late) based on the interval between initiating or increasing the dose of the medication and their onset. In this classification, *acute dyskinesias* develop within days and *tardive (late) dyskinesias* at 6 months or longer, but almost always within 12 months of starting the medication (Box 18.2). Psychiatrists tend to use the term "extrapyramidal symptoms" to describe any involuntary movements due to these medications.

Acute Dyskinesias

When it occurs, acute dyskinesia develops in about 90% of cases within the first 5 days and 50% of cases within the first 2 days of initiating or increasing the dose of the medication. Dyskinesias complicate the use of second-generation antipsychotics less frequently than the use of first-generation neuroleptics. They also complicate the use of dopamine receptor-blocking medications to treat nonpsychiatric conditions, such as metoclopramide (Reglan) as an antiemetic or antimigraine therapy.

Parenteral administration and combinations of offending agents are more likely to precipitate acute dyskinesias.

BOX 18.2	Neuroleptic-Induced Movement Disorders

Acute dyskinesias
   Akathisia
   Neuroleptic-malignant syndrome
   Oculogyric crisis and other dystonias
Tardive dyskinesias
   Akathisia
   Dystonia
   Oral-buccal-lingual dyskinesia*
   Tics
   Tremor
   Stereotypies
Dose-dependent dyskinesia
   Parkinsonism
Withdrawal-emergent dyskinesias

*Commonly referred to as "tardive dyskinesia"

Other risk factors include youth, male gender, comorbid substance abuse, prior electroconvulsive therapy, and pre-existing brain damage. In particular, individuals who have abused cocaine place themselves at a 40-fold increased risk of developing acute dystonic reactions to antipsychotics.

With the exception of NMS, acute dyskinesias usually spontaneously subside or respond to parenteral anticholinergics or antihistamines. Sometimes acute dyskinesias persist indefinitely despite appropriate treatment.

Acute dyskinesias fall into three categories:
* Oculogyric crisis and other acute dystonias
* Akathisia
* NMS (see Chapter 6)

In addition, dopamine receptor-blocking agents can induce parkinsonism (see earlier) in a dose-dependent manner.

Oculogyric Crisis and Other Acute Dystonias

Acute dystonic reactions consist of the abrupt development of limb or trunk dystonic postures, repetitive jaw and face muscle contractions, tongue protrusion, torticollis, or, in special cases, oculogyric crisis (Fig. 18.39). These dyskinesias may occur alone or in combinations, but typically facial, cervical, and/or jaw dystonia accompany oculogyric crisis. Physicians must keep in mind that several serious neurologic disorders – seizures, tetanus, drugs of abuse, and strychnine poisoning – can cause similar movements. For example, in large urban hospitals, patients who present with oculogyric crisis or other acute dystonia and do not respond to anticholinergics and antihistaminics are often experiencing phencyclidine (PCP) intoxication.

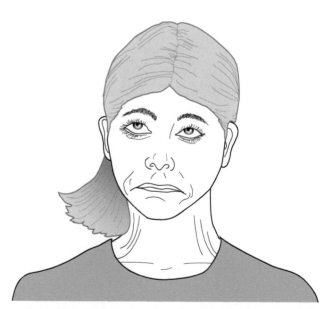

FIGURE 18.39 ■ During an oculogyric crisis, the eyes forcefully roll upward and sometimes sideways but always conjugately. This patient also exhibits contraction of the platysma. Elements of mandibular and cervical dystonia also may be present, with opening or closing of the jaw and extension of the neck. Parenteral anticholinergics almost always abort this frightening dystonia.

The pathophysiology of acute dystonic reactions remains unknown. Of course, their temporal relationship to dopamine-blockade suggests that lack of dopamine activity causes them. In the opposite scenario, because of the drug-induced blockade of dopamine receptors, a feedback loop may provoke an increased secretion of dopamine or a dopamine-like neurotransmitter that causes the movement. Another theory suggests that the movements' favorable response to anticholinergics shows that they result from excessive cholinergic activity.

Akathisia

In akathisia, nearly regular limb and trunk movements continually plague the patient (Fig. 18.40). Although akathisia can involve the trunk and arms, it predominantly affects the legs. Most importantly, it forces patients to move about and prohibits their sitting still or lying quietly in bed. When standing, patients tend to shuffle, march in place, or rock on their heels and toes. When sitting, which they find difficult, patients squirm, sway back and forth, or rub their feet on the floor – hence the origin of the term "akathisia" (Greek, *a*, without + *kathisis*, sitting).

A subjective component of akathisia frequently disturbs the patient as much as the movements. As with tics, a psychic urge drives akathisia; however, moving does not relieve the urge. For example, patients with akathisia may experience intense restlessness, a need or compulsion to move, or even an irresistible desire to walk. This component of the problem sometimes forces patients to abandon their medical regimen.

In subtle cases, akathisia often remains undetected because the movements are mostly an exaggeration of normal movements. In a more problematic situation, physicians may reasonably confuse akathisia with insufficiently treated anxiety, psychosis, or agitated depression. Thus, psychiatrists must often decide either to increase or reduce an antipsychotic medicine for a restless patient with psychosis.

Akathisia also resembles movements induced by fluoxetine, cocaine ("crack dancing"), or excessive levodopa. In addition, although RLS looks like akathisia and RLS patients share the urge to move their legs, akathisia patients do not experience the paresthesias that characterize RLS and their movements are not specifically related to sleep. To emphasize that akathisia, tics, and RLS stem in part from uncomfortable sensations, one neurologist quipped that patients with these disorders move because they are distressed, but patients with most other movement disorders are distressed because they move.

Propranolol (a β-blocker), clonidine (an α-2 agonist), and mirtazapine may suppress the movements, but anticholinergics will not help. When the physician cannot distinguish between akathisia and restlessness from undertreated psychosis, prescribing a benzodiazepine until the diagnosis emerges is a credible strategy.

Tardive Dyskinesia

Oral-Buccal-Lingual Dyskinesias

Some physicians use the term "tardive dyskinesia" in a narrow sense to refer to the common antipsychotic-induced *oral-buccal-lingual* (also called *choreic* or *orofacial*) *dyskinesia*, which consists of stereotyped tongue, jaw, and face movements (Fig. 18.41). Others employ the term "tardive dyskinesia" more broadly by applying it to all types of abnormal movements due to dopamine receptor-blocking agents (see Box 18.2), and reserve the specific label "classic tardive dyskinesias" to describe the oral-buccal-lingual movements.

Clinicians use the *Abnormal Involuntary Movement Scale (AIMS)* to describe the presence, locations, and severity of abnormal movements (Fig. 18.42). It provides a global rating scale that allows physicians to assess pretreatment status and subsequent changes. However, even assuming interrater reliability, the AIMS has several drawbacks. It does not capture the fact that movements may vary in intensity over time. The rating of severity from 1 to 5 is subjective and gross. The AIMS does not recognize akinesia (lack of movement), which should carry as much diagnostic weight as hyperkinesia. It does not distinguish among chorea, dystonia, tics, and stereotypies. Finally, it omits several important movements, such as tremor, dysarthria, and respiratory tics.

Most, but not all, studies have concluded that the overall incidence of tardive dyskinesia is higher with first- than second-generation antipsychotics. Explanations for

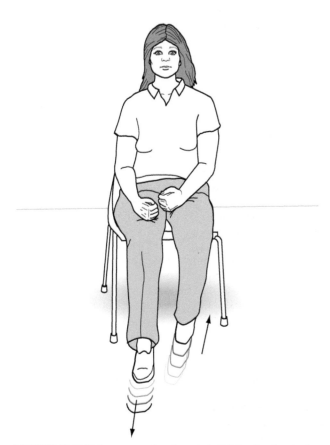

FIGURE 18.40 ■ This woman developed akathisia after beginning a regimen of antipsychotic medicines. She feels driven to move her legs and continually shuffles them in regular to-and-fro sliding movements. Although akathisia can lead to repetitive semipurposeful arm movements, such as scratching, hair smoothing, and rubbing, it predominantly affects the legs.

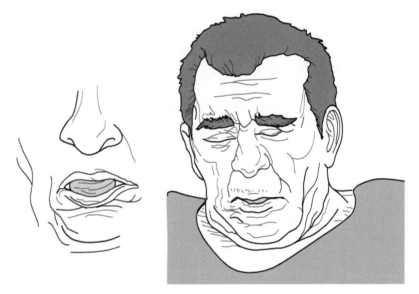

FIGURE 18.41 ■ The oral-buccal-lingual type of tardive dyskinesia consists of repetitive tongue movements accompanied by continual jaw and facial muscle contractions. These movements typically include tongue darting, lip smacking, kissing, lip puckering, and chewing; sometimes blepharospasm also is present. Unlike the movements in chorea and cranial dystonias, tongue movements in oral-buccal-lingual tardive dyskinesia are not only prominent, but they may lead to tongue enlargement (macroglossia).

that finding include the facts that dopamine receptor-blocking antipsychotic agents with a high affinity for D2 receptors, which are mostly the first-generation neuroleptics, remain the strongest risk factor for tardive dyskinesia; second-generation antipsychotics act primarily on $5HT_{2A}$ receptors and produce a high $5HT_{2A}$/D2 blockade ratio; second-generation antipsychotics adhere either weakly or transiently to the D2 receptor; and some, such as aripiprazole, partially agonize as well as block the D2 receptor. Quetiapine and clozapine, which have negligible affinity for dopamine receptors, are not associated with tardive dyskinesia. Other powerful risk factors include the duration of treatment and total medication dosage, age greater than 60 years, and female gender (especially for patients older than 65 years). Interesting but less powerful risk factors include prior history of medication-induced extrapyramidal side effects, dementia or other sign of brain damage, underlying affective rather than psychotic illness, and certain genes.

Some studies have found that the yearly incidence of tardive dyskinesia remained constant throughout medication exposure and concluded that patients have the same chance of developing this complication during the first year as during the fifth year of treatment. Others have reported that the incidence increases slightly with longer duration of treatment.

Etiology

Despite its limitations, the classic *dopamine receptor supersensitivity theory* remains consistent with several of the condition's major clinical features (Fig. 18.43). Tardive dyskinesia begins after 6 months or more from the initiation of dopamine receptor-blocking medicines. The dyskinesias resemble movements produced by excessive levodopa. Maneuvers that expose the postsynaptic neuron to increased dopamine activity – reducing the dosage of the dopamine receptor blocker, stopping it, or adding levodopa – intensify the movements. Likewise, increasing the medication dosage, which reduces dopamine activity,

suppresses the movements. The traditional theory views tardive dyskinesia as the result of upregulation of D2 receptors, but evidence from a capuchin monkey model has suggested that it is D3 receptors rather than D2 receptors that become supersensitive.

An alternate theory attributes the disorder to deficient or abnormal GABA activity in the striatum. Another posits that the glutamate system triggers excitotoxicity through NMDA receptors. Still another suggests that catecholamine metabolism creates neurotoxic free radicals. It is likely that a combination of mechanisms contribute to the development of tardive dyskinesia.

Treatment

The best treatment is prevention. Physicians should endeavor to avoid prescribing antipsychotic and other medications associated with tardive dyskinesias. When their use is warranted, physicians should prescribe minimal doses. Once tardive dyskinesia appears, physicians should resist a natural temptation to abruptly stop the medicine. They should taper it – over weeks or months – because abruptly stopping it may unmask the withdrawal-emergent syndrome (see later).

Alternatively, switching from a first- to a second-generation antipsychotic or from one second-generation agent to another sometimes helps. Although the benefit may take months to materialize, switching to clozapine in cases of refractory, disabling tardive dyskinesia is a standard strategy.

Studies have found that tetrabenazine reduces tardive dyskinesias, undoubtedly by reducing dopamine activity. However, depression and suicidal ideation may complicate its use. Moreover, it has not received an FDA indication for use in tardive dyskinesia. As a last resort, the physician can reduce dopamine activity by restarting or increasing the dosage of a typical dopamine-blocking medication or substituting a more potent one. This strategy risks creating a vicious cycle where recurrence of the dyskinesia requires additional medication.

EXAMINATION PROCEDURE

Either before or after completing the Examination Procedure observe the patient unobtrusively, at rest (e.g., in waiting room).

The chair to be used in this examination should be a hard, firm one without arms.

___

1. Ask patient to remove shoes and socks.

2. Ask patient whether there is anything in his/her mouth (i.e., gum, candy, etc.) and if there is, to remove it.

3. Ask patient about the <u>current</u> condition of his/her teeth. Ask patient if he/she wears dentures. Do teeth or dentures bother patient <u>now</u>?

4. Ask patient whether he/she notices any movements in mouth, face, hands, or feet. If yes, ask to describe and to what extent they <u>currently</u> bother patient or interfere with his/her activities.

5. Have patient sit in chair with hands on knees, legs slightly apart, and feet flat on floor. (Look at entire body for movements while in this position.)

6. Ask patient to sit with hands hanging unsupported, if male, between legs, if female and wearing a dress, hanging over knees. (Observe hands and other body areas.)

7. Ask patient to open mouth. (Observe tongue at rest within mouth.) Do this twice.

8. Ask patient to protrude tongue. (Observe abnormalities of tongue movement.) Do this twice.

9. Ask patient to tap thumb, with each finger, as rapidly as possible for 10–15 seconds; separately with right hand, then with left hand. (Observe facial and leg movements.)

10. Flex and extend patient's left and right arms (one at a time). (Note any rigidity.)

11. Ask patient to stand up. (Observe in profile. Observe all body areas again, hips included.)

12. Ask patient to extend both arms outstretched in front with palms down. (Observe trunk, legs, and mouth.)

13. Have patients walk a few paces, turn, and walk back to chair. (Observe hands and gait.) Do this twice.

FIGURE 18.42 ■ The Abnormal Involuntary Movement Scale (AIMS) guides the examiner through inspection for dyskinesias of the face, jaw, tongue, trunk, and limbs. The examiner records observations when the patient is at rest, extending the tongue or limbs, or performing certain activities, such as finger tapping, standing, or walking. In addition, the examiner checks for rigidity. This revision of the original (Guy, 1976) requests that patients remove their shoes and socks, and it does not rate as less severe those movements that are activated by voluntary movements.

DEPARTMENT OF HEALTH AND HUMAN SERVICES PUBLIC HEALTH SERVICE Alcohol, Drug Abuse, and Mental Health Administration NIMH Treatment Strategies in Schizophrenia Study	PATIENT NUMBER	DATA GROUP	EVALUATION DATE
	— — — —	aims	— — — — — — M M D D Y Y

ABNORMAL INVOLUNTARY MOVEMENT SCALE (AIMS)

PATIENT NAME

RATER NAME

RATER NUMBER	EVALUATION TYPE (Circle)
— — —	1 Baseline 4 Start double-blind 7 Start open meds 10 Early termination 2 2-week minor 5 Major evaluation 8 During open meds 11 Study completion 3 6 Other 9 Stop open meds

INSTRUCTIONS: Complete Examination Procedure (reverse side) before making ratings.
MOVEMENT RATINGS: Rate highest severity observed.

Code: 1 = None
2 = Minimal, may be extreme normal
3 = Mild
4 = Moderate
5 = Severe

			(Circle One)			
FACIAL AND ORAL MOVEMENTS:	1.	**Muscles of Facial Expression** e.g., movements of forehead, eyebrows, periorbital area, cheeks; include frowning, blinking, smiling, grimacing	1	2	3	4	5
	2.	**Lips and Perioral Area** e.g., puckering, pouting, smacking	1	2	3	4	5
	3.	**Jaw** e.g., biting, clenching, chewing, mouth opening, lateral movement	1	2	3	4	5
	4.	**Tongue** Rate only increase in movement both in and out of mouth. NOT inability to sustain movement	1	2	3	4	5
EXTREMITY MOVEMENTS:	5.	**Upper** (arms, wrists, hands, fingers) Include choreic movements, (i.e., rapid, objectively purposeless irregular, spontaneous), athetoid movements (i.e., slow, irregular, complex, serpentine). Do NOT include tremor (i.e., repetitive, regular, rhythmic)	1	2	3	4	5
	6.	**Lower** (legs, knees, ankles, toes) e.g., lateral knee movement, foot tapping, heel dropping, foot squirming, inversion and eversion of foot	1	2	3	4	5
TRUNK MOVEMENTS:	7.	**Neck, shoulders, hips** e.g., rocking, twisting, squirming, pelvic gyrations	1	2	3	4	5
GLOBAL JUDGMENTS:	8.	**Severity of abnormal movements**	None, normal 1 Minimal 2 Mild 3 Moderate 4 Severe 5			
	9.	**Incapacitation due to abnormal movements**	None, normal 1 Minimal 2 Mild 3 Moderate 4 Severe 5			
	10.	**Patient's awareness of abnormal movements** Rate only patient's report	No awareness 1 Aware, no distress 2 Aware, mild distress 3 Aware, moderate distress 4 Aware, severe distress 5			
DENTAL STATUS:	11.	**Current problems with teeth and/or dentures**	No 1 Yes 2			
	12.	**Does patient usually wear dentures?**	No 1 Yes 2			

FIGURE 18.42, cont'd

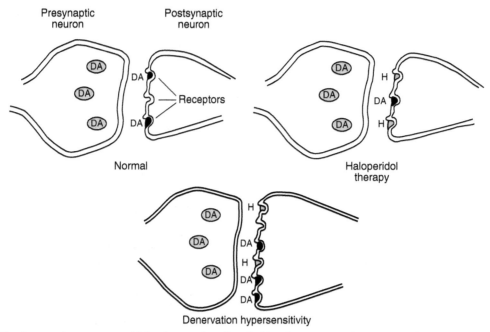

FIGURE 18.43 ■ The denervation supersensitivity theory of tardive dyskinesia proposes that when antipsychotic agents such as haloperidol bind to postsynaptic dopamine receptors, the remaining receptors become particularly sensitive and new ones develop. As a result dopamine released from the presynaptic neuron or present in the synaptic cleft triggers these supersensitive receptors and elicits hyperkinesia. DA, dopamine; H, haloperidol.

A different approach counterbalances enhanced dopamine activity by increasing acetylcholine (ACh) activity (see Fig. 18.13). Despite the credibility of the theory, physostigmine, which prolongs ACh activity, and ACh precursors, such as deanol (Deaner), lecithin, or choline, help for only brief periods. Rigorous studies of a possible role for the anticholinesterase medications approved for Alzheimer disease – donepezil, rivastigmine, and galantamine – to treat tardive dyskinesia are lacking. The opposite approach, giving anticholinergics, also does not help.

Medications that affect other neurotransmitters also fail to help. For example, GABA agonists, such as baclofen, calcium-channel blockers, such as diltiazem (Cardizem), lithium, and opiates, provide no consistent relief. Medications with some evidence of benefit are benzodiazepines and vitamin E, but the effects are mild.

Neurologists have hesitated to use botulinum injections for tongue dyskinesias. Injecting the tongue's main muscles (the genioglossus and geniohyoid) would require a needle to pass through their rich vascular supply and risk an uncontrollable hemorrhage. Moreover, botulinum might weaken tongue or throat muscles enough to occlude the airway.

Preliminary studies found that DBS directed at the GPi ameliorates oral-buccal-lingual and other varieties of tardive dyskinesia. Moreover, patients may discontinue the medicines that physicians prescribed to reduce the movements and enjoy an improved quality of life. DBS causes no cognitive impairment or exacerbation of depression.

A 2013 guideline from the American Academy of Neurology offers evidence-based recommendations regarding various treatments for tardive syndromes. The strongest evidence supports a probable benefit of clonazepam for short-term treatment of oral-buccal-lingual dyskinesias, and probable benefit of ginkgo biloba extract – an antioxidant – for treating tardive dyskinesia in inpatients with schizophrenia. The authors also deemed amantadine and tetrabenazine to be options, though the evidence for their beneficial effect is weaker. While risperidone may mask tardive dyskinesias, it can also cause them and therefore was not recommended. The guideline examined many other interventions – including numerous medications and supplements, GPi DBS, and withdrawal or switching of neuroleptics – but found data to be insufficient to recommend any of them.

Pharmacotherapy for tardive dyskinesia may not be necessary. Even without intervention, approximately 33% of oral-buccal-lingual cases undergo remission spontaneously.

Tardive Dystonia

Another type of tardive dyskinesia, *tardive dystonia*, consists of sustained, powerful, twisting movements predominantly of the neck, upper arms, and trunk (Fig. 18.44). Retrocollis, reflecting contraction of the extensor neck muscles, is a common pattern. It is more typical of tardive dystonia than of primary cervical dystonia in which torticollis and laterocollis are usually more prominent. Related movements, including oral-buccal-lingual dyskinesia, blepharospasm, and akathisia, often accompany tardive dystonia. Otherwise, tardive dystonia resembles the dystonia of Wilson disease, juvenile Huntington disease, or DYT1 dystonia.

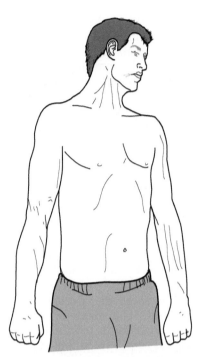

FIGURE 18.44 ■ After receiving neuroleptic treatment for 6 years, this 25-year-old man began to develop prolonged, forceful twisting (torsion) and extension of his arms, extension of his head and neck (retrocollis), and exaggerated arching of his back. Subsequently, subtle oral-buccal-lingual choreiform movements, blepharospasm, and other varieties of tardive dyskinesia arose. His physicians diagnosed his condition as tardive dystonia. Had there been no history of exposure to neuroleptic medications, they would have considered Wilson disease and DYT1 dystonia as potential diagnoses.

A relatively short exposure to dopamine-blocking agents, sometimes as brief as 3 months, can cause tardive dystonia. Thereafter, it complicates exposure at a low but constant yearly rate. Spontaneous remissions occur in about 12% of cases.

Several entirely different medicines may suppress tardive dystonia. In contrast to their lack of benefit in oral-buccal-lingual dyskinesia, anticholinergics sometimes reduce tardive dystonia, as they do other forms of dystonia. Clozapine and tetrabenazine, which each reduce dopamine activity through different mechanisms, often help. Botulinum injections may alleviate dystonia in severely involved specific muscle groups, such as the neck extensors.

DBS alleviates tardive dystonia just as it does DYT1 dystonia. It provides the same benefits and safety margin as when used for oral-buccal-lingual dyskinesia.

Other Tardive Dyskinesias

Tardive akathisia, which resembles the acutely developing disorder, persists by definition for longer than 6 months after the medication is begun. In addition, it may appear only after the patient has stopped the offending medication. As with tardive dystonia, other tardive dyskinesias often accompany tardive akathisia.

Opioids, benzodiazepines, and propranolol can sometimes alleviate tardive akathisia. Reported benefits from reserpine, tetrabenazine, amantadine, anticholinergics, and other medications remain unconfirmed.

Tardive tics, another variety of tardive dyskinesia, include vocal tics, which consist of persistent simple vocalizations, such as grunts, and respiratory tics, which consist of sudden, loud, irregular gasps. Tardive dyskinesias also include *tardive tremors* and other persistent movements. As in cases of tardive dystonia and akathisia, oral-buccal-lingual movements often accompany each of these varieties of tardive dyskinesia.

Withdrawal-Emergent Syndrome

Involuntary movements sometimes appear after sudden cessation of prolonged treatment with dopamine-blocking agents. This condition, the *withdrawal-emergent syndrome*, usually consists of mild to moderately severe chorea with motor impersistence and restlessness. The explanation for the withdrawal-emergent syndrome – a variation of that for tardive dyskinesias – is that removal of a dopamine receptor-blocking medication suddenly exposes supersensitive dopamine receptors to relatively high concentrations of dopamine.

The withdrawal-emergent syndrome typically affects children and lasts 4 to 12 weeks. Episodes longer than 6 months in duration probably represent tardive dyskinesia. Intolerable withdrawal dyskinesias may force physicians to reinstitute the offending medication and then taper it more slowly.

MOVEMENT DISORDERS FROM OTHER PSYCHIATRIC MEDICATIONS

As SSRIs elevate a patient's mood, they may also increase motor activity to abnormal levels, inducing myoclonus, tremor, or akathisia-like leg movements. As discussed previously, SSRIs may cause the serotonin syndrome (see also Chapter 6). Despite these caveats, serious adverse reactions to SSRIs occur in only a small proportion of patients – usually when SSRIs are administered in extraordinarily high doses, in combination with other medications (such as nonselective monoamine oxidase inhibitors), or in patients with a preexisting neurologic disorder.

About 10% of patients taking TCAs develop a fine, rapid tremor that resembles essential tremor and also responds to propranolol. The antidepressant amoxapine, which has dopamine antagonist properties, can induce parkinsonism; however, almost no other antidepressant causes parkinsonism or other signs of extrapyramidal dysfunction.

Lithium at high therapeutic serum concentrations can also induce a tremor that resembles essential tremor. At toxic concentrations, it produces a severe, coarse intention tremor often accompanied by ataxia of the trunk, i.e., signs of cerebellar dysfunction. Sometimes lithium toxicity causes extrapyramidal signs. Although adding propranolol may suppress a mild tremor, reducing the lithium dose is usually preferable.

Antiepileptic drugs often cause tremors, ataxia, and other movement disorders, but generally only at toxic serum concentrations. As an exception, valproate may cause a tremor independent of dose.

Noniatrogenic Movements

Physicians must pause before attributing every case of involuntary facial, tongue, and jaw movement to a complication of an antipsychotic. As already discussed, physicians might observe similar movements in Huntington disease, cranial dystonia, tics, and stereotypies.

Stereotyped movements of the face, mouth, or tongue appear sporadically in medication-naïve schizophrenic patients and were even described before the introduction of antipsychotics. Similarly, in *buccolingual dyskinesia of the elderly*, older unmedicated individuals, especially those with dementia, develop these movements. In another condition with a predilection for the elderly, *edentulous orofacial dyskinesia*, individuals develop chorea of the tongue as if the absence of teeth deprives the tongue of its normal proprioceptive feedback. Properly fitting dentures usually stop edentulous dyskinesia.

PSYCHOGENIC MOVEMENTS

The diagnosis of psychogenic movements usually relies on several factors: (1) the movements' abrupt onset and subsequent intermittent occurrence; (2) incongruency, inconsistency, and multiplicity of the movements (variability in location, pattern, and number); (3) presence of astasia-abasia (see Fig. 3.4); and (4) certain characteristics of particular movements (see below). Psychogenic movements and other psychogenic neurologic disorders appear to cause greater disability than the neurologic versions. Some authors have advocated use of the term "functional movement disorders" rather than "psychogenic movement disorders"; others feel that the former name is vague and confusing to both patients and physicians. The term "nonorganic" also is unsatisfactory to the majority of psychiatrists and neurologists, who believe that mental disorders originate in the nervous system and eschew separation of the mind and brain. Likewise, the adjective "hysterical" is inaccurate (movement disorders do not relate to the uterus) and potentially offensive (these disorders afflict men as well as women). Overall, neurologists continue to favor the label "psychogenic" for clarity of communication. Psychiatrists may wish to further categorize these conditions by DSM-5 criteria as Conversion Disorder (Functional Neurological Symptom Disorder), Factitious Disorder, or Malingering.

Neurologists find that psychogenic movements assume almost any pattern and that two or more often simultaneously occur. The majority of psychogenic movements simulate tremor, dystonia, gait impairment, or myoclonus, but may also present as chorea or tics. Psychiatric comorbidity (especially depression or panic attacks) is frequent, and family history of neuropsychiatric disease – or even the same psychogenic movement disorder – may be present.

Children and adolescents are subject to developing psychogenic movement disorders. One study showed that in patients older than 13 years, females had a four-fold greater incidence than males, but in patients younger than 13 years the incidence was equal for girls and boys. Pediatric patients may have a better prognosis than adults. Favorable outcomes are associated with a multidisciplinary approach involving specialists from neurology, psychiatry, psychology, and social work as well as with actively engaging the family. Despite a common misconception, psychogenic movement disorders also can emerge in the elderly.

Psychogenic tremor characteristically oscillates in two or more planes and has a variable frequency. In addition, because of fatigue, the tremor wanes in amplitude during long examinations. Several maneuvers support a diagnosis of psychogenic tremor. When a psychogenic tremor affects one arm, it often switches sides when the physician restrains that arm. In addition to forcing the tremor to switch sides, the examiner can *entrain* the frequency of a psychogenic tremor by employing the following maneuver: the examiner asks the patient to move the affected hand first at a slow speed, then fast speed, and finally back to the slow speed. The examiner often must set an example. The variability in tremor frequency that this maneuver induces reveals its willful origin. Also, placing weights on the wrist of patients with other types of tremor dampens the amplitude and slows the frequency of their tremor, but weights usually magnify the force and amplitude of psychogenic tremor.

Psychogenic myoclonus imitates jerks that randomly strike different muscle groups. As with true myoclonus, the movements have variable velocity and intensity. In contrast, psychogenic myoclonus recedes after a few minutes, presumably as patients tire, but returns after a rest period.

In *psychogenic dystonia*, the movements appear unique, inconsistent in location, and paroxysmal. Moreover, unlike patients with either genuine focal or generalized dystonia, those with psychogenic dystonia give the impression of having pain, weakness, and sensory loss.

Psychogenic gaits feature slowness and knee buckling. In addition, trembling and dystonic posturing sometimes disrupt normal walking. However, patients may merely exaggerate their effort or demonstrate inefficient movement. Whatever the pattern, the impairment often "forces" patients into wheelchairs, keeps them at bedrest, or allows them to ambulate, but only with grimacing and apparently great effort. Their unsteadiness threatens to topple them (see astasia-abasia, Fig. 3.4). Some neurologists point out that crutches, neck braces, and lumbar supports do not speed recovery and serve only to advertise patients' disability.

Some movements, while also psychogenic in the larger sense of the word, are culturally sanctioned and thus the DSM-5 would not include them as a Conversion Disorder or other psychiatric illness. Anthropologists and other authorities classify them as "folk illnesses" or "culture-bound" behaviors. The *jumping Frenchmen of Maine*, the best known example, consists of a group of otherwise healthy citizens of French-Canadian descent who respond to unexpected, loud noises by leaping upward, screaming, or throwing any object in their hand. Unlike a normal response, this behavior does not attenuate with repeated stimulation, i.e., does not exhibit habituation. Some of their descendants in Louisiana, the *Raging Cajuns*, display the same excessive startle response. Similarly, certain residents of rural Malaysia and Indonesia, *latahs*, overreact to trivial stimuli by suddenly cursing, laughing convulsively, or performing dancelike movements. Usually only one member of a group displays the behavior.

Movements as a Manifestation of Psychiatric Illnesses

Abnormal involuntary movement disorders often constitute a component of certain psychiatric disturbances. For example, stereotypies are present very frequently in autism; a fine tremor is a common manifestation of anxiety; bradykinetic, slow voluntary movement (*psychomotor retardation*) characterizes depression; and, judging by historical records, tardive dyskinesia-like movements may appear before any medication exposure in schizophrenic patients.

The DSM-5 has demoted *catatonia* from an independent class to a feature of Psychotic, Bipolar Depressive, or Medical Disorder. Its diagnosis requires at least three symptoms from a list of 12, including catalepsy, waxy flexibility, stereotypy, grimacing, echolalia, and echopraxia.

Neurologists diagnose catatonia when patients with psychosis or major depression remain uncommunicative and stare vacantly, motionless, and in fixed natural or unnatural postures, but amenable to examiners' placing them in different positions, i.e., catalepsy. Despite patients' mutism and immobility, their consciousness persists. They should have a normal or near-normal EEG. Their differential diagnosis includes neuroleptic malignant syndrome (see Chapter 6), PCP intoxication, parkinsonism, and dystonia. When catatonia occurs as a manifestation of psychosis or a mood disorder, an intravenously administered benzodiazepine may interrupt it and provide diagnostic as well as therapeutic help. Administration of ECT also reportedly aborts catatonia.

A florid example of psychogenic movement disorder occurs in *mass hysteria* or *mass psychogenic illness*, in which many individuals – small groups to almost 1000 people – suddenly display the same bizarre behavior. Even in present-day United States and other developed countries, the behavior spreads rapidly and extensively in an epidemic pattern. The "victims" are so consistently primarily or exclusively adolescent females that the demography is diagnostically crucial. Depending on the episode, victims have imitated seizures, stridor, fainting, or tics. In instances of mass hysteria, groups of individuals have complained of entirely subjective problems, such as itching, dizziness, and "sick building" symptoms.

Even with Sydenham chorea, which can appear in mini-epidemics among adolescent women living in the same community, affected individuals have set off exaggerated psychologic responses and elicited movements in healthy adolescents throughout the entire community. Episodes have also included normal activities taken to excess, such as uncontrollable dancing, laughing, or singing. Reports of "dancing mania" (or St. Vitus' dance) from medieval Europe describe hundreds of people dancing to the point of exhaustion and even death.

Caveats

Despite an obvious psychiatric explanation, making a diagnosis of psychogenic movement disorder carries a risk. As discussed previously (see earlier and Chapter 3), neurologists and other physicians may easily misdiagnose movements as psychogenic when they are either bizarre or they respond to tricks, concentration, anxiety-producing situations, or other environmental factors. In another problem, psychotropic medications may induce unusual yet partly controllable side effects, such as acute dystonic reactions, tardive dystonia, tremors, and akathisia. Moreover, medication-induced movements, such as akathisia or oculogyric crisis, may exacerbate psychiatric disturbances that the medications were intended to treat.

Another caveat concerns the high incidence of psychogenic movement disorders reported by movement disorder centers. Their finding of a large proportion of patients with psychogenic movement disorders is partly attributable to their attracting unique cases, having the clinical experience and technology to diagnose rare disorders, and willingness to assume the burden of making a possibly unwelcome diagnosis. Outside of such centers, the incidence of psychogenic movement disorders is actually low. In addition, few patients have seen movement disorders, other than tremor, that might serve as a model. Even fewer patients have the stamina and determination to sustain a consistent, voluntary movement. (Try it yourself!)

Physicians make use of all aspects of a patient's clinical history when diagnosing a specific movement disorder. Boxes 18.2, 18.3, and 18.4 emphasize the importance of neuroleptic exposure, age at onset, and presence of cognitive impairment in narrowing the differential diagnosis.

BOX 18.3	Commonly Cited Movement Disorders That May Begin in Childhood or Adolescence

EARLY CHILDHOOD

Athetosis or choreoathetosis
Lesch–Nyhan syndrome*

CHILDHOOD

Dopa-responsive dystonia*
Dystonia associated with *DYT1* gene*
Myoclonus from subacute sclerosing panencephalitis (SSPE)
Parkinson disease
Sydenham chorea
Tourette disorder*
Withdrawal-emergent dyskinesia

ADOLESCENCE

Essential tremor*
Huntington disease (juvenile Huntington disease)*
Medication- and drug-induced movements
Tardive dyskinesias
Wilson disease*

---

*Genetic transmission.

BOX 18.4	Movement Disorders Associated with Cognitive Impairment

YOUNG CHILDREN

Athetosis or choreoathetosis*
Lesch–Nyhan syndrome
Rett syndrome

OLDER CHILDREN AND ADOLESCENTS

Huntington disease
Subacute sclerosing panencephalitis
Wilson disease

ADULTS

Creutzfeldt-Jakob disease[†]
Huntington disease
Parkinson disease

*Despite incapacitating movements, many choreoathetosis patients have no mental retardation (see Chapter 13).
[†]Myoclonus.

REFERENCES

Parkinson Disease and Parkinsonism

Appleby, B. S., Duggan, P. S., Regenberg, A., et al. (2007). Psychiatric and neuropsychiatric adverse events associated with deep brain stimulation: A meta-analysis of ten years' experience. *Movement Disorders: Official Journal of the Movement Disorder Society, 22,* 1722–1728.

Derkinderen, P., Shannon, K. M., & Brundin, P. (2014). Gut feelings about smoking and coffee in Parkinson's disease. *Movement Disorders: Official Journal of the Movement Disorder Society, 29,* 976–979.

Dissanayaka, N. N. N. W., White, E., O'Sullivan, J. D., et al. (2014). The clinical spectrum of anxiety in Parkinson's disease. *Movement Disorders: Official Journal of the Movement Disorder Society, 29,* 967–975.

Dujardin, K., Langlois, C., Plomhause, L., et al. (2014). Apathy in untreated early-stage Parkinson disease: Relationship with other non-motor symptoms. *Movement Disorders: Official Journal of the Movement Disorder Society, 29,* 1796–1801.

Emre, M., Aarsland, D., Brown, R., et al. (2007). Clinical diagnostic criteria for dementia associated with Parkinson's disease. *Movement Disorders: Official Journal of the Movement Disorder Society, 22,* 1689–1707.

Erro, R., Bhatia, K. P., & Tinazzi, M. (2015). Parkinsonism following neuroleptic exposure: A double-hit hypothesis? *Movement Disorders: Official Journal of the Movement Disorder Society, 30,* 780–784.

Fasano, A., Barra, A., Nicosia, P., et al. (2008). Cocaine addiction: From habits to stereotypical-repetitive behaviors and punding. *Drug and Alcohol Dependence, 96,* 178–182.

Forsaa, E. B., Larsen, J. P., Wentzel-Larsen, T., et al. (2010). A 12-year population-based study of psychosis in Parkinson disease. *Archives of Neurology, 67,* 996–1001.

Foubert-Samier, A., Helmer, C., Perez, F., et al. (2012). Past exposure to neuroleptic drugs and risk of Parkinson disease in an elderly cohort. *Neurology, 79,* 1615–1621.

Friedman, J. H., & Weintraub, D. (2012). Glad about SAD (PD). *Neurology, 78,* 1198–1199.

Fox, S. H., Katzenschlanger, R., Lim, S. Y., et al. (2011). The Movement Disorder Society Evidence-Based Medicine Review Update: Treatments for the motor symptoms of Parkinson's disease. *Movement Disorders: Official Journal of the Movement Disorder Society, 26*(Suppl. 3), S2–S41.

Hu, M. T., Szewczyk-Królikowski, K., Tomlinson, P., et al. (2014). Predictors of cognitive impairment in an early-stage Parkinson's disease cohort. *Movement Disorders: Official Journal of the Movement Disorder Society, 29,* 351–359.

Kim, Y. E., Kang, S. Y., Ma, H. I., et al. (2015). A visual rating scale for the hummingbird sign with adjustable diagnostic validity. *Journal of Parkinson's Disease, 5,* 605–612.

Lang, A. E. (2014). Clinical heterogeneity in progressive supranuclear palsy: Challenges to diagnosis, pathogenesis and future therapies. *Movement Disorders: Official Journal of the Movement Disorder Society, 29,* 1707–1709.

Lee, A. H., & Weintraub, D. (2012). Psychosis in Parkinson's disease without dementia: Common and comorbid with other non-motor symptoms. *Movement Disorders: Official Journal of the Movement Disorder Society, 27,* 858–863.

Marras, C., & Lang, A. (2008). Changing concepts in Parkinson disease: Moving beyond the Decade of the Brain. *Neurology, 70,* 1996–2003.

Martinez-Martin, P., Arroyo, S., Rojo-Abuin, J. M., et al. (2008). Burden, perceived health status, and mood among caregivers of Parkinson's disease patients. *Movement Disorders: Official Journal of the Movement Disorder Society, 23,* 1673–1680.

Menza, M., Dobkin, R. D., Marin, H., et al. (2009). The impact of treatment of depression on quality of life, disability and relapse in patients in Parkinson's disease. *Movement Disorders: Official Journal of the Movement Disorder Society, 24,* 1325–1322.

Menza, M., Dobkin, R. D., Marin, H., et al. (2009). A controlled trial of antidepressants in patients with Parkinson disease and depression. *Neurology, 72,* 886–892.

Merola, A., Zibetti, M., Angrisano, S., et al. (2011). Parkinson's disease progression at 30 years: A study of subthalamic deep brain-stimulated patients. *Brain: A Journal of Neurology, 134,* 2074–2084.

Miyasaki, J. M., Shannon, K., Voon, V., et al. (2006). Practice parameter: Evaluation and treatment of depression, psychosis, and dementia in Parkinson disease (an evidence-based review): Report of the Quality Standards Subcommittee of the American Academy of Neurology. *Neurology, 66,* 996–1002.

Moro, E., Lozano, A. M., Pollak, P., et al. (2010). Long-term results of a multicenter study on subthalamic and pallidal stimulation in Parkinson's disease. *Movement Disorders: Official Journal of the Movement Disorder Society, 25,* 578–586.

Mortimer, J. A., Borenstein, A. R., & Nelson, L. M. (2012). Associations of welding and manganese exposure with Parkinson disease: Review and meta-analysis. *Neurology, 79,* 1174–1180.

Olanow, C. W., & Brundin, P. (2013). Parkinson's disease and alpha synuclein: is Parkinson's disease a prion-like disorder? *Movement Disorders: Official Journal of the Movement Disorder Society, 28,* 31–40.

Olanow, C. W., Wakeman, D. R., & Kordower, J. H. (2014). Peripheral alpha-synuclein and Parkinson's disease. *Movement Disorders: Official Journal of the Movement Disorder Society, 29,* 963–966.

Okai, D., Askey-Jones, S., Samuel, M., et al. (2013). Trial of CBT for impulse control behaviors affecting Parkinson patients and their caregivers. *Neurology, 80,* 792–799.

Pezzoli, G., & Cereda, E. (2013). Exposure to pesticides or solvents and risk of Parkinson disease. *Neurology, 80,* 2035–2041.

Ravina, B., Marder, K., Fernandez, H. H., et al. (2007). Diagnostic criteria for psychosis in Parkinson's disease: Report of an NINDS, NIMH work group. *Movement Disorders: Official Journal of the Movement Disorder Society, 22,* 1061–1068.

Ravina, B., Elm, J., Camicioli, R., et al. (2009). The course of depressive symptoms in early Parkinson's disease. *Movement Disorders: Official Journal of the Movement Disorder Society, 24,* 1306–1311.

Richard, I. H., McDermott, M. P., Kurlan, R., et al. (2012). A randomized, double-blind, placebo-controlled trial of antidepressants in Parkinson disease. *Neurology, 78,* 1229–1236.

Soulas, T., Gurrucha, J. M., Palfi, S., et al. (2008). Attempted and completed suicide after subthalamic nucleus stimulation for Parkinson's disease. *Journal of Neurology, Neurosurgery, and Psychiatry, 79,* 952–954.

Spencer, A. H., Rickards, H., Fasano, A., et al. (2011). The prevalence and clinical characteristics of punding in Parkinson's disease. *Movement Disorders: Official Journal of the Movement Disorder Society, 26,* 578–586.

Stocchi, F., Abbruzzese, G., Ceravolo, R., et al. (2014). Prevalence of fatigue in Parkinson disease and its clinical correlates. *Neurology, 83,* 215–220.

Weintraub, D., Koester, J., Potenza, M. N., et al. (2010). Impulse control disorders in Parkinson disease. *Archives of Neurology, 67,* 589–595.

Weintraub, D., David, A. S., Evans, A. H., et al. (2015). Clinical spectrum of impulse control disorders in Parkinson's disease. *Movement Disorders: Official Journal of the Movement Disorder Society, 30,* 121–127.

Willis, A. W., Evanoff, B. A., Lian, M., et al. (2010). Metal emissions and urban incident Parkinson disease: A community health study of Medicare beneficiaries by using geographic information systems. *American Journal of Epidemiology, 172,* 1357–1363.

Chorea

Jankovic, J., & Clarence-Smith, K. (2011). Tetrabenazine for the treatment of chorea and other hyperkinetic movement disorders. *Expert Review of Neurotherapeutics, 11*, 1509–1523.

Killoran, A., & Biglan, K. M. (2014). Current therapeutic options for Huntington's disease: Good clinical practice versus evidence-based approaches. *Movement Disorders: Official Journal of the Movement Disorder Society, 29*, 1404–1413.

Kranick, S. M., Mowry, E. M., Colcher, A., et al. (2010). Movement disorders and pregnancy: A review of the literature. *Movement Disorders: Official Journal of the Movement Disorder Society, 25*, 665–671.

Maia, D. P., Teixeria, A. L., Cunningham, M. C. Q., et al. (2005). Obsessive compulsive behavior, hyperactivity, and attention deficit disorder in Sydenham chorea. *Neurology, 64*, 1799–1801.

O'Toole, O., Lennon, V. A., Ahlskog, J. E., et al. (2013). Autoimmune chorea in adults. *Neurology, 80*, 1133–1144.

Paulsen, J. (2011). Cognitive impairment in Huntington disease: Diagnosis and treatment. *Current Neurology and Neuroscience Reports, 11*, 474–483.

Paulsen, J. S., Hoth, K. F., Nehl, C., et al. (2005). Critical periods of suicide risk in Huntington's disease. *The American Journal of Psychiatry, 162*, 725–731.

Philips, W., Shannon, K. M., & Barker, R. A. (2008). The current clinical management of Huntington's disease. *Movement Disorders: Official Journal of the Movement Disorder Society, 23*, 1491–1504.

Wilson Disease

Machado, A., Chien, H. F., Deguti, M. M., et al. (2006). Neurologic manifestations in Wilson's disease: Report of 119 cases. *Movement Disorders: Official Journal of the Movement Disorder Society, 21*, 2192–2196.

Portala, K., Westermark, K., von Knorring, L., et al. (2000). Psychopathology in treated Wilson's disease determined by means of CPRS expert and self-ratings. *Acta Psychiatrica Scandinavica, 101*, 104–109.

Sidiropoulos, C., Hutchison, W., Mestre, T., et al. (2013). Bilateral pallidal stimulation for Wilson's disease. *Movement Disorders: Official Journal of the Movement Disorder Society, 28*, 1292–1295.

Soltanzadeh, A., Soltanzadeh, P., Nafissi, S., et al. (2007). Wilson's disease: A great masquerader. *European Neurology, 57*, 80–85.

Dystonia (Nonmedication Induced)

Altenmüeller, E., & Jabusch, H. C. (2010). Focal dystonia in musicians: phenomenology, pathophysiology, triggering factors, and treatment. *Medical Problems of Performing Artists, 25*, 3–9.

Borggraefe, I., Mehrkens, J. H., Telegravciska, M., et al. (2010). Bilateral pallidal stimulation in children and adolescents with primary generalized dystonia. *Brain and Development, 32*, 223–228.

Conti, A. M., Pullman, S., & Frucht, S. J. (2008). The hand that has forgotten its cunning – lessons from musicians' hand dystonia. *Movement Disorders: Official Journal of the Movement Disorder Society, 23*, 1398–1406.

Geyer, H. L., & Bressman, S. B. (2006). The diagnosis of dystonia. *The Lancet. Neurology, 5*, 780–790.

Hallett, M., Evinger, C., Jankovic, J., et al. (2008). Update in blepharospasm. *Neurology, 71*, 1275–1282.

Heiman, G. A., Ottman, R., Saunders-Pullman, R. J., et al. (2004). Increased risk for recurrent major depression in DYT1 dystonia mutation carriers. *Neurology, 63*, 631–637.

Isaias, I. U., Alterman, R. L., & Tagliati, M. (2009). Deep brain stimulation for primary generalized dystonia: Long term outcomes. *Archives of Neurology, 66*, 465–470.

Jankovic, J. (2013). Medical treatment of dystonia. *Movement Disorders: Official Journal of the Movement Disorder Society, 28*, 1001–1012.

Jhanshahi, M., Czernecki, V., & Zurowski, A. M. (2011). Neuropsychological, neuropsychiatric, and quality of life issues in DMS for dystonia. *Movement Disorders: Official Journal of the Movement Disorder Society, 26*(Suppl. 1), S63–S78.

Jinnah, H. A., Visser, J. E., Harris, J. C., et al. (2006). Delineation of the motor disorder of Lesch-Nyhan disease. *Brain: A Journal of Neurology, 129*, 1201–1217.

Moro, E., Gross, R. E., & Krauss, J. K. (2013). What's new in surgical treatment for dystonia? *Movement Disorders: Official Journal of the Movement Disorder Society, 38*, 1013–1020.

Schretlen, D. J., Ward, J., Meyer, S. M., et al. (2005). Behavioral aspects of Lesch-Nyhan disease and its variants. *Developmental Medicine and Child Neurology, 47*, 673–677.

Schuele, S., & Lederman, R. J. (2003). Long-term outcome of focal dystonia in string instrumentalists. *Movement Disorders: Official Journal of the Movement Disorder Society, 19*, 43–48.

Essential Tremor

Deuschl, G., Raethjen, J., Hellriegel, H., et al. (2011). Treatment of patients with essential tremor. *The Lancet. Neurology, 10*, 148–161.

Elias, W. J., Huss, D., Voss, T., et al. (2013). A pilot study of focused ultrasound thalamotomy for essential tremor. *The New England Journal of Medicine, 369*, 640–648.

Jellinger, K. A. (2014). Is there cerebellar pathology in essential tremor? *Movement Disorders: Official Journal of the Movement Disorder Society, 29*, 435–436.

Lorenz, D., Poremba, C., Papengut, F., et al. (2011). The psychological burden of essential tremor in an outpatient- and a community-based cohort. *European Journal of Neurology, 18*, 972–979.

Sadeghi, R., & Ondo, W. G. (2010). Pharmacological management of essential tremor. *Drugs, 70*, 2215–2228.

Witjas, T., Carron, R., Krack, P., et al. (2015). A prospective single-blind study of Gamma Knife thalamotomy for tremor. *Neurology, 85*, 1562–1568.

Zhang, K., Bhatia, S., Oh, M. Y., et al. (2010). Long-term results of thalamic deep brain stimulation for essential tremor. *Journal of Neurosurgery, 112*, 1271–1276.

Tics, Tourette Disorder, and Related Disorders

Ackerman, L., Duits, A., van der Linden, C., et al. (2011). Double-blind clinical trial of thalamic stimulation in patients with Tourette syndrome. *Brain: A Journal of Neurology, 134*, 832–844.

Barry, S., Baird, G., Lascelles, K., et al. (2011). Neurodevelopmental movement disorders: An update on childhood motor stereotypies. *Developmental Medicine and Child Neurology, 53*, 979–985.

Bernard, B. A., Stebbins, G. T., Siegel, S., et al. (2009). Determinants of quality of life in children with Gilles de la Tourette syndrome. *Movement Disorders: Official Journal of the Movement Disorder Society, 24*, 1070–1073.

Church, J. A., & Schlaggar, B. L. (2014). Pediatric Tourette syndrome: insights from recent neuroimaging studies. *Journal of Obsessive-Compulsive and Related Disorders, 3*, 386–393.

Cubo, E., Chmura, T., & Goetz, C. (2008). Comparison of tic characteristics between children and adults. *Movement Disorders: Official Journal of the Movement Disorder Society, 23*, 2407–2411.

Eddy, C. M., & Cavanna, A. E. (2013). "It's a curse!" Coprolalia in Tourette syndrome. *European Journal of Neurology, 20*, 1467–1470.

Ehrlich, D., Swan, M., Robbins, M. S., et al. Demographics, comorbidities and clinical features in hospitalized patients with myoclonus. Poster presented at the American Academy of Neurology Annual Scientific Meeting, 2015.

Fraint, A., & Pal, G. (2015). Deep brain stimulation in Tourette's syndrome. *Frontiers in Neurology, 6*, 170.

Jankovic, J., Gelineau-Kattner, R., & Davidson, A. (2010). Tourette's syndrome in adults. *Movement Disorders: Official Journal of the Movement Disorder Society, 25*, 2171–2175.

Kurlan, R. (2010). Tourette's syndrome. *The New England Journal of Medicine, 363*, 2332–2338.

Kurlan, R., Johnson, D., & Kaplan, E. L. (2008). Streptococcal infection and exacerbations of childhood tics and obsessive-compulsive symptoms: A prospective blinded cohort study. *Pediatrics, 121*, 1188–1197.

Martin-Fernandez, R., Zrinzo, L., Aviles-Olmos, I., et al. (2011). Deep brain stimulation for Gilles de la Tourette syndrome. *Movement Disorders: Official Journal of the Movement Disorder Society, 26*, 1922–1930.

McNaught, K. S., & Mink, J. W. (2011). Advances in understanding and treatment of Tourette syndrome. *Nature Reviews. Neurology, 7*, 667–676.

Muller-Vahl, K. R., & Krueger, D. (2011). Does Tourette syndrome prevent tardive dyskinesia? *Movement Disorders: Official Journal of the Movement Disorder Society, 26*, 2442–2444.

Scahill, L., Woods, D. W., Himle, M. B., et al. (2013). Current controversies on the role of behavior therapy in Tourette syndrome. *Movement Disorders: Official Journal of the Movement Disorder Society, 28*, 1179–1183.

Schrag, A., Gilbert, R., & Giovannoni, G. (2009). at al. Streptococcal infection, Tourette syndrome, and OCD. *Neurology, 73*, 1256–1263.

Shprecher, D., & Kurlan, R. (2009). The management of tics. *Movement Disorders: Official Journal of the Movement Disorder Society, 24,* 15–24.

Swedo, S. E., Garvey, M., Snider, L., et al. (2001). The PANDAS subgroup: Recognition and treatment. *CNS Spectrums, 6,* 419–426.

Wijemanne, S., Wu, L. J. C., & Jankovic, J. (2014). Long-term efficacy and safety of fluphenazine in patients with Tourette syndrome. *Movement Disorders: Official Journal of the Movement Disorder Society, 29,* 126–130.

Yaltho, T. C., & Jankovic, J. (2011). The many faces of hemifacial spasm: Differential diagnosis of unilateral facial spasms. *Movement Disorders: Official Journal of the Movement Disorder Society, 26,* 1582–1592.

Medication-Induced and Related Movement Disorders

Bhidayasiri, R., Fahn, S., Weiner, W. J., et al. (2013). Evidence-based guideline: Treatment of tardive syndromes: Report of the Guideline Development Subcommittee of the American Academy of Neurology. *Neurology, 81,* 463–469.

Bondon-Guitton, E., Perez-Lloret, S., Bagheri, H., et al. (2011). Drug-induced Parkinsonism: A review of 17 years' experience in a regional pharmacovigilance center in France. *Movement Disorders: Official Journal of the Movement Disorder Society, 26,* 2226–2231.

Brust, J. C. M. (2010). Substance abuse and movement disorders. *Movement Disorders: Official Journal of the Movement Disorder Society, 25,* 2010–2020.

Capelle, H. H., Blahak, C., Schrader, C., et al. (2010). Chronic deep brain stimulation in patients with tardive dystonia without a history of major psychosis. *Movement Disorders: Official Journal of the Movement Disorder Society, 25,* 1477–1481.

Caroff, S. N., Hurford, I., Lybrand, J., et al. (2011). Movement disorders induced by antipsychotic drugs: Implications of the CATIE Schizophrenia Trial. *Neurologic Clinics, 29,* 127–viii.

Chang, E. F., Schrock, L. E., Starr, P. A., et al. (2010). Long-term benefit sustained after bilateral pallidal deep brain stimulation in patients with refractory tardive dyskinesia. *Stereotactic and Functional Neurosurgery, 88,* 304–310.

Correll, C. U., & Schenk, E. M. (2008). Tardive dyskinesia and new antipsychotics. *Current Opinion in Psychiatry, 21,* 151–156.

Guy, W. (1976). Abnormal Involuntary Movement Scale (AIMS). In *ECDEU Assessment Manual for Psychopharmacology, U.S. Department of Health, Education, and Welfare,* pp. 534–537.

Kane, J. M., Fleischhacker, W. W., Hansen, L., et al. (2009). Akathisia: An updated review focusing on second-generation antipsychotics. *The Journal of Clinical Psychiatry, 70,* 627–643.

Mahmoudi, S., Lévesque, D., & Blanchet, P. J. (2014). Upregulation of dopamine D3, not D2, receptors correlates with tardive dyskinesia in a primate model. *Movement Disorders: Official Journal of the Movement Disorder Society, 29,* 1125–1133.

Mejia, N. I., & Jankovic, J. (2010). Tardive dyskinesia and withdrawal emergent syndrome in children. *Expert Review of Neurotherapeutics, 10,* 893–901.

Niethammer, M., & Ford, B. (2007). Permanent lithium-induced cerebellar toxicity. *Movement Disorders: Official Journal of the Movement Disorder Society, 22,* 570–573.

Soares-Weiser, K., Maayan, N., & McGrath, J. (2011). Vitamin E for neuroleptic-induced tardive dyskinesia. *The Cochrane Database of Systematic Reviews,* (2), Art. No.: CD000209, doi:10.1002/14651858. CD000209.pub2.

Teo, J. T., Edwards, M. J., & Bhatia, K. (2012). Tardive dyskinesia is caused by maladaptive synaptic plasticity: A hypothesis. *Movement Disorders: Official Journal of the Movement Disorder Society, 27,* 1205–1215.

Psychogenic Movement Disorders

Baik, J. S., & Lang, A. E. (2007). Gait abnormalities in psychogenic movement disorders. *Movement Disorders: Official Journal of the Movement Disorder Society, 22,* 395–399.

Baizabal-Carvallo, J. F., & Jankovic, J. (2014). The clinical features of psychogenic movement disorders resembling tics. *Journal of Neurology, Neurosurgery, and Psychiatry, 85,* 573–575.

Bartlesman, M., & Eckhardt, P. P. (2007). Mental illness in the former Dutch Indies – four psychiatric syndromes: amok, latah, koro, and neurasthenia. *Nederlands Tijdschrift Voor Geneeskunde, 151,* 2845–2851.

Batla, A., Stamelou, M., Edwards, M. J., et al. (2013). Functional movement disorders are not uncommon in the elderly. *Movement Disorders: Official Journal of the Movement Disorder Society, 38,* 540–543.

Canavese, C., Ciano, C., Zibordi, F., et al. (2012). Phenomenology of psychogenic movement disorders in children. *Movement Disorders: Official Journal of the Movement Disorder Society, 27,* 1153–1157.

Daniels, J. (2009). Catatonia: Clinical aspects and neurobiological correlates. *The Journal of Neuropsychiatry and Clinical Neurosciences, 21,* 371–380.

Espay, A. J., Goldenhar, L. M., Voon, V., et al. (2009). Opinions and clinical practices related to diagnosing and managing patients with psychogenic movement disorders. *Movement Disorders: Official Journal of the Movement Disorder Society, 24,* 1366–1374.

Fahn, S., & Olanow, C. W. (2014). "Psychogenic movement disorders": They are what they are. *Movement Disorders: Official Journal of the Movement Disorder Society, 29,* 853–856.

Faust, J., & Soman, T. B. (2012). Psychogenic movement disorders in children: Characteristics and predictors of outcome. *Journal of Child Neurology, 27,* 610–614.

Ferrara, J., & Jankovic, J. (2008). Psychogenic movement disorders in children. *Movement Disorders: Official Journal of the Movement Disorder Society, 23,* 1875–1881.

Fink, M., & Taylor, M. A. (2009). The catatonia syndrome. *Archives of General Psychiatry, 66,* 1173–1177.

Hallett, M., Fahn, S., Jankovic, J., et al. (2006). *Psychogenic Movement Disorders.* Philadelphia: Lippincott Williams & Wilkins.

Jankovic, J., Vuong, K. D., & Thomas, M. (2006). Psychogenic tremor: Long-term outcome. *CNS Spectrums, 11,* 501–508.

Lees, A. (2001). Jumpers. *Movement Disorders: Official Journal of the Movement Disorder Society, 16,* 403–404.

Massey, E. W. (1984). Goosey patients: Relationship to jumping Frenchmen, Myriachit, Latah, and tic convulsif. *North Carolina Medical Journal, 45,* 556–558.

McKeon, A., Ahlskog, J. E., Bower, J. H., et al. (2009). Psychogenic tremor. *Movement Disorders: Official Journal of the Movement Disorder Society, 24,* 72–76.

Schwingenschuh, P., Pont-Sunyer, C., Surtees, R., et al. (2008). Psychogenic movement in children: A report of 15 cases and a review of the literature. *Movement Disorders: Official Journal of the Movement Disorder Society, 13,* 1882–1888.

Shill, H., & Gerber, P. (2006). Evaluation of clinical diagnostic criteria for psychogenic movement disorders. *Movement Disorders: Official Journal of the Movement Disorder Society, 21,* 1163–1168.

Saint-Hilaire, M. H., & Saint-Hilaire, J. M. (2001). Jumping Frenchmen of Maine. *Movement Disorders: Official Journal of the Movement Disorder Society, 16,* 530.

Stamelou, M., Cossu, G., Edwards, M. J., et al. (2013). Familial psychogenic movement disorders. *Movement Disorders: Official Journal of the Movement Disorder Society, 28,* 1295–1298.

Tanner, C. M., & Chamberland, J. (2001). Latah in Jakarta, Indonesia. *Movement Disorders: Official Journal of the Movement Disorder Society, 16,* 526–529.

Waller, J. (2009). A forgotten plague: making sense of dancing mania. *Lancet, 373,* 624–625.

QUESTIONS AND ANSWERS

1. Which of the following statements concerning obsessive-compulsive symptoms and obsessive-compulsive disorder (OCD) in Tourette disorder is *false*?
   a. Symptoms generally occur in about one-quarter of both males and females.
   b. Obsessions and compulsions as a manifestation of Tourette disorder are indistinguishable from those in pure OCD.
   c. Selective serotonin reuptake inhibitors (SSRIs) and clomipramine help alleviate obsessive-compulsive symptoms and OCD in Tourette disorder.
   d. Obsessive-compulsive symptoms and OCD emerge several years after the onset of motor tics, generally in late adolescence.

Answer: b. Obsessions and compulsions as a manifestation of Tourette disorder differ somewhat from those that are manifestations of pure OCD. For example, obsessions in Tourette disorder typically relate to sex, violence, and aggression, but those in pure OCD typically relate to dirt, germs, and illness. Similarly, compulsions in Tourette disorders often consist of checking and ordering, but those of pure OCD usually consist of more elaborate activities, such as handwashing or housecleaning.

2. In a child with Tourette disorder, what is the effect of treating ADHD with stimulants?
   a. Stimulants will have no effect on either the tics or ADHD.
   b. Whatever effect stimulants have on the tics, they will worsen the ADHD.
   c. Whatever effect stimulants have on ADHD, they will worsen the tics.
   d. After a brief exacerbation of tics, stimulants will suppress ADHD.

Answer: d. ADHD is the most frequently occurring and disruptive comorbid psychiatric condition in Tourette disorder. It requires aggressive treatment. When physicians prescribe stimulants for ADHD in Tourette disorder, the medicines may cause a transient, mild flare-up of the tics, but they suppress ADHD. This is a similar conundrum and solution facing physicians treating children with ADHD comorbid with epilepsy: stimulants suppress ADHD and have little or no effect on epilepsy.

3. Which *three* descriptions pertain to obscenities in Tourette disorder?
   a. Vocalizations include only scatological terms.
   b. About 15% or less of patients make obscene vocal tics (coprolalia).
   c. Obscene vocal tics usually develop as an initial symptom.

   d. When they occur, obscene vocal tics develop late in the course.
   e. Occasionally patients make obscene gestures (copropraxia).

Answer: b, d, e.

4. When its comorbidities complicate Tourette disorder, in which sequence do they unfold?
   a. ADHD, then motor tics, then vocal tics, then OCD symptoms.
   b. OCD symptoms, then motor tics, then vocal tics, then ADHD.
   c. Tics, ADHD, and OCD symptoms occur randomly.
   d. All manifestations arise together.

Answer: a. ADHD precedes motor tics. Obsessive-compulsive symptoms and OCD, when they occur, are a late complication.

5. In Huntington disease, which protein does the *huntingtin* gene transcribe?
   a. Huntingtin
   b. Orexin (hypocretin)
   c. Dystrophin
   d. Cytosine-adenine-guanine

Answer: a. The *huntingtin* (*HTT*) gene codes for the cytoplasmic protein, huntingtin. Patients with narcolepsy-cataplexy have a deficiency of orexin (hypocretin) in their cerebrospinal fluid (CSF) and hypothalamus. The muscle protein dystrophin is abnormal or absent in certain muscular dystrophies such as Duchenne muscular dystrophy. Cytosine-adenine-guanine (CAG) constitutes the trinucleotide base that occurs in excess in the huntingtin gene.

6. Which of the following statements concerning punding is *false*?
   a. Punding consists of an all-consuming complex repetitive stereotyped behavior, such as tirelessly arranging silverware in certain patterns.
   b. It is a manifestation of amphetamine intoxication as well as a complication of Parkinson disease overtreatment.
   c. No treatment strategy will reverse this complication.
   d. While punding, patients are oblivious to their daily activities.

Answer: c. Reducing dopaminergic medications or adding an antipsychotic agent will reduce the abnormal behavior. Of course, reducing dopaminergic activity is likely to lead to recurrence or worsening of patients' tremor, rigidity, and bradykinesia.

7. What percent of Parkinson disease patients have anosmia?
   a. 100%
   b. 90%
   c. 50%
   d. 10%

Answer: b. As with other neurodegenerative illnesses, particularly Alzheimer disease, Parkinson patients have a high incidence of anosmia. Some researchers contend that a patient's intact smell sensation almost eliminates Parkinson disease as a diagnostic consideration. Schizophrenic patients also have an increased incidence of anosmia, but not in the proportion of those with the neurodegenerative diseases.

8. A 69-year-old retired dentist with advanced Parkinson disease underwent emergency abdominal surgery. The surgery and immediate postoperative period were uncomplicated, but the next day he developed agitation and confusion. A psychiatrist found that the patient was disoriented, incoherent, febrile, and rigid. Which is the most appropriate diagnosis?
   a. Delirium
   b. Persistent anesthesia and analgesia effect
   c. Intraabdominal infection
   d. Neuroleptic malignant syndrome (NMS)

Answer: d. Because his surgeons withheld his dopaminergic and other medications for the surgery, the Parkinson disease was untreated and the patient developed NMS. Although the diagnosis of delirium may be technically correct, the more inclusive and helpful diagnosis is NMS.

9. Which illnesses do neurologists term "polyglutamine"? (More than one answer may be correct.)
   a. Spinocerebellar ataxia (SCA) subtypes
   b. Amyotrophic lateral sclerosis (ALS)
   c. Huntington disease
   d. Parkinson disease

Answer: a, c. Certain SCAs and Huntington disease are characterized by excessive production of polyglutamines.

10–15. Match the tremor variety (10–15) with effective medicine(s) (a–f). (More than one answer may be correct for each tremor diagnosis.)

10. Essential tremor
11. Cerebellar tremor
12. Parkinson disease
13. Stage-fright (performance anxiety)
14. Hyperthyroidism
15. Delirium tremens
   a. Levodopa (L-dopa)
   b. Propranolol (Inderal)
   c. Amantadine (Symmetrel)
   d. Trihexyphenidyl (Artane)
   e. Primidone (Mysoline)
   f. None of the above

Answers: 10–b, e; 11–f; 12–a, c, d; 13–b; 14–b; 15–f. Deep brain stimulation suppresses Parkinson disease and essential tremors.

16. Which *three* of these statements apply to spasmodic torticollis?
   a. It may consist of any combination of laterocollis, retrocollis, and anterocollis as well as torticollis.
   b. It develops in childhood.
   c. Surgical sectioning of the sternocleidomastoid and adjacent muscles relieves it.
   d. Light pressure to the chin in a counter-rotational direction may transiently overcome it.
   e. Whether a manifestation of tardive dystonia or an idiopathic condition, botulinum toxin injections greatly reduce torticollis.

Answer: a, d, e.

17. A psychiatrist is asked to evaluate an immobile, expressionless, mute 21-year-old woman who stares straight ahead. The psychiatrist cannot engage her but is able to position her limbs in a variety of positions that she holds for at least 10 minutes. The patient's records reveal a history of a mood disorder. While awaiting a neurology consultation, which of the following is the best initial management of this patient?
   a. Order magnetic resonance imaging (MRI).
   b. Give a therapeutic trial of a benzodiazepine.
   c. Obtain a blood test and slit-lamp examination to exclude Wilson disease.
   d. Administer an antipsychotic drug because the patient probably has catatonic schizophrenia.

Answer: b. Catatonia is usually a manifestation of schizophrenia or, more likely, a mood disorder. However, the following neurologic conditions may be responsible: methyl-phenyl-tetrahydro-pyridine (MPTP) exposure, antipsychotic-induced parkinsonism, severe Parkinson disease, NMS, phencyclidine (PCP) intoxication, juvenile Huntington disease, Wilson disease, and nonconvulsive status epilepticus. When psychiatric disorders cause catatonia, benzodiazepines will briefly reverse it and, with underlying neurologic causes, do no harm.

18. Which statement is *true* regarding early-onset primary (DYT1) dystonia?
   a. As with Huntington disease, excessive trinucleotide repeats cause early-onset primary dystonia.
   b. Affected individuals typically develop cognitive impairment.
   c. The inheritance is sex-linked dominant with relatively low penetrance.
   d. The disease is most frequent among Ashkenazi (Central and Eastern European) Jews.

Answer: d. DYT1 dystonia – like Tay–Sachs, some varieties of Parkinson disease, and Gaucher diseases – occurs most frequently among Ashkenazic (Central and Eastern European) Jews. The illness usually first causes dystonia of the muscles of one leg, but patients may present with tortipelvis. It does not affect cognition. Unlike Huntington disease, which results from excessive trinucleotide repeats and exhibits complete penetrance, the inheritance of DYT1 follows a pattern of autosomal dominant inheritance, with relatively low penetrance, from a mutation that involves deletion of a trinucleotide sequence in the *TOR1A* gene.

19. Which feature characterizes the childhood variety of Huntington disease?
    a. Chorea
    b. Rigidity
    c. Prolonged course
    d. Maternal inheritance

Answer: b. Rather than chorea, rigidity along with akinesia characterizes the childhood variety of Huntington disease. The responsible mutation consists of an excessively long sequence of trinucleotide repeats, which is even greater than in the adult variety. Childhood Huntington disease usually follows inheritance from the father and pursues a rapid demise. Because of rigidity, the childhood variety of Huntington disease mimics Wilson disease, DYT1 dystonia, tardive dystonia, and dopamine-responsive dystonia.

20. The family of a patient with Parkinson disease brings him to a physician because of frightening nightmares. Another problem is that, despite taking a long-acting, controlled-release levodopa preparation (Sinemet CR) at bedtime, he awakes in the morning with rigidity. What change in medication would be most helpful?
    a. Increase the dose of Sinemet CR at bedtime.
    b. Add a second-generation antipsychotic at bedtime.
    c. Take only a regular levodopa preparation in the early evening and another immediately upon awakening in the morning 20–30 minutes before getting out of bed.
    d. Take only a regular levodopa preparation at bedtime.

Answer: c. The frightening nightmares are actually nocturnal hallucinations, which are a side effect of levodopa. Stopping the bedtime long-acting levodopa preparation dose should eliminate them. The levodopa probably is unnecessary when the patient sleeps. Leaving a pill on a night stand and taking it 20–30 minutes before arising can circumvent the problem of morning rigidity.

21. For patients with depression comorbid with Parkinson disease, which treatment will be *least* effective?
    a. SSRIs
    b. Tricyclic antidepressants
    c. Electroconvulsive therapy (ECT)
    d. Dopamine agonists

Answer: d. Providing normal or even excessive dopamine concentrations does not alleviate depression comorbid with Parkinson disease. Deep-brain stimulation (DBS) usually greatly improves the motor impairments but does not alleviate depression. SSRIs, tricyclic antidepressants, and ECT all alleviate depression in Parkinson disease.

22. Which is the expected benefit of DBS in Parkinson disease patients?
    a. Improves postural instability
    b. Reverses cognitive impairment
    c. Reduces psychiatric comorbidity
    d. Reverses bradykinesia and tremor
    e. All of the above

Answer: d. DBS improves the tremor, rigidity, and bradykinesia of Parkinson disease. It also allows for a reduction in medications, which eliminates many medication-induced problems, including dyskinesia and nocturnal hallucinations. However, DBS does not improve postural instability, cognitive impairment, or any psychiatric comorbidity. In fact, DBS occasionally precipitates or worsens comorbid dementia or depression. These neuropsychiatric complications are surprising in view of the electrodes' usual location in the GPi (globus pallidus internal segment) or subthalamic nuclei, areas not usually associated with either depression or dementia. In any case, if Parkinson disease patients have either dementia or severe depression, they are usually not accepted as candidates for DBS.

23. Which feature distinguishes dementia as a symptom of Parkinson disease from dementia as a symptom of dementia with Lewy body disease?
    a. Dementia is one of the first symptoms of Parkinson disease but not Lewy bodies disease.
    b. Dementia is one of the first symptoms of Lewy bodies disease but not Parkinson disease.
    c. The dementia of Parkinson disease correlates with the tremor.
    d. The dementia of Lewy bodies disease correlates with aggression and loss of inhibition.

Answer: b. While dementia is characteristically the presenting feature of Lewy bodies disease, it usually does not complicate Parkinson disease until at least 5 years after the onset of the disease. When dementia complicates Parkinson disease, it correlates with rigidity and bradykinesia, but not tremor. Aggression and loss of inhibition are manifestations of frontotemporal dementia, but not of Parkinson or Lewy bodies diseases.

24. Which one of the following is *not* a Parkinson-plus syndrome?
    a. Multiple system atrophy
    b. Corticobasal degeneration
    c. Progressive supranuclear palsy
    d. MPTP-induced parkinsonism

Answer: d. A group of several illnesses – loosely termed "Parkinson-plus" illnesses – manifests other disturbances in addition to parkinsonism. Multiple system atrophy subsumes a set of disorders which neurologists subcategorize based on their most prominent feature: ataxia (olivopontocerebellar degeneration), hypotension and incontinence (Shy–Drager syndrome), or parkinsonism (striatonigral degeneration). Symptoms of corticobasal degeneration are variable but may include asymmetric parkinsonism, apraxia, myoclonus, alien limb phenomenon, dysarthria, dysphagia, and loss of cortical sensory modalities such as graphesthesia and stereognosis. Limited vertical ocular motility characterizes progressive supranuclear palsy. However, MPTP induces parkinsonism without other pronounced findings.

25. A previously well 8-year-old girl, who was a gifted chess player, began to develop dystonic movements of her legs that interfered with her after-school athletic activities and incapacitated her every evening. She remained undiagnosed for 18 months. By then, she clearly had dystonia that was present almost throughout the entire day but still worse at night. No family member has a similar problem. Of the following, which is the most likely diagnosis?
    a. Duchenne muscular dystrophy
    b. Dopa-responsive dystonia
    c. Cerebral palsy
    d. DYT1 dystonia

Answer: b. Dystonia that interferes with gait and, unlike primary dystonia, has a characteristic diurnal pattern characterizes dopa-responsive dystonia (DRD). Small doses of levodopa correct the gait impairment and involuntary movements. DRD may mimic cerebral palsy (CP), especially the athetotic variety, but CP is apparent within the first 1 to 2 years of life and does not fluctuate. To exclude DRD, neurologists often give children a therapeutic trial of levodopa. Children with DRD will improve while those with athetotic CP will not. Duchenne muscular dystrophy affects only boys and does not cause involuntary movements or fluctuate.

26. What is the biochemical deficiency in dopa-responsive dystonia?
    a. Deficiency of the cofactor for synthesis of tyrosine hydroxylase
    b. Deficiency of dopa-decarboxylase
    c. Deficiency of the substrate phenylalanine
    d. Abnormal L-DOPA

Answer: a. Dopamine responsive dystonia is due to insufficient synthesis of tetrahydrobiopterin, which is an essential cofactor for phenylalanine hydroxylase and tyrosine hydroxylase.

27. Which is the most sensitive screening test for the onset of dementia in Parkinson disease patients?
    a. The Mini-Mental State Examination (MMSE)
    b. Montreal Cognitive Assessment (MoCA)
    c. Abnormal Involuntary Movement Scale (AIMS)

d. Determining the patient's apolipoprotein E (APOE) status

Answer: b. The MoCA is more sensitive than the MMSE in screening for early dementia in either Parkinson or Huntington disease. The AIMS assesses only involuntary movements. APOE status is not a criterion for diagnosing dementia (see Chapter 7).

28. A psychiatrist is asked to evaluate a 70-year-old retired waiter who has developed visual hallucinations. An ophthalmologist had found only mild visual impairment. During the past year, the patient had developed cognitive impairments that, according to his family, fluctuate from day to day. The patient has mild slowness of movement and generally increased muscle tone. His neurologic examination is otherwise normal. The psychiatrist prescribes small doses of haloperidol. Several days later, the patient becomes rigid, akinetic, and unable to speak or eat. Of the following, which is the most likely underlying scenario?
    a. He has been overmedicated with haloperidol, relative to the requirements of older patients.
    b. The haloperidol converted mild to severe Parkinson disease.
    c. He has Alzheimer disease.
    d. He has dementia with Lewy bodies disease.

Answer: d. The patient probably has dementia with Lewy bodies disease, which causes fluctuating cognitive impairment, visual hallucinations, and mild parkinsonism. Because the illness renders patients unusually sensitive to dopamine-blocking medications, the haloperidol induced severe parkinsonism.

29. Which one of the following enzymes increases the concentration of L-DOPA?
    a. Catechol-O-methyltransferase (COMT)
    b. Monoamine oxidase (MAO)
    c. Dopa-decarboxylase
    d. Tyrosine hydroxylase

Answer: d. Tyrosine hydroxylase converts tyrosine to L-DOPA, but the other enzymes reduce L-DOPA by metabolizing it. In Parkinson disease, an absence of tyrosine hydroxylase leads to dopamine deficiency and insufficient dopamine. Neurologists use inhibitors of COMT and of MAO to treat Parkinson disease.

30. Which one of the following characterizes necrosis but not apoptosis?
    a. Energy-requiring
    b. Programmed pattern of death
    c. Infiltration of mononuclear cells into the area of cell death
    d. Normal mechanism of development for some organs
    e. Cell death

Answer: c. Both apoptosis and necrosis are forms or mechanisms of cell death. Apoptosis is programmed cell death, which occurs in the normal evolution of certain organs, such as the thymus gland, as well as in several degenerative illnesses, such as Huntington disease and ALS. Apoptosis is also orderly and requires energy. Necrosis, in contrast, is characterized by infiltration of mononuclear cells into the area of cell death (inflammation), does not require energy, and is not programmed or normally occurring. It follows a stroke, trauma, or other physical insult. Neurologists sometimes call it "cell death by destruction."

31. A 67-year-old man is comatose 1 week after sustaining a brainstem infarction. Among other abnormalities, his palate spontaneously elevates symmetrically – as though he were saying "ah" – at a regular rate of 120 times per minute. What is the origin of this movement disorder?
    a. An infarction in the medulla's inferior olivary nuclei, midbrain's red nuclei, or cerebellum's dentate nuclei, or their connections.
    b. Parkinson disease
    c. A toxic-metabolic aberration
    d. Nonspecific myoclonus

Answer: a. He has palatal tremor, which was reclassified from myoclonus, because it consists of regular, rhythmic movements in a single plane. Palatal tremor results from lesions in the anatomic triangle composed of the inferior olivary, dentate, and red nuclei. Unlike most movement disorders, palatal tremor is entirely regular and persists during sleep and coma.

32–35. Match the illness (32–35) with its inheritance pattern (a–d).

32. Huntington disease
33. Red–green color blindness
34. Wilson disease
35. DYT1 dystonia
    a. Recessive sex-linked
    b. Autosomal recessive
    c. Autosomal dominant
    d. None of the above

Answers: 32–c, 33–a, 34–b, 35–c. Though both Huntington disease and DYT1 dystonia show autosomal dominance inheritance, the penetrance in Huntington disease is almost 100% while penetrance in DYT1 dystonia is only about 30%.

36. Which medication will deplete dopamine from its presynaptic neurons and reduce hyperkinetic movement disorders, such as tics, chorea, and varieties of tardive dyskinesia?
    a. Carbidopa
    b. COMT inhibitors
    c. Tetrabenazine
    d. Risperidone

Answer: c. Tetrabenazine depletes dopamine from its storage vesicles in presynaptic neurons and thereby reduces many hyperkinetic movement disorders. Unfortunately, tetrabenazine potentially causes parkinsonism, depression, and suicidal ideation. Carbidopa blocks the synthesis of dopamine from L-DOPA; however, because it does not cross the blood–brain barrier, carbidopa works only in the periphery and not in the basal ganglia. COMT inhibitors increase dopamine concentration. Although they help in Parkinson disease, COMT inhibitors provide no benefit in the hyperkinetic disorders. Risperidone may reduce hyperkinetic movement disorders but does so by blocking the postsynaptic dopamine receptors and thereby leads to parkinsonism.

37. What is the implication of a patient's falling backward during the pull test?
    a. Cerebellar dysfunction
    b. Gait apraxia
    c. Gait ataxia
    d. Impaired postural reflexes

Answer: d. During the pull test, a patient falling backward, like spontaneous retropulsion, indicates impaired postural reflexes. This finding is typical of Parkinson disease and other parkinsonian conditions.

38. Which of the following statements regarding dementia in Parkinson disease is *true*?
    a. The prevalence of dementia is unrelated to the illness' physical manifestations.
    b. Once dementia complicates Parkinson disease, cognition declines precipitously.
    c. Rapid, almost manic, thinking is a component of Parkinson disease dementia.
    d. Parkinson disease dementia is an example of cortical dementia.
    e. Dementia is more likely to complicate "non-tremor-predominant" than "tremor-predominant" Parkinson disease.

Answer: e. Dementia is more likely to complicate Parkinson disease when rigidity and bradykinesia are prominent, i.e., dementia is more prevalent in "nontremor-predominant" than "tremor-predominant" Parkinson disease. The prevalence of dementia increases in proportion to physical impairments, especially bradykinesia, and eventually reaches 80%. Affected patients lose 2.3 points annually on the Mini-Mental State Examination. The gait impairment, bradyphrenia, and lack of language impairment render Parkinson disease a prime example of subcortical dementia.

39. Which is the rate-limiting step in dopamine synthesis?
    a. Phenylalanine to tyrosine
    b. Tyrosine to L-DOPA
    c. Tyrosine to dopamine
    d. L-DOPA to dopamine
    e. Dopamine to norepinephrine
    f. None of the above

Answer: b. The rate-limiting step in dopamine synthesis is the conversion of tyrosine to L-DOPA, catalyzed by tyrosine hydroxylase.

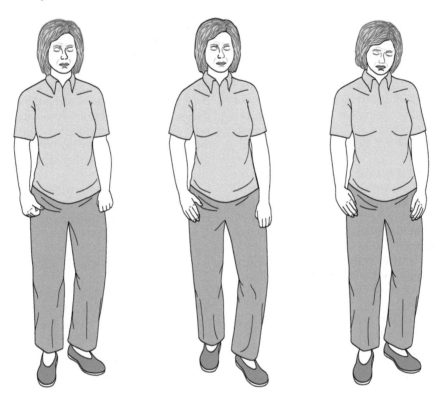

40. A 30-year-old woman admitted for cocaine intoxication has incessant movements of her feet (see figure). She claims that she "must" walk constantly. When forced to sit, she continually abducts and adducts her legs and shuffles her feet. She is belligerent, but alert and without cognitive impairment. Which of the following is the most likely cause of her leg movements and walking?
a. Sydenham chorea
b. Excitement from bipolar disorder
c. Huntington chorea
d. Persistent cocaine effect

Answer: d. She has cocaine-induced "crack dancing," in which an urge to walk compels incessant lower-extremity movements. Her movements stem from cocaine triggering the release of dopamine from presynaptic storage sites and thus increasing dopamine activity. Akathisia and restless leg syndrome cause similar involuntary leg movements and a compulsion to walk. Chorea causes arm and trunk as well as leg movements, but neither in such a stereotyped pattern nor with an urge to move.

41–49. Match the underlying abnormality (41–49) with the associated condition (a–g).

41. Uremia or cerebral anoxia
42. Toxoplasmosis
43. Perinatal kernicterus
44. Low serum ceruloplasmin
45. Infarction of the subthalamic nucleus
46. Nigrostriatal depigmentation
47. Prion infection
48. Atrophy of the caudate heads

49. Cavitary lesions of the globus pallidus and putamen
a. Huntington disease
b. Wilson disease
c. Hemiballismus
d. Creutzfeldt–Jakob disease
e. Choreoathetotic cerebral palsy
f. Parkinson disease
g. Myoclonus

Answers: 41–g; 42–c; 43–e; 44–b; 45–c; 46–f; 47–d (and, based on recent findings, perhaps f!); 48–a; 49–b.

50. A nursing home's medical director sought a psychiatry consultation for a resident – a 70-year-old retired disc jockey with moderately severe Parkinson disease – who recently had been refusing to attend rehabilitation and occupational therapy. On questioning by the psychiatrist, the patient was alert and generally oriented with preserved cognitive ability; however, she judged that he had depression. Which of the following statements regarding depression in this situation is most correct?
a. When comorbid with Parkinson disease, depression worsens cognitive impairment.
b. Comorbid depression is a potential explanation for this patient's responding poorly to medical and physical therapy.
c. Comorbid depression interferes with Parkinson disease patients' sleep.
d. Comorbid depression interferes with Parkinson disease patients' ability to adjust to limitations imposed by the illness.
e. All of the above.

Answer: e. Depression frequently complicates Parkinson disease and worsens patients' mood, sleep cycle, cognitive capacity, and motor function.

51. After admission to a psychiatric unit for the onset of major depression with suicidal ideation, a 78-year-old man was found to have continuous, aimless tongue protrusion and some lip smacking. He had lost all of his teeth when he was a young man. Because of his recent weight loss, his dentures no longer fit and he had given up wearing them. Before diagnosing tardive dyskinesia, which treatment should the medical staff institute?
    a. A therapeutic trial of a second-generation antipsychotic
    b. Anticholinergic treatment
    c. Beginning a dopamine agonist
    d. Obtaining properly fitting dentures

Answer: d. The patient probably has edentulous oral dyskinesia (edentulous chorea). Correctly fitting dentures will stop the tongue and lip movements and thereby provide a diagnosis as well as treatment.

52. Which of the following statements regarding genetically determined Parkinson disease is *false*?
    a. Mutations in the *parkin* and *α-synuclein* genes give rise to familial Parkinson disease.
    b. Unlike in sporadic, commonly occurring cases, the basal ganglia in genetically determined Parkinson disease cases lack Lewy bodies.
    c. The majority of Parkinson disease patients younger than 20 years harbor the *parkin* mutation.
    d. Genetically determined Parkinson disease cases comprise less than 1% of the total cases.

Answer: d. Genetically determined Parkinson disease cases comprise up to 10% – not 1% – of the total cases. When mutations are responsible, they typically lead to the onset of Parkinson disease before age 50 years. In fact, the majority of Parkinson disease patients younger than 20 years harbor the *parkin* mutation on chromosome 6.

53. Hospitalized on several occasions during the previous 3 years for progressively severe schizophrenia, a 29-year-old man has been readmitted because of paranoid hallucinations and general deterioration. His psychiatrists reinstituted second-generation antipsychotics. Several months later, a psychiatrist notices that the patient's neck spontaneously retroverts (extends) and his limbs straighten. Which is the most appropriate description of this man's movements?
    a. Tics
    b. Tardive dystonia
    c. Cervical dystonia
    d. A psychogenic disorder

Answer: b. He has retrocollis, extension of his arms, and probably unobserved extension of his trunk as manifestations of tardive dystonia. Second- as well as first-generation antipsychotics cause this variety of tardive dyskinesia. The involvement of the limbs signifies that he has more than cervical dystonia, which is a focal dystonia of the neck. The retrocollis is the most troublesome aspect of tardive dystonia. Botulinum treatment may alleviate it without causing systemic side effects.

54. Which *three* of the following neurodegenerative disorders do neurologists label "tauopathies"?
    a. Alzheimer disease
    b. Frontotemporal dementia
    c. Progressive supranuclear palsy (PSP)
    d. Dementia with Lewy bodies disease
    e. Parkinson disease

Answer: a, b, c.

55. In the above question, which *two* of the disorders do neurologists label "synucleinopathies"?

Answer: d, e.

56. Which single statement is *true* regarding the CAG trinucleotide repeats in Huntington disease?
    a. The pathologic sequence is located on chromosome 4.
    b. Normal individuals do not have CAG trinucleotide repeats.
    c. The number of repeats in patients' sperm and eggs remain stable.
    d. An affected mother's gene would be more unstable than an affected father's.

Answer: a. Normal individuals have fewer than 36 CAG trinucleotide repeats and Huntington disease patients usually have more than 39 repeats. Individuals who have 36 to 39 repeats – the "indeterminate" range – may show few if any stigmata of the illness, but their children who inherit the mutation often have overt disease because of its tendency to expand. A father with Huntington disease is more apt to cause an earlier-appearing, more severe case in his children who inherit the mutation because DNA in sperm is particularly unstable.

57. Which *four* illnesses result from excessive trinucleotide repeats?
    a. Myotonic dystrophy
    b. Depression
    c. Fragile X syndrome
    d. Alzheimer disease
    e. Huntington disease
    f. Duchenne muscular dystrophy
    g. Certain spinocerebellar ataxias (SCAs)

Answer: a, c, e, g. Because excess CAG repeats causes transcription of proteins with abnormally long strings of the amino acid glutamine, neurologists call Huntington disease and many SCAs polyglutamine diseases. In myotonic dystrophy the repeated trinucleotide is CTG, while in fragile X it is CGG.

58. Which is the most appropriate term for the tendency of a genetic illness to produce symptoms in increasingly younger victims in successive generations?
a. Anticipation
b. Suppression
c. Disinhibition
d. None of the above because it does not happen

Answer: a. Anticipation occurs in Huntington disease, myotonic dystrophy, and several other illnesses. This phenomenon characterizes illnesses transmitted by excess trinucleotide repeats.

59. Which *four* disorders cause dementia in adolescents?
a. Creutzfeldt–Jakob disease
b. Wilson disease
c. Choreoathetotic cerebral palsy
d. Huntington disease
e. Subacute sclerosing panencephalitis (SSPE)
f. Variant Creutzfeldt–Jakob disease
g. Dopamine-responsive dystonia

Answer: b, d, e, f. These illnesses cause dementia in adolescents, but personality change or behavioral disturbances – rather than academic difficulties – often is the presenting symptom.

60. Which Parkinson disease patients are most apt to cause depression in their caregivers?
a. Patients with depression
b. Patients with acute, devastating illness
c. Patients with physical impairments
d. Patients who require complicated medical regimens

Answer: a. In general, caregivers also have a reduced quality of life. Caregivers of Parkinson disease patients are most apt to develop depression when the patient has depression. Women caregivers also show high anxiety scores.

61–65. Match the patient's description (61–65) with the neurologic disturbances (a–g).

61. A 70-year-old man develops a high-pitched, squeaky voice that forces him to whisper. Nevertheless, he can sing with a normal volume and pitch.
62. An actor begins to have bilateral hand tremor while on stage.
63. Continual forced bilateral eyelid closure prevents a 70-year-old man from reading and driving.
64. A middle-aged woman develops continual face, eyelid, and jaw contractions.
65. An author develops hand cramps when writing with a pen, but he can use a computer keyboard and button his shirts.
a. Blepharospasm
b. Writer's cramp
c. Spasmodic dysphonia
d. Meige syndrome (cranial dystonia)
e. Oromandibular dystonia
f. Anxiety-induced tremor
g. Aphasia
h. Spasmodic torticollis

Answers: 61–c, 62–f, 63–a, 64–d, 65–b. Blepharospasm, Meige syndrome, oromandibular dystonia, and spasmodic dysphonia are varieties of cranial dystonia. Spasmodic torticollis is classified as cervical dystonia. Writer's cramp also is a type of focal dystonia. Antipsychotic exposure often precedes the development of cranial and cervical dystonias; however, most patients have no history of medicine exposure or psychiatric illness. For neurologists, stage fright represents an anxiety-induced tremor. The DSM-5 would include stage fright as Social Anxiety Disorder (social phobia), performance only.

66. Which *two* structures comprise the striatum?
a. Caudate
b. Putamen
c. Globus pallidus
d. Subthalamic nucleus
e. Substantia nigra

Answer: a, b.

67. Which one of the following statements is *true* regarding psychogenic movement disorders in children?
a. Psychogenic movement disorders do not occur in children.
b. When psychogenic movement disorders occur in children, they usually mimic tremor, dystonia, myoclonus, or gait impairment.
c. If a psychogenic movement disorder were to occur in a child, it would be pure rather than one of several movements.

Answer: b. As when they occur in adults, psychogenic movement disorders in children tend to mimic tremor, dystonia, myoclonus, or gait impairment. Moreover, as with adults who have them, multiple movements occur simultaneously.

68. Why is carbidopa combined with levodopa for treatment of Parkinson disease?
a. Carbidopa acts as a dopamine agonist.
b. Carbidopa enhances metabolism of levodopa.
c. Carbidopa inhibits metabolism of levodopa.
d. Carbidopa is a COMT inhibitor.

Answer: c. Carbidopa, a dopa decarboxylase inhibitor, impedes metabolism of levodopa in the systemic circulation, but, because it cannot cross the blood–brain barrier, does not interfere with the nigrostriatal tract conversion of levodopa to dopamine in the substantia nigra. The combination allows for the use of lower doses of levodopa. Also, because dopamine in the periphery would cause hypotension, nausea, and vomiting, combining it with carbidopa avoids nausea and vomiting. Entacapone is a COMT inhibitor.

69. Since infancy, a 25-year-old man has had involuntary slow, twisting movements of his face, mouth, trunk, and limbs (see figure below). The neck muscles have hypertrophied. He performs poorly on standard intelligence tests. Which *two* of the following statements regarding his condition are *true*?

a. His children might inherit this condition.

b. He probably performs poorly on standard intelligence tests, in part, because he is dysarthric and unable to use his hands.

c. He probably has congenital abnormalities in the basal ganglia.

d. His condition is not associated with cognitive impairments.

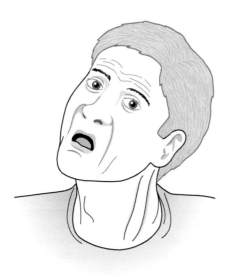

Answer: b, c. He probably has athetosis, which is a type of cerebral palsy (CP) that becomes apparent between infancy and ages 2 and 4 years. Athetotic CP usually results from perinatal injuries to the basal ganglia. It is often, but not necessarily, associated with mental retardation. Superficial clinical examinations and standard intelligence tests tend to underestimate children with cerebral palsy, especially those with the athetotic and choreoathetotic varieties, because of their motor impairments and dysarthria. Early-onset primary dystonia, which usually appears in childhood, is carried on the DYT1 gene and inherited as an autosomal dominant condition. It is not associated with cognitive dysfunction.

70. Which of the following statements concerning Lesch–Nyhan syndrome is *false*?

a. Its symptoms include dystonia and other movements in children aged 2 to 6 years.

b. It is transmitted as an autosomal dominant genetic illness.

c. Boys with Lesch–Nyhan syndrome have bitten off parts of their lips and fingertips.

d. The basic deficit is a deficiency of the enzyme HGPRT1.

e. The enzyme deficiency often leads to renal failure.

Answer: b. Lesch–Nyhan syndrome, characterized by self-mutilation, is transmitted as an X-linked recessive illness. Its underlying HGPRT deficiency (due to mutation in the *HPRT1* gene) causes hyperuricemia, which often leads to fatal renal failure.

71. A 79-year-old man under treatment with lithium for bipolar disorder has a fine, rapid tremor of his outstretched hands. What action should the psychiatrist take?

a. The psychiatrist must immediately stop the lithium because the patient has reached a toxic serum concentration.

b. The psychiatrist should check the serum concentration of lithium because the patient may have reached a toxic serum concentration.

c. The psychiatrist should add a β-blocker to suppress the tremor.

d. None of the above is correct.

Answer: b. Such a tremor is not necessarily a sign of lithium toxicity and may occur at therapeutic serum concentrations. Nevertheless, because the lithium serum concentrations closely correlate with toxicity and the elderly are especially vulnerable, the psychiatrist should immediately check its level. Lithium toxicity may damage the cerebellum, cause seizures, or lead to diabetes insipidus. If patients with cluster headache, bipolar disease, or other conditions require lithium and therapeutic levels cause a tremor, a β-blocker will suppress the tremor and allow the patient to continue the medicine.

72. What is the mechanism of action that permits propranolol to suppress essential tremor?

a. It reduces cardiac output.

b. It is a mild sedative.

c. It blocks adrenergic sympathetic nervous system receptors.

d. It suppresses synthesis of norepinephrine.

Answer: c. Propranolol is a relatively nonspecific adrenergic sympathetic receptor blocker that suppresses essential tremor. It also is a preventative therapy for migraine and reduces hypertension and angina. However, because it blocks sympathetic receptors, propranolol may precipitate asthma and congestive heart failure. If prescribed for a patient with history of affective disorder, physicians should monitor for worsening of depression.

73. When neurosurgeons place the electrodes for DBS in Parkinson disease, which region is the target?

a. Ventral intermediate (VIM) nucleus of the thalamus

b. Anterior cingulate gyrus or anterior limb of the internal capsule

c. GPi or subthalamic nucleus

d. Cerebellum

Answer: c. For DBS in Parkinson disease, the target is usually either the GPi or subthalamic nucleus. For DBS in essential tremor, they usually target the VIM nucleus of the thalamus. For refractory depression, they usually target the anterior cingulate gyrus or anterior limb of the internal capsule, but DBS is not FDA-approved for treatment of depression.

74. By which mechanism does botulinum toxin treat blepharospasm and other focal dystonias?
    a. Botulinum toxin, like tetrabenazine, depletes dopamine.
    b. Botulinum toxin reduces synthesis of dopamine by inhibiting tyrosine hydroxylase.
    c. Botulinum toxin impedes release of acetylcholine (ACh) from the presynaptic neuron at the neuromuscular junction neuron.
    d. Botulinum toxin, like myasthenia gravis antibodies, binds to the postsynaptic ACh receptors.

Answer: c. Botulinum toxin blocks release of ACh from the presynaptic neuron in the neuromuscular junction by cleaving a protein necessary for exocytosis of the ACh from the motor nerve terminal. It thus reduces contraction of overactive muscles, thereby decreasing dystonia and spasticity. Lambert–Eaton myasthenic syndrome (see Chapter 6) also causes weakness due to decreased ACh release from the presynaptic nerve terminal, but it is an autoimmune disease with antibodies directed against the voltage-gated calcium channel.

75. After developing personality changes and slowed thinking for 1 to 2 years, a 39-year-old high school music teacher presents for evaluation. He relates that his father died at age 65 years from Huntington disease, but his mother is alive and well. A neurologic examination shows subtle chorea, motor impersistence, and jerky saccades. After the neurologist offers a clinical diagnosis of Huntington disease, the patient agrees to undergo genetic testing. Which of the following patterns will the test most likely show?
    a. Maternal gene, 20 CAG repeats; paternal gene, 45 CAG repeats
    b. Maternal gene, 30 CAG repeats; paternal gene, 30 CAG repeats
    c. Maternal gene, 45 CAG repeats; paternal gene, 20 CAG repeats
    d. Maternal gene, 20 CAG repeats; paternal gene, 80 CAG repeats
    e. Maternal gene, 80 CAG repeats; paternal gene, 20 CAG repeats

Answer: a. The patient's father, who died relatively late in life from Huntington disease, probably had a relatively low elevation of CAG repeats, i.e., 45 instead of 80 repeats. Because the mother is not affected, her CAG complement level must have been normal. Had the father carried a gene with more than 60 repeats (answer d), he would have developed the juvenile variety of the illness and died at a young age, probably

before fathering any children. If the mother's CAG complement had been elevated (answers c and e), she would have been the affected parent. Had both sets of genes shown normal CAG repeats (answer b), the neurologist would have been obligated to consider other diagnoses (or an alternative parentage).

76. Which statement about saccades is *false*?
    a. Saccades are rapid, accurate, conjugate eye movements.
    b. Saccadic eye movements are abnormal in Huntington disease and schizophrenia.
    c. Abnormal saccades are an early sign of Huntington disease.
    d. In Huntington disease, patients may initiate saccades by jerking their head or blinking.
    e. Saccadic eye movements in Huntington disease saccades are jerky.
    f. Neurologists consider saccadic eye movements to be normal if fixation eventually comes to rest on the target, whether or not it initially undershoots or overshoots it.

Answer: f. Normal saccades shoot smoothly, directly, and accurately from one target to another, and they show no under- or overshooting.

77. A neurologist evaluates a 70-year-old retired bandleader because he has fallen many times during the previous 6 months. The examination reveals axial rigidity and limb bradykinesia but no tremor. The patient cannot voluntarily look upward or downward, but when the neurologist rocks the patient's head in a "yes–yes" pattern, the patient's eyes move vertically relative to the head. Which is the most likely diagnosis?
    a. Parkinson disease
    b. Lewy bodies disease
    c. Progressive supranuclear palsy (PSP)
    d. Frontotemporal lobar degeneration

Answer: c. This man has PSP. He has fallen because he cannot look downward and his rigidity and bradykinesia prevent him from catching himself if he begins to fall. The signature of PSP is loss of voluntary vertical ocular movement but intact reflex movements.

78. When they hear deliberate or accidental noises, certain members of a large family living in Maine respond by leaping upwards, screaming, and throwing any object from their hands. Which is the most likely explanation for their response?
    a. Culture-bound behavior
    b. Stimulus-sensitive myoclonus
    c. Anxiety
    d. Hyperacusis
    e. Akathisia

Answer: a. Probably of French-Canadian descent, these individuals with exaggerated startle responses are the jumping Frenchmen of Maine demonstrating a culture-bound behavior or folk-illness. Similarly, latahs of rural Malaysia and Indonesia and *myriachit* of Siberia overreact to trivial stimuli by suddenly cursing, laughing convulsively, or moving in dance-like patterns.

79. Shortly after the emergency room physicians administered a small intramuscular dose of haloperidol to an intravenous drug addict with dangerous agitation and psychotic thinking, the physicians noticed that muscles throughout his entire body were having intermittent but powerful contractions. His temperature was 103°F. His creatine kinase (CK) was 350 mg/dl. The physicians found an abscess deep in his left thigh. As the evaluation continued, laryngeal and pharyngeal contractions made his breathing difficult, his face intermittently grimaced, and his jaw clenched. Touching the patient triggered intense muscle contractions. They administered broad-spectrum antibiotics for the infection, but anticholinergics and antihistamines did not correct the muscle contractions. Which condition best explains muscle contractions?
    a. Acute dystonic reaction to haloperidol
    b. Seizures
    c. Cranial dystonia
    d. The thigh infection

Answer: d. Trismus (lockjaw), prominent involuntary face and jaw muscle contractions, and the examination provoking muscle contractions indicate that he has tetanus from the thigh infection. Drug addicts are prone to tetanus because they use contaminated needles. Tetanus immunization lasts for only about 10 years. When the immunity wears off, patients are vulnerable to either generalized tetanus or more often "regional tetanus," where only the infected body region, such as one arm or leg, is affected. The neuroleptic-malignant syndrome is possible, but it is less likely because the emergency room staff administered only a small dose of haloperidol, the CK elevation was modest, and the abscess explained the rise in temperature.

80. Which of the following medicines is most likely to elevate the serum prolactin concentration?
    a. Clozapine
    b. Ropinirole
    c. Haloperidol
    d. Levodopa

Answer: c. Dopamine-blocking antipsychotic agents provoke prolactin release and elevate its serum concentration. In addition, primary generalized seizures, some partial complex seizures, and pituitary adenomas also provoke prolactin release and elevate its serum concentration.

81. A 50-year-old systems analyst, who has been taking various SSRIs for 10 years, states that her face pulls to the left and her left eyelid closes (see figure below). The movements are more intense during anxiety and appear in bursts lasting several seconds to a few minutes, but they are not painful. The eyelid closure interferes with her driving her car.

Which one of the following conditions is probably responsible for her movements?
    a. An aberrant blood vessel at the cerebellopontine angle
    b. Focal seizures
    c. Dopamine-blocking antipsychotics
    d. Anxiety
    e. Antidepressants

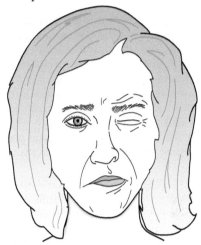

Answer: a. She has hemifacial spasm. In many cases, the cause is an aberrant blood vessel that compresses the facial nerve as it exits from the brainstem. Sometimes, aberrant nerve regeneration from a prior facial nerve trauma or Bell's palsy causes hemifacial spasm. However, it is almost never psychogenic.

82. Which *two* structures constitute the lenticular nuclei?
    a. Caudate
    b. Putamen
    c. Globus pallidus
    d. Subthalamic nucleus
    e. Substantia nigra

Answer: b, c. The putamen and globus pallidus form the lenticular nuclei. This nuclear complex bears the brunt of hepatolenticular degeneration (Wilson disease).

83. Which one of the following nuclei is unpigmented?
    a. Substantia nigra
    b. Locus ceruleus
    c. Dorsal motor X
    d. Anterior thalamic

Answer: d. Thalamic nuclei, which are mostly sensory relay nuclei, are not pigmented. Substantia nigra, locus ceruleus, and dorsal motor nuclei, which are constituents of the motor system, normally are pigmented. They lose their color in Parkinson disease.

84. A family brings its 72-year-old patriarch for evaluation of dementia that developed during the previous 4–6 months. The neurologic examination reveals mild rigidity and bradykinesia, as well as a dysfunction in multiple cognitive domains. Which

one of the following statements is best applied to this case?
a. His substantia nigra probably contains Lewy bodies.
b. His cerebral cortex, as well as substantia nigra, probably contains Lewy bodies.
c. He probably has depression.
d. He probably has Alzheimer disease.

Answer: b. He probably has dementia from Lewy bodies disease in view of the extrapyramidal signs (rigidity and bradykinesia). Parkinson disease (answer a), at its onset, generally does not cause depression or dementia. Alzheimer disease does not present with either pyramidal or extrapyramidal signs. Physicians should question the patient's family about visual hallucinations, which are typically an early or initial symptom in dementia from Lewy bodies disease (see Chapter 7) and possible exposure to dopamine receptor-blocking agents.

85. In the treatment of depression in Parkinson disease patients, which of the following statements is *true*?
   a. Insight psychotherapy is not only essential, it is usually sufficient.
   b. ECT is contraindicated.
   c. Selegiline may have an activating effect.
   d. Tocopherol is often helpful.

Answer: c. Selegiline is metabolized, in part, to amphetamine and methamphetamine. Although physicians should avoid administering an SSRI together with selegiline, the actual incidence of serotonin syndrome is very low because selegiline at the usual doses selectively inhibits MAO-B, which metabolizes dopamine. In actuality, the serotonin syndrome is a complication of inhibitors of MAO-A, which metabolize serotonin, or MAO-B inhibitors at very high doses, at which they lose their selectivity for the MAO-B isoform. ECT is helpful for depression in Parkinson disease patients, in whom it will temporarily relieve the motor symptoms as well as the depression. Tocopherol (vitamin E) has no proven benefit on either the mental or physical manifestations of Parkinson disease.

86. Which of the following complications is the most common reason why families place Parkinson disease patients in nursing homes?
   a. Hallucinations and delusions
   b. Depression
   c. Rigidity
   d. Akinesia

Answer: a. Psychosis, not physical incapacity or incontinence, is the most frequent reason that families place Parkinson disease patients in nursing homes. The family's disturbed sleep, which usually results from the patient's behavior, is the most common reason.

87. With which of the following dopamine receptor subtypes do all antiparkinson dopamine agonists interact?
   a. D1
   b. D2
   c. Both
   d. Neither

Answer: b. Effective antiparkinson dopamine agonists stimulate D2. They may either stimulate or inhibit D1.

88. Which Parkinson disease feature has the *least* correlation with dementia?
   a. Old age at onset
   b. Rapid progression of the illness
   c. Poor response to dopamine medications
   d. Tremor
   e. Akinesia

Answer: d. Dementia is least closely correlated with tremor. If dementia develops simultaneously with parkinsonism consider conditions other than Parkinson disease. For example, in individuals older than 50 years, consider dementia from Lewy bodies disease. In adolescents and young adults, consider Wilson disease, juvenile Huntington disease, and drug abuse.

89. A 70-year-old man, under treatment for depression for 10 years, has begun to develop intermittent bilateral contractions of the orbicularis oculi (see figure). His medications included a tricyclic antidepressant until 2 years ago, when physicians substituted a SSRI. He had a good response to the change. He has undergone two courses of ECT. The involuntary movements impair his ability to read and intensify the depression. What would be the best treatment?
   a. Return to a TCA
   b. Prohibit any further ECT
   c. Reduce the dose of the serotonin re-uptake inhibitors
   d. Add anticholinergic medications
   e. Administer injections of botulinum toxin

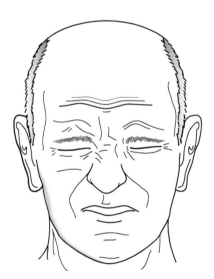

Answer: e. The patient has developed blepharospasm, but it is probably not a side effect of either the antidepressants or ECT. Although blepharospasm may follow treatment with dopamine-blocking antipsychotic agents, it is usually an idiopathic condition. Regardless of its cause, botulinum toxin injections into the affected muscles will alleviate the blepharospasm and allow antidepressant treatment to continue.

90–92. Match the neurotransmitter (90–92) with its metabolic product (a–c).

90. Norepinephrine
91. Dopamine
92. Serotonin
   a. Homovanillic acid (HVA)
   b. 5-Hydroxyindoleacetic acid (5-HIAA)
   c. Vanillylmandelic acid (VMA)

Answer: 90–c, 91–a, 92–b.

93. Which one of the following movement disorders is *not* accompanied or preceded by an urge to move?
   a. Tics
   b. Akathisia
   c. Tremor
   d. Restless leg syndrome movements

Answer: c. Urges to move do not precede tremor or most other movements. In contrast, irrepressible, indescribable sensations, psychic tension, or urges precede or trigger tics, akathisia, and restless leg movements. Patients can suppress these movements for several minutes, but when the movements break through, they often return in a flurry. Neurologists sometimes, perhaps inaccurately, term these movements "compulsions."

94. After 6 weeks of change in personality, characterized by fearfulness, hyperreligiosity, and easily provoked anger, a 70-year-old anesthesiologist consulted a neurologist, who found mild cognitive impairment but no abnormal physical neurologic findings. Routine blood tests, MRI, CSF analysis, and positron emission tomography disclosed no abnormalities. After another 6 weeks, the neurologist found that the patient had cognitive decline to the point of dementia and small, rapid contractions of the patient's limb and trunk muscles. Which is the most likely explanation for the rapidly progressive dementia?
   a. Demerol (meperidine) abuse
   b. Bismuth intoxication
   c. Creutzfeldt–Jakob disease
   d. Delirium

Answer: c. The patient has developed myoclonus as well as rapidly progressive dementia. In its initial stages, Creutzfeldt–Jakob disease – the prototypical prion disease – may not produce the characteristic CSF finding (14-3-3 protein) or abnormalities on imaging studies. Abuse of opioids, such as Demerol (meperidine), an occupational hazard for anesthesiologists, and bismuth intoxication may each cause myoclonus and cognitive impairment. Delirium would have caused a fluctuating level of consciousness and, at its onset, EEG abnormalities, particularly slowing and disorganized background activity.

95. Which of the following conditions will the Abnormal Involuntary Movement Scale (AIMS) capture?
   a. Oral-bucco-lingual dyskinesia
   b. Bradykinesia
   c. Tremor
   d. Dysarthria

Answer: a. Developed primarily to detect the oral-bucco-lingual dyskinesia variety of tardive dyskinesia, the AIMS rates dyskinesias of the face, jaw, tongue, trunk, and limbs. It is not applicable to tremor, dystonia, tics, stereotypies, or varieties of tardive dyskinesia other than oral-bucco-lingual dyskinesia.

96. Which of the following does *not* describe free radicals?
   a. They contain single, unpaired electrons.
   b. They are stable.
   c. They snatch away single electrons from neighboring atoms or molecules.
   d. Removal of electrons from atoms or molecules oxidizes them.
   e. Methylphenylpyridinium (MMP+) is a free radical.

Answer: b. Free radicals are unstable because they contain an unpaired electron. To complete themselves, free radicals capture single electrons from neighboring atoms, which leads to oxidation of the atom or molecule.

97. Which of the following predisposes to Parkinson disease?
   a. Cigarette smoking
   b. High caffeine consumption
   c. Drinking well water
   d. Taking nonsteroidal anti-inflammatory agents (NSAIDs)

Answer: c. Epidemiologic studies have shown that consumption of well water is a risk factor for developing Parkinson disease. Other studies have shown that the incidence of Parkinson disease varies *inversely* with cigarette smoking, high caffeine consumption, taking NSAIDs, and having an elevated uric acid serum concentration – but whether these activities actually protect individuals against Parkinson disease or are associated with decreased risk through some confounding factor is unclear.

98. Which *two* of the following characteristics accurately describe dementia in Parkinson disease?
   a. It responds to levodopa.
   b. It responds to dopamine agonists.
   c. Thought processes are typically slow.
   d. Patients have difficulty shifting mental sets.
   e. Aphasia and apraxia are typical manifestations of the dementia.

Answer: c, d. Bradyphrenia, lack of initiative, and depression are comorbid with dementia in Parkinson disease. These manifestations of the disease do not respond to dopaminergic medications. The dementia of Parkinson disease is a subcortical dementia, while features like aphasia and apraxia are typical of cortical dementia.

99. Which *three* of the following Parkinson disease symptoms will *not* respond to an increase in dopaminergic medications?
    a. Dementia
    b. Tremor
    c. Rigidity
    d. Bradykinesia
    e. Depression
    f. Hallucinations

Answer: a, e, f. Mental aberrations are unaffected by restoring dopamine activity. In fact, excessive dopamine activity precipitates hallucinations, especially in the later stages of the illness.

100. A neurologic examination of a 17-year-old boy, who has had declining schoolwork, reveals dysarthria, tremor, and a brown–green ring at the periphery of each cornea. Which of the following laboratory abnormalities is most likely to be found?
    a. Little or no copper-transporting serum protein
    b. Metachromatic granules in the urine
    c. Periodic EEG complexes
    d. MPTP metabolic products in the urine

Answer: a. In view of the history, tremor, and Kayser–Fleisher ring, he probably has Wilson disease (hepatolenticular degeneration). This illness is an autosomal recessive disorder associated with a marked reduction in serum ceruloplasmin, which is a copper-transporting protein, and visible copper deposits in the periphery of the cornea (the Kayser–Fleisher ring).

101. Which is the effect of stimulation of D1 receptors in the striatum by dopamine?
    a. The interaction stimulates adenylate cyclase activity.
    b. The interaction inhibits adenylate cyclase activity.
    c. The interaction has no effect on adenylate cyclase activity.

Answer: a. Interaction of dopamine with striatal D1 receptors stimulates adenylate cyclase activity and gives rise to the *direct pathway* from the striatum to the output nuclei of the basal ganglia, while dopamine–D2 receptor interaction inhibits adenylate cyclase activity in the first step of the *indirect pathway*.

102. What is the most likely outcome if an asymptomatic individual with a family history of Huntington disease undergoes testing for the Huntington disease mutation and the result indicates that he carries more than 40 alleles?
    a. He will attempt suicide.
    b. He will develop depression.
    c. His emotional state will be neutral or he will have some reduced anxiety.

Answer: c. The peak of anxiety and depression occurs in potential carriers of Huntington disease before they undergo testing. Even after learning that they carry the mutation, carriers often have no change in their emotional state or may enjoy some reduction in anxiety. Huntington disease mutation carriers commit suicide most often later in their course, but before they are physically impaired. Similarly, individuals learning that they carry two apolipoprotein E4 alleles, which greatly predisposes them to Alzheimer disease, generally have a reduction in anxiety compared to their pretest situation.

103. Which is the essential neurotransmitter feature of the globus pallidus?
    a. An inhibitory gamma-aminobutyric acid (GABA)-based nucleus
    b. An acetylcholine-generating structure
    c. An excitatory, glutamate-based nucleus.

Answer: a. In contrast, the subthalamic nucleus is an excitatory, glutamate-based nucleus, and the nucleus basalis of Meynert is an acetylcholine-generating structure.

104. During one weekend, a group of 10 high-school freshmen – the entire women's cheerleader team – developed tremulousness of their arms and legs whenever they walked. Also, they began to stutter when they spoke. None of them had fever or any other systemic symptom. Neurologists found no abnormality other than the movements. Which is the most likely diagnosis?
    a. Drug abuse
    b. Psychosis
    c. Mass hysteria
    d. Environmental intoxication

Answer: c. The simultaneous development of incapacitating, apparently involuntary movements or seizures in a group of adolescent girls suggests mass hysteria or mass psychogenic illness. Also, the acute development of stuttering in adults is usually psychogenic. Physicians should consider Sydenham chorea because it is a life-threatening condition that affects groups and females are more susceptible, but these girls simultaneously rather than sequentially developed the movements, which were tremulous and accompanied by stuttering.

105. A 60-year-old priest who has had Parkinson disease for 4 years has begun to develop episodes of kicking and punching lasting several minutes during his sleep. The episodes differ from each other and do not include incontinence or tongue biting. The man has no recollection of them in the morning. Which of the following tests would most likely reveal the diagnosis?
    a. Electroencephalogram (EEG)
    b. MRI
    c. Polysomnogram (PSG)
    d. None of the above

Answer: c. A PSG would probably show that he has REM sleep behavior disorder, which is a common comorbidity of Parkinson disease (see Chapter 17). REM sleep behavior disorder is also a cardinal sign of dementia from

Lewy bodies disease. Both Parkinson disease and Lewy bodies disease are synucleinopathies. This patient's episodes are probably not seizures because they vary and the activity is semipurposeful.

106. In the preceding question, which would be the best treatment?
  a. Clonazepam
  b. Phenytoin
  c. Carbamazepine
  d. Choral hydrate
  e. Clonidine

Answer: a. Clonazepam is highly effective for REM sleep behavior disorder. Given at bedtime, a small dose of clonazepam suppresses most episodes. Antiepileptic drugs produce little or no benefit.

107. A 70-year-old engineer with Parkinson disease for about 5 years has begun to gamble for the first time in his life. Although he has neither won nor lost much money, he has spent inordinate amounts of time in casinos. He feels compelled to gamble, but he enjoys all of its aspects. He had depression 10 years ago, but currently has no disturbance in his mood. Which is the most likely explanation for his new pastime?
  a. Impulse control disorder
  b. Depression
  c. Dementia
  d. Bipolar disorder

Answer: a. Impulse control disorders in Parkinson disease usually entail compulsive self-gratifying behavior, such as pathologic gambling, compulsive sexual behavior, compulsive buying, or binge-eating disorder. Dopamine agonist treatment of Parkinson disease is the most powerful risk factor. Others risk factors include being unmarried, cigarette smoking, and a family history of gambling. It probably stems from dopaminergic medicines' ability to stimulate reward systems. Reducing or stopping dopamine agonists or treating appropriate patients with DBS eliminates the impulse control disorder.

108. Which of the following observations would indicate essential tremor rather than psychogenic tremor in a patient's hand?
  a. The tremor disappears during sleep.
  b. Following the example of the examiner, the patient's affected hand oscillates at a slow speed, then fast speed, and then back to the slow speed.
  c. Administration of a propranolol (a β-blocker) or primidone (a congener of phenobarbital) reduces the tremor.
  d. A physician holding the arm affected by a tremor may see it shift to the other, previously unaffected arm.

Answer: c. Neurologists often have difficulty distinguishing between essential and psychogenic tremor. Also, Parkinson, essential, and psychogenic tremors all stop during sleep. Psychogenic tremors, when *coherent*, affect both arms with identical movements. The examiner can frequently *entrain* a psychogenic tremor to follow a variable frequency. Also, a psychogenic tremor often switches sides when the physician restrains the affected arm. Propranolol or primidone reduces essential tremor but usually not psychogenic tremor.

109. What is the effect of administering allopurinol to Lesch–Nyhan syndrome patients?
  a. Allopurinol decreases serum uric acid concentrations and reduces the dystonia and self-injurious behavior.
  b. Allopurinol decreases serum uric acid concentrations, but it has no effect on the dystonia or self-injurious behavior.
  c. Allopurinol has no effect on serum uric acid concentrations, dystonia, or self-injurious behavior.
  d. Allopurinol has no effect on serum uric acid concentrations, but it reduces the dystonia and self-injurious behavior.

Answer: b. Although allopurinol reduces the serum uric acid concentrations and thus protects the kidneys, it does not alter the neurologic manifestations of Lesch–Nyhan.

Brain Tumors, Metastatic Cancer, and Paraneoplastic Syndromes

With their unpredictable onset and frequently tragic course, brain tumors command unique attention. Moreover, they seem to arise in children and adults in the prime of their life. Because brain tumors may produce depression, thought disorders, or cognitive impairment without any accompanying physical symptoms, they occasionally mimic psychiatric disturbances. Brain tumors remain the *bête noir* of psychiatry.

VARIETIES

Primary Brain Tumors

Primary brain and spinal tumors may arise within the brain or spinal cord tissue (*parenchyma*) itself or from their membrane coverings (*meninges*) (Box 19.1). Pathologists have named the largest group of parenchymal tumors, *gliomas*, after their original cell line, *glial cells*, which normally provide the structural, biochemical, and immunologic support for the central nervous system (CNS). Growing in the substance of the brain, gliomas are described as intraparenchymal (or intra-axial). *Meningeal cells* give rise to the most common primary brain tumors, *meningiomas*. Because these tumors arise from the coverings of the CNS, rather than from actual brain or spinal cord tissue, they grow outside of the brain, i.e., in extraparenchymal (extra-axial) locations. In contrast, CNS neurons rarely form tumors in adults.

Of the various potential etiologies of primary brain tumors, studies have established that only ionizing radiation, certain neurocutaneous disorders (see Chapter 13), and various genetic mutations constitute risk factors. So far, data have not proven that cellphone use constitutes a risk factor.

Gliomas

Gliomas include tumors named for specific cell types: *oligodendrogliomas*, *ependymomas*, and *astrocytomas*. *Oligodendrocytes*, which normally produce the myelin covering that insulates CNS neurons,* may give rise to *oligodendrogliomas*. These tumors, which occur infrequently and

grow slowly, produce manifestations similar to those caused by the more commonly occurring astrocytomas (see later).

Ependymomas arise from *ependymal cells*, which are cells that line the ventricles of the brain and the central canal of the spinal cord. In general, ependymomas arise in the brain of adults, but in the spinal cord of children. When ependymomas arise in the brain, because of their inopportune location, they may obstruct cerebrospinal fluid (CSF) flow and cause hydrocephalus (see later). Depending on type and malignant grade, ependymomas may be treated with surgery, radiation therapy, chemotherapy, or a combination of therapies.

Astrocytomas, which arise from *astrocytes*, originate anywhere in the CNS. When they are low-grade, these tumors do not invade surrounding tissue. They strike children as well as adults and are the most common tumor in children. In children, astrocytomas tend to be relatively benign cystic, noninvasive tumors in the cerebellum. Because neurosurgeons can readily remove an entire cerebellar astrocytoma without causing appreciable sequelae, their cure rate approaches 90%. Sometimes astrocytomas arise in children's brainstems where they invade cranial nerve nuclei and long tracts. Brainstem astrocytomas tend to be highly malignant and not amenable to surgery.

For adults, astrocytomas occur predominantly in the cerebrum, infiltrate extensively, and often degenerate into an even more malignant form: glioblastomas. Total surgical removal of astrocytomas is practical only when the surrounding brain can be sacrificed. For low-grade astrocytomas, combined surgery and radiotherapy prolong life for approximately 10 years.

Glioblastomas, the most malignant variety of astrocytoma, are the most frequently occurring brain tumor. Most importantly, they arise in relatively young individuals: the age of patients at the time of a glioblastoma diagnosis averages only 54 years. Moreover, they notoriously present with changes in personality or behavior rather than physical deficits or seizures, and thus psychiatrists are sometimes the first physicians to encounter an individual who is later found to have a glioblastoma.

Glioblastomas develop almost exclusively in the cerebrum. They not only grow rapidly and relentlessly, they infiltrate widely. Glioblastomas frequently cross the anterior portion of the corpus callosum, the *genu*, and infiltrate the frontal lobes to produce the infamous "butterfly

---

*Schwann cells produce the myelin insulation for the peripheral nervous system (PNS) (see Chapter 5).

glioma" (Figs. 19.1A, 20.8, and 20.20). Their tendency to involve the frontal lobes explains their causing personality or behavior changes.

Radiotherapy, steroids, and chemotherapy may slow the growth of glioblastoma and provide a brief physically comfortable period. Surgical excision rarely eliminates these tumors. In fact, many patients, especially the elderly and those with pronounced neurologic deficits, gain little from treatment. Glioblastoma patients survive for only about 15 months. Moreover, persistence of the tumor and side effects of treatment often produce

incapacitating cognitive and emotional deterioration long before death.

Meningiomas

Arising independently or as an integral part of neurofibromatosis type 1 (see Chapter 13), meningiomas usually create symptoms by compressing the underlying brain or spinal cord (Figs. 19.1B and 20.10). They predominate in middle-aged women. Because they expand slowly, meningiomas often grow quite large before they produce symptoms.

Neurologists frequently detect small meningiomas as an incidental finding on imaging studies of the brain. Small cerebral meningiomas usually remain asymptomatic and innocuous. They rarely require surgical removal. Neurologists generally follow patients harboring meningiomas with periodic clinical evaluation and MRI or CT. Even moderate-sized meningiomas located in certain areas may not produce symptoms. For example, meningiomas over the right frontal lobe can grow to an extraordinary size before they cause problems.

Primary Central Nervous System Lymphoma

In contrast to systemic lymphoma, which commonly spreads to the CNS, *primary central nervous system*

BOX 19.1	Primary Brain Tumors

Gliomas
  Astrocyte tumors
    Astrocytoma
    Glioblastoma
  Oligodendroglioma
  Ependymomas
Meningioma*
Lymphoma
Medulloblastoma
Pituitary adenoma*
Acoustic neuroma*

*Relatively benign histology

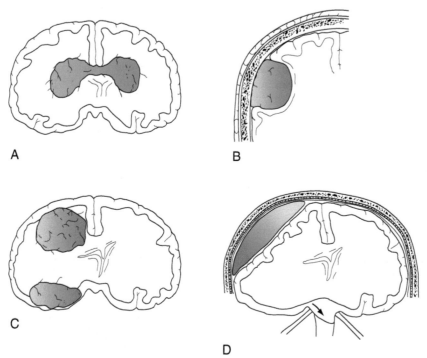

A   B

C   D

FIGURE 19.1 ■ A, A *glioblastoma* – the most malignant form of glioma – typically infiltrates along white matter tracts. Sometimes it spreads through the heavily myelinated corpus callosum in a "butterfly" pattern (see Figs. 20.8 and 20.20). B, Meningiomas arise from the meninges overlying the brain or spinal cord and grow slowly (see Fig. 20.10). They compress and irritate the CNS but almost never infiltrate it. C, *Metastatic tumors*, usually multiple and surrounded by edema, destroy large areas of brain and raise intracranial pressure (see Fig. 20.8). D, A *subdural hematoma*, typically located over one cerebral hemisphere (see Fig. 20.9), compresses the underlying brain and ventricles, and pushes away (shifts) midline structures. Large, acute, rapidly expanding subdural hematomas force the brainstem and ipsilateral oculomotor (third cranial) nerve through the tentorial notch. Such *transtentorial herniation*, which occurs with epidural as well as subdural hematomas (see Chapter 22), constitutes an immediately life-threatening condition. In contrast, small meningiomas and chronic subdural hematomas cause relatively few symptoms because they are extra-axial and exert little mass effect.

lymphoma (*PCNSL*) arises exclusively within the brain or occasionally the spinal cord. An impaired immune system is a powerful risk factor for development of *PCNSL*. Thus, these tumors complicate ataxia-telangiectasia and immunosuppressive therapy for organ transplant as well as acquired immune deficiency syndrome (AIDS).

PCNSL resembles cerebral toxoplasmosis and malignant gliomas in its clinical features, particularly focal neurologic deficits and seizures, and appearance on computed tomography (CT) and magnetic resonance imaging (MRI) (see Fig. 20.11). Steroids, methotrexate, and other chemotherapeutic agents often produce dramatic remissions.

Metastatic Tumors

Systemic tumors metastasize to the brain and spinal cord by hematogenous routes. They cannot spread through a lymphatic system because the brain, unlike almost all other organs, does not have a lymphatic system. Metastatic tumors tend to be multiple, surrounded by edema, and rapidly growing. Although individual tumors may each be small, their combined mass constitutes an oppressive intracerebral burden (Figs. 19.1C and 20.8).

Cancers of the lung, breast, kidney, and skin (malignant melanomas) most often give rise to cerebral metastases. In contrast, because the portal vein diverts metastases to the liver, gastrointestinal, pelvic, and prostatic cancers spread to the brain rarely or only late in their course.

Approximately 15% of all cancer patients initially present with symptoms of cerebral metastases; however, as treatment drives systemic tumors into long remissions, cerebral metastases, which often do not respond to therapy, cause symptoms in a greater proportion of patients. Metastases resist systemic chemotherapy because the blood–brain barrier blocks most medications from attacking them. Moreover, chemotherapy and radiotherapy have relatively little effect against metastatic tumors because, compared to a primary tumor, they are poorly differentiated. On the other hand, the discovery of a metastatic brain tumor is occasionally the first indication that a person has cancer and leads to an earlier diagnosis.

Whatever the origin of cerebral metastases, conventional treatments, such as steroids and radiotherapy, provide palliative care. Stereotactic radiosurgery, which consists of a cobalt device, linear accelerator, or a cyclotron delivering a highly focused beam of radiation to metastases, alone or in conjunction with whole-brain radiation, usually shrinks the tumors. In cases involving a single metastasis, surgeons can help the patient, at least temporarily, by removing it. Nevertheless, most patients with metastatic brain tumors survive less than 9 months.

INITIAL SYMPTOMS

Local Signs

By damaging surrounding tissue, brain tumors usually produce lateralized neurologic deficits, often called "focal signs," such as hemiparesis and dominant or nondominant

hemisphere neuropsychologic disorders (see Chapter 8). Tumors arising in "eloquent" regions – cerebral cortex areas critical to motor or neuropsychologic function, such as Broca's or Wernicke's areas – produce obvious impairments. Tumors that are small, slow-growing, or located in "silent" regions of the brain, such as the right frontal lobe or either of the anterior temporal lobes, notoriously fail to produce symptoms. Tumors that arise from cranial nerves, although rare, almost immediately result in readily recognizable deficits. For example, optic nerve gliomas cause visual loss, and acoustic neuromas cause unilateral progressive hearing loss and tinnitus (see later).

A first-time seizure in an individual older than 60 years frequently heralds the presence of a cerebral tumor. However, because strokes cause seizures nearly as often as tumors, a 60-year-old individual presenting with a first seizure is approximately equally likely to have sustained a stroke as to have developed a brain tumor. Regardless of whether the etiology is a brain tumor or stroke, seizures typically begin as a focal seizure that subsequently undergoes secondary generalization (see Chapter 10).

A brain tumor's tendency to cause seizures also pertains to electroconvulsive therapy (ECT). For example, if a patient harboring a brain tumor were to undergo ECT, the procedure might give rise to multiple, uninterrupted, life-threatening seizures (*status epilepticus*). However, the benefits of ECT might outweigh the risks if the tumor were small enough not to cause neurologic deficits or surrounding cerebral edema. Large brain tumors, on the other hand, constitute an unequivocal problem regarding ECT. Large brain tumors might not only account for depressive symptoms, but also precipitate transtentorial herniation during ECT (Fig. 19.1D). Thus, before their patients undergo ECT, neurologists should order either an MRI or CT.

Signs of Increased Intracranial Pressure

In addition to damaging brain tissue, tumors may raise intracranial pressure (ICP) through many mechanisms. They grow rapidly, occupy a large volume, provoke surrounding edema, obstruct the flow of CSF through the ventricles, or impede CSF reabsorption through the arachnoid villi. Whatever the cause, increased pressure (pressures exceeding 200 mm H_2O) creates symptoms and signs that may add to or supersede local effects.

Headache, while the most common symptom of increased ICP, actually occurs in only one-half of patients. Usually resembling tension-type headache, it most often consists of diffuse, dull, relatively mild pain that initially responds to mild analgesics, including aspirin. Sometimes, a localized or unilateral headache points to a tumor's location and mimics migraine. In any case, as pressure rises, headaches worsen, especially in the early morning hours, and the pain begins to awaken patients from sleep. Increasing ICP eventually produces nausea and vomiting, as well as an intense headache.

Despite the statistic that less than 1 out of 1000 people with headache harbors a brain tumor, both patient and physician frequently have great concerns – spoken or unspoken – that any headache may indicate a brain

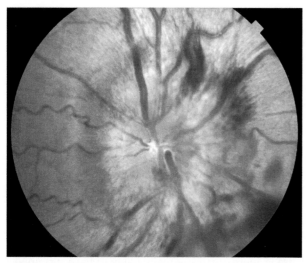

FIGURE 19.2 ■ Papilledema's main features consist of reddening of the optic disk, which loses its distinct margin, and distention of the retinal veins. In addition, the disk is elevated and hemorrhages appear at its edge. (Compare this disk to the normal optic disk in Figure 4.4 and another one with less severe papilledema in Chapter 9, Question 72.)

tumor. These concerns sometimes thwart diagnosis of a less threatening disorder, such as migraine or depression. Neurologists, dispensing with lengthy explanations or reassurances, often simply order a CT or MRI to exclude a tumor and move on with their evaluation and treatment plan.

Another sign of increased intracranial pressure, *papilledema*, occurs as pressure is transmitted along the optic nerves to the optic disks (Fig. 19.2). Although papilledema has a notorious association with brain tumors, it occurs late, if at all. Thus, because only a small proportion of brain tumor patients have papilledema during an initial examination, its absence should not be taken as evidence against the presence of a brain tumor. In fact, among young adults, especially overweight females with menstrual irregularity, *idiopathic intracranial hypertension* (*pseudotumor cerebri*) is much more likely than a brain tumor to explain papilledema (see Chapter 9).

In considering manifestations of brain tumors, meningiomas constitute a special category. Unlike gliomas, as discussed previously, meningiomas are common and usually small; even large ones may remain asymptomatic. Also, they arise and usually remain entirely in extra-axial locations and, when symptomatic, produce characteristic syndromes. For example, a meningioma arising from the falx, a *parasagittal meningioma*, can compress the medial motor cortex and cause spastic paresis of one or both legs. A meningioma arising from the sphenoid wing can damage the adjacent temporal lobe and, because of its proximity to the orbit, cause proptosis and paresis of eye movement. Likewise, an *olfactory groove meningioma* can compress the adjacent olfactory and optic nerves and the overlying frontal lobe (see Foster–Kennedy syndrome, Chapter 4), causing anosmia, unilateral blindness, and, when large, frontal lobe dysfunction (see Chapter 7).

COGNITIVE AND PERSONALITY CHANGES

Direct Effects of Tumors

As a preliminary practical point, most rapidly evolving tumor-related cognitive impairments or personality changes result from a glioblastoma. Another point is that tumors in the frontal lobe produce personality changes consisting of psychomotor retardation, emotional dulling, loss of initiative, poor insight, and reduced capacity to execute complex mental tasks. This clinical picture, like that of frontotemporal dementia (see Chapter 7), consists of disturbances in behavior and affect that overshadow cognitive impairments, and those disturbances in turn overshadow physical impairments.

In a somewhat opposite effect, frontal lobe tumors sometimes impair normal inhibitory systems. Patients with lack of inhibition (*disinhibition*) may overreact to an irritation, liberally use profanities, cry with little provocation, jump excitedly from topic to topic, and speak without tolerating interruptions. By way of contrast, parietal or occipital lobe tumors, as well as right-sided far anterior frontal lesions, unless they cause increased ICP, have relatively little effect on mood or cognitive function.

Overall, with numerous potential causes, depression is a frequent comorbidity of a brain tumor. When thought to be directly secondary to the effects of neoplasm, a difficult determination to make, the DSM-5 classifies this as Depressive Disorder Due to Another Medical Condition. Depressive symptoms not only arise soon after diagnosis, but they increase in prevalence and severity during the ensuing illness, and predict a poor quality of life.

In brain tumor cases, a psychiatrist might attempt to determine the patient's mood, cognitive capacity, neurologic deficits, and iatrogenic factors. With no standard guidelines for prescribing antidepressants or other psychotropics, psychiatrists must approach each situation entirely on an individual basis. In addition to prescribing a psychotropic and precluding ECT, psychiatrists might offer advice on alterations in mental status, guide pain management, assist in appointing a health-care proxy, and help with decisions about end-of-life care.

Medication and Other Treatment

Opioids for cancer-related pain can cause delirium and undesirable changes in mood. On the other hand, insufficient opioids can lead to suffering, insomnia, and drug-seeking behavior. Benzodiazepines and hypnotics help control pain, anxiety, and insomnia, but may themselves cause mental dullness, confusion, and disruption of the sleep–wake cycle.

Other medications likely to induce mental status changes in cancer patients are antiepileptic drugs (AEDs), steroids, antiemetics, and antihistamines. Although physicians can usually predict potential physical side effects of common medications, their mental side effects in cancer patients often arise insidiously and unexpectedly. For example, patients with undiagnosed liver metastases may have slowed metabolism of medications leading to their unexpected accumulation. Similarly, because cancer patients often have lost body mass, physicians may inadvertently prescribe relatively large doses of a medicine. When cancer involves several organs, various specialists may each order different medicines that not only cause mental status abnormalities, but also may adversely interact.

Many chemotherapy agents do not cause mental status changes because they cannot penetrate the blood–brain barrier. A notable exception occurs when physicians administer methotrexate intrathecally (into the subarachnoid space, usually through a lumbar puncture [LP] or into the ventricular space through a special catheter called an *Ommaya reservoir*) because it often causes adverse CNS effects. Although intrathecal methotrexate, which is frequently administered in conjunction with cranial radiotherapy, may protect children from leukemic cells invading the CNS, it often induces short-term confusional states and occasionally permanent learning disabilities and personality changes. Other systemic chemotherapies, such as temozolomide for glioblastoma, are able to cross the blood–brain barrier in order to reach their target cells.

When chemotherapy penetrates the barrier and damages oligodendrocytes, the most vulnerable CNS cells, short- and long-term sequelae can evolve. After 3 months to 5 years following treatment, loss of the oligodendrocytes leads to demyelination. Cancer survivors who sustain chemotherapy-induced CNS demyelination typically have cognitive decline and personality changes, paresis and spasticity, and ataxia and gait impairment – alone or in combination. Their MRIs show the demyelination.

Radiotherapy sometimes causes inflammatory arteritis and necrosis, depending on the total dose and rapidity with which it is administered. Small strokes, which begin to accumulate 6 to 18 months after a course of radiotherapy, lead to a stepwise progression of cognitive impairments and personality changes resembling vascular cognitive impairment (see Chapter 7). Hemiparesis and dysarthria often accompany neuropsychologic changes. MRIs of patients with radiation-induced cognitive impairments typically reveal white matter changes (*leukoencephalopathy*). Overall, radiotherapy induces more cognitive impairment than most chemotherapy agents.

Whole-brain radiation administered to children for acute leukemia or brain tumors may result not only in cognitive impairment, but also in problems from hypothalamic–pituitary deficiency, particularly growth retardation, developmental delay, and late, incomplete puberty. Compared to young and middle-aged adults, children are more susceptible to radiation-induced cognitive impairment. Current experimental protocols are investigating protection (shielding) of the hippocampi during radiotherapy as well as the use of memantine (Namenda) for postradiotherapy cognitive impairment.

Infections and Organ Failure

Immunosuppressive agents, radiotherapy, and various open ports, such as intravenous lines and urinary catheters, leave cancer patients susceptible to systemic infection. Bacteria, fungi, and opportunistic organisms invade and proliferate, without provoking an immunologic response, and cause sepsis.

In addition, systemic cancer, infections, and various treatments often cause renal, pulmonary, or hepatic failure. Alone or together, sepsis and organ failure often lead to delirium. Perhaps owing to comorbid depression, delirium in cancer patients may consist primarily of apathy, reticence, and sleep disturbance.

Infective agents sometimes invade the CNS while sparing other organs. Because cancer patients often cannot respond with fever or leukocytosis to an infection, they may not show the usual markers. In fact, only 5% of cancer patients with meningitis will have the classic triad of fever, nuchal rigidity, and encephalopathy. Also, because of their immunocompromised state, cancer patients are susceptible to opportunistic infections. For example, *progressive multifocal leukoencephalopathy* (*PML*) results from a polyomavirus that attacks CNS myelin. Indeed, CSF analysis in PML cases yields JC virus DNA. Usually complicating the late course of an illness, PML causes dementia and variable physical impairments, but not delirium, fever, or leukocytosis. PML has also complicated AIDS and immunosuppression therapy, including the MS treatment natalizumab (see Chapters 7, 15, and 20).

Ectopic Hormone Production

Sometimes tumors synthesize and excrete hormones, *ectopic hormones*, in unregulated, large quantities. For example, tumors may produce parathyroid hormone that causes hypercalcemia, or produce antidiuretic hormone secretion (SIADH) that causes hyponatremia. Ectopic hormone-induced metabolic aberrations often cause delirium and, if severe enough, seizures.

OTHER TREATMENT-INDUCED SYMPTOMS

In contrast to chemotherapy-induced CNS demyelination, chemotherapy-induced peripheral neuropathy, from damage to either axons or the myelin-generating Schwann cells, usually occurs during or shortly after chemotherapy. Although severe enough at times to cause paresis and painful sensory impairment, chemotherapy-induced neuropathy tends to improve after exposure ceases.

In an acute, often debilitating side effect, chemotherapy induces nausea and vomiting (*chemotherapy-induced emesis*). This problem usually stems from chemotherapy agents' triggering the brain's *chemoreceptor zone* and its adjacent *vomiting center*. These zones are located in the *area postrema* of the medulla, which is one of the few regions of the brain unprotected by the blood–brain barrier. The absence of a blood–brain barrier leaves the chemoreceptor zone freely accessible to any blood-borne substance. Thus, if people inadvertently ingest toxins, such as in poisonous mushrooms, they will immediately vomit. From a medical perspective, morphine, heroin, and high doses of levodopa, as well as several chemotherapeutic agents, activate the chemoreceptor zone and induce vomiting. On the other hand, both dopamine receptor-blocking agents and 5-HT$_3$ antagonists prevent chemotherapy-induced nausea and vomiting (see Chapter 21).

Radiotherapy of the spine or mediastinum can strike the spinal cord and cause spinal cord radiation necrosis (*radiation myelitis*). Similarly, radiation of pituitary tumors may lead to necrosis of the adjacent pituitary gland. In this situation, radiation scatter may also cause necrosis of the nearby medial-inferior temporal lobes. Young adult survivors of childhood non-CNS cancers, such as Hodgkin disease that required radiation of the chest and neck, also have an increased incidence of stroke. Their strokes occur because the extracranial portions of the carotid and vertebral arteries develop radiation-induced fibrosis that occludes the vessels.

PARANEOPLASTIC SYNDROMES

Systemic cancer sometimes causes neurologic syndromes not by directly invading the nervous system, but by inciting antibody-mediated immune responses directed against the CNS, PNS, or neuromuscular junction. Neurologists previously aptly called these disorders "remote effects of carcinoma," but now they term them *paraneoplastic syndromes*. Paraneoplastic syndromes probably begin with the patients generating antibodies directed against a tumor's antigens. The antibodies cross-react with neurons' intracellular components, cell surfaces, or synaptic receptors. Antibodies involved in paraneoplastic syndromes include, among others, those directed against voltage-gated potassium channels (VGKC) and N-methyl-d-aspartate (NMDA) receptors (Table 19.1). Of the numerous paraneoplastic syndromes, three are particularly relevant: cerebellar degeneration, limbic encephalitis, and Lambert–Eaton myasthenic syndrome (LEMS). Their pathophysiology likely represents "molecular mimicry" that is analogous to anti-streptococcal antibodies cross-reacting with basal ganglia to cause Sydenham chorea (see Chapter 18). Other paraneoplastic syndromes include sensory *neuronopathy*, which is dysfunction of the peripheral sensory nerve cell body; *stiff-person syndrome* (see Chapter 21); *opsoclonus-myoclonus*, a unique syndrome of eye, limb, and truncal movement abnormalities most commonly associated with the pediatric tumor *neuroblastoma*; and *dermatomyositis* and *polymyositis* (see Chapter 6).

Symptoms of paraneoplastic syndromes often appear several months before or after the discovery of an underlying tumor. When neurologists diagnose a paraneoplastic syndrome in a patient without a known malignancy, they order tests to search for one. Their evaluation may include blood tests for known tumor markers; CT of the chest, abdomen, and pelvis; colonoscopy; mammography or testicular ultrasound; and even positron emission tomography (PET), a nuclear medicine study that may identify very small tumors not seen on other imaging modalities. If physicians detect an underlying tumor and patients undergo surgery or chemotherapy that removes or shrinks it, paraneoplastic syndromes usually subside. Alternatively, immunosuppressive treatments, such as steroids, plasmapheresis, or intravenous immunoglobulin, may reduce the symptoms.

TABLE 19.1 Paraneoplastic Syndromes

Syndrome	Tumor	Associated Antibodies
Cerebellar degeneration	SCLC Gynecologic Breast Lymphoma Thymoma	Anti-Hu Anti-Yo Anti-Ri Anti-CV2
Limbic encephalitis	SCLC Testes Breast Ovarian teratoma Thymoma	Anti-Hu Anti-Ma Anti-Amphiphysin Anti-NMDA receptor Anti-VGKC Anti-GAD
Lambert–Eaton myasthenic syndrome	SCLC	Anti-VGCC
Sensory neuronopathy	SCLC	Anti-Hu
Stiff-person syndrome	SCLC Breast Thymoma	Anti-GAD Anti-Amphiphysin
Opsoclonus-myoclonus	Neuroblastoma SCLC Gynecologic Breast	Anti-Ri
Dermatomyositis/polymyositis	Ovary Pancreas Stomach Colorectal Non-Hodgkin lymphoma	No associated antibody

Abbreviations: SCLC – small-cell lung cancer; NMDA – N-methyl-D-aspartate; VGKC – voltage-gated potassium channel; GAD – glutamic acid decarboxylase; VGCC – voltage-gated calcium channel.

Cerebellar Degeneration

The most well-established paraneoplastic syndrome consists of ataxia, dysmetria, dysarthria, and/or nystagmus attributable to cerebellar degeneration due to an underlying neoplasm. A gynecologic cancer, lymphoma, or, most often, small-cell tumor of the lung usually incites it. In fact, cerebellar degeneration and other paraneoplastic syndromes complicate 1% to 3% of cases of small-cell lung cancer. In paraneoplastic cerebellar degeneration, blood tests reveal *antineuronal antibodies*, such as anti-Yo, anti-Hu or anti-CV2 antibodies, directed against the relevant CNS neurons.

Paraneoplastic Limbic Encephalitis

Limbic encephalitis, as a paraneoplastic phenomenon, results from antibody-mediated limbic system inflammation. As its clinical hallmark, over several days to several weeks, individuals develop pronounced memory impairment (amnesia) often accompanied by irritability and behavioral disturbances. In addition, temporal lobe inflammation causes focal seizures with impairment of consciousness or awareness. Limbic encephalitis often heralds small-cell carcinoma of the lung or testicular cancer, but it may also be a manifestation of occult, non-malignant disorders.

Whatever the underlying disorder, neurologic tests usually reflect temporal lobe abnormalities. MRI may show atrophy of the mesial temporal lobes and an electroencephalogram (EEG) should show spikes or slow-waves emanating from the temporal lobes. Serum often contains anti-VGKC, anti-Hu, anti-Ma2, or other antibodies that react with limbic system neurons.

Anti-NMDA Receptor Encephalitis

Anti-NMDA receptor encephalitis, which results from antibodies directed against NMDA receptors, is a variety of paraneoplastic limbic encephalitis. It typically presents, like other forms of limbic encephalitis, with several days of progressively severe amnesia and behavioral disturbances. Then psychosis, seizures, involuntary movements, and autonomic instability often occur and eclipse the prodrome. This disorder typically occurs in young adult women. Neurologists might initially suspect herpes simplex encephalitis, phencyclidine (PCP) or other illicit drug intoxication, an anti-VGKC antibody paraneoplastic syndrome, or variant Creutzfeldt–Jakob – or an acute psychosis. To confuse the diagnostic picture further, a small minority of patients may present with isolated psychiatric episodes.

In most cases the MRI initially shows no abnormalities; however, the CSF shows a lymphocytic pleocytosis. The CSF and serum contain antibodies to NMDA receptors. The antibody concentration, greater in the serum than CSF, roughly correlates with the severity of the illness. The CSF also contains oligoclonal bands, as it does in the CSF of cases of multiple sclerosis and other CNS inflammatory illnesses (see Chapter 15).

The classic example of anti-NMDA receptor encephalitis consists of amnesia with mood change and depersonalization, involuntary movements, and seizures in a young woman eventually found to be harboring an ovarian teratoma. Overall, almost 50% of young adult women with this disorder harbor an ovarian teratoma, which presumably has triggered an antibody response to its neural tissue. While an ovarian teratoma is the most common neoplasm associated with anti-NMDA receptor encephalitis, physicians have implicated other neoplasms in a minority of patients. Finally, this syndrome can appear as a pure autoimmune disorder without any underlying tumor. Some case series have linked this diagnosis to prior herpes simplex encephalitis. However, like other paraneoplastic conditions, anti-NMDA receptor encephalitis usually presents before the discovery of a patient's neoplasm. Thus, close surveillance for a tumor is warranted in patients who initially seem to be cancer-free.

Lambert–Eaton Myasthenic Syndrome

In *Lambert–Eaton myasthenic syndrome* (*LEMS*), small-cell lung cancer or occasionally a different neoplasm, provokes antibodies directed against voltage-gated calcium channels (VGCC) on the presynaptic side of the neuromuscular junction. Influx of calcium ions through VGCC

into the motor nerve terminal is required for release of acetylcholine (ACh) (see Chapter 6); by blocking these channels, the antibodies prevent release of ACh and cause proximal limb muscle weakness, which patients briefly overcome with repetitive actions. Their weakness has different qualities and different distribution than myasthenia gravis – the well-known disorder of the ACh receptors on the postsynaptic side of the neuromuscular junction (see Chapter 6). Patients with myasthenia primarily have facial and extraocular muscle weakness that worsens on exertion. The presence of antibodies to VGCC and nerve conduction studies that show an incremental response with exercise readily distinguish LEMS from myasthenia.

DIAGNOSTIC TESTS FOR BRAIN TUMORS

Physicians should consider brain tumors and related conditions without waiting for a patient to have deficits. They should not rely exclusively on the mental status examination to distinguish between psychiatric disorders and brain tumors. In addition, commonplace complaints of fatigue, weight loss, menstrual irregularity, or infertility might prompt evaluation for pituitary insufficiency.

Neurologists generally order CT or MRI of the brain, admittedly liberally, for patients who have intellectual decline, those over 50 years who show substantial emotional changes, most adults with headaches not attributable to migraine, cluster, or giant-cell arteritis (see Chapter 9), or, as previously discussed, those who are particularly concerned. Neurologists often also suggest CT or MRI for patients with any new psychiatric illness severe enough to warrant hospitalization or ECT.

CT remains a satisfactory screening procedure in many situations (see Chapter 20). It is sensitive to most tumors and other mass lesions, rapidly performed, relatively inexpensive, permissible for patients with pacemakers, and tolerable for most with claustrophobia. It remains preferable for detecting acute intracranial bleeding, including subarachnoid hemorrhage, subdural hematomas, and intracerebral hemorrhages. CT will also detect fractures and other abnormalities of the skull. On the other hand, its ionizing radiation, certainly in children, carries a risk of inducing a malignancy (see Chapter 20).

MRI, especially with gadolinium infusion, remains superior in detecting lesions that are small or located in areas encased by bone, such as optic gliomas, acoustic neuromas, pituitary adenomas, and some posterior fossa tumors. It can readily demonstrate white matter abnormalities associated with brain tumors, such as radiation necrosis, chemotherapy-induced leukoencephalopathy, and PML. If CT suggests a tumor, MRI still remains necessary to determine its exact location, internal structure, and involvement of surrounding brain. PET can help differentiate cerebral radiation necrosis from tumor recurrence.

For detecting tumors or other mass lesions, an EEG, especially in comparison to CT and MRI, is simply inappropriate. Nevertheless, in patients with brain tumors or other cancers, it remains a good diagnostic test for

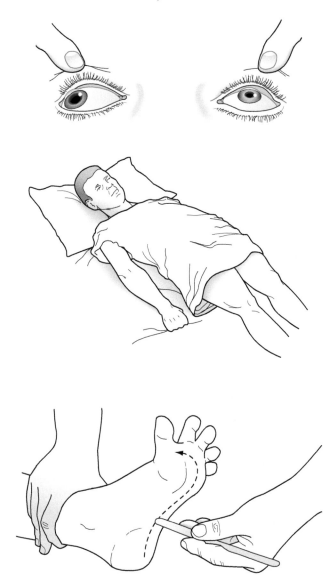

FIGURE 19.3 ■ A patient with *transtentorial herniation* from a right-sided subdural hematoma (Fig. 19.1D) has coma, decerebrate (extensor) posture, Babinski signs, and a dilated right pupil. The right temporal lobe compressing the right (ipsilateral) oculomotor nerve and brainstem through the tentorial notch causes this catastrophe.

delirium, particularly hepatic encephalopathy. An EEG may also assist in the diagnosis of seizures.

Neurologists generally do not perform an LP to analyze CSF when they suspect a brain tumor or other intracranial mass lesion because, in such cases, the CSF profile lacks a distinctive profile and rarely reveals malignant cells (see Chapter 20). More important, with large, expanding supratentorial mass lesions, an LP can precipitate transtentorial herniation (Figs. 19.1D and 19.3). Neurologists perform an LP when patients may have carcinomatous or chronic infectious meningitis. Testing requires large volumes of CSF for cytology, chemistry studies, and microbial antigens, cultures, and polymerase chain reaction. In an exception to the general rule of not performing an LP in patients with a cerebral mass lesion, neurologists may perform one to test the CSF for Epstein–Barr (EB) virus in an AIDS patient found to have

a cerebral tumor because a positive result would be suggestive of cerebral lymphoma and potentially obviate surgery. Similarly, they may perform one in cases of suspected PML to look for JC virus DNA.

RELATED CONDITIONS

Pituitary Adenomas

Although clinicians often view *pituitary adenomas* as brain tumors, their symptoms, histology, and treatment differ considerably from those of glioblastomas, astrocytomas, and meningiomas. In classic studies, the usual manifestations of pituitary adenomas included profound mental, physical, and visual loss; however, those studies reported on patients whose symptoms resulted from large pituitary tumors that produced extraordinary levels of hormones, expanded out of the sella to encroach on the adjacent temporal lobes and optic chiasm, and obstructed the flow of CSF through the third ventricle. Physicians now routinely diagnose pituitary adenomas early in their course, while they remain microscopic in size, by using MRI and blood tests for hormone levels.

In both men and women, prolactinomas produce infertility, decreased libido, headache, and eventually characteristic visual field deficits. Additionally, in women, they produce amenorrhea and galactorrhea, and in men, erectile dysfunction and gynecomastia. Because loss of libido encompasses the nonsexual as well as sexual aspects of their lives, patients with pituitary adenomas may appear depressed or cognitively impaired.

Most pituitary adenomas are either prolactinomas, which secrete prolactin, or *chromophobe adenomas*, which do not. Although prolactinomas usually remain microscopic, they sometimes grow larger than 10 mm, in which case neurologists consider them macroadenomas. Pituitary adenomas of that size may exert pressure on surrounding structures (Fig. 19.4). Their upward pressure on the diaphragma sellae usually causes bitemporal and generalized headache. Compressing the optic chiasm, which is above the diaphragma sellae, causes the visual field deficits. Initially they cause bitemporal superior quadrantanopia and, with further enlargement, bitemporal hemianopia (see Fig. 12.8).

MRI reveals almost all pituitary adenomas. Serum prolactin level determination usually shows elevations with prolactinomas and some chromophobe adenomas. Visual field testing helps detect those that have expanded out of the sella. Treatment varies with tumor type and size, presence of visual deficit, and institutional expertise, but the usual options include radiation, trans-sphenoidal microsurgery, and, with prolactin-secreting tumors, a dopamine agonist, such as bromocriptine or cabergoline. As in a previous caveat, treating large tumors with radiation or craniotomy risks causing panhypopituitarism and, from temporal lobe damage, memory impairment and seizures.

Less commonly occurring pituitary growths secrete *growth hormone*, which can cause *acromegaly*, or *adrenocorticotropin hormone (ACTH)*, which can lead to *Cushing syndrome*. In addition to disfiguring patients, these tumors

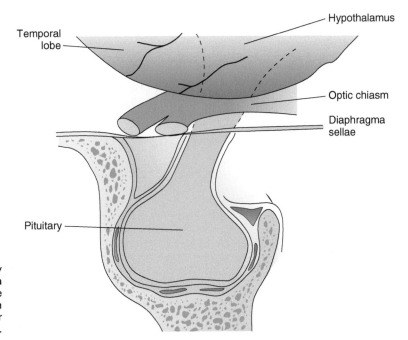

FIGURE 19.4 ■ Pituitary adenomas grow laterally and inferiorly against the walls of the sella turcica and upward against the *diaphragma sellae*. Large adenomas compress the optic chiasm, which causes a distinctive bitemporal hemianopia or bitemporal superior quadrantanopia (see Fig. 12.8).

may cause endocrine changes that produce depression and, rarely, psychosis. These tumors usually remain as collections of hyperplastic cells rather than forming adenoma-like masses that encroach on the optic chiasm or cause headache.

In contrast to these relatively benign pituitary lesions, *craniopharyngiomas* are large, calcified, cystic, congenital lesion derived from Rathke's pouch that arise in children as well as in adults. Unlike pituitary adenomas, craniopharyngiomas grow within the hypothalamus, which is located above the diaphragma sellae (see Fig. 19.4). Because craniopharyngiomas cause endocrine deficiency, affected children routinely have delayed or incomplete physical, sexual, and mental maturation; adults tend to have impaired libido, amenorrhea, and apathy; and both children and adults develop diabetes insipidus. When craniopharyngiomas press downward on the optic chiasm, the pressure causes optic atrophy and, as with pituitary tumors, bitemporal hemianopia. If the tumors completely compress the third ventricle, the obstructive hydrocephalus that ensues leads to papilledema with headache, nausea, and vomiting – classic signs of increased intracranial pressure. Removing these lesions frequently requires extensive surgery and radiotherapy.

Postpartum pituitary necrosis, widely known as *Sheehan syndrome*, also causes pituitary insufficiency. Although radiotherapy and several other conditions might cause pituitary infarction, Sheehan syndrome typically results from obstetric deliveries complicated by massive blood loss. In overt cases of Sheehan syndrome, postpartum women fail to lactate, remain hypotensive, lose weight, and undergo regression of secondary sexual characteristics. In subtle cases, which are more common, several months to several years after delivering, women have only scant menses, diminished libido, and constant weakness. Physicians may misinterpret their symptoms as postpartum depression or chronic fatigue syndrome.

Acoustic Neuromas

When cells covering the acoustic (eighth cranial) nerve proliferate, they form a distinctive tumor – the *acoustic neuroma* or *schwannoma*. (The term "acoustic neuroma," however, is a misnomer because Schwann cells, not neurons, proliferate.) Growing from the vestibular division of the acoustic nerve, schwannomas usually arise between the internal auditory canal and cerebellopontine angle where they may compress adjacent structures, particularly the fifth (trigeminal) and seventh (facial) cranial nerves as well as damage the eight nerve. Although relatively benign, these tumors cause hearing impairment – predominantly loss of speech discrimination – and tinnitus. Although they usually arise from the vestibular division of the nerve, these tumors rarely cause imbalance or vertigo. If acoustic neuromas grow to compress the fifth cranial nerve, patients experience sensory symptoms in their face, ranging from tingling to trigeminal neuralgia-like pain. If these tumors compress the seventh cranial nerve, patients lose facial muscle strength.

Most acoustic neuromas grow unilaterally and spontaneously. Bilateral acoustic neuromas, in contrast, characteristically are a manifestation of neurofibromatosis type 2 (NF2), an autosomal dominant disorder of chromosome 22 (see Chapter 13). Gadolinium-enhanced MRI (see Fig. 20.27), auditory tests, and brainstem auditory evoked responses (see BAERs, Chapter 15) detect acoustic neuromas. Stereotactic radiosurgery with a gamma knife or linear accelerator treatments can remove acoustic neuromas while preserving most if not all hearing and facial strength.

Spine Metastases

Lung, breast, and other cancers often metastasize to the vertebrae and then grow into the spinal epidural space

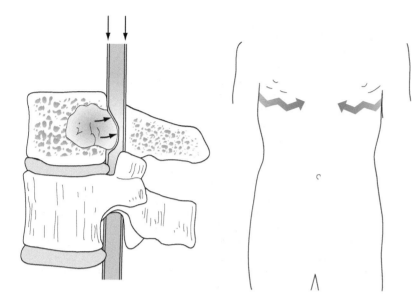

FIGURE 19.5 ■ *Left,* Vertebral metastases typically grow posteriorly to encroach on the spinal *epidural space* (*arrows*). *Epidural metastases* in the cervical and thoracic regions may cause spinal cord compression, which can result in paraplegia or quadriplegia, loss of sensation (hypesthesia) below the level of the lesion, and incontinence. Epidural metastases in the lumbar region may compress the cauda equina (see Fig. 5.12). *Right,* Patients have "local pain" from destruction of the vertebrae and band-like "radiating pain," in the dermatome of the affected nerve root (*jagged arrows*). The location of the pain and level of the hypalgesia indicate the site of an epidural metastatic tumor (see Fig. 2.16).

(Fig. 19.5). *Epidural metastases* characteristically cause severe pain not only in the affected region (local pain), but also along the path of the affected nerve roots (radicular pain). For example, patients with thoracic spine metastases typically have interscapular spine pain that radiates around the chest in a bandlike pattern. Similarly, patients with lumbar spine metastases suffer from lower back pain that, unlike simple musculoskeletal pain, radiates down the legs.

If cervical or thoracic epidural metastases grow large enough, they compress the spinal cord. Metastatic spinal cord compression causes not only local and radicular pain, but also quadriplegia or paraplegia, loss of sensation below the lesion, and urinary and fecal incontinence (see Chapters 2 and 16). In addition, although patients typically retain their cognitive capacity, their pain, physical incapacity, and the undeniable progression of their illness often lead to depression.

Early diagnosis and treatment may prevent paraplegia; however, once this dreaded complication sets in, patients almost never regain their ability to walk. Neurologists usually rely on an MRI to confirm their clinical impression. Therapy consists of steroids, radiation, and, sometimes, decompressive laminectomy.

Other Causes of Limb Weakness in Cancer Patients

Certain cancers trigger paraneoplastic inflammatory conditions that affect the PNS solely, such as LEMS. In addition, lung, breast, ovarian, gastric, and other solid tumors provoke *dermatomyositis,* which consists of diffuse, proximal muscle weakness, muscle tenderness, and a heliotrope rash on the face and extensor skin surfaces. While no antibody is associated with dermatomyositis, its appearance often heralds the diagnosis of neoplastic disease, making it another example of a paraneoplastic condition.

Sometimes weakness is iatrogenic. For example, prolonged use of steroids, whether as a medication or an illicit bodybuilding supplement, may result in *steroid*

myopathy or collapse of a hip or vertebrae. Similarly, long-term use of diuretics without potassium supplements results in *hypokalemic myopathy.* Various chemotherapy agents, such as vincristine, cause *polyneuropathy* that often includes a disturbing sensory component (see Chapter 5). Radiation therapy also can be injurious to neural tissues.

In contrast to the generalized weakness of these polyneuropathies, cancer-induced *mononeuropathies* – injuries of individual peripheral nerves – cause paresis and sensory loss limited to the distribution of those nerves (see Table 5.1). With cancer-induced loss of muscle bulk and subcutaneous fat, mild to moderate pressure – even the patient's own weight – compresses peripheral nerves deprived of their protective cushions. Compression injuries most often damage the sciatic, fibular, and radial nerves when bedridden patients remain in one position in bed or secured in a wheelchair for prolonged periods, or are pulled onto stretchers. Sometimes misplaced injections or other accidents injure these nerves.

When lung or breast cancer invades the nearby brachial plexus or pelvic cancer invades the neighboring lumbosacral plexus, patients suffer excruciating pain as well as paresis. Because tumor cells have actually invaded the nerves, routine treatments, such as radiotherapy and opioids, will provide only limited analgesia. Physicians must prescribe treatments for neuropathic pain (see Chapter 14).

DISORDERS THAT RESEMBLE BRAIN TUMORS

Strokes, like tumors, occur predominantly in older people and cause physical deficits, seizures, and cognitive impairment. Nevertheless, the course, many symptoms, and results of imaging studies of strokes and tumors differ so much that, in the final analysis, physicians almost always arrive at the correct diagnosis.

Subdural hematomas also occur frequently and mimic brain tumors. Head trauma is the most common cause of intracranial bleeding in the potential space between the dura (the thick layer of the meninges) and the underlying brain – the subdural space (Figs. 19.1D and 20.9). Because subdural bleeding originates from veins, its pressure is low and volume relatively small. After the bleeding forms a hematoma, fluid accumulates and the collection enlarges. During subsequent weeks, subdural hematomas exert an increasingly greater mass effect that presses broadly against one or both cerebral hemispheres. Subdural hematomas produce headaches, confusion, personality change, dementia, and other nonspecific symptoms of generalized cerebral dysfunction – much more than lateralized signs.

For several reasons, older individuals are especially vulnerable to subdural hematomas. They tend to fall and suffer head injury. They often take aspirin or other medicines that have an anticoagulant effect. Once intracranial bleeding starts, it continues unchecked because an atrophied brain cannot compress the bleeding vessels. Also, because subdural hematomas typically produce insidious nonspecific symptoms and signs rather than lateralized ones, the patient and family may fail to appreciate the significance of headaches and nonspecific symptoms.

Neurosurgeons are able to easily evacuate subdural hematomas, but frequently a conservative approach suffices. Prompt diagnosis and treatment usually restore cerebral function. In other words, subdural hematomas represent a correctable form of dementia.

Arteriovenous malformations (*AVMs*) – a potential source of headaches and seizures, as well as intracerebral hemorrhage – consist of congenital vascular anomalies of large veins and arteries directly joined without the normal intervening capillary bed. Although a neurosurgeon might be able to resect the AVM, the surgery generally requires removal of the normal surrounding brain. Interventional neuroradiologists may obliterate the malformation by infusing epoxies or solid particles. If that procedure only shrinks the AVM, it will still be more amenable to neurosurgical resection.

Because intracranial bleeding is common and an emergency situation, physicians should know the causes and implications of bleeding into the different intracranial regions: Venous bleeding, usually under low pressure, generally accumulates in the subdural space. Head trauma-induced arterial bleeding, which is under high pressure, collects in the epidural space. Rupture of a berry aneurysm, which is also under high pressure, leads to bleeding in the subarachnoid hemorrhage. Uncontrolled hypertension or cocaine use may lead to bleeding in the basal ganglia, thalamus, pons, or cerebellum. AVMs may bleed into any part of the brain.

Bacterial *abscesses* usually result from sepsis originating in intravenous drug abuse, dental procedures, sinusitis, endocarditis, or immunodeficiency. They typically present with signs of a cerebral mass lesion rather than a systemic infection. In their clinical presentation and imaging studies, abscesses resemble brain tumors (see Fig. 20.15).

Although bacteria are the infecting organisms in most abscesses, *toxoplasmosis* is usually responsible in patients with AIDS. Cerebral toxoplasmosis differs from bacterial abscesses in that it occurs in multiple sites, but concentrates in the basal ganglia. Thus, unlike almost all other mass lesions, toxoplasmosis routinely presents with chorea, hemiballismus, or other involuntary movement disorder.

Patients with *neurocysticercosis* usually have multiple intracerebral cysts that have originated from a gastrointestinal tapeworm (*Taenia solium*) infestation. Although each cyst may be small, their total number occupies a considerable space. They also tend to block CSF flow and thus cause obstructive hydrocephalus. Moreover, as they die, their fluid contents leak and provoke an inflammatory response in the surrounding brain. This irritation, as well as their mass effect, often causes seizures. Almost all patients show cognitive impairment and about 13% have dementia. Because cysticercosis is endemic in Central and South America and the Indian subcontinent, immigrants from these regions often harbor neurocysticercosis. CT and MRI readily detect the cysts (see Fig. 20.12). Whatever the antibiotic regimen, neurologists almost always add AEDs.

Tuberculosis causes intracerebral masses, *tuberculomas*, particularly in AIDS patients and citizens of the Indian subcontinent. CT and MRI can also detect tuberculomas, even when the clinical evaluation does not suggest the diagnosis.

As another disorder that mimics brain tumor, *idiopathic intracranial hypertension* (*pseudotumor cerebri*) produces headache, papilledema, and, in severe cases, sixth cranial nerve palsies; however, it does not affect cognitive capacity or produce seizures (see above and Chapter 9).

REFERENCES

Barry, H., Hardiman, O., Healy, D. G., et al. (2011). Anti-NMDA receptor encephalitis: an important differential diagnosis in psychosis. *The British Journal of Psychiatry*, Epub, 1–2.

Darnell, R. B., & Posner, J. B. (2003). Paraneoplastic syndromes involving the nervous system. *The New England Journal of Medicine, 349*, 1543–1554.

DeAndrade, D. C., Rodrigues, C. I., & Abraham, R. (2010). Cognitive impairment and dementia in neurocysticercosis. *Neurology, 74*, 1288–1295.

DeSena, A., Graves, D., Warnack, W., et al. (2014). Herpes simplex encephalitis as a potential cause of anti-*N*-methyl-D-aspartate receptor antibody encephalitis. *Journal of the American Medical Association Neurology, 71*, 344–346.

Duffner, P. K. (2004). Long-term effects of radiation therapy on cognitive and endocrine function in children with leukemia and brain tumors. *Neurology, 10*, 293–310.

Grauss, F., & Dalmau, J. (2012). Paraneoplastic neurological syndromes. *Current Opinion in Neurology, 25*, 795–801.

Kayser, M. S., Kohler, C. G., & Dalmau, J. (2010). Psychiatric manifestations of paraneoplastic disorders. *The American Journal of Psychiatry, 16667*, 1039–1050.

Kayser, M. S., Titulaer, M. J., Gresa-Aribas, N., et al. (2013). Frequency and characteristics of isolated psychiatric episodes in anti-*N*-methyl-D-aspartate receptor encephalitis. *Journal of the American Medical Association Neurology, 70*, 1133–1139.

Litofsky, N. S., Farace, E., Anderson, F., et al. (2004). Depression in patients with high-grade glioma: Results of the Glioma Outcomes Project. *Neurosurgery, 54*, 358–366.

Martel, S., De Angelis, F., Lapointe, E., et al. (2014). Paraneoplastic neurologic syndromes: clinical presentation and management. *Current Problems in Cancer, 38*, 115–134.

Morris, B., Partap, S., Yeom, K., et al. (2009). Cerebrovascular disease in childhood cancer survivors. *Neurology, 73*, 1906–1913.

Pelletier, G., Verhoef, M. J., Khatri, N., et al. (2002). Quality of life in brain tumor patients: The relative contributions of depression, fatigue, emotional distress, and existential issues. *Journal of Neuro-Oncology, 57*, 41–49.

Raizer, J., & Parsa, A. (2015). Current understanding and treatment of gliomas. *Cancer Treatment and Research, 163,* 1–184.

Ross, L., Johansen, C., Dalton, S. O., et al. (2003). Psychiatric hospitalization among survivors of cancer in childhood or adolescence. *The New England Journal of Medicine, 349,* 650–657.

Safdieh, J. E., Mead, P. A., Sepkowitz, K. A., et al. (2008). Bacterial and fungal meningitis in patients with cancer. *Neurology, 70,* 943–947.

Tess, A. V., & Smetna, G. W. (2009). Medical evaluation of patients undergoing electroconvulsive therapy. *The New England Journal of Medicine, 360,* 1437–1444.

Torres, I. J., Mundt, A. J., Sweeney, P. J., et al. (2003). A longitudinal neuropsychological study of partial brain radiation in adults with brain tumors. *Neurology, 60,* 1113–1118.

Zaidat, O. O., & Ruff, R. L. (2002). Treatment of spinal epidural metastasis improves patient survival and functional state. *Neurology, 58,* 1360–1366.

CHAPTER 19

QUESTIONS AND ANSWERS

1. After 2 weeks of progressively greater difficulty playing soccer and paying attention in school, a 7-year-old boy develops a severe headache, nausea, and vomiting. His examination shows papilledema and ataxia. Of the following, which is the most likely cause?
   a. Migraine
   b. Idiopathic intracranial hypertension (pseudotumor cerebri)
   c. Glioblastoma
   d. Astrocytoma of the cerebellum

Answer: d. The combination of headache, nausea, vomiting, and, most significantly, papilledema suggests hydrocephalus. The preceding ataxia, indicated by his diminished athletic ability, suggests that the problem originated in the cerebellum. Most likely, a cerebellar astrocytoma grew large enough to block cerebrospinal fluid (CSF) flow through the fourth ventricle, causing obstructive hydrocephalus. Among children with brain tumors, cerebellar astrocytomas occur frequently. Although basilar migraine attacks can cause nausea, vomiting, and ataxia, they do not last for 6 weeks or cause papilledema. Idiopathic intracranial hypertension (pseudotumor cerebri) occurs more commonly in obese young women and is unlikely to present with ataxia or vomiting. Glioblastomas develop almost only in older adults. A traumatic subdural hematoma, from an athletic injury or conceivably child abuse, is also a credible explanation for the child's symptoms and signs.

2. A primary care physician referred a 60-year-old construction worker for evaluation of episodes of impaired consciousness lasting 1 to 3 minutes. During these, the patient mutters nonsensically and makes kissing movements. He has diabetes and hypertension, and has smoked two packs of cigarettes daily since enlisting in the Navy at 17 years. A neurologist finds that the patient has a left superior quadrantanopia, right dysmetria, and right intention tremor. Electroencephalographic monitoring confirms that the episodes represent partial complex seizures originating from the right temporal lobe. Of the following conditions, which is the most likely illness?
   a. Subdural hematomas
   b. Metastatic carcinoma in the right temporal lobe and right cerebellar hemisphere
   c. Glioblastoma of the left temporal lobe
   d. Strokes in the right temporal lobe and right cerebellar hemisphere
   e. Multiple sclerosis

Answer: b. Although neurologists try to attribute all of a patient's symptoms and signs to a single location, this patient's clinical picture suggests a multifocal process. The seizures and superior quadrantanopsia are attributable to the right temporal lobe. The right-sided dysmetria and intention tremor are referable to the right cerebellum. These multiple lesions are probably manifestations of metastatic cancer, but alternative explanations include multiple embolic strokes and abscesses. Strokes may cause mild, transient headaches. While subdural hematomas often occur over both cerebral hemispheres, they rarely cause seizures or occur in the posterior fossa. At his age, he is unlikely to have developed multiple sclerosis (MS). Moreover, headaches and seizures are not initial symptoms of MS.

3. Which of the following patients is most likely to develop cerebral gliomas?
   a. A 30-year-old woman with multiple *café-au-lait* spots
   b. A 21-year-old woman with bilateral acoustic neuromas
   c. A 21-year-old man with mental retardation, epilepsy, and adenoma sebaceum
   d. A 30-year-old man with a vascular malformation in the distribution of the trigeminal nerve

Answer: c. The patient with the mental retardation, epilepsy, and adenoma sebaceum has tuberous sclerosis. The cerebral tubers, which are a component of this illness, are composed of large astrocytes, giant cells and dysmorphic neurons. About 10% of patients with tuberous sclerosis develop subependymal giant-cell astrocytomas. The woman with the *café-au-lait* spots has neurofibromatosis type 1 (NF1), which is often complicated by meningiomas, as well as neuromas of peripheral nerves. The woman with the acoustic neuromas probably has neurofibromatosis type 2 (NF2). The man with the vascular malformation has Sturge–Weber syndrome, which is not associated with neoplasms.

4. A 50-year-old woman has impaired ability to hear when she places her telephone receiver against her right ear. She also has right-sided tinnitus and loss of auditory acuity. Her neurologic examination is otherwise normal. Of the following, which one is the most likely illness?
   a. Left temporal lobe meningioma
   b. Psychogenic factors
   c. MS
   d. A cerebellopontine angle tumor

Answer: d. Acoustic neuromas, the most common cerebellopontine angle tumor, typically cause speech discrimination impairment, tinnitus, and the gradual loss of auditory acuity. Because acoustic neuromas develop slowly, they do not cause vertigo. Lesions of the cerebral hemispheres or the brainstem, including MS plaques, do not cause auditory disturbances. As discussed in the previous case, bilateral acoustic neuromas are a typical manifestation of NF2.

5. During the previous 2 years, a 55-year-old woman with multiple *café-au-lait* spots developed slowly increasing severe paresis of the left leg, which had hyperactive DTRs and a Babinski sign. Before undergoing further evaluation, she had a seizure that began with clonic movements of the left foot, then leg, and finally the arm. On examination, she has left hemiparesis, hyperactive DTRs, and a Babinski sign. Of the following, which is the most likely illness?
    a. Right cerebral glioblastoma
    b. Right cerebral meningioma
    c. Left cerebral glioblastoma
    d. Left cerebral meningioma

Answer: b. The evolution of a hemiparesis over a relatively long time, especially when it is accompanied by a partial (motor) seizure, suggests a cerebral tumor. A meningioma is more likely than a glioblastoma in view of the chronicity of the hemiparesis and her probably having NF1.

6. Which of the following is *least* likely to cause headaches in the elderly?
    a. Subdural hematoma
    b. Open-angle glaucoma
    c. Brain tumors
    d. Temporal arteritis
    e. Nitroglycerin and other vasodilator medications

Answer: b. Open-angle glaucoma is not associated with headaches, but closed or narrow-angle glaucoma is associated with headache, as well as eye pain, and blurred vision. The other conditions often cause headaches in the elderly. In addition, headache may be a symptom of depression and other psychiatric disorders.

7. Brain tumors often produce headaches that are worse in the early morning, waking patients from sleep. Which *five* of the following headaches also typically begin in the early morning?
    a. Tension headache
    b. Idiopathic intracranial hypertension
    c. Migraine
    d. Trigeminal neuralgia
    e. Postconcussive syndrome
    f. Cluster headache
    g. Sleep apnea-induced headache
    h. Caffeine withdrawal

Answer: b, c, f, g, h. Idiopathic intracranial hypertension (pseudotumor) headaches are usually worse in the morning because the symptoms of increased ICP are worse in the supine position. Migraine and cluster headaches characteristically develop during REM sleep, which occurs predominantly in the early morning. Hypoxia and carbon dioxide retention also cause headache.

8. An obese 22-year-old woman has moderately severe generalized headaches. She has papilledema and paresis of abduction of her right eye but no other neurologic abnormalities. Routine blood and chemistry tests are normal. A CT shows small ventricles but no mass lesion. What would be the most appropriate next step?
    a. MRI
    b. EEG
    c. Lumbar puncture (LP) to measure the opening pressure and withdraw CSF
    d. None of the above

Answer: c. The patient almost certainly has idiopathic intracranial hypertension (IIH), which is classically referred to as pseudotumor cerebri. The increased intracranial pressure stretches the sixth nerve and weakens the abducens muscle. Because the sixth nerve problem does not reflect a mass lesion, neurologists often call it a "false localizing sign." Given the clinical picture and normal CT, MRI is not necessary. Instead, physicians should perform an LP to diagnose IIH and exclude the unlikely possibility of chronic meningitis. In IIH, the CSF pressure is usually above 300 mm H_2O, which is a marked elevation. Chronic papilledema, from this or any other condition, may lead to optic atrophy and then blindness. IIH is one of the rare situations where an LP is performed despite papilledema or suspicion of increased intracranial pressure.

9. A 45-year-old police officer suffering from alcohol abuse and personality disturbances has become obsessed with the idea that he has a brain tumor. Careful medical and neurologic examinations are normal. What would most neurologists do next?
    a. Offer reassurance
    b. Suggest psychotherapy
    c. Give an antidepressant
    d. Treat him for obsession
    e. Order an MRI

Answer: e. Even though brain tumors are rare in middle-aged people with a normal neurologic examination, especially when psychiatric disturbances can explain the symptom, most neurologists would order a MRI or CT for several reasons. At the onset, about 50% of the patients with tumors have no overt physical neurologic deficits. Other structural lesions, such as an AVM or subdural hematoma, could be responsible for the patient's symptoms. Furthermore, with a normal study, a neurologist can give more secure reassurance, feel protected in the event of a medical-legal problem, and refer the patient to a psychiatrist who, in turn, will probably feel more confident in accepting the patient.

10. A psychiatrist was asked to consult on a 60-year-old retired sanitation truck driver with lung cancer who developed confusion, disorientation, and agitation during his second week of hospitalization. He resisted a full neurologic examination, but a neurologist determined that he had no hemiparesis, papilledema, or nuchal rigidity. A noncontrast head CT was normal. The psychiatrist diagnosed delirium. Which one of the following is its *least* likely cause?
   a. Hyperkalemia
   b. Pneumonia
   c. Liver metastases with hepatic encephalopathy
   d. Withdrawal from alcohol or other substance
   e. Inappropriate ADH secretion
   f. Hypercalcemia
   g. Liver metastases with slowed metabolism of medications

Answer: a. The psychiatrist was correct: The patient has delirium. However, that diagnosis requires a physician to determine its cause. Numerous conditions may cause delirium in cancer patients. The normal neurologic examination, although rudimentary, and normal noncontrast head CT indicate that he does not have cerebral metastases. Except for hyperkalemia, the other disorders frequently complicate lung cancer, even when it has not spread to the brain, and cause delirium. In addition, hospitalization of individuals who abuse alcohol or other substances may lead to withdrawal symptoms that can reach the point of delirium.

11. In the above case (Question 10), a chest X-ray revealed pneumonia. After a course of antibiotics, his delirium resolved. One month later, his delirium recurred and was more threatening than the previous time. A CT revealed two ring-shaped lesions with surrounding edema in his cerebral hemispheres. An extensive evaluation found no other potential explanation. His primary care team solicited a psychiatry consultation. Which medication regimen should the psychiatrist recommend?
   a. A major neuroleptic and steroids
   b. A minor tranquilizer and steroids
   c. Steroids
   d. Hypnotics
   e. An antiepileptic drug

Answer: a. In this situation, a small dose of a neuroleptic will reduce the patient's behavioral disturbances and reduce the risk of harm. Steroids such as dexamethasone will reduce the edema and thus the volume of the lesions, and thereby will bring about a rapid and dramatic, although temporary, improvement.

12. A 65-year-old woman with the onset of dementia over 9 months has no physical or neurologic abnormalities except for frontal release signs and hyperactive DTRs. A complete laboratory evaluation and EEG reveal no specific abnormality. A CT shows atrophy and a small meningioma in the right parietal convexity. Which would be the most appropriate next step?
   a. Have the tumor removed.
   b. Tentatively diagnose Alzheimer disease and repeat the clinical evaluation and CT in 6 to 12 months.
   c. Obtain an MRI.

Answer: b. Her meningioma is irrelevant to her dementia. Meningiomas grow so slowly that they can be followed by periodic clinical examinations and scans. However, if meningiomas grow large enough to compress brain tissue or cause symptoms, neurosurgeons can remove them. Because a meningioma has a paucity of water and a great deal of calcium, MRI is unlikely to provide more useful information than already provided by the CT.

13. A 75-year-old man who has had dementia for 6 years suddenly develops increased irritability and behavioral disturbances. He has no lateralized signs or indications of increased intracranial pressure. He is treated with a major tranquilizer. One week later, he becomes somnolent and has a seizure. He remains comatose with a left hemiparesis. No abnormalities are found on a general medical examination or routine laboratory tests, but a CT shows an extra-axial curved lucency and a shift of midline cerebral structures. Before any treatment can be instituted, the patient dies. An autopsy discloses cerebral atrophy and a large chronic subdural hematoma. Which of the following statements concerning subdural hematomas is *false*?
   a. Subdural hematomas are apt to occur in the elderly, especially in those individuals who have a history of dementia and cerebral atrophy.
   b. Subdural hematomas are usually located outside or overlying the brain, i.e., in an extra-axial compartment.
   c. Unless they are large or rapidly expanding, subdural hematomas may not cause lateralized signs or greatly raise intracranial pressure.
   d. In chronic subdurals, CT portrays aged blood as less radiodense than brain, and in acute subdurals, fresh blood is more radiodense than brain. In other words, chronic hematomas are black (radiolucent) and fresh ones are white (radiodense). With acute bleeding into chronic subdurals, densities appear within lucent regions.
   e. The trauma required to cause a subdural hematoma is usually so great that it causes loss of consciousness for 1 hour or longer.

Answer: e. The elderly are more susceptible than young adults to developing subdurals for several reasons. Minimal or no trauma tears apart the delicate bridging veins of their meninges. With cerebral atrophy, the cerebral cortex cannot dampen overlying bleeding. The elderly often take aspirin, warfarin, or other medicines that impede clotting. Finally, elder abuse may cause the head trauma.

14. Which structure is *not* located in the posterior fossa?
   a. Sphenoid wing
   b. Chemoreceptors for vomiting

c. Vertebrobasilar artery system
d. Cerebellum
e. Fourth ventricle

Answer: a.

15. Match the brain lesion (1–6) with the group(s) at the greatest risk (a–j).
1. Chronic subdural hematoma
2. Cerebellar astrocytoma
3. Cerebral lymphomas
4. Neurocysticercosis
5. Tuberculomas
6. Acoustic neuromas
    a. Elderly individuals
    b. Children
    c. Residents of Central America
    d. Residents of the Indian subcontinent
    e. Neurofibromatosis type 1
    f. Neurofibromatosis type 2
    g. Trisomy 21
    h. Acquired immunodeficiency syndrome (AIDS) patients

Answer: 1–a; 2–b; 3–h; 4–c and d; 5–d; 6–f.

16. Which one of the following does *not* usually indicate a pituitary adenoma?
    a. Increased serum prolactin level
    b. Cognitive impairment
    c. Galactorrhea
    d. Bitemporal hemianopia
    e. Decreased libido
    f. Menstrual irregularity
    g. Headaches
    h. Bitemporal superior quadrantanopia
    i. Infertility

Answer: b. Because pituitary tumors can grow upwards to compress the optic chiasm and hypothalamus, they lead to headaches, visual field impairments, and pan-hypopituitarism. Also, certain pituitary tumors secrete prolactin.

17. Which of the following pituitary conditions is most likely to emerge in a 12-year-old child with delayed growth, puberty, and social maturity?
    a. Chromophobe adenoma
    b. Prolactinoma
    c. Cushing syndrome
    d. Craniopharyngioma

Answer: d. Unlike other pituitary region tumors, craniopharyngiomas are congenital lesions that produce symptoms in children and adults. These tumors are typically cystic and located in the hypothalamic region. Because of their high calcium content, skull X-rays as well as CT readily identify them. In children, craniopharyngiomas cause delayed puberty and poor school performance. When craniopharyngiomas are large, they cause visual impairments characteristic of pituitary tumors

(e.g., bitemporal hemianopia or superior quadrantanopia) and optic atrophy. They may also cause diabetes insipidus if they grow into the hypothalamus and obstructive hydrocephalus if they grow to occlude outflow from the third ventricle.

18. Of the following statements regarding paraneoplastic syndromes, which is *true*?
    a. They only appear after the underlying cancer has metastasized.
    b. They are only associated with small-cell carcinoma of the lung and gynecologic cancers.
    c. Immunosuppression often relieves the symptoms.
    d. Neurologic paraneoplastic syndromes, such as Lambert–Eaton syndrome, cerebellar degeneration, and limbic encephalitis, result from antibodies directed against cell surface antigens.

Answer: c. Immunosuppression, as well as chemotherapy, radiation, and other cancer treatments, frequently relieve paraneoplastic syndromes. If the underlying cancer is cured, they may completely remit. Paraneoplastic syndromes often appear weeks to months before a cancer is detectable and are associated with a wide variety of malignancies. Antineuronal antibodies probably cause Lambert–Eaton syndrome, cerebellar degeneration, and limbic encephalitis.

19. A 65-year-old man with metastatic prostate carcinoma has been in agony from bone metastases. He is agitated, verbose, and threatening in his demands for morphine. His behavior has become a major management problem, and his family is also becoming disruptive. CT, MRI, and blood tests have shown that the patient has no cerebral metastases, infection, hypercalcemia, or other metabolic aberrations. Which *two* recommendations should a psychiatry consultant make in response to this situation?
    a. Help the primary physicians control the patient's pain with as much narcotic (opioid medication) as he requires. Once the pain is controlled, the situation can be reassessed.
    b. Stop all medications because they can be the cause of the behavioral disorder.
    c. Immediately administer minor or major tranquilizers.
    d. Before treating further, perform an MRI and LP for signs of opportunistic infections.

Answer: a and possibly c. Prostatic cancer rarely spreads to the brain, but it commonly spreads to bone where metastases cause agonizing pain. However, hormone manipulation, radiotherapy, and opioids can partly or fully control the pain. If medicines do not adequately alleviate it, drug-seeking behavior will persist. Long-acting opioids, such as methadone, and others delivered by patch or continuous intravenous infusion are particularly effective. Breakthrough pain may be alleviated by rescue doses of parenteral opioids, such as morphine. Judicious use of antidepressants, antiepileptic drugs, and tranquilizers may provide additional analgesia, mood improvement, and restful sleep.

20. What mechanism has been proposed to explain limbic encephalitis and other paraneoplastic syndromes?
   a. Antibody formation
   b. Viral infection
   c. Endocrine disturbance
   d. Toxins secreted by the tumor

Answer: a. The etiology of paraneoplastic cerebellar degeneration, limbic encephalitis, and other paraneoplastic syndromes has been attributed to antibodies that react with neurons, i.e., antineuronal antibodies.

21. Which *three* lesions tend to arise in the extra-axial space?
   a. Butterfly gliomas
   b. Astrocytomas
   c. Meningiomas
   d. Epidural hematomas
   e. Subdural hematomas
   f. Medulloblastomas

Answer: c, d, e.

22. Which *two* of the following are *not* functions of glial cells?
   a. To provide structure for the spinal cord.
   b. To provide structure for the brain.
   c. To clear debris from infections and strokes.
   d. To generate a myelin coat for CNS neurons.
   e. To generate a myelin coat for PNS neurons.
   f. To generate electrochemical potentials.

Answer: e, f. Glial cells, such as astrocytes, normally provide physical structure, a nutritional network, and response to inflammation and cell death. Schwann cells generate the myelin coat for PNS neurons. Neurons generate electrochemical potentials.

23. Which *three* are actions of oligodendrocytes?
   a. Occasionally become oligodendrogliomas
   b. Generate myelin for the CNS
   c. Generate myelin for the PNS
   d. Generate action potentials
   e. Act as a glial cell

Answer: a, b, e. Oligodendrocytes are also the target of the demyelinating process in multiple sclerosis.

24. In which *three* aspects do brain tumors in children differ from those in adults?
   a. Childhood tumors more often develop in posterior fossa structures.
   b. Childhood astrocytomas are usually resectable.
   c. In children, tumors often present with signs of hydrocephalus.
   d. Metastatic tumors in children are as common as primary brain tumors.
   e. Meningiomas are relatively common in children.
   f. Pituitary adenomas are relatively common in children.

Answer: a, b, c. Childhood astrocytomas often develop in the cerebellum, block CSF flow through the fourth ventricle, and thus cause hydrocephalus. Neurosurgeons routinely resect them and effect a complete cure. Medulloblastomas, which develop in the medulla, are unresectable. They remain resistant to chemotherapy and radiotherapy.

25. Match the condition that causes weakness (1–5) with the impairment of ACh transmission at neuromuscular junctions (a–d).
1. Myasthenia gravis
2. Lambert–Eaton syndrome
3. Botulism
4. Guillain–Barré syndrome
5. Botulinum toxin
   a. Impaired release of ACh quanta from presynaptic neurons
   b. Abnormalities of the ACh receptor on postsynaptic neurons
   c. Enhanced re-uptake of ACh into the presynaptic neurons
   d. None of the above

Answer: 1–b, 2–a, 3–a, 4–d, 5–a.

26. Which statement is *false* regarding the chemoreceptor area of the brain?
   a. It is located in the superior surface of the medulla.
   b. It is located in the area postrema.
   c. It is unprotected by the blood–brain barrier.
   d. The area is inaccessible to most chemicals.

Answer: d. The chemoreceptor area of the brain is situated on the superior surface of the medulla. Because it is devoid of the blood–brain barrier, it is immediately exposed to blood-borne substances. Morphine, heroin, many chemotherapeutic agents, numerous toxins and, in large doses, levodopa provoke vomiting as soon as they contact it.

27. Serum prolactin levels that are transiently elevated above the baseline are a useful diagnostic test for seizures. Which *five* of the following conditions or medicines elevate the baseline serum prolactin level?
   a. Chromophobe adenoma
   b. Prolactinoma
   c. Phenothiazines
   d. Butyrophenones
   e. Estrogens
   f. Bromocriptine
   g. Dopamine
   h. Propranolol
   i. Levodopa
   j. Cabergoline

Answer: a–e. Numerous medications and prolactinomas raise serum prolactin concentrations. Generalized and some partial seizures increase the serum prolactin concentration – at least temporarily. Bromocriptine, cabergoline, dopamine, and L-dopa, in contrast, reduce it. Propranolol has no effect on prolactin levels.

28. Which *two* are potential complications of performing ECT on a patient with an undetected meningioma?
    a. Skin necrosis
    b. Status epilepticus
    c. Transtentorial herniation
    d. Exacerbating Parkinson disease

Answer: b, c. With proper precautions, including obtaining either a CT or MRI, ECT carries few neurologic risks. Brain tumors are an important neurologic contraindication, although it may not be an absolute one. The importance of a brain tumor in respect to ECT is that it might be the cause of the depression or other indication for ECT, it might lead to status epilepticus, and, if large, a tumor may cause swelling and transtentorial herniation.

29–31. Match the varieties of hemorrhage (29–31) with the most likely cause (a–c):

29. Subarachnoid hemorrhage
30. Subdural hematoma
31. Epidural hematoma
    a. Middle meningeal artery laceration
    b. Rupture of a berry aneurysm
    c. Trauma of bridging meningeal veins

Answers:

29–b. Although trauma and mycotic aneurysms may cause a subarachnoid hemorrhage, the most frequent and important cause is rupture of an aneurysm arising from one of the arteries that comprise the circle of Willis.
30–c. Bleeding from small meningeal veins is the usual cause of subdural hematomas.
31–a. Lacerations of the middle meningeal artery, which often result from a fracture of the temporal bone, are usually the cause of epidural hematomas.

32. A 46-year-old woman with metastatic breast cancer develops a disconcerting numbness in the skin over the right lower chin. She has no weakness of face or jaw muscles and the remainder of her neurologic examination is normal. However, X-rays of her jaw reveal a lytic lesion in the right lower mandible. What is the diagnosis?
    a. Mental neuropathy
    b. Mononeuritis multiplex
    c. A remote effect of carcinoma
    d. A facial nerve injury

Answer: a. The mental nerve, a branch of the trigeminal nerve, provides sensation from the skin overlying the chin. Damage to this nerve, "mental neuropathy" – an

unfortunate coincidence of words – causes numbness of the skin of one side of the chin, i.e., the "numb chin sign." In this case, a metastasis to the mandible at the site where the mental nerve passes through its foramen has caused the mental neuropathy. Trauma to the same site could also produce mental neuropathy.

33. A family brings a 59-year-old high-school basketball coach for psychiatric consultation because he has become apathetic and markedly forgetful, but intermittently he becomes loud and inexplicably angry. An examination confirms that he has amnesia and personality changes. One month before this consultation, his physicians diagnosed small-cell carcinoma of the lung. An MRI with and without gadolinium of the head is normal and 3 LPs show normal CSF chemistries, absence of cells, and an opening pressure of 150 mmH$_2$O. The results of all his blood tests are also within normal limits. However, an EEG shows focal slowing and spikes over the temporal lobes. Which is the most likely explanation for his memory deficit and other abnormalities?
    a. A depressive disorder
    b. An inflammatory condition affecting the temporal lobes
    c. Temporal lobe metastases that have remained undetected by the MRI
    d. Partial complex seizures

Answer: b. He probably has limbic encephalitis, which is a paraneoplastic syndrome associated with small-cell carcinoma of the lung and several other neoplasms. Limbic encephalitis is characterized by memory impairment and personality changes, but it may also lead to generalized cognitive impairment and seizures. Without the underlying lung carcinoma, herpes simplex encephalitis would be a credible diagnosis.

34. Which of the following organs is most resistant to ionizing radiation?
    a. Bone marrow
    b. Brain
    c. Gastrointestinal tract
    d. Lung

Answer: b. The brain and other regions of the CNS are relatively resistant to ionizing radiation; however, ionizing radiation, in large or sustained doses, may lead to radiation necrosis or, in the long term, development of brain tumors. On the other hand, evidence so far does not implicate cell phone use as a cause of brain tumors.

35. A 59-year-old active professor of English presents with a 3-week history of dulled affect, sleeplessness, and mild morning headaches. Aspirin relieves the headaches. Six years before, following the death of his mother, he had prolonged mourning. On examination, he scores 28/30 on the MMSE, but he is inattentive and reticent. He has psychomotor impersistence, but no lateralized neurologic deficit. An

MRI reveals a single large ring-shaped mass lesion in the right frontal lobe that compresses the anterior horn of the lateral ventricle and shifts midline structures to the left. Which is the most likely nature of the lesion?

a. Glioblastoma
b. Meningioma
c. Bacterial abscess
d. None of the above

Answer: a. The large ring-shaped mass lesion revealed by the MRI indicates that his symptoms and signs are attributable to a glioblastoma. The possible episode of depression 6 years before is too distant to be relevant. A meningioma is unlikely in view of the rapidity of his symptoms and the MRI shows an intra-axial lesion. Although the MRI features are consistent with a bacterial abscess, he has no systemic symptoms of one. Nevertheless, many neurologists would request a biopsy. When the lesion is situated in the nondominant frontal lobe, as this one is, a generous excision would provide the patient with a definite diagnosis and additional months of life with reduction of his headaches and other symptoms.

36. Eight months after completing whole-brain radiotherapy for metastatic lung cancer, a 47-year-old former newspaper reporter suddenly developed aphasia and right-sided hemiparesis. Her MRI showed an acute infarction in the distribution of a branch of her left middle cerebral artery and small residual metastatic tumors in the right frontal lobe and left cerebellum. Which is the most likely cause of the stroke?

a. Another metastatic tumor
b. Chemotherapy
c. Atherosclerosis
d. Radiation arteritis or necrosis

Answer: d. Radiotherapy damages intracerebral arteries as well as the malignant tumor cells. Because of radiation arteritis, patients sometimes sustain one or more small strokes that cause combinations of cognitive, personality, and motor impairments between 6 and 18 months after completion of the treatment. The history, MRI appearance, and routine tests usually distinguish this condition from other causes of stroke in this age group, such as use of cocaine, hypertension, cardiac valvular disease, atrial fibrillation, and blood dyscrasias.

37. Which of the following statements concerning depression comorbid with brain tumors is *true*?

a. Depression develops before surgery and subsides after tumor resection.
b. Depression rarely occurs in brain-tumor patients.
c. Depression arises immediately after surgery and subsequently increases in severity.
d. The presence of comorbid depression does not affect the patient's quality of life.

Answer: c. In brain-tumor patients, depression not only arises immediately after surgery, but increases in severity during the ensuing course. Along with physical debility, treatment-induced fatigue, cognitive impairments, and other emotional changes, depressive symptoms predict a poor quality of life.

38. The surgical service solicits a psychiatric consultation because a 79-year-old man suddenly became "depressed." The psychiatrist determines that he had been making an uneventful recovery for the preceding 3 weeks following resection of extensive colon cancer. When the psychiatrist examines the patient, she finds that he is intermittently lethargic and often inattentive. When she captures his attention, she finds that he is incompletely oriented and has a poor memory. Although his white blood cell count is elevated, he has no fever, asterixis, nuchal rigidity, papilledema, or lateralized neurologic findings. A head CT shows no abnormality. Which is most likely responsible for his change in mental state?

a. Toxic-metabolic encephalopathy
b. Paraneoplastic limbic encephalitis
c. Cerebral metastases
d. Major depression

Answer: a. The patient probably has delirium from a toxic-metabolic encephalopathy, which has several potential explanations: sepsis, electrolyte imbalance, and metastases to the liver. Even minimal toxic-metabolic aberrations in elderly patients cause marked changes in their mood and level of consciousness. A potentially misleading aspect is that overwhelming sepsis sometimes fails to raise the white blood count. After his primary physicians correct the encephalopathy and determine the extent of tumor spread, they can reconsult the psychiatrist to evaluate the patient for depression.

39. A family brings their 74-year-old patriarch, a diner owner, to a neurologist because he began offending his customers and forgetting their orders. Although he rarely drinks alcohol, he has smoked two packs of cigarettes daily since he came to this country as a teenager. He takes no medications. He has lost 20 lb. His neurologic examination shows pronounced memory impairment, but no lateralized signs or papilledema. An MRI detected no mass lesions, but the medial temporal lobes are smaller than normal. Routine blood tests show mild anemia, but no other abnormality. An EEG contains temporal spikes. Which test should the neurologist now order?

a. CT of the head
b. CT of the chest
c. CSF analysis by a spinal tap
d. Brain biopsy

Answer: b. A man with a more than a 100 pack-year history of smoking cigarettes and an unexplained 20-lb weight loss deserves a CT of the chest for investigation of lung cancer – no matter the particular symptoms. His amnesia, MRI, and EEG point to temporal lobe damage. Most likely he has developed limbic encephalitis as the presenting feature of a small-cell carcinoma of the lung.

In addition to ordering the chest CT, his physician should order a paraneoplastic encephalitis panel. In contrast, CSF analysis would probably not reveal useful information in this situation, except possibly for suggesting Creutzfeldt–Jakob disease (in which case it may detect 14-3-3 protein). Creutzfeldt–Jakob disease is a reasonable alternative diagnosis, but he has no myoclonus.

40. A 29-year-old intravenous drug addict with AIDS comes to the emergency room with uncontrollable involuntary, uncoordinated, large-scale jerky movements of his left arm and leg. He remains alert and free of headache. An MRI shows multiple small ring-enhancing lesions predominantly in the basal ganglia. Which is the most likely etiology of the cerebral lesions?
    a. Cerebral abscesses
    b. Neurocysticercosis
    c. Multiple cerebral hemorrhages
    d. Multiple strokes

    Answer: a. He probably has toxoplasmosis, which has a predilection for the basal ganglia. Unlike other cerebral mass lesions, toxoplasmosis causes movement disorders, including, as in the case, hemiballismus. A mass lesion tracking across the corpus callosum and infiltrating both frontal lobes in a "butterfly" pattern suggests a glioblastoma invading both frontal lobes. Multiple cerebral cortical cysts indicate neurocysticercosis, but AIDS patients are not particularly vulnerable to this CNS infection.

41. While resecting a cerebral seizure focus or tumor, neurosurgeons are naturally reluctant to excise "eloquent" cerebral cortex – areas of the cortex critical for physical or neuropsychological function. Which of the following is the most eloquent region of the brain?
    a. The anterior section of the right frontal lobe
    b. The posterior section of the left frontal lobe
    c. The anterior section of the right occipital lobe
    d. The posterior section of the left occipital lobe

    Answer: b. Broca's area, one of the most eloquent areas of the brain, is situated in the posterior section of the left frontal lobe. The occipital lobes contain the visual cortex, which is important but not as critical as the language cortex. Almost the entire right frontal lobe, anterior to the motor strip, and the anterior tips of the temporal lobes are "silent" – devoid of readily recognizable cognitive, sensory, or motor function. Surgeons may remove these areas with little overt consequence, although neuropsychologic testing may show mood and personality change.

42. Which is the most frequently occurring complication of radiation leukoencephalopathy in adults?
    a. Cognitive impairment
    b. Psychosis
    c. Convulsions
    d. None of the above

Answer: a. Sometimes immediately but more frequently after an interval of several years, whole-brain radiotherapy causes cognitive and physical impairments because it induces leukoencephalopathy.

43. When administered to children, radiation therapy may prevent the spread of acute leukemia to the CNS or obliterate unresectable tumors. However, the treatment has many potential complications. Which of the following is *false*?
    a. Young children, compared to young and middle-aged adults, are resistant to radiation-induced cognitive impairment.
    b. In young children, radiation therapy may lead to Intellectual Disability.
    c. In children, radiation therapy may lead to panhypopituitarism.
    d. In children, radiation therapy may lead to growth retardation.

    Answer: a. Compared to adults, children are more vulnerable to radiation-induced cognitive impairment.

44. A close friend brings a 68-year-old retired nurse for psychiatric evaluation for depression. The patient explains that she has lost her liveliness, energy, and interest in other people during the previous 3–6 months. However, she denies memory and other cognitive impairments, headaches, and systemic symptoms. On examination, she scores 28 on the MMSE and has no physical neurologic abnormalities, but she has psychomotor retardation, emotional dulling, and reduced capacity to execute complex mental tasks. During the examination and more so afterwards, she speaks excessively, loudly, and aggressively. With which *two* conditions is her clinical presentation most consistent?
    a. Frontal lobe tumor
    b. Alzheimer disease
    c. Dementia with Lewy bodies
    d. Frontotemporal dementia
    e. Creutzfeldt–Jakob disease
    f. Vascular dementia

    Answer: a, d. Her dulling of affect, loss of inhibition, and loquaciousness, with relatively normal memory and cognitive capacity, indicate frontal lobe dysfunction rather than simply dementia. Also, she has no physical abnormalities that would point to Creutzfeldt–Jakob diseases, dementia with Lewy bodies, or vascular cognitive impairment. MRI would distinguish a frontal lobe tumor from frontotemporal dementia.

45. Which electrolyte disturbance is most likely to complicate the course of a patient who presents with a previously undiagnosed, rapidly expanding metastatic brain tumor?
    a. Hypernatremia
    b. Hyponatremia

c. Hyperkalemia

d. Hypokalemia

Answer: b. Patients who sustain intracranial catastrophes, such as major traumatic brain injury, subarachnoid hemorrhage, or sudden elevation in intracranial pressure from a rapidly growing brain tumor typically develop the syndrome of inappropriate antidiuretic hormone (SIADH) secretion. SIADH essentially dilutes the electrolytes and lowers the serum osmolality. Hyponatremia, the most pronounced effect, may lead to delirium or seizures. Physicians must slowly correct hyponatremia because overly rapid correction may lead to demyelination of the pons, i.e., central pontine myelinolysis.

46. Which of the following is the most commonly occurring brain tumor in middle-aged women?
    a. Glioblastoma
    b. Meningioma
    c. Acoustic neuroma
    d. Astrocytoma

Answer: b. Small meningiomas are commonplace in middle-aged individuals. Because they grow slowly and remain asymptomatic, they pose no immediate threat. Small meningiomas do not cause psychiatric symptoms. Neurologists generally follow them rather than immediately recommend surgery.

47. With which condition is the JC virus associated?
    a. Progressive multifocal leukoencephalopathy (PML)
    b. Primary cerebral lymphoma
    c. Glioblastoma
    d. Meningioma

Answer: a. The JC virus is closely and probably causally related to PML. When CSF studies detect evidence of JC virus, neurologists usually omit a cerebral biopsy in the diagnosis of PML. The virus is named after John Cunningham, an afflicted patient, and has no relation with Jakob–Creutzfeldt disease.

48. With which condition is Epstein–Barr (EB) virus associated?
    a. Progressive multifocal leukoencephalopathy (PML)
    b. Primary cerebral lymphoma
    c. Glioblastoma
    d. Meningioma

Answer: b. The EB virus is associated with primary cerebral lymphoma in AIDS patients. The association is close, but before instituting radiation therapy, neurologists often insist on a biopsy of the lesion.

49. Six months after delivering her third child, a 28-year-old woman seeks a psychiatric consultation for "depression." She reports loss of interest in her husband and their children. She describes having little appetite or energy, sleeping poorly, and losing interest in sex. Her weight has fallen to below her prepregnancy level. Her menses initially returned, but were scant. Then, 2 months before the visit, her menses stopped. Two weeks before the psychiatric consultation, a neurologic evaluation showed no visual field or visual acuity deficits, or other abnormalities. A head MRI, with views of the sella, was normal. Routine blood tests were normal except that the serum prolactin level was slightly elevated. Which is the most likely diagnosis?
    a. Major depression
    b. Postpartum pituitary insufficiency
    c. Prolactinoma
    d. None of the above

Answer: b. Except for not having an obstetric complication, such as hemorrhage, this patient has typical pituitary insufficiency. Her symptoms mimic, to a certain extent, postpartum depression. Thus, endocrinologic evaluation is generally indicated in women who seem to have postpartum depression. With all the potential medical explanations for her symptoms and lack of some criteria, major depression is not a tenable diagnosis. The modest prolactin elevation and lack of a visible abnormality on MRI speak against a prolactinoma. Despite the indications of pituitary insufficiency, the presence of amenorrhea and elevated prolactin level indicate that another pregnancy may have occurred. In any case, she should undergo testing for pregnancy and use of birth control before the psychiatrist prescribes an antidepressant or the endocrinologist prescribes hormone replacement.

50. During a week-long vacation, after a strenuous first semester of college, a 19-year-old woman developed involuntary right arm and leg movements and then unexplained anxiety. While undergoing a medical evaluation, she developed partial complex seizures. Aside from a temperature of 100.0 degrees, she had no general medical abnormalities. She was confused and disoriented, and had poor memory, but she had no meningeal or lateralized findings. Her CSF showed 25 lymphocytes and a slightly elevated protein concentration, but no antibodies to herpes simplex virus or any common bacteria. Toxicology studies were consistently negative. A transvaginal ultrasound detected an ovarian lesion. Which is the most likely diagnosis?
    a. Anti-NMDA receptor encephalitis
    b. Herpes simplex virus encephalitis
    c. Metastatic ovarian carcinoma
    d. Voltage-gated potassium channel (VGKC) antibody encephalitis

Answer: a. She has a syndrome of the rapid onset of involuntary movements, seizures, and encephalopathy with CSF lymphocytic pleocytosis. With the finding of an ovarian lesion in a young adult woman without evidence of an infection, anti-NMDA receptor encephalitis is the most likely diagnosis. Detecting serum and CSF anti-NMDA antibodies would confirm the diagnosis. Because of its neuropsychiatric features, patients with anti-NMDA receptor antibodies are first apt to present to psychiatrists. VGKC antibody encephalitis may also cause neuropsychiatric symptoms of a quality and severity that mimic acute schizophrenia; however, VGKC antibody encephalitis is not associated with ovarian lesions.

51. In the previous case, which is the most likely ovarian pathology?
    a. Ectopic pregnancy
    b. Ovarian cancer
    c. Teratoma
    d. Cyst

Answer: c. Teratomas most often underlie anti-NMDA antibody encephalitis in young women. When it is present, removing the teratoma typically reverses the condition.

LUMBAR PUNCTURE AND IMAGING STUDIES

LUMBAR PUNCTURE

Neurologists often obtain cerebrospinal fluid (CSF) by performing a lumbar puncture (LP) – one of the oldest neurologic tests still employed – in a variety of clinical circumstances. When patients have at least two elements of the relatively common triad of headache, fever, and nuchal rigidity, neurologists usually perform an LP to look for meningitis, subarachnoid hemorrhage, or other inflammatory conditions affecting the central nervous system (CNS). They also perform an LP in cases of dementia attributable to infectious illnesses. In Creutzfeldt–Jakob disease (CJD), the CSF almost always contains 14-3-3 protein; in subacute sclerosing panencephalitis (SSPE), antimeasles antibodies; in acquired immunodeficiency syndrome (AIDS), retrovirus markers; and other infectious illnesses, such as cryptococcal or tuberculous meningitis, herpes simplex encephalitis, or neurosyphilis, specific antigens or DNA detectable by polymerase chain reaction (PCR). In another particularly useful test, neurologists send CSF for the JC virus in patients with AIDS who have a cerebral white matter lesion. If present, the JC virus indicates that the diagnosis is progressive multifocal leukoencephalopathy (PML) (see Fig. 15.11). Moreover, a positive test obviates the need for a brain biopsy. Neurologists also test the CSF of patients suspected of having multiple sclerosis (MS) for oligoclonal bands and myelin basic protein (see Chapter 15). In Alzheimer disease, the CSF contains increased levels of tau protein but decreased levels of β-amyloid and Aβ42 peptide.

Diagnosing neurologic illnesses sometimes rests on abnormalities of the CSF profile, which comprises the CSF color, red and white blood cell count, and concentrations of protein and glucose (Table 20.1). For example, most infectious or inflammatory CNS illnesses cause a CSF *pleocytosis* (increase in the CSF white blood cell count). In these illnesses, a rise in protein concentration parallels CSF pleocytosis, and, in their hallmark sign, glucose concentration falls to abnormally low levels. Bacterial meningitis accentuates that profile: CSF pleocytosis is markedly elevated, with a predominance of polymorphonuclear instead of lymphocytic cells, and the glucose concentration can fall to undetectable levels. Cultures of virus, fungus, and *Mycobacterium* may require 1 to 3 weeks to identify an organism, but sometimes antigen testing can immediately indicate bacterial and nonbacterial organisms. As an exception to the general observation that infectious and inflammatory conditions produce CSF pleocytosis, in Guillain–Barré syndrome, CSF contains a markedly elevated protein concentration but little or no increase in the white cell content (the "albuminocytologic disassociation," see Chapter 5).

Despite the potential contribution of CSF examination, certain circumstances contraindicate an LP. For example, neurologists do not perform one when patients have a sacral decubitus ulcer because the LP needle might drive bacteria into the spinal canal and infect the CSF. In addition, neurologists insert the LP needle only below the first lumbar vertebra, the lower boundary of the spinal cord, to prevent spinal cord injury.

An intracranial mass lesion is one of the most common contraindications to an LP. This prohibition is based on the fear that an LP could suddenly reduce pressure in the spinal canal, allowing the unopposed force of a cerebral mass to lead to transtentorial herniation (see Fig. 19.3). Moreover, a CSF examination would not help in diagnosing most mass lesions because their CSF profiles are not distinctive. Although increased intracranial pressure without an associated mass lesion defines idiopathic intracranial hypertension (pseudotumor cerebri, see Chapter 9), in this setting neurologists perform LPs with impunity for diagnosis and occasionally for treatment. Overall, unless neurologists suspect acute bacterial meningitis or subarachnoid hemorrhage, in which case rapid diagnosis is crucial, they usually do not perform an LP or they postpone it until after imaging studies have excluded an intracranial lesion.

Another potential problem with an LP occurs when trauma during the procedure allows blood to mix with the CSF, which may falsely indicate a subarachnoid hemorrhage or other intracranial source. To distinguish blood induced by the procedure, laboratories centrifuge bloody CSF. Xanthochromia (Greek, *xanthos* yellow + *chroma* color) in the supernatant means that bleeding into the CSF space took place several hours before the LP and that red blood cells gave rise to the yellow pigment, which actually represents degraded heme molecules. In contrast, a clear supernatant means that the LP procedure itself gave rise to the blood in the CSF.

IMAGING STUDIES

Although computed tomography (CT) and magnetic resonance imaging (MRI) should not supplant physicians' clinical judgment, they undeniably provide extraordinarily accurate diagnoses. Each technique has given

TABLE 20.1 Cerebrospinal Fluid (CSF) Profiles*

	COLOR	WBC/ml	Protein (mg/dL)	Glucose (mg/dL)	MISCELLANEOUS
Normal	Clear	0–4[+]	30–45	60–100	
Bacterial meningitis	*Turbid*	100–500°	75–200	*0–40*	Gram stain may reveal organisms
Viral meningitis	*Turbid*	*50–100*[+&]	50–100	0–60	
TB and fungal meningitis^	*Turbid*	*100–500*[+]	100–500	40–60	*Cryptococcus* antigen should be ordered
Neurosyphilis	Clear	5–200[+]	45–100	40–80	VDRL positive[$]
Guillain–Barré syndrome	Clear	*5–20*	*80–200*	60–100	
Subarachnoid hemorrhage	*Bloody*	#	45–80	60–100	Supernatant usually xanthochromic if not bloody

*Characteristic abnormalities in italics
[+]Mostly lymphocytes
[&]In encephalitis from herpes simplex virus, the CSF also contains red blood cells
°Mostly polymorphonuclear cells
^In carcinomatous meningitis, the CSF profile is similar to fungal meningitis but malignant cells may be detected on cytologic examination
[$]Up to 40% of neurosyphilis cases have a false-negative VDRL CSF test (see Chapter 7)
#White and red cells are in the same proportion as in blood (1:1000)

clinical neurology a quantum leap forward. In fact, Drs. Allan M. Cormack and Godfrey N. Hounsfield garnered Nobel prizes in 1979 for development of CT, and Dr. Paul C. Lauterbur and Sir Peter Mansfield, the Nobel prizes in 2003 for discoveries fundamental to MRI.

Conceding that in many situations these imaging studies surpass the reliability of their neurologic examination, neurologists routinely order CT and MRI to evaluate patients' dementia, aphasia, neuropsychologic deficits, seizures, and other conditions. Even in cases of apparent delirium, they order it to exclude an underlying structural lesion. Neurologists also use imaging studies to follow the course of certain illnesses, such as brain tumors and multiple sclerosis, because their clinical manifestations often fail to reflect disease activity as reliably as imaging studies.

On the other hand, neurologists do not routinely order imaging studies in evaluating patients with sleep disturbances, absence seizures, cluster and migraine headaches, Parkinson disease, tics, or essential tremor. They also find that imaging studies, while revealing a neurologic aspect of the disorder, do not help with patients' diagnosis or management. For example, in autism, dyslexia and other learning disabilities, attention deficit hyperactivity disorder (ADHD), Tourette disorder, and Rett syndrome, imaging studies usually show normal brains, small brains, or regional variations, such as cerebellar atrophy.

When neurologists consult on psychiatric patients, they often recommend imaging studies, among other tests, for patients who have a first episode of psychosis, atypical psychosis, major depression after age 50 years, episodic behavioral disturbances, and, in some cases, anorexia. They also suggest imaging studies for patients prior to electroconvulsive treatment (ECT) for several reasons. A CT or MRI might detect lesions that could explain the psychiatric symptoms without producing overt physical deficits, such as neurocysticercosis or extensive cerebral demyelination. Likewise, cerebral lesions may provoke status epilepticus or transtentorial herniation. Although helpful in many circumstances, imaging studies often fail to clarify the relationships, if any, between psychiatric symptoms and many common abnormalities that the studies uncover, such as cerebral atrophy, mild communicating hydrocephalus, small cerebral lesions, subcortical hyperintensities, and congenital abnormalities.

COMPUTED TOMOGRAPHY

Using beams of ionizing radiation, which are essentially X-rays, CT generates images of the brain, other soft tissues, and skull. CT displays structures increasingly *more* radiodense than brain, such as tumors, blood, bone, calcifications, and surgical devices, in gradations increasingly closer to white than black. Similarly, it shows structures increasingly *less* radiodense than the brain, particularly the CSF-filled ventricles, in gradations increasingly closer to black. Thus, it shows in dark to black gradations several common lesions characterized by the absence of acute blood, such as cerebral infarctions, chronic subdural hematomas, edema surrounding tumors, and the center of cystic lesions. Likewise, it shows in light to white gradations several common lesions characterized by calcium or excessive blood, such as calcifications in the choroid plexus or meningiomas, acute subarachnoid, subdural, or intracerebral hemorrhages, and radiopaque intraventricular shunts. By manipulating the software, CT and MRI can display the brain from three major perspectives: axial (or horizontal, the conventional top-down view), coronal (front-to-back view), and sagittal (side view).

Although lacking fine detail, CT clearly reveals changes in major structures (Fig. 20.1). It shows generalized cerebral atrophy, such as occurs in advanced age or Alzheimer disease (Figs. 20.2 and 20.3), and atrophy of a particular region, such as with porencephaly (Fig. 20.4),

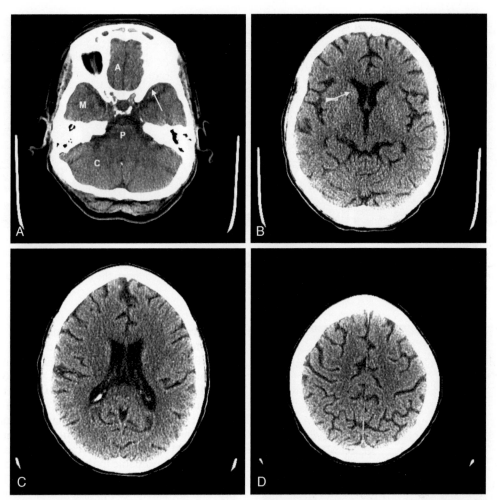

FIGURE 20.1 ■ These computed tomography (CT) scans show progressively higher axial images of a normal brain. *A,* The anterior cranial fossae (*A*) contain the anterior frontal lobes and the olfactory nerves. The middle fossae (*M*) contain the anterior temporal lobes, which are situated behind the bony sphenoid wing (*arrow*). The posterior fossa contains the cerebellum (*C*) and the medulla and pons (*P*) – major components of the *bulb. B,* The head of the caudate nucleus (*arrow*) indents the anterior horn of the lateral ventricle. *C,* The lateral ventricles extend lengthwise in the hemispheres. *D,* The cerebral cortex rests against the inner table of the skull. Thin sulci separate the gyri.

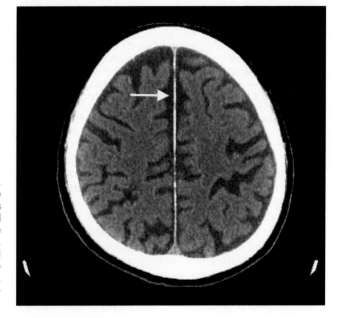

FIGURE 20.2 ■ This CT illustrates generalized cerebral atrophy. (See Fig. 20.18 for MRI appearance of cerebral atrophy.) Because of atrophy, the gyri shrink, sulci expand, cerebral cortex retracts from the inner table of the skull and from the falx (*arrow*), and ventricles expand (not seen on this image, which is above the level of the ventricles). Cerebral atrophy, as pictured in this case, represents a normal concomitant of old age. Although cerebral atrophy is associated with Alzheimer disease, vascular cognitive impairment, trisomy 21, alcoholism, neurodegenerative illnesses, and treatment-resistant schizophrenia, it is not invariably associated with dementia.

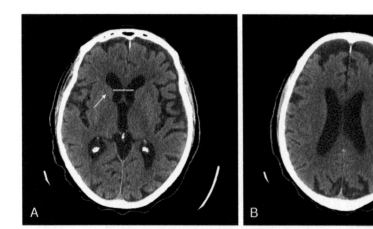
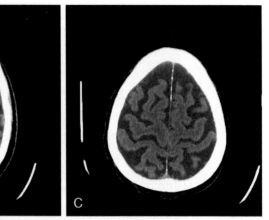

FIGURE 20.3 ■ These three progressively higher (left to right) CT images show that cerebral atrophy leads to expansion of the lateral ventricles (horizontal line) and widening of the third ventricle – *hydrocephalus ex vacuo* – as well as thinning of cerebral gyri and widening of sulci (*C*). Nevertheless, as *A* shows, the head of the caudate nucleus (arrow) maintains its normal volume and continues to indent the lateral border of the lateral ventricle. In Huntington disease, by way of contrast, the characteristic atrophy of the head of the caudate nuclei allows the ventricles to bow outward (see Fig. 20.5).

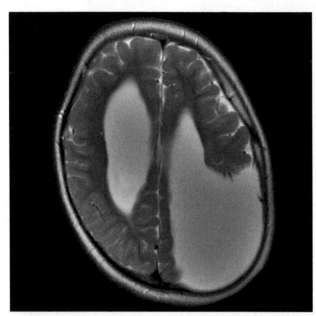

FIGURE 20.4 ■ CT and MRI, by convention, display the brain with its lateral sides reversed. For example, the left cerebral hemisphere appears on the right side of the CT image. Nevertheless, the frontal lobes still appear on the top on the image. In this MRI, the misshapen region filled with CSF in the parietal lobe represents a congenital absence of brain tissue, *porencephaly*, in the patient's left parietal lobe. The porencephaly displays the opposite effect of a mass lesion: the cystic lesion draws the adjacent lateral ventricle and midline structures toward it.

Huntington disease (Fig. 20.5), and frontotemporal dementia (Fig. 20.6). Similarly, it shows expansion of the ventricles – hydrocephalus – not only as a consequence of generalized atrophy (hydrocephalus ex vacuo) (see Fig. 20.3), but also from normal-pressure hydrocephalus (Fig. 20.7) and CSF obstructions (obstructive hydrocephalus) (see later). CT readily detects large lesions, such as primary and metastatic tumors (Fig. 20.8). CT will also reveal subdural hematomas, except perhaps for isodense ones (Fig. 20.9). CT is even superior at finding

dense, calcium-laden meningiomas (Fig. 20.10). It can show numerous small lesions, such as in toxoplasmosis (Fig. 20.11) and cysticercosis (Fig. 20.12), with the detail necessary for a firm diagnosis. (Cysticercosis, which is caused by the parasite *Taenia solium*, is the most common cerebral mass lesion in South and Central America.)

CT can also show strokes that are large established infarctions and those that are hemorrhagic (Fig. 20.13); however, MRI can better locate those that are small or acute. CT is invaluable in the special situation of cerebellar hemorrhage, where rapid diagnosis is essential to prevent brainstem compression and obstructive hydrocephalus (Fig. 20.14).

Despite the small risk of pediatric cerebral radiation exposure (see later), physicians routinely obtain head CT in suspected child abuse because 80% of cases include *nonaccidental head injury* (*NAHI*). Moreover, up to 50% of cases of NAHI result in neurologic deficits and 30% in fatality. CTs and MRIs are able to detect skull fractures and subdural hematomas that are bilateral and of different ages, which are the hallmark of NAHI.

The administration of an intravenous contrast agent during CT increases the density of blood-filled structures and whitens their image. This technique, *contrast enhancement*, highlights vascular structures, such as arteriovenous malformations (AVMs), glioblastomas, and membranes surrounding chronic subdural hematomas and cystic lesions (Fig. 20.15).

Although MRI holds many advantages, CT remains less expensive than MRI, highly reliable, and available in movable compact machines. It is particularly valuable during emergencies, when speed is critical and gross anatomical pictures suffice. For example, the procedure, which takes less than 5 minutes, satisfactorily reveals lesions that require immediate attention, such as epidural and acute subdural hematomas, large cerebellar hemorrhages, obstructive hydrocephalus, and subarachnoid hemorrhage. Also, patients with pacemakers, defibrillators, and other indwelling metallic devices, and those with claustrophobia can undergo CT but not MRI.

Text continued on p. 479

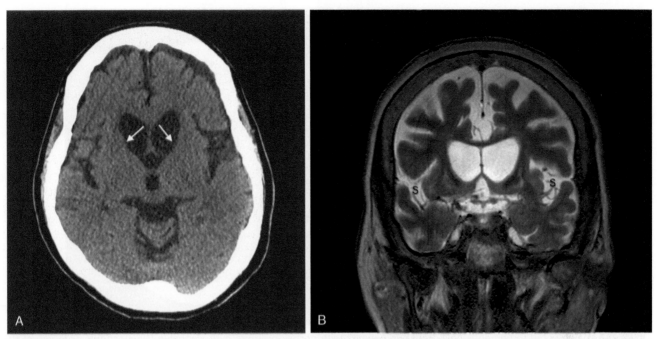

FIGURE 20.5 ■ *A*, This CT shows the characteristic abnormality of Huntington disease: the anterior horns of the lateral ventricles are convex (bowed outward) because of atrophy of the caudate nuclei (*arrows*). The convex shape of the ventricles in Huntington disease contrasts with the concave shape seen in normal individuals (see Figs. 20.1B and 20.17) and in those with cerebral atrophy and hydrocephalus ex vacuo (see Figs. 20.2, 20.3, and 20.18). In addition to the caudate atrophy, Huntington disease, like many other neurodegenerative illnesses, is associated with cortical atrophy with widened sulci and enlarged ventricles. *B*, This *coronal* view of the MRI of the same patient also shows the convex expansion of the lateral ventricles, large sulci, and widened Sylvian fissures (*S*).

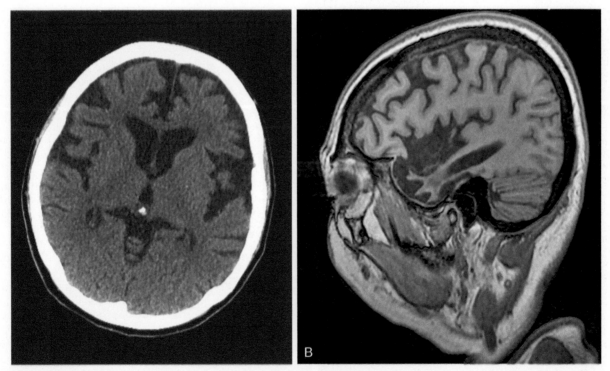

FIGURE 20.6 ■ *A*, This CT from a patient with frontotemporal dementia shows atrophy of the frontal and temporal lobes. Characteristically, the parietal and occipital lobes remain unchanged. *B*, Sagittal MRI from another patient with frontotemporal dementia clearly demonstrates the selective frontal and temporal lobe atrophy.

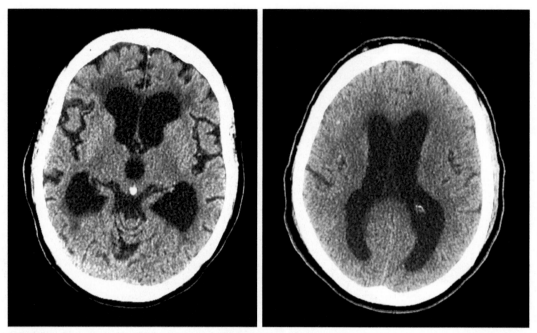

FIGURE 20.7 ■ Computed tomography (CT), from two patients with normal-pressure hydrocephalus (NPH), shows widening of the third and lateral ventricles with little or no cerebral atrophy. (See Fig. 20.19 for MRI of NPH.)

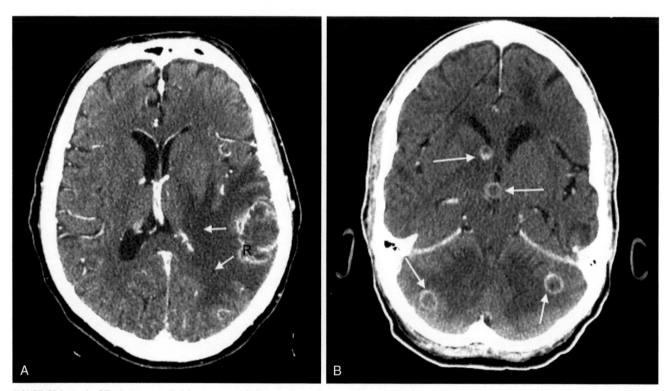

FIGURE 20.8 ■ *A,* CT shows a glioblastoma with its characteristic white, contrast-enhanced ring (R) and black border of edema (*arrows*). (See Fig. 20.20 for MRI showing a glioblastoma.) *B,* In another patient, CT shows several metastatic cerebral tumors that enhance with contrast (*arrows*).

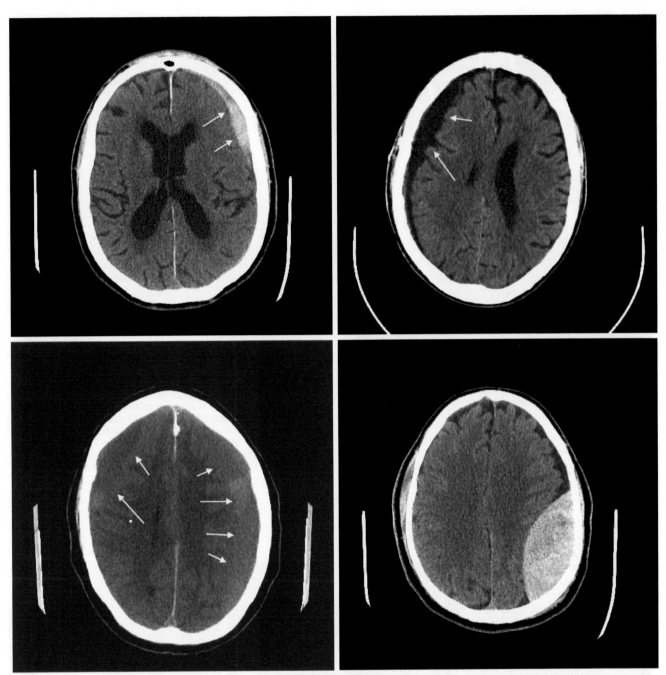

FIGURE 20.9 ■ *A,* The *acute* subdural hematoma (*arrows*) overlying the patient's left frontal lobe contains fresh blood, which is radiodense compared to normal brain tissue. *B,* The *chronic* subdural hematoma (*arrows*), overlying this patient's right cerebral hemisphere, contains aged, liquefied blood that is less radiodense than brain. Chronic subdural hematomas are typically black on a CT and often bordered by a radiodense, contrast-enhancing membrane, not well seen here. *C,* As acute subdural hematomas evolve into chronic ones, their density decreases to that of the underlying brain's density. When they become isodense, subdurals may be indistinguishable from the underlying brain tissue. This CT shows a barely visible isodense subdural overlying both of this patient's cerebral hemispheres. However, the membrane, compression of the gyri-sulci pattern, and shift of midline structures reveal its presence. *D,* This CT shows an epidural hematoma, which almost always represents acute intracranial bleed and therefore appears white. In the majority of cases, the CT shows a skull fracture, which is not seen in this view, as well as blood under the scalp. Note the hematoma's classic elliptical shape and, because of compression, shift of the underlying brain.

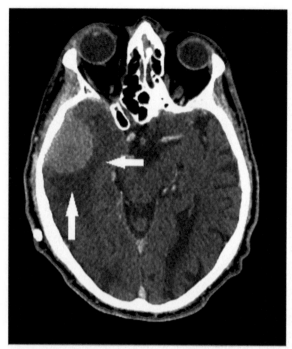

FIGURE 20.10 ■ This axial CT of a previously healthy 59-year-old man shows a large, rounded radiodense right temporal lesion, with a dural margin and some local edema (*arrows*). This image was obtained after the administration of intravenous iodinated contrast, and the lesion enhances uniformly. The lesion is typical for a chronic, slowly growing meningioma. As in this patient, meningiomas often reach a large size before producing seizures, neuropsychologic changes, or other symptoms.

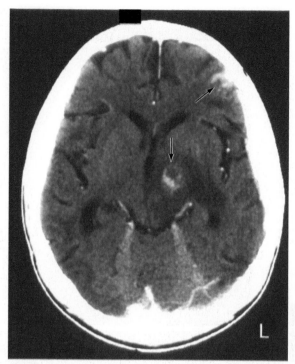

FIGURE 20.11 ■ A CT shows two toxoplasmosis lesions (*arrows*) enhanced by contrast infusion in the left cerebrum in a patient with AIDS. As in this study, toxoplasmosis has a predilection for developing in the basal ganglia in AIDS patients with CD4 counts below 200 cells/mm³. The infection's propensity to develop in the basal ganglia explains why AIDS patients who develop involuntary movement disorders, such as hemiballismus or chorea, are likely to harbor toxoplasmosis.

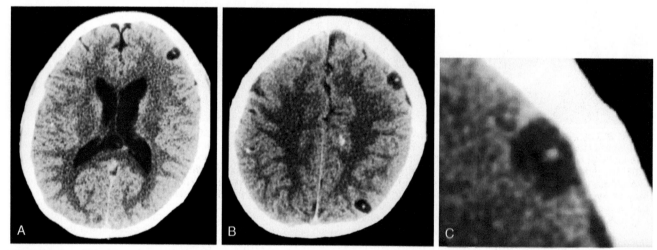

FIGURE 20.12 ■ This CT shows multiple cerebral cysticercosis lesions at two levels in the cerebrum (*A* and *B*) and an enlargement of the frontal cortex lesion (*C*). These lesions, in contrast to toxoplasmosis (see Fig. 20.11), are usually situated in the cerebral cortex, contain calcification, and lack surrounding edema. Even though each cyst is small, together they exert a substantial cumulative mass effect and irritate the surrounding cerebral cortex. Their tendency to irritate the cerebral cortex explains why patients with cysticercosis often first come to medical attention because of seizures.

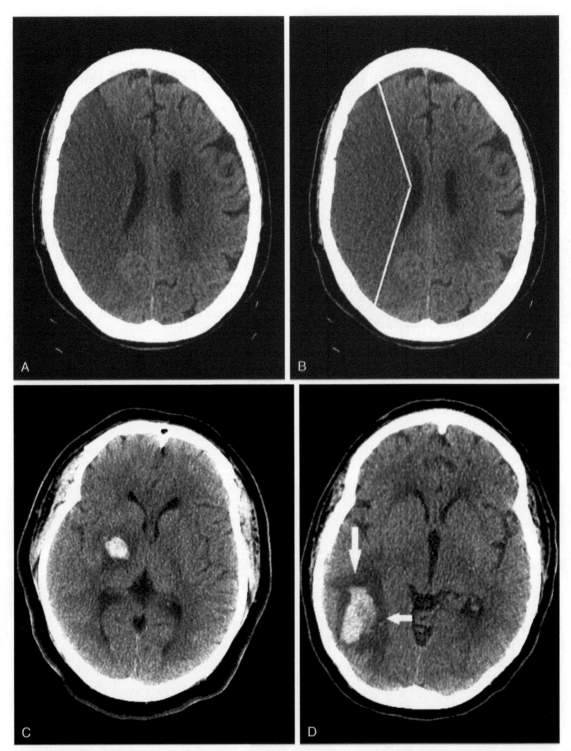

FIGURE 20.13 ■ *A*, This CT image shows an acute stroke from occlusion of the *right* middle cerebral artery. Because the infarcted area of the brain is deprived of blood, which is normally radiodense, it is darker (more hypodense) than the adjacent normal brain. In addition, its mass effect compresses the adjacent lateral ventricle and shifts midline structures. *B*, An outline of the stroke on the same image shows its wedge-shaped area in the lateral portion of the right cerebral hemisphere, containing the origin of the corticospinal tract for the left face and arm. *C*, This image shows a cerebral hemorrhage, likely from uncontrolled hypertension, which originated in the right thalamus. The blood, denser than the brain, forms the hyperdensity in the shape of a white plume. *D*, In this image, a hemorrhage (*arrows*) involves the right parietal lobe and compresses the occipital horn of the right lateral ventricle.

On the other hand, undergoing a CT exposes any patient to ionizing radiation. This radiation exposure potentially endangers children and adolescents because their dosage is relatively greater than for adults and their skull is thinner. Giving roughly the radiation of a skull X-ray series, a single head CT adds a measurable risk (0.07%) to the child's lifetime cancer risk. Furthermore, dental X-rays and, more so, dental CTs add to their lifetime radiation exposure. Another consideration in children is that because ocular lenses are highly susceptible

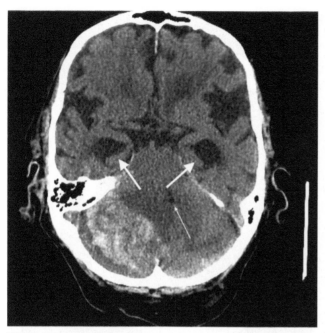

FIGURE 20.14 ■ This CT shows a large hyperdense, white mass lesion in the posterior fossa. The lesion is a cerebellar hemorrhage that has compressed and shifted the fourth ventricle (thin arrow), blocking CSF passage. The resulting obstructive hydrocephalus has caused dilation of the temporal horns of the lateral ventricles (*arrows*).

to radiation, CT adds to the risk of developing radiation-induced cataracts.

MAGNETIC RESONANCE IMAGING

In MRI, a powerful magnet forces protons to spin with their axes parallel to the magnetic field. Then radiofrequency (RF) pulses align the axes. After each RF pulse, the protons resume their original alignment ("relax") within the magnetic field and thereby emit energy. Different tissues emit characteristic, identifiable energy signals.

In the brain, hydrogen nuclei (protons) in water-containing tissues emit most of the signal. The differences in water content of tissues in various areas of the brain result in signals of different intensity. Sophisticated software converts them into images (the scans).

MRI offers several advantages over CT in addition to not exposing the patient to ionizing radiation. Because the resolution of MRI surpasses that of CT, its images provide finer detail (Fig. 20.16), more vivid displays of neuroanatomy (Fig. 20.17), and better illustrations of large common structural changes, such as atrophy (Fig. 20.18) and hydrocephalus (see Figs. 20.5, 20.7, and 20.19). It also shows fine detail of mass lesions, such as glioblastomas and strokes (Figs. 20.20 through 20.24). With *diffusion-weighted images* (*DWI*), a standard sequence

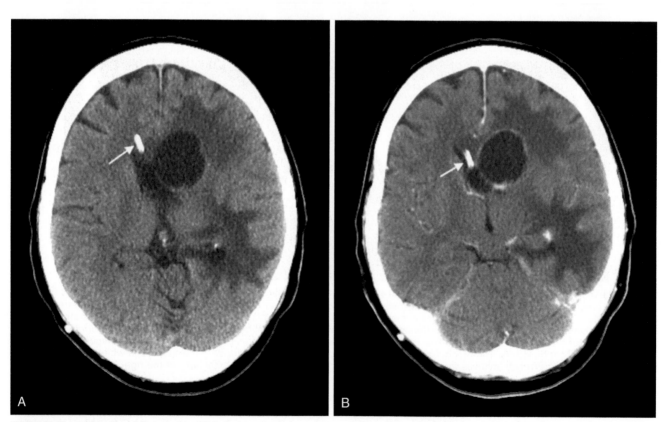

FIGURE 20.15 ■ CT before (*A*) and after (*B*) infusion of contrast material highlights an abscess in a patient's left frontal region. Disruption of the blood–brain barrier allows the contrast material to concentrate in the lesion's membranes. In both images, a radio-opaque ventricular catheter can be visualized (arrow).

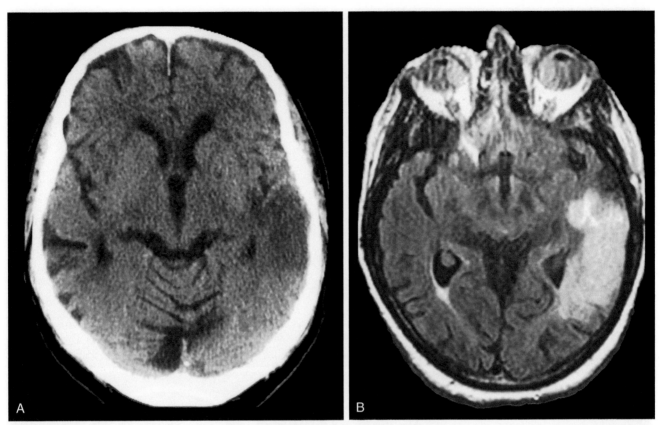

FIGURE 20.16 ■ CT (*A*) and MRI (*B*) showing MRI's superior resolution and ability to detect acute cerebral infarctions. In this case, a left temporal lobe infarction, barely discernible on CT, is obvious on MRI.

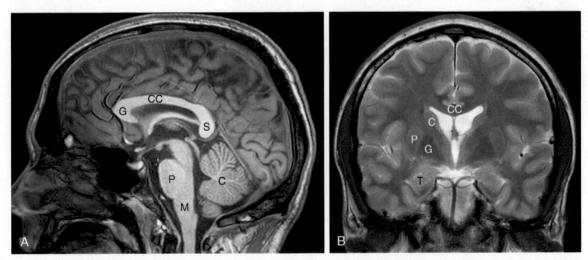

FIGURE 20.17 ■ *A,* An MRI *sagittal* view of a normal brain reveals exquisitely detailed cerebral gyri and sulci, the corpus callosum (*CC*) (the "great commissure"), and three major structures of the posterior fossa: the pons (*P*), medulla (*M*), and cerebellum (*C*). The anterior portion of the corpus callosum is the genu (*G*), and its posterior portion, the splenium (*S*). In addition, it shows the cervical–medullary junction and various nonneurologic soft tissue structures. Note that the medulla remains above the foramen magnum. *B,* The coronal view reveals the corpus callosum (*CC*), which connects the cerebral hemispheres. The white matter of the corpus callosum and subcortical cerebral hemispheres is distinct from the ribbon of overlying gray matter. The anterior horns of the lateral ventricles, with their concave lateral borders, are beneath the corpus callosum and indented by the caudate nuclei (*C*) (see Fig. 18.1A). The putamen (*P*) sits lateral to the globus pallidus (*G*). The frontal lobe is above the Sylvian fissure, and the temporal lobe (T) is below.

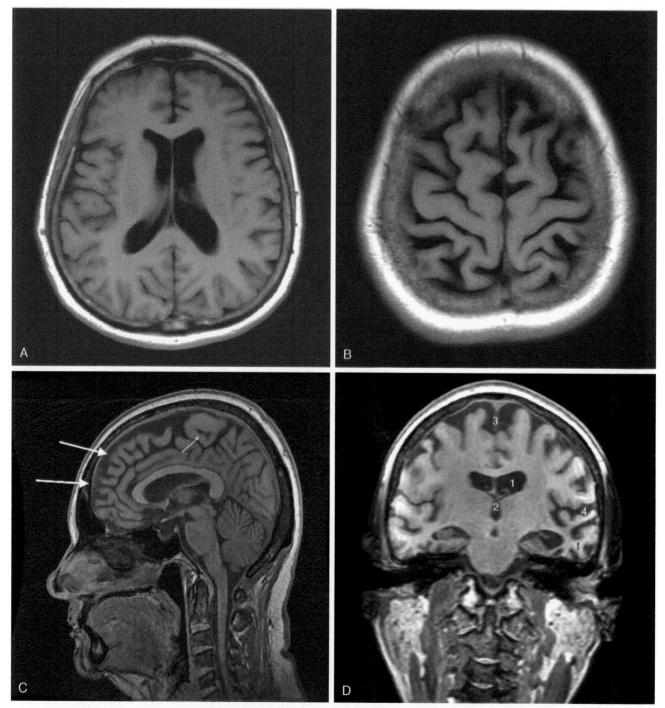

FIGURE 20.18 ■ Four MRI images of cerebral atrophy can be contrasted to the normal brain (see Fig. 20.17). MRI emphasizes cerebral atrophy because it does not detect the cortical bone of the skull, which emits almost no signal because it contains virtually no water. However, the scalp emits a signal because it contains blood, fat, and other water-containing soft tissues. *A*, In this axial view through the cerebral hemispheres, the CSF, which is dark, fills the dilated lateral ventricles and sulci. In other MRI sequences (not shown), CSF appears bright. *B*, In a view that shows the surface of the brain, MRI demonstrates the thin gyri. To fill the void left by the atrophied gyri, copious amounts of CSF fill the sulci and cover the cortex. *C*, In a sagittal view, the MRI shows thin, ribbon-like frontal lobe gyri (*large arrows*) and less atrophied parietal lobe gyri (*small arrow*). The corpus callosum, pons, and cerebellum stand out. The tentorium, appearing as a straight line, is situated above the cerebellum. *D*, This coronal view through the frontal lobes shows typical manifestations of cerebral atrophy: (1) dilated lateral ventricles, (2) an enlarged third ventricle, (3) enlargement of the anterior interhemispheric fissure because of separation of the medial surfaces of the frontal lobes, and (4) dilated Sylvian fissures with the atrophic temporal lobe (t) below and the atrophic frontal lobe above.

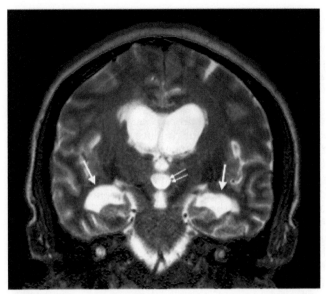

FIGURE 20.19 ■ This MRI study shows a coronal view of the brain of a patient with NPH. It demonstrates the classic findings: dilation of the lateral ventricles, their temporal horns (*large arrows*), and the third ventricle (*pair of arrows*), and absence of cerebral atrophy.

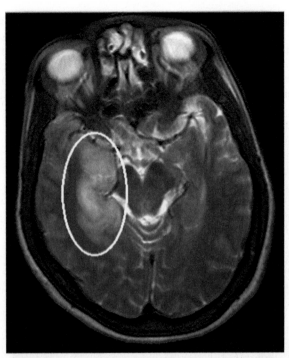

FIGURE 20.21 ■ An axial projection of an MRI of a young man with acute herpes simplex encephalitis shows hyperintensity in inferior gyri of the right temporal lobe (*circled*). As in this case, herpes simplex infection typically causes hemorrhagic inflammation in the inferior surface of the temporal and frontal lobes. Permanent temporal lobe damage, which is often bilateral, subjects survivors to memory impairment (amnesia), partial complex seizures, and the Klüver–Bucy syndrome.

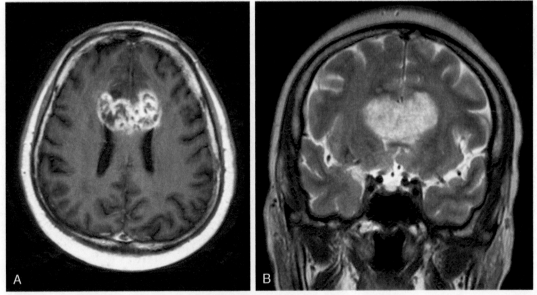

FIGURE 20.20 ■ Axial (*A*) and coronal (*B*) projections of an MRI show a large lobulated hyperintense lesion that, on biopsy, proved to be a glioblastoma. This aggressive, deadly tumor often develops in one frontal lobe and infiltrates through the genu of the corpus callosum to invade the other. It first caused personality changes and cognitive impairments, but no physical deficits. Neurologists often describe the MRI appearance of such tumors as "butterfly gliomas."

of a routine study, MRI can show cerebral infarctions not only with fine detail, but, unlike CT, also almost immediately after their onset (see Fig. 20.24). MRI, but not CT, can support the diagnosis of illnesses that alter cerebral or spinal cord white matter, i.e., leukoencephalopathies, such as many congenital storage diseases, MS

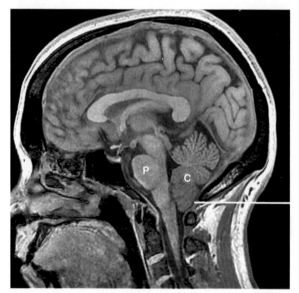

FIGURE 20.22 ■ In this sagittal MRI view of an Arnold–Chiari malformation, the cerebellar tonsils (C) and the medulla, caudal to the pons (P), are situated below the foramen magnum (*line*). The malformation has also caused aqueductal stenosis that will lead to hydrocephalus (not seen).

(Fig. 20.25), PML, and hydrocarbon solvent abuse. In MS, neurologists rely on MRI to confirm the diagnosis, establish the extent, and subsequently detect new, often clinically silent lesions. MRI also shows abnormalities, although not specific, in prion illnesses, such as CJD and fatal familial insomnia (see Chapter 17).

MRI holds another advantage because most of the skull is composed of cortical bone, which contains no water: the skull does not produce linear streak artifacts that obscure images – a common problem in CT. The lack of artifact allows MRI to generate detailed images of structures in bony casings, such as the acoustic nerves, cerebellum and other posterior fossa contents, the pituitary gland, and the spinal cord. Neurologists require MRI in diagnosing mesial temporal sclerosis (Fig. 20.26) and planning epilepsy surgery. MRI is also indispensable in identifying acoustic neuromas (Fig. 20.27). However, because it does not detect lesions with little or no water content, MRI may fail to display skull fractures. MRI is used safely in pediatric populations, and neurologists order this test for the evaluation of children with milestone regression, significantly increased head circumference for age, and epilepsy.

Administration of paramagnetic contrast solutions, such as gadopentetate (gadolinium), can enhance intracranial abnormalities. Although they do not cross the intact blood–brain barrier, contrast solutions highlight lesions that disrupt the barrier, such as neoplasms, abscesses, active MS plaques, and acute infarctions. Gadolinium, once thought to be universally safe, is avoided in patients with renal insufficiency or failure, as there is

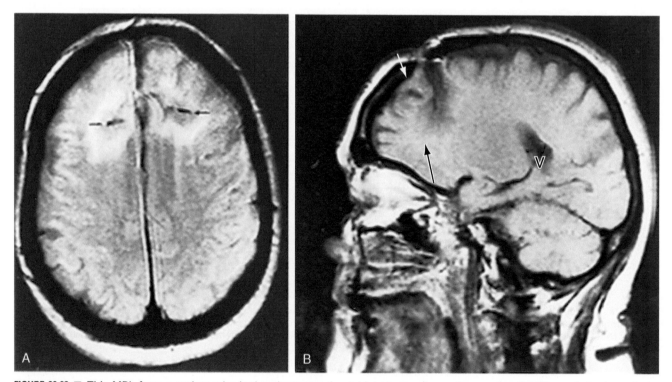

FIGURE 20.23 ■ This MRI, from a patient who had undergone a frontal lobotomy, shows the results of drilling a hole through the skull above each frontal lobe and severing their white matter tracts. *A*, The axial view shows black horizontal slits, which represent the incisions and their surrounding scar tissue. *B*, The sagittal view through the right cerebral hemisphere shows the skull defect (*white arrow*) and lowermost extent of the incision (*black arrow*). The frontal lobe anterior to the incision has undergone atrophy. The radiolucent area in the posterior cerebrum (*V*) is the right posterior lateral ventricle.

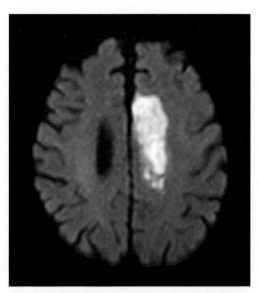

FIGURE 20.24 ■ This diffusion-weighted image (DWI) sequence on MRI shows an acute stroke in the left anterior cerebral artery territory. This finding was not apparent on CT done shortly after onset of symptoms.

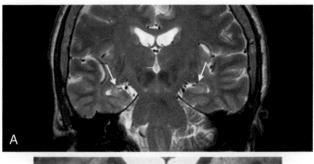

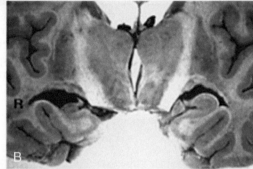

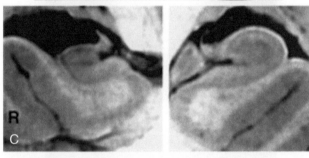

FIGURE 20.26 ■ *A,* This coronal view of an MRI shows right-sided mesial temporal sclerosis, which consists of shrinkage and scarring of the hippocampus and underlying amygdala. Comparing the medial temporal lobes (*arrows*), the patient's left-sided medial temporal lobe is round and broad, but the right-sided one, beset by sclerosis, is contracted and poorly demarcated. Moreover, because of the sclerosis, it emits a slightly brighter (*white*) signal. *B,* The brain, at approximately the comparable level as the MRI, shows that the patient's normal left medial temporal lobe is round and has a well-demarcated cortex. In the enlarged sections (*C*), the patient's left medial temporal lobe appears as a duck's head facing medially. The lateral ventricle's rounded temporal horn overlies the temporal lobe. In contrast, the patient's right medial temporal lobe is shrunken and contracted inferiorly and laterally. The overlying ventricle's temporal horn is much larger than its counterpart because atrophy allowed it to expand.

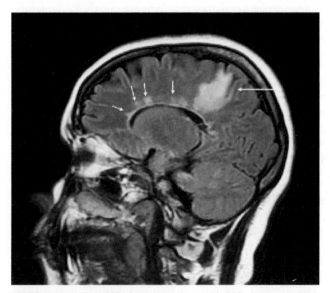

FIGURE 20.25 ■ This MRI from a patient with MS shows multiple areas of demyelination. MS lesions, often called plaques, are typically high signal (*white*) and clustered in the deep white matter of the cerebral hemispheres, and tend to spread outward from the ventricles ("Dawson's fingers"). In this sagittal view image, a large lesion is situated in the patient's right parietal lobe, posterior to the lateral ventricle (*arrow*). Multiple lesions arise periventricularly (small arrows) and may also involve the corpus callosum. Because MS plaques generally first develop in the periventricular white matter and spare the cerebral cortex, cognitive impairments are not an early manifestation of MS.

an association between gadolinium exposure in such patients and a rare but debilitating and generally irreversible condition, *nephrogenic sclerosing fibrosis,* in which skin, muscle, and other tissues become fibrotic and indurated.

Despite its greater resolution, MRI is no more effective than CT in diagnosing several important illnesses,

including Alzheimer disease and childhood neuropsychiatric conditions. Moreover, it has some disadvantages. One problem is that for 30 to 40 minutes, patients remain entirely within the bore of the MRI magnet – an intimidating long, narrow tunnel, with a diameter only slightly wider than their body. Even excluding patients with known claustrophobia, at least 10% of the remainder, sometimes in utter panic, abort the procedure. Taking a benzodiazepine and wearing a sleep mask may alleviate enough anxiety to allow many mildly claustrophobic patients to remain in the machine.

A potentially life-threatening problem with MRI is that the magnet forcefully attracts ferrous metals.

Metallic objects inadvertently brought into the room have formed deadly missiles. Pacemakers, implanted hearing devices, intracranial aneurysm clips manufactured before 1993, and other medical devices might be dislodged or destroyed if the patient were exposed to the intense magnetic field.

As an expectable corollary of the large number of MRI studies performed and the high resolution of MRI, many scans detect abnormalities that have no established clinical significance. For example, brain MRI in 4% of asymptomatic individuals aged 45 to 60 years old and in almost 20% of those 75 to 97 years old shows small hyperintense lesions, which neurologists dub "unidentified bright objects (UBOs)." Neurologists variously attribute these UBOs to migraine, small strokes, small MS plaques, dilated CSF spaces, or normal aged-related changes.

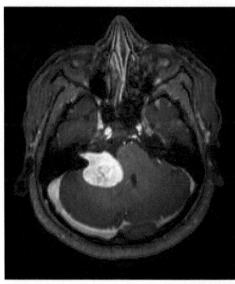

FIGURE 20.27 ■ A large acoustic neuroma, originating from the patient's right cerebellopontine angle, compresses the pons and shifts the fourth ventricle. In contrast to being obvious on this MRI, cerebellopontine angle lesions may escape detection on CT because they are usually small and sequestered in a corner of the skull base where artifacts obscure them. Neurofibromatosis type 2 patients, who tend to develop bilateral acoustic neuromas, routinely undergo MRI with views of the internal auditory canals.

MRI also detects small cerebral artery aneurysms and meningiomas that are innocuous and bear no relationship to patients' symptoms.

Other Applications of Magnetic Resonance

With the appropriate software, magnetic resonance can generate images of intracranial and extracranial cerebral vessels. This technique, magnetic resonance angiography (MRA), can display highly accurate images of the carotid and vertebral arteries (Fig. 11.2). It can detect aneurysms, AVMs, and other vascular malformations. Because it can outline internal carotid artery stenosis, plaques, and dissections, MRA eliminates the need for conventional carotid angiography (Fig. 20.28), which can be hazardous and painful.

The remarkable sensitivity of MRI has led to *functional MRI (fMRI)*, a technique that displays gross metabolic activity. Based on different properties of blood in its oxygenated and deoxygenated states, fMRI exploits small increases in blood flow and oxygen metabolism during cerebral activity. It highlights regions of the brain receiving sensory stimuli, initiating physical activity, imagining sensory or physical experiences, and performing cognitive processes – activities that increase metabolic demands. For example, it can detect language circuits. Thus, fMRI may eventually replace the Wada test in epilepsy surgery candidates (see Chapter 8).

Magnetic resonance spectroscopy (MRS) detects the chemical composition of cerebral tissues and lesions. The technique's software suppresses water-generated signals and then analyzes the remaining ones to determine the presence and concentration of choline, creatine, N-acetyl aspartate, lactic acid, lipids, and other chemicals. Preliminary work has shown that MRS can characterize tumors, abscesses, other lesions, mitochondrial encephalopathies, and degenerative diseases by the presence and relative concentrations of these substrates.

Another application of magnetic resonance, *diffusion tensor imaging (DTI)*, contrasts normal and abnormal flow of water molecules. DTI measures *anisotropy*, which consists of the greater diffusion of water molecule motion in certain directions than in others. Among its many uses, DTI dramatically and in multiple colors shows white matter tracts. It readily detects traumatic brain injury

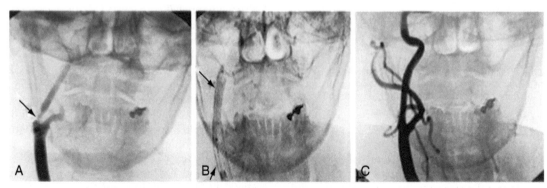

FIGURE 20.28 ■ This angiogram shows how insertion and deployment of a carotid stent form a tubular scaffold that reduces stenosis. *A,* The angiogram demonstrates the right common carotid artery ascending and dividing into the external and internal carotid artery, which has a severe stenosis (arrow). *B,* The stent (*arrows*) has been inserted and expanded. *C,* A follow-up angiogram shows a patent and smooth internal carotid artery.

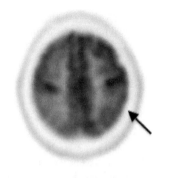 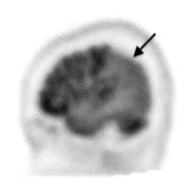 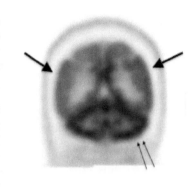

FIGURE 20.29 ■ This PET scan of the brain of a patient with Alzheimer disease dementia demonstrates the typical decreased metabolic activity in the parietal lobes (large arrows) but normal metabolic activity in the occipital lobes (small double arrows).

(TBI), even in cases without abnormality on neurologic physical examination or conventional MRI. DTI is useful in finding TBI in closed head injuries, such as warfare blast injuries. What might be helpful to therapists is that in patients with posttraumatic stress disorder who possibly have comorbid TBI, DTI will detect the presence and extent of the TBI.

POSITRON EMISSION TOMOGRAPHY

In contrast to CT and MRI, which can provide exquisitely detailed images of CNS anatomy, *positron emission tomography* (*PET*) provides a rough, relatively low-resolution picture of metabolic activity in various regions of the brain. In other words, PET illustrates brain function rather than structure. PET relies on positron-emitting, biologically active radioisotopes (*radioligands*) produced in cyclotrons and incorporated into organic molecules. The radioligands, which are inhaled or injected intravenously, undergo metabolism in the brain and emit positrons. The reaction between positrons and electrons produces photons, which PET detects and transforms into images.

Most PET studies measure the metabolism of a substitute for glucose, fluorine-18-labeled fluorodeoxyglucose (FDG). Like glucose, FDG is absorbed into the brain and metabolized. The metabolism of FDG emits positrons at a rate that parallels cerebral glucose metabolism. Similarly, metabolism of oxygen-15-labeled water reflects cerebral blood flow and metabolism of fluorine-18-labeled fluorodopa reflects dopamine metabolism. PET using radioligands for serotonin, gamma-aminobutyric acid (GABA), and acetylcholine (ACh) permits visualization of the distribution and activity of their receptors. All these radioligands have a brief half-life. For example, oxygen-15 has a half-life of 2 minutes, and fluorine-18 less than 2 hours.

Neuroscientists use PET to analyze cerebral metabolism during normal activities, administration of medications, and several illnesses. It offers valuable imaging in some varieties of epilepsy, neurodegenerative illnesses, and structural lesions. In epilepsy, PET images show that in focal epilepsy with impaired awareness (formerly complex partial epilepsy), the affected temporal lobe is generally hypoactive during the interictal period but hyperactive during seizures. Determining whether the temporal lobe is epileptogenic by this method, which is complementary to electroencephalography and fMRI, helps decide if a temporal lobectomy would benefit a patient with intractable epilepsy (see Chapter 10).

PET is also helpful in studying several neurodegenerative illnesses. In Alzheimer disease, PET shows decreased cerebral metabolism, especially in the parietal and frontal lobes' association areas (Fig. 20.29). It can also help distinguish vascular neurocognitive disorder and frontotemporal dementia from Alzheimer disease. More importantly, using one of several amyloid-binding ligands, PET can localize and quantitate amyloid deposition, which allows for a diagnosis of Alzheimer disease in its presymptomatic as well as symptomatic stages (see Chapter 7). The implication of positive findings in presymptomatic individuals is that neurologists may diagnose Alzheimer disease long before patients fulfill *Diagnostic and Statistical Manual of Mental Disorders, 5th Edition* (DSM-5) criteria for the disease. PET may also detect abnormalities that appear before either clinical signs or MRI abnormalities in Parkinson and Huntington diseases, and it can monitor the progression of these illnesses.

Although useful when the diagnosis rests on regional changes in metabolic activity, PET cannot reliably detect or classify brain tumors because the brain is so highly metabolic that any increased activity generated by a tumor would be lost in the background levels. Moreover, its resolution is too low to allow precise delineation of a lesion's anatomy. However, PET can make valuable contributions in certain situations because it can distinguish between tumors and some nonmalignant conditions. For example, PET can distinguish between recurrent brain tumors and radiation necrosis. Also, as a complement to CSF testing for the JC virus in the diagnosis of PML, PET can also distinguish PML from lymphoma because PML lesions are typically hypometabolic while lymphomas are typically hypermetabolic.

SINGLE-PHOTON EMISSION COMPUTED TOMOGRAPHY

Single-photon emission computed tomography (*SPECT*), like PET, portrays changes in cerebral function. It can map cerebral blood flow and, to a certain extent, neurotransmitter receptor activity. It can show major changes in cerebral blood flow – which reflects metabolic activity – in stroke, seizures, migraine, recurrent brain tumors, and neurodegenerative diseases.

Like PET, SPECT lacks precision and fine spatial resolution. However, it is simpler to operate, less expensive, and suitable for many clinical studies. SPECT uses readily available, stable radioligands, such as radioactive xenon, which do not require a cyclotron for preparation. The radioligands emit only a single easily detectable photon.

Although SPECT demonstrates somewhat different patterns in dementia due to Alzheimer disease, vascular disease, or head injury, neurologists do not consider it a part of a routine evaluation of patients with dementia.

INTERVENTIONAL RADIOLOGY

In the past decade, neuroradiologists have introduced dramatic therapies for several neurologic diseases. They offer MRI-guided needle biopsies of cerebral and spinal lesions, which are often deep-seated or otherwise unapproachable, that spare patients invasive and painful surgery. Neuroradiologists have been able to dilate stenoses of external carotid arteries and insert stents to maintain their patency (see Chapter 11), but treating stenoses in small intracerebral vessels remains unsafe. They can float epoxy resins or particles into inoperable AVMs or aneurysms. Similarly, they can direct catheters to deliver chemotherapy to brain tumors.

REFERENCES

Allison, K., Miller, T., & Bello, J. (2008). Neuroradiological imaging in children. In A. M. Walker, D. M. Kaufman, C. Pfeffer, et al. (Eds.), *Child and Adolescent Neurology for Psychiatrists*. Philadelphia: Lippincott Williams & Wilkins.

Fazel, R., Krumholz, H., Wang, S. M. Y., et al. (2009). Exposure to low-dose ionizing radiation from medical imaging procedures. *The New England Journal of Medicine, 361,* 849–857.

Giedd, J. N. (2006). Anatomic imaging of the developing brain. In C. E. Coffey & R. A. Brumback (Eds.), *Pediatric Neuropsychiatry*. Philadelphia: Lippincott Williams & Wilkins.

Johnson, K. A., & Becker, J. A. The Whole Brain Atlas: <http://www.med.harvard.edu/AANLIB/home.html>.

Miglioretti, D. L., Johnson, E., Williams, A., et al. (2013). The use of computed tomography in pediatrics and the associated radiation exposure and estimated cancer risk. *JAMA Pediatrics, 167,* 700–707.

Ong, K. T., Villemagne, V. L., Bahar-Fuchs, A., et al. (2015). Aβ imaging with 18-F-florbetaben in prodromal Alzheimer's disease: a prospective outcome study. *Journal of Neurology, Neurosurgery, and Psychiatry., 86,* 431–436.

Runge, V. M., Smoker, W. R. K., & Valavanis, A. (2015). *Neuroradiology: The Essentials with MR and CT*. New York: Thieme.

Tocchio, S., Kline-Fath, B., Kanal, E., et al. (2015). MRI evaluation and safety in the developing brain. *Seminars in Perinatology, 39,* 73–104.

Vernooij, M., Ikram, M. A., Tanghe, H. L., et al. (2007). Incidental findings on brain MRI in the general population. *The New England Journal of Medicine, 357,* 1821–1828.

QUESTIONS AND ANSWERS

1. Why do laboratories centrifuge blood-tinged CSF?
   a. Concentrating cells allows for easier counting.
   b. It permits detection of xanthochromia.
   c. It restores the balance between cells and protein.
   d. The proteins separate from the glucose.

Answer: b. Centrifuging separates the cells from the CSF to allow detection of xanthochromia in the CSF supernatant. If present, xanthochromia indicates that bleeding occurred in the CSF several hours before a spinal tap. The origin of xanthochromia is usually head trauma or a subarachnoid hemorrhage, as opposed to merely a traumatic spinal tap. Excessively eating carrots or very high CSF protein, which retains bilirubin, lends a yellow or orange hue to CSF that mimics xanthochromia.

2–3. During the 12 hours before his family brought him for evaluation, a 50-year-old man developed fever, confusion, headache, and lethargy. His neurologic examination showed memory loss and inattention, but no nuchal rigidity or lateralized findings. During his general medical examination, which revealed no abnormalities, he had repetitive lip-smacking movements, shaking movements of his right hand, and then loss of consciousness for 15 minutes. A chest X-ray and head CT showed no abnormalities.

2. Which profile is his CSF apt to show?
   a. WBC 80/mL, 90% lymphocytes; glucose 50 mg/dL; protein 60 mg/dL
   b. WBC 200/mL, 80% polymorphonuclear cells; glucose 15 mg/dL; protein 90 mg/dL
   c. WBC 3/mL; glucose 80 mg/dL; protein 35 mg/dL
   d. WBC 300/mL, 100% lymphocytes; glucose 5 mg/dL; protein 300 mg/dL

Answer: a. He probably has developed herpes simplex encephalitis in view of the amnesia and partial complex seizure, which reflect temporal lobe damage. The lack of nuchal rigidity indicates the absence of meningitis. Profile *b* indicates bacterial meningitis; profile *c* is normal; and profile *d* suggests a chronic nonbacterial process, such as tuberculous or carcinomatous meningitis.

3. If further testing confirms the clinical diagnosis of herpes simplex encephalitis, which is the most common

variety of nonepidemic encephalitis, what is the magnetic resonance imaging (MRI) most likely to show?
   a. No abnormalities
   b. Hemorrhagic regions in one or both temporal lobes
   c. Multiple circular lesions in the cerebral cortex
   d. Multiple circular lesions in the deep cerebrum

Answer: b. Herpes simplex causes hemorrhagic encephalitis that affects the base of the brain, particularly the inferior temporal and frontal lobes.

4–7. Match the disease with the CSF marker:

4. Alzheimer disease
5. Creutzfeldt–Jakob
6. Multiple sclerosis
7. Subacute sclerosing panencephalitis
   a. 14-3-3 protein
   b. Antimeasles antibodies
   c. Increased levels of tau protein and decreased levels of Aβ42 peptide
   d. Oligoclonal bands

Answers: 4–c, 5–a, 6–d, 7–b.

8. A 30-year-old woman with a history of depression develops increasingly severe generalized headaches. Neurologic examination shows florid papilledema and bilateral sixth cranial nerve palsies, but she remains fully alert and without cognitive impairment, paresis, or ataxia. An MRI shows small ventricles and no mass lesions. Which profile is her CSF apt to show?
   a. Pressure 300 mm H_2O; WBC 80/mL, 90% lymphocytes; glucose 50 mg/dL; protein 60 mg/dL
   b. Pressure 200 mm H_2O; WBC 200/mL, 80% polymorphonuclear cells; glucose 15 mg/dL; protein 90 mg/dL
   c. Pressure 450 mm H_2O; WBC 1/mL; glucose 65 mg/dL; protein 20 mg/dL
   d. Pressure 100 mm H_2O; WBC 300/mL, 100% lymphocytes; glucose 5 mg/dL; protein 300 mg/dL

Answer: c. She probably has idiopathic intracranial hypertension (pseudotumor cerebri) with high enough pressure to stretch the sixth nerves, creating a classic false localizing sign. In this condition, the CSF protein and glucose concentrations are often lower than normal, as if by dilution.

9. Why does contrast infusion during CT highlight brain tumors and abscesses?
   a. Inflammatory cells absorb contrast material.
   b. Osmotic forces pull the material into the lesion.
   c. Breakdown of the blood–brain barrier surrounding the lesion allows contrast material to highlight its boundaries.
   d. Neoplastic and infectious cells metabolize contrast material.

Answer: c. Brain tumors, abscesses, and other lesions disrupt the blood–brain barrier and allow contrast material to surround and penetrate at least their perimeter.

10. Which one of the following intracranial structures will be readily recognizable on CT but almost invisible on MRI?
    a. Temporal lobe hematoma
    b. Porencephaly
    c. Calcified pineal gland
    d. Toxoplasmosis

Answer: c. Calcified objects that lack water, such as calcium in a choroid plexus, congenital infections, and a calcified pineal gland, will emit little or no signal on MRI without using special sequences. However, their calcium, which is radiodense, blocks the ionizing radiation of CT and thus allows for detection of these anatomic and pathologic findings.

11–12. Below is the MRI of a 30-year-old man with progressive cognitive impairment for 2 years and a family history of a similar disorder.

11. Which view of the brain does this scan portray?
    a. Axial
    b. Transaxial
    c. Coronal
    d. Sagittal

Answer: c. This is a *coronal* view, which is readily identifiable by displaying simultaneously the frontal and temporal lobes and the lateral and third ventricles. *Axial* and *transaxial* are synonymous with each other.

12. Although the image is not definitive, which cause of dementia does it suggest?
    a. Alzheimer disease
    b. Frontotemporal dementia
    c. Huntington disease
    d. Diffuse Lewy bodies disease
    e. A structural lesion

Answer: c. This image shows diffuse cerebral atrophy, which is nonspecific. More strikingly, it shows convex expansion of the lateral ventricles because of atrophy of the head of the caudate nuclei. That abnormality strongly suggests Huntington disease.

13–14. The wife of a 65-year-old man reports that over 6 months he has lost his liveliness. She states, "The situation has gone from dumb to dementia." He sold his business 4 months before the visit because of his lack of interest and then financial miscalculations. On examination, he has mild cognitive impairment and apathy, but no lateral signs. Below is his CT.

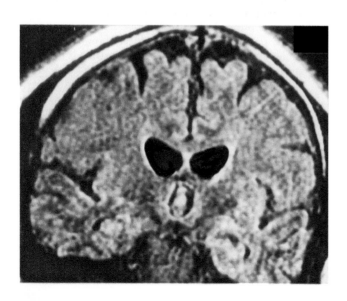

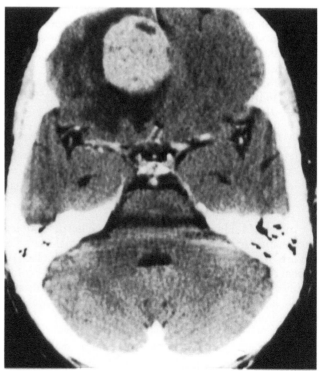

13. Where is the lesion located?
  a. Left frontal
  b. Right frontal
  c. At the junction of the middle and anterior fossae
  d. None of the above

Answer: b. In this CT axial view, as is customary, the left side of the brain is displayed on the right. A large radiodense (white) circular lesion sits in the medial portion of the patient's right frontal lobe. The black hypodensity, posterior and lateral to the lesion, indicates edema. Structural lesions of the frontal lobes, especially those that grow slowly on the right side, may reach extraordinary size before they produce symptoms. Frontal lobe lesions frequently dull the patient's personality, drain initiative, and diminish creativity. Alternatively, frontal lesions may reduce inhibition. Compared to their effect on mood and behavior, frontal lobe lesions may cause little or no cognitive impairment or physical abnormality.

14. What is the most likely etiology of the lesion?
  a. Abscess
  b. Glioblastoma
  c. Meningioma
  d. Stroke

Answer: c. The lesion's extra-axial location, circular shape, and relatively uniform, high density indicate that it is a meningioma. Adjusting the displayed image would reveal that it contains calcium, which is characteristic of meningiomas. The condition's relatively long course also suggests a slowly developing lesion, such as a meningioma, rather than an abscess or glioblastoma. Also, abscesses and glioblastomas usually have hyperintense borders and heterogeneous density. Large strokes generally conform to the distribution of a cerebral artery and have a wedge-shaped appearance.

15–16. Performed as part of the evaluation of a 30-year-old man who presented after his first seizure, an MRI showed several ring-shaped lesions.

15. Which of the following conditions do not typically cause multiple ring-shaped lesions?

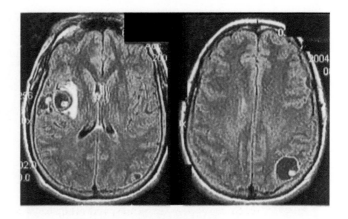

  a. Abscess
  b. Toxoplasmosis
  c. Cysticercosis
  d. Metastases
  e. Primary brain tumors

Answer: e. Primary brain tumors, such as glioblastomas and astrocytomas, typically cause only single lesions, which may have a ring shape. The other conditions typically cause multiple ring-shaped lesions. The history, nonneurologic findings, blood tests, or, if necessary, a biopsy usually allow a diagnosis.

16. In this case, which is the most likely diagnosis?
  a. Abscess
  b. Toxoplasmosis
  c. Cysticercosis
  d. Metastases
  e. Primary brain tumors

Answer: c. The two MRI images show three ring-shaped lesions at the gray–white matter junction. The lesions have a rim with a high signal and a small area of high signal in their periphery. In the left image, the broad white streak medial to the lesion is edema. The appearance of these lesions is characteristic of cysticercosis, which is one of the most common causes of seizures among recent immigrants from South and Central America.

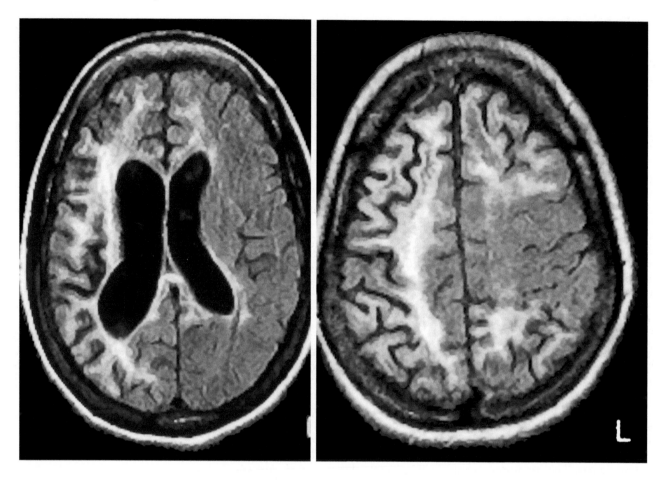

17. A 39-year-old man has developed cognitive impairment and mild left hemiparesis. He has been under immunosuppressive treatment for 12 years to preserve a renal transplant. Based on the history and MRIs, which of the following is the most likely diagnosis?
a. Multiple sclerosis (MS)
b. Progressive multifocal leukoencephalopathy (PML)
c. Toluene abuse
d. Metachromatic leukodystrophy (MLD)

Answer: b. The MRI images show multiple regions of high signal intensity in the white matter in both cerebral hemispheres, but in his right more so than in his left hemisphere. The lower cut (*left*) shows an enlarged right lateral ventricle and high signal in the subcortical white matter. The higher cut (*right*) shows the cerebral cortex with signal changes in the subcortical white matter of the patient's right hemisphere and anterior and posterior regions of the left hemisphere. The images also show cerebral atrophy, which has led to ventricular enlargement and loss of cerebral volume. Patients with chronic immunosuppression from medication or acquired immunodeficiency syndrome (AIDS) are at risk of developing PML and cerebral atrophy. MS, toluene abuse, and MLD also cause white matter damage, but the patient's history more strongly suggests PML.

18. A 75-year-old man came to his physician because of 6 weeks of increasingly severe left-sided headache. A neurologic examination showed inattention, apathy, word-finding difficulties, and a mild right-sided hemiparesis. Before the onset of these symptoms, he had been in good health and a general medical examination disclosed no significant abnormalities. Which condition does the CT indicate?
a. Glioblastoma
b. Acute subdural hematoma
c. Chronic subdural hematoma
d. Stroke
e. Porencephaly

Answer: c. The CT reveals a large, concave radiolucent mass lesion, with a surrounding radiodense membrane, overlying the left cerebral hemisphere. The lesion compresses and shifts structures contralaterally. This appearance and the extra-axial location help identify it as a subdural hematoma. A radiolucent hematoma is likely to be chronic. Subdural hematomas are relatively common

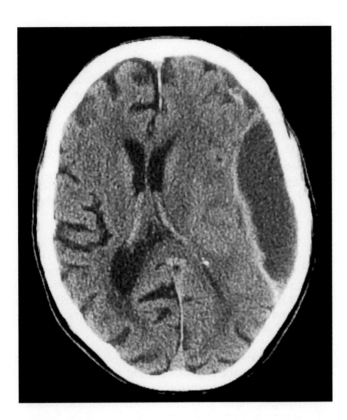

21. A medical student was watching her father and his friends play baseball in a senior citizen's league. A foul ball struck one of her father's teammates in his left forehead and knocked him unconscious. He recovered after a minute and waved off suggestions for medical evaluation. The student felt reassured when she found that he was alert, oriented, had equal and reactive pupils, and was able to ambulate. However, 20 minutes later, he suddenly lapsed into coma. In the emergency room, the staff obtained this CT. What is the abnormality?

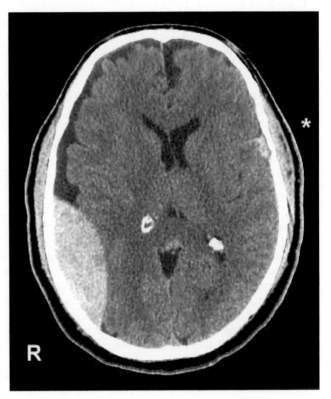

in older individuals because they often fall and strike their head, cerebral atrophy stretches bridging veins and makes them especially vulnerable to trauma, and the atrophy does not allow the brain to compress any bleeding that might occur. In addition, older individuals often take aspirin or other medicine that inhibits coagulation.

19. Which technique is most diagnostically valuable in cases of closed head injury in which patients have prolonged postconcussion symptoms?
   a. MRI
   b. fMRI
   c. DTI
   d. PET

   Answer: c. DTI readily detects traumatic brain injury, including axonal shear injury, even in cases without overt abnormality on conventional MRI sequences.

20. Which structure constitutes the lateral border of the lateral ventricle?
   a. Corpus callosum
   b. Caudate nucleus
   c. Hypothalamus
   d. Amygdala

   Answer: b. The corpus callosum is the roof; the hypothalamus, the floor; and the caudate, the lateral borders of the lateral ventricles (see Figs. 18.1 and 20.17). Atrophy of the caudate, which is characteristic of Huntington disease, allows the lateral ventricles to expand and assume a convex, "bat-wing" appearance (see Fig. 20.5 and Questions 11 and 12).

   a. Subarachnoid hemorrhage
   b. Acute subdural hematoma
   c. Chronic subdural hematoma
   d. Epidural hematoma

   Answer: d. The large, convex, uniformly dense white mass is fresh blood. Its elliptical shape indicates that it is located in the epidural rather than the subdural space. The mass effect of the hemorrhage has caused compression of the right lateral ventricle's anterior and occipital horns and right-to-left shift of the calcified choroid plexuses (the white globule-shaped structures). Note the contralateral scalp hematoma and small intracranial bleeding (*) at the site of impact. Thus, the epidural hematoma is a contrecoup injury.

22. CTs and MRIs of schizophrenic patients are most apt to show enlargement of which of the following structures?
   a. Amygdala
   b. Hippocampus

c. Caudate nucleus
d. Ventricles
e. Cerebral cortex

Answer: d.

23. Which of the following tissues is the most sensitive to radiation?
   a. Peripheral nerve
   b. Cerebral neuron
   c. Ocular lens
   d. Cerebellar neurons

Answer: c. Ocular lenses are more sensitive than brain tissue to radiation. Either radiotherapy or diagnostic imaging that uses ionizing radiation, particularly CT, may induce cataracts.

24. CT and MRI reveal the fine structure of the brain. In diagnosing which of the following conditions would these imaging studies show the most useful information?
   a. Autism
   b. Dyslexia
   c. Attention deficit hyperactivity disorder (ADHD)
   d. Nonaccidental head injury (NAHI)

Answer: d. In classic cases of NAHI, CT or MRI may reveal intracranial bleeding in different compartments (the epidural, subdural, or subarachnoid spaces), different ages of residual blood collections, and skull fractures. The imaging studies in most neuropsychiatric conditions, including autism, ADHD, and learning disabilities, show few changes and those are minimal and nonspecific. Moreover, in most neuropsychiatric conditions, the information that CT scans provide does not justify the radiation exposure.

25. Which technique is most helpful in diagnosing Alzheimer disease?
   a. MRI
   b. Functional magnetic resonance imaging (fMRI)
   c. Diffusion tensor imaging (DTI)
   d. Positron emission tomography (PET)

Answer: d. Using ligands that bind to amyloid, PET can reliably detect the characteristic amyloid accumulation. The other studies show inconsistent or nonspecific abnormalities.

26. Which technique measures anisotropy?
   a. MRI
   b. fMRI
   c. DTI
   d. PET

Answer: c. In the context of DTI, anisotropy refers to the diffusion of water molecules in some directions more than others. Anisotropy is most apparent in white matter tracts.

27. What causes multiple small hyperintense cerebral lesions on MRI?
   a. Lyme disease
   b. Migraine
   c. Age-related changes
   d. Dilated CSF spaces
   e. Any of the above

Answer: e. Any of these conditions may cause multiple small cerebral hyperintense MRI lesions, which neurologists call *unidentified bright objects* (*UBOs*). UBOs are common, lack a consistent source, and carry no implication of serious illness.

28. A 58-year-old man with uncontrolled hypertension presents to the ER with a blood pressure of 240/110 and new left hemiparesis and dysarthria. The neurologist wants to obtain an MRI, but the patient's severe claustrophobia prevents him from being in the machine for more than 2 to 3 minutes. The radiologists report that this is enough time to obtain only one sequence. Which one should his physicians select?
   a. T1
   b. T2
   c. T2 FLAIR
   d. DWI
   e. DTI

Answer: d. DWI, or diffusion-weighted imaging, is extraordinarily sensitive for the abnormal diffusion of water molecules characteristic of acute cerebral ischemia. T1 sequences are appropriate for examining general anatomy and T2 and T2 FLAIR (*FL*uid *A*ttenuated *I*nversion *R*ecovery) sequences are important for examining acute and chronic cerebral lesions. In FLAIR sequences, the CSF is dark instead of bright. DTI is not a standard sequence, and performing it requires more than a few minutes.

NEUROTRANSMITTERS AND DRUG ABUSE

Neurologists traditionally attribute neurologic symptoms and signs to a lesion in a certain area of the central nervous system (CNS) and use imaging studies such as computed tomography (CT) and magnetic resonance imaging (MRI) to confirm their clinical localization. Another way to envision neurologic illnesses is in terms of disruptions in CNS neurotransmitters. This chapter reviews the synthesis, metabolism, and anatomic pathways of the most important neurotransmitters, and their altered activity in common neurologic disorders:

- Monoamines:
  - Catecholamines: dopamine, norepinephrine (noradrenaline), and epinephrine (adrenaline)
  - Indolamines: serotonin
- Acetylcholine
- Neuropeptides:
  - Inhibitory amino acids: gamma-aminobutyric acid (GABA), glycine
  - Excitatory amino acids: glutamate
- Nitric oxide.

MONOAMINES

Dopamine

Synthesis and Metabolism

Phenylalanine $\xrightarrow{\textit{Phenylalanine hydroxylase}}$ Tyrosine
$\xrightarrow{\textit{Tyrosine hydroxylase}}$ DOPA
$\xrightarrow{\textit{DOPA decarboxylase}}$ Dopamine

Neurologists hold dopamine synthesis in preeminent regard and treasure each substrate, enzyme, and byproduct. They capitalize on its synthesis and storage when they treat Parkinson disease and several other neurologic illnesses.

Dopamine synthesis begins with the amino acid phenylalanine, and proceeds sequentially through tyrosine, DOPA, and then dopamine. *Tyrosine hydroxylase* is the rate-limiting enzyme in this pathway. Another important enzyme is *DOPA decarboxylase*, which decarboxylates DOPA to form dopamine. That same enzyme acts on both naturally occurring DOPA and the Parkinson disease medicine, levodopa (L-dopa).

The primary termination process consists of dopamine reuptake into the presynaptic neuron. In addition, two different enzymes metabolize dopamine: *catechol-O-methyltransferase* (*COMT*), mostly an extracellular enzyme, and *monoamine oxidase-B* (*MAO-B*), mostly an intracellular enzyme. Certain medicines for Parkinson disease and other illnesses preserve dopamine by inhibiting these enzymes (see later and Chapter 18).

Dopamine metabolism by COMT and MAO-B yields *homovanillic acid* (*HVA*). Cerebrospinal fluid (CSF) concentration of HVA corresponds roughly to dopaminergic activity in the brain.

Anatomy

Three "long dopamine tracts" hold great clinical importance in neurology:

1. The *nigrostriatal tract*, the major component of the extrapyramidal motor system, synthesizes most dopamine in the brain. This tract projects from the substantia nigra, the crescentic pigmented nuclei in the midbrain (Fig. 21.1), to the predominantly D2 receptors of the striatum (the caudate nucleus and putamen [see Chapter 18]).
2. The *mesolimbic tract* projects from the ventral tegmental area, situated in the inferior medial portion of the midbrain, to the amygdala and other portions of the limbic system. Its receptors are predominantly D4. The mesolimbic tract appears to propagate the positive symptoms of psychosis; many antipsychotic agents block dopamine transmission in this tract, thereby reducing dopamine activity in the limbic system and thus suppressing psychotic symptoms.
3. The *mesocortical tract* also projects from the ventral tegmental area, but it terminates primarily in the frontal cortex. It also terminates in the cingulate and prefrontal gyrus, creating an overlap with the mesolimbic system. The mesocortical tract likely propagates negative symptoms of psychosis. Because illicit drugs affect both the mesolimbic and mesocortical tracts, these tracts also serve as neural conduits for drug addiction.

In addition to these long tracts, several "short dopamine tracts" hold clinical significance. The *tubero-infundibular tract* connects the hypothalamic region with the pituitary

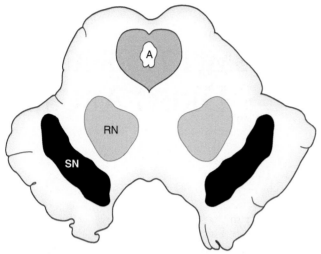

FIGURE 21.1 ■ This sketch shows the midbrain, which gives rise to several dopamine-producing tracts – including the nigrostriatal, mesolimbic, and mesocortical. The nigrostriatal tract begins in the substantia nigra (*SN*), the large curved black structures in the base of the midbrain (also see Fig. 18.2). The red nuclei (*RN*), which receive cerebellar outflow tracts, sit above the substantia nigra. The upper portion of the midbrain, the tectum (Latin, roof; *tegere*, to cover), contains the aqueduct of Sylvius (*A*) surrounded by the periaqueductal gray matter.

TABLE 21.1	Pharmacology of D1 and D2 Receptors	
	D1	**D2**
Effect of stimulation on cyclic AMP production	Increased	Decreased
Greatest concentrations	Striatum, limbic system, cerebral cortex	Striatum, substantia nigra
Effect of dopamine	Weak agonist	Strong agonist
Effect of phenothiazines	Strong antagonist	Strong antagonist
Effect of butyrophenones	Weak antagonist	Strong antagonist
Effect of clozapine	Weak antagonist	Weak antagonist

gland. Dopamine in the *tubero-infundibular* tract suppresses prolactin secretion and thus inhibits galactorrhea. As a corollary, blockade of the *tubero-infundibular* tract promotes galactorrhea, as seen with many antipsychotic agents. Another short tract exists within the retina.

Receptors

Although neuroscientists have identified numerous dopamine receptors, the most important ones are the D1, D2, and closely related receptors. The D1 receptor group includes both the D1 and D5 receptor subtypes. The D2 receptor group includes the D2, D3, and D4 receptor subtypes. These dopamine receptors are coupled to guanine nucleotide-binding proteins (G proteins). Because they exert their effects through second messengers such as cyclic AMP, neuroscientists consider them "slow" neurotransmitters. Brian K. Kobilka and Robert J. Lefkowitz, who elucidated G protein-coupled receptors, received the Nobel Prize in Chemistry in 2012.

The D1 and D2 receptors remain the most important in extrapyramidal disorders and psychosis (Table 21.1). With several exceptions, the effectiveness of antipsychotic agents hinges on their ability to block D2 receptors. Clozapine and quetiapine, in contrast, bind more strongly to D1 than D2 receptors. Some second-generation antipsychotic agents, such as quetiapine, risperidone, and ziprasidone, block serotonin as well as dopamine receptors, but aripiprazole and brexpiprazole stimulate D2 and one serotonin receptor while blocking another.

When antipsychotics block D2 receptors, the reduced dopamine activity potentially induces parkinsonism, raises prolactin production (inducing galactorrhea), and places patients at risk for tardive dyskinesia. Some atypical antipsychotic agents, particularly risperidone and its

active metabolite paliperidone (Invega), raise prolactin serum concentration. The nonpsychiatric medications metoclopramide (Reglan), which blocks D2 receptors, and tetrabenazine (see Chapter 18), which depletes dopamine from its presynaptic storage vesicles, also increase serum prolactin concentration and induce parkinsonism. On the other hand, aripiprazole, clozapine, and ziprasidone reduce or only slightly increase prolactin concentrations.

Physicians should bear in mind that finding an elevated serum prolactin level does not always indicate use of a dopamine-blocking medication or the presence of a pituitary tumor (see Chapter 19). The most common cause of serum prolactin elevation is pregnancy. Generalized tonic-clonic seizures raise serum prolactin concentrations during the postictal period. Detection of a prolactin elevation helps distinguish these seizures from *psychogenic nonepileptic seizures* (see Chapter 10).

Conditions Due to Reduced Dopamine Activity

Deficiencies in dopamine synthesis enzymes underlie several well-known neurologic disorders. A genetically determined absence of *phenylalanine hydroxylase*, the initial enzyme in catecholamine synthesis, leads to *phenylketonuria* (*PKU*) (see Chapter 13). A multifactorial genetic deficiency of a cofactor for both phenylalanine hydroxylase and tyrosine hydroxylase leads to *dopa-responsive dystonia* (*DRD*) (see Chapter 18). Although studies have not yet established the definitive basis of restless legs syndrome, dopamine agonists are an effective treatment (see Chapter 17).

In Parkinson disease, the progressive degeneration of dopamine-synthesizing neurons in the substantia nigra leads to increasingly severe dopamine deficiency. Neurologists treating Parkinson disease patients attempt to enhance dopamine activity in three ways:

1. They administer the *dopamine precursor* levodopa. As long as enough nigrostriatal (presynaptic) neurons remain intact, which is generally the

case during the first 5 years of the illness, DOPA decarboxylase converts levodopa to dopamine in sufficient quantities to reverse the symptoms (see Fig. 18.3).

2. As the disease progresses, the presynaptic neurons degenerate and can no longer synthesize, store, and appropriately release dopamine. At this time, if not as a first-line treatment, neurologists may prescribe a *dopamine agonist*, such as pramipexole, ropinirole, or rotigotine, to stimulate dopamine receptors.

3. As long as dopamine synthesis continues, neurologists prescribe medicines that slow its metabolism. Two medications – *carbidopa* and *entacapone* – inactivate enzymes that metabolize levodopa and thereby enhance dopamine activity (see Fig. 18.12). Carbidopa inactivates DOPA decarboxylase. Entacapone inhibits COMT, which normally inactivates levodopa by converting it to 3-O-methyldopa. Both enzyme inhibitors act almost entirely outside the CNS because they have little ability to penetrate the blood–brain barrier. Administering these enzyme-inhibitors along with levodopa enables small doses of levodopa to be effective. Another therapeutic option entails protecting dopamine from MAO-B. To enact this strategy, neurologists prescribe selegiline (Eldepryl), or rasagiline (Azilect), which are inhibitors of MAO-B.

Medication-Induced Parkinsonism

In contrast to Parkinson disease, where presynaptic neurons have degenerated, medication-induced blockade of basal ganglia D2 receptors causes parkinsonism. This distinction holds great clinical importance when a patient who is under treatment with an antipsychotic agent develops Parkinson disease-like symptoms. Giving levodopa at the same time as antipsychotic agents that block D2 receptors may still increase dopamine concentrations, but the dopamine will not stimulate its receptors or correct the symptoms. More important, excess dopamine may over-stimulate frontal cortex and limbic system dopamine receptors to provoke or exacerbate a psychosis. Thus, when a patient who has been treated with an antipsychotic agent – even for as briefly as 1 month – appears to have developed Parkinson disease, physicians should generally maintain that the patient has iatrogenic parkinsonism; search for alternative diagnoses that can cause both psychosis and parkinsonism, such as dementia with Lewy bodies or Wilson disease; and postpone administering medicines that enhance dopamine.

Neuroleptic Malignant Syndrome

An acute absence of dopamine activity causes the parkinson-hyperpyrexia or central dopaminergic syndrome, which neurologists still call the neuroleptic malignant syndrome (NMS) (see Chapter 6). Administering dopamine agonists, such as bromocriptine, may compensate for the absence of dopamine activity and alleviate some of the symptoms, but treatment is generally supportive.

Conditions Due to Excessive Dopamine Activity

Of the several mechanisms that might lead to excessive dopamine activity, the most common is the administration of levodopa. Stimulants also cause excessive dopamine activity by provoking dopamine release from its presynaptic storage sites, blocking its reuptake, or both (see later). Some psychiatric medications, such as bupropion (Wellbutrin), also block dopamine reuptake. In a different mechanism that possibly underlies tardive dyskinesia and Tourette disorder, increased sensitivity of the postsynaptic receptors results in excessive dopaminergic activity.

Whatever the cause, excessive dopamine activity produces a range of side effects from psychosis to hyperkinetic movement disorders. For example, Parkinson disease patients taking levodopa develop visual hallucinations, paranoia, and thought disorders that can reach psychotic proportions. Excessive dopamine activity also produces hyperkinetic movement disorders, such as chorea, tremor, tics, dystonia, and tardive dyskinesia.

As a less dramatic example of the effects of excessive dopamine, some Parkinson disease patients become overly involved with stimulating activities, such as sex and gambling. In these cases, neurologists diagnose the *dopamine dysregulation syndrome* or *impulse control disorder* (see Chapter 18). They usually ascribe the aberrant behavior to dopamine-induced novelty-seeking and inattention.

On the other hand, with a small increase in dopamine activity, individuals enjoy a sense of well-being. That sensation is but a mere glimmer of a cocaine or amphetamine rush.

In addition to their effects on movements, dopamine and its agonists, acting through the tubero-infundibular tract, inhibit prolactin release from the pituitary gland. Neurologists and endocrinologists prescribe bromocriptine and cabergoline, both dopamine agonists, to shrink and inactivate prolactinomas. In the opposite situation, when typical or atypical neuroleptics – but not clozapine or quetiapine – block tubero-infundibular tract receptors, they enhance prolactin release. Patient taking these medicines often report decreased sexual drive and galactorrhea.

Norepinephrine and Epinephrine

Synthesis and Metabolism

$$Dopamine \xrightarrow{\textit{Dopamine β-hydroxylase}} Norepinephrine$$
$$\xrightarrow{\textit{Phenylethanolamine N-methyl-transferase}} Epinephrine$$

After the catecholamine pathway yields dopamine, it goes on to yield norepinephrine and finally epinephrine. As with dopamine synthesis, tyrosine hydroxylase remains the ratelimiting enzyme in the synthesis. Also, as with dopamine, reuptake and metabolism by COMT and MAO terminate their actions. However, because the MAO-A variety of MAO metabolizes norepinephrine, most norepinephrine metabolism takes place outside the

CNS. Norepinephrine's primary metabolic byproduct, which appears in the urine, is *vanillylmandelic acid* (*VMA*).

Anatomy

CNS norepinephrine synthesis takes place primarily in the *locus ceruleus*, which is located in the dorsal portion of the pons (Fig. 21.2). Neurons from the locus ceruleus project to the cerebral cortex, limbic system, and reticular activating system. In addition, whereas dopamine tracts remain confined to the brain, norepinephrine tracts project down into the spinal cord.

Also unlike dopamine, norepinephrine serves as the neurotransmitter for the sympathetic nervous system's postganglionic neurons. In the adrenal gland, a pathway converts norepinephrine (noradrenaline) to epinephrine (adrenaline).

Receptors

Norepinephrine receptors are located in the cerebral cortex, brainstem, and spinal cord. The α_2 and β_2 receptors,

termed "autoreceptors," are situated on presynaptic neurons. Through a feedback mechanism, these presynaptic receptors modulate norepinephrine synthesis and release (Fig. 21.3). Postsynaptic receptors are also of two varieties, α_1 and β_1, and they produce varied and sometimes almost opposite effects (Table 21.2).

Conditions Due to Alterations in Norepinephrine Activity

In Parkinson disease, the locus ceruleus, just like the substantia nigra, degenerates and loses its pigment. Loss of norepinephrine typically leads to orthostatic hypotension, sleep disturbances, and depression. Droxidopa (Northera), which the body metabolizes to norepinephrine, recently became available for treatment of symptomatic orthostatic hypotension in Parkinson disease and related illnesses.

In the opposite situation, excessive stimulation of β_2 adrenergic sites leads to tremor and bronchodilation. For example, isoproterenol and epinephrine, particularly when used for asthma, cause tremor as they alleviate bronchospasm. Conversely, β-blockers, which are contraindicated in asthma patients, suppress essential tremor (see Chapter 18).

Pheochromocytomas secrete norepinephrine or epinephrine, which causes hypertension, tachycardia, and sometimes convulsions. A similar response – the tyramine reaction – could occur when patients who are taking a MAO-A inhibitor or a very large dose of an MAO-B inhibitor consume large amounts of certain tyramine-containing foods or wine.

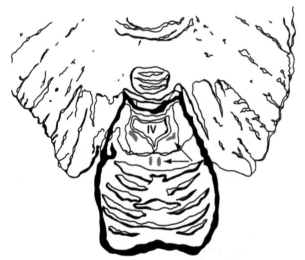

FIGURE 21.2 ■ This sketch shows the pons, fourth ventricle (IV), and the overlying cerebellum. The pons contains paired locus ceruleus (*diagonal arrow*) and dorsal raphe nucleus (*horizontal arrow*). The locus ceruleus gives rise to norepinephrine tracts. The dorsal raphe nucleus gives rise to serotonin tracts that spread upwards to the diencephalon and cerebrum. A caudal raphe nucleus, in the pons and medulla (not pictured), gives rise to serotonin tracts that spread downward in the spinal cord.

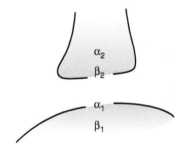

FIGURE 21.3 ■ In norepinephrine synapses, the postsynaptic neuron has α_1 and β_1 receptors that initiate the sympathetic "flight or fight" response. The presynaptic neuron has α_2 and β_2 autoreceptors that modulate sympathetic responses (see Table 21.2).

TABLE 21.2	**Pharmacology of Norepinephrine Receptors**		
Receptor*	**Effect of Stimulation**	**Agonists**	**Antagonists**
Presynaptic			
α_2	Vasodilation, hypotension	Clonidine	Yohimbine
β_2	Bronchodilation	Isoproterenol	Propranolol
Postsynaptic			
α_1	Vasoconstriction	Phenylephrine	Phenoxybenzamine, phentolamine
β_1	Cardiac stimulation	Dobutamine	Metoprolol

*See Figure 21.3

Serotonin

Synthesis and Metabolism

$$\text{Tryptophan} \xrightarrow[\text{hydroxylase}]{\text{Tryptophan}} \text{5-hydroxytryptophan}$$

$$\xrightarrow[\text{decarboxylase}]{\text{Amino acid}} \text{5-hydroxytryptamine}$$

$$\text{(5-HT, Serotonin)} \xrightarrow{\text{MAO-A}} \text{5-Hydroxyindoleacetic acid}$$

$$\text{(5HIAA)}$$

Serotonin (5-hydroxytryptamine, 5-HT) is another monoamine, but an *indolamine* rather than a catecholamine. Serotonin synthesis parallels dopamine synthesis: hydroxylation then decarboxylation. However, the rate-limiting factor in serotonin synthesis is the concentration of *tryptophan* rather than the hydroxylase enzyme. Re-uptake and, to a lesser extent, oxidation terminate serotonin's activity.

One metabolic pathway converts serotonin to melatonin, which is also an indolamine. In another pathway, MAO-A metabolizes serotonin to 5-hydroxyindoleacetic acid (5-HIAA). In short, MAO-A metabolizes norepinephrine and serotonin, but MAO-B metabolizes dopamine. Although platelets, gastrointestinal cells, and other nonneurologic cells synthesize more than 98% of the body's *total* serotonin, this nonneurologic serotonin does not penetrate the blood–brain barrier. Thus, CSF concentrations of HIAA reflect CNS serotonin activity.

Anatomy

Serotonin-producing CNS neurons reside predominantly in the *dorsal raphe nuclei*, which are located in the midline of the dorsal midbrain and pons (see Fig. 21.2). Serotonin tracts project rostrally (upward) to innervate the cortex, limbic system, striatum, and cerebellum. They also innervate intracranial blood vessels, particularly those around the trigeminal nerve.

Another serotonin-producing center, the *caudal raphe nuclei*, is located in the midline of the lower pons and medulla. It projects caudally (downward) to the dorsal horn of the spinal cord to reduce pain (see Chapter 14).

Receptors

Studies have identified numerous CNS serotonin receptors ($5HT_1$–$5HT_7$) and many subtypes. Serotonin receptors differ in their function, response to medications, effect on second-messenger systems, and excitatory or inhibitory capacity. Several serotonin receptors, such as $5HT_{1D}$, are presynaptic autoreceptors that suppress serotonin synthesis or block its release. $5HT_1$ promotes production of adenyl cyclase and is inhibitory, but $5HT_2$ promotes production of phosphatidyl inositol and is excitatory. Other serotonin receptors are usually G protein-linked and excitatory.

Conditions Due to Alterations in Serotonin Activity

Serotonin plays a major role in the daily sleep–wake cycle. The activity of serotonin-producing cells reaches its highest level during arousal, drops to quiescent levels during slow-wave sleep, and disappears during REM sleep (see Chapter 17).

More than in any other disorder, low serotonin activity is associated with depression. In one of the most consistent findings in biologic psychiatry, low postmortem CSF concentrations of HIAA, the major serotonin metabolite, characterize suicides by violent means. Similarly, individuals with poorly controlled violent tendencies, even those without a history of depression, have low concentrations of CSF HIAA.

Serotonin levels are also low in individuals with Parkinson or Alzheimer disease. Among Parkinson disease patients, the decrease is more pronounced in those with comorbid depression.

Sumatriptan and other triptans, a mainstay of migraine therapy, are selective $5\text{-}HT_{1D}$ receptor agonists. Once stimulated, these serotonin receptors inhibit the release of pain-producing vasoactive and inflammatory substances from trigeminal nerve endings.

A series of powerful antiemetics, including dolasetron (Anzemet) and ondansetron (Zofran), are $5HT_3$ antagonists. By affecting the medulla's *area postrema*, one of the few areas of the brain unprotected by the blood–brain barrier, they reduce chemotherapy-induced nausea and vomiting. Similarly, second-generation antipsychotics typically act as antagonists of $5HT_{2A}$ as well as D2 receptors.

Although increased serotonin activity is often therapeutic, excessive activity poses a danger. For example, combinations of medicines that simultaneously block serotonin reuptake and inhibit its metabolism lead to toxic serotonin concentrations and the *serotonin syndrome* (see Chapters 6 and 18).

In another situation characterized by excessive serotonin activity, LSD (D-lysergic acid diethylamide) induces hallucinations and euphoria by stimulating $5\text{-}HT_2$ receptors. Similarly, "ecstasy" (methylenedioxymethamphetamine [MDMA]), although it also stimulates dopaminergic activity, greatly enhances serotonin activity by triggering a presynaptic outpouring. Ecstasy surpasses LSD in stimulating serotonin activity.

ACETYLCHOLINE (ACh)

Synthesis and Metabolism

$$\text{Acetyl CoA} + \text{Choline} \xrightarrow{\text{Choline acetyltransferase}} \text{ACh}$$

The combination of acetyl co-enzyme A and choline forms acetylcholine (ACh). Although ACh synthesis depends on the enzyme *choline acetyltransferase* (*ChAT*), the rate-limiting factor is the concentration of choline.

Unlike monoamines, ACh does not undergo reuptake. Instead, *cholinesterase* (the common shorthand for acetylcholinesterase) terminates its action in the synaptic cleft. This enzyme hydrolyzes ACh back to acetyl coenzyme A and choline.

Anatomy

In the CNS, most ACh tracts originate in the *nucleus basalis of Meynert* (located in the *substantia innominata*) and adjacent nuclei situated in the *basal forebrain* (a rostral portion of the brainstem) (Fig. 21.4). These nuclei send

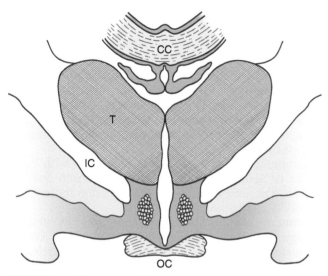

FIGURE 21.4 ■ This coronal view of the diencephalon, the region just rostral to the brainstem region, shows the nucleus basalis of Meynert (pictured as a grape-like cluster) situated adjacent to the third ventricle. Note the corpus callosum (CC), internal capsule (IC), and the optic chiasm (OC), which are all heavily myelinated structures, and thalamus (T).

TABLE 21.3	Cerebral Cortex and Neuromuscular Junction ACh Receptors	
	Cerebral Cortex	Neuromuscular Junction
Predominant ACh receptors	Muscarinic	Nicotinic
Main action	Excitatory or inhibitory	Excitatory
Agents that block receptor	Atropine, scopolamine	Curare, α-bungarotoxin

cholinergic projections throughout the cerebral cortex but particularly to the hippocampus, amygdala, and cortical association areas. In addition, ACh serves as the neurotransmitter in the autonomic nervous system and at the neuromuscular junction (see Fig. 6.1).

Receptors

ACh receptors fall into two categories, *nicotinic* and *muscarinic*. They differ in their anatomic distribution, effect (excitatory or inhibitory), and susceptibility to different blocking agents (Table 21.3).

Conditions Due to Reduced ACh Activity at the Neuromuscular Junction

In the PNS, decreased neuromuscular ACh activity – from either impaired presynaptic ACh release or blockade of postsynaptic ACh receptors – leads to muscle paralysis. Conditions that interfere with ACh activity have different etiologies and induce distinct patterns of weakness. For example, in Lambert–Eaton syndrome, a paraneoplastic disorder, antibodies impair the release of ACh from presynaptic neurons in the neuromuscular

junction and cause weakness of limbs (see Chapters 6 and 19). Botulinum toxin also impairs ACh release from the presynaptic neuron. When ingested as a food poison, the toxin causes potentially fatal weakness of ocular, facial, limb, and respiratory muscles (botulism). When injected into affected muscles for treatment of focal dystonia, pharmacologic botulinum toxin inhibits forceful muscle contractions because it slows or prevents ACh release from the presynaptic neuron (see Chapter 18).

Curare and many other poisons, and antibodies such as those associated with myasthenia gravis block ACh receptors at the postsynaptic neuron of the neuromuscular junction. The pattern of weakness in myasthenia gravis is distinctive: patients have asymmetric paresis of the extraocular and facial muscles, but not the pupils. To overcome the ACh receptor blockade in myasthenia gravis, neurologists administer an *anticholinesterase* (the common contraction of antiacetylcholinesterase), such as edrophonium (Tensilon) and pyridostigmine (Mestinon) to inhibit cholinesterase and thereby reduce the breakdown of ACh in the synaptic cleft (see Chapter 6 and Fig. 7.6). The ability of edrophonium to effectively but temporarily reverse myasthenia-induced paralysis, led to the "Tensilon Test" (see Fig. 6.3). Neurologists prescribe pyridostigmine, a longer-acting anticholinesterase, for therapeutic use in patients with myasthenia.

Conditions Due to Reduced ACh Activity in the CNS

In Alzheimer disease, trisomy 21, and some cases of Parkinson disease, the cerebral cortex has markedly reduced cerebral ACh concentrations, ChAT activity, and muscarinic receptors (see Chapter 7). In addition, some nicotinic receptors are depleted.

To counteract the ACh deficiency in Alzheimer disease, neurologists have attempted several strategies to enhance its synthesis or slow its metabolism. In hopes of enhancing ACh synthesis, they have administered precursors, such as choline and lecithin (phosphatidylcholine). Although analogous to providing a dopamine precursor (levodopa) in Parkinson disease treatment, this strategy fails to reverse the symptoms of Alzheimer disease. A complementary strategy has been to slow ACh metabolism by administering long-acting cholinesterase inhibitors that cross the blood–brain barrier, such as donepezil (see Chapter 7).

Reduced ACh concentrations also characterize trisomy 21, which shares many clinical and pathologic features of Alzheimer disease. Also, in Parkinson disease and progressive supranuclear palsy (PSP) the cortex has reduced ACh concentrations.

Many studies have suggested that an absolute ACh deficiency or a relative ACh deficiency compared to dopamine activity causes delirium. Reduced ACh activity leading to cognitive impairment or delirium may occasionally have an iatrogenic basis. For example, scopolamine and other drugs that block muscarinic ACh receptors interfere with memory, learning, attention, and level of consciousness – even in normal individuals. In fact, scopolamine, which readily crosses the blood–brain barrier, induces a transient amnesia that has been a laboratory model for Alzheimer disease dementia.

Anticholinergic Syndrome

Chlorpromazine, other antipsychotic agents, and tricyclic antidepressants may block muscarinic ACh receptors and cause anticholinergic side effects, including drowsiness, dry mouth, urinary hesitancy, constipation, and accommodation paresis (see Chapter 12). Nonpsychiatric medicines such as atropine, scopolamine, benztropine, and trihexyphenidyl, may also cause troublesome anticholinergic side effects. With enough anticholinergic activity, individuals develop the *anticholinergic syndrome*: dilated pupils, elevated pulse and blood pressure, dry skin and hyperthermia, and delirium that may progress to coma. In this situation physicians may administer physostigmine, an anticholinesterase that crosses the blood–brain barrier, to restore ACh activity.

Conditions Due to Excessive ACh Activity

Individuals may be victims of ACh intoxication not because they ingest ACh but because they are exposed to substances that inactivate cholinesterase. Unmetabolized, excessive ACh leads to a *cholinergic crisis* – predominantly a muscarinic parasympathetic discharge – that consists of bradycardia, hypotension, miosis, and a characteristic outpouring of bodily fluids in the form of excess lacrimation, salivation, bronchial secretions, and diarrhea. Toxic levels in the peripheral nervous system (PNS) cause flaccid quadriparesis and fasciculations. Toxic levels of ACh in the CNS cause delirium, slurred speech, and seizures.

Cholinergic crises have occurred in patients with dementia who accidentally take too many donepezil pills or apply rivastigmine patches without removing the old ones. Similarly, eating certain mushrooms will cause ACh toxicity. Individuals may suffer from exposure to organophosphorus insecticides, such as parathion and malathion, or they may swallow a Latin American rat poison, *Tres Pasitos*, which looks like grains of rice. Ingestion of these poisons may be the result of suicide, homicide attempts, or occupational exposure.

Many poison gases, such as the terrorist gas sarin, are organophosphates that raise ACh concentrations to toxic levels. They cause such copious bronchial secretions and weakness of the chest and airway muscles that victims drown in their own secretions. The immediate treatment of poison gas exposure is atropine. It reverses the parasympathetic overactivity by competitively inhibiting ACh at muscarinic receptors. Pralidoxime, a complementary treatment, reactivates cholinesterase activity.

NEUROPEPTIDES

Gamma-Aminobutyric Acid (GABA) – An Inhibitory Amino Acid Neurotransmitter

Synthesis and Metabolism

$$\text{Glutamate} \xrightarrow{\text{GAD} + B_6} \text{GABA}$$

Glutamic acid decarboxylase (GAD) with its cofactor, vitamin B_6 (pyridoxine), decarboxylates glutamate to produce GABA. GABA and, to a lesser extent, glycine are the brain's major inhibitory neurotransmitters. GABA undergoes re-uptake and metabolism principally by GABA transaminase.

Anatomy

Reflecting its widespread and critical role, GABA is distributed throughout the entire CNS. However, it is concentrated in the striatum, hypothalamus, spinal cord, and temporal lobes.

Receptors

Of the two GABA receptors subtypes – $GABA_A$ and $GABA_B$ – $GABA_A$ receptors are more numerous and important. $GABA_A$ receptors have binding sites for benzodiazepines, barbiturates, ethanol, hypnotics, propofol, certain steroids (neurosteroids) and some antiepileptic drugs (AEDs), as well as GABA.

When stimulated, $GABA_A$ receptors open chloride channels that allow negatively charged chloride ions (Cl-) to flow into the cell. The influx of these negative-charged ions lowers (makes more negative) the neuron's resting potential, which is normally –70 mV. Because the hyperpolarization occurs rapidly, neurologists term GABA and several other neurotransmitters "fast."

The GABA-induced lowering of the resting potential hyperpolarizes the membrane, which inhibits the neuron. Not surprisingly, alcohol and most of the medicines that act on $GABA_A$ receptors are CNS depressants.

The $GABA_B$ receptor, a G protein coupled to calcium and potassium channels, is also inhibitory. In contrast to the large numbers of medicines that bind to the $GABA_A$ receptor, few bind to the $GABA_B$ receptor. The best known is baclofen (Lioresal), which counteracts spasticity. Other medicines that alleviate spasticity act through different mechanisms. For example, tizanidine (Zanaflex) acts as an α_2 adrenergic agonist and dantrolene (Dantrium) acts directly on muscles.

Conditions Due to Alterations in GABA Activity

GABA deficiency is characterized by a lack of inhibition, which leads to excessive activity. For example, in Huntington disease, depleted GABA reduces inhibition in the basal ganglia. The loss of inhibition probably leads to the chorea. Tetanus and strychnine poisoning, which are characterized by muscle spasms, each reflects decreased GABA activity (see later). Several studies have attributed the restlessness of alcohol withdrawal to a deficiency in $GABA_A$ activity. That theory is consistent with the improvement that benzodiazepines produce, presumably through stimulation of $GABA_A$ receptors.

In the *stiff-person syndrome*, formerly known as the stiff-man syndrome, anti-GAD antibodies reduce GABA activity, leading to muscle stiffness and gait impairment. Physicians might mistake this disorder for catatonia or an antipsychotic-induced acute dystonic reaction. Neurologists usually diagnose the stiff-person syndrome by finding anti-GAD antibodies in the serum and CSF.

In many cases, the stiff-person syndrome is associated with an underlying neoplasm, such as breast cancer, or various autoimmune diseases. Whatever the cause might be, immunomodulation and diazepam usually reduce the stiffness.

Diets deficient in pyridoxine, the cofactor for GAD, impair GABA synthesis and cause seizures. Likewise, an overdose of isoniazid (INH), which interferes with pyridoxine, occasionally leads to seizures. In both cases, the seizures respond to intravenous pyridoxine.

In the opposite direction, several AEDs are effective, in part, because they increase GABA activity. For example, valproate (Depakote) increases brain GABA concentration. Topiramate (Topamax) enhances GABA$_A$ receptor activity. Vigabatrin (Sabril) increases GABA concentrations by reducing its metabolic enzyme, GABA transaminase.

In certain situations, flumazenil, a benzodiazepine antagonist, blocks GABA receptors. Flumazenil is thus useful for benzodiazepine overdose. Flumazenil also reverses some of the symptoms of hepatic encephalopathy because it displaces false benzodiazepine-like neurotransmitters from GABA receptors (see Chapter 7).

Glycine – Another Inhibitory Amino Acid Neurotransmitter

Synthesis, Metabolism, and Anatomy

Glycine, a simple amino acid not essential to the human diet, acts not only as a powerful inhibitory neurotransmitter but also paradoxically as a co-agonist or modulator of the excitatory neurotransmitter glutamate at NMDA receptors. Hydroxymethyl transferase converts the amino acid serine to glycine.

$$\text{Serine} \xrightarrow{\text{Hydroxymethyl transferase}} \text{Glycine}$$

Glycine's inhibitory activity acts on the motor neurons of the ventral horn of the spinal cord and the brainstem. Under normal circumstances, glycine provides inhibition of muscle tone that balances the excitation of muscle tone provided by other neurotransmitters. Several different metabolic pathways inactivate it.

Conditions Due to Alterations in Glycine Activity

Tetanus and strychnine poisonings reduce glycine activity. In both poisonings, loss of inhibitory muscle activity causes unrelenting, powerful, potentially fatal spasms. In tetanus (see Chapter 6), the toxin (tetanospasmin) prevents the *presynaptic* release of glycine and GABA. Due mostly to the loss of glycine-induced muscle inhibition, tetanus patients suffer "tetanic contractions" of limb, facial, and jaw muscles, typically manifest as "lockjaw." Through a different mechanism of action, but with similar results, strychnine blocks the *postsynaptic* glycine receptor and causes fatal limb, larynx, and trunk muscle spasms.

Glutamate – An Excitatory Amino Acid Neurotransmitter

Synthesis, Metabolism, and Anatomy

$$\text{Glutamine} \xrightarrow{\text{Glutaminase}} \text{Glutamate}$$

Glutamate, a simple amino acid synthesized from glutamine, is the most important excitatory neurotransmitter. Its tracts project throughout the brain and spinal cord. Re-uptake into presynaptic neurons and adjacent support cells terminate glutamate activity. To a lesser extent, glutamate undergoes nonspecific metabolism.

Aspartate is another excitatory amino acid. Compared to glutamate, its anatomy and clinical roles are less well established.

Receptors

Of several glutamate receptors, the *N-methyl-D-aspartate* (*NMDA*) subtype is the most important. The NMDA receptor has binding sites for glycine, phencyclidine (PCP), and a PCP congener, ketamine (see later), as well as glutamate. In its interactions with NMDA receptors, glutamate acts as a fast neurotransmitter.

Conditions Due to Alterations in NMDA Activity

In several disorders, excessive NMDA activity floods the neuron with potentially lethal concentrations of calcium and sodium. Through this process, *excitotoxicity*, glutamate–NMDA interactions lead to neuron death through apoptosis. Excitotoxicity may be intimately involved in the pathophysiology of epilepsy, stroke, Parkinson and Huntington diseases, and traumatic brain injury. In addition, in a paraneoplastic syndrome triggered by ovarian teratomas in young women, antibodies directed toward NMDA receptors give rise to an autoimmune limbic encephalitis that may mimic schizophrenia (see Chapter 19).

One approach to stemming the progression of these diseases has been to use medicines that block glutamate–NMDA interactions. For example, memantine (Namenda), an NMDA receptor antagonist, blocks deleterious excitatory neurotransmission and temporarily slows the progression of Alzheimer disease. Neurologists have tried a similar strategy in amyotrophic lateral sclerosis (ALS), stroke, cerebral anoxia, and acute head trauma. Also, the AEDs gabapentin and lamotrigine are partly glutamate antagonists.

On the other hand, deficient NMDA activity can also be harmful. For example, PCP and ketamine, which cause psychosis, appear to block the NMDA calcium channel (see later).

Other Neuropeptides

Endorphins, enkephalins, and substance P, which are situated in the spinal cord and brain, provide endogenous analgesia in response to painful stimuli (see Chapter 14). Substance P and, to a lesser degree, other neuropeptides are depleted in Alzheimer disease. The neuropeptide hypocretin (also known as orexin) plays a crucial role in the normal sleep–wake cycle and its absence in the CSF characterizes narcolepsy with cataplexy (see Chapter 17).

NITRIC OXIDE

Synthesis and Metabolism

$$\text{Arginine} + \text{Oxygen} \xrightarrow{\textit{Nitric oxide synthase}} \text{Nitric oxide} + \text{Citrulline}$$

Nitric oxide (NO) is an important neurotransmitter for endothelial cells and the immunologic system. NO inhibits platelet aggregation, dilates blood vessels, and boosts host defenses against infections and tumors. NO diffuses into cells and interacts directly with enzymes and iron–sulfur complexes; however, it has no specific membrane receptors. From a neurologic viewpoint, its main functions include regulating cerebral blood flow and facilitating penile erections. NO is so important to the functioning of the human body that the journal *Science* named NO the Molecule of the Year in 1992 and three scientists – Robert F. Furchgott, Louis J. Ignore, and Ferid Murad – won the Nobel Prize in 1998 for elucidating its functions.

Do not confuse nitric oxide (NO) with nitrous oxide (N_2O), which is a gaseous anesthetic ("laughing gas"). When inhaled as a form of drug abuse, N_2O leads to vitamin B_{12} deficiency, which results in cognitive impairment and spinal cord damage.

Conditions Due to Alterations in NO Activity

The best-known role of NO is in generating erections (see Chapter 16). With sexual stimulation of the penis, parasympathetic neurons produce and release NO. NO then promotes the production of cyclic guanosine monophosphate (cGMP), which dilates the vascular system and creates an erection. Sildenafil (Viagra), for example, slows the metabolism of cGMP and increases blood flow in the penis, which, in turn, produces, strengthens, and prolongs erections.

NEUROLOGIC ASPECTS OF DRUG ABUSE

Cocaine

Pharmacology

Cocaine and amphetamines (see later) primarily act through the sympathetic nervous system to stimulate the CNS, i.e., they are sympathomimetic agents. Cocaine provokes a discharge of dopamine from its presynaptic storage vesicles and then blocks its re-uptake, in large part by inhibiting the dopamine transporter (DaT). Resulting mostly from blocked re-uptake, a greatly increased dopamine synaptic concentration over-stimulates its receptors, especially those in the mesolimbic system.

In addition, cocaine blocks the reuptake of serotonin and norepinephrine. The resulting enhanced serotonin activity produces euphoria. The enhanced norepinephrine activity causes systemic sympathomimetic effects, including arrhythmias, hypertension, vasospasm, and pupillary dilation. (Similarly, 2% to 10% cocaine eye drops dilate normal pupils because the cocaine stimulates α_1 receptors in the ciliary muscles.)

Cocaine also blocks transmission in the PNS. For example, cocaine applied or injected at a specific site produces local anesthesia. Although it may stem from CNS rather than PNS dysfunction, habitual cocaine users often experience a paresthesia of ants crawling on or under their skin. Neurologists call this sensation *formication* (Latin, *formica*, ant), but cocaine users call it "coke bugs."

Plasma and liver enzymes rapidly metabolize cocaine, giving it a half-life as brief as 30 to 90 minutes. Nevertheless, urine toxicology screens may detect cocaine's major metabolic product – benzoylecgonine – for 2–5 days.

Clinical Effects

The immediate effect of cocaine typically consists of a brief period of euphoria accompanied by a sense of increased sexual, physical, and mental power. By way of contrast to heroin and other opioids (see later), cocaine leaves users fully alert – even hypervigilant – with enlarged, although reactive, pupils.

Cocaine, like other stimulants, not only reduces sleep time, it suppresses or even eliminates the rapid eye movement (REM) phase. As would be expected, discontinuing chronic cocaine use leads to a rebound in REM sleep as if to compensate for a loss of REM during intoxication (see Chapter 17).

Overdose

After taking cocaine, users may become agitated, irrational, hallucinatory, and paranoid. Moreover, cocaine's sympathomimetic and dopaminergic effects cause strokes, cardiac arrhythmias, myocardial infarctions, and seizures.

Cocaine-induced strokes usually occur within two hours of cocaine use. They may take the form of non-hemorrhagic (ischemic) cerebral infarctions or, as a reflection of cocaine-induced hypertension or vasculitis, cerebral hemorrhage. Similarly, physicians have attributed hypertensive cerebral hemorrhages to the use of performance-enhancing and body-building over-the-counter supplements, such as dimethylamylamine (DMAA).

Cocaine-induced seizures, which usually occur within 2 hours of use, disproportionately follow first-time exposure. Sometimes they are the presenting sign of a cocaine-induced stroke. For practical purposes, a seizure in a young adult should prompt an investigation for drug abuse.

In contrast, use or even an overdose of barbiturates, benzodiazepines, or alcohol rarely causes strokes or seizures. However, withdrawal from any of these substances frequently precipitates not only seizures but also status epilepticus (see Chapter 10).

Probably because cocaine suddenly increases dopamine activity, its use also produces or exacerbates involuntary movements, such as facial tics, chorea, tremor, dystonia, and repetitive, purposeless behavior (stereotypies, see Chapter 18). When cocaine induces chorea, patients' legs and feet typically move incessantly, and they cannot stand at attention. Neurologists label these involuntary movements "crack dancing," and point out that they mimic chorea, restless legs syndrome, akathisia, and undertreated agitation. Cocaine addiction causes abnormal, repetitive behavior and preoccupation with useless activities, such as hoarding, adjusting electronic equipment, and sorting similar objects. Neurologists call these activities, which are similar to stereotypies, "punding."

Studies have not established the frequency, nature, or severity of cocaine-induced cognitive impairment. However, some studies indicate that individuals repeatedly using cocaine have cognitive defects that consist of impairments in attention, verbal learning, and memory. When present, strokes and other forms of brain damage are probably responsible, at least in part, for the cognitive impairment.

Computed tomography (CT) of habitual cocaine users shows cerebral atrophy. With its superior resolution, magnetic resonance imaging (MRI) also shows demyelination, hyperintensities, vasospasm, and stroke-like defects. Functional imaging, such as single-photon emission computed tomography (SPECT), shows multiple patchy areas of hypoperfusion (a "Swiss cheese" pattern).

Treatment of Intoxication and Overdose

Behavioral and cognitive aspects of cocaine overdose generally resolve spontaneously; however, co-intoxication with alcohol potentiates the adverse effects of cocaine. Rest, seclusion, and, if necessary, benzodiazepines will suppress agitation and related symptoms. Antipsychotic agents will reduce psychosis and violent behavior, but some of them, like cocaine itself, may lower the seizure threshold. Life-threatening hypertension, another hazard of cocaine, may require an α-blocker antihypertensive medication, such as phentolamine (see Table 21.2).

Withdrawal

When deprived of cocaine, habitual users often rapidly lose their energy and ability to appreciate their normally pleasurable activities and languish in a dysphoric mood, i.e., they "crash." Vivid, disturbing dreams, which probably represent REM rebound, disturb their sleep. However, they do not suffer the physical tortures – wrenching bone pain or autonomic disturbances – of heroin withdrawal.

Amphetamine

The term "amphetamine" commonly refers to illicit stimulants, particularly methamphetamine ("crystal," "ice," "speed"), as well as stimulant medications, such as dextroamphetamine (Dexedrine) and methylphenidate (Ritalin). In contrast to cocaine, which predominantly blocks dopamine re-uptake, amphetamines provoke a presynaptic dopamine discharge. Amphetamines also increase norepinephrine activity that produces sympathomimetic effects and their complications, including stroke. Chronic amphetamine use may lead to long-lasting cognitive impairment and psychiatric disturbances.

Paradoxically, in controlled situations, amphetamines increase concentration and improve standard test scores. They also suppress physical and mental hyperactivity in children and adults with attention deficit hyperactivity disorder (ADHD). Notably, stimulants neither increase the risk of tics in children with ADHD nor exacerbate tics in children with Tourette disorder. Partly on the basis of these observations, one theory proposes that amphetamines stimulate inhibitory neurons but not excitatory neurons.

When abused, amphetamines produce cocaine-like effects, including a hyperalert state, decreased total sleep time, and reduced REM phase sleep. Because the half-life of amphetamines is generally about 8 hours and the half-life of methamphetamine is as long as 12 hours, and because methamphetamines are lipophilic and therefore readily cross the blood–brain barrier, these stimulants' effects persist much longer than cocaine's. Nevertheless, when used as a treatment for ADHD, narcolepsy, or other indication, patients may need to take amphetamines several times a day or use an extended-release preparation. Routine urine toxicology can detect amphetamines for only about 24 hours and many medications, such as selegiline (see Chapter 18), produce a false-positive result.

Overdose and Withdrawal

Because of their shared pharmacology, treatment of amphetamine and cocaine intoxication and withdrawal is similar for the two substances.

Ecstasy

Whereas cocaine, amphetamines, and other stimulants greatly increase dopamine and other catecholamine activity, ecstasy (MDMA) greatly increases serotonin activity. By rapidly releasing presynaptic serotonin stores, ecstasy prompts waves of serotonin that create euphoria, emotional closeness, and, at high doses, psychedelic experiences and agitation. Ecstasy often causes dry mouth, bruxism (jaw clenching), sweating, hyperthermia, and other components of the serotonin syndrome. These reactions have prompted compensatory water drinking that lead to hyponatremia.

Opioids

Pharmacology

Opioid is a broad term encompassing medical and "street" narcotics, as well as endogenous opiate-like substances (see endorphins, Chapter 14). Although opioids may inhibit the reuptake of monoamines and affect other neurotransmitters, their primary action is directly on a group of receptors that are situated in the brain and spinal cord.

Of several opioid receptors, the μ (mu) receptors mediate opioid-induced euphoria.

Clinical Effects

Medical opioids may lessen pain, ease suffering, reduce anxiety, and induce a sense of well-being. Parenterally administered opioids routinely lead to nausea and vomiting, which probably result from opioids' directly stimulating the medulla's chemoreceptor trigger zone. Either directly related to intravenous drug abuse or indirectly to their life style, opioid abusers place themselves at risk of brain damage from vasospasm, bacterial endocarditis, foreign particle emboli, head trauma, and complications of human immunodeficiency virus (HIV) infection.

Overdose

Opioid overdose causes a characteristic triad of coma, miosis, and respiratory depression. The respiratory depression, which is potentially fatal, takes the form of a slow rate rather than shallow depth of breathing. It often precipitates pulmonary edema. The coma routinely leads to radial or sciatic nerve compression from lying for prolonged periods in unnatural positions (see Chapter 5). Unlike cocaine intoxication, heroin and morphine overdoses rarely cause seizures. Urine tests for opioids can detect heroin and morphine for up to 2 days, and methadone, which has a longer half-life, for up to 5 days.

If an overdose leads to hypoxia, patients suffer damage of the basal ganglia and cerebral cortex that can result in cognitive impairment. However, formal studies have failed to demonstrate cognitive impairment with chronic, well-controlled opioid use. For example, individuals on methadone maintenance programs, patients treated with opioids for chronic pain, and several famous physicians who abused opioids did not show cognitive decline.

The opioid antagonist naloxone (Narcan) displaces heroin, morphine, and other opioids from their receptors and reverses opioid-induced respiratory depression. Another antagonist, naltrexone (ReVia), which is an oral agent for maintenance or detoxification, prevents opioids from reaching their receptors. Physicians should be aware that for patients treated with opioids for chronic pain, opioid antagonists alone or combined with an opioid, such as nalbuphine (Nubain) and butorphanol (Stadol), might reverse the analgesia, allow patients' pain and agony to return, and precipitate withdrawal symptoms.

Withdrawal From Chronic Use

Prominent features of opioid withdrawal typically include drug- or medication-seeking behavior, dysphoric mood, lacrimation, abdominal cramps, piloerection, and autonomic hyperactivity. Heroin withdrawal symptoms begin within several hours after the last dose and peak at 1 to 3 days. Because of methadone's longer half-life, its withdrawal symptoms begin 1 to 2 days after the last dose and peak at about 6 days. Clonidine, the α_2 norepinephrine agonist, may alleviate autonomic symptoms of opioid withdrawal.

Other Clinical Aspects

Medical personnel – including anesthesiologists, other physicians, and dentists – are particularly at risk for surreptitious opioid abuse. Physicians should avoid prescribing certain medicines to patients enrolled in methadone-maintenance programs. For example, phenytoin (Dilantin), carbamazepine (Tegretol), and efavirenz (Sustiva) enhance methadone metabolism or compete for its receptor. Thus, these medicines may precipitate opioid withdrawal symptoms. Increasing the methadone dose when these medicines are added will reduce or even prevent withdrawal. Certain medicines will cause the opposite situation. For example, giving erythromycin or fluvoxamine to someone in a methadone maintenance program will slow the methadone metabolism and may increase its serum concentration to a clinically significant extent.

Heroin does not have a specific CNS receptor, but, like morphine, attaches to the μ receptor and produces the same effects. Compared to morphine, it more easily penetrates the blood–brain barrier. Contrary to some popular pronouncements, heroin holds no medically distinguishable advantage as a treatment for cancer pain.

Phencyclidine

Phencyclidine (PCP) acts simultaneously as a central analgesic, depressant, and hallucinogen. In its primary mechanism of action, PCP blocks glutamate from interacting with NMDA receptors, which prevents normal glutamate-induced excitation.

In small doses, PCP use mimics alcohol intoxication in that it causes euphoria, dysarthria, ataxia, and nystagmus. At high doses, PCP causes paranoia, delusions, and hallucinations (the positive symptoms of schizophrenia) and psychomotor retardation and emotional withdrawal (the negative symptoms). With its capacity to produce the full range of schizophrenia symptoms, PCP stands apart from LSD and other psychomimetic drugs that produce only the positive symptoms. Because PCP use produces both the positive and negative symptoms, it serves as a laboratory model of schizophrenia.

Intoxication

In addition to causing symptoms of schizophrenia, PCP intoxication causes combinations of muscle rigidity, bursts of horizontal, vertical, and rotatory nystagmus, stereotypies, and a blank stare. PCP-induced muscle rigidity may cause rhabdomyolysis and other features of NMS, but physicians rarely confuse these two conditions. PCP-intoxicated individuals typically lie with their eyes open, unaware of their surroundings, and oblivious to pain. Neurologists describe them as being in "PCP coma." Sometimes PCP causes seizures that progress to status epilepticus; however, PCP rarely causes stroke. Another important aspect of PCP intoxication is that the drug-induced psychosis often leads to violent incidents, such as motor vehicle crashes, confrontations with police, and drowning.

Multiple exposures to PCP, according to several reports, produce chronic memory impairment and confusion. One study found that about one-quarter of individuals who experienced a PCP-induced psychosis returned in about 1 year with the diagnosis of schizophrenia.

Treatment

Unlike for opioid antagonists, no particular medicine acts as an antagonist for PCP. Treatment is symptomatic and may include seclusion and sedation with benzodiazepines. Because PCP often causes muscle rigidity, physicians should reserve dopamine-blocking antipsychotic agents for extreme cases, as they might further increase muscle rigidity. If muscle rigidity develops, muscle relaxants such as dantrolene may prevent rhabdomyolysis. Benzodiazepines will abort PCP-induced seizures.

Ketamine

Ketamine is a legitimate veterinary anesthetic. It has a chemical structure similar to PCP and also blocks NMDA receptors. Although ketamine produces many of the same mood and thought alterations as PCP, its effects are briefer, milder, and less likely to include hallucinations, agitation, and violence. In fact, researchers are testing ketamine as an antidepressant.

Gamma-Hydroxybutyrate

Metabolism of GABA yields, in part, gamma-hydroxybutyrate (GHB), which releases endogenous opioids. The sodium salt of GHB is sodium oxybate (Xyrem), which is useful in the treatment of narcolepsy-cataplexy and excessive daytime sleepiness (see Chapter 17). GHB and sodium oxybate probably activate $GABA_B$ receptors and thereby reduce dopamine activity.

In small doses, GHB causes relaxation and mild euphoria, but in intoxicating doses it induces an almost immediate deep sleep-like state for several hours. When victims return to full consciousness, they have little or no recall, i.e., they experience temporary but profound amnesia. GHB has gained notoriety as the agent involved in drug-facilitated sexual assault (date rape). Physicians and pharmacies must monitor prescriptions and distribution for sodium oxybate because of its potential nefarious use.

Marijuana and Synthetic Marijuana

Marijuana (cannabis) contains numerous chemicals, but from a psychoactive perspective, the most potent is delta-9-tetrahydrocannabinol (Δ9-THC). The hippocampus, basal ganglia, cerebellum, and to a less extent, cerebral cortex all contain G protein-coupled Δ9-THC receptors. Marijuana contains many compounds that have negligible psychoactive effects, such as cannabidiol. Urine toxicology can detect marijuana use.

Intoxication

In mild, recreational doses, marijuana produces euphoria and pleasantly altered perceptions for 1 to 3 hours. Curiously, while reducing many desires, it often increases the appetite for food. At these levels, marijuana may impair coordination, judgment, cognition, and perception. As with many hypnotics, marijuana reduces REM sleep.

Unlike small doses of marijuana, which produce sedation, large doses may cause anxiety, panic, and psychosis accompanied by physical signs, characteristically dilated conjunctiva vessels and tachycardia – in DSM-5 terminology, Cannabis Intoxication. If disturbing psychologic symptoms persist, benzodiazepines or, if necessary, antipsychotic agents can suppress them. In contrast to many other drugs, marijuana intoxication is not fatal and rarely, if ever, causes seizures or stroke.

Withdrawal, which the DSM-5 labels Cannabis Withdrawal in its Substance-Related Disorders section, causes anxiety, irritability, and inattention, although not seizures or hallucinations. The medical community and the legislators of states that have legalized marijuana have not paid adequate attention to the existence and treatment of marijuana withdrawal symptoms.

Efficacy in Neurologic Disorders

By patient-centered measures, oral THC probably reduces multiple sclerosis-induced spasticity, central pain, and painful spasms. However, no studies have shown clear benefit in tremor, levodopa-induced dyskinesias, or behavioral disturbances in dementia. While studies so far have been inconclusive, neurologists are studying THC compounds for the treatment of intractable epilepsy syndromes. Conventional medicines are more effective for each of its purported benefits. For example, antagonists of D2 receptors, such as metoclopramide (Reglan), and $5HT_3$ serotonin receptors, such as ondansetron, are much more effective antiemetics than marijuana. Similarly, although marijuana lowers intraocular pressure, its effect is too mild and short-lived to constitute a useful treatment for glaucoma. In multiple sclerosis, the prolonged use of the drug impairs cognition to a much greater degree than it relieves spasticity and pain. Finally, when contemplating prescribing marijuana for treatment for a chronic illness, physicians must consider the consequences of eventual withdrawal, which include insomnia and mental and physical agitation.

Synthetic Marijuana

Amateur or professional chemists have skirted the law by synthesizing and distributing marijuana-like cannabinoids with street names such as "Spice" or "K2." Users often add them to tobacco or actual marijuana, e-cigarettes, energy drinks, or illicit drugs. Depending on the specific product and method of delivery, synthetic marijuanas may have different, more profound, or dangerous effects. Whether from contaminants or the synthetic marijuana itself, users have frequently developed delirium, psychotic reactions, seizures, and stroke. Also, they have developed renal disease and cardiac arrhythmias. Toxicology tests cannot keep up with the numerous substances that the chemists supply.

Nicotine

Nicotine binds to nicotinic cholinergic receptors, particularly in the mesolimbic system. In addition, nicotine provokes the release of dopamine in the mesolimbic system and frontal cortex. Almost all individuals who use nicotine obtain it from cigarettes, which, as the tobacco industry has acknowledged, serve primarily as nicotine delivery devices. The main impetus for smoking cigarettes ironically lies more in suppressing withdrawal symptoms – anxiety, insomnia, restlessness, tremulousness, craving, and weight gain – than deriving pleasure. Nicotine in cigarettes has no appreciable cognitive effect, but individuals going through withdrawal typically suffer from anxiety, poor concentration, and preoccupation with their lack of cigarettes.

Although stopping tobacco use is usually voluntary, it is often coerced, involuntary, and unexpected as when smokers are hospitalized. Nicotine replacement with gum, patches, or e-cigarettes may alleviate withdrawal symptoms. Varenicline (Chantix), a tobacco-cessation medicine, acts as a partial agonist of certain nicotinic ACh receptors. Cytisine has a similar mechanism of action and benefit. A different antitobacco product, bupropion (Zyban and Wellbutrin) acts a nicotine receptor antagonist and an inhibitor of dopamine reuptake in the mesolimbic system.

"Bath Salts"

Clearly not a bathing or beauty product, "bath salts" or "psychoactive bath salts" (PABS) are a group of stimulants with benign names, such as Ivory Wave and White Horse. Their active ingredient, methylenedioxyprovalerone (MDPV), inhibits dopamine and norepinephrine reuptake. Thus, they cause cocaine-like effects: agitated delirium, often with paranoid aspects and hallucinations, and sympathetic overstimulation with tachycardia, hypertension, and enlarged pupils. They also cause cocaine-like vascular complications: stroke and myocardial infarction.

Routine urine toxicology tests cannot readily detect this category of stimulants. Physicians may be forced to initiate treatment, especially to support vital function and quell dangerous activity, without having an exact diagnosis. Severe tachycardia and other signs of sympathetic overstimulation may require an intravenous benzodiazepine, which will also help reduce the likelihood of seizures. Dangerous behavior or thinking may require small doses of antipsychotic agents.

REFERENCES

Neurotransmitters

Beaulieu-Boire, I., & Lang, A. E. (2015). Behavioral effects of levodopa. *Movement Disorders: Official Journal of the Movement Disorder Society*, *30*, 90–102.

Benarroch, E. E. (2012). GABA$_B$ receptors. *Neurology*, *78*, 578–584.

McKeon, A., Robinson, M. T., McEvoy, K. M., et al. (2012). Stiff-man syndrome and variants: Clinical course, treatments, and outcomes. *Archives of Neurology*, *69*, 230–238.

Stahl, S. M. (2013). *Stahl's Essential Psychopharmacology: Neuroscientific Basis and Practical Applications* (4th ed.). Cambridge: Cambridge University Press.

Drug Abuse

Abramowicz, M. (2015). (Ed). Abuse-deterrent opioid formulations. *Medical Letter*, *57*, 119–120.

Benowitz, N. L. (2010). Nicotine addiction. *The New England Journal of Medicine*, *362*, 2295–2303.

Brust, J. C. (2014). Neurologic complications of illicit drug abuse. *Continuum*, *20*, 642–656.

Derlet, R. W., Rice, P., Horowitz, B. Z., et al. (1989). Amphetamine toxicity: Experience with 127 cases. *The Journal of Emergency Medicine*, *7*, 157–161.

Dobbs, M. R. (2009). *Clinical Neurotoxicology*. Philadelphia: Saunders.

Fasano, A., Barra, A., Nicosia, P., et al. (2008). Cocaine addiction: From habits to stereotypical-repetitive behaviors and punding. *Drug and Alcohol Dependence*, *96*, 178–182.

Geke, A. H., Ahmed, A. I. A., Verkes, R. J., et al. (2015). Tetrahydrocannabinol for neuropsychiatric symptoms in dementia. *Neurology*, *84*, 2338–2346.

Herning, R. I., Better, W., Tate, K., et al. (2005). Neuropsychiatric alterations in MDMA users. *Annals of the New York Academy of Sciences*, *1053*, 20–27.

Hoffman, R. S., Howland, M. A., Lewin, N. A., et al. (Eds.), (2014). *Goldfrank's Toxicologic Emergencies* (10th ed.). New York: McGraw-Hill.

Koppel, B. S., Brust, J. C. M., Fife, T., et al. (2014). Efficacy and safety of medical marijuana in selected neurologic disorders: Report of the Guideline Development Subcommittee of the American Academy of Neurology. *Neurology*, *82*, 1556–1563.

Majlesi, N., Shih, R., Fiesseler, F. W., et al. (2010). Cocaine-associated seizures and incidence of status epilepticus. *West Journal Emergency Medicine*, *11*, 157–160.

McCarron, M. M., Schulze, B. W., Thompson, G. A., et al. (1981). Acute phencyclidine intoxication: Incidence of clinical findings in 1,000 cases. *Annals of Emergency Medicine*, *10*, 237–242.

Miotto, K., Striebel, J., Cho, A. K., et al. (2013). Clinical and pharmacological aspects of bath salts: A review of the literature and case reports. *Drug and Alcohol Dependence*, *132*, 1–12.

Nadeau, S. E. (2015). Opioids for chronic pain: To prescribe or not to prescribe – What is the question? *Neurology*, *85*, 646–651.

Penders, T. M., & Gestring, R. (2011). Hallucinatory delirium following use of MDPV: "Bath salts". *General Hospital Psychiatry*, *33*, 525–526.

Schweinsburg, A. D., Brown, S. A., & Tapert, S. F. (2008). The influence of marijuana use on neurocognitive functioning in adolescents. *Current Drug Abuse Reviews*, *1*, 99–111.

Snead, O. C., & Gibson, K. M. (2005). γ-hydroxybutyric acid. *The New England Journal of Medicine*, *352*, 2721–2732.

Tait, R. J., Mackinnon, A., & Christensen, H. (2011). Cannabis use and cognitive function: 8-year trajectory in a young adult cohort. *Addiction (Abingdon, England)*, *106*, 2195–2203.

Trecki, J., Gerona, R. R., & Schwartz, M. D. (2015). Synthetic cannabinoid-related illness and deaths. *The New England Journal of Medicine*, *373*, 103–106.

CHAPTER 21

QUESTIONS AND ANSWERS

1. Why do parenterally administered opioids induce vomiting?
   a. They block re-uptake of dopamine into presynaptic neurons.
   b. They stimulate the area postrema.
   c. They induce hypertension.
   d. They provoke a discharge of dopamine from presynaptic storage vesicles.

Answer: b. Intravenous injections of heroin or morphine characteristically lead to vomiting because they stimulate the *area postrema*, one of the few areas of the brain unprotected by the blood–brain barrier. The *area postrema* is situated on the dorsal surface of the medulla and contains the chemoreceptor trigger zone. When opioids strike the adjacent respiratory area, which is similarly unprotected, they depress the rate of respirations, which may lead to potentially fatal anoxia. The combination of opioid-induced vomiting and a depressed level of consciousness often leads to potentially fatal aspiration.

2. Which are features of opioid overdose?
   a. Seizures and strokes
   b. Hallucinations and delusions
   c. Mydriasis, agitation, and tachycardia
   d. Miosis, apnea, and pulmonary edema

Answer: d. Opioid overdose causes miosis and depresses the level of consciousness. Depression of respirations causes pulmonary edema that appears as foam from the mouth and throat.

3. A physician who prescribed donepezil (Aricept) to a patient with Alzheimer disease was unaware that the patient was taking bethanechol (Urecholine and others) for urinary retention. The electronic medical record system (EMR) alerted the physician to a potential drug interaction and blocked the prescription. Which problems did the EMR's intercession likely avoid?
   a. Hypotension, bradycardia, abdominal cramps
   b. Depression, delirium
   c. Hypertension, tachycardia
   d. Constipation, dry mouth

Answer: a. Both donepezil and bethanechol are commonly used cholinergic medicines. Physicians prescribe bethanechol to counteract urinary retention due to diabetic autonomic neuropathy and the side effects of tricyclic antidepressants and other medicines. The combination of donepezil and bethanechol would have placed the patient at risk for a cholinergic crisis. The excess cholinergic parasympathetic activity could have led to bronchospasm and seizures as well as hypotension, bradycardia, and abdominal cramps.

4. Which substance's primary active constituent is delta-9-tetrahydrocannabinol (Δ9-THC)?
   a. Cocaine
   b. Phencyclidine (PCP)
   c. Amphetamine
   d. Cannabis

Answer: d. Cannabis is the primary constituent of marijuana, and its primary active constituent is Δ9-THC.

5. Which enzyme metabolizes norepinephrine?
   a. MAO-A
   b. MAO-B
   c. Tyrosine hydroxylase
   d. Phenylalanine hydroxylase

Answer: a.

6. A former heroin addict had epilepsy as a teenager. While attending his methadone maintenance program, he developed a flurry of seizures. ER physicians immediately administered phenytoin (Dilantin). Although it controlled the seizures, the patient became agitated and combative. He also reported nausea and abdominal pain. A psychiatrist found piloerection and muscle cramps. Which is the best course of action?
   a. Administer a benzodiazepine.
   b. Administer naloxone (Narcan).
   c. Increase the dose of phenytoin.
   d. Increase the dose of methadone.

Answer: d. Phenytoin, efavirenz (Sustiva), and other medicines enhance methadone metabolism or compete for its receptor. When physicians administer them to individuals in methadone maintenance programs, the adverse interaction may be so powerful that the individuals go into withdrawal – as in this case. Withdrawal more frequently occurs when physicians prescribe inadequate doses of methadone to opioid users (such as when they are hospitalized or incarcerated). In these scenarios, raising the dose of methadone will alleviate the symptoms. On the other hand, erythromycin and fluvoxamine slow the metabolism of methadone and increase its serum concentration.

7. After eating a meal that included fruits and vegetables gathered from the nearby woods, almost all members of a commune developed abdominal cramps, diarrhea, salivation, tearing, and blurred vision. Some also had delirium and others had recurrence of asthma. Emergency medical service workers

found bradycardia and hypotension in all of them. Which is the most likely toxin?
a. Ricin
b. Muscarine from mushrooms
c. LSD
d. Marijuana

Answer: b. Wild mushrooms may contain the poison muscarine. Mushroom poisoning (mycetism) typically causes a cholinergic crisis from overstimulation of muscarinic receptors.

8. For the victims in the previous question, which is the best treatment?
a. Atropine
b. Naloxone
c. Pyridostigmine
d. Edrophonium

Answer: a. Atropine will displace the excess acetylcholine from its receptors and thereby restore a normal heart rate, reduce bronchospasm, and stop the excessive gastrointestinal hypermotility. Pyridostigmine and edrophonium, in contrast, will inactivate acetylcholinesterase and further increase cholinergic activity.

9. Police brought a 24-year-old man and his similarly aged girlfriend to the psychiatry ER because they were walking rapidly but aimlessly about the town center and speaking nonsense about various threats to the country. The medical resident found both of their pulses to be 100–120 beats per minute and respiratory rates 36 per minute, but their temperatures to be normal. Their pupils were 7 mm. Urine tests on each detected benzoylecgonine. Which is the most likely intoxicant?
a. Amphetamine
b. Cocaine
c. Methamphetamine
d. Phencyclidine

Answer: b. With some variations, the clinical presentation of this pair is consistent with intoxication with any of these stimulants. However, detecting benzoylecgonine indicates that the responsible agent was cocaine. Testing may detect benzoylecgonine for 2–5 days after cocaine use.

10. Which is *not* a sign of excessive sympathetic activity?
a. Tachycardia
b. Eyelid retraction
c. Hypertension
d. Miosis

Answer: d. With excessive sympathetic activity, pupils dilate.

11. Which substance has the weakest antiemetic effect?
a. Marijuana
b. D2 dopamine blockers
c. 5HT$_3$ antagonists

Answer: a. D2 dopamine blockers and 5HT$_3$ antagonists have substantial antiemetic effects. Marijuana has relatively weak antiemetic effects that do not justify its reputation as a chemotherapy adjunct.

12. Each of the following medicines alleviates spasticity. Which one acts as an α_2 adrenergic agonist?
a. Baclofen
b. Tizanidine
c. Dantrolene
d. Benzodiazepines

Answer: b. Tizanidine (Zanaflex) acts as an α_2 adrenergic agonist. Baclofen binds to GABA$_B$ receptors, dantrolene acts directly on muscles, and benzodiazepines act on GABA$_A$ receptors.

13. Which product of dopamine metabolism is measurable in the CSF?
a. Monoamine oxidase (MAO)
b. Homovanillic acid (HVA)
c. Catechol-O-methyltransferase (COMT)
d. Vanillylmandelic acid (VMA)

Answer: b. MAO and COMT are enzymes that metabolize dopamine. VMA, which is excreted in the urine, is a metabolic product of norepinephrine.

14. Which of the following statements is true regarding synthetic marijuana?
a. Synthetic marijuana is a benign drug.
b. Commercial laboratories produce a uniform substance marketed as "spice" or "K2."
c. It is illegal.
d. Unlike marijuana, synthetic marijuana frequently causes delirium, psychotic reactions, seizures, and strokes.

Answer: d. Amateur and professional chemists synthesize a variety of compounds that they sell as synthetic marijuana. Until law enforcement officials identify each substance and enact regulations prohibiting its manufacture and sale, the compounds remain legal. Many of them cause a wide variety of neurologic and psychiatric problems.

15. Which is the rate-limiting enzyme in the synthesis of dopamine?
a. DOPA decarboxylase
b. Tyrosine hydroxylase
c. MAO
d. Dopamine β-hydroxylase

Answer: b.

16. Of the choices listed in Question 15, which is the rate-limiting enzyme in the synthesis of norepinephrine?

Answer: b. As a general rule, tyrosine hydroxylase is the rate-limiting enzyme in catecholamine synthesis.

17. Which statement regarding stimulating D1 and D2 dopamine receptors is correct?

a. Stimulation of the D1 receptor increases cyclic AMP activity and stimulation of the D2 receptor decreases cyclic AMP activity.
b. Stimulation of the D1 receptor decreases ATP to cyclic AMP production and stimulation of the D2 receptor increases cyclic AMP activity.

Answer: a.

18. Which dopamine tract is responsible for the elevated prolactin concentration induced by many antipsychotic agents?
    a. Nigrostriatal
    b. Mesolimbic
    c. Tubero-infundibular
    d. None of the above

Answer: c. The tubero-infundibular tract connects the hypothalamus and the pituitary gland. Dopamine D2 blockade provokes prolactin release and elevates serum prolactin concentration. By way of contrast, the strength of a medicine's dopamine blockade of the mesolimbic system usually correlates with its antipsychotic effect.

19. Which is the primary site for conversion of norepinephrine to epinephrine?
    a. Locus ceruleus
    b. Striatum
    c. Adrenal medulla
    d. Nigrostriatal tact

Answer: c. The alternate name for epinephrine – *adrenaline* – reflects the location of its synthesis.

20. Which is the major metabolic pathway for serotonin?
    a. Metabolism by COMT to 5-hydroxyindoleacetic acid (5-HIAA)
    b. Metabolism by MAO to 5-HIAA
    c. Metabolism by decarboxylase to HVA
    d. Metabolism by HVA to 5-HIAA

Answer: b. Serotonin, like dopamine, mostly undergoes reuptake. MAO metabolizes available serotonin to 5-HIAA. CSF concentrations of HIAA reflect CNS serotonin activity.

21. Where is the main site of serotonin production?
    a. Dorsal raphe nuclei
    b. Regions adjacent to the aqueduct in the midbrain
    c. Striatum
    d. None of the above

Answer: d. Almost all serotonin is produced in platelets, the gastrointestinal tract, and other nonneurologic organs. Within the brain, serotonin-producing neurons are located predominantly in the dorsal raphe nuclei, which are near the aqueduct in the dorsal midbrain. These neurons produce only 2% of the body's total serotonin.

22. A 48-year-old man with a history of major depression commits suicide by igniting several sticks of dynamite. Which neurotransmitter abnormality would investigators most likely find on postmortem examination?
    a. Low concentrations of CSF HVA
    b. Low concentrations of CSF HIAA
    c. Low GABA concentrations in the basal ganglia
    d. High dopamine concentrations

Answer: b. Low concentration of CSF HIAA characterizes violent suicides and reflects decreased CNS serotonin activity. Low GABA concentrations in the basal ganglia are characteristic of Huntington disease.

23. A counselor found her former cocaine addict client shuffling and reshuffling a deck of cards with no intent to play a card game. The client barked at the counselor when she tried to engage him. Then he remained mute. This behavior continued for several hours and then he went to sleep. What term do neurologists apply to this behavior?
    a. Punding
    b. Obsessive-compulsive behavior
    c. Withdrawal
    d. Depression

Answer: a. Cocaine use sometimes causes abnormal, repetitive behavior and preoccupation with useless activities. These activities, which are similar to stereotypies, include hoarding, adjusting electronic equipment, and sorting similar objects. Punding also occurs in Parkinson disease patients. When an examiner attempts to distract patients from their task while they are punding they become irritable. Punding does not correlate with mood or anxiety disorders.

24. In the synthesis of acetylcholine from acetyl-CoA and choline, which is the rate-limiting factor?
    a. Choline acetyltransferase (ChAT)
    b. Acetyl CoA
    c. Choline
    d. None of the above

Answer: c.

25. Which comparison between Lambert–Eaton syndrome and myasthenia gravis is true?
    a. Lambert–Eaton syndrome is a paraneoplastic syndrome, whereas myasthenia gravis is an autoimmune disorder.
    b. Lambert–Eaton syndrome is associated with decreased ACh production, whereas myasthenia gravis is associated with excess ACh production.
    c. Lambert–Eaton syndrome is characterized by defective ACh receptors, whereas myasthenia gravis is characterized by impaired presynaptic ACh release.
    d. Lambert–Eaton syndrome is alleviated by botulism, whereas myasthenia gravis is alleviated by cholinesterases.

Answer: a. In both illnesses, impaired ACh activity at the neuromuscular junction causes muscle weakness. Impaired presynaptic ACh release characterizes Lambert–Eaton syndrome. Although usually a paraneoplastic syndrome, Lambert–Eaton may represent a purely autoimmune disorder. In contrast, myasthenia gravis is an autoimmune disorder characterized by defective ACh receptors on the postsynaptic membrane. Anticholinesterases, which preserve acetylcholine, usually improve the weakness in myasthenia gravis.

26. When GABA interacts with GABA$_A$ receptors, which event is most likely to occur?
    a. Sodium channels are opened and the neuron's membrane becomes hyperpolarized.
    b. Chloride channels are opened and the neuron's membrane becomes hyperpolarized.
    c. An influx of ions depolarizes the neuron.
    d. An influx of ions leads to excitation.

Answer: b. The GABA$_A$ receptor is ubiquitous, multifaceted, and sensitive to benzodiazepines and barbiturates as well as GABA. When stimulated, the GABA$_A$ receptor permits the influx of chloride. The influx of negatively charged ions hyperpolarizes the membrane and inhibits depolarization.

27. Which is the approximate normal resting potential of neurons?
    a. +100 mV
    b. +70 mV
    c. 0 mV
    d. –70 mV
    e. –100 mV

Answer: d. The normal resting potential is –70 mV. When the resting potential is –100 mV, the neuron is hyperpolarized and thereby inhibited.

28. Which role does glycine play?
    a. Glycine is an inhibitory amino acid neurotransmitter.
    b. Glycine modulates the N-methyl-D-aspartate (NMDA) receptor.
    c. Glycine raises the resting potential (i.e., makes it less negative).
    d. a and b

Answer: d. Glycine is primarily an inhibitory amino acid neurotransmitter, but it also modulates the NMDA receptor. Inhibitory neurotransmitters generally make the resting potential more negative.

29. Of the following, which method terminates most dopamine activity?
    a. Decarboxylation
    b. Oxidation
    c. Reuptake
    d. Hydroxylation

Answer: c. Most dopamine undergoes reuptake, but monoamine oxidase (MAO) and catechol-O-methyl-transferase (COMT) metabolize the remainder, intracellularly and extracellularly, respectively.

30. Which neurotransmitter is confined almost entirely to the brain?
    a. Dopamine
    b. Glutamate
    c. Glycine
    d. Norepinephrine
    e. Serotonin

Answer: a. Dopamine is found in the adrenal medulla and retina, but primarily is confined to the brain. The other neurotransmitters may be found in the spinal cord or autonomic nervous system as well as the brain.

31. Which is the effect of glutamate–NMDA interaction under normal circumstances?
    a. Inhibition
    b. Inhibition through hyperpolarization
    c. Excitation
    d. Excitotoxicity

Answer: c. Glutamate, the principal CNS excitatory neurotransmitter, interacts with the NMDA and other receptors to open calcium channels. With excessive activity, the calcium influx raises intracellular concentrations to lethal levels, i.e., excitotoxicity.

32. Of the following, which is the best treatment for atropine poisoning?
    a. Scopolamine
    b. Edrophonium
    c. Neostigmine
    d. Physostigmine

Answer: d. Atropine is an inhibitor of muscarinic cholinergic receptors. Physostigmine, an anticholinesterase, crosses the blood–brain barrier and elevates acetylcholine concentration.

33. In Alzheimer disease, which of the following receptors is most depleted?
    a. Muscarinic acetylcholine
    b. Nicotinic acetylcholine
    c. Nigrostriatal dopamine
    d. Frontal dopamine

Answer: a. In Alzheimer disease, muscarinic acetylcholine receptors are depleted, especially in the limbic system and association areas.

34. Which one of the following inhibits dopamine metabolism and yields amphetamine-like metabolites?
    a. Haloperidol
    b. Selegiline
    c. Amitriptyline
    d. Ropinirole

Answer: b. Although the neuroprotective role of selegiline remains unproven, it inhibits dopamine metabolism and improves parkinsonism. Selegiline also provides an antidepressant effect partly through its metabolic products, amphetamine and methamphetamine.

35. What effect does tetrabenazine have on dopamine transmission?
    a. It stimulates dopamine transmission by acting as a precursor.
    b. It substitutes for dopamine by acting as an agonist.
    c. It interferes with dopamine transmission by blocking D2 receptors.
    d. It reduces dopamine transmission by depleting dopamine from its presynaptic storage sites.

Answer: d. Tetrabenazine depletes dopamine from its presynaptic storage sites and thereby reduces involuntary movements. Tetrabenazine is useful in the treatment of hyperkinetic movement disorders, such as chorea, Tourette syndrome, and oral-bucco-lingual tardive dyskinesia. Unfortunately, tetrabenazine-induced dopamine reduction may lead to parkinsonism and depression with suicidal ideation. It also leads to an innocuous elevation of serum prolactin.

36. A 50-year-old man is hospitalized for alcohol withdrawal. His physicians prophylactically order clonidine and propranolol. This treatment will not help prevent which of the following potential complications of alcohol withdrawal?
    a. Tachycardia
    b. Tremor
    c. Agitation
    d. Seizures

Answer: d. During alcohol withdrawal, clonidine, an α_2 norepinephrine agonist, and propranolol, a β-blocker, will reduce many physical and some psychological manifestations; however, they will not help prevent alcohol-withdrawal seizures. Although benzodiazepines may raise the seizure threshold and help in other ways, neurologists generally do not prophylactically administer antiepileptic drugs in alcohol withdrawal.

37. After 1 week of progressively severe delirium, a 23-year-old woman developed myoclonus and then had a flurry of seizures. An exhaustive evaluation found only that her serum contained antibodies to the NMDA receptor. Which is the most likely underlying pathology?
    a. Huntington disease
    b. PCP intoxication
    c. Ovarian teratoma
    d. Memantine (Namenda) intoxication

Answer: c. In a paraneoplastic syndrome, particularly the one triggered by ovarian teratomas in young women, antibodies directed toward NMDA receptors cause an autoimmune limbic encephalitis.

38. Which one of the following characterizes fast neurotransmitters?
    a. They work through ion channels.
    b. They work through G proteins.
    c. They work through second messengers.
    d. They include dopamine and norepinephrine.

Answer: a. Fast neurotransmitters, such as GABA and glutamate, work through ion channels. Slow neurotransmitters, such as the catecholamines, work through G proteins and second messengers such as cAMP.

39. To which process do excessive glutamate–NMDA receptor interactions lead?
    a. Hyperpolarization
    b. Excitotoxicity
    c. Apoptosis
    d. Involution

Answer: b. Excessive NMDA activation leads to flooding of the neurons with potentially lethal concentrations of calcium – excitotoxicity.

40. Frank, a 40-year-old semi-retired rock musician, has been smoking marijuana on a daily basis for more than 20 years. Unexpectedly institutionalized, he is cut off from his supply. Which will be the predominant withdrawal symptom?
    a. Seizures
    b. Yawning
    c. Irritability
    d. Hallucinations

Answer: c. Unlike abrupt withdrawal from alcohol or benzodiazepines, withdrawal from marijuana, like withdrawal from tobacco, causes irritability and inattentiveness. Yawning characterizes heroin withdrawal. Hallucinations characterize alcohol withdrawal.

41. Which one of the following statements concerning neurotransmission is *false*?
    a. Glutamate–NMDA receptor interactions are fast and excitatory.
    b. Glutamate–NMDA receptor interactions affect the calcium channel.
    c. Benzodiazepine–GABA_A receptor interactions are fast and inhibitory.
    d. Benzodiazepine–GABA_A receptor interactions, which promote the influx of chloride, reduce the polarization of the resting potential.

Answer: d. Benzodiazepine–GABA_A receptor interactions promote the influx of chloride ion (Cl⁻), making the resting potential more negative. The more negative resting potential hyperpolarizes the membrane and inhibits the neuron.

42. Which of the following is a second messenger?
    a. Cyclic AMP
    b. Serotonin
    c. Endorphins
    d. Thyroid hormone

Answer: a. Cyclic AMP, like phosphatidyl inositol, is a second messenger.

43. Which dopamine tract is most likely responsible for positive symptoms in psychosis?
a. Nigrostriatal
b. Mesolimbic
c. Tubero-infundibular
d. Mesocortical

Answer: b.

44. Which dopamine tract is most likely responsible for negative symptoms in psychosis?
a. Nigrostriatal
b. Mesolimbic
c. Tubero-infundibular
d. Mesocortical

Answer: d.

45. Which of the following pairs are inhibitory amino acid neurotransmitters?
a. GABA and glycine
b. Glutamate and aspartate
c. Epinephrine and norepinephrine
d. L-dopa (levodopa) and carbidopa

Answer: a. GABA and glycine are inhibitory amino acid neurotransmitters. Glutamate and aspartate are excitatory amino acid neurotransmitters.

46–51. Match the medication (46–51) with the enzyme (a–e) that it inhibits.

46. Selegiline
47. Carbidopa
48. Entacapone
49. Edrophonium
50. Tranylcypromine
51. Pyridostigmine
a. DOPA decarboxylase
b. COMT
c. MAO-B
d. Acetylcholinesterase
e. MAO-A

Answers: 46–c, 47–a, 48–b, 49–d, 50–e, 51–d.

52–56. Match the illness (52–56) with the deficient enzyme(s) (a–e).

52. Phenylketonuria
53. Parkinson disease
54. Tay–Sachs disease
55. Alzheimer disease
56. Huntington disease
a. Phenylalanine hydroxylase
b. Tyrosine hydroxylase
c. Glutamate decarboxylase
d. Choline acetyltransferase
e. Hexosaminidase-A

Answers: 52–a, 53–b, 54–e, 55–d, 56–c.

57. A 75-year-old retired policeman's family abruptly discontinued all his Parkinson disease medicines after he began to yell about vivid, frightening nocturnal visual hallucinations. His yelling prevented the entire household from sleeping. Two days later he became "stiff as a board," febrile, and delirious. His family brought him to the ER where the staff found him stuporous, febrile, and rigid. While awaiting blood test results, which treatments should the staff administer in addition to providing fluids, glucose, and electrolytes?
a. A second-generation antipsychotic
b. Dantrolene and his usual Parkinson disease medicines
c. Aspirin
d. A first-generation antipsychotic

Answer: b. Most likely the patient has developed the neuroleptic malignant syndrome (dopamine depletion syndrome) because of the abrupt loss of dopaminergic activity. An infection may be the cause of his delirium and fever, but probably not the rigidity. The medical staff should administer dantrolene and reinstitute his usual Parkinson disease medicines. A benzodiazepine might reduce his agitation, give him some rest, and allow him to cooperate with treatment.

58. A young man is brought to the psychiatric ER after he wandered away from an all-night dance party. He appears anxious, but he repeats that he feels "close to everyone." His pupils have a normal diameter and reactivity to light. His eyes have full, conjugate movement without nystagmus. He grinds his teeth. Which is the most likely intoxicant?
a. A dopamine-blocking antipsychotic agent
b. PCP
c. Heroin
d. Ecstasy

Answer: d. Ecstasy is a stimulant that typically induces a sense of empathy, but paradoxically, in many cases, it induces anxiety. Intoxication characteristically causes bruxism (teeth grinding), which may mimic the dystonic jaw movements from antipsychotics. Alcohol, hypnotics, and other substances cause nystagmus, but PCP causes prominent, coarse, multidirectional nystagmus accompanied by generalized muscle rigidity. Heroin causes miosis and a depressed level of consciousness.

59. Of the following atypical antipsychotics, which raises the serum prolactin concentration to its highest level?
a. Aripiprazole
b. Ziprasidone
c. Risperidone
d. Clozapine
e. Olanzapine

Answer: c. Of these agents, risperidone raises the prolactin level to the greatest extent and is also the most likely to cause galactorrhea. Clozapine is least likely to raise the prolactin level.

60. Which of the following is *false* regarding the GABA$_B$ receptor?
    a. GABA$_B$ receptors are more numerous and more widely distributed than GABA$_A$ receptors.
    b. GABA$_B$ receptors are G protein-linked channel inhibitors.
    c. Baclofen binds to GABA$_B$ receptors.
    d. Like GABA$_A$ receptors, GABA$_B$ receptors are complex molecules.

Answer: a. GABA$_A$ receptors are more numerous and more widely distributed than GABA$_B$ receptors.

61. In a suicide attempt, a 40-year-old man who had been under treatment for tuberculosis (TB) and major depression for several years took an overdose of isoniazid (INH). Shortly afterwards, he developed status epilepticus. Which would be the most specific, effective treatment?
    a. Topiramate
    b. Thiamine
    c. Lorazepam
    d. Pyridoxine (vitamin B$_6$)

Answer: d. INH, a treatment for TB, possesses some antidepressant properties and interferes with pyridoxine. Pyridoxine is the cofactor for glutamate decarboxylase, which is a crucial enzyme in GABA synthesis. Thus, large doses of INH create a GABA deficiency. The loss of this inhibitory neurotransmitter causes seizures. Doctors prescribing INH should add pyridoxine.

62. Which of the following statements concerning "bath salts" is true?
    a. They block the reuptake of dopamine and norepinephrine.
    b. They lead to a surge of parasympathetic activity.
    c. They act like opioids and induce a sense of calm but also depress respirations.
    d. They are naturally occurring psychoactive drugs found in Baden Baden and Wiesbaden.

Answer: a. Methylenedioxypyrovalerone (MDPV) is the active ingredient of the synthetic stimulants "bath salts." These drugs block the reuptake of dopamine and norepinephrine and induce hallucinatory delirium and a sympathetic surge.

63. A psychiatry consultant was requested to evaluate Tony, a 55-year-old bartender, who insisted on being discharged against medical advice. He had been admitted for pneumonia superimposed on chronic obstructive lung disease. In the hospital, after his pneumonia began to respond to treatment, he became cantankerous and then agitated and sullen. Tony stated that he has smoked two packs of cigarettes each day, but denied ever drinking alcohol. His physical neurologic examination, routine blood tests, and head CT were all normal. Tony demanded cigarettes or an immediate discharge. Which would be the first, best treatment?
    a. Varenicline (Chantix)
    b. Selegiline
    c. Alprazolam
    d. Haloperidol

Answer: a. Tony is going through nicotine withdrawal. In some cases, alprazolam may be helpful on a temporary basis to reduce physical and mental agitation, but it may have an adverse effect in patients with chronic obstructive lung disease. Varenicline, a nicotine ACh receptor agonist, would be a good treatment in most cases. Alternatively the patient may benefit from bupropion, a nicotine antagonist and inhibitor of dopamine reuptake, or a nicotine patch.

64. A 67-year-old woman, a recent immigrant from Central America, received fluoxetine for depression. After drinking tea made from various herbs sold in the local bodega, she developed anxiety and tremulousness. Which medication should ER psychiatrists administer?
    a. A benzodiazepine
    b. Physostigmine
    c. An atypical neuroleptic
    d. None of the above

Answer: d. The woman is experiencing a mild serotonin syndrome. Her physicians should keep her calm and hydrated, and allow it to pass. In Latino communities, bodegas and botanicas sell, among other products, religious icons and folk medicines, including herbs. Some folk medicines contain St. John's wort (*Hypericum perforatum*, a genus of flowering plants), mercury, and other potentially harmful substances. The combination of St. John's wort and an SSRI may lead to the serotonin syndrome.

65. Which of the following medicines would most likely reduce hyperkinetic involuntary movement disorders?
    a. Tetrabenazine
    b. Levodopa
    c. Benzodiazepine
    d. Carbidopa

Answer: a. Tetrabenazine, which depletes dopamine from presynaptic storage vesicles in the nigrostriatal tract, reduces chorea, tics, and medication-induced dyskinesias.

66. On which receptors do second-generation antipsychotics act?
    a. D1 and 5HT$_{2A}$ receptors
    b. D2 and 5HT$_{2A}$ receptors
    c. D2 and 5-HT$_{1D}$ receptors
    d. D2 and 5HT$_3$ receptors

Answer: b. Second-generation antipsychotics act as antagonists of 5HT$_{2A}$ as well as D2 receptors. Triptans used to treat migraine are selective 5-HT$_{1D}$ receptor agonists. Dolasetron and ondansetron, which are antiemetics used in conjunction with chemotherapy agents, are 5HT$_3$ antagonists.

67. Which drug of abuse most increases serotonin activity?
    a. PCP
    b. Amphetamine
    c. LSD
    d. Ecstasy
    e. Cocaine

Answer: d. Ecstasy greatly increases CNS serotonin activity by releasing it from its presynaptic storage vesicles. LSD stimulates serotonin receptors, but its effects are less pronounced than those of ecstasy. Amphetamine and cocaine act primarily on the dopamine system, and PCP on NMDA receptors.

68–73. Match the site of neurotransmitter synthesis (68–73) with the region(s) of the nervous system (a–e) where it is located. More than one answer may be appropriate.

68. Locus ceruleus
69. Dorsal raphe nuclei
70. Adrenal medulla
71. Substantia nigra
72. Nucleus basalis of Meynert
73. Caudal raphe nuclei
    a. Basal forebrain
    b. Midbrain
    c. Pons
    d. Medulla
    e. Adrenal gland

Answers: 68–c, 69–b and c, 70–e, 71–b, 72–a, 73–c and d.

74. A woman, 5 months pregnant, asks for methadone maintenance because federal agents have interrupted her heroin supply. Which action would best preserve the health of the patient and the fetus?
    a. Do not accept her into a methadone maintenance program until after she delivers.
    b. Have her undergo heroin detoxification to avoid exposing the fetus to methadone.
    c. Enroll her in a methadone maintenance program as soon as possible.
    d. Have her stop all opioids, i.e., "go cold turkey."

Answer: c. Both the fetus and the mother are probably dependent on heroin. Physicians should probably switch the mother from heroin to methadone. After she delivers, physicians can detoxify both the mother and infant.

75. To which receptors do ketamine and PCP bind?
    a. NMDA
    b. Norepinephrine
    c. Serotonin
    d. GABA$_A$

Answer: a. Ketamine, a legitimate veterinary anesthetic, and PCP have a similar chemical structure and both block NMDA receptors.

76. What is the effect of the binding of ketamine and PCP to the NMDA receptor?
    a. Inhibition of the influx of calcium
    b. Promotion of the influx of calcium
    c. Inhibition of the influx of chloride
    d. Promotion of the influx of chloride

Answer: a. Ketamine and PCP inhibit the influx of calcium, which is usually provoked by interactions of glutamate or aspartate with the NMDA receptor.

77. Which of the following statements concerning sodium oxybate (Xyrem) is *false*?
    a. It is indicated for the treatment of cataplexy in narcolepsy.
    b. It is indicated for the treatment of excessive daytime sleepiness in narcolepsy.
    c. It is the sodium salt of gamma-hydroxybutyrate (GHB).
    d. Because it has been implicated as the agent in drug-facilitated sexual assault (date rape), the manufacture and sale of sodium oxybate are illegal.

Answer: d. Sodium oxybate is indicated for the treatment of narcolepsy with cataplexy. Because sodium oxybate has been implicated in date rape, its manufacture and distribution are closely monitored.

78. Of the following dopamine receptors, which is most stimulated by cocaine?
    a. D1
    b. D2 mesocortical
    c. D2 mesolimbic
    d. D3

Answer: c. Cocaine mostly affects the D2 mesolimbic receptors.

79. Which is the best treatment for cocaine-induced psychosis with dangerous, violent behavior?
    a. Dopamine-blocking neuroleptics
    b. Benzodiazepines
    c. Seclusion and, if necessary, restraints
    d. None of the above

Answer: a. Because the main effect of cocaine is to increase dopamine activity by blocking its reuptake, dopamine-blocking neuroleptics are the best short-term treatment. However, in this situation, physicians should cautiously use these neuroleptics because they may lower the seizure threshold.

80. When used in the treatment of Alzheimer disease, what is the mechanism of action of memantine?
    a. It interferes with cholinesterase.
    b. It antagonizes NMDA receptors.
    c. It mimics ACh's actions, i.e., it is a cholinomimetic.
    d. It dissolves amyloid.

Answer: b. Unlike anticholinesterase therapy for Alzheimer disease, which attempts to preserve ACh by inhibiting cholinesterase, memantine antagonizes NMDA receptors.

81. Which is the best treatment for cocaine-induced severe hypertension?
    a. Diuretics
    b. Calcium channel blockers
    c. ACE inhibitors
    d. Phentolamine

Answer: d. An α-blocker, such as phentolamine, is probably the most rapid and effective antihypertensive therapy. Controlling blood pressure may forestall a cerebral hemorrhage.

82. Which is the effect of amphetamine on sleep?
    a. Decreases light sleep
    b. Decreases slow-wave sleep
    c. Decreases proportion of REM
    d. Displaces REM from nighttime to daytime

Answer: c. Amphetamines not only reduce total sleep time, but they also particularly suppress the REM phase.

83. What is the primary effect of opioids on respiration?
    a. They reduce the respiratory rate.
    b. They reduce the depth of respirations.
    c. They increase the rate but reduce the depth of respirations.
    d. They increase the depth and rate of respirations.

Answer: a. Opioids primarily reduce the respiratory rate. In an overdose, opioids lead to respiratory arrest and pulmonary edema.

84. What is the effect of interaction of PCP with the NMDA receptor?
    a. It stabilizes the ion channel.
    b. It leads to an influx of negatively charged chloride ions, which hyperpolarizes the neuron.
    c. It triggers an influx of calcium, which leads to excitotoxicity.
    d. It prevents the influx of calcium that glutamate induces.

Answer: d. Glutamate ordinarily triggers an influx of calcium, but interactions of PCP with NMDA receptors prevent it. PCP elicits both the positive and negative symptoms of schizophrenia – unlike amphetamine and other stimulants.

85. Which of the following is a common effect of marijuana use?
    a. Fatal intoxication
    b. Seizures
    c. Stroke
    d. Reduced REM sleep

Answer: d.

86. Which of the following statements concerning nicotine is *false*?
    a. Nicotine affects CNS cholinergic receptors.
    b. Nicotine receptors are located in the mesolimbic pathway.
    c. Bupropion may help smokers through withdrawal because, like nicotine, it increases dopamine concentrations.
    d. Nicotine receptors are the predominant cholinergic receptors in the CNS.

Answer: d. Although both muscarinic and nicotinic receptors are present in the CNS, muscarinic receptors predominate. In the PNS, nicotinic receptors predominate at the neuromuscular junction.

87. A 40-year-old man presented to a neurologist because of increasingly severe lumbar back pain. When upright, he had hyperlordosis and limited range of movement about the low back and legs. He had begun to walk like a "tin soldier." Extensive testing revealed antibodies to glutamic acid decarboxylase (GAD) in the serum and spinal fluid. What is his most likely diagnosis?
    a. Parkinson disease
    b. Tetanus
    c. Stiff-person syndrome
    d. Catatonia

Answer: c. He has stiff-person syndrome, which neurologists previously called "stiff-man" syndrome. This disorder is often – but not always – a paraneoplastic syndrome associated with anti-GAD antibodies that reduce the synthesis of GABA. Decreased GABA activity results in abnormally increased muscular tone.

88. What is the mechanism of action of methylenedioxymethamphetamine (MDMA), also known as ecstasy, in producing euphoria?
    a. Dopamine release and blocked reuptake
    b. Serotonin surge
    c. Mild glutamate toxicity
    d. Stimulation of μ (mu) receptors

Answer: b. MDMA provokes release of presynaptic serotonin stores, which leads to euphoria. In high doses, it also provokes hallucinations and overstimulation.

89. Which is the most prevalent excitatory neurotransmitter?
    a. Norepinephrine
    b. GABA
    c. Glutamate
    d. Dopamine

Answer: c.

90. Which neurotransmitter imbalance most likely underlies delirium?
    a. Excessive dopamine activity
    b. Deficient dopamine activity

c. Excessive ACh activity
d. Deficient ACh activity

Answer: d. Delirium is most closely associated with an absolute or, compared to dopamine activity, relative ACh deficiency.

91. Which of these medicines is *not* like the others?
    a. Apomorphine
    b. Ropinirole
    c. Pramipexole
    d. Levodopa

Answer: d. Although all these medicines alleviate the symptoms of Parkinson disease, only levodopa is a dopamine precursor. The others are dopamine agonists.

92. Serotonin activity fluctuates during the sleep–wake cycle. When is its activity greatest?
    a. Slow-wave sleep
    b. REM sleep
    c. Arousal
    d. None of the above

Answer: c.

93. In its fluctuations during the sleep–wake cycle, when is serotonin concentration lowest?
    a. Slow-wave sleep
    b. REM sleep
    c. Arousal
    d. None of the above

Answer: b. Serotonin concentration falls during slow-wave sleep and almost disappears during REM sleep.

94. Which enzyme predominates in serotonin metabolism?
    a. MAO-A
    b. MAO-B
    c. COMT
    d. DOPA decarboxylase

Answer: a. In general, MAO-A metabolizes serotonin and MAO-B metabolizes dopamine. The Parkinson disease medicine selegiline at the usual dose (10 mg daily) inhibits only MAO-B and does not pose significant risk of hypertensive crisis or serotonin syndrome.

95. Which of the following is *not* a manifestation of anticholinergic medicines?
    a. Miosis
    b. Tachycardia and hypertension
    c. Dry skin and low-grade fever
    d. Constipation and urinary retention
    e. Toxic encephalopathy (with high doses)

Answers: a. Because anticholinergic medications reduce parasympathetic activity and thereby allow sympathetic activity to predominate, they dilate pupils, cause tachycardia and hypertension, and reduce bowel and bladder activity. At high concentrations, anticholinergic medications interfere with CNS cholinergic (ACh) transmission and thereby produce memory impairment, confusion, hallucinations, and depression of the sensorium. Pharmacologic agents that might cause toxic levels of anticholinergic activity include atropine, trihexyphenidyl, benztropine, tricyclic antidepressants, and certain dopamine-blocking antipsychotic agents. Physostigmine, a cholinesterase inhibitor that crosses the blood–brain barrier, can restore CNS ACh activity.

96. Which of the following is a nicotinic ACh receptor agonist?
    a. Varenicline
    b. Bupropion
    c. Donepezil
    d. Selegiline

Answer: a. Varenicline (Chantix) is an agonist of certain nicotinic ACh receptors. In contrast, bupropion is an antagonist of nicotinic ACh receptors. Donepezil enhances ACh activity by reducing cholinesterase, but not by interacting with ACh receptors. Selegiline inhibits MAO-B.

TRAUMATIC BRAIN INJURY

Neurologists divide *traumatic brain injury* (*TBI*) into *mild* and *severe* categories. Following the classification scheme of the American Academy of Neurology, which is one of many, neurologists define mild TBI as "a trauma-induced alteration in mental status that may or may not involve loss of consciousness." Typically, this altered mental status consists of confusion and amnesia that lasts seconds to minutes. Neurologists expect that the patient will have no focal neurologic signs, such as hemiparesis, cranial nerve abnormalities, or incoordination. Physicians sometimes use the term *concussion* to refer to mild TBI.

In contrast, neurologists define severe TBI as post-traumatic prolonged loss of consciousness (more than 12 hours) with radiographic signs of injury to brain, skull, or intracranial blood vessels. Civilians most at risk for severe TBI are 15-to-24-year-old men and individuals older than 75 years. For them, common causes of TBI include motor vehicle crashes (MVCs), athletic and recreational accidents, on-the-job injuries, falls, and violent assaults. At any age, alcohol plays a major role in TBI because it impairs judgment, coordination, and wakefulness. In the elderly, falls not only commonly cause TBI, but they also pose several clinical problems. Strokes often cause the patient to fall and thereby sustain TBI deficits superimposed on those that are stroke-induced. Falls may also cause bodily injury, such as a hip fracture, which leads to nonneurologic deficits. Also, fall-induced impairments and TBI in general may represent *elder abuse*.

Historically, head injuries from shrapnel and bullets have been the typical causes of wartime TBI. In modern warfare, however, such as the Iraq and Afghanistan conflicts, blast injuries are much more common than penetrating wounds.

MAJOR HEAD TRAUMA

How Does Head Trauma Cause TBI?

Direct Force

A blow to the head – by its direct mechanical force (a *coup* injury) – disrupts the underlying, delicate brain tissue (the *parenchyma*). As with strokes, trauma causes cell death by necrosis and its accompanying inflammatory changes, particularly mononuclear cell infiltration. (In contrast, neurodegenerative diseases, such as Huntington disease and amyotrophic lateral sclerosis [ALS], cause cell death by apoptosis [see Chapter 18].)

In addition to causing the coup injury, head trauma throws the brain against the opposite inner surface (table) of the skull, which causes a *contrecoup* injury of that surface of the brain. Damage from contrecoup injuries frequently surpasses that from the coup injury. Contrecoup injuries frequently damage the temporal and frontal lobes because their anterior surfaces abut the sharp edges of the skull's anterior and middle cranial fossae (Fig. 22.1). Depending on its severity, damage to the frontal and temporal lobes characteristically leads to memory impairment and personality changes. In one exception to this mechanism, frontal trauma rarely leads to countercoup occipital lobe injuries because the occipital skull is relatively flat and smooth.

Diffuse Axonal Shearing

Diffuse axonal shearing, another potential consequence of TBI, consists not only of trauma to long subcortical white matter axons, but also damage to cytoskeletal elements and a fatal intracellular influx of calcium. Although neither computed tomography (CT) nor magnetic resonance imaging (MRI) can reliably illustrate diffuse axonal shearing, particularly in milder cases, diffusion tensor imaging (DTI) readily detects it by showing traumatic disruption of white matter tracts (see Chapter 20). Secondary effects of axonal shearing, such as cerebral contusion and petechial hemorrhage, may be more readily visualized on neuroimaging, particularly MRI.

Intracerebral Bleeding

Blunt trauma causes intraparenchymal bleeding that ranges in severity from petechiae to hematomas. In addition, it causes diffuse *cerebral edema*, which increases intracranial pressure. Hematomas within the brain and over its surface exert pressure on adjacent brain tissue. If they expand beyond a certain size, they force transtentorial herniation (see later).

Bleeding Within the Skull but Outside the Brain

Head injury, ruptured aneurysms, and other insults often cause bleeding in the spaces between the three meninges, which are readily recalled using the mnemonic *PAD*: *pia*, *arachnoid*, and *dura mater*:

- Pia mater, the innermost layer, is a thin, translucent, vascular membrane adherent to the cerebral gyri. It follows gyri into sulci and thus allows for a generous region, the *subarachnoid space*, between it and the immediately overlying layer – the arachnoid mater.
- Arachnoid mater, also thin, spans the tops of gyri, capping the sulci. The subarachnoid space, which contains the cerebrospinal fluid (CSF), envelops the brain and, continuing downward within the spinal

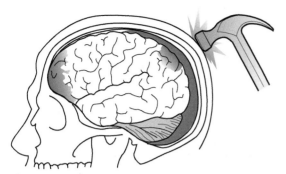

FIGURE 22.1 ■ In this drawing, a hammer blow to the back of the head inflicts a *coup* injury to the occipital region and, as is typical, a more extensive *contrecoup* injury to the inferior surface of the frontal and anterior tips of the temporal lobes.

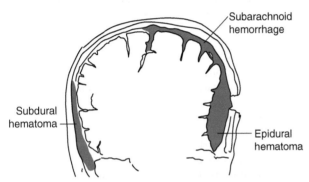

FIGURE 22.2 ■ Meningeal arterial bleeding, which usually results from a blow forceful enough to fracture the skull, causes an *epidural hematoma*. In contrast, venous bleeding, usually slower and under less pressure, causes a *subdural hematoma*. Ruptured aneurysms and head trauma often cause *subarachnoid hemorrhage (SAH)*. In SAH, blood spreads within the subarachnoid space over the convexities, between the gyri, into the interhemispheric fissure, and down into the spinal canal.

canal to the sacrum, the spinal cord and cauda equina. Neurologists performing a spinal tap or lumbar puncture (LP) insert a needle into the subarachnoid space below the *conus medullaris* (lower end of the spinal cord), which is situated between the T12 and L1 vertebrae, to sample CSF.

- *Dura mater*, the outermost layer of the meninges, is a thick fibrous tissue adherent to the interior surface of the skull. Two of its infoldings, the *falx* and *tentorium*, support the brain and house most of its venous drainage. Neurologists designate the space between the skull and the underlying dura as the *epidural space*, and between the dura and the underlying arachnoid as the *subdural space*. Major head trauma may cause hematomas in either or both of these areas.

Epidural hematomas, which typically result from temporal bone fractures with concomitant middle meningeal artery lacerations, are essentially rapidly expanding, high-pressure, fresh blood clots (Fig. 22.2). They compress the underlying brain and force it through the tentorial notch, producing *transtentorial herniation* (see Fig. 19.3). Unless

surgery can immediately arrest the bleeding, epidural hematomas are usually fatal.

As an example, a victim of an assault with a baseball bat lost consciousness when struck. After regaining consciousness for 1 hour, the victim lapsed into coma and developed fatal decerebrate posturing (see Fig. 19.3). A CT showed a temporal skull fracture and an underlying epidural hematoma (see Fig. 20.9D). Neurologists label the period when the victim transiently regained consciousness, the *lucid interval*.

In contrast, *subdural hematomas* usually result from slowly bleeding bridging veins, which are under relatively low pressure, into the subdural space (see Fig. 20.9). Dark venous blood generally oozes into the extensive subdural space until the expanding hematoma encounters underlying brain. The brain dampens bleeding and suppresses further expansion of the subdural. However, if the hematoma continues to expand, it may lead to cerebral transtentorial herniation or cerebellar herniation through the foramen magnum. Survivors often have permanent brain damage from the initial trauma and the pressure from the subdural hematoma.

Acute subdural hematomas, which are most apt to occur in alcoholics, individuals medicated with anticoagulants, or the elderly (see later), produce headache, confusion, and a deteriorating level of consciousness over several hours to 1 or 2 days. Depending on the extent of the bleeding and time until the diagnosis, patients may develop focal signs and herniation. A history of head trauma does not necessarily precede the symptoms. CT shows acute, dense blood in the subdural space (see Fig. 20.9).

Chronic subdural hematomas that have developed and persisted for weeks, usually have spread extensively in the subdural space (see Fig. 20.9). They typically give rise to an insidiously developing headache, change in personality, and cognitive impairment, but only subtle focal physical deficits (see Chapters 19 and 20). Although subdural hematomas may spontaneously resolve, they sometimes require surgical evacuation. Because subdural hematomas cause cognitive decline that is rapid but treatable, neurologists often include subdural hematomas as an potential explanation for "rapidly developing dementia" and a "reversible cause of dementia" (see Chapter 7).

People older than 65 years are susceptible to chronic subdural hematomas for several reasons. They have a tendency to fall. They often take aspirin, anticoagulants, and other medications that increase their tendency to bleed. Most important, age-related cerebral atrophy results in increased tension on the bridging veins.

Once enough blood has collected, whether epidural, subdural, or even subarachnoid, signs of increased intracranial pressure may develop, including headache, confusion, nausea, vomiting, and focal neurologic signs. To avoid the often-fatal complication of herniation, neurologists try hyperventilation and infusions of hypertonic saline or mannitol to reduce cerebral blood volume. While controversial, they will even induce mild hypothermia, which may further reduce intracranial pressure. These measures are usually temporary and help to slow progression while the patient is being prepared for surgical intervention, either to evacuate a blood collection or to remove cerebrospinal fluid through a shunt mechanism.

Foreign Bodies

In addition to the disruption of brain tissue and intraparenchymal bleeding, gun-shot wounds and other penetrating injuries leave bone, shrapnel, and other foreign bodies in the brain. These foreign bodies act as a focus that may generate seizures and a nidus for brain abscesses. Although desirable, neurosurgeons cannot remove all foreign bodies because many lodge in inaccessible areas.

Posttraumatic Coma and Delirium

Neurologists find it useful to classify the level of consciousness of TBI patients (and others) as *alert, lethargic, stuporous,* or *comatose.* They may also use the *Glasgow Coma Scale (GCS),* which measures three readily apparent neurologic functions: eye opening, speaking, and moving (Table 22.1). In major head trauma the GCS correlates closely with survival and neurologic sequelae; however, in minor head trauma it correlates poorly. Moreover, physicians cannot appropriately include the GCS as part of a standard mental status examination for patients suspected of having dementia or circumscribed neuropsychologic deficits.

By the first day after TBI, 90% of patients with a GCS score of 3 (the lowest possible score) have a fatal outcome, and most of the remaining never regain consciousness. By 4 weeks, almost all TBI comatose patients die, partially recover and regain consciousness, or evolve into the vegetative state (see Chapter 11). When in coma or the vegetative state, individuals cannot perceive pain and do not suffer.

As patients surviving major TBI emerge from coma, their mental state usually fluctuates, and cognitive and personality changes emerge. In this twilight zone, they are often confused, disoriented, agitated, and combative. Their mental processes may be so disrupted and their behavior so counterproductive that they warrant treatment with antipsychotic agents.

During this time, physicians must keep in mind the possible role of drug and alcohol use in the trauma and its aftermath. Not only may substance abuse have caused the trauma, but also because the effects of drugs and alcohol may persist for several days, patients may have substance-induced delirium comorbid with TBI. During the recovery phase, alcohol or drug withdrawal may cause seizures and a markedly lower pain threshold, as well as abnormal behavior from substance-withdrawal delirium superimposed on TBI.

Even after recovery from TBI, alcohol abuse stalks survivors. It and other substance abuse often remain a source of continued disability. Binge drinking complicates the life of major TBI survivors 18 times more often than age-matched controls.

Preexisting dementia also leaves patients particularly susceptible to posttraumatic delirium. In fact, dementia may have led to the trauma, as when a patient with Alzheimer disease causes a MVC. Also, numerous trauma-related conditions may produce posttraumatic delirium, such as painful injuries, adverse reactions to antiepileptic drugs (AEDs), opioids, and other medications, and systemic complications, such as hypoxia, sepsis, electrolyte disturbances, and fat emboli.

Physical Sequelae

TBI characteristically causes focal neurologic deficits such as hemiparesis, spasticity, and ataxia. Some studies, which remain controversial, assert that TBI may also lead to involuntary movement disorders similar to Parkinson disease.

Recovery from physical deficits, to the extent that it occurs, usually reaches a maximum within 6 months. During the recovery period and afterwards, patients can increase their functional abilities with physical and occupational therapy, braces, other mechanical devices, and modifications of their environment.

Any damage to the special sensory organs, such as the eye, ear, or nose and their cranial nerves, although not strictly speaking a "brain injury," adds to a patient's neurologic disability. It may also lead to sensory deprivation, disfigurement, and functional impairment. Frontal head trauma, which is probably the most common injury, often shears the filaments of the olfactory nerves as they pass through the cribriform plate. Thus, patients sustaining frontal head trauma often develop combinations of anosmia and personality and cognitive impairments. In addition, TBI that damages a patient's hypothalamus disrupts their sleep–wake cycle, resulting in insomnia, inattention, and sometimes a requirement for additional medicines (see later).

TABLE 22.1	The Glasgow Coma Scale (GCS)	
Category		**Score**
Eyes opening	Never	1
	To pain	2
	To verbal stimuli	3
	Spontaneously	4
Best verbal response	None	1
	Incomprehensible sounds	2
	Inappropriate words	3
	Disoriented and converses	4
	Oriented and converses	5
Best motor response	None	1
	Extension*	2
	Flexion^	3
	Flexion withdrawal	4
	Patient localizes pain	5
	Patient obeys	6
Total		3–15

*Decerebrate rigidity (see Fig. 19.3)
^Decorticate rigidity (see Fig. 11.5)
This standard scale quantitates the level of consciousness, with lower scores indicating poorer neurologic function. Neurologists interpret scores of 3–8 as signifying severe TBI or coma; 9–12, moderate TBI; and 13–15, mild TBI. However, the GCS is not readily applicable to patients who have sustained cerebral hypoxia and, because they cannot make a verbal response, those who are intubated. Adapted with kind permission from Teasdale G, Jennett B: Assessment of coma and impaired consciousness: A practical scale. Lancet 1974;2:81-84.

Posttraumatic Epilepsy

Cerebral scars and residual foreign bodies routinely form epileptic foci. They generate posttraumatic epilepsy (PTE), which is one of the most commonly occurring complications of major TBI. As time passes after an injury the prevalence of PTE increases; eventually reaching 50%. The prevalence is greater following penetrating rather than blunt or blast injury, and among patients who abuse alcohol. In contrast, PTE rarely complicates minor head trauma.

Seizures that occur either within the first 24 hours (immediate posttraumatic seizures) or the first 7 days (early posttraumatic seizures) do not fall within the definition of PTE because neurologists label them "provoked seizures." Only seizures that occur (and recur) more than 7 days after the traumatic injury fall into the definition of PTE. Of note, 1 week of phenytoin or levetiracetam prophylaxis following severe TBI reduces early posttraumatic seizures, but no AED clearly reduces the prevalence of PTE, which may account for 5–6% of all epilepsy. PTE remits in only 25–50% of cases. PTE usually takes the form of complex partial seizures that undergo secondary generalization (see Chapter 10). Not only does PTE cause disability and carry the risk of further head injury, AEDs may exacerbate TBI-induced cognitive and personality changes. Complicating the treatment of these patients is the fact that some studies have shown an increase of psychogenic nonepileptic seizures (see Chapter 10) in patients with milder TBI.

Cognitive Impairment

TBI-induced coma usually lasts, at most, 4 weeks. By then, most patients have either succumbed to their injuries or recovered at least some cognition. However, many patients remain in a twilight state with their eyes open, but unconscious. These patients are incapable of thinking, communicating, or deliberately moving. They cannot perceive pain and do not suffer. Most of them linger in the *persistent vegetative state* (see Chapter 11). Neurologists use the term *permanent* vegetative state once 3 months have passed without change.

Of those TBI patients who regain consciousness, many still have residual incapacitating cognitive impairments. They remain reticent, responsive to only simple requests, and capable of initiating only rudimentary bodily functions. Moreover, physical deficits and PTE accompany their cognitive impairments.

The *Diagnostic and Statistical Manual of Mental Disorders, 5th Edition* (DSM-5) has replaced its previous edition's term "dementia due to head trauma" with the label Neurocognitive Disorder Due to Traumatic Brain Injury.

As a general rule, severely injured patients have profound cognitive deficits. To some extent their deficits correlate with the depth of their immediate posttraumatic coma, as measured by the GCS. However, their deficits more strongly correlate with the duration of the posttraumatic amnesia, which includes the patient's time in coma. Cognitive deficits include not only memory impairment (see later), but also apraxia, impulsivity, inattention, and slowed information processing. One important caveat remains: self-reported cognitive complaints correlate more closely with premorbid low educational status, emotional stress, and poor physical condition than with neuropsychological test results.

Surprisingly, the location of the trauma, with one important exception, correlates inconsistently with cognitive impairment. Left temporal lobe injuries, the exception, routinely produce vocabulary deficits similar to anomic aphasia (see Chapter 8).

Just as medications may cause or add to delirium in the immediate posttraumatic period, numerous AEDs, muscle relaxants, and opioids may further depress cognitive function. These medicines may also alter the patient's personality, mood, and sleep–wake cycle. Similarly, comorbid posttraumatic stress disorder (PTSD) may worsen cognitive impairment.

Recovery of motor and language skills usually reaches a maximum within 6 months, but intellectual recovery may not peak until 18 months. Older patients generally recover more slowly and less completely than younger patients.

In addition to causing debilitating cognitive impairments, some epidemiologic studies suggest that TBI also constitutes a risk factor for Alzheimer disease. Studies have shown that severe head trauma causes increased levels of insoluble amyloid with deposition into amyloid plaques, one of the hallmarks of Alzheimer disease. Several studies also suggest that moderate and severe head trauma in individuals with two ApoE4 alleles correlates with a marked increased risk of developing Alzheimer disease (see Chapter 7). Individuals with two ApoE4 alleles who survive moderate TBI may have double the risk of developing Alzheimer disease, and those surviving severe TBI may have four times the risk. (A confounding issue for some of these studies is that individuals with Alzheimer disease are prone to accidents in which they sustain TBI and come to medical attention.) Studies of veterans with a history of TBI revealed a 60% increase in the risk of developing dementia in comparison to veterans without a TBI history.

TBI-induced memory impairment, *posttraumatic amnesia*, is the most consistent neuropsychologic TBI-induced deficit. It includes memory loss for the trauma and immediately preceding events (*retrograde amnesia*); this period of amnestic time diminishes during recovery to the point where patients will frequently remember all preceding details except for the actual traumatic event. Amnesia of newly presented information (*anterograde amnesia*) is uncommon with mild TBI, but very common with moderate-to-severe TBI. Because this period of time represents information that has failed to encode in a patient's memory, this period of time is never recovered. Even compared to the depth or duration of coma, the duration of posttraumatic amnesia provides the most reliable predictor for overall neuropsychological outcome, including cognitive impairments.

Treatment Strategies for Posttraumatic Cognitive Impairment

Neurologists and other physicians who work with cognitively impaired TBI patients administer medications in hopes of increasing their attentiveness if not reversing their learning and memory impairments. Of the numerous medicines that purportedly help, few have undergone rigorous trials that have documented their value. For example, many trials have indicated that methylphenidate and other dopamine-enhancing medications increase patients' attention and, directly or indirectly, memory. Anticholinesterases may also improve TBI patients' memory; at least those who have suffered severe memory deficits (see Chapter 7). Treatment of comorbid PTSD, if present, may improve cognitive impairments and other posttraumatic neuropsychological changes. At the same time, physicians should, if possible, reduce or eliminate medicines that may interfere with attention and memory, such as AEDs, antipsychotics, and minor tranquilizers. They should always bear in mind that multiple medicines are likely to lead to adverse interactions and unwanted, occasionally fatal, outcomes.

Patients do well with cognitive, behavioral, physical, and occupational rehabilitation, i.e., nonpharmacologic treatment. Exposure therapy, for example, may provide greater benefit for PTSD than psychotropics. Multidisciplinary teams have a role in restoring patients' intellectual functioning and returning them to their place in the family and work. Classic strategies – physical, occupational, and speech therapy, identification and treatment of depression, anxiety, and insomnia, and social interactions with peers – enhance remaining functions, reduce impediments, and provide compensatory mechanisms for injured ones.

Other Mental Disturbances

Aggression

Many severe TBI patients, particularly those with frontal lobe damage, remain reticent, docile, and dependent. On the other hand, some patients tend toward either verbal or physical aggression.

Premorbid factors as well as the location of the injury and its other sequelae are risk factors for posttraumatic aggression. These include premorbid poor social functioning and, in some studies, substance abuse. Injury of the frontal lobes more than other brain regions is a risk factor. The most powerful risk factor is probably TBI-induced depression.

Although antidepressants usually have a therapeutic role, alone they may be insufficient. β-Blockers more reliably suppress aggressive behavior. AEDs, especially those with mood-stabilizing effects, such as valproate and carbamazepine, reportedly suppress violent outbursts.

Personality Changes

Frontal and temporal lobe damage may lead to personality changes in which patients develop an abrupt, suspicious, or argumentative manner. Because frontal lobe damage may impair inhibitory centers, the resulting lack of inhibition – *disinhibition* – allows unbridled aggressiveness, loquaciousness, impulsivity, and hyperactivity.

In addition to altering patients' personality and possibly cognitive capacity, frontal lobe injury may disable their executive abilities. Just as with patients who sustain anterior cerebral artery infarctions, those who sustain frontal lobe trauma have impaired ability to solve abstract problems, plan sequenced actions, or execute responses. Moreover, patients who develop pseudobulbar palsy, another complication of frontal lobe trauma, may display emotional incontinence with easily precipitated fits of *pathologic laughing* or *crying*, and unpredictable sudden switches between them (see Chapter 4).

Depression

Posttraumatic depression comprises an ill-defined combination of depressive symptoms. Developing in 25–50% of TBI patients, posttraumatic depression has a weak correlation with the severity of TBI. Several preinjury factors – substance abuse, depression, and poor social functioning – predispose TBI patients to posttraumatic depression. Several trauma-induced factors – cognitive impairments, PTE, and impaired physical, occupational, and social skills – further increase its incidence. Once present, posttraumatic depression predicts poor quality of life.

If depression complicates trauma, it interferes with patient rehabilitation and compliance. It also reduces patients' chances of making a complete recovery and is a risk factor for comorbid PTSD. Moreover, depression following TBI represents a risk factor for aggression.

Depressed TBI patients invariably require psychopharmacology. They may benefit from selective serotonin reuptake inhibitors (SSRIs), mood stabilizers, and anxiolytics. They also often need a full array of ancillary services, including physical and occupational therapy, financial assistance, and psychologic support.

Psychosis

Posttraumatic psychosis takes the form primarily of delusions, paranoia, and auditory hallucinations. Impairments in cognition, especially memory, and executive ability are frequent comorbidities of posttraumatic psychotic disorder.

Most cases of TBI-induced psychosis develop in males. There is a bimodal distribution of time to onset, either within the first 2 years after the trauma or after 5 years. Contrary to previously held beliefs, psychosis occurs equally as often in the aftermath of mild TBI as it does following moderate-to-severe TBI. Risk factors include a family history of psychosis and a long duration of unconsciousness. Overall, about 20% of severe TBI survivors develop psychosis.

Treatment usually entails not only typical or atypical antipsychotics, but also the addition of antidepressants or AEDs. As with depressed TBI patients, those with psychosis require extensive ancillary services.

Trauma in Childhood

Compared to TBI in adults, TBI in children has somewhat different features. For example, children are frequent victims of deliberately inflicted (nonaccidental) head injury. Also, children with attention deficit hyperactivity disorder (ADHD) or behavior disorder, compared to unaffected ones, are more likely to have engaged in dangerous activities and to have suffered non-accidental injuries. Similarly, children with learning disabilities, compared to those without such disabilities, are more apt to sustain sports-related TBI. Then, in a reciprocal relationship, TBI is likely to exacerbate learning disabilities.

The prognosis for children with TBI generally surpasses that for adults with comparable TBI. The severity and extent of brain damage in children largely determine their prognosis, but the GCS is not a suitable guide. Other prognostic factors include the family's socioeconomic status and psychiatric history.

As with adults, children's memory is particularly vulnerable to TBI and the duration of their posttraumatic amnesia correlates with their ultimate cognitive impairment and behavioral disturbances. In addition, TBI-induced social problems and behavioral disturbances handicap children as well as adults. Sometimes their residual injuries do not appear until they confront the academic and social demands of successive school years. In this case, as children "grow into their deficits," TBI may limit their cognitive and psychosocial development.

When TBI occurs before growth spurts, affected limbs may fail to achieve their normal expected size. The limbs' growth arrest resembles the limb foreshortening that accompanies spastic hemiparesis in congenital cerebral injuries (see Fig. 13.4). If dominant hemisphere injury were to occur before age 5 years, the opposite hemisphere would usually assume control of language. For example, a left-sided cerebral injury in a 4-year-old child will probably not result in aphasia because the plasticity of the brain allows the right cerebral hemisphere to develop language centers. If TBI affects the dominant hemisphere of someone age 5 years old or older, it is likely to cause language impairments, if not clear-cut aphasia.

In another potential scenario, TBI in children may damage the hypothalamic–pituitary axis. Resulting endocrine disturbances may lead to obesity, precocious puberty, or delayed puberty.

Nonaccidental Head Injury

Nonaccidental head injury (NAHI) and abusive head trauma are more legally acceptable terms meaning child abuse. An infant's brain, compared to one of an adult, is especially vulnerable to trauma because it has greater water content, much less myelin, and a covering of only the soft, thin skull. NAHI often leaves no external sign of trauma, such as face or scalp abrasions or burns. Rages of violent shaking or even direct blows typically injure only the brain, retinae, and internal organs.

The *shaken baby syndrome*, another form of abusive head trauma, consists of the injuries inflicted by violent back-and-forth throws, without direct impact. In this violent act, rotational (angular) deceleration produces diffuse axonal shearing, hemorrhages in the brain's delicate parenchyma and subdural space, and retinal hemorrhages (Fig. 22.3).

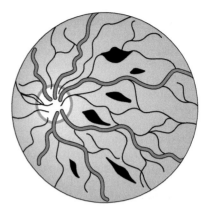

FIGURE 22.3 ■ Head trauma causes small hemorrhages throughout the retina – not just around the disk as in papilledema.

Although children may accidentally fall backward and injure their occiput, if they fall forward, they reflexively extend their arms to shield their face and eyes. Therefore facial, ocular, and anterior skull injuries more strongly suggest NAHI than occipital injuries. Spiral fractures of long bones and fractures of different ages, when accompanying head trauma, certainly suggest NAHI.

Physicians must perform a fundoscopic examination to find retinal hemorrhages. In the absence of external injuries, retinal hemorrhages may be the sole clinical indication that a child has sustained NAHI; however, they are not pathognomonic. For example, bleeding diatheses, spontaneous subarachnoid hemorrhages, arteriovenous malformations, and sepsis, as well as genuine accidental trauma, also cause retinal hemorrhages.

MRIs may detect and approximate the chronicity of intracranial bleeding. They can show hemorrhages in the subarachnoid, subdural, and epidural spaces and in the cerebrum and brainstem. Nevertheless, as in most acute head trauma, neurologists and neurosurgeons usually immediately obtain a head CT because, compared to MRI, hospitals can perform it rapidly with little or no sedation, and it shows the skull.

Children who survive NAHI often have residual cognitive impairment, behavioral difficulties, learning disabilities, developmental delay, and seizures. Sometimes neuropsychologic sequelae may not appear for several years. As discussed above, many NAHI survivors have either had ADHD before abuse or develop it afterwards.

Elder Abuse

Elder abuse, child abuse's geriatric counterpart, usually results from family members or other caregivers mistreating older individuals. Chronic neurologic and psychiatric disorders, particularly dementia, are risk factors. Physicians must be cautious: even without mistreatment, older individuals are prone to falls, fractures, and subdural hematomas.

MINOR HEAD TRAUMA

Neurologists usually define minor TBI, including *concussions*, as trauma-induced alteration in mental status with or without impairment of consciousness for less than 30 minutes and a GCS no lower than 13. If amnesia also occurs, it must last less than 24 hours. Although MVCs and occupational injuries frequently cause minor TBI, neurologic studies have concentrated on sports-induced TBIs because they are numerous, predictable, and, by studying pre-injury academic records, readily amenable to analysis.

Head Trauma in Sports

Sports-induced TBIs usually consist of concussions, the most common form of minor head trauma. When assessing injured athletes, neurologists classify concussions based on two factors: whether confusion lasts more or less than 15 minutes, and whether or not the athlete lost consciousness.

After a concussion, athletes' confusion usually consists of inattention, slowed responses to inquiries, disorientation, and impaired memory. They frequently report headache and nausea, and, on examination, have dysarthria, impairment of tandem gait, and loss of dexterity. However, neurologists do not require that the athlete have physical symptoms or signs to diagnose a concussion.

Sometimes the head trauma damages one or both trochlear (fourth) cranial nerves, causing diplopia (see Chapters 4 and 12). Head trauma may also damage the inner ear's vestibular system. This injury causes vertigo, which patients may describe as "dizziness." Patients' rapidly moving their head or changing position induces vertigo. Neurologic examination of the affected athlete may show nystagmus.

These physical deficits usually diminish by 1 week after the injury. Afterwards, mostly subjective problems comprise the postconcussion picture.

At 1 week, athletes with a headache, the most common postconcussion symptom, will usually still show impairments in memory and other neuropsychologic functions. Their other postconcussion symptoms may include irritability, mood changes, and sleep disturbances. Physicians assess injured athletes with various screening or computerized tests, but the Mini-Mental Status Examination (MMSE) (see Chapter 7) is not helpful.

During the time that postconcussion symptoms persist, which may extend for several months, neurologists routinely bar athletes from returning to play. For concussions that involve loss of consciousness, neurologists may bar athletes from playing for the entire season.

Studies justify such a stringent policy. They show that athletes who sustain a concussion are more apt than uninjured ones to have additional concussions. Even allowing for a full recovery from a concussion, subsequent concussions have a cumulative or multiplicative effect. Athletes cannot decide for themselves if they are ready to return to play. For a variety of reasons, athletes tend to underreport symptoms. Many are too young to have good judgment. They may deny injuries so that they remain eligible. The injury itself may not allow them to appreciate it.

Physicians and other supervisors must enforce a stringent policy mostly because athletes who have received a concussion are vulnerable to the *second impact syndrome*. In this condition, an additional blow, received within days of the original injury, leads to destructive and potentially fatal cerebral edema. It affects children and teenagers more frequently and more severely than adults, and leads to death in almost 50% of cases.

The intercollegiate sports with the greatest risk of concussion are ice hockey, football, and both men's and women's soccer. High school TBI risks are greatest for football, but also significant for wrestling, basketball, field hockey, and soccer. The risk in soccer probably relates to players' not wearing helmets despite their routine head-to-head collisions and heading the soccer ball.

Professional and amateur soccer players have subtle but undeniable impairments in memory, visual perception, and other cognitive functions. College football players develop neuropsychological impairments and exacerbation of preexisting learning disabilities. Professional football players who sustain concussions are 1.5 to 3 times more likely to develop depression than their teammates who do not have head injuries. Results of brain imaging and neuropsychiatric testing in retired players are similar to the results in TBI patients. There is growing evidence that even with repeated subconcussive injuries, permanent changes can occur in the brain (see *chronic traumatic encephalopathy*, below).

The American Academy of Neurology, which released a Position Statement on Sports Concussion in 2013, recommends immediate removal of an athlete who has sustained a concussion until all symptoms have abated and a licensed health-care professional has performed an evaluation.

Patients, parents, and psychiatrists should weigh the risks of TBI in contact sports against those in equally vigorous noncontact sports. At the least, parents and psychiatrists should steer children with learning disabilities and other academic impediments away from the risk of TBI.

Chronic Traumatic Encephalopathy

Boxers (pugilists) receive blows to the head that frequently leave them dazed. Repeated episodes of such TBI lead to cognitive impairment, often reaching the severity of dementia, and Parkinson disease-like physical deficits (see Chapter 18). Overall, depending on the length of their career, boxers have approximately a 20% risk of dementia. Dementia pugilistica falls under the larger umbrella category of *chronic traumatic encephalopathy* (*CTE*), which encompasses all progressive neurodegenerative conditions related to repeated TBI. Autopsies of deceased football players show excess cerebral tau protein and plaques and tangles – a pattern similar to that present in brains of Alzheimer disease patients. The mortality of professional football players in the National Football League from neurodegenerative disease is three times higher than the general US population. Before their death, these players develop a constellation of symptoms, consisting of memory loss, depression, aggressive behavior, and executive dysfunction.

Postconcussion Syndrome

The most common sequelae of minor head trauma comprise an admixture of symptoms that neurologists place into a catch-all term, *postconcussion syndrome*. This disorder probably falls under the rubric of the DSM-5 term, Neurocognitive Disorder Due to Traumatic Brain Injury. Lacking a strict definition, neurologists base a diagnosis of postconcussion syndrome on one or more core symptoms – headache, memory impairment, and insomnia – lasting more than 2 to 3 months. These and other symptoms of postconcussion syndrome remain entirely subjective and often nonspecific, variable, and occasionally unending.

Neurologists find that postconcussion syndrome patients have a normal physical and neurologic examination, CT, and MRI. Although the EEG often shows minor abnormalities, the changes are generally inconsistent, insignificant, and often attributable to medications. Similarly, neuropsychological tests often reveal minor and uneven abnormalities, and those changes may be attributable to inattention, depression, exaggeration, lack of education, or even malingering.

Proposed etiologies of the postconcussion syndrome include diffuse axonal shearing, excitatory neurotransmitter imbalance, and subtle cerebral contusions. In addition, any coexistent whiplash injury (see later) may cause head and neck pain. No matter which postconcussion symptoms predominate, they distract patients, interfere with their sleep, and require them to take medicines that may impair their mood and cognition.

Although neurologists routinely diagnose and treat patients with the postconcussion syndrome, individual patients regularly provoke skepticism. Prolonged symptoms are associated with psychiatric and socioeconomic factors as much as with neurologic injury. They do not correlate with either the estimated force of impact or the usual neurologic parameters of TBI – i.e., GCS scores and duration of amnesia. Among compensation claimants undergoing neuropsychological tests, their effort or socioeconomic status often has more of an effect than the severity of the TBI on their scores. For example, assembly-line workers dissatisfied with their workplace typically fare poorly after head trauma; however, children, soldiers, self-employed workers, and professionals rarely report prolonged or incapacitating symptoms. Finally, treatment that is usually effective for headache and insomnia generally fails to alleviate these symptoms in posttraumatic patients.

The postconcussion syndrome may last inordinately long. Patients with premorbid intellectual and personality abnormalities tend to have permanent symptoms. For some patients, symptoms seem inextricably linked to litigation and other unsettled issues.

On the other hand, some reports indicate that the postconcussion syndrome results predominantly from neurologic injury. Support for this position is the finding that postconcussion symptoms are similar from patient to patient. In addition, the syndrome strikes many self-employed and highly motivated people, including physicians. In addition, according to some data, symptoms correlate poorly with outstanding litigation and persist after legal claims are settled.

Many children and some adults may not report postconcussion symptoms because they are unable to describe them, have a stoic disposition, or substitute other symptoms. For example, rather than complaining of posttraumatic headaches, children may have somnolence, inattention, or hyperactivity. Professionals unable to describe their feelings may develop unusual irritability.

Headache

The signature of postconcussion syndrome is a dull, generalized, endless headache. Movement, bending, work, and alcohol use usually worsen it. In 50% of patients, postconcussion headache lasts longer than 1 year, and in 25%, longer than 3 years. Surprisingly, postconcussion headache occurs more frequently in mildly injured individuals than in moderately or severely injured individuals. One consideration in patients with continuous postconcussion headache is that the trauma may have exacerbated preexisting migraine. Another is that use of analgesics, prescribed for any aspect of the injury, for as few as 15 days each month for 3 months has created chronic daily headache (see Chapter 9).

Memory Impairment

Patients with postconcussion syndrome characteristically describe mild amnesia accompanied by inattention or easy distractibility, slowed information processing, and difficulty completing complex mental tasks. As with other postconcussion symptoms, the amnesia shows little correlation with the severity of trauma.

One potential explanation for amnesia in postconcussion syndrome is that the trauma may have propelled the anterior poles of the frontal and temporal lobes against the rough, bony inner surfaces and edges of the anterior and middle cranial fossae. Comorbid PTSD, depression, anxiety, treatment with opioids and other medications, and substance abuse might also contribute to postconcussion amnesia.

Insomnia

Postconcussion syndrome patients regularly report inability to fall or remain asleep. They also describe excessive daytime sleepiness (EDS), but neither nighttime sleep nor daytime naps restore their full normal wakefulness. For patients with postconcussion insomnia, comorbid physical and psychiatric conditions – pain, anxiety, depression, and PTSD – sometimes exacerbate if not cause the insomnia. Also, patients' tendency to consume excessive caffeine, alcohol, opioids, and other medications makes the problem worse.

On the other hand, whatever the cause, physicians might consider that a pre-existing sleep disorder actually led to the TBI. For example, patients with sleep apnea, narcolepsy, or sleep deprivation might have EDS that contributes to causing an MVC (see Chapter 17).

Other Symptoms

Postconcussion syndrome patients often report that they have "dizziness." In most cases, their symptom is not authentic vertigo, but a nonspecific subjective experience with variable, idiosyncratic meanings that substitutes for lightheadedness, anxiety, unsteadiness, or lassitude. Except for patients who have vertigo because they sustained labyrinth damage, posttraumatic dizziness remains difficult to define and almost impossible to treat.

Patients also commonly have exquisite sensitivity to light (photophobia) and sound (phonophobia). They cannot tolerate even everyday levels of sunlight, street noise, or workplace activity. The hypersensitivity intensifies patients' headaches, distracts them from work-related tasks, and pushes them into seclusion.

In addition, patients often describe symptoms of depression, anxiety, irritability, and moodiness, but perhaps not in a few words. They also frequently report that their injuries reduce their desire for sex and other previously enjoyable activities.

In contrast, some patients with the postconcussion syndrome may minimize their symptoms. Whether stoic or in denial, they fail to acknowledge memory impairments, other cognitive deficits, personality changes, or physical impediments. Using poor judgment, they may resume their work at demanding jobs.

Mild TBI has a complex relationship with PTSD. For one thing, the incidence of PTSD is similar among individuals who have sustained mild TBI and those who have not. Also, the most powerful risk factor for PTSD is not TBI, but pre-TBI affective or anxiety disorder.

Treatment and Recovery

Almost all patients improve to a greater or lesser extent. About 85% fully recover and none deteriorate. Although recovery from postconcussion symptoms often follows a nonlinear and uncertain course, it should take place by 3 months in uncomplicated cases.

Neurologists attempt to educate and reassure the patient and family about the nature, extent, and course of postconcussion syndrome. Many urge patients with minor or vague symptoms to attempt to return to work with a reduced load, but patients with demanding or dangerous jobs to take a medical leave. With symptoms refractory to treatment and the passage of time, neurologists often find it fruitless to dissuade patients' and families' beliefs that the symptoms are the result of the TBI; instead, they focus on ameliorating the symptoms.

Perhaps more than in other syndromes, the symptoms of postconcussive syndrome seem to present in an inextricable group. No single medicine or other treatment relieves all elements of the syndrome. Moreover, many medicines directed at one symptom, such as analgesics, may exacerbate another symptom, such as sleepiness. One strategy is to work with the patient to identify the most troublesome symptom and target it for treatment with specific medicines.

For headaches, neurologists often prescribe mild, nonaddicting analgesics similar to those used for tension-type headaches. They typically prescribe nonsteroidal anti-inflammatory drugs (NSAIDs) and tricyclic antidepressants. These medications may alleviate insomnia and neck pain as well as headaches. Even when only a minimal migraine component exists or the patient has a history of migraine, antimigraine medicines may help (see Chapter 9).

Physicians must cautiously treat insomnia. They should avoid prescribing hypnotics because they easily lead to EDS, mimic symptoms of TBI, or worsen depression and cognitive impairment. They may prescribe modafinil to counteract excessive daytime sleepiness, but it will not alleviate fatigue. Whatever medicines physicians prescribe, they should prohibit alcohol because it may induce disturbances in personality, behavior, sleep, and judgment. Nonpharmacologic strategies, which have some advocates, include relaxation training, cognitive behavioral therapy, and instituting basic memory devices, such as checklists.

Some patients have symptoms that persist or, in a small proportion of cases, incapacitate the patient. Risk factors for incomplete recovery from postconcussion syndrome include the following:

- The patient has a history of attention deficit disorder, learning disability, or neurosis.
- Before the accident, the patient was in a low socioeconomic status, an unskilled or semiskilled worker, dissatisfied with the job, or in danger of being fired.
- An MVC caused the concussion.
- The symptoms are multiple and include bodily pains.
- Comorbidities – psychiatric conditions, medications especially polypharmacy, substance abuse, and PTSD – impair diagnosis and treatment.

WHIPLASH

Mechanism of Action

The common MVC is the rear-end collision. In these MVCs, the sudden impact snaps the driver's and passengers' head and neck backwards and then forwards. It causes a *flexion–extension* neck injury (*whiplash*) (Fig. 22.4) because it wrenches the neck's soft tissues, including ligaments, tendons, and the trapezius, paraspinal, and numerous small delicate muscles.

Whiplash may also aggravate degenerative spine disease and herniate cervical intervertebral disks (see Chapter 5). A severe rear-end MVC may fracture or dislocate cervical vertebrae, which can even transect the spinal cord.

MVC victims wearing their seatbelt should not sustain concomitant direct head trauma. However, because whiplash often jostles the brain within the skull, some MVC patients develop postconcussion syndrome as well as a whiplash.

Symptoms

As in the postconcussion syndrome, the development, severity, and duration of whiplash symptoms do not correlate with the MVC's forcefulness, as calculated from its speed. The primary symptom of whiplash is neck pain. It typically radiates upward towards the head and downward to the shoulders, arms, and lower back. With

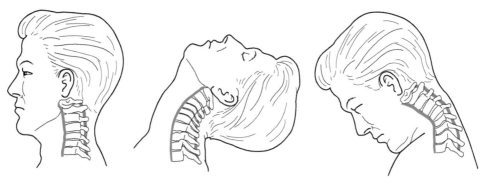

FIGURE 22.4 ■ Cervical flexion–extension injuries, popularly called "whiplash," may tear the anterior and posterior longitudinal ligaments (*red*) and other soft tissues, herniate intervertebral disks, and exacerbate cervical spondylosis (see Chapter 5).

simultaneous head trauma and whiplash, the symptoms of each exacerbate those of the other.

Even without head trauma, whiplash patients often report suffering from cognitive impairments, mood changes, inattention, and dizziness. (Despite the large number of individuals who sustain whiplash injury and the regularity of their cognitive and mood symptoms, the DSM-5 does not explicitly define this disorder. Psychiatrists might consider it as a variety of Neurocognitive Disorder Due to Traumatic Brain Injury.) When trauma results in herniation of cervical intervertebral disks, patients typically have radicular pain (pain that radiates into the dermatomes of the affected nerve roots), weakness, and loss of deep tendon reflexes in their arms. MRI can detect herniated disks as well as fractures and vertebral dislocations. Electromyography (EMG) may establish the presence of a nerve root injury. However, numerous other techniques which have crept into practice, including thermography, surface EMG, and ultrasound, lack diagnostic reliability.

Approximately 50% of whiplash patients recover by 3 months and 75% by 6 months, which is approximately the course of postconcussive symptoms. Still, 20% have symptoms for 2 years or longer. Risk factors for prolonged disability include middle age, preexisting degenerative spine disease, persistent headache, and psychiatric comorbidity, particularly anxiety, depression, and PTSD. In addition, compensation and other forms of litigation, looking at the population at large, constitute one of the most powerful risk factors in the United States. As an example of the effects of litigation, after Saskatchewan, Canada converted its tort-compensation system to a no-fault plan, its citizens enjoyed a markedly reduced incidence of whiplash and, when it developed, a better prognosis.

Treatment

Treatment of whiplash remains largely empiric and variable. In fact, patients may improve with little or no treatment. Many respond to reassurance, rest, at-home exercise, or simple physical measures, such as massage and heat. Patients should avoid vigorous cervical manipulation, such as that which occurs as part of chiropractic treatment, because it may lead to spinal cord injury or vertebral artery dissection. Although protecting the head and neck from further abrupt movement is obviously reasonable, the purported benefits of a restraining soft cervical collar remain controversial. Medications for whiplash include muscle relaxants, NSAIDs, nonopioid analgesics, and – for their analgesic and sedative, as well as their mood-elevating, effects – antidepressants. Migraine medications, according to some reports, may help.

REFERENCES

Amen, D., Newberg, A., Thatcher, R., et al. (2011). Impact of playing American professional football on long-term brain function. *The Journal of Neuropsychiatry and Clinical Neurosciences, 23*, 98–106.

Barnes, D. E., Kaup, A., Kirby, K. A., et al. (2014). Traumatic brain injury and risk of dementia in older veterans. *Neurol, 83*, 312–319.

Bombardier, C. H., Fann, J. R., Temkin, N. R., et al. (2010). Rates of major depressive disorder and clinical outcomes following traumatic brain injury. *JAMA: The Journal of the American Medical Association, 303*, 1938–1945.

Cassidy, J. D., Carroll, L. J., Côté, P., et al. (2000). Effect of eliminating compensation for pain and suffering on the outcome of insurance claims for whiplash injury. *The New England Journal of Medicine, 342*, 1179–1186.

Faul, M., Xu, L., Wald, M. M., et al.: Traumatic Brain Injury in the United States: Emergency Department Visits, Hospitalizations, and Deaths 2002–2006. US Department of Health and Human Services Centers for Disease Control and Prevention 2010.

Fleminger, S., Oliver, D. L., Lovestone, S., et al. (2003). Head injury as a risk factor for Alzheimer's disease. *Journal of Neurology, Neurosurgery, and Psychiatry, 74*, 857–862.

Fujii, D., & Fujii, D. C. (2012). Psychotic disorder due to traumatic brain injury: analysis of case studies in the literature. *The Journal of Neuropsychiatry and Clinical Neurosciences, 24*, 278–289.

Giza, C. G., Kutcher, J. S., Ashwal, S., et al. (2013). Summary of evidence-based guideline update: evaluation and management of concussion in sports (Report of the Guideline Development Subcommittee of the American Academy of Neurology). *Neurology, 80*, 2250–2257.

Green, P., Rohling, M. L., Lees-Haley, P. R., et al. (2001). Effort has a greater effect on test scores than severe brain injury in compensation claimants. *Brain Injury, 15*, 1045–1060.

Hoge, C. W., McGurk, D., Thomas, J. L., et al. (2008). Mild traumatic brain injury in U.S. soldiers returning from Iraq. *The New England Journal of Medicine, 358*, 453–463.

Koponen, S., Taiminen, T., Kairisto, V., et al. (2004). APO-e4 predicts dementia but not other psychiatric disorders after traumatic brain injury. *Neurology, 63*, 749–750.

Lachs, M. S., & Pillemer, K. A. (2015). Elder abuse. *The New England Journal of Medicine, 373*, 1947–1956.

Lehman, E. J., Hein, M. J., Baron, S. L., et al. (2012). Neurodegenerative causes of death among retired National Football League players. *Neurology, 79*, 1970–1974.

Levin, H., Wilde, E., Troyanskaya, M., et al. (2010). Diffusion tensor imaging of mild to moderate blast-related traumatic brain injury and its sequelae. *Journal of Neurotrauma, 27*, 683–694.

McCrea, M., Guskiewicz, K. M., Marshall, S. W., et al. (2003). Acute effects and recovery time following concussion in collegiate football players: The NCAA Concussion Study. *JAMA: The Journal of the American Medical Association, 290,* 2556–2563.

McKee, A. C., Thor, S. T., Kierman, P. T., et al. (2015). The neuropathology of chronic traumatic encephalopathy. *Brain Path, 25*(3), 350–364.

Mears, S., Shores, E. A., Taylor, A. J., et al. (2008). Mild traumatic brain injury does not predict acute postconcussion syndrome. *J Neurol Neurol Psychiatry, 79,* 300–306.

Mechtler, L. L., Kalyan, S. K., & Crutchfield, K. E. (2014). Advanced neuroimaging of mild traumatic brain injury. *Neurologic Clinics, 32,* 31–58.

Montenigro, P. H., Bernick, C., & Cantu, R. C. (2015). Clinical features of repetitive traumatic brain injury and chronic traumatic encephalopathy. *Brain Path, 25*(3), 304–317.

Rao, V. R., & Parko, K. L. (2015). Clinical approach to post-traumatic epilepsy. *Seminars in Neurology, 35,* 57–63.

Rao, V., Rosenberg, P., Bertrand, M., et al. (2009). Aggression after traumatic brain injury: Prevalence and correlates. *The Journal of Neuropsychiatry and Clinical Neurosciences, 21,* 420–429.

Rohling, M. L., Allen, L. M., & Green, P. (2002). Who is exaggerating cognitive impairment and who is not? *CNS Spectrums, 7,* 387–395.

Salinsky, M., Storzbach, D., Goy, E., et al. (2015). Traumatic brain injury and psychogenic seizures in veterans. *The Journal of Head Trauma Rehabilitation, 30,* E65–E70.

Schmans, B., Lindboom, J., Schagen, S., et al. (1998). Cognitive complaints in patients after whiplash injury: The impact of malingering. *Journal of Neurology, Neurosurgery, and Psychiatry, 64,* 339–343.

Siddall, O. M. (2005). Use of methylphenidate in traumatic brain injury. *The Annals of Pharmacotherapy, 39,* 1309–1313.

Silver, J. M., McAllister, R. W., & Yudofsky, S. C. (2011). *Textbook of Traumatic Brain Injury* (2nd ed.). Washington DC: American Psychiatric Publishing.

Stocchetti, N., & Mass, A. I. R. (2014). Traumatic intracranial hypertension. *The New England Journal of Medicine, 370*(22), 2121–2130.

Stulemeijer, M., Vos, P. E., Bleijenberg, G., et al. (2007). Cognitive complaints after mild traumatic brain injury: Things are not always what they seem. *J Psychosomatic Res, 63,* 637–645.

Tateno, A., Jorge, R. E., & Robinson, R. G. (2004). Pathologic laughing and crying following traumatic brain injury. *The Journal of Neuropsychiatry and Clinical Neurosciences, 16,* 426–434.

Warden, D. L., Gordon, B., & McAllister, T. W. (2006). Neurobehavioral guidelines for the pharmacologic treatment of neurobehavioral sequelae of traumatic brain injury. *Journal of Neurotrauma, 23,* 1468–1501.

Wenzel, H. G., Haug, T. T., Mykletun, A., et al. (2002). A population study of anxiety and depression among persons who report whiplash traumas. *J Psychsom Res, 53,* 831–835.

Writer, B. W., & Schillerstrom, J. E. (2009). Psychopharmacological treatment for cognitive impairment in survivors of traumatic brain injury: A critical review. *The Journal of Neuropsychiatry and Clinical Neurosciences, 21,* 362–370.

QUESTIONS AND ANSWERS

1. Physicians use the Glasgow Coma Scale (GCS) to assess three manifestations of a patient's level of consciousness following TBI. Which of the following functions is *not* assessed by the GCS?
   a. Vital signs
   b. Eye opening
   c. Speaking (best verbal response)
   d. Moving (best motor response)

Answer: a. Vital signs, except for respirations, vary independently of the level of consciousness. Physicians using the GCS rate three functions that reflect responsiveness and score patients on a scale of 3 to 15.

2. At the scene of a high-speed, single-vehicle, motor vehicle crash (MVC), emergency workers found a stuporous 24-year-old man and judged him to have a GCS score of 9. They dressed his head and bodily wounds and supported his circulation. During transfer to the hospital, he lapsed into coma and developed decerebrate posture and a left third cranial nerve palsy. On arrival, his GCS had fallen to 3. X-rays showed a fracture through his left temporal bone of the skull. Which is the most likely cause of his deterioration?
   a. Subdural hematoma
   b. Alcohol intoxication
   c. Middle meningeal artery laceration
   d. Subarachnoid hemorrhage

Answer: c. The temporal skull fracture probably lacerated the middle meningeal artery and led to an epidural hematoma. His GCS score of 3 predicts a fatal outcome. In another aspect of this case, a high-speed single-driver single-vehicle MVC may represent a suicide.

3. Which statement is *false* regarding chronic subdural hematomas?
   a. On computed tomography (CT), they frequently appear as extra-axial, long, curved, radiodense (white) mass lesions.
   b. They are a correctable cause of dementia.
   c. They cause few lateralized deficits, such as hemiparesis, compared to nonspecific generalized symptoms, such as headaches and personality changes.
   d. The elderly are prone to subdural hematomas because they have cerebral atrophy and a tendency to fall.
   e. Many chronic subdural hematomas are reabsorbed without the need for surgery.

Answer: a. *Acute* subdural hematomas, which contain fresh blood, are radiodense (white). Chronic ones, where the blood cells have lysed, are radiolucent (black). At some time between their acute and chronic stages, they may reach the same density (isodense) as the brain and become indistinguishable from it. Like other mass lesions, subdurals may compress the adjacent ventricles and shift midline structures to the opposite side (See Fig. 20.9).

4. Which condition is most likely to follow TBI causing a GCS score of 7?
   a. Anterograde amnesia
   b. Postconcussion syndrome
   c. Retrograde amnesia
   d. Seizures

Answer: a. The most common sequela of moderately severe TBI consists of a period of anterograde amnesia. TBI less often and less severely produces fixed retrograde amnesia. Seizures, postconcussion syndrome, and neck pain are also associated, but less closely.

5. To which injury does the term *contrecoup* most appropriately apply?
   a. Injury of the temporal lobe, especially its anterior surface, after an occipital blow
   b. Blindness after an occipital lobe blow
   c. Diffuse axonal shearing after localized head trauma
   d. Injury of the occipital lobe after an occipital blow

Answer: a. Head trauma that damages the opposite side of the brain is a *contrecoup* injury. These injuries can be envisioned as resulting from the brain's "bouncing against the other side of the skull." The surface of the brain – its cortex – bears the brunt. Brain damage is most pronounced where the brain strikes the rough or sharpened inner surfaces of the skull, such as in the anterior fossa, which cradles the anterior-inferior frontal lobes and the middle fossa, which cradles the anterior temporal lobes.

6. Neurosurgeons frequently cannot remove all shrapnel and other fragments from penetrating head wounds. Which *two* are consequences of retained foreign bodies?
   a. They may act as a scar focus for posttraumatic epilepsy (PTE).
   b. They envelop themselves with calcium and remain as benign scars.
   c. They may act as a nidus for a brain abscess.

d. They can dislodge and enter the general circulation.

Answer: a, c. Foreign bodies may be so numerous or situated in inoperable areas that neurosurgeons cannot remove all of them. Each retained foreign body may act as a nidus for an abscess or a scar focus for PTE.

7. Which injury suggests the shaken baby syndrome (abusive head trauma) in infants and young children?
   a. Periventricular intracranial calcifications
   b. Retinal hemorrhages
   c. Tram track calcifications
   d. Dislocated optic lens

Answer: b. Violent shaking of infants and young children causes nonaccidental head injury (NAHI), a common form of child abuse. Shaken babies or those who have sustained abusive head trauma often develop raised intracranial pressure and intracranial bleeding; however, the only visible sign on clinical evaluation may be retinal hemorrhages, which require fundoscopic examination for detection. Periventricular intracranial calcifications are a sign of in utero infection with cytomegalovirus. Scattered intracranial calcifications are a sign of in utero infection with toxoplasmosis. Calcifications in layers of the cerebral cortex, tram track calcifications, are a manifestation of Sturge–Weber syndrome. Homocystinuria may lead to lens dislocation.

8. Which cognitive function is most susceptible to head trauma?
   a. Judgment
   b. Language function
   c. Memory
   d. Constructional ability

Answer: c. Head trauma typically causes amnesia. Causes of isolated, acutely occurring amnesia include various substances (scopolamine, GHB, alcohol), seizures with altered awareness, and transient global amnesia, as well as head trauma.

9. Of the following varieties of seizure, which is the most common sequela of TBI?
   a. Psychogenic
   b. Partial with secondary generalization
   c. Absence
   d. Primary generalized

Answer: b. Posttraumatic epilepsy (PTE) is common. TBI typically causes partial (focal) seizures, especially complex partial seizures, which undergo secondary generalization. TBI does not cause primary generalized seizures, e.g., absence (petit mal) or tonic-clonic seizures without initial focal onset.

10. After falling forward and striking his head, a 72-year-old gentleman describes being unable to read because he sees double. To alleviate the problem, he covers one eye, avoids looking at closely held objects, or tilts his head to the left. The visual acuity in each eye is normal. Which is the most likely site of injury?
    a. Medial longitudinal fasciculus
    b. Left trochlear nerve
    c. Right trochlear nerve
    d. Left abducens nerve

Answer: c. Head trauma may damage one or both trochlear (fourth) cranial nerves. Each trochlear nerve supplies the ipsilateral superior oblique muscle. Affected individuals cannot intort the eye when it is adducted. Thus, they have diplopia when looking at a closely held object, such as a newspaper. With unilateral nerve damage, tilting the head away from the injured side reduces the diplopia.

11. Of the following, which is the most reliable indicator of TBI sequelae?
    a. GCS score at first evaluation
    b. Duration of retrograde amnesia
    c. Duration of anterograde amnesia
    d. Blood alcohol level

Answer: b. The duration of retrograde amnesia, which includes the duration of any coma, correlates with the functional and neuropsychologic outcome. It provides a more reliable prognosis than either the first GCS or duration of coma.

12. Which of the following is *not* a characteristic of TBI-induced psychosis?
    a. Moderate-to-severe TBI
    b. Family history of psychosis
    c. Long duration of unconsciousness
    d. Usually appears 5 years after TBI
    e. Delusion, paranoia, and auditory hallucinations

Answer: d. When it complicates head trauma, TBI-induced psychosis usually appears within 2 years. The other features commonly occur.

13. Which *three* of the following are typically located in the subarachnoid space?
    a. Cerebrospinal fluid (CSF)
    b. Lymph
    c. Purulent CSF in cases of meningitis
    d. Epidural hematomas in cases of major head trauma
    e. Blood from ruptured berry aneurysms
    f. Aqueous humor

Answer: a, c, e. The subarachnoid space, which is situated between the arachnoid and the pia layers of the meninges, normally contains crystal-clear CSF. However, the CSF becomes purulent in bacterial meningitis, bloody with subarachnoid hemorrhage from ruptured berry aneurysms or trauma, and filled with mononuclear cells in viral meningitis. The subarachnoid space surrounds the brain and extends down into the lumbar sac. To sample the CSF, neurologists insert LP needles into the lumbar subarachnoid space. Epidural hematomas are located outside of the thick dura matter; however, severe

TBI may cause both subarachnoid and intraparenchymal bleeding. The brain has no lymphatic system. Aqueous humor is confined to the eye.

14. Regarding posttraumatic cognitive impairment, which of these statements is *false*?
    a. Cognitive recovery is slower and less complete in patients older than 65 years compared to younger patients.
    b. Recovery of motor and language skills usually reaches a maximum within 6 months after the injury.
    c. Cognitive recovery, to the extent that it occurs, takes place sooner than motor recovery.
    d. Cognitive impairment correlates with low GCS scores.

Answer: c. Maximum motor recovery usually is completed during the first 6 months after trauma, but cognitive recovery does not reach its maximum until 18 months. Cognitive recovery may be further delayed in individuals older than 65 years.

15. Regarding posttraumatic cognitive impairment, which statement is *false*?
    a. The severity of cognitive impairment correlates with the lesion's size.
    b. The severity of cognitive impairment correlates with the lesion's location.
    c. Use of alcohol may add to posttraumatic cognitive impairment.
    d. Use of antiepileptic drugs may add to posttraumatic cognitive impairment.

Answer: b. With few exceptions, the traumatic lesion's location does not correlate with the presence or severity of cognitive impairment. Left temporal lesions, an exception, often produce aphasia.

16. Of the following statements, which one best describes postconcussive headaches?
    a. Their severity is proportional to the duration of unconsciousness.
    b. Their severity is proportional to the severity of the head trauma.
    c. Of common postconcussive symptoms, headaches are most closely associated with memory and concentration impairment.
    d. They are a risk factor for PTE.

Answer: c. Postconcussive headaches are most closely associated with memory and concentration impairment. However, as with the other postconcussive symptoms, they show little correlation with the duration of unconsciousness or severity of trauma. Concussions, in contrast to penetrating TBI, carry a negligible risk for posttraumatic epilepsy. In other words, the prevalence of PTE increases with the severity of TBI.

17. Regarding nonaccidental head injury (NAHI) or abusive head trauma, which of the following statements is *false*?
    a. Survivors have an increased incidence of developmental delay and learning disabilities.
    b. Survivors have an increased incidence of epilepsy.
    c. Neuropsychologic sequelae are always detectable during the period of abuse.
    d. Many survivors have preexisting attention deficit hyperactivity disorder (ADHD).
    e. Many survivors develop posttraumatic ADHD.

Answer: c. Neuropsychologic sequelae may not appear for several years.

18. Which of the following statements best describes diffuse axonal shearing?
    a. Head magnetic resonance imaging (MRI), but not CT, can readily detect diffuse axonal shearing.
    b. It predominantly affects long subcortical white matter axons.
    c. It explains posttraumatic headache.
    d. The EEG can reliably diagnose diffuse axonal shearing.
    e. It predominantly affects long cortical gray matter neurons.

Answer: b. Diffuse axonal shearing, which predominantly affects long subcortical white matter axons, is a pathologic diagnosis that includes much more than shearing of long axons. It includes damage to cytoskeletal structures and causes an intracellular influx of calcium. Although MRI may show petechiae, they are not a diagnostic finding. Similarly, EEG, and neuropsychologic testing cannot reliably diagnose diffuse axonal shearing. Of note, diffusion tensor imaging may show areas of white tract abnormality. Only an autopsy can confirm the diagnosis.

19. Which is the order of the layers of the meningeal mater, from innermost to outermost?
    a. Arachnoid, pia, dura
    b. Dura, pia, arachnoid
    c. Pia, arachnoid, dura
    d. Pia, dura, arachnoid

Answer: c. The mnemonic is PAD.

20. Of the following statements, which one most accurately describes posttraumatic depression?
    a. It develops in almost all patients who have had a GCS score of 3 to 7.
    b. Preexisting drug and alcohol abuse, depression, and poor social functioning are risk factors for posttraumatic depression.
    c. It closely correlates with the severity of the head trauma.
    d. Although posttraumatic depression affects mood, it does not impede recovery of function.

Answer: b. Posttraumatic depression develops in about 25% of TBI patients, but its occurrence correlates weakly with the severity of the head trauma and the GCS score. Risk factors include the usual ones for depression: drug and alcohol abuse, previous depression, and poor social functioning. Risk factors also include TBI-induced ones: cognitive impairment, PTE, physical deficits, occupational incapacity, and loss of social skills. TBI-related depression interferes with patients' rehabilitation, compliance, and socialization. It also reduces patients' likelihood of making a recovery.

21. Which histologic change characterizes TBI?
    a. Vacuoles in the cerebral cortex
    b. Infiltration of mononuclear cells and other inflammatory changes
    c. Degenerating neurons without a monocular infiltrate
    d. Loss of myelin in the periventricular region

Answer: b. Inflammatory changes are associated with TBI and strokes. In both, neurons die by necrosis. Vacuoles characterize spongiform changes, the hallmark of prion infections, such as Creutzfeldt–Jakob disease. Dying neurons without a mononuclear infiltrate signify apoptosis, which occurs in amyotrophic lateral sclerosis and other neurodegenerative conditions. Demyelination, especially in the periventricular region, characterizes multiple sclerosis.

22. Of the following complications of TBI, which is the *least* frequent?
    a. Depression
    b. Substance abuse
    c. Personality disorders
    d. Psychosis

Answer: c. As TBI sequelae, personality changes are common, but personality disorders are rare. Also, post-traumatic depression and substance abuse are common, while psychosis is uncommon.

23. Regarding TBI, what is the *second impact syndrome*?
    a. Contrecoup injuries causing greater damage than coup injuries
    b. Frontal head injuries causing cervical spine injuries that may sever the spinal cord
    c. A second head injury occurring several days to several weeks after a concussion, causing catastrophic brain swelling
    d. Head trauma causing intracerebral and subarachnoid hemorrhage

Answer: c. Although all of these combinations occur, the second impact refers to a subsequent head injury, occurring several days to several weeks after a concussion. Occasionally it causes catastrophic, potentially fatal brain swelling – the *second impact syndrome*. Even though this syndrome rarely occurs, its effects are so devastating that neurologists and other physicians forbid athletes from returning to play for weeks to months following a concussion.

24. Which of the following does Battle's sign indicate?
    a. Subarachnoid hemorrhage
    b. Basilar skull fracture
    c. Increased intracranial pressure
    d. Shaken baby syndrome

Answer: b. Battle's sign, ecchymosis over the mastoid, indicates a skull fracture, usually involving the temporal

bone. Physicians named this finding after the 19th century surgeon, William Henry Battle.

25. Which of the following do periorbital ecchymoses indicate?
    a. Subarachnoid hemorrhage
    b. Basilar skull fracture
    c. Increased intracranial pressure
    d. Shaken baby syndrome

Answer: b. Periorbital ecchymoses (raccoon eyes), like Battle's sign, usually indicate a basilar skull fracture. However, traumatic or surgical nasal bone fractures and scalp lacerations can also produce the same picture.

26. Of the following, which is the most common sequela of TBI?
    a. Personality disorder
    b. Personality changes
    c. Depression
    d. Anxiety disorder

Answer: b.

27. Which was the most common TBI in the Iraq war?
    a. Penetrating injury
    b. Blast injury
    c. Thermal exposure
    d. Toxicity

Answer: b.

28. Which statement most accurately compares the risk of developing Alzheimer disease among TBI survivors carrying two ApoE4 alleles compared to those carrying none?
    a. Carrying two ApoE4 alleles does not affect the risk of developing Alzheimer disease.
    b. Carrying two ApoE4 alleles increases the risk of developing Alzheimer disease following only severe TBI.
    c. Carrying two ApoE4 alleles increases the risk of developing Alzheimer disease following moderate as well as severe, but not mild, TBI.
    d. Among TBI survivors, carrying two ApoE4 alleles increases the risk of developing Alzheimer disease equally among all severities of TBI.

Answer: c. Compared to TBI survivors carrying no ApoE4 alleles, survivors of moderate TBI carrying two ApoE4 alleles have a more than two-fold increased risk of developing Alzheimer disease and survivors of severe TBI carrying two ApoE4 alleles have a more than four-fold increased risk; however, survivors of mild TBI have no increased risk.

29. After the emergency room staff evaluated a 77-year-old widow who had sustained a fall but did not fracture any bones, she refused to return home to her family. Her objections were unclear, but they were so vocal and adamant that the staff solicited a psychiatry consultation. The psychiatrist found that during the previous 3 months, the ER staff had

evaluated her on different occasions for diabetic ketoacidosis, hypoglycemia, a wrist fracture, and rib fractures. For which condition should the staff evaluate the patient before sending her home?
a. Alzheimer disease
b. Frontotemporal dementia
c. Anosognosia
d. Pituitary tumor
e. None of the above

Answer: e. Physicians should consider elder abuse. It may be subtle, taking the form of administering more than or less than prescribed medications, allowing the person to fall, and inappropriate restraints, as well as actual blows.

30. A well-kicked soccer ball struck the head of a 16-year-old high school freshman who was not a particularly good athlete or student. The blow stunned him, but did not cause a loss of consciousness. For the next week he blamed the injury for his inability to learn new material in school. Of the following deficits, which one would neuropsychologic testing most likely reveal?
a. Depression
b. Inattention
c. Dyslexia
d. Constructional apraxia

Answer: b. He probably has inattention and memory impairment (amnesia) that impair his ability to learn new material. Students are particularly sensitive to TBI-induced inattention and amnesia. Physicians should direct students with learning disabilities away from sports that entail head trauma.

31. Which of the following statements is *true* regarding diffusion tensor imaging (DTI)?
a. It is a commonly used imaging technique for diagnosing ischemic strokes.
b. Thalamic injuries are well identified.
c. Subtle asymmetries of white matter tracts may be appreciated.
d. DTI is a standard part of TBI evaluation.

Answer: c. DTI visualizes white matter tracts. Its greatest usefulness is in assessing injury to these tracts, such as in TBI. MRI cannot detect such damage.

32. A 32-year-old Marine who witnessed the violent death of men in his company has flashbacks and other symptoms of posttraumatic stress disorder (PTSD). He also sustained low back injury from a fall. His neurologic examination and MRIs of his head and low back are normal. His physicians have prescribed hypnotics, benzodiazepines, antidepressants, and, for low back pain, opioids, but he remains incapacitated. Which strategy would probably produce the greatest benefit with least risk and side effect?
a. Switch to an antipsychotic
b. Use only a single medicine that would target the primary symptom

c. Reduce the number and dosage of medicines, and initiate nonpharmacologic treatments
d. Switch to long-acting preparations, such as methadone, to reduce the "ups and downs"

Answer: c. Independent, uncoordinated treatment by psychiatrists, neurologists, surgeons, and physiatrists often leads to polypharmacy, which is often counterproductive and dangerous. A single physician should supervise the medication regimen to avoid cumulative adverse effects, medicines that counteract each other, and combinations that lead to toxicity. That physician should generally curtail the medicine regimen and substitute nonpharmacologic treatments, such as exposure therapy, psychotherapy, and various forms of rehabilitation.

33. Which sequela has the closest correlation with the severity of TBI?
a. Posttraumatic epilepsy (PTE)
b. Depression
c. PTSD
d. Postconcussion syndrome

Answer: a. PTE clearly increases in proportion to the severity of TBI; however, the other symptoms have remarkably little correlation with TBI severity.

34. Which of the following is the most powerful risk factor for TBI-induced aggression?
a. Depression
b. Premorbid poor social functioning
c. Premorbid substance abuse
d. Posttraumatic poor social functioning

Answer: a. All are risk factors, but the presence of posttraumatic depression has the closest correlation with TBI-induced aggression. Notably, the aggression may be verbal as well as physical.

35. A 37-year-old woman sustained a concussion in a rear-end motor vehicle crash. She sought medical attention primarily for posttraumatic headaches that plagued her three times a week. Because she carried a history of migraine since she was a teenager, the neurologist prescribed an aspirin-butalbital-caffeine compound. When that medication proved inadequate, he added an acetaminophen-codeine compound. After 4 months, she stated that she was suffering from almost daily headaches. A repeat neurologic examination, MRI of her head, and routine tests showed no abnormality. At this time, which is the most likely cause of her headaches?
a. Depression
b. PTSD
c. Migraine
d. Medication overuse

Answer: d. Constant use of analgesics, particularly aspirin-butalbital-caffeine compounds and opioids, leads to chronic daily headache. Moreover, polypharmacy is often counterproductive. Although TBI can exacerbate migraine and antimigraine medicines are indicated in this situation, these particular medicines carry more potential harm than expectable benefits. Preventative antimigraine medicines, such as a tricyclic antidepressant or topiramate, would reduce these headaches. In addition, tricyclic antidepressants may reduce posttraumatic insomnia, depression, and bodily pains.

36. The autopsy findings of deceased retired professional football players most closely resemble the pathologic findings in which of the following neurodegenerative diseases?
    a. Parkinson disease
    b. Amyotrophic lateral sclerosis
    c. Huntington disease
    d. Alzheimer disease

Answer: d. Increased cerebral accumulation of tau protein and plaques and tangles in the brains of the football players resembles the abnormality of Alzheimer disease.

37. Is the following statement *true* or *false*? Post-TBI therapy with 7 days of phenytoin or levetiracetam will prevent the development of posttraumatic epilepsy.
    a. True
    b. False

Answer: False. One week of phenytoin or levetiracetam will prevent early posttraumatic seizures only during that week. The presence or absence of this therapy does not correlate with the development of posttraumatic epilepsy.

38. Which of the following is *false* about chronic traumatic encephalopathy (CTE)?
    a. Autopsied brains of patients with CTE reveal pathology similar to Alzheimer dementia.
    b. Mortality of former NFL players is three times higher than age-matched controls in the general population.
    c. Patients show symptoms of memory loss, depression, aggression, and executive dysfunction.
    d. CTE is only associated with professional football and boxing.

Answer: d. CTE has been associated with multiple professional and amateur sports, including, football, boxing, rugby, ice hockey, soccer, and cheerleading.

PATIENT AND FAMILY SUPPORT GROUPS

The following organizations provide patients and their families with educational, legal, medical, and personal assistance. Some of them also provide educational materials for physicians.

GENERAL RESOURCES

American Academy of Neurology
https://patients.aan.com/

Neurology: Official Journal of the American Academy of Neurology
www.neurology.org

National Institutes of Health
www.nih.gov

National Institutes of Health Clinical Trials:
www.ClinicalTrials.gov

ACQUIRED IMMUNE DEFICIENCY SYNDROME (AIDS)

Gay Men's Health Crisis
www.gmhc.org

ALZHEIMER DISEASE

Alzheimer's Association
www.alz.org

AMYOTROPHIC LATERAL SCLEROSIS (ALS)

Amyotrophic Lateral Sclerosis Association
www.alsa.org

APHASIA AND RELATED DISORDERS

American Speech-Language Hearing Association
www.asha.org

AUTISM

Autism Society of America
www.autism-society.org

BLEPHAROSPASM

Benign Essential Blepharospasm Research Foundation
www.blepharospasm.org

BLINDNESS

American Foundation for the Blind
www.afb.org

Lighthouse Guild
www.lighthouseguild.org

BRAIN TUMORS

American Brain Tumor Association
www.abta.org

Children's Brain Tumor Foundation
www.cbtf.org

National Brain Tumor Society
www.braintumor.org

CEREBRAL PALSY

March of Dimes
www.marchofdimes.org

United Cerebral Palsy Association
www.ucp.org

DYSTONIA

Musicians with Dystonia
https://www.dystonia-foundation.org/about-us/people/musicianswithdystonia

Dystonia Medical Research Foundation
www.dystonia-foundation.org

EPILEPSY

Epilepsy Foundation of America
www.epilepsyfoundation.org

FRAUDULENT THERAPIES

Quakwatch
www.quackwatch.org

GUILLAIN–BARRÉ SYNDROME

Guillain–Barré Syndrome Foundation International
www.guillain-barre.com

HUNTINGTON DISEASE

Huntington's Disease Society of American
www.hdsa.org

MIGRAINE AND HEADACHE

American Council for Headache Education
www.achenet.org

American Headache Society
www.americanheadachesociety.org

National Headache Foundation
www.headaches.org

MULTIPLE SCLEROSIS

National Multiple Sclerosis Association of America (MSAA)
www.msaa.com

National Multiple Sclerosis Society
www.nmss.org

MUSCULAR DYSTROPHY AND RELATED DISORDERS

Muscular Dystrophy Association, Inc.
www.mdausa.org

MYASTHENIA GRAVIS

Myasthenia Gravis Foundation of America
www.myasthenia.org

NEUROFIBROMATOSIS

Neurofibromatosis Network
www.nfnetwork.org

PAIN

American Chronic Pain Association
www.theacpa.org

International Association for the Study of Pain
http://www.iasp-pain.org/index.aspx

American Pain Foundation
www.painfoundation.org

American Academy of Pain Medicine
www.painmed.org

PARAPLEGIA

See spinal cord injury

PARKINSON DISEASE

National Parkinson Foundation
www.parkinson.org

Parkinson's Disease Foundation
www.pdf.org

POSTPOLIO SYNDROME

International Polio Network
www.post-polio.org

RETT SYNDROME

International Rett Syndrome Association
www.rettsyndrome.org

SLEEP DISORDERS

American Academy of Sleep Medicine
www.aasmnet.org

American Board of Sleep Medicine
http://www.absm.org

SPASMODIC DYSPHONIA

See dystonia

SPASMODIC TORTICOLLIS

National Spasmodic Torticollis Association
www.torticollis.org

SPINA BIFIDA

Spina Bifida Association of America
www.spinabifidaassociation.org

SPINAL CORD INJURY

National Spinal Cord Injury Association
www.spinalcord.org

Paralyzed Veterans of America
www.pva.org

STROKE

American Heart Association
www.americanheart.org

National Stroke Association
www.stroke.org

STUTTERING

The Stuttering Foundation
www.stutteringhelp.org

TOURETTE SYNDROME

Tourette Syndrome Association
www.tourette.org

TRAUMATIC BRAIN INJURY

Brain Injury Association
www.biausa.org

TUBEROUS SCLEROSIS

Tuberous Sclerosis Alliance
www.tsalliance.org

Tuberous Sclerosis Association
www.tuberous-sclerosis.org

TREMOR

International Tremor Foundation
www.essentialtremor.org

WILSON DISEASE

Wilson's Disease Association International
www.wilsonsdisease.org

Costs of Various Tests and Treatments*

Tests	Cost in US$
Genetic tests	
APO genotype	900
Duchenne muscular dystrophy	3,400
Dystonia (DYT1)	1,100
Fragile X DNA sequence	3,000
Huntington disease	530
Neurofibromatosis type 1 (NF1)	5,700
Rett syndrome (MECP2) duplication/deletion	880
Electroencephalogram (EEG)	
Routine EEG	500
EEG video monitoring per day	4,200
Electromyography (EMG)/Nerve conduction velocity (NCV)	
For carpal tunnel	1,200
For radiculopathy	1,500
Evoked response testing	750
Imaging	
Computed tomography (CT)	
Head	1,600
Cervical spine	2,400
Diffusion tensor imaging (DTI)	3,000
Dopamine transporter scan (DaTscan)	5,000
Magnetic resonance imaging (MRI)	
Head	2,900
Cervical spine	2,900
Positron emission tomography (PET)	4,200
Lumbar puncture (spinal tap)	450
Sleep studies	
Multiple sleep latency test (MSLT)	4,200
Polysomnography (PSG) per night	8,500

Treatments	Cost in US$
Deep brain stimulation for essential tremor or Parkinson disease	42,000
Medications' monthly wholesale cost from on-line discount pharmacy	
Alzheimer disease	
Donepezil 10 mg 30 pills	9
Memantine 10 mg 60 pills	15
Rivastigmine 3 mg 60 pills	95
Epilepsy	
Lamotrigine 100 mg 60 pills	16
Levetiracetam 500 mg 90 pills	35
Phenytoin 100 mg 90 pills	12
Topiramate 100 mg 90 pills	35
Valproate 500 mg 90 pills	30
Erectile dysfunction	
Sildenafil 100 mg 10 pills	385
Tadalafil 10 mg 10 pills	465
Inflammatory diseases	
Intravenous gammaglobulin infusions (six)	60,000
Migraine	
Sumatriptan 100 mg 9 pills	15
Multiple sclerosis medications	
Copaxone 30 syringes	2,400
Fingolimod 0.5 mg 30 pills	5,400
Interferon beta-1a 4 syringes	5,300
Dimethyl fumarate 240 mg 60 pills	5,800
Parkinson disease	
L-dopa with carbidopa 25/250 90 pills	27
Ropinirole 1 mg 120 pills	50
Huntington disease chorea	
Tetrabenazine 12.5 mg 70 pills	3,700
Rehabilitation/nursing home care	
Acute rehabilitation inpatient/day	1,000
Assisted living, monthly	3,500
Nursing home care, monthly	11,000
Skilled nursing facility/day	9,000
Plasmapheresis (for Guillain–Barré syndrome or myasthenia gravis)	
Six-exchange course	7,000

*Approximate charges in US$ for representative tests and treatments in New York City in 2016. Prices vary notoriously. Moreover, the charge to Medicare and commercial insurers hides behind the price to consumers.

DISEASES TRANSMITTED BY CHROMOSOME OR MITOCHONDRIA ABNORMALITIES

A. Chromosomes and the Diseases They Transmit*

1	Alzheimer disease, Presenillin 2
3	von Hippel–Lindau sydrome
4	Huntington disease Parkinson disease α-synuclein gene
5	Infantile and juvenile spinal muscular atrophy (Werdnig–Hoffman and Kugelberg–Welander diseases)
6	Creutzfeldt–Jakob disease Parkinson disease, Parkin Spinocerebellar ataxia Type 1
7	Williams syndrome
9	Dystonia (early-onset primary dystonia [DYT1]) Friedreich ataxia Tuberous sclerosis complex 2 (TSC1)
12	Phenylketonuria (PKU)
13	Wilson disease
14	Alzheimer disease, Presenillin 1 Dopamine responsive dystonia
15	Angelman syndrome Dyslexia, susceptibilty to (and other genes) Prader–Willi syndrome Tay–Sachs disease (hexosaminidase A deficiency)
16	Tuberous sclerosis complex 2 (TSC2)
17	Charcot–Marie–Tooth disease, Type 1A Frontotemporal lobar degeneration Narcolepsy-Cataplexy Neurofibromatosis Type 1
19	Apolipoprotein E (ApoE) Familial hemiplegic migraine Malignant hyperthermia susceptibility (ryanodine receptor) Myotonic dystrophy
20	Fatal familial insomnia
21	Homocystinura due to cystanthione beta-synthase deficiency Myoclonic epilepsy of Unverricht and Lundborg Trisomy 21 (Down syndrome)
22	Metachromatic leukodystrophy due to arylsulfatase A deficiency Neurofibromatosis Type 2 Velocardiofacial and DiGeorge syndromes
X	Adrenoleukodystrophy Duchenne muscular dystrophy Fragile X syndrome Lesch–Nyhan syndrome Rett syndrome (MECP2)

For additional and continually updated information visit:
www.genetests.org/
http://omim.org/
*This table presents the most common associations. Often, several different mutations may produce similar clinical features and some mutations provide only susceptibility to an illness.

B. Diseases Transmitted by Mitochondria

Cytochrome c oxidase deficiency
Leigh syndrome
MELAS (mitochondrial encephalomyopathy, lactic acidosis, stroke)
MERRF (myoclonic epilepsy, ragged red fibers)
Progressive external ophthalmoplegia

C. Diseases Transmitted by Excessive Trinucleotide Repeats

Disease	Transmission	Chromosome	Trinucleotide
Fragile X syndrome	Sex linked	X	CGG
Friedreich ataxia	Autosomal recessive	9	GAA
Huntington disease	Autosomal dominant	4	CAG
Myotonic dystrophy	Autosomal dominant	19	CTG
Oculopharyngeal dystrophy	Autosomal dominant	14	GCC
Spinocerebellar atrophies (SCAs)			
Type 1	Autosomal dominant	6	CAG
Type 2	Autosomal dominant	12	CAG
Type 3*	Autosomal dominant	14	CAG

*Machado–Joseph disease

CHEMICAL AND BIOLOGICAL NEUROTOXINS

Condition	Mechanism of Action	Effects
Atropine, scopolamine	Blocks cerebral ACh* receptors	Delirium, amnesia, systemic autonomic anticholinergic effects
Botulinum toxin poisoning	Impairs release of ACh from *presynaptic* neurons	Paresis, especially of ocular, pharyngeal, and respiratory muscles
Curare, α-bungarotoxin	Blocks neuromuscular ACh receptor	Paralysis of voluntary muscle
Ciguatera fish poisoning	Prolongs opening of voltage-gated Na^+ channels in nerves and muscles	Acute painful neuropathy, loss of sensation in limbs, victims perceive hot objects as cold
Lambert–Eaton syndrome	Impairs release of ACh from *presynaptic* neurons	Weakness of limb muscles
Myasthenia gravis	Impairs function of *postsynaptic* ACh receptors	Weakness of ocular, bulbar, and proximal limb muscles
Organophosphate insecticides/nerve gas exposure	Inhibits cholinesterase, which increases ACh concentration, causing *postsynaptic* dysfunction	Brief stimulation then paresis of all muscles; increased parasympathetic activity; confusion, seizures
Tetanus or strychnine poisoning	Inhibits GABA$^\$$ and glycine$^\$$ receptors	Spasmodic, tetanic muscle contractions from uninhibited motor system

*Acetylcholine
$^\$$Inhibitory neurotransmitters

ADDITIONAL REVIEW QUESTIONS AND ANSWERS

1. Which portion of the brainstem is shown in this myelin-stained section?
a. Diencephalon
b. Midbrain
c. Pons
d. Medulla

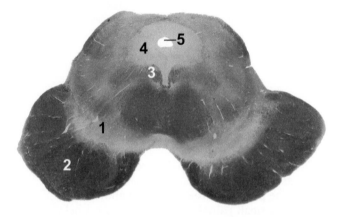

Answer: b. The midbrain, the uppermost section of the brainstem, is situated between the diencephalon and the pons. Neurologists identify the midbrain by its silhouette and sometimes quip that the midbrain, held upside-down, looks like Mickey Mouse.

2. Match each description (a–j) to one or two areas of the midbrain (1–5) pictured above. Some structures are not pictured.
a. Origin of the nigrostriatal tract
b. Conduit for cerebrospinal fluid (CSF)
c. Periaqueductal gray matter
d. Sixth cranial nerve nucleus
e. Third cranial nerve nucleus
f. Descending corticospinal tract
g. Site of dopamine synthesis
h. Aqueduct of Sylvius
i. Cerebral peduncle

Answers:
a–1: The curved area, unstained in this myelin-stained preparation, is the substantia nigra, which gives rise to the nigrostriatal tract.
b–5: This is the aqueduct of Sylvius, which is the CSF passageway from the third to fourth ventricles.
c–4: The gray area surrounding the aqueduct (5) is the periaqueductal gray matter.
d: The sixth cranial nerve nuclei are located in the pons and thus are not included in this picture of the midbrain.

e–3: The third cranial nerve nuclei, like most other brainstem motor nuclei, are paired and midline. The third and fourth cranial nerve nuclei are situated in the midbrain.
f–2: The corticospinal tracts descend in the dark, heavily myelinated cerebral peduncle. In the midbrain they are ipsilateral to their origin, but they cross in the medulla's pyramids.
g–1: This is the substantia nigra, superior to the cerebral peduncles.
h–5: This is the aqueduct of Sylvius, the CSF conduit between the third and fourth ventricles, which is surrounded by the periaqueductal gray matter.
i–2: This is the cerebral peduncle, which contains the corticospinal tract.

3. Which portion of the brainstem is shown in this myelin-stained section?
a. Diencephalon
b. Midbrain
c. Pons
d. Medulla

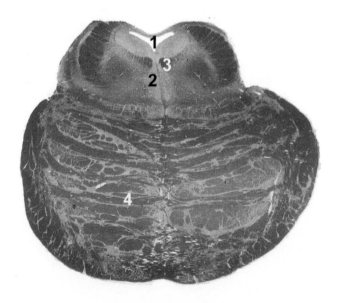

Answer: c. The pons is the section of the brainstem situated between the midbrain and the medulla. Neurologists identify the pons by its bulbous silhouette, large CSF passageway dorsally, and prominent crossing fibers in its lower portion.

545

4. Match the description (a–h) to the area of the pons (1–4) pictured above. Some structures are not pictured.
   a. Corticobulbar and corticospinal tract fibers
   b. Basis pontis
   c. Seventh cranial nerve exiting the brainstem
   d. Upper portion of the fourth ventricle
   e. Medial longitudinal fasciculus (MLF)
   f. Third cranial nerve nucleus
   g. Sixth cranial nerve nucleus
   h. Site of norepinephrine synthesis

Answers:
a and b–4: The basis pontis, the large bulbous lower portion of the pons, contains the corticobulbar tract, corticospinal tract, and cerebellar fibers.

   c: The seventh cranial nerves (not pictured) exit ventrolaterally from the pons and join the fifth and eighth cranial nerves in the cerebellopontine angle. Consequently, a tumor or other lesion in the cerebellopontine angle can disrupt cranial nerves V, VII, and VIII.

d–1: The fourth ventricle overlies the pons and medulla.

e–2: The MLF, which is a heavily myelinated longitudinal tract, traverses the pons in the dorsal midline (see Fig. 12.11).

   f: The third cranial nerve nuclei are located in the midbrain and thus are not included in this picture of the pons.

g–3: The sixth (abducens) cranial nerve nuclei are paired dorsal midline structures.

   h: Each locus ceruleus, sites of norepinephrine synthesis, is situated inferiorly and laterally to the fourth ventricle in the pons, but they are not identifiable in this picture.

5. Which portion of the brain is shown in this myelin-stained section?
   a. Diencephalon
   b. Midbrain
   c. Pons
   d. Medulla

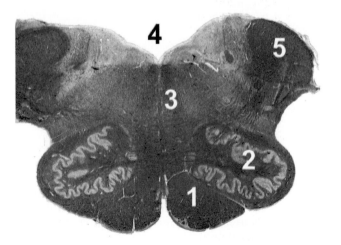

Answer: d. The medulla, the most caudal (lowermost) section of the brainstem, is readily identifiable by its bilateral, scalloped structures (the inferior olivary nuclei).

6. Match each description (a–h) to an area of the medulla (1–5) pictured above.
   a. Cerebellar inflow tract
   b. Inferior olivary nuclei
   c. Fourth ventricle
   d. Decussation of the medial lemniscus
   e. Corticospinal tracts
   f. Pyramids

Answers:
   a–5: Cerebellar inflow tracts pass through the medulla.
   b–2: The inferior olivary nuclei are the prominent scalloped structures.
   c–4: The fourth ventricle sits above the medulla and below the cerebellum.
   d–3: The posterior columns of the spinal cord, conveying position and vibration sensation, ascend into the medulla, where they cross in the decussation of the medial lemniscus.
e and f–1: The corticospinal tracts descend into the medulla and cross in its pyramids.

7. Which structures (a–h) are labeled (1–3) in this axial magnetic resonance image (MRI).
   1. The portion of the brainstem above #1
   2. The small paired gray oval structures below #2.
   3. The serpiginous dark lines seeming to emanate laterally from #2
   4. The almost vertical dark tracts designated #3
   a. Diencephalon
   b. Midbrain
   c. Pons
   d. Medulla
   e. Mammillary bodies
   f. Optic nerves

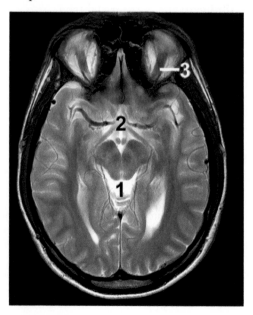

g. Anterior cerebral arteries
h. Middle cerebral arteries

Answers:

1–b: This slice shows the midbrain with its Mickey Mouse silhouette.

2–e: The small, paired gray oval structures are the mammillary bodies.

3–h: Because this sequence portrays blood flowing though arteries as black, the middle cerebral arteries appear black.

4–f: The structures are the optic nerves.

8. Match each number (1–5) with a structure (a–j) shown on this MRI.

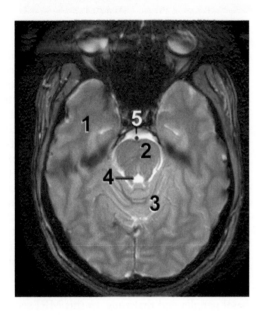

a. Midbrain
b. Pons
c. Medulla
d. Cerebellum
e. Frontal lobe
f. Temporal lobe
g. Occipital lobe
h. Third ventricle
i. Fourth ventricle
j. Basilar artery

Answers: Compared to the MRI shown in Question 7, this one shows a more caudal (lower) slice of brain.

1–f: The temporal lobe, which sits mostly in the middle fossa.

2–b: The bulbous shape defines the pons.

3–d: The cerebellum, with its gyri much thinner than cerebral gyri, is posterior to the pons.

4–i: The fourth ventricle sits above and posterior to the pons and below the cerebellum. It contains CSF, which appears white in this sequence.

5–j. The small, black circular structure anterior to the pons is the basilar artery. As in Question 7, the MRI shows blood flowing though arteries as black.

9. Match the number (1–4) with one or two structures (a–r) shown on this MRI.

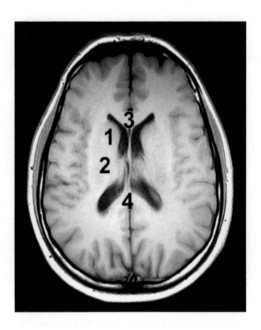

a. Diencephalon
b. Midbrain
c. Pons
d. Medulla
e. Thalamus
f. Globus pallidus
g. Putamen
h. Head of the caudate nucleus
i. Genu of the corpus callosum
j. Splenium of the corpus callosum
k. Planum temporale
l. Prefrontal cortex
m. Parietal lobe
n. Cingulate gyrus
o. Cerebellum
p. Optic chiasm
q. Fourth ventricle
r. Occipital lobe

Answers: Cutting through the cerebrum and lateral ventricles, this MRI shows a more rostral (higher) axial slice of brain.

1–h: The head of the caudate nucleus indents the lateral ventricle and forms its lateral border. In Huntington disease, it atrophies.

2–a, e: The thalamus forms the lateral border of the third ventricle. It is a major component of the diencephalon, which also includes hypothalamus and subthalamus.

3–i, 4j: This slice captures both the genu (anterior portion) (3) and splenium (posterior portion) (4) of the corpus callosum, "the great white commissure."

10. Match the numbers (1–11) on this MRI with the structures (a–r) listed in the previous question.

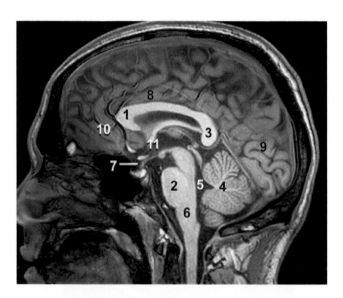

Answers: This is a sagittal midline view of the brain.
1–i, 3–j: These structures are the genu and splenium of the corpus callosum.
2–c, 6–d: The pons and the medulla are the two caudal components of the brainstem.
4–o, 5–q: The cerebellum, occupying most of the posterior fossa, overlies the fourth ventricle (5) and sits above the foramen magnum (not labeled).
   7–p: The optic chiasm sits superior to the sella, which holds the pituitary gland.
   8–n: The cingulate gyrus is a component of the limbic system. Notably, a portion of the cingulate gyrus sweeps under the genu. Neurologists call this portion the "subcingulate gyrus." It has been the target for deep brain stimulation for refractory depression.
   9–r: The occipital lobe houses primary visual cortex.
 10–l: Notably, a portion of the cingulate gyrus sweeps under the genu.
 11–a: The diencephalon sits just rostral to the brainstem

11. In this coronal view match the numbers (1–6) with the structures (a–h).
  a. Lateral ventricle
  b. Third ventricle
  c. Fourth ventricle
  d. Globus pallidus
  e. Putamen
  f. Caudate nucleus

  g. Vermis
  h. Corpus callosum

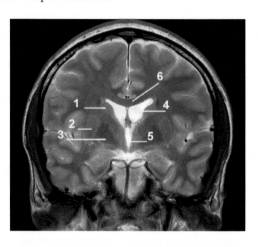

Answers:
1–f: The caudate nucleus indents the lateral-inferior wall of the third ventricle. As a distinctive feature of Huntington disease, the caudate nucleus undergoes atrophy, allowing the lateral ventricle to expand (see Fig. 20.5).
2–e: The putamen is lateral to the globus pallidus (see Fig. 18.1). Neurologists consider the putamen and caudate together to constitute the (corpus) striatum or neostriatum.
3–d: The globus pallidus is medial to the putamen. Neurologists consider the globus pallidus and putamen to be the lenticular nuclei. In hepatolenticular degeneration (Wilson disease) the lenticular nuclei degenerate. It has been the target of deep-brain stimulation for involuntary movement disorders.
4–a: The wing-shaped lateral ventricles extend over the basal ganglia and thalamus. In this MRI sequence, the CSF is hyperintense (bright white).
5–b: The third ventricle, which also contains CSF, is vertical.
6–h: The corpus callosum, the thick commissure passing between the hemispheres, sits above the lateral ventricles.

12. Three years following kidney transplantation, the 44-year-old recipient required constant immunosuppression. After he developed malaise, headache, and confusion, his nephrologist solicited a neurologic consultation. In addition to cognitive impairment, the neurologic examination showed fever, blurred optic disk margins, nuchal rigidity, and bilateral sixth cranial nerve palsies. Computed tomography (CT) showed hydrocephalus, but no mass lesions. The CSF, under a pressure of 400 mm H_2O, was turbid. It contained 400 WBC/ml (86% lymphocytes), 250 mg/dL protein, and 40 mg/dL glucose. Under microscopic inspection of the CSF, special stains revealed encapsulated organisms. Which organism has most likely caused the meningitis?
  a. *Cryptococcus*
  b. *Streptococcus pneumoniae*

c. herpes simplex

d. Tuberculosis

Answer: a. Immunosuppressed or immunodeficient patients are susceptible to opportunistic infections, such as fungal or tuberculous meningitis. These and other forms of meningitis, which are typically chronic, have a predilection to accumulate at the base of the brain and prevent CSF reabsorption through the arachnoid villi. Impaired CSF reabsorption leads to communicating hydrocephalus. The resulting increased intracranial pressure stretches the sixth cranial nerves to give a "false localizing sign." The CSF profile suggests a tuberculous or fungal rather than a bacterial or viral infection (see Table 20.1). The finding of encapsulated organisms indicates that *Cryptococcus* was the infective agent. Detecting *Cryptococcus* antigen in the CSF would confirm the diagnosis of cryptococcal meningitis.

13. Which of the following antiepileptic drugs (AEDs) undergoes renal clearance rather than hepatic metabolism?
    a. Valproate (Depakote)
    b. Lamotrigine (Lamictal)
    c. Levetiracetam (Keppra)
    d. Carbamazepine (Tegretol)

Answer: c. Most AEDs that physicians use for mood stabilization or pain suppression undergo hepatic metabolism. However, levetiracetam (Keppra), topiramate (Topamax), and gabapentin (Neurontin) undergo renal clearance.

14. A 51-year-old retired businessman has shown progressively more severe erratic uninhibited behavior, a ravenous appetite, and inability to manage the family's finances. His family finally brought him for a psychiatric consultation when he displayed no interest in attending his best friend's funeral. The physical portion of his neurologic examination was normal. His Mini Mental Status Examination (MMSE) score was 25. This is his head CT.

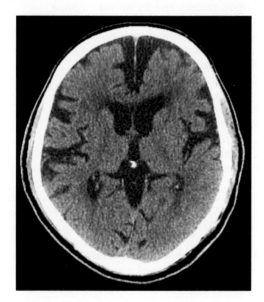

Which of the following conditions is most likely responsible for his neurocognitive disorder?
a. Alzheimer disease
b. Bipolar disorder
c. Frontotemporal lobar degeneration (frontotemporal dementia)
d. Vascular disease (vascular neurocognitive disorder)
e. Prion disease

Answer: c. Uninhibited behavior, hyperorality, lack of empathy, impaired executive function, and lack of sympathy with underlying mild cognitive impairment in this relatively young patient indicate that his diagnosis is major neurocognitive disorder due to frontotemporal lobar degeneration. This illness is the most common cause of dementia in adults younger than 60 years. His CT showing atrophy of the frontal lobes confirms the diagnosis and excludes mass lesions and hydrocephalus. The patient probably does not have Creutzfeldt–Jakob, the most common prion disease, because his course has been too slowly progressive, no physician detected myoclonus, and the CT is inconsistent. Because the MMSE does not include an assessment for impaired executive function, it may not detect changes indicative of frontotemporal lobar degeneration. In this regard, the Montreal Cognitive Assessment (MoCA) is probably a better bedside test than the MMSE.

15. A 70-year-old man said that he suddenly developed trouble seeing. His CT is shown below. What will a clinical examination most likely reveal?

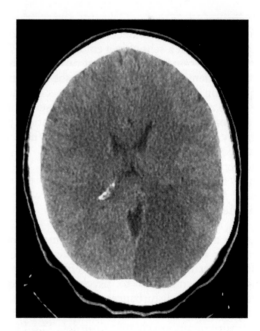

a. Left homonymous hemianopia
b. Right homonymous hemianopia
c. Aphasia
d. Dementia

Answer: b. The CT shows an infarction in the distribution of the left posterior cerebral artery (PCA), which includes the left occipital lobe. The left occipital infarction will cause a right homonymous hemianopia.

16–19. Match the visual field loss (16–20) to the condition most closely associated with it (a–k). For each number, one letter is sufficient, except for 19, which allows for three answers.

16. Left homonymous hemianopia with macular sparing
17. Fortification scotoma
18. Central scotoma, lasting for 2 weeks
19. Bitemporal hemianopia
  a. Retinal injury, for example retinal detachment or embolus from carotid artery
  b. Psychogenic disturbance
  c. Migraine with aura
  d. Diabetes insipidus
  e. Loss of libido
  f. Optic chiasm compression
  g. Amaurosis fugax
  h. Internal capsule infarction
  i. Aphasia
  j. Occipital infarction
  k. Optic or retrobulbar neuritis

Answers:
    16–j:
    17–c:
    18–k:
  19–d, e, f: Diabetes insipidus and loss of libido are associated with pituitary tumors.

20. Pollyanna, a 28-year-old health-care worker who has had a life-long tendency toward depression, set off to establish a school in a country where *Plasmodium falciparum* and less virulent varieties of malaria were endemic. As a precaution, she took mefloquine on the prescribed once-a-week schedule. After 6 months of mild to moderately severe symptoms of depression, she developed agitation, persecutory delusions, and hallucinations. Which is the most likely cause?
  a. Separation anxiety
  b. *P. vivax* infection
  c. *P. falciparum* infection
  d. Mefloquine toxicity

Answer: d. Initially marketed as Lariam, mefloquine is a synthetic analog of quinine that, like quinine, may prevent or treat malaria. Its adverse effects range from depression and confusion to psychosis. Mefloquine-induced psychiatric disturbances may last for years or become permanent. Its use is contraindicated in patients with a history of any psychiatric disorder. The FDA has issued a boxed warning about the adverse psychiatric effects of mefloquine. Although all varieties of malaria may cause delirium, *P. falciparum* is the most likely to cause central nervous system (CNS) damage.

21. An 80-year-old man being treated for depression has developed right-sided frontal headaches, pain on chewing, diffuse muscle aches, and intermittent low-grade fevers. Examination shows that the vision in his right eye is 20/200, but in the left eye 20/30. His temporal arteries are prominent and tender. There is no papilledema, hemiparesis, or other neurologic sign. Which condition is most likely?
  a. Open-angle glaucoma
  b. Optic neuritis
  c. Giant-cell arteritis
  d. Narrow-angle glaucoma

Answer: c. The headache, jaw claudication, and systemic symptoms indicate giant-cell arteritis (temporal arteritis). Physicians should diagnose this condition rapidly because, if untreated, it can cause blindness and strokes. The diagnostic tests are the sedimentation rate and temporal artery biopsy. Recent studies have suggested that varicella zoster infection may be causally related. Untreated glaucoma (both narrow- and open-angle) can also lead to blindness and narrow-angle glaucoma is associated with pain, but neither is associated with jaw claudication or systemic symptoms.

22–30. Match the ocular abnormality (22–30) with the most probable cause (a–k). One letter for each number is sufficient.

22. Right third cranial nerve paresis and left hemiparesis
23. Left sixth cranial nerve paresis and right hemiparesis
24. Right Horner syndrome, right facial hypalgesia, right limb ataxia, and left limb and trunk hypalgesia
25. Internuclear ophthalmoplegia
26. Right sixth and seventh cranial nerve paresis and left hemiparesis
27. Ptosis, facial diplegia, and ophthalmoplegia with normally reactive pupils
28. Small, irregular pupils that accommodate but do not react
29. Fever, agitated confusion, and dilated pupils
30. Stupor, miosis, and pulmonary edema
  a. Neuromuscular junction impairment
  b. Anticholinergic intoxication
  c. Right pontine lesion
  d. Left pontine lesion
  e. Left midbrain lesion
  f. Right midbrain lesion
  g. Midline dorsal brainstem lesion
  h. Left lateral medullary lesion
  i. Right lateral medullary lesion
  j. Syphilis
  k. Opioids

Answer: 22–f, 23–d, 24–i, 25–g, 26–c, 27–a (myasthenia gravis), 28–j (Argyll–Robertson pupils), 29–b (scopolamine intoxication), 30–k (heroin or methadone overdose).

31. A 30-year-old highly competitive, anxious and neurotic person sustained a compound fracture of his tibia and fibula while skiing above his ability. One year after an open reduction and fixation of the fractures he complained not only of incessant pain at the site of the surgery, he insisted that his clothing and casual touching of his entire lower leg bring on excruciating, burning pain. What do neurologists term this symptom?

a. Allodynia
b. Analgesia
c. Dysesthesia
d. Hyperpathia

Answer: a. When patients report that a neutral stimulus such as a cotton wisp or finger touch provokes pain, neurologists term the symptom *allodynia*. Examples include scalp allodynia in migraine; thigh allodynia in meralgia paresthetica; and allodynia in body parts affected by complex regional pain syndrome (CRPS). When patients report that a mildly painful stimulus provokes disproportionately great pain, neurologists term the symptom *hyperpathia*. When patients report that an area is numb to painful stimuli, neurologists term the symptom *analgesia*. When patients report that they have an altered perception of a stimulus, neurologists term the symptom or finding *dysesthesia*. All of these symptoms are, of course, subjective and potentially modified by the patient's psychological, financial, and medical context.

32. A 60-year-old man with dementia has a gait abnormality in which he excessively raises his legs. He seems to climb as he walks. His pupils are small (miotic), poorly reactive, and irregular. What is the gait abnormality?

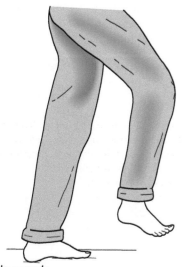

a. Gait apraxia
b. Congenital spastic paraparesis
c. Steppage gait from tabes dorsalis
d. Astasia-abasia

Answer: c. The patient has a steppage gait because he has lost position sense (proprioception). He instinctively raises his legs to avoid catching the tips of his toes when he walks, especially when he steps onto curbs. He has tertiary syphilis that has caused loss of position sense and Argyll–Robertson pupils. Steppage gait is also a

manifestation of a combined system disease (vitamin B_{12} deficiency), spinocerebellar ataxia, and, if it impairs position sense, neuropathy.

33–35. Match the confabulation (33–35) with the lesion (a–c) that might produce it.

33. A blind patient "describes" the physician's clothing. His pupils are round, equal, and reactive to light.
34. A man with recent onset of left hemiparesis claims that he cannot move his left arm and leg because he is too tired.
35. An agitated, diaphoretic middle-aged man describes bizarre occurrences and experiences visual hallucinations. When asked to repeat six digits, he says random numbers.
    a. Nondominant parietal lobe infarction
    b. Bilateral occipital lobe infarctions
    c. Hemorrhage into the limbic system

Answers:

33–b: Cortical blindness usually results from infarction or trauma of both occipital lobes. The pupils react normally because the optic and oculomotor nerves and their interconnections in the brainstem are unaffected. Most patients with cortical blindness are aware of their deficit and accept it. However, some explicitly deny their loss of vision and others implicitly deny it by confabulating, as in this case, or using other defense mechanisms. Neurologists diagnose Anton's syndrome in patients who explicitly or implicitly deny blindness from either ocular or cortical injury.

34–a: In anosognosia, patients with hemiparesis from a nondominant hemisphere infarct also often confabulate, deny, and use other defense mechanisms in response to their hemiparesis. The lesion typically involves the right parietal lobe.

35–c: In alcohol withdrawal, often as part of delirium tremens (DTs), patients may confabulate. Hemorrhage into the limbic system underlies Wernicke–Korsakoff syndrome, which may be comorbid with DTs.

36. A disheveled, disoriented young man staggers into the emergency room (ER). The medical staff finds that he is somnolent and, when awakened, he has nystagmus and gait ataxia. Which is the most likely illness?
    a. Subdural hematoma
    b. Cerebral infarction
    c. Wernicke–Korsakoff syndrome
    d. Psychogenic disturbance

Answer: c. He displays several of the major features of Wernicke–Korsakoff syndrome, which classically consists of nystagmus with or without other oculomotor abnormalities, ataxia, and either anterograde amnesia or depressed level of consciousness. In practice, neurologists often invoke less stringent criteria and make a clinical diagnosis in individuals presenting with any of those findings in the context of nutritional deficiency. More important, neurologists treat patients with suspected Wernicke–Korsakoff syndrome with thiamine IV because it is harmless, painless, and potentially capable of sparing them from permanent neurocognitive impairment. They do not wait for a determination of serum thiamine levels because the test is time-consuming and not readily available.

37. Neurologists admit an 11-year-old boy because of headache, nausea, and vomiting following 2 weeks of clumsiness. They find that he has papilledema, ataxia, bilateral hyperactive DTRs, and Babinski signs. Which is the most likely diagnosis?
    a. Multiple sclerosis (MS)
    b. Drug abuse
    c. Cerebellar tumor
    d. Spinocerebellar degeneration

Answer: c. Cerebellar astrocytomas, a relatively common brain tumor in children, block the aqueduct of Sylvius and compress or infiltrate the cerebellum. Blockage of CSF flow creates obstructive hydrocephalus, which causes symptoms and signs of increased intracranial pressure: headache, nausea, vomiting, and papilledema.

38. Which *four* of the following symptoms constitute the narcoleptic tetrad?
    a. Inability to move on awakening (hypnopompic sleep paralysis)
    b. Hunger or anorexia
    c. Vivid dreams when falling asleep (hypnagogic hallucinations)
    d. Excessive daytime sleepiness
    e. Night terrors (pavor nocturnus)
    f. Episodic loss of muscle tone (cataplexy)
    g. Snoring

Answer: a, c, d, f.

39. During the first week of hospitalization for acute psychosis, an adolescent male began to drink large quantities of water and other fluids. After 1 week he developed a seizure. Which one of the following conditions is most likely to have caused the seizure?
    a. Steroid abuse
    b. Diabetes insipidus
    c. Hyponatremia
    d. Parkinson disease
    e. Haloperidol

Answer: c. Whether psychiatric illness or another disorder causes excessive water intake (polydipsia), the resulting dilutional hyponatremia may cause seizures. Alternatively, routine use of AEDs (carbamazepine and oxcarbazepine), antipsychotic agents, SSRIs, and tricyclic antidepressants may lead to hyponatremia, particularly in patients older than 65 years and those taking diuretics. These AEDs cause hyponatremia because they interfere with renal reabsorption of sodium.

40. Whenever a 40-year-old man hears a good joke or is surprised, his jaw drops open, his neck muscles lose their tone, and his head falls forward. When frightened or very excited, his entire body feels weak. Aside from excessive daytime sleepiness (EDS), obesity, and mild hypertension, he is in good health. Which is probably the best medicine for this patient?
    a. An anxiolytic
    b. Sodium oxybate
    c. Modafinil
    d. β-Blocker

Answer: b. He probably has cataplexy, which warrants a diagnosis of narcolepsy. As in this patient's case, cataplexy sometimes consists only of momentary loss of tone in a single muscle group, such as the jaw or neck muscles. A powerful hypnotic, sodium oxybate (Xyrem), which is gamma-hydroxybutyrate (GHB, often called the "date-rape drug"), will help suppress cataplexy. Modafinil reduces EDS. In combination, oxybate and modafinil are helpful in narcolepsy with cataplexy.

41. A 23-year-old woman presents to a neurologist with a 6-year history of a progressively severe involuntary movement disorder in which her limbs, trunk, and neck contort into twisted and grotesque postures. Her muscles are hypertrophied. She has lost her body fat. In contrast to her physical disability, her cognitive function remains normal. She has no history of exposure to neuroleptics and no family member has a similar symptom. Of the following, which is the most likely cause of her movement disorder?
    a. Huntington disease
    b. Cerebral palsy
    c. DYT1 dystonia
    d. Tardive dystonia

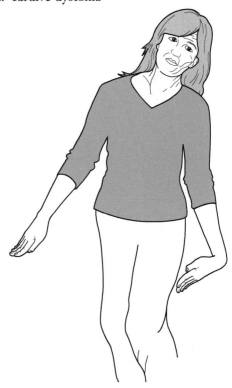

Answer: c. She has dystonia. The muscle hypertrophy and lack of body fat indicate its chronicity and neurologic basis. Of the many causes of dystonia in young adults, the most common are DYT1 early-onset primary dystonia (torsion dystonia), tardive dystonia, Wilson disease, the juvenile form of Huntington disease, and, in children, DOPA-responsive dystonia. Of the choices offered, the most likely is DYT1 dystonia. Her physicians should inquire if her relatives are Ashkenazi (Central and Eastern European Jews), which is the population that most carries the DYT1 gene, and, if she wishes, send a blood specimen for genetic testing.

42. A 20-year-old assembly-line worker in a heavy equipment factory, who indulges in "glue sniffing," reports numbness, tingling sensations, and mild hand and feet weakness. Which of the following portions of the nervous system has the glue sniffing damaged?
    a. Neuromuscular junction
    b. Corpus callosum
    c. Peripheral nerves
    d. Basal ganglia

Answer: c. Glue contains n-hexane and other volatile hydrocarbon solvents. These chemicals carry a great potential for abuse because they induce a mild euphoria. Chronic exposure causes peripheral neuropathy that typically presents with numbness, paresthesias, and weakness of the distal extremities. Some hydrocarbons, such as toluene, penetrate the blood–brain barrier and damage cerebral and cerebellar myelin.

43. Three weeks after recovering from a frontal craniotomy for a ruptured anterior communicating artery aneurysm, a patient remains apathetic and almost mute; however, when urged, he can name objects, follow requests, and repeat phrases. When walking, his steps are short and hesitant. He has lost bladder control. A CT shows lucencies in both frontal lobes, but normal-size ventricles. Which one of the following is most likely to have complicated the aneurysm or surgery?
    a. After surviving the rupture of an aneurysm and the neurosurgery, he has developed posttraumatic stress disorder.
    b. Brain damage from the aneurysm and the surgery has led to dementia.
    c. Subarachnoid hemorrhage-induced vasospasm or the surgery occluded both anterior cerebral arteries and caused bifrontal infarctions.
    d. The hemorrhage has led to communicating hydrocephalus.

Answer: c. The anterior communicating arteries supply the anterior and medial portions of the frontal lobes, including the medial surface of the motor cortex, which controls the voluntary function of the legs and bladder. Infarction of frontal lobes creates personality changes, gait impairment, and urinary incontinence. Communicating hydrocephalus sometimes follows subarachnoid hemorrhage because blood in the subarachnoid space impairs reabsorption of CSF.

44. Which *three* of the following conditions often lead to a patient's reporting "putrid smells" that the physician cannot detect?
    a. Seizures that originate in the uncus
    b. Sinusitis
    c. Migraines
    d. Seizures that originate in the parietal lobe
    e. Valproic acid
    f. Dental infections

Answer: a, b, f. Infections in the sinuses and mouth are the most common causes of putrid smells. Migraines often include visual but rarely auditory or olfactory auras.

45. For which *five* conditions might a lumbar puncture (LP) be indicated?
    a. Subdural hematoma
    b. Strokes
    c. Posterior fossa brain tumor
    d. Unruptured arteriovenous malformation (AVM)
    e. Idiopathic intracranial hypertension (pseudotumor cerebri)
    f. MS
    g. Bacterial meningitis
    h. Subacute sclerosing panencephalitis
    i. Viral encephalitis

Answer: e, f, g, h, i. Intracranial mass lesions usually preclude an LP because it might precipitate transtentorial or tonsillar herniation. In addition, with solid primary CNS tumors, CSF analysis is usually not diagnostically helpful.

46. A 68-year-old man with metastatic prostate cancer controls his pain with morphine tablets that he takes every 6 hours. When leaving the house for a daytime trip with his family, he counts his pills. During the trip, he frequently recounts the remaining pills. Which term would most accurately describe his behavior?
    a. Obsessive-compulsive ritual
    b. Hoarding
    c. Addiction
    d. Pseudoaddiction

Answer: d. Anticipating a recurrence of severe pain from metastatic cancer if he exhausts his supply of opioids, the patient carefully schedules himself. Although his behavior appears to reflect addiction or obsessive-compulsive behavior, neurologists term it *pseudoaddiction*. His behavior also suggests that his morphine dose is too meager and the interval between doses too great. With such tight restrictions, he is constantly on the verge of recurrence of pain. His physicians should prescribe more generous doses and decrease the time between medication administration. They might switch him to long-acting oral or transdermal opioids.

47. In which *three* of the following illnesses do patients usually retain decisional capacity despite quadriparesis and respiratory failure?
    a. Guillain–Barré syndrome
    b. Locked-in syndrome

c. Persistent vegetative state

d. Cervical spinal cord gunshot wound

Answer: a, b, d.

48. The parents of an 13-year-old girl bring her to the pediatrician because she has developed twitchy, restless movements. The parents, more so than the girl, are distraught. The pediatrician determines that she has normal orientation, judgment, and language function. When her arms are extended at his request, her fingers show individual flexion or extension movements, as if playing a piano. Her face grimaces and smirks. She walks in an irregular and clumsy pattern. She is unable to protrude her tongue or stand at attention for 10 seconds. Which test would have the *lowest* yield?
   a. Venereal Disease Research Laboratory (VDRL)
   b. Inquiries about oral contraceptives
   c. Antistreptolysin O (ASLO) titer
   d. Pregnancy
   e. Anti-nuclear antibody (ANA) titer

Answer: a. She has chorea. In adolescents, it is usually a sign of rheumatic fever (Sydenham chorea), lupus, pregnancy (chorea gravidarum), or a side effect of oral contraceptives. In older children, cocaine use sometimes causes acute chorea (crack dancing).

49. Which *two* procedures would be most helpful in determining the dominant hemisphere?
   a. Brainstem auditory-evoked responses (BAER)
   b. CT
   c. Electroencephalograph (EEG) with sphenoidal electrodes
   d. Functional magnetic resonance imaging (fMRI)
   e. Intracarotid sodium amobarbital injection (Wada test)
   f. Visual-evoked responses (VER)

Answer: d, e. The Wada test (intracarotid amobarbital injection) determines the dominant hemisphere by producing aphasia. Functional but not standard MRI can detect the dominant hemisphere.

50. When women take nonsteroidal anti-inflammatory drugs (NSAIDs) for menstrual cramps, which substances do these medicines inhibit?
   a. Enkephalins
   b. Endorphins
   c. Prostaglandins
   d. Serotonin

Answer: c. NSAIDs alleviate pain and inflammation by reducing prostaglandins.

51. Which *two* statements are true regarding the dorsal raphe nucleus?
   a. It contains high concentrations of endorphins.
   b. Stimulating it causes pain.
   c. Stimulating it produces analgesia.

d. Stimulating it produces behavioral changes.

e. It contains a high serotonin concentration.

Answer: c, e.

52. Several friends bring a stuporous 14-year-old boy to the ER. The physicians find that he is apneic and his pupils are miotic. A froth bubbles from his nostrils and mouth. Which condition is the most likely responsible?
   a. Cocaine intoxication
   b. Heroin overdose
   c. Methamphetamine intoxication
   d. 3,4-methylenedioxy-methamphetamine (MDMA, Ecstasy)

Answer: b. Heroin overdose typically causes stupor, miosis, apnea, and, in severe cases, pulmonary edema. Respiratory support and administering naloxone (Narcan) are the best treatments. While physicians usually administer naloxone intravenously in the emergency room, a newly developed nasal spray of naloxone allows medical personnel to administer it in locations where intravenous administration would be impossible. Moreover, the nasal spray allows administration to addicts without intravenous access because of scar tissue. Cocaine, methamphetamine, and MDMA are stimulants that generally cause excitement, hypertension, and enlarged pupils.

53–55. A 29-year-old woman reports that she has developed a tremor when she writes, drinks coffee, and lights a cigarette.

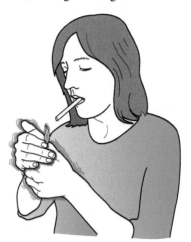

53. Which *four* of the following conditions can lead to such a tremor?
   a. Essential tremor
   b. Wilson disease
   c. Anxiety
   d. Huntington chorea
   e. Athetosis
   f. Use of valproate
   g. Dystonia
   h. Rett syndrome

Answer: a, b, c, f. Essential tremor causes tremor that is worst with action. Wilson disease is a rare but important condition that should be considered in young adults who develop a tremor. Anxiety can produce a tremor that is indistinguishable from essential tremor and also responds to β-adrenergic blockers. Numerous medications, including tricyclic antidepressants and valproate, cause or exacerbate tremor.

54. Physicians caring for the patient in the previous question want to exclude Wilson disease. Which *two* tests should they order?
    a. MRI
    b. Slit-lamp examination
    c. Positron emission tomography (PET)
    d. Serum ceruloplasmin
    e. Serum copper concentration

Answer: b, d. Slit-lamp examination to look for a Kayser–Fleisher ring and determination of the serum ceruloplasmin, which is low in the illness, are the best initial tests. Positive results may indicate further testing, such as 24-hour urinary copper determination and genetic analysis. MRI and PET will detect Wilson disease, but only in advanced cases. Random serum copper concentrations reflect only the individual's recent meals' copper content.

55. Of the following medications, which is most effective for essential tremor?
    a. Anticholinergics
    b. Dopamine agonists
    c. α-Adrenergic blockers
    d. Propranolol

Answer: d. Propranolol and perhaps some other β-blockers suppress the tremor in about 50% of patients. Alternatively, primidone (Mysoline), which undergoes metabolism to phenobarbital, may suppress the tremor. Deep-brain stimulation is dramatically effective.

56. Of the following, which *two* characteristics distinguish classic neurotransmitters from endocrine hormones, such as thyroxine?
    a. Classic neurotransmitters or their metabolic products circulate in detectable quantities in the blood.
    b. Classic neurotransmitters are produced and stored at a site adjacent to the target organ.
    c. Classic neurotransmitters or their metabolic products are often present in detectable concentrations in the CSF, but not in the blood.
    d. Classic neurotransmitters are steroids.

Answer: b, c.

57. To which feature of neurons does the term "plasticity" refer?
    a. Mechanical properties
    b. Ability to reorganize
    c. Ability to resist change
    d. Chemical constituents

Answer: b. *Plasticity* means the capacity to be altered or molded. In neurologic terms, plasticity refers to the ability of the CNS to undergo reorganization. Several studies have purportedly demonstrated that CNS plasticity occurs in partial recovery after strokes and chronic pain.

58. Which of the following techniques is the most sensitive in detecting an acute stroke?
    a. MRI
    b. fMRI
    c. MRI with diffusion-weighted images (DWI) sequences
    d. PET

Answer: c. DWI is the most sensitive study for detecting acute strokes. PET lacks resolution as well as the ability to detect acute ischemic changes.

59. A 68-year-old house painter has weakness, atrophy, and areflexic DTRs in his arms. The biceps and triceps muscles have fasciculations. He has sensory loss in his right hand, brisk DTRs in his legs, and a right Babinski sign. Which one of the following features suggests that he has cervical spondylosis rather than amyotrophic lateral sclerosis (ALS)?
    a. Hand atrophy
    b. Hyperactive DTRs
    c. Sensory loss
    d. Babinski sign

Answer: c. House painting requires prolonged neck hyperextension, which often leads to cervical spondylosis. In turn, cervical spondylosis leads to cervical nerve root compression that causes sensory impairment along with fasciculations and loss of strength and DTRs – lower motor neuron signs – in the arms and hands. In addition, cervical spondylosis leads to weakness, spasticity, hyperactive DTRs, and Babinski signs – upper motor neuron signs – in the legs. Cervical spondylosis, a much more frequently occurring condition than ALS, is an occupational hazard of jobs, such as house painting, that require prolonged neck hyperextension. A clear-cut distinguishing feature is that ALS, like other motor neuron diseases, does not cause sensory loss, but cervical spondylosis does.

60. A 70-year-old man with no known family or friends wandered into the psychiatry ER for no apparent reason. He was dull and apathetic. However, he knew the month, year, place, his address, and his social security number. He seemed well-nourished and clean. Although reticent, he was able to name objects, repeat phrases, and follow two-step requests. His neurologic examination showed no lateralized signs or indications of increased intracranial pressure. Routine blood tests showed no abnormalities. His head CT showed striking changes in the frontal lobes. Judging from these representative slices of the CT and the clinical presentation, which is his most likely underlying disorder?
    a. Frontotemporal lobar degeneration
    b. Vascular disease
    c. Traumatic brain injury
    d. Postsurgical personality change

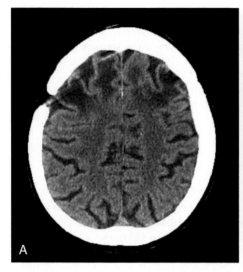 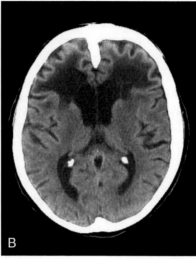 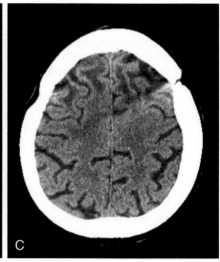

Answer: d. This patient displays a muted affect, not dementia, aphasia, or any psychiatric illness. The central CT slice shows loss of frontal lobe white matter with preserved cerebral cortex. The pattern excludes frontotemporal, vascular, and traumatic dementia because those conditions obliterate the cortex as well as the underlying white matter. Although CTs of patients with schizophrenia show cerebral atrophy and compensatory ventricular enlargement, the frontal lobe destruction in these slices is inconsistent with psychiatric disorders.

Note the skull defect in the temples. Further investigation established that this patient had undergone a *frontal lobotomy*, which typically consisted of a neurosurgeon drilling burr holes through the skull at the temples, inserting a scalpel or other instrument, and then blindly severing the frontal lobe's white matter tracts. Because the frontal lobotomy involved severing the white matter tracts, physicians sometimes called the procedure a *leucotomy* (see also Fig. 20.23.) In a simplification of the procedure, the transorbital lobotomy, the surgeon thrust an ice pick-like instrument through the orbit of the skull, under the upper eyelid, to sever the white matter tracts. The introduction of chlorpromazine eliminated the indication for the procedure. In the interim, the neurosurgeon who promulgated the frontal lobotomy, Antonio Moniz, won a Nobel Prize.

61. Which condition has the highest incidence of comorbid depression or depressive symptoms?
    a. Parkinson disease
    b. Multiple sclerosis
    c. Epilepsy
    d. Alzheimer disease

Answer: c. Physicians find depression or depressive symptoms in all of the disorders but most frequently with epilepsy. This association is strongest for focal seizures with altered awareness, which neurologists previously called complex partial seizures. Neurologists frequently attribute depression or depressive symptoms in epilepsy patients to the underlying brain damage, seizures, AEDs, and epilepsy surgery.

62. As people age, what is the most common EEG change?
    a. Loss of amplitude
    b. Slowing of the background activity
    c. Fragmentation of background
    d. Episodic β-activity

Answer: b.

63. At the suggestion of his mistress, a 55-year-old man with testicular cancer consulted a neurologist because, although the tumor was in remission, he had developed a short temper, apathy, and irritability. He was taking no medications and did not use alcohol or illicit drugs. His neurologic examination found pronounced memory loss and a flattened affect. An MRI with gadolinium showed atrophy of the mesial temporal lobes and an EEG showed spikes and slow-waves emanating from that same region. Routine blood tests, including for human immunodeficiency virus (HIV), showed no abnormalities. Which of the following tests is most likely to reveal the diagnosis?
    a. Serum anti-Ma2 antibodies
    b. CSF for 14-3-3 protein
    c. Acetylcholine (ACh) receptor antibodies
    d. CT of the head

Answer: a. Even though the tumor may be in remission, the patient seems to have developed limbic encephalitis. This paraneoplastic syndrome often represents the initial symptom or sign of recurrence of testicular or small-cell lung carcinoma. Individuals with this disorder develop pronounced memory impairment combined with irritability, behavioral disturbances, personality changes, and focal seizures. Their serum typically contains antibodies, usually of the anti-Ma2 or anti-Hu variety, which react with limbic system neurons.

64. Which structure contains 80% of the brain's dopamine content?
    a. Third ventricle
    b. Thalamus

c. Cerebral cortex

d. Corpus striatum

Answer: d. The corpus striatum, which is the terminus of the nigrostriatal tract, consists of the caudate nucleus and putamen.

65. In which condition do patients perform the Gowers maneuver?
    a. Psychogenic weakness
    b. Duchenne dystrophy
    c. Myotonic dystrophy
    d. Myasthenia gravis

Answer: b. Boys with Duchenne muscular dystrophy, because of their proximal leg weakness, use their arms and hands to push themselves upright to stand (see Gowers maneuver, see Fig. 6.4).

66. One month after a right cerebral infarction that caused a mild left hemiparesis, a 60-year-old man describes an intense burning sensation in the left side of his face and arm. A neurologic examination discloses that he has lost sensations in these areas for touch, warm, and cold. What is the origin of the patient's symptom?
    a. Parietal lobe injury
    b. Brachial plexus injury
    c. Lateral spinothalamic injury
    d. Thalamic injury

Answer: d. This characteristically burning sensation is thalamic pain, a type of central pain. It is usually a consequence of an infarction of the contralateral thalamus because of loss of sensory input to the brain (*deafferentation*). Amputations (phantom limb) and brachial plexus avulsion cause similar deafferentation pain. Thalamic pain frequently responds to gabapentin, carbamazepine, other AED, or to tricyclic antidepressants but not to analgesics.

67. Which *two* of the following tests rely on ionizing radiation?
    a. CT
    b. MRI
    c. Isotopic brain scan
    d. EEG

Answer: a, c.

68. In individuals with the human variety of the Klüver–Bucy syndrome, which symptom is *least* common?
    a. Oral exploration
    b. Amnesia
    c. Uncontrollable sexual activity
    d. Placid demeanor
    e. Anger

Answer: c. All these symptoms may occur as features of the Klüver–Bucy syndrome in humans, as well as monkeys. However, although humans may have increased sexual desire, they usually express it only in inappropriate verbal outbursts and abide by most social conventions. Herpes encephalitis, contusion of the temporal lobes, and multiple strokes are the most common causes of the Klüver–Bucy syndrome in humans.

69. A mother brought her 10-year-old daughter for a psychiatric consultation after the teacher reported that her lack of facial expressivity indicates depression. The girl, however, had been doing well academically and socially, and she seemed cheerful to her parents. The psychiatrist observed that she lacked facial expression and had labial dysarthria. Which of the following should the psychiatrist do to begin the diagnostic evaluation?
    a. Ask the mother to bring in early childhood photographs.
    b. Send the child for neuropsychologic testing.
    c. Send the child for a neurologic consultation.
    d. Send the child for a speech and hearing consultation.

Answer: a. Bilateral facial weakness, which deprives the person of expressivity, may give the appearance of depression. Comparing the child to early childhood photographs, the first step in the diagnosis, should determine if facial weakness is congenital or acquired. Congenital disorders include obstetrical forceps facial damage, velocardiofacial syndrome, and congenital absence of the 7th cranial nerve nuclei, which may be accompanied by absence of the 6th cranial nerve nuclei (*Möbius syndrome*). Although myotonic dystrophy and myasthenia gravis typically appear in young adults, they may appear in prepubescent children.

70. REM sleep behavior disorder is often a precursor of which illness category?
    a. Synucleinopathies
    b. Tauopathies
    c. Cerebral neoplasms
    d. Prion illnesses

Answer: a. REM sleep behavior disorder often precedes Parkinson disease and dementia with Lewy bodies disease, which are both synucleinopathies. The relationship is bidirectional: REM sleep behavior disorder often develops in the course of either of these diseases. In contrast, REM sleep behavior disorder rarely complicates either Alzheimer disease or frontotemporal dementia, each of which is a tauopathy.

71. With which condition is slow gait (≤0.7 m/s) *least* closely associated?
    a. Dementia, in general
    b. Parkinson disease after 5 years
    c. Alzheimer disease, in the first 5 years
    d. Falls

Answer: c. Slow gait is associated with strokes, hospitalization, falls, disability, death, and dementia due to most dementia-producing illnesses, except for the initial stage of Alzheimer disease.

72. A 25-year-old waiter has episodes of feeling dizzy and dreamy that last 3 to 5 minutes. During them, he also has paresthesias in his fingertips and around his mouth. Sometimes his wrists bend, his fingers cramp together, and his foot flexes. An EEG during an episode showed slowing of the background activity. Of the following conditions, which one is the most likely diagnosis?
a. Focal seizures with altered awareness
b. Focal dystonia
c. Absence seizures
d. Hyperventilation

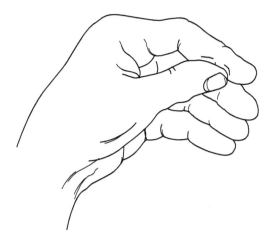

Answer: d. He is probably having episodes of hyperventilation causing carpopedal spasm and EEG slowing. This impression can be confirmed if hyperventilating for 2 to 4 minutes reproduces the patient's symptoms.

73. A retired shoe salesman was hospitalized for a stroke that caused a moderately severe left-hemiparesis. He complained to his children that his nurse had placed a plastic hand on his chest the previous night. He also related that when he buttons his shirt with his right hand, his left hand immediately unbuttons it. When his children asked their father to show them the plastic hand, he groped with his right hand and naively lifted his own left hand. In addition, even though his own watch and wedding ring were in the appropriate place on the left side, he denied that the wrist and finger were his own. Instead, he insisted that they belonged to "Plasticman," who would be returning for his missing limb. Which syndrome does the patient *not* demonstrate?
a. Anosognosia
b. Alien hand syndrome
c. Anton syndrome
d. Denial

Answer: c. Anton syndrome consists of explicit or implicit denial of blindness. This patient, using classic defense mechanisms, shows all the features of the *alien hand syndrome* (or *alien limb syndrome*). He projects his defective left arm and hand to another individual, the alien, Plasticman. The left hand's undoing the right hand's work, "intermanual conflict," is a frequent manifestation of the alien hand syndrome. Patients can assign the role of the controller of the limb to either real or imaginary (confabulated) individuals. This patient is displaying implicit denial. In addition, his failure to acknowledge his hemiparesis is a form of anosognosia.

74. A 32-year-old dentist is referred to a psychiatrist for management of postpartum depression. For 5 months after the delivery of her fifth child, which was complicated by a placental hemorrhage, she finds herself unable to cope with her family. She describes having insufficient energy to do her share of the housework. She is unable to return to work. She never resumed her menses or regained her libido. She has anorexia and has lost 10 lb. Her obstetrician, internist, and a neurologic consultant find no physical signs of illness. Nevertheless, which condition is most likely responsible?
a. MS
b. Lupus
c. Sheehan syndrome
d. Pregnancy

Answer: c. Deliveries complicated by hypotension may cause postpartum pituitary necrosis (Sheehan syndrome). The manifestations of the resulting panhypopituitarism, which may not develop for several months to several years after delivery, include failure of lactation, scanty or no menses, generalized indifference, loss of libido, and easily fatigability. Except for loss of some secondary sexual characteristics, patients usually have no physical abnormalities. The symptoms of postpartum panhypopituitarism may mimic those of postpartum depression.

75. After attempting to conceive for several years, a 33-year-old woman consults a neurologist because she has developed a chronic daily generalized dull headache. Her neurologic examination is normal, but an MRI discloses a small area of increased signal in her pituitary gland. Her serum prolactin concentration is greatly elevated. Which is the most likely cause of her infertility and headaches?
a. Migraine
b. Tension-type headache
c. Prolactinoma
d. Chronic daily headache

Answer: c. A prolactinoma explains the symptoms, MRI abnormality, and elevated prolactin level. If her prolactin level were normal and blood tests disclosed antiphospholipid antibodies, physicians might attribute her headache and infertility to the antiphospholipid syndrome. This disorder is a lupus-like condition that may lead to headache, multiple miscarriages, and strokes or chorea.

76. A 45-year-old woman, pictured below, has developed frequent blinking and intermittent involuntarily closures of her left eye. She has no ocular abnormality or change in intellectual capacity.

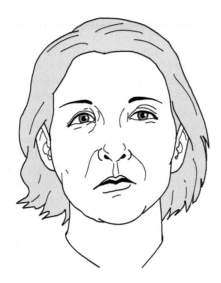 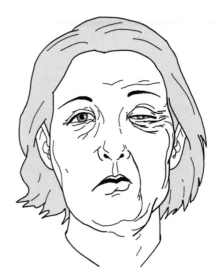

Which area of her nervous system is responsible for her problem?
a. Trigeminal nerve at the cerebellopontine angle
b. Left cerebral cortex
c. Facial nerve at the cerebellopontine angle
d. Autonomic nervous system

Answer: c. The patient has left-sided hemifacial spasm, not blepharospasm or seizures. Note that in addition to the closure of her left upper and lower eyelids, the muscles of the left side of her mouth contract, pulling the mouth laterally and deepening the nasolabial fold. Hemifacial spasm is frequently associated with an aberrant blood vessel compressing the facial nerve as it emerges from the brainstem. Treatment options are botulinum toxin injections and neurosurgical microvascular decompression of the facial nerve as it exits from the brainstem at the cerebellopontine angle.

77. A teenage couple attempted suicide by sitting in a car with the engine running in a closed garage. They were discovered in a comatose state. The young woman recovered. After spending several weeks in coma, the young man began to open his eyes and no longer required a ventilator. Three months later, he was awake but still bedridden. At 1 year, he remains in a flexed posture, mute, and unresponsive to stimulation. From which condition does he most likely suffer?
a. Dementia
b. Global aphasia
c. Persistent vegetative state
d. Isolation aphasia

Answer: c. Carbon monoxide poisoning probably caused generalized cerebral cortex destruction that led to coma and, after 3 months, persistent vegetative state (PVS). PVS is characterized by permanent dementia, unconsciousness, unresponsiveness, and lack of voluntary movement.

78. In which condition is myoclonus rarely if ever observed?
a. Normeperidine toxicity
b. SSPE
c. Neuroleptic malignant syndrome (NMS)
d. Serotonin syndrome
e. Creutzfeldt–Jakob disease (CJD)
f. Mitochondrial disorders

Answer: c. Patients with NMS are frequently tremulous, but myoclonus is much more characteristic of the serotonin syndrome. All of the other syndromes include myoclonus as a common clinical feature.

79. While recovering from abdominal surgery for a gunshot wound, a 25-year-old drug addict complains of incessant severe postoperative abdominal pain. When moderate doses of various opioids fail to alleviate the pain, his surgeons administer pentazocine (Talwin). Afterwards, instead of becoming painfree and calm, he becomes severely anxious, agitated, irrational, and diaphoretic. Which one of the following medicines would reduce the symptoms and allow further investigation?
a. A dopamine-blocking antipsychotic
b. Methadone
c. Butorphanol
d. Benadryl

Answer: b. Pentazocine and butorphanol (Stadol) are mixed opioid agonist–antagonist preparations that may precipitate withdrawal in opioid addicts. Being aware of their vulnerability, opioid addicts often claim, with some justification, that they are allergic to mixed opioid agonist–antagonists. Methadone or other opioids will abort the withdrawal symptoms and alleviate the pain.

80. Physicians hospitalized a 22-year-old previously healthy nurse for the sudden onset of generalized muscle weakness. An internist diagnosed

hypokalemic myopathy. What are *three* causes of hypokalemic myopathy that develop in young adults?
a. Adrenal insufficiency
b. Pernicious anemia
c. Diuretic use or abuse
d. Excessive vitamin use
e. Diarrhea from laxative abuse
f. Steroid use

Answer: c, e, f. Hypokalemic myopathy in previously healthy young adults may be iatrogenic, a manifestation of underlying illness, or self-induced. Hypokalemia is especially likely to be self-induced by health-care workers who surreptitiously take diuretics. Steroids may cause weakness by a direct muscle injury (steroid myopathy) or indirectly by depleting serum potassium (hypokalemic myopathy). Weakness from steroid myopathy is an occasional unintended consequence of bodybuilders using steroids.

81. Which *two* of the following statements concerning prions are true?
a. They contain RNA.
b. They contain reverse transcriptase.
c. They are infectious agents.
d. They cause CJD.

Answer: c, d. Prions are protein-containing infective agents that contain neither DNA nor RNA. They cause CJD and other spongiform encephalopathies. Prions or prion-markers can be identified in cerebral biopsies of patients with Creutzfeldt–Jakob disease (CJD). HIV is an RNA virus that contains reverse transcriptase. Some research has suggested that prions cause several neurodegenerative illnesses, including Parkinson and Alzheimer diseases.

82. During a recent hospitalization for liver failure, a 44-year-old former bartender was anxious, unable to sleep, and fearful of seeing new physicians. He repeatedly asked about the side effects of all medicines, including ones that he had taken for years. He was intermittently lethargic and disoriented. He was always easily distractible and was unable to concentrate on mental status testing. After treatment restored his liver function to normal levels, those symptoms spontaneously resolved. However, several months later, following gastrointestinal bleeding, he had recurrence of the same symptoms, which also resolved when his liver function returned to normal levels. Regarding his being anxious, unable to sleep, and fearful of seeing new physicians, which is the most accurate diagnosis?
a. Anxiety disorder due to another medical condition (hepatic encephalopathy)
b. Substance (alcohol) withdrawal delirium
c. Acute stress disorder
d. Delirium due to another medical condition (hepatic encephalopathy)

Answer: d. Symptoms of delirium often include anxiety, insomnia, unfounded fears, and cognitive impairments, such as disorientation. When the medical condition underlying the delirium resolves, as in this case, those symptoms remit. Anxiety disorder due to another medical condition must not occur exclusively during the course of delirium. Although substance withdrawal may play a role in some cases, there is no historical or clinical evidence that this patient was going through withdrawal during either of his two hospitalizations. Although hospitalization for a serious illness is stressful, this patient does not fulfill the criteria for acute stress disorder because he has a chronic condition rather than exposure to a single event and he lacks the usual manifestations, such as intrusion and dissociative symptoms.

83. A 54-year-old friend of the bartender described in the previous question was brought to the ER after almost a week of binge drinking. He was boisterous and combative. Although he denied having visual hallucinations, he behaved as though he did. He was unaware that he was in an ER and was unable to state the month or year. He could not recall four digits, the current president, or his recent whereabouts. He had tachycardia, mild hypertension, and a low-grade fever, but no nystagmus or extraocular muscle palsy. He was treated with thiamine, other vitamins, and glucose. His blood alcohol level was greatly elevated, and tests for other substances of abuse were negative. Which is his most likely diagnosis?
a. Substance intoxication delirium
b. Substance (alcohol) withdrawal delirium
c. Substance intoxication
d. Delirium due to another medical condition

Answer: a. Granted that the distinction is subtle, but this patient's diagnosis is more likely substance intoxication delirium than substance intoxication because of his disturbance in awareness with disorientation. His cognitive impairment is pronounced and warrants immediate medical attention.

84. The patient described in the previous question underwent a full evaluation that failed to find an alternative diagnosis. Because of his abnormal vital signs and his belligerence, the medical staff admitted him to the medical service. Even with optimum medical care, which condition is most likely to threaten his life?
a. Petechiae in the limbic system
b. Seizures
c. Sepsis
d. Cardiac arrhythmias or cardiovascular shock

Answer: d. Patients with untreated Wernicke–Korsakoff syndrome may develop petechiae (minute hemorrhages) in the limbic system structures, such as the mammillary bodies and periaqueductal gray matter. Individuals may develop seizures either when heavily intoxicated with alcohol or going through alcohol withdrawal, but they are rarely fatal. Sepsis usually follows aspiration pneumonia, but when diagnosed it usually responds to antibiotics. However, cardiac arrhythmias and cardiovascular shock occur frequently with severe alcohol intoxication as well as DTs and are often refractory to treatment.

85. By the time Johnny reached the third grade he was still struggling with simple reading. For example, he confused "b" with "v" and could not grasp the meaning of many of the words that he read. His grammar and spelling were poor when he wrote. Nevertheless, he was above grade level in arithmetic and vocabulary. Also, he was verbal, affable, and quick to respond to almost all the teacher's questions. Which is his most likely diagnosis?
    a. Language disorder
    b. Aphasia
    c. Intellectual disability, mild
    d. Specific learning disorder

Answer: d. Johnny's impairment is limited to reading and writing. Previously called Dyslexia, his disorder would fall into the category of specific learning disorder with impairment in reading and impairment of written expression. The diagnosis of Language Disorder, which is another development disorder, requires a reduced vocabulary, limited sentence structure, and impaired discourse (essentially inability to use words and sentences). Aphasia is an acquired disorder of verbal expression that usually, but not always, includes impairments in reading. The diagnosis of Intellectual Disability, previously called Mental Retardation, requires impairments in all areas of intellectual function and deficits in adaptive functioning.

86. During an evaluation for the learning disability, a school psychologist found that Johnny's father, who was a physician, and one of his sisters also struggled with reading. His other sister, a brother, and their mother all had no particular academic problems. Why can't Johnny read?
    a. He has an inherited left cerebral lesion that should be evaluated with a head CT.
    b. He inherited a genetic mutation specific for dyslexia.
    c. He inherited the fragile X mutation.
    d. He and his father have a deficiency in phenylalanine hydroxylase (PAH).

Answer: b. Inherited genetic mutations underlie many cases of dyslexia. If only for research purposes, genetic testing may be appropriate in Johnny's family. Performing a head CT, however, would be inappropriate because it would detect only large congenital cerebral cortical abnormalities, such as cortical dysplasia, and it exposes children to significant levels of ionizing radiation. An MRI might show a small area of cortical dysplasia and a relatively smooth left-sided planum temporale. Johnny probably does not carry the fragile X mutation, even with a low number of trinucleotide repeats, because this mutation causes global rather than a specific intellectual impairment. Although the fragile X mutation usually causes pronounced intellectual disability in boys, it may cause subclinical cognitive problems in girls. An absence of PAH leads to phenylketonuria (PKU). If untreated,

PKU leads to progressively greater global cognitive impairment and death. Incidentally, many children with dyslexia who receive academic intervention and learn to circumvent their impediment become successful in medicine or another profession.

87. Which of the following disorders is *not* transmitted in an autosomal recessive pattern?
    a. Ataxia-telangiectasia
    b. Homocystinuria
    c. Phenylketonuria
    d. Lesch–Nyhan

Answer: d. Lesch–Nyhan syndrome is a sex-linked recessively inherited disorder. The others are autosomal recessive disorders. They are so uncommon, especially in the case of homocystinuria, that the family history may reveal consanguinity.

88–89. A neurologist is called to see a retired colleague who has suddenly developed severe headache, nausea, and vomiting. He is 82 years old and has a history of hypertension and depression. She finds that he is stuporous and diaphoretic with nuchal rigidity and bilateral Babinski signs. His blood pressure is 210/130 mm Hg. His family reports finding bottles of chlorpromazine, isocarboxazid, propranolol, and meperidine.

88. Of the following, which are the *two* most likely diagnoses?
    a. Adverse medication interaction
    b. Meningitis
    c. Intracranial hemorrhage
    d. Migraine

Answer: a, c. The patient has classic signs of an intracranial hemorrhage: headache, stupor, nausea, vomiting, and nuchal rigidity. He may have suffered a hypertensive cerebral hemorrhage even assuming that he complied with his prescription for antihypertensive medications. Alternatively, he may have experienced a drug-induced hemorrhage primarily from the isocarboxazid (Marplan). That medication, like tranylcypromine (Parnate), phenelzine (Nardil), and others, is a monoamine oxidase inhibitor (MAOI). Meperidine (Demerol) and dextromethorphan will cause similar, potentially fatal interactions with MAOIs. If people who take MAOIs eat certain foods, such as liver or aged cheese, they are liable to develop acute, severe hypertension. Sometimes people purposefully take mixtures of prohibited foods and medicines in suicide attempts.

89. If an MAOI caused a hypertensive reaction, which of the following medications might reduce the blood pressure?
    a. Phentolamine
    b. Chlorpromazine
    c. Propranolol
    d. Dibenzoxazepine

Answer: a. The most specific treatment for an MAOI-induced hypertensive reaction is the α-adrenergic blocking agent, phentolamine (Regitine), at a dose of 5 mg, given slowly and intravenously.

90. Which structure connects the hippocampus and the hypothalamus?
    a. Corpus callosum
    b. Cingulate gyrus
    c. Fornix
    d. None of the above

Answer: c. The fornix connects the hippocampus and mammillary bodies, which are an extension of the hypothalamus. The mammillary bodies, in turn, connect via the mammillothalamic tract to the anterior nucleus of the thalamus.

91. Rescued from a high-speed motor vehicle crash, the driver was stuporous and had forehead lacerations. After he regained consciousness, neurologists found that he had paresis of his right arm and leg and a right-sided Babinski sign. In addition, he had no position sensation in his fingers and toes on the right. The left arm and leg had normal strength and position sensation but decreased pin-prick sensation. He had no language, ocular, or visual impairment. Where is the lesion that is causing his paresis?
    a. Frontal lobe
    b. Brainstem
    c. Cervical spinal cord
    d. Lumbar spinal cord

Answer: c. He has hemisection of the cervical spinal cord resulting in the Brown–Séquard syndrome. The cervical spinal cord is vulnerable in motor vehicle crashes because, when the forehead strikes the wheel or dashboard, the head and neck snap backward (hyperextend). Physicians should evaluate drivers involved in a high-speed motor vehicle crash, especially if they display behavioral abnormalities, for drug and alcohol intoxication as well as head trauma.

92. Of the following, which is the most common cause of acquired intellectual disability?
    a. Angelman syndrome
    b. Down syndrome
    c. Fragile X syndrome
    d. Fetal alcohol syndrome

Answer: d. Although studies have identified risk factors for fetal alcohol syndrome, it is basically the result of the mother's consuming alcohol during and perhaps also before her pregnancy. It is also the most readily preventable cause of intellectual disability.

93. Of the choices offered in the previous question, which is the most common inherited cause of intellectual disability?

Answer: c. The mutation causing fragile X syndrome is passed from parent to child. Although the mother transmitting the mutation is likely to be asymptomatic and fully functional, neuropsychologic testing may reveal learning disabilities. Down syndrome (trisomy 21) is, of course, a genetic disorder, but it is never inherited from a parent, i.e., neither parent has carried the mutation and neither is affected.

94. Of those choices, which is the most common diagnosable cause of autistic spectrum disorder (ASD) symptoms?

Answer: c. Of the several well-known syndromes that include ASD symptoms – Angelman, fragile X syndrome, Landau–Kleffner, Rett, neurofibromatosis type 1, and tuberous sclerosis – fragile X syndrome is the most common.

95. Of the following substances, which one is most likely to produce seizures during an acute intoxication?
    a. Cocaine
    b. Phencyclidine (PCP)
    c. D9-THC
    d. Heroin
    e. Benzodiazepine
    f. Amphetamine
    g. Alcohol
    h. Morphine

Answer: a. Cocaine, whether smoked, inhaled, injected, or swallowed, readily causes seizures. Almost one-half of the cases of cocaine-induced seizures occur in first-time users. PCP and amphetamine cause seizures but less frequently than cocaine. An overdose of heroin or another opioid usually does not cause seizures, except if it leads to hypoxia. The active agent in marijuana, Δ9-THC, actually has a mild AED effect. Just as syphilis was the "great imitator" of 19th century medicine, cocaine intoxication – because it can cause seizures, strokes, involuntary movements, psychosis, bizarre behavior, and myocardial infarction – might be the great imitator of the current era.

96. Which *two* of the substances listed in Question 95 are associated with seizures after several days of abstinence?

Answer: e, g. Benzodiazepines and alcohol generally do not cause seizures during intoxication; however, withdrawal from these substances often produces seizures that are sometimes intractable. Although adult opiate addicts do not develop seizures during either withdrawal or detoxification, babies born of drug-addicted mothers often develop seizures because of opiate withdrawal during their immediate neonatal period.

97. Which one of the substances listed in Question 95 is most likely to cause a stroke?

Answer: a. Cocaine frequently causes cerebral hemorrhages and ischemic infarctions. Furthermore, seizures often complicate cocaine-induced strokes. Amphetamine produces similar mental changes, but it infrequently causes strokes or seizures. In urban young and middle-aged populations, cocaine is the most common cause of stroke. Neurologists in urban areas sometimes quip that cocaine is also the second and third most common cause of stroke.

98. After a 19-year-old college student developed physical and mental agitation, vivid hallucinations, and combative behavior, her roommates brought her to the ER. Although groggy and largely incoherent, she denied use of drugs and alcohol, other than smoking marijuana before her change in mental status. When she previously used marijuana, she never developed such a reaction. She was hypertensive, oblivious to a laceration, and kept her eyes wide open. She made repetitive, purposeless kissing movements. She had three-directional nystagmus. Which of the substances listed in Question 95 is probably responsible?

Answer: b. Pronounced nystagmus is characteristic of PCP intoxication. Somebody probably laced her marijuana with PCP.

99. Which are *two* effects of the normal gamma-aminobutyric acid (GABA)-induced influx of chloride ions?
    a. Neurons are inhibited.
    b. Neurons are excited.
    c. The resting potential is made more negative.
    d. The resting potential is made more positive.
    e. NMDA receptors are activated.

Answer: a, c. The normal resting potential is –70 mV. An influx of chloride ion (Cl⁻), which makes the resting potential more negative, inhibits neuron activity.

100. One dozen unrelated middle-aged individuals have found that, when exposed to various everyday chemicals or merely their odors, they develop asthma-like reactions, skin rashes or pruritus, anxiety, seizures, migraine headaches, paresthesias, and other neurologic problems. They have banded together and formed a community that prohibits the use of perfumes, carpet and other fabric cleaners, dry cleaning, deodorants, and other synthetic and some naturally occurring volatile chemicals. When encountered individually, each seems thoughtful, reasonable, friendly, and well dressed. Which condition would best describe these individuals' condition?
    a. Mass hysteria
    b. Multiple chemical sensitivity syndrome
    c. Neurotoxic exposure
    d. Asthma

Answer: b. *Pseudoneurotoxic* conditions are neurologic disorders that develop or worsen coincident with exposure to a chemical, but the chemical neither causes nor worsens the underlying disorder. Multiple chemical sensitivity syndrome is a prime example of a pseudoneurotoxic condition. Studies have shown that when odors are masked or presented unknowingly to "victims," they cause no reaction. Individuals with multiple chemical sensitivity syndrome tend to band together. Sometimes they establish communities that outlaw as many chemicals as possible. In matters unrelated to chemical exposure, they manifest no overt psychiatric symptoms.

101. Insert the proper enzyme (a–d) into the synthetic steps for epinephrine synthesis.

$$\text{Tyrosine} \xrightarrow{1} \text{DOPA} \xrightarrow{2} \text{Dopamine} \xrightarrow{3} \text{Norepinephrine} \xrightarrow{4} \text{Epinephrine}$$

    a. DOPA decarboxylase
    b. Phenylethanolamine N-methyl-transferase
    c. Dopamine β-hydroxylase
    d. Tyrosine hydroxylase

Answer: 1–d, 2–a, 3–c, 4–b.

$$\text{Tyrosine} \xrightarrow{\text{tyrosine hydroxylase}} \text{DOPA} \xrightarrow{\text{DOPA decarboxylase}}$$
$$\text{Dopamine} \xrightarrow{\text{dopamine-β-hydroxylase}} \text{Norepinephrine}$$
$$\xrightarrow{\text{phenylethanolamine N-methyl-transferase}} \text{Epinephrine}$$

102. In Question 101, which is the rate-limiting enzyme?

Answer: d. Tyrosine hydroxylase.

103. A 28-year-old man has a history of schizophrenia, for which he has been receiving dopamine-blocking antipsychotics. He also uses illicit intravenous drugs. He comes to the ER because he has developed involuntary, intermittent spasmodic muscle contractions in his left arm. The examiner's touching the arm or even loud noises precipitate the arm movements. Physicians find a deep skin infection in the patient's left forearm. His examination is otherwise normal. Which condition is most likely responsible for the left arm movements?
    a. Localized neuroleptic-induced dystonia
    b. Partial status epilepticus
    c. Drug-seeking behavior
    d. Tetanus

Answer: d. The localized form of tetanus occurs in individuals who have partial immunity due to distant or ineffective immunizations. The generalized form of tetanus, which develops in individuals who have never been immunized, causes the muscles of the entire body to have contractions and the jaw to close forcefully (trismus). Tetanus is a hazard of using needles contaminated by soil or rusted metal.

104. Which symptom is the *least* frequent manifestation of Alzheimer disease?
    a. Delusions
    b. Suicide ideation
    c. Hallucinations
    d. Anxiety

Answer: b. With the onset of dementia, Alzheimer disease patients frequently develop anxiety or depression.

Delusions and hallucinations are symptoms of moderate-to-severe dementia. Remarkably few Alzheimer disease patients have suicidal ideation.

105. Which *two* of the following conditions are likely to cause spasticity?
   a. MS that affects the spinal cord
   b. Parkinson disease
   c. Cerebellar degeneration
   d. Poliomyelitis
   e. HTLV-1 myelitis
   f. Myotonic dystrophy

Answer: a, e. Spasticity – increased muscle tone elicited by the examiner rapidly stretching the limb – is a sign of injury to the upper motor neurons of the corticospinal tract. The injury can affect the corticospinal tract anywhere along its path from the cerebrum, through the brainstem, and down the spinal cord. Spasticity is characteristic of MS which affects the brain or the spinal cord, HTLV-1 myelitis (a spinal cord infection), stroke, and many other conditions (see Box 15.1). In contrast, muscle rigidity – inflexibility of muscle – is a sign of basal ganglia disorders, such as dystonia or Parkinson disease. Cerebellar degeneration leads to muscle hypotonia. Poliomyelitis is an infection of the lower motor neurons that leads to muscle flaccidity and atrophy. Myotonic dystrophy induces myotonia, which is delayed muscle relaxation after a contraction or after percussion.

106. In the preceding question, which *two* of the choices are associated with clonus?

Answer: a, e. Clonus, like spasticity, is a manifestation of upper motor neuron injury.

107. In which of the following structures do the lower motor neurons of the limbs originate?
   a. White matter of the spinal cord
   b. Cauda equina
   c. Anterior horn cells of the spinal cord
   d. Neuromuscular junction
   e. Corticospinal tract

Answer: c. The cell bodies of the lower motor neurons of the limbs reside in the anterior horn of the spinal cord and give rise to the motor axons of peripheral nerves. Similarly, the lower motor neurons of the brainstem originate in the motor cranial nerve nuclei, such as the facial nerve (cranial nerve VII) and the hypoglossal nerve (XII).

108. Where do the corticobulbar fibers terminate?
   a. Anterior horn cells of the spinal cord
   b. Cranial nerve nuclei I to XII
   c. Lower cranial nerve nuclei
   d. Autonomic nervous system pathways

Answer: c. Like the corticospinal tract, the corticobulbar tract also contains upper motor neurons; however, it conveys motor impulses from the cerebral cortex to the motor nuclei of the brainstem. The corticobulbar tract innervates nuclei of cranial nerves that supply muscles of the jaw, face, nasopharynx, and tongue.

109. Which of the following substances is particularly toxic to the spinal cord?
   a. *n*-Hexane
   b. Nitrous oxide
   c. Vincristine
   d. Ciguatoxin
   e. Venlafaxine

Answer: b. All these disorders are neurotoxins – some to the spinal cord and some to the peripheral nerves. Nitrous oxide, often a substance of abuse, causes spinal cord damage (myelopathy) because it interferes with vitamin B$_{12}$ metabolism. The others – *n*-hexane (a hydrocarbon solvent), vincristine (a chemotherapy agent), and ciguatoxin (a fish toxin) – cause peripheral nerve damage (neuropathy). Standard antipsychotic agents, selective serotonin reuptake inhibitors (SSRIs), and selective norepinephrine reuptake inhibitors (SNRIs) do not cause either myelopathy or neuropathy.

110. In an attempt to control his bedwetting before a sleep-over, the parents of 8-year-old Richard gave him his usual desmopressin (DDAVP) nasal inhalant treatment. At the sleepover, all the children drank several large cups of soda. By midnight, Richard was stuporous. What is the most likely explanation?
   a. Diabetic coma
   b. Hypoglycemia
   c. Water intoxication with hypernatremia
   d. Water intoxication with hyponatremia

Answer: d. DDAVP is a synthetic form of the antidiuretic hormone (ADH) vasopressin that promotes water retention. Given by injection or nasal inhalation, it prevents enuresis for a single night. Excessive DDAVP, too great fluid intake, or both may lead to water retention, water intoxication, and, by dilution, hyponatremia.

111. Which structure forms the roof of lateral ventricles?
   a. Caudate nuclei
   b. Corpus callosum
   c. Pons
   d. Medulla
   e. Cerebellum

Answer: b. The corpus callosum forms the roof and the caudate nuclei form the lateral walls of the lateral ventricles. The cerebellum forms the roof of the fourth ventricle.

112. Following a firefight where he sustained a blast injury that caused mild but definite traumatic brain injury (TBI), a Marine developed intrusive recollections of firefights, distress, and over-reactions to loud noises. Which of the following sleep disorders is he most apt to experience?
   a. Insomnia
   b. Recurrent distressing dreams
   c. Excessive daytime sleepiness
   d. Multiple awakenings

Answer: b. He has post-traumatic stress disorder (PTSD) in which dreams with affect or content related to the trauma constitute a DSM-5 intrusion symptom. The other symptoms also occur in PTSD but do not fulfill DSM-5 criteria.

113. A veteran sustained a shrapnel wound that transected his thoracic spinal cord 10 years before death. This is a sketch of an upper level of his cervical spinal cord, representing a histologic stain that blackens normal myelin. Which condition does this pattern exemplify?
    a. Wallerian degeneration
    b. Combined system disease
    c. Multiple sclerosis
    d. Tabes dorsalis

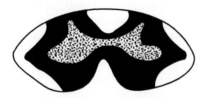

Answer: a. Following an injury, portions of nerve fibers disconnected from their cell bodies undergo Wallerian degeneration. Those tracts lose their myelin and ability to absorb standard histologic stains. (Compare this figure to Figs. 2.15 and 2.18, which map the ascending and descending tracts, and Fig. 2.19, which shows combined system disease, tabes dorsalis, and multiple sclerosis.) The salient feature in this case is that certain ascending tracts, which are sensory, remain unstained and presumably demyelinated because of the thoracic spinal cord injury. In particular, the spinothalamic tracts (anterolateral) and the spinocerebellar tracts (posterolateral) are both mostly unstained. The medial portion of the posterior column, the *fasciculus gracilis*, is also unstained. In contrast, the lateral segment of the posterior column, which consists of the *fasciculus cuneatus*, is stained. The difference occurs because the *fasciculus gracilis* originates in the legs and was interrupted by the gunshot wound and therefore is unstained. However, the *fasciculus cuneatus* remains undamaged and its myelin is normally stained. This man's deficits must have consisted of paraplegia, incontinence, and loss of all sensory modalities in his trunk and in his legs.

114. Which substance is absent in biopsies of voluntary muscles of Duchenne dystrophy patients?
    a. Dystrophin
    b. Acetylcholine (ACh)
    c. Ion channels
    d. Insulin

Answer: a. The muscle cell-membrane protein *dystrophin* is absent in Duchenne dystrophy.

115. A patient who sustained a left cerebral embolus has left–right confusion, finger agnosia, and agraphia. Which other neuropsychologic abnormality is expectable?
    a. Alexia
    b. Dementia
    c. Acalculia
    d. Amnesia

Answer: c. Gerstmann's syndrome, which is usually caused by a dominant parietal lobe lesion, comprises left–right confusion, finger agnosia, agraphia, and acalculia; however, all four components are rarely found together in a single patient, and each component may be incomplete. For example, patients may show dysgraphia and dyscalculia rather than agraphia and acalculia.

116. In the limbic system, which tract conveys impulses between the hippocampus and the mammillary bodies?
    a. Mammillothalamic tract
    b. Cingulate gyrus
    c. Fornix
    d. None of the above

Answer: c. The trajectory of the limbic system is hippocampus and adjacent amygdala; fornix; mammillary bodies; mammillothalamic tract; anterior nucleus of the thalamus; cingulate gyrus.

117. Which chromosome contains the gene responsible for formation of the protein from which Aβ (beta-amyloid) is cleaved?
    a. 4
    b. 14
    c. 21
    d. X

Answer: c. Chromosome 21 contains the gene for amyloid precursor protein, which is cleaved by secretases into Aβ. Thus, trisomy 21 (Down syndrome) individuals, who have three genes for amyloid precursor protein, routinely develop Alzheimer disease.

118. At birth, a male infant is found to have a delicate sac-like protrusion at the base of his spine. His legs have flaccid areflexic paraplegia, and urine dribbles continually from his penis, which never has erections. Which condition do these findings indicate?
    a. Cerebral diplegia
    b. Meningomyelocele
    c. Dandy–Walker malformation
    d. Arnold–Chiari malformation
    e. Spina bifida

Answer: b. The baby has a meningomyelocele. This congenital abnormality usually consists of a deformed lumbosacral spinal cord and cauda equina protruding through a defect in the lumbosacral spine. It causes paraplegia with bladder, bowel, and sexual dysfunction. Studies have implicated maternal exposure to environmental toxins, such as potato blight, and several medications, including valproic acid and carbamazepine. Taking folic acid and other supplements before and during pregnancy reduces the risk of this malformation.

119. Narcolepsy–cataplexy patients are deficient in the neuropeptide transmitter orexin, also known as

hypocretin. Which of the following statements about it is *false*?
a. The lateral hypothalamus is completely or almost completely devoid of orexin-producing cells in narcolepsy patients.
b. Orexin inhibits NREM sleep.
c. Orexin inhibits REM sleep.
d. Orexin promotes wakefulness.
e. Orexin stimulates the appetite.

Answer: b. Orexin actually inhibits REM sleep. In the standard model of narcolepsy–cataplexy, REM sleep intrudes into daytime wakefulness and causes flaccid, areflexic paralysis and sleep attacks. Normal amounts of orexin activity prevent REM sleep from intruding into daytime wakefulness.

120. Which of the following is *not* a feature of ataxia-telangiectasia?
a. Deficiency in IgA
b. Autosomal dominant inheritance
c. Onset of ataxia in childhood
d. Dilated vessels on the conjunctiva
e. Death from sinus or respiratory infection

Answer: b. Ataxia-telangiectasia is a neurocutaneous disorder that is inherited in an autosomal recessive pattern. Children with this disorder have telangiectasias of conjunctival blood vessels, ataxia, IgA deficiencies that often lead to the development of recurrent sinopulmonary infection, lymphomas, and often cognitive impairment.

121. After several years of dementia, a family placed their 80-year-old grandfather in a nursing home. He remained alert and happy in his new surroundings until, over a 3-day period, he became lethargic and then stuporous. Once transferred to a hospital, he was febrile and comatose. A neurologist reported no lateralized findings, indications of meningeal irritation, or signs of increased intracranial pressure. The blood urea nitrogen was 40, the creatinine was 3.0, and the white blood count was 17,000 cells/mL. A head CT showed only age-appropriate atrophy. What would an EEG most likely show?
a. Sleep spindles
b. Diffuse background slowing and disorganization
c. Continual triphasic waves
d. β-Activity

Answer: b. The patient has developed delirium (toxic-metabolic encephalopathy) superimposed on dementia. Dementia is the most statistically powerful risk factor for delirium. The background EEG in dementia may be disorganized and slower than normal, i.e., in the theta or delta range. Sleep spindles characterize the normal NREM sleep phase N2. Triphasic waves develop in hepatic encephalopathy and several other toxic-metabolic encephalopathies, such as severe uremia (more severe than in this vignette). When patients take sedatives, including benzodiazepines, or are anxious, their EEG typically shows β-activity.

122. Which *two* of the following areas of the brain are most vulnerable to chronic alcoholism?
a. Cerebellar hemispheres
b. Optic nerves
c. Cerebellar vermis
d. Corpus callosum
e. Mammillary bodies

Answer: c, e. Although alcohol may damage any of these areas, chronic alcoholism is most likely to cause atrophy of the cerebellar vermis, which in turn causes gait ataxia. Repeated bouts of alcohol consumption lead to damage of the mammillary bodies and other areas of the limbic system.

123. A 66-year-old hypertensive businesswoman had the sudden painless onset of left-sided hemiparesis. She remains fully alert, comfortable, oriented, and with good memory and judgment. In addition, she has right-sided ptosis, the right pupil is dilated, and the right eye is laterally deviated. Which of the following events probably developed?
a. Periaqueductal petechial hemorrhages
b. Subdural hematoma with herniation
c. Midbrain arterial thrombosis
d. Cerebral hemorrhage

Answer: c. She sustained a right-sided midbrain infarction that damaged her third cranial nerve and adjacent corticospinal tract (Weber's syndrome). Because midbrain, pons, and medulla lesions are distant from the cerebrum, cognitive functions are almost always preserved in brainstem infarctions. Of the other possible answers, periaqueductal petechial hemorrhages are indicative of Wernicke's encephalopathy, a condition in which patients have anterograde amnesia, nystagmus, and ataxia, as well as oculomotor paresis. Subdural hematoma with herniation causes brainstem compression that leads to stupor or coma and decerebrate posturing. A cerebral hemorrhage can cause stupor or coma and a third cranial nerve palsy if it compresses the nerve and brainstem.

124. A patient developed areflexic quadriplegia and required intubation and mechanical ventilation. His physicians correctly diagnosed Guillain–Barré syndrome. Although the blood oxygenation was normal, the blood pressure was labile and a generalized seizure complicated his course. A head CT was normal, but the serum sodium was 116 mmol/L. A neurologist attributed the seizure to the hyponatremia. Which is the most likely cause of the hyponatremia?
a. Fluctuating blood pressure
b. Syndrome of inappropriate antidiuretic hormone secretion (SIADH)
c. Cerebritis
d. Central pontine myelinolysis

Answer: b. SIADH often complicates severe Guillain–Barré syndrome. The SIADH causes hyponatremia so severe as to cause seizures. Too rapid correction of hyponatremia might cause central pontine myelinolysis (CPM). Recent studies have shown that too rapid correction of either hypernatremia or hyponatremia leads to demyelination in the cerebrum as well as the pons. These findings have prompted some neurologists to rename the disorder "osmotic demyelination syndrome."

125. Having suffered from well-documented focal seizures with altered awareness (complex partial seizures), since late childhood, a 29-year-old computer programmer began to have a seizure every 2 to 3 months. Most seizures disabled her for at least a day and some had placed her in danger. She has dutifully taken many AED regimens during the previous decades. Her serum AED concentrations were always in the therapeutic range. Because of her uncontrolled epilepsy, she had few friends and she had difficulty completing her work. She consulted a psychiatrist for depression. Which would be the best overall strategy?
    a. Add a third AED
    b. Add an antidepressant to the AED regimen
    c. Change one of the conventional AEDs to a mood-stabilizing AED, such as valproate
    d. Seek consultation regarding epilepsy surgery

Answer: d. She has refractory epilepsy and comorbid depression. Adding a third AED adds only about an 8% chance of suppressing the seizures and its side effects will impose an additional burden. Also, some studies suggest that AEDs entail a risk of suicide. Surgical resection of an identifiable cortical focus offers her the best chance for epilepsy control and improvement in her quality of life. In carefully selected patients, epilepsy surgery is routine, highly effective, and reasonably safe. For this patient, surgery would have been appropriate years before – even after briefer trials of two AEDs. If surgery is feasible, it should greatly reduce if not eliminate her seizures and decrease her AED requirements. Successful surgery will probably alleviate her depression and improve her cognitive function. An antidepressant and psychotherapy may provide additional help. In general, seizure control should be the primary treatment for depression comorbid with epilepsy.

126. A 19-year-old woman with anorexia seeks medical evaluation when she unexpectedly loses additional weight and appears cachectic. She also starts to experience bloating and abdominal distension after meals, diarrhea, and, most disturbingly to her, numbness in her feet. Her neurologic examination shows mild lower leg weakness and sensory loss, and absent ankle DTRs. Routine blood tests, including a glucose tolerance test, are normal. Electrical tests confirm a clinical suspicion of a peripheral neuropathy. Which should be the next procedure?
    a. Pregnancy testing
    b. Serum 5-aminolevulinic acid (ALA) determination
    c. Anti-transglutaminase antibody determination
    d. Skin tests for tuberculosis

Answer: c. She may have celiac disease, which is a gastrointestinal malabsorption disorder characterized by gluten intolerance, malnutrition, weight loss, abdominal bloating, and diarrhea. Without proper diagnosis and treatment, patients eventually develop CNS and PNS complications, most frequently peripheral neuropathy and ataxia. Switching to a gluten-free diet usually resolves the neurologic and other symptoms. Diabetes can cause many of these symptoms, but this patient's normal blood tests exclude it. Pregnancy might be considered as a cause of nausea and vomiting, but not peripheral neuropathy. Urine and serum porphobilinogen and ALA are present in attacks of acute intermittent porphyria, which causes abdominal pain and neuropathy. Tuberculosis (TB) may cause cachexia, but usually fever, cough, and other symptoms of a system infection are also present. Some medicines used to treat TB, such as isoniazid or ethambutol, may cause a peripheral neuropathy.

127. Which one of the following is more characteristic of nightmares than sleep terrors?
    a. They occur in N3 (slow-wave or deep NREM) sleep.
    b. The events are actually frightening dreams with contents that are often recalled on awakening.
    c. They are associated with sleepwalking.
    d. They follow a partial awakening or arousal.
    e. Sweating and tachycardia accompany them.

Answer: b. Sleep terrors are a variety of parasomnia, but nightmares are actually dreams with a frightening content (see Table 17.2: Sleep Terrors Compared to Nightmares).

128. After a minor motor vehicle crash, a 21-year-old waitress presents to the ER with left-hemiparesis. She is alert but distraught. Her visual fields, facial strength, sensation, and deep tendon and plantar reflexes are normal. When the neurologist asks her to elevate and then abduct her left leg against his resistance, the leg has no movement. However, when the neurologist asks her to abduct her right leg, she pushes outward with both legs. What does this demonstration signify?
    a. Peripheral nerve rather than CNS injury
    b. Spinal cord injury
    c. Muscle injury
    d. Cauda equina injury
    e. None of the above

Answer: e. Her left leg, which seems to have no strength, reflexively abducts when she forcefully abducts the right leg. This disparity, the abductor sign, indicates psychogenic weakness. The abductor sign is comparable to the Hoover sign, in which the leg with psychogenic paresis will forcefully push downward or elevate when the patient's efforts are directed toward moving the unaffected leg in the opposite direction. Although the examination indicates psychogenic weakness, this situation lends itself to various interpretations. For example, she may be embellishing a minor physical injury, such as a muscle strain. If she has no injury, she still may be suffering from posttraumatic stress or, for a variety of reasons, completely malingering. As initial steps, neurologists might give a mild analgesic or muscle relaxant and, if the symptoms persist, they might send her for physical therapy.

129. On several occasions, a 21-year-old college student has been unable to rise from bed upon awakening in the morning. In addition, when seemingly paralyzed, the student twice found himself having visual hallucinations. He is otherwise in good mental and physical health. Which one of the following conditions is the most likely cause of his symptoms?
  a. Incipient psychosis
  b. A paroxysm of spikes and waves from the mesial temporal cortex
  c. An intrusion or persistence of REM sleep into wakefulness
  d. Cerebral artery vasospasm

Answer: c. He is probably having sleep paralysis and sleep hallucinations, which are often manifestations of narcolepsy. His physicians should seek other manifestations of narcolepsy, such as fits of daytime sleepiness and cataplexy. In addition, they should consider periodic paralysis (such as from hypokalemia), sleep deprivation, alcohol abuse, and illicit drug use.

130. Which of the following conditions is *not* a common manifestation of trisomy 21 (Down) syndrome?
  a. Neurocognitive disorder
  b. Intellectual disability
  c. Central sleep apnea
  d. Obstructive sleep apnea

Answer: c. Obstructive sleep apnea, not central sleep apnea, is common in trisomy 21 syndrome because of the lax oropharyngeal muscles and large tongue.

131. Six weeks after a cardiac arrest, a 48-year-old man is able to open his eyes, but he is mute and unresponsive to verbal and gestured requests. Although he breathes normally, he has flexion of his limbs, cannot eat or swallow food placed in his mouth, and remains incontinent of urine. An EEG shows slow, low-voltage, disorganized activity. An additional month passes and he does not improve. Which of the following terms best describes his condition?
  a. Persistent vegetative state
  b. Coma
  c. Stupor
  d. Locked-in syndrome

Answer: a. He is in a persistent vegetative state with no consciousness or ability to feel pain or to suffer. He has no cognition or purposeful movements. His prognosis for a functional recovery is less than one in a thousand.

132. Six months after surviving a stroke in which his basilar artery was occluded, a 75-year-old retired merchant seaman remains quadriplegic, mute,

unable to follow verbal or gestured requests, and unable to breathe, eat, or swallow. Nevertheless, through eyelid blinks, he can communicate using Morse code, which he had learned in the Navy. An EEG shows 10-Hz activity over the occipital area. Which of the following terms best describes his condition?
  a. Persistent vegetative state
  b. Coma
  c. Stupor
  d. Locked-in syndrome

Answer: d. In contrast to the prior case, this man has intact cognition. Damage to the base of his pons and medulla impairs his breathing, swallowing, speaking, and movement of his limbs, but he has characteristically retained his ability to communicate. He has preserved decisional capacity.

133. Match the cell type (a–e) with its function (1–5).
  a. Microglia
  b. Astrocytes
  c. Oligodendrocytes
  d. Schwann cells
  e. Ependymal cells
    1. Generate myelin for the CNS
    2. Provide chemical and physical supportive role for neurons
    3. Acting most often as macrophages, perform the primary immunologic defense
    4. Generate myelin for the peripheral nervous system
    5. Line the ventricles

Answer: a–3, b–2, c–1, d–4, e–5.

134. Which of the following statements is *true* concerning steroid-induced psychosis?
  a. It generally occurs only when the dose exceeds 100 mg/day of prednisone or the equivalent of another steroid.
  b. Neuropsychiatric manifestations are usually permanent.
  c. It may induce depressive symptoms rather than euphoria or mania.
  d. EDS occurs more commonly than insomnia.

Answer: c. Steroid-induced psychosis, commonly known as steroid psychosis, usually first causes insomnia, then pronounced euphoria, and eventually a thought disorder, but sometimes depressive symptoms. The critical dose of prednisone is 40 mg/day: lower doses rarely cause steroid psychosis, but higher doses frequently cause it.

135. A cardiologist admitted a 54-year-old man with a history of chronic schizophrenia because he had an acute myocardial infarction. His medications had included a first-generation antipsychotic, but his physicians, surmising that it played a role in causing the infarction, discontinued it. His mental status remained stable and he recovered enough

to enter cardiac rehabilitation. His cardiologist placed him on aspirin and a statin, and withheld all antipsychotics. However, shortly after entering the rehabilitation program, he developed muscle pains and weakness. His creatine kinase (CK) rose to 4000 U/L and his temperature rose to 100.5. His blood pressure rose and his urine turned dark. Which process was most likely to have occurred?
a. He developed neuroleptic malignant syndrome.
b. He developed severe statin-induced myopathy.
c. He overexerted himself in the rehabilitation program.
d. He suffered a seizure.

Answer: b. Statins occasionally cause myonecrosis that bears some resemblance to neuroleptic malignant syndrome.

136. Which one of the following neurologic infections is caused by a spirochete?
a. AIDS encephalitis
b. Meningococcal meningitis
c. Herpes simplex encephalitis
d. Lyme disease

Answer: d. Syphilis is not the only spirochete infection. *Borrelia burgdorferi*, a different spirochete, causes Lyme disease. Its neurologic manifestations include meningitis, encephalitis, bilateral or unilateral facial weakness (which mimics Bell palsy), and polyneuropathy.

137. Which *three* of the following individuals might have an EEG showing electrocerebral silence?
a. A 10-year-old boy underwater for 10 minutes in an icy pond
b. A 60-year-old man, comatose and apneic, from taking an overdose of barbiturates
c. A 55-year-old woman with the locked-in syndrome for 1 year
d. A 65-year-old man with a decade of Alzheimer disease dementia
e. A 17-year-old boy who sustained massive head trauma in a motor vehicle crash has a Glasgow Coma Scale of 3
f. A 79-year-old man in a persistent vegetative state

Answer: a, b, e. EEG electrocerebral silence, a "flat" EEG, usually indicates brain death. Head trauma in an organ donor candidate is the most common circumstance when an EEG is performed to confirm a clinical diagnosis of brain death. A Glasgow Coma Scale of 3 indicates no brainstem or cerebral function, but additional testing is required to document brain death. On the other hand, an EEG showing electrocerebral silence cannot confirm brain death in individuals who have either hypothermia, such as occurs in children who have drowned in icy ponds, or anyone who has taken a barbiturate overdose. Although these individuals often have no clinical sign of brain activity and their EEGs show electrocerebral silence, they may make a full recovery.

138. Which *three* of the following are effects of caffeine consumption?
a. Headaches
b. Bradycardia
c. Prolonged sleep latency
d. Sleep fragmentation
e. Urinary retention
f. Tremor

Answer: c, d, f. Although it is one of the world's most popular drugs, caffeine impairs sleep, induces diuresis, provokes tremor in susceptible individuals, and causes tachycardia, palpitations, and other cardiac disturbances. Its mental effects sometimes mimic anxiety. Moreover, caffeine withdrawal, even from missing a customary morning coffee, may produce headache and anxiety.

139. Which *four* of the following headaches occur predominantly in the morning?
a. Tension headaches
b. Sleep apnea
c. Brain tumors
d. Chronic obstructive lung disease
e. Sleeping in a warm room with no fresh air
f. Trigeminal neuralgia

Answer: b, c, d, e. Increased carbon dioxide blood levels from pulmonary dysfunction or absence of circulating air leads to painful cerebral vasodilation. At their onset, brain tumors cause increased intracranial pressure when the patient is recumbent.

140. Insert the proper substrates (a–e) into the synthesis and metabolism of dopamine.

$$1 \xrightarrow{\text{tyrosine hydroxylase}} 2 \xrightarrow{\text{DOPA decarboxylase}}$$
$$3 \xrightarrow{\text{dopamine-}\beta\text{-hydroxylase}}$$
$$4 \xrightarrow{\text{phenylethanolamine N-methyl-transferase}} 5$$

a. Dopamine
b. Epinephrine
c. DOPA
d. Norepinephrine
e. Tyrosine

Answer: 1–e, 2–c, 3–a, 4–d, 5–b.

$$\text{Tyrosine} \xrightarrow{\text{tyrosine hydroxylase}} \text{DOPA} \xrightarrow{\text{DOPA decarboxylase}}$$
$$\text{Dopamine} \xrightarrow{\text{dopamine }\beta\text{-hydroxylase}} \text{Norepinephrine}$$
$$\xrightarrow{\text{phenylethanolamine N-methyl-transferase}} \text{Epinephrine}$$

141. Complete the indolamine pathway.

$$\text{Tryptophan} \xrightarrow{\text{tryptophan hydroxylase}}$$
$$5\text{-X} \xrightarrow{\text{amino acid decarboxylase}} 5\text{-Y}$$
$$\xrightarrow{\text{MAO}} 5\text{-Z}$$

Answer: X = hydroxytryptophan, Y = hydroxytryptamine, Z = Hydroxyindoleacetic acid

142. What will the olfactory bulb show in a patient with Alzheimer disease?
    a. Plaques and tangles
    b. Lewy bodies
    c. Spongiform changes
    d. No abnormality

Answer: a. In neurodegenerative diseases, the olfactory bulb tends to show the same pathology as the cerebral cortex. Examination of the olfactory bulb in Alzheimer disease shows plaques and tangles; in Parkinson disease and dementia with Lewy bodies, it shows Lewy bodies; in Creutzfeldt–Jakob disease it shows spongiform changes.

143. A neurologist examined a 70-year-old man who sustained a right cerebral infarction resulting in left hemiplegia. As the neurologist was washing her hands at a bedside sink, the patient pointed to his own left arm and asked her, "Doc! Did you break your arm? Here it is." What disturbance probably gave rise to that question?
    a. Inappropriate humor
    b. Dementia
    c. Neglect
    d. A psychogenic disturbance

Answer: c. Patients with nondominant hemisphere lesions, unable to comprehend or accept their left hemiplegia, often disown their body parts and, as a defense mechanism, project them to others. As in this case, patients with anosognosia use projection.

144. Which of the following tastes is based on L-glutamate?
    a. Sweet
    b. Sour
    c. Salty
    d. Bitter
    e. Umami

Answer: e. Umami, the "fifth taste," is the detection of L-glutamate, which people perceive as "richness." For example, foods flavored with monosodium glutamate (MSG) taste flavorful and satisfying.

145. During which period of gestation is the neural tube formed?
    a. First trimester
    b. Second trimester
    c. Third trimester
    d. Variable time
    e. At the moment of conception

Answer: a. During the third and fourth weeks of gestation, the dorsal ectoderm invaginates to form a closed, midline neural tube that eventually gives rise to the spinal cord and other elements of the neural tube. This is an intricate maneuver that is susceptible to disruption by toxins and medications, including AEDs. Improper neural tube closure leads to neural tube defects such as meningomyelocele.

146. Match the medication category with its potential adverse reaction or side effects.
    1. β-Blocker
    2. Phenytoin
    3. Caffeine
    4. Anticholinergics
    5. SSRIs with MAO inhibitors
    a. Agitation, myoclonus, fever, diarrhea
    b. Blurred vision, urinary difficulty, forgetfulness
    c. Palpitations, tachycardia, anxiety
    d. Exfoliative dermatitis, especially at mucocutaneous boarders
    e. Bradycardia, orthostatic hypotension, fatigue

Answer: 1–e, 2–d (Stevens–Johnson syndrome), 3–c (caffeinism), 4–b (anticholinergic effects), 5–a (serotonin syndrome).

147. After falling down a flight of stairs, a 37-year-old woman came to the ER with severe low back pain. She reports numbness in her vagina and rectum. After several hours of urinary retention, she saw that she had urinary incontinence. She was unable to walk because of weakness of her left leg and ankle. Both Achilles' DTRs were absent. Her bladder was distended. Which is the most accurate diagnosis?
    a. Psychogenic paresis
    b. Herniated lumbosacral disk
    c. Cauda equina syndrome
    d. Peripheral neuropathy

Answer: c. She has saddle anesthesia, overflow urinary incontinence, and areflexic paresis of at least one distal lower extremity – the triad of the cauda equina syndrome. As in her case, the cause is often an acute, massively herniated disk compressing the lower lumbar and sacral nerve roots within the spinal canal. Other causes include penetrating wounds and metastatic tumors of the lumbosacral spine.

148. A 44-year-old Connecticut housewife reports that she cannot recall her day-to-day activities, has become forgetful, feels "tired all the time," and suffers from incessant neck and low back pain. She recalls that her symptoms began 1 year before the visit. They persist despite a course of an appropriate intravenous antibiotic for a diagnosis of Lyme disease. A neurologist found no abnormalities. She has asked her internist to administer a second course of antibiotics, especially to reverse her cognitive impairment. In this situation, which of the following strategies rests on the best medical evidence?
    a. Administer another course of antibiotics.
    b. Only if a repeat Lyme titer is elevated, administer another course of antibiotics.
    c. For the next 6 months, administer a weekly course of antibiotics.
    d. Do none of the above.

Answer: d. Six months after a course of antibiotic treatment for Lyme disease, a small percent of patients describe having persistent, often incapacitating, cognitive impairment, other neuropsychologic symptoms, and fatigue. These symptoms fall under the rubric of chronic Lyme disease or post-Lyme disease syndrome. Some physicians diagnose this disorder on clinical grounds despite the absence of both objective findings and the fact that serologies remain positive for an extended period, even after treatment. Additional courses of antibiotic treatment will not improve patients' cognitive function. Of course, evaluation for chronic fatigue syndrome may help.

149. A 19-year-old female college student, who was diagnosed as having chronic noninfectious hepatitis the preceding year, began to have a subtle decline in her grades. A neurologic examination found dysarthria, tremor, and depression. Except for abnormal liver function tests, routine laboratory testing, MRI, CSF, and EEG revealed no abnormalities. Which test should the neurologist order?
    a. HIV
    b. HTLV-1
    c. MS evaluation
    d. Antistreptolysin O titer
    e. Serum ceruloplasmin

Answer: e. In summary, this patient has hepatic dysfunction, cognitive impairment, depression, tremor, and dysarthria. She may have Wilson disease (hepatolenticular degeneration). A low serum concentration of ceruloplasmin, the copper-carrying serum protein, is indicative of Wilson disease. This illness, which is transmitted in an autosomal recessive pattern, may affect only the liver, but when it has neurologic manifestations, a slit-lamp examination of the cornea should reveal a Kayser–Fleischer ring. Wilson disease is the quintessential "correctable cause of dementia" in adolescents and teenagers. Other causes of hepatic dysfunction and mental changes include mononucleosis, alcoholism, industrial toxin exposure, and illicit substance use. Although MS also often causes tremor and dysarthria, it is unlikely to be present in this case because of her young age, progressive course, early onset of cognitive impairment, and normal MRI.

150. Match the spinal cord tract with its function.
    a. Pyramidal
    b. Spinothalamic
    c. *Fasciculus gracilis*
    d. Spinocerebellar
    e. *Fasciculus cuneatus*
       1. Ascends in the spinal cord to the cerebellum to assist with coordination
       2. Descends as the corticospinal tract to innervate the anterior horn cells
       3. Ascends to convey pain sensation to the brain
       4. Transmits position sense from the upper extremities
       5. Transmits position sense from the lower extremities

Answer: a–2, b–3, c–5, d–1, e–4.

151. Which *four* characteristics indicate that facial weakness is attributable to a seventh cranial nerve lesion rather than a cerebral lesion?
    a. Only flattening of the nasolabial fold
    b. Loss or alteration of taste sensation
    c. Inability to close the eyelid muscles
    d. Hyperacusis or tinnitus ipsilateral to the facial weakness
    e. Aphasia
    f. Mastoid pain

Answer: b, c, d, f. Weakness of upper as well as lower facial muscles and the disruption of hearing and taste sensations characterize a cranial nerve VII injury. When the facial nerve is inflamed, pain is referred to the mastoid region.

152. A 35-year-old woman reports episodes of visual obscuration followed by a throbbing, generalized headache that occurs several times yearly and lasts 5–6 hours each time. Medical and neurologic evaluations and a head CT with and without contrast are normal. Which one of the following conditions is most likely?
    a. Migraine without aura
    b. Transient ischemic attacks (TIAs) from basilar artery stenosis
    c. Migraine with aura
    d. TIAs from carotid artery stenosis
    e. MS

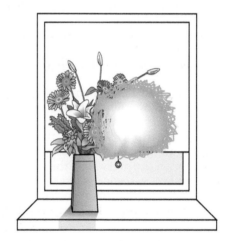

Answer: c. Visual loss or hallucination typically precedes a headache or occurs as a separate symptom in migraine with aura; however, symptomatology of migraine without aura, by definition, does not include sensory disturbances. Although tension headaches are frequently episodic, they are not accompanied by visual symptoms. TIAs of the ophthalmic artery, the first branch of the internal carotid artery, often cause transient loss of vision (amaurosis fugax) in one eye. The visual impairment in such cases usually lasts for less than 20 minutes and has no accompanying headache. Basilar artery TIAs typically cause bilateral visual changes accompanied by vertigo and ataxia, but no headache. MS may cause episodes of unilateral visual loss and pain in or around the eye (optic neuritis), but the symptoms last several days to weeks and usually other neurologic deficits accompany the visual ones.

153. Which symptom is *not* a side effect of treatment for Parkinson disease?
  a. Dyskinesias
  b. Vivid dreams
  c. Sleep attacks
  d. Galactorrhea

Answer: d. Galactorrhea, which is often accompanied by amenorrhea, is a manifestation of excessive prolactin concentration. Increased dopamine activity from precursors or agonists suppresses serum prolactin concentration, but that change produces no symptoms.

154. A 21-year-old woman who was diagnosed at birth as having phenylketonuria (PKU) maintained herself successfully by following a strict phenylalanine-free diet. Once away from home, she deviated from her diet, particularly by drinking diet sodas. She also recently conceived. The father was found not to be a carrier of PKU. Which one of the following statements regarding the fetus is *false*?
  a. In all likelihood, the fetus will be heterozygote for the PKU gene.
  b. In affected (homozygote) individuals, the blood tyrosine level is low and phenylalanine level is elevated.
  c. Although the woman may sustain brain damage by her deviation from the diet, the fetus, which has normal metabolic enzymes, will be unharmed.
  d. PKU infants appear normal at birth.

Answer: c. Because PKU is an autosomal recessive disorder, the mother must be carrying two mutations. Assuming that the father has no mutations, all of their progeny will be heterozygotes. Even though the fetus is heterozygous, an affected mother's excessive phenylalanine consumption can overwhelm the fetus' metabolic systems and produce excessive in utero concentrations of phenylalanine and its toxic metabolic products. When pregnant, women with PKU must strictly adhere to their diet.

155. Which *five* varieties of tremor may be suppressed with β-blocker medication?
  a. Essential
  b. Performance anxiety
  c. Resting
  d. Lithium-induced
  e. Wilson disease
  f. Cerebellar
  g. Hyperthyroid
  h. Psychogenic

Answer: a, b, d, g, h. β-blockers suppress the tremor associated with excessive autonomic nervous system activity that may result from anxiety, medications, or genetic factors.

156. Match the pathologic lesion (a–g) with the associated movement disorder (1–6).
  a. Atrophy of the caudate nuclei heads
  b. Lewy bodies
  c. Depigmentation of the substantia nigra
  d. Infarction of the contralateral subthalamic nucleus
  e. Compression of the seventh cranial nerve by an aberrant vessel
  f. Depigmentation of the locus ceruleus
  g. DYT1 gene
    1. Parkinson disease
    2. Huntington disease
    3. Early-onset primary (torsion) dystonia
    4. Hemifacial spasm
    5. Meige syndrome
    6. Hemiballismus

Answer: a–2, b–1, c–1, d–6, e–4, f–1, g–3.

157. Several days after an automobile accident in which he sustained a whiplash injury, a 16-year-old boy begins to notice neck pain and weakness in his fingers. He has lost pin sensation in a shawl pattern over his shoulder, upper arms, and hands, but vibration and joint position sensation are preserved. DTRs in his arms are diminished, but those in his legs are brisk. Plantar reflexes are equivocal. Which one of the following processes most likely developed?
  a. Worsening of the whiplash symptoms
  b. Development of a herniated cervical intervertebral disk
  c. Bleeding into the center of the spinal cord
  d. Emergence of poststress symptoms

Answer: c. Forceful flexion–extension cervical movement may lead to hemorrhage in the center of the cervical spinal cord – hematomyelia. Its most common causes are motor vehicle, trampoline, horseback riding, and diving accidents. Once it has begun, hematomyelia stretches and disrupts the crossing fibers of the lateral spinothalamic tract, impairing pin and temperature sensation in the arms. The lesion compresses the anterior horn cells of the cervical spinal cord, which contain lower motor neurons that innervate the arms and hands. It also compresses the corticospinal tracts, which cause long tract motor signs in the legs. Syringomyelia (syrinx), the nontraumatic variety of this disorder, develops more insidiously, but the symptoms and signs are similar (see Fig. 2.18).

158. Which medication for treatment of Parkinson disease produces amphetamine or amphetamine-like substances?
  a. Levodopa-carbidopa
  b. Selegiline
  c. COMT inhibitors
  d. Tocopherol

Answer: b. Selegiline (Eldepryl, Deprenyl), an inhibitor of MAO-B, retards dopamine metabolism. Selegiline metabolism yields small, but possibly clinically significant, amounts of amphetamine and methamphetamine. COMT inhibitors produce no such effect.

159. Which of the following is *absent* in patients in the persistent vegetative state?
   a. Quadriparesis
   b. Sleep–wake cycling
   c. Withdrawal of limbs to noxious stimuli
   d. Sustained, meaningful eye contact
   e. Breathing and swallowing

Answer: d. Although patients in the persistent vegetative state may briefly follow (track) individuals or objects, they do not establish sustained, meaningful eye contact. Only vital functions – digesting food, sleeping, and maintaining temperature – persist in the vegetative state. Confusion sometimes arises when family members misinterpret patients' random or reflex eye movements, which remain conjugate, for genuine eye contact and a form of communication.

160. The parents of an 8-year-old girl report that she has episodes of confusion and headache lasting between 1 and 2 days. Her neurologic examination and all routine blood tests were normal. During EEG-CCTV monitoring for epilepsy, the EEG showed no epileptiform discharges during three episodes. However, her serum lactic and pyruvate acids levels rose fourfold. A muscle biopsy showed ragged red fibers and absence of respiratory enzymes. Which should be the next test?
   a. Glucose tolerance test
   b. Chromosome analysis for trinucleotide repeats
   c. Analysis of her mitochondrial DNA (mtDNA)
   d. Polysomnography

Answer: c. Although other causes of episodic confusion – migraines, epilepsy, sleep disorders, and TIAs – might be considered, she probably has a mitochondrial encephalopathy in view of her episodes of confusion with lactic acidosis and the muscle biopsy's abnormalities.

161. A 40-year-old man was struck on the back of his head with a baseball bat. He sustained a skull fracture and was rendered comatose for 2 days. When he became conversant, he confabulated about visitors, was unable to identify his family, and stumbled around his room. He could not count fingers or read the "big E." His pupils were round and reactive to light. Fundoscopic examination revealed no abnormalities. Extraocular movements were normal. He acted as though his vision was intact and explicitly denied that he had visual impairment. What is the nature of his visual impairment?
   a. Retinal detachments
   b. Gerstmann syndrome
   c. Ocular blindness
   d. Cortical blindness

Answer: d. Trauma to his visual cortex has led to cortical blindness. His eyes, optic nerves, oculomotor nerves, and midbrain – which form the light reflex arc – remain normal. His implicit and explicit denial of blindness, with a tendency to confabulate, is a variety of anosognosia (Anton's syndrome). Cortical blindness, complicated or not by Anton's syndrome, may result from occlusion of both posterior cerebral arteries as well as occipital lobe trauma.

162. Match the system (a–d) with the associated structures (1–4).
   a. Cholinergic
   b. Serotonergic
   c. Noradrenergic (norepinephrine-containing)
   d. Dopaminergic
   1. Nucleus basalis of Meynert
   2. Dorsal raphe nucleus
   3. Locus ceruleus
   4. Mesolimbic and mesocortical tracts

Answer: a–1, b–2, c–3, d–4.

163. What is the cardinal feature of conduction aphasia?
   a. Patients cannot name objects
   b. Patients cannot follow simple requests
   c. Patients cannot repeat
   d. Patients have diffuse cognitive impairment
   e. Patients cannot lead a symphony orchestra

Answer: c. Patients with conduction aphasia cannot repeat what they hear; however, they can comprehend and follow requests, and they can name objects. They also may make paraphasic errors. Conduction aphasia results from a lesion interrupting the arcuate fasciculus, which normally connects Wernicke's and Broca's areas (see Fig. 8.3). Because the lesion severs the connecting fibers between two intact centers, neurologists consider conduction aphasia a disconnection syndrome.

164. Which one of the following conditions is *not* a disconnection syndrome?
   a. Alexia without agraphia
   b. Conduction aphasia
   c. Split-brain syndrome
   d. Gerstmann syndrome
   e. Ideomotor apraxia

Answer: d. Except for Gerstmann syndrome, these conditions are disconnection syndromes. Another distinction is that dominant hemisphere lesions cause all but one of these neuropsychologic syndromes: the exception is the split-brain syndrome, which results from a long, lengthwise corpus callosum lesion.

165. Which part of the body is most commonly involved in tardive akathisia?
   a. Head
   b. Arms
   c. Legs
   d. Trunk

Answer: c. Tardive akathisia frequently, most severely, and usually exclusively involves the legs; however, it may also involve the trunk, head, neck, and arms. When akathisia is extensive, it resembles chorea.

166. Which are the *two* most common movements in akathisia?
  a. Walking or marching in place
  b. Tremor of legs
  c. Crossing or rapidly adducting and abducting the legs
  d. Periodic flexion at the hip and ankle, especially when asleep

Answer: a, c.

167. Which statement is *false* regarding most cases of neuropathy associated with HIV?
  a. It is distal and symmetric.
  b. The sensory symptoms, including painful dysesthesias, are more bothersome and more pronounced than motor symptoms, such as weakness and areflexia.
  c. It is associated with depression.
  d. It develops early in the course of the illness.

Answer: d. HIV neuropathy is typically distal, painful, and sensory. It is associated with a high viral load and low CD4 count, and occurs late in the course.

168. A neurologist is consulted for a 37-year-old woman who has seemingly lost her ability to move her left arm and leg during the previous 3 weeks. Although she has gait impairment and has become unable to use utensils with her left hand, she appears unconcerned. Her face is symmetric and her visual fields intact. Her DTRs are symmetric and she does not have a Babinski sign. When asked to abduct her legs against the examiner's hands, the right leg abducts against the force of the examiner's hand. At the same time, the examiner's hand meets considerable resistance when trying to push the left leg medially. Then, the patient is asked to abduct her left leg against the examiner's hand. That leg fails to abduct and, at the same time, the right leg exerts so little force that the examiner easily pushes it medially. Which two of the following statements concerning this case are *false*?
  a. This patient's abductor test suggests a psychogenic basis.
  b. Her lack of obvious concern is strong, reliable evidence of a psychogenic basis.
  c. Patients with left-sided neglect or hemiparkinsonism may have left-sided hypokinesia that might reasonably be mistaken for hemiparesis.
  d. Recent studies have confirmed that psychogenic hemiparesis much more often affects the left than right side.

Answer: b, d. Recent studies have failed to confirm earlier observations that psychogenic hemiparesis is associated with *la belle indifférence* or that it involves the left much more than the right side of the body. If this patient has psychogenic hemiparesis, physicians would probably be able to elicit a Hoover's as well as an adductor sign (see Figs. 3.2 and 3.3). In examining patients with unilateral immobility, physicians should consider neglect and hemiparkinsonism, which can cause hypokinesia without paresis.

169. A medical resident suddenly awakens from a deep sleep intensely fearful, with her heart racing and sweat running down her back. The interruptions do not follow sleep deprivation, alcohol use, or any particular event. Once awake, she worries very little about her patients, but is terribly fearful of her parents' health, her social relationships, and her next job. Whether or not she is able to return to sleep, she can recall her fears in the morning. Which of the following conditions is the most likely explanation for these episodes?
  a. REM sleep behavior disorder
  b. Sleep terrors
  c. Nightmares
  d. Nocturnal panic attacks
  e. Focal seizures with altered awareness originating in a frontal lobe

Answer: d. Panic attacks may arise primarily or exclusively during sleep. In addition to expressing frightening ideas, panic attacks trigger autonomic responses, particularly tachycardia and sweating.

170. A 55-year-old woman and her twin brother, who live hundreds of miles apart, have each developed insomnia that has not responded to several medications. An examination of the siblings reveals inattentiveness and mild confusion, labile hypertension and tachycardia, and myoclonus. MRIs show atrophy of the thalamus. Which illness has developed?
  a. A prion disease
  b. Alzheimer disease
  c. Lewy bodies disease
  d. VCI
  e. Manic-depressive illness

Answer: a. They have developed fatal familial insomnia, a prion illness, because of a genetic susceptibility. This rapidly fatal illness is characterized by cognitive impairment, personality changes, autonomic hyperactivity, and myoclonus as well as refractory insomnia.

171. What is the most caudal (lowermost) level of the body to which upper motor neurons descend?
  a. Foramen magnum
  b. Medulla
  c. Thoracic spine
  d. First lumbar vertebrae (L1)

Answer: d. The spinal cord carries axons of upper motor neurons in the corticospinal tracts. The lowest level of the CNS, which is the lowermost extent of upper motor neurons, is at the first lumbar vertebra (L1). Neurologists perform spinal taps at the L2–L3 level or lower to avoid striking the spinal cord.

172. In which condition does Horner's syndrome fail to appear?
a. Migraines
b. Pancoast tumors
c. Dissection of the carotid artery
d. Lateral medullary (Wallenberg) syndrome
e. Cluster headaches
f. Cervical syringomyelia

Answer: a. Horner's syndrome – miosis, ptosis, and anhidrosis – is found in conditions that interrupt the sympathetic fibers anywhere along their course in the brainstem, cervical spinal cord, superior cervical ganglion, or the cervical chain wrapped around the internal carotid artery (see Fig. 12.14).

173. Of the following, which is the most significant risk factor for stroke?
a. Type A personality
b. Race
c. Hypertension
d. Obesity

Answer: c. Of the numerous risk factors for strokes, hypertension and advanced age are, by far, the two most powerful. Other stroke risk factors include obesity, diabetes, race, and elevated cholesterol levels. All these risk factors tend to be comorbid, but statistical methods such as regression analysis can isolate the individual impact of each.

174. A 50-year-old policeman has developed diplopia on looking to the left. His right pupil is dilated and poorly reactive to light. He has right-sided ptosis. Which injury is most likely to have occurred?
a. Left sixth cranial nerve palsy
b. Right third cranial nerve palsy
c. Right transtentorial herniation
d. Left third cranial nerve palsy
e. Left transtentorial herniation
f. Myasthenia-induced paresis

Answer: b. Although diplopia on left lateral gaze might be attributable to either a left sixth or right third cranial nerve palsy, his ptosis and pupil dilation indicate that the right third cranial nerve is responsible. Patients with herniation are stuporous or comatose. Although myasthenia may cause medial rectus palsy and ptosis, those findings fluctuate and the illness does not affect the pupil.

175. Which finding is most closely associated with tremor on intention?
a. Dysdiadochokinesia
b. Rigidity
c. Bradykinesia
d. Tremor at rest

Answer: a. Tremor on intention and other limb coordination problems, particularly dysdiadochokinesia (impaired rapid alternating movements), are associated with cerebellar hemisphere injury. Tremor at rest, rigidity, and bradykinesia are features of Parkinson disease.

176. Which medicines are appropriate in the treatment of painful diabetic neuropathy?
a. AEDs, such as gabapentin
b. Duloxetine
c. Tricyclic antidepressants
d. Opioids
e. All of the above

Answer: e. Conditions that may induce neuropathic pain include thalamic infarctions, postherpetic neuralgia, trauma, and diabetic neuropathy. Although stemming from different etiologies, the pain usually responds to the same set of medicines, which includes gabapentin, pregabalin, tricyclic antidepressants, and some AEDs. Although SSRIs usually produce little analgesia, an SNRI like duloxetine or venlafaxine is sometimes helpful.

177. Which of the following medications does *not* lower the seizure threshold?
a. Maprotiline (Ludiomil)
b. Diazepam (Valium)
c. Clomipramine (Anafranil)
d. Chlorpromazine (Thorazine)

Answer: b.

178. The family of a 75-year-old man brought him for evaluation for depression because he seemed apathetic, inattentive, and unresponsive. The psychiatrist found that he had marked memory problems and impairments in calculations and construction. The psychiatrist also elicited a history of vivid hallucinations at night and during the day. In fact, the patient seemed to report getting physically involved in his dreams. His wife confirmed hitting and running movements during his sleep. Several months previously, a neurologist had offered a tentative diagnosis of early Parkinson disease because the patient had a slow gait; however, because the signs were subtle and the patient had no functional impairment, he prescribed no medicines. What is the most likely underlying condition?
a. Depression
b. Alzheimer disease
c. Dementia with Lewy bodies
d. Medication-induced hallucinations

Answer: c. The patient has the major features of dementia with Lewy bodies (Major neurocognitive impairment due to Lewy body disease): dementia, fluctuating levels of consciousness, hallucinations, and Parkinsonism. In addition, his sleep behavior suggests *dream enactment*, which is a hallmark of REM sleep behavior disorder. Lewy body disease and REM sleep behavior disorder have a bidirectional relationship: one often follows the other.

179. Video-EEG monitoring is helpful in diagnosing which of the following conditions?
a. The type or frequency of the seizures
b. The presence of psychogenic seizures
c. The origin of seizures

d. Correlation of seizures with AED blood levels

e. All of the above

Answer: e. Video-EEG monitoring has become the standard in diagnosing, classifying, and treating epilepsy. Depending on the circumstances, it also reliably diagnoses nonseizure disorders, including sleep disturbances and psychogenic episodes.

180. Which of the following illnesses is transmitted by a retrovirus?

a. CJD

b. Kuru

c. Gerstmann–Sträussler–Scheinker (GSS)

d. Fatal familial insomnia

e. HIV disease

Answer: e. A retrovirus transmits HIV. Prions transmit the other illnesses.

181. Which of the following medications inhibits HIV reverse transcriptase?

a. Trimethoprim-sulfamethoxazole (Bactrim, Septra, and others)

b. Pyrimethamine (Daraprim)

c. Ganciclovir (Cytovene)

d. Zidovudine (Retrovir)

e. Pentamidine

Answer: d. Previously known as AZT and often given when HIV infection is first detected, zidovudine has increased median survival after diagnosis. Side effects include myopathy, headache, fatigue, malaise, and confusion. Trimethoprim-sulfamethoxazole and pentamidine are each effective for *Pneumocystis jirovecii* (formerly called *P. carinii*) pneumonia. Pyrimethamine (Daraprim) is the treatment of choice for cerebral toxoplasmosis. Ganciclovir (Cytovene) is useful for cytomegalovirus (CMV) infections, especially CMV retinitis and colitis.

182. Which condition constitutes a risk factor for dementia following TBI?

a. Blood type A

b. Apolipoprotein E4 (ApoE4)

c. Rheumatoid arthritis

d. Periodontal disease

Answer: b. Carrying two alleles of ApoE4 predisposes individuals who have sustained TBI to posttraumatic dementia; however, the risk pertains only to moderate or severe injury. Carrying two alleles of ApoE4 also predisposes HIV-infected individuals to HIV-associated neurocognitive disorder (HAND) or neurocognitive disorders due to HIV infection. Periodontal disease is a risk factor for stroke.

183. Which of the following areas of the brain is most susceptible to anoxia?

a. Medulla

b. Wernicke's area

c. Globus pallidus

d. Hippocampus

Answer: d. Although the entire cerebral cortex is vulnerable to anoxia, the hippocampus is the most sensitive. Carbon monoxide poisoning leads to anoxic damage of the globus pallidus.

184. A 55-year-old retired steelworker under treatment for epilepsy reports that he awoke with the worst headache of his life. He developed a throbbing pain centered in and around his right eye and then lost vision in that eye. Its pupil is oval and unreactive to light and accommodation. The entire conjunctiva is red and injected. The left eye is entirely normal and extraocular movements are full. The remainder of his neurologic examination is normal and he has no nuchal rigidity. Which should be the next test?

a. MRI of the head

b. CT of the head

c. LP

d. Determining intraocular pressure

Answer: d. This patient has symptoms and signs of acute angle-closure glaucoma. Physicians must diagnose this disorder by determining intraocular pressure and treat it as promptly as possible. Although many cases have no apparent cause, the use of the AED topiramate led to glaucoma in this patient. Although developing the "worst headache of one's life" suggests a subarachnoid hemorrhage from a ruptured aneurysm, other conditions produce this symptom.

185. Which laboratory abnormality characterizes cyanide poisoning?

a. Marked serum lactic acidosis

b. Arterial methemoglobinemia

c. Serum porphobilinogen elevation

d. Marked arterial carbon dioxide elevation

Answer: a. Cyanide poisons cellular respiratory enzymes. The interruption of their aerobic metabolism leads to marked elevations in lactic and pyruvate acids along with death of highly metabolically active cells, particularly those in the brain. Carbon monoxide poisoning causes arterial methemoglobinemia. Acute intermittent porphyria leads to excretion of porphobilinogen and ALA. Patients with chronic obstructive pulmonary disease characteristically retain carbon dioxide. Carbon dioxide intoxication causes coma.

186. What is the mechanism of action of botulinum toxin when used to treat focal dystonias such as spasmodic torticollis?

a. Like curare, botulinum toxin blocks ACh neuromuscular receptors.

b. Botulinum toxin impairs ACh presynaptic release at the neuromuscular junction.

c. Botulinum toxin depletes dopamine.

d. Like pyridostigmine (Mestinon), botulinum enhances ACh activity.

e. Like nerve gas, botulinum toxin creates a depolarization of the postsynaptic ACh receptor site.

f. Botulinum toxin blocks reuptake of ACh.

Answer: b. Botulinum toxin impairs ACh release from the presynaptic neuron at the neuromuscular junction and thereby reduces the force of muscle contraction. Although botulinum toxin may cause weakness, it greatly reduces the involuntary, forceful, prolonged contractions of dystonia. Curare and many nerve gases block the ACh neuromuscular receptors and thus induce lethal paralysis. In contrast to dopamine and many other neurotransmitters whose activity is largely terminated by reuptake, ACh activity is terminated entirely by cholinesterase metabolism.

187. A 27-year-old actress has excessive sweating in her axilla and profound sweating of her palms. She dreads shaking hands and has even had water glasses slip from her hands because of the moisture. She must change her clothes several times a day. This problem is independent of her stage appearances, but it threatens to exclude her from stage work. She has tried β-blockers as well as antiperspirants and talcum powder. All of them failed to stop or hide the problem. At this point, which would be next best treatment?
    a. Radiation
    b. Botulinum toxin injections
    c. Atropine
    d. Benzodiazepine

Answer: b. Hyperhidrosis responds to intradermal botulinum toxin injections into the affected areas. The toxin reduces the excessive cholinergic activity responsible for the condition. The injections, while painful and requiring repetition every 3 months, are highly effective and rarely produce side effects. Botulinum toxin also reduces excessive salivation when neurologists inject it into the parotid and salivary glands. Radiation will stop sweating, but malignancies may complicate its use. Atropine provides little benefit for hyperhidrosis and produces systemic side effects.

188. Match the brainstem region (a–l) with its location (1–5).
    a. Cranial nerve nucleus that innervates the jaw muscles
    b. Cranial nerve that adducts each eye
    c. Trochlear nerve
    d. Cranial nerves that move eyes laterally
    e. Origins of the nigrostriatal tract
    f. Cranial nerves that innervate the tongue muscles
    g. Cranial nerves that govern speech and swallowing
    h. Thalamus
    i. Hypothalamus
    j. Locus ceruleus
    k. Crossing of the pyramids
    l. Cranial nerve that innervates the upper and lower face muscles
        1. Diencephalon
        2. Midbrain
        3. Pons
        4. Medulla
        5. None of the above

Answer: a–3, b–2, c–2, d–3, e–2, f–4, g–4, h–1, i–1, j–3, k–4, l–3.

189. Which *two* statements concerning syphilis and neurosyphilis are *true*?
    a. In an appropriate clinical setting, a positive CSF-VDRL test confirms the diagnosis of neurosyphilis.
    b. The incidence of syphilis has risen during the AIDS epidemic.
    c. A negative CSF-VDRL test is strong evidence against a diagnosis of neurosyphilis.
    d. A positive serum VDRL or RPR at a dilution of 1:2 is strong evidence of syphilis.

Answer: a, b. Although a positive CSF-VDRL is strong evidence of neurosyphilis, a large proportion of patients with neurosyphilis – 40% in one study – have a negative CSF-VDRL. False-positive serum results, which are generally 1:4 or less, are attributable to other infections, rheumatologic diseases, drug addiction, and changes in serum proteins found with old age. False-negative serum results may be found when the disease is "burnt out," the infectious activity is low, or in rare cases when the antibody concentration is so great that a visible reaction is prevented (prozone inhibition phenomenon).

190. Match the skin lesions (a–k) with its associated neurologic features (1–11).
    a. Adenoma sebaceum
    b. Kaposi sarcoma
    c. Vaginal chancre
    d. Congenital facial angioma in the distribution of the first division of the trigeminal nerve
    e. Acute eruption of vesicles in the distribution of the first division trigeminal nerve
    f. *Café-au-lait* spots
    g. Protuberance of hair tuft, skin, and soft tissue over the lumbar spine
    h. Erythema migrans
    i. Anesthetic, depigmented patches on the coolest regions of the face and body
    j. Dermatitis, diarrhea, and dementia
    k. White lines across the nails (Mees' lines)
        1. Possible later treponema infection of the CNS
        2. Round growths in the brain that cause dementia and seizures
        3. Two layers of calcified cerebral cortical angioma that causes seizures
        4. CNS lymphoma
        5. Neurofibromas
        6. Lancinating pain in the distribution of the skin lesion
        7. Impotence and leg weakness
        8. Pellagra
        9. Bell's palsy-like facial weakness
        10. Leprosy
        11. Arsenic poisoning

Answer: a–2, b–4, c–1, d–3, e–6, f–5, g–7, h–9, i–10, j–8, k–11.

191. Identify the structures (1–6) on this MRI of a normal brain:

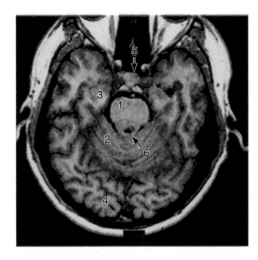

a. Mesial temporal lobe
b. Third ventricle
c. Upper (rostral) portion of the fourth ventricle
d. Midbrain
e. Pons
f. Medulla
g. Pituitary gland
h. Occipital cortex
i. Cerebellum

Answer: 1–e, 2–i, 3–a, 4–h, 5–g, 6–c.

192. In retrospect, the parents of a 4-year-old girl saw that she was losing her ability to speak and had regressed in social interactions during the previous year. When she had a seizure during her sleep, they brought her for an evaluation. No relative had any neurologic or psychiatric disorder. A pediatrician and pediatric neurologist found no physical abnormalities. Routine blood tests and an MRI also showed no abnormalities. Before making a diagnosis of autism spectrum disorder (ASD), which should be the next test?
a. Genome sequencing
b. Audiometry
c. Exploration of why it took the parent a year to recognize their child's regression.
d. CSF analysis for antimeasles antibodies

Answer: b. The first order of business is to see if the child has lost hearing because deafness may explain a child's social withdrawal and apparent cognitive decline as well as lack of communication. Moreover, cochlear implants and learning sign language may ameliorate the problem. Genomic sequencing remains too costly and nonspecific; however, girls who lose milestones and communication abilities should usually undergo genetic testing for MECP2 and other mutations associated with Rett syndrome. CSF analysis for antimeasles antibodies is a good test for subacute sclerosis panencephalitis, but this girl's course was too long and she lacked myoclonus.

193. The girl in the previous question underwent audiometry and related testing which showed no loss of hearing. Genetic testing excluded Rett syndrome. She underwent a 24-hour EEG that captured epileptiform activity, especially during slow-wave sleep. Which of the following disorders is the most likely diagnosis?
a. ASD
b. Landau–Kleffner syndrome (LKS)
c. Elective mutism
d. Fragile X syndrome

Answer: b. Although boys outnumber girls by 2:1, this girl has LKS or acquired epileptic aphasia. This disorder is characterized by regression in verbal communication – aphasia – followed by seizures – especially during slow-wave sleep – in children who have normal development until the age of 2 to 8 years. Physicians should distinguish LKS from deafness, Rett syndrome, and idiopathic ASD. The distinction is sometimes difficult because seizures complicate Rett syndrome and ASD. In LKS, antiepileptic drugs suppress the seizures and many children stabilize and some improve.

194. Which *three* of the following conditions are associated with meningomyeloceles?
a. Intellectual disability
b. Hydrocephalus
c. Neurofibromatosis
d. Intravenous drug abuse
e. Flaccid paraparesis with incontinence

Answer: a, b, e. The primary manifestations of meningomyeloceles are paraparesis and incontinence. They are associated with hydrocephalus and intellectual disability.

195. About 10 days after beginning treatment with phenytoin, a 10-year-old boy developed blister-like lesions on the conjunctiva, mouth, and other mucocutaneous regions. Which condition is most likely?
a. Meningococcal meningitis
b. Child abuse
c. Allergy
d. Seizure-associated trauma

Answer: c. He has developed Stevens–Johnson syndrome, which is a rare, life-threatening, allergic reaction. This adverse reaction has a predilection for mucocutaneous regions, but may involve the entire skin.

196. Which AED has a chemical structure that most closely resembles a tricyclic antidepressant?
a. Phenytoin
b. Phenobarbital
c. Carbamazepine
d. Valproic acid

Answer: c. In their chemical structures, carbamazepine closely resembles imipramine.

197. Which is the best study to identify mesial temporal sclerosis?
a. CT
b. MRI
c. EEG
d. Routine X-rays

Answer: b. MRI provides better resolution than CT and does not produce signal artifacts from the skull.

198. Which cell transmits congenital illnesses attributable to mutations in mtDNA?
a. The egg and the sperm in equal proportion
b. The egg exclusively
c. The sperm exclusively
d. The amniotic fluid

Answer: b. The egg supplies all mtDNA for the embryo. The tail of the sperm contains all of the sperm's mitochondria. After propelling the sperm to the egg, the tail drops off.

199. In testing a 35-year-old man with gait impairment, the neurologist asked him to stand with his feet together with his eyes open and then closed. With his eyes open, the patient was stable. When his eyes were closed, the patient began to topple, but to avoid falling he separated his feet to steady himself. In which *two* regions of the nervous system would damage most likely cause this test result?
a. Peripheral nervous system
b. Cerebellum
c. Posterior columns of the spinal cord
d. Labyrinthine system
e. Corticospinal tracts

Answer: a, c. The neurologist has subjected the patient to the Romberg test, in which a positive (abnormal) result consists of inability to stand erect with closed eyes and the feet held closely together. The explanation is that maintaining a standing position requires intact vision and joint position sensation. An intact sensory system permits continual monitoring and, if necessary, compensatory motor adjustments. Closing the eyes eliminates visual input and forces patients to rely entirely on joint position sensation, which is normally conveyed through peripheral nerves to the posterior columns of the spinal cord to the brain. The Romberg sign is present in both peripheral sensory neuropathies, such as diabetic neuropathy, and diseases that damage the posterior columns of the spinal cord, such as MS, combined system disease, tabes dorsalis, and certain spinocerebellar ataxias.

200. A 50-year-old Caribbean woman walks without bending her hips or knees. She holds her legs straight and closely together with her feet pointed inward. She tends to walk on the balls of her feet and sometimes trips on inclines and when walking up a curb. Tests of her mental status, cranial nerves, and upper extremities show no abnormalities. However, her legs have mild weakness and abnormally brisk DTRs. She has clonus and bilateral Babinski signs, but no sensory loss. MRIs of her brain and spinal cord are normal. Her vitamin B_{12} and copper levels are normal. Which of the following serologies is most likely to be positive?
a. HTLV-III (human T-lymphotropic virus type III)
b. Antiparietal cell and antiintrinsic factor antibodies
c. HTLV-1 (human T-lymphotropic virus type 1)
d. RPR (rapid plasma reagin)

Answer: c. She walks abnormally because her legs are spastic and mildly paretic, which indicates that she has a myelopathy. When caused by HTLV-1, as in this case, the infection is called tropical spastic paraparesis or HTLV-1-associated myelopathy. It occurs in a worldwide swath straddling the equator and is endemic in the Caribbean islands. In contrast, antiparietal cell and antiintrinsic factor antibodies are findings in vitamin B_{12} deficiency, which is the primary cause of combined system disease. Posterior column sensory loss, as well as spasticity, characterizes B_{12} deficiency-induced combined system disease. Positive tests for RPR would indicate syphilis. Tabes dorsalis, a manifestation of tertiary syphilis, produces a steppage gait (see Fig. 2.20) that is almost always accompanied by posterior column sensory loss, areflexia in the legs, and Argyll–Robinson pupils. HTLV-III is an older name for HIV. HIV spinal cord infections produce a clinical picture similar to combined system disease. HTLV-1-associated myelopathy also mimics MS when it involves the spinal cord and the CSF of these patients contains oligoclonal bands; however, MS uncommonly develops in individuals raised in the Caribbean islands.

201. The parents of a 5-year-old boy report that after a normal first 5 years of growth and development, their son has been withdrawing from them and has begun to flap his hands. During a preliminary evaluation, he seems to have below average intelligence and pronounced loss of language skills. He has spasticity. Which of the following illnesses is *least* likely?
a. Autism
b. Rett syndrome
c. Angelman syndrome
d. Cerebral palsy/intellectual disability
e. Lesch–Nyhan syndrome

Answer: d. Except for cerebral palsy/intellectual disability, which is evident by late infancy and nonprogressive, all the conditions have symptoms that appear in childhood and include abnormal hand movements. Although Rett syndrome typically develops in girls, cases – mostly *forme frustes* – have occurred in boys.

202. Of the following, which one is the most common form of inherited intellectual disability?
a. Alzheimer disease
b. Rett syndrome
c. Trisomy 18
d. Fragile X syndrome
e. Turner syndrome
f. Trisomy 21

Answer: d. Of the choices, the fragile X syndrome is the most common cause of inherited intellectual disability. The fragile X syndrome causes retardation in 1 in 1000 to 1500 boys. Fragile X boys tend to have a long, thin face, large ears, and large testes (see Fig. 13.18). The fragile X syndrome occurs in 1 girl in 2000 to 2500, though the intellectual disability is milder than in boys. Although fragile X may cause features of autism in both genders, it has no specific clinical signs. DNA analysis demonstrates excessive CGG trinucleotide repeats on the X chromosome. Neurologists do not consider trisomy 21 (Down syndrome) an inherited condition because the parents of a trisomy 21 patient do not have the mutation and the patients generally do not reproduce.

203. Why is carbidopa administered along with levodopa in the treatment of Parkinson disease?
    a. Carbidopa is a decarboxylase inhibitor that retards the metabolism of CNS L-DOPA.
    b. Carbidopa maximizes the nigrostriatal L-DOPA concentration.
    c. Carbidopa is a MAOI.
    d. Carbidopa is a dopamine agonist.

Answer: b. Carbidopa is a decarboxylase inhibitor that is administered in fixed combinations with levodopa (as in Sinemet). Because carbidopa does not cross the blood–brain barrier, it slows only systemic levodopa metabolism, and thereby maximizes nigrostriatal levodopa concentration. Because small doses of levodopa are effective when administered with carbidopa, patients have relatively few dopaminergic side effects.

204. In evaluating a 68-year-old woman who has begun to have problems walking and performing her activities of daily living, a neurologist tests the patient by asking her to remain in place while she pulls her backward by the shoulders. On one try, the patient involuntarily takes three steps backward. On another, she seems to fall backward "en bloc" (see the figure below). What is the significance of the patient's response?

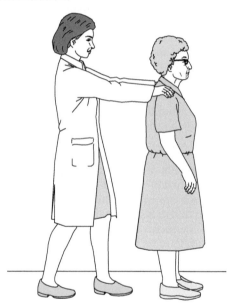

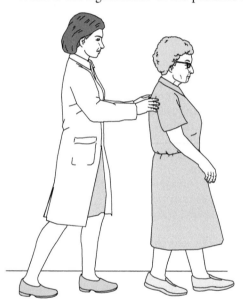

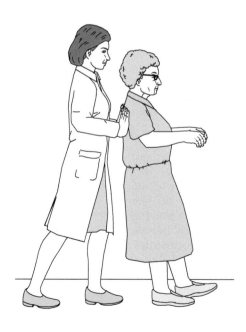

a. She has paresis of all her limbs, as though she had bilateral cerebral infarctions.
b. She has lost cerebellar function.
c. She has impaired postural reflexes.
d. Although the CNS may be normal, the labyrinthine system has been damaged.

Answer: c. She first had retropulsion and then an unequivocally positive pull test. These responses are a result of basal ganglia dysfunction impairing postural reflexes. The pull test (pictured above) is positive in parkinsonism from any cause.

205. Match the treatment of Parkinson disease (a–e) with its mechanism of action (1–4).
   a. Ropinirole
   b. Levodopa
   c. Selegiline
   d. Pramipexole
   e. Rasagiline
      1. A dopamine precursor
      2. A dopamine agonist
      3. An MAO-A inhibitor
      4. An MAO-B inhibitor

Answer: a–2, b–1, c–4, d–2, e–4.

206. Which neuropsychiatric deficit is a manifestation of both transient global amnesia (TGA) and Wernicke–Korsakoff syndrome?
   a. Anterograde amnesia
   b. Retrograde amnesia
   c. Global amnesia
   d. Dementia

Answer: a.

207. An 80-year-old woman who was under the care of a psychiatrist for depression reported the development of apathy, fatigue, and weight loss. Her mood was stable and her medications had not been changed. The psychiatrist found that she had tachycardia and an enlarged thyroid but no tremor, heat intolerance, or sweaty palms. Of the following, which is the most likely diagnosis?
   a. Hypothyroidism
   b. Hyperthyroidism
   c. An occult infection
   d. Renal failure

Answer: b. Hyperthyroidism in individuals aged 80 years or older sometimes presents with apathy, inattention, fatigue, and weight loss rather than with the classic signs of hyperthyroidism: tremor, heat intolerance, sweaty palms, increased appetite, and goiter. In other words, hyperthyroidism in the elderly may present with depressive symptoms and subtle, nonspecific physical signs.

208. Of the following, which feature is most closely associated with dementia in Alzheimer disease?
   a. Cerebral atrophy
   b. Senile plaques

c. Neurofibrillary tangles
d. Pick bodies

Answer: c. Although the initial studies indicated that plaques were the abnormality most closely associated with dementia, recent work indicates that the tangles are even more closely associated. Because tau is the major constituent of neurofibrillary tangles, neurologists sometimes refer to Alzheimer disease as a tauopathy. Cerebral atrophy, which is the only one of these items apparent on MRI and CT, is an age-related change.

209. Match the FDA pharmaceutical pregnancy categories with the fetal risks due to pharmaceuticals.
   a. Pregnancy Category A
   b. Pregnancy Category B
   c. Pregnancy Category C
   d. Pregnancy Category D
   e. Pregnancy Category X
      1. Adequate and well-controlled human studies have failed to demonstrate a risk to the fetus in the first trimester of pregnancy (and there is no evidence of risk in later trimesters).
      2. Either animal reproduction studies have failed to demonstrate a risk to the fetus but there are no adequate and well-controlled studies in pregnant women *or* animal studies have shown an adverse effect (other than a decrease in fertility), but adequate and well-controlled studies in pregnant women have failed to demonstrate a risk to the fetus in any trimester.
      3. Animal reproduction studies have shown an adverse effect on the fetus and there are no adequate and well-controlled studies in humans, but potential benefits may warrant use of the drug in pregnant women despite potential risk.
      4. There is positive evidence of human fetal risk based on adverse reaction data from investigational or marketing experience or studies in humans, but potential benefits may warrant use of the drug in pregnant woman despite potential risk.
      5. Studies in animals or humans have demonstrated fetal abnormalities and/or there is positive evidence of human fetal risk based on adverse reaction data from investigational or marketing experience, and the risks involved in use of the drug in pregnant women clearly outweigh potential benefits.

Answer: a–1, b–2, c–3, d–4, e–5.

210. Which of the following conditions does a positive response to the Tensilon (edrophonium) test indicate?
   a. Muscular dystrophy
   b. Myasthenia gravis
   c. Myotonic dystrophy
   d. None of the above

Answer: b. Tensilon (edrophonium) is a cholinesterase inhibitor that prolongs the effectiveness of ACh at the neuromuscular junction. Edrophonium temporarily reverses ocular and facial weakness in an individual with myasthenia gravis; however, its side effects include bradycardia and excessive salivation. Neurologists sometimes substitute the "ice pack test" for diagnosing myasthenia presenting with ptosis. In this test, the neurologist holds a glove filled with crushed ice against the weak eyelid for 60 seconds. If the cooling, which improves signal transmission across the neuromuscular junction, restores the eyelid's strength and corrects the ptosis, neurologists interpret the response as support for a diagnosis of myasthenia.

211. Which *two* of the following neurotransmitters project from the brainstem to the spinal cord?
   a. Norepinephrine
   b. Dopamine
   c. Serotonin

Answer: a, c. Norepinephrine and serotonin tracts project through the length of the spinal cord as well as to the cerebral cortex. Dopamine tracts also project to the cerebral cortex, but they are confined to the brain.

212. Which of the following neurotransmitters is an indolamine?
   a. Norepinephrine
   b. Dopamine
   c. Serotonin
   d. Epinephrine

Answer: c. Serotonin is an indolamine, which is a five-member ring containing nitrogen joined to a benzene (six-member) ring with an amine group. The other neurotransmitters are catecholamines, structures with a benzene ring with two hydroxyl groups and an amine group.

213. In the preceding question, which neurotransmitter's synthesis begins with tryptophan?

Answer: c. Tryptophan is the precursor for serotonin. Tyrosine is the precursor for the catecholamines.

214. Which EEG activity do benzodiazepines induce?
   a. α
   b. β
   c. θ
   d. Δ

Answer: b. Benzodiazepines induce β-activity. The presence of β-activity may indicate surreptitious benzodiazepine use.

215. Where does the corticospinal tract cross as it descends?
   a. Internal capsule
   b. Base of the pons
   c. Pyramids of the medulla
   d. Anterior horns cells

Answer: c. The corticospinal tract crosses in the pyramids of the medulla, giving rise to its alternative name, the pyramidal tract.

216. Which artery supplies Broca's area?
   a. Anterior cerebral
   b. Middle cerebral
   c. Posterior cerebral
   d. Basilar

Answer: b. The left middle cerebral artery supplies Broca's area.

217. Seizures routinely complicate intoxication or overdose of all but which one of the following substances?
   a. Heroin
   b. Cocaine
   c. Methamphetamine
   d. Alcohol

Answer: a. Heroin overdose rarely, if ever, causes seizures.

218. A 20-year-old woman, who had been in psychotherapy for the recent onset of marked, unexplained anxiety, developed memory impairment, myoclonus, and then focal seizures. An extensive evaluation, including an EEG, MRI, and LP disclosed only a lymphocytic pleocytosis in her CSF. At the suggestion of an astute medical student, further testing detected NMDA receptor antibodies. Which of the following abnormalities is likely to underlie her disorder?
   a. A low CD4 count
   b. An ovarian teratoma
   c. Illicit drug use
   d. AIDS

Answer: b. She probably has NMDA receptor encephalitis, which is frequently a paraneoplastic syndrome. The classic presentation involving NMDA receptor antibodies consists of a young woman who presents with acute neuropsychiatric symptoms and then develops seizures or involuntary movements. The first clue is usually the presence of serum NMDA receptor antibodies. Then transvaginal ultrasound detects an ovarian teratoma. Removing the ovary and initiating immunosuppression usually resolves the problem.

219. An individual with bipolar disorder began to stare into space, stopped speaking, and maintained a fixed posture where he sat with his hands on his hips. The staff was still able to move him into other positions, which he maintained for hours. His blood pressure, pulse, temperature, and CPK levels were normal. Urine analysis detected no illicit substances, particularly PCP. An EEG revealed only beta activity. Which would be the next best test?
   a. CT
   b. MRI
   c. Intravenous lorazepam
   d. Lumbar puncture

Answer: c. This patient has developed, in DSM-5 terminology, Catatonia associated with another mental disorder. Benzodiazepines will briefly reverse it. His normal vital signs and CPK argue against neuroleptic malignant syndrome and the negative urine toxicology excludes drug-induced catatonia. In DSM-5, not all patients with catatonia show its classic signs: catalepsy, waxy flexibility, and mutism. The DSM-5 offers, among the 12 possible signs of catatonia, several that reflect mental or physical hyperactivity, including stereotypy, agitation, grimacing, echolalia, and echopraxia. The DSM-5 also defines another category based on cause: Catatonia associated with another medical condition. It applies the same diagnostic criteria. Catatonia from drug intoxication, especially with PCP, NMDA receptor antibody encephalitis, and other toxic-metabolic aberrations would fall into this category. In contrast, the DSM-5 – somewhat arbitrarily – excludes cases of rigidity and mutism that develop during delirium, neuroleptic malignant syndrome, or treatment with a dopamine-blocking medicine from the diagnosis of Catatonia associated with another medical condition.

220. Which is the most characteristic change in Huntington disease?
    a. D2 dopamine receptors are hypoactive.
    b. D2 dopamine receptors are hyperactive.
    c. ACh receptors are reduced in the nucleus basalis of Meynert.
    d. Gamma-aminobutyric acid (GABA) concentrations are reduced to less than 50% of normal in the corpus striatum.

Answer: d. GABA concentrations are reduced to less than 50% of normal in the caudate nuclei, which is a major component of the corpus striatum.

221. In asymptomatic individuals, which substance will bind to cerebral amyloid to assist in the diagnosis of Alzheimer disease?
    a. Pittsburgh compound B
    b. Antibodies to α-synuclein
    c. Serum anti-amyloid antibodies
    d. ApoE

Answer: a. In PET studies, Pittsburgh compound B binds to amyloid, as do florbetapir, flumetamol, and florbetaben. The quantity and distribution of amyloid assists in the diagnosis of Alzheimer disease, even in its presymptomatic stage. Antibodies to α-synuclein in histologic preparations can support a diagnosis of Parkinson disease or dementia with Lewy bodies. Serum anti-amyloid antibodies do not have the specificity or sensitivity for clinical usefulness. ApoE promotes amyloid deposition, but it does not adhere to cerebral amyloid.

222. Of the following tests, which one provides the most reliable confirmation of the clinical diagnosis of MS when it is in a quiescent state?
    a. MRI of the brain
    b. VERs
    c. CT of the head
    d. Testing CSF for oligoclonal bands

Answer: a. In the appropriate sequences, MRI portrays MS plaques as hyperintense white patches. Gadolinium infusion enhances acute plaques, which are associated with MS flare-ups. In addition to distinguishing between acute and chronic plaques, MRI can determine total lesion load and lesion location. Oligoclonal bands in the CSF are only suggestive of the illness. CT is too insensitive for diagnostic purposes.

223. When is MS most likely to be exacerbated?
    a. During pregnancy
    b. During times of psychologic stress
    c. In adolescence
    d. After trauma
    e. During the first 3 postpartum months

Answer: e. Although pregnancy is associated with reduction in MS attacks, women with MS frequently experience exacerbations during the first 3 postpartum months. The other factors are unproven precipitants of MS exacerbations.

224. When contemplating having a second child, a young mother who had developed MS during the postpartum period of her first delivery inquires about the effect of a second or third pregnancy on her MS. Which *two* statements reflect current thinking?
    a. Deliveries are almost always more complicated when the mother has MS.
    b. MS worsens in a stepwise pattern with each succeeding pregnancy.
    c. The number of pregnancies has little or no effect on the ultimate outcome of MS.
    d. Her offspring, compared to the general population, will have a slightly increased risk of developing MS.

Answer: c, d.

225. Once every 1 to 3 months, a 13-year-old girl experiences unilateral throbbing headaches associated with nausea and vomiting. Until the previous year, scintillating scotomata preceded the headaches. Now, she sees distortions of her father, whether or not he is in the room. She sees him expand and contract with his head disproportionately larger or smaller than his body. After 2 to 10 minutes, this visual hallucination disappears. Several minutes afterwards, the headache ensues. Which is the most likely explanation for the visual hallucination?
    a. It is an aura of a seizure.
    b. It is an aura of migraine.
    c. It is an indication of abuse.
    d. It results from hallucinogen use.

Answer: b. She has a well-known migraine aura, the "Alice-in-Wonderland" syndrome, which consists of seeing enlarged (macropsia) or shrunken (micropsia) versions of oneself, other individuals, or objects. Some body elements, especially the head or an eye, will change disproportionately. Visual hallucinations occur in all of the other conditions, but not with the stereotyped features, regularity, or the subsequent headache.

226. A 32-year-old woman under treatment for depression and obesity reports to her psychiatrist that she frequently awakes at night, goes to her kitchen, cooks and eats bacon and eggs, and returns to sleep. She recalls the events in the morning and days later during her psychiatric visits. Which is the best term for her behavior?
    a. Nocturnal seizure disorder
    b. Nightmares
    c. Sleep-related eating
    d. Kleine–Levin syndrome

Answer: c. Sleep-related eating consists of partly or fully awakening from sleep – usually NREM but occasionally REM sleep – and consuming large amounts of high-calorie food. Sometimes the meal entails elaborate preparation. Reflecting their having been at least partially awake, patients typically recall the eating. Not surprisingly, sleep-related eating is associated with obesity and depression. Because people with this disorder are not fully awake, they sometimes injure themselves when toasting, cooking, or slicing their food. This case probably does not represent seizure activity because the woman reported herself to be fully alert and her activities were thoughtful. Kleine–Levin syndrome is also unlikely because she was alert both during the episodes and during the daytime. Her behavior is unlikely to represent nightmares or other dreams because she has organized, relatively complex behavior and activities. If she had been taking a benzodiazepine receptor agonist, that medicine might have been responsible.

227. Which one of the following is characteristic of the N-methyl-D-aspartate receptor?
    a. It is usually called the NMDA receptor.
    b. It regulates channels that transmit cations.
    c. Excitatory neurotransmitters, such as glutamate, bind to this receptor.
    d. Overstimulation of the receptor leads to cell death by calcium flooding.
    e. The NMDA receptor may be excitotoxic in strokes, epilepsy, and Huntington disease.
    f. All of the above.

Answer: f.

228. A psychiatrist is asked to evaluate a 45-year-old inpatient because she paces incessantly. Following a review of the chart, he found that she had been admitted 3 days before with a diagnosis of major depression with psychomotor agitation. Her treatment regimen included antipsychotic as well as antidepressant medications. Except for her psychiatric condition, she had been in good health. When the psychiatrist asked her why she was pacing about, she told him that she was forcing herself to move and that she was unable to rest.

She had no oral-bucco-lingual movements and no dystonia. Which is the most likely diagnosis?
    a. Akathisia
    b. Huntington disease
    c. Crack dancing
    d. Undertreated major depression
    e. Restless leg syndrome

Answer: a. Although all of these conditions may cause excessive leg movement or pacing, this case's setting and the psychologic drive indicate that the patient has akathisia, which is an acute reaction to dopamine receptor-blocking neuroleptics. Other acute reactions to dopamine-blocking neuroleptics include dystonia of limb muscles, dystonic extraocular muscle movements (oculogyric crises), parkinsonism, and neuroleptic malignant syndrome.

229. What is the pattern of innervation of the anal and urinary bladder sphincters?
    a. The internal sphincter is innervated by the peripheral nervous system, and the external sphincter is innervated by the autonomic nervous system.
    b. The internal sphincter is innervated by the autonomic nervous system, and the external sphincter is innervated by the peripheral nervous system.
    c. The CNS innervates the internal sphincter, and the autonomic nervous system innervates the external sphincter.
    d. The peripheral nervous system innervates the internal sphincter, and the CNS innervates the external sphincter.

Answer: b. The autonomic nervous system innervates the internal sphincter and the peripheral nervous system innervates the external sphincter. The internal sphincter is thus under involuntary control, but the external sphincter is under voluntary control. The internal sphincter is stronger than the external sphincter.

230. Of the following regions of the brain, which *two* are most likely to be damaged by a *coup–contrecoup* blow?
    a. Frontal lobe
    b. Parietal lobe
    c. Occipital lobe
    d. Temporal lobe poles
    e. Cerebellum
    f. Brainstem

Answer: a, d. *Coup–contrecoup* injuries have their greatest impact on the temporal and frontal lobes' anterior–inferior surfaces because they abut the hard bony surfaces of the anterior and middle cranial fossae.

231. Through which structure is CSF normally absorbed?
    a. Spinal cord
    b. Inner surface of the lateral ventricles
    c. Choroid plexus
    d. Arachnoid granulations
    e. Cerebral hemisphere tissue

Answer: d. CSF is normally secreted by the choroid plexus and absorbed through the arachnoid granulations (or arachnoid villi), predominantly at the base of the brain. When meningitis or subarachnoid hemorrhage inflames the arachnoid membrane, CSF absorption is impaired and communicating or normal-pressure hydro-cephalus develops. In those conditions, some CSF may be absorbed through the inner surface of the ventricles.

232. After she underwent vigorous hair washing at her local beauty parlor, a 75-year-old woman developed vertigo, nausea, and diplopia. On examination, she has ataxia and nystagmus. A CT shows no abnormalities. What is the most likely cause of her disturbance?
    a. Cerebral ischemia
    b. Brainstem ischemia
    c. A chemical in the hair wash
    d. Labyrinthitis

Answer: b. Elderly individuals typically have osteophytes that press against their vertebral arteries as they pass upward through the cervical spine. If the neck were hyperextended, as may occur during hair washing, constriction of the vertebral arteries may interrupt blood flow and lead to ischemia or infarction of the brainstem or cerebellum.

233. A 35-year-old psychiatrist in her last trimester of pregnancy has painful tingling in her palms, thumbs, and adjacent two or three fingers. She also loses her grasp of small objects, which seem to drop from her fingers. She has no objective abnormalities. Percussion of the wrist reproduces the paresthesias. What is the cause of her problem?
    a. Entrapment of the median nerve in each wrist
    b. Peripheral neuropathy
    c. Cervical spondylosis
    d. Guillain–Barré syndrome
    e. Lyme disease

Answer: a. She has bilateral carpal tunnel syndrome, which is median nerve compression or entrapment at the wrist. The usual distribution of the median nerve is the palmar surface of the thumb, adjacent two fingers, and the lateral portion of the palm, but many people with carpal tunnel syndrome have sensory disturbances that do not conform to the textbook's map. Paresthesias in the median nerve distribution produced by tapping the (ventral) flexor surface of the wrist – Tinel's sign – are almost pathognomonic (see Fig. 5.3). Carpal tunnel syndrome may occur during pregnancy, before menses, and after trauma to the wrist. "Repetitive stress" during wrist exercising, excessive driving, or construction work, such as jackhammer use, may cause it. Nerve conduction velocity studies that demonstrate slowing in the median nerve across the wrist support a clinical diagnosis. This patient's carpal tunnel syndrome will probably resolve after delivery. Most patients respond to wrist splints, diuretics, or change in activities. Individuals who do not respond to these conservative measures may benefit from steroid injections into the carpal tunnel or surgery.

234. A 19-year-old student at a small New England college was hospitalized after she developed ascending, flaccid, and areflexic weakness of her legs, trunk, and then arms. MRIs of her head and cervical spine were normal. Her CSF contained 5 lymphocytes/mL, a glucose concentration of 55 mg/dL, and a protein concentration of 105 mg/dL. Then she developed ocular, facial, and pharyngeal weakness. When she developed periods of agitation, the intensive care unit physicians solicited a psychiatry consultation. Which of the following conditions is the most likely cause of her disorder?
    a. MS
    b. Botulism
    c. Poliomyelitis
    d. Guillain–Barré syndrome

Answer: d. Her extensive, rapidly advancing peripheral neuropathy and the albumino-cytologic dissociation in the CSF indicate that she has Guillain–Barré syndrome. Neurologists sometimes call this disorder "acute inflammatory demyelinating polyradiculoneuropathy" (AIDP). In contrast, MS produces signs of corticospinal tract paresis; poliomyelitis is asymmetric and does not involve ocular motility; and botulism begins with bulbar palsy. Moreover, those illnesses do not cause albumino-cytologic disassociation in the CSF. On the other hand, many infectious illnesses – *Campylobacter jejuni* infection, mononucleosis, Lyme disease, AIDS, and hepatitis, – can "trigger" Guillain–Barré syndrome. Although several of these illnesses may affect the CNS as well as the PNS, physicians should first assume that hypoxia rather than direct cerebral involvement has caused the periods of agitation. After physicians secure proper ventilation, they can search for the specific etiology.

Botulism usually begins with dysphagia and dysarthria that expands into respiratory insufficiency. Examination of a botulism patient usually reveals large and unreactive pupils, and ptosis. If the attack progresses, victims develop generalized flaccid paresis. Infants sometimes develop botulism by swallowing botulinum toxin-producing spores in unpasteurized honey. In contrast, adults usually develop botulism by ingesting the actual toxin produced by spores in improperly preserved canned foods or occasionally by deliberate poisoning, i.e., attempted homicide. Victims often live near construction sites where spores become airborne or farms where workers and machinery accidentally toss contaminated soil onto food. They require supportive care.

235. Which *three* of the following statements about CNS and PNS myelin are true?
    a. The same cells produce CNS and PNS myelin.
    b. Oligodendrocytes produce CNS myelin and Schwann cells produce PNS myelin.
    c. Both CNS and PNS myelin insulate electrochemical transmissions.
    d. The same illnesses affect both CNS and PNS myelin.
    e. The optic nerves are covered by CNS myelin.

Answer: b, c, e.

236. If a neurologist examines an individual who sustained damage to the left lateral geniculate body, which will be the most prominent finding?
   a. Loss of the ipsilateral pupillary light reflex
   b. Loss of the contralateral pupillary light reflex
   c. Impaired ipsilateral hearing
   d. Impaired contralateral hearing
   e. None of the above

Answer: e. The lateral geniculate body is the origin of the geniculocalcarine tract. The patient will have a contralateral homonymous hemianopia or, if the damage does not affect the entire lateral geniculate body, partial visual loss in the contralateral visual hemifield.

237. The police brought a 31-year-old man to the ER because he had been in a "zombie-like rage" running through a dance club. He was disoriented and combative, and seemed to be hallucinating. His blood pressure was 146/102 and his pulse 132. His pupils were dilated but reactive. He had no nystagmus, muscle rigidity, or lateralized neurologic signs. While the patient underwent testing, physicians provided supportive care and administered a benzodiazepine and small doses of an antipsychotic agent. When he responded, the patient claimed that he had been smoking "bad cocaine." Which is the most likely intoxicant?
   a. PCP
   b. Methylenedioxypyrovalerone (MDPV)
   c. Cannabis
   d. Methylenedioxymethamphetamine (MDMA)

Answer: b. MDPV, commonly known as "bath salts," is a synthetic psychoactive drug that blocks the reuptake of both dopamine and norepinephrine. Like synthetic cocaine, MDPV causes an agitated, hallucinatory, and often paranoid delirium accompanied by signs of a sympathetic surge, such as hypertension and tachycardia. PCP would have caused nystagmus and muscle rigidity. Neither cannabis nor MDMA (ecstasy) would have caused violence or signs of a sympathetic surge.

238. Following vigorous treatment with dopamine-blocking antipsychotic agents for a recurrence of schizophrenia, a 29-year-old man lapses into stupor. His temperature rises to 104° F and his pulse increases to 130 bpm. Neurologists find generalized muscle rigidity. Which one of the following strategies would be *least* helpful?
   a. Treatment with dopamine agonists, such as bromocriptine
   b. Administration of intravenous fluids
   c. Halting further administration of antipsychotic agents
   d. Administration of muscle relaxants, such as dantrolene
   e. Administration of dopamine precursors, such as L-DOPA with carbidopa

Answer: e. He has developed the neuroleptic malignant syndrome. Physicians should attempt to restore dopamine activity, but administering levodopa will not stimulate the receptors because the antipsychotic agents are blocking the dopamine receptors. Supportive treatment should correct the dehydration, fever, and muscle rigidity. Some reports describe success with electroconvulsive therapy (ECT).

239. Which *two* of the following statements are *true* regarding ACh?
   a. It is a neurotransmitter at the neuromuscular junction.
   b. It is a neurotransmitter in the CNS.
   c. Like GABA, ACh is an inhibitory neurotransmitter.
   d. ACh is deactivated equally by re-uptake and by metabolism.

Answer: a, b.

240. The wife of a 65-year-old retired furniture salesman brings him for psychiatric evaluation because she believes that he is depressed. The psychiatrist determines that he shows apathy rather than change in mood or vegetative symptoms. On testing, she finds that he has mild dementia and notes that he walks in an erect, stiff posture and would fall if his wife did not support him. A neurologist finds rigidity and bradykinesia, as well as dementia, but no tremor. In response to the pull test, the salesman has retropulsion. Then, after he trips and falls when walking, the neurologist checks his eye movements and finds that he is unable to look downward or upward, but when the neurologist rocks his head, his eyes move much more fully in these directions. Which is the most likely diagnosis?
   a. Normal-pressure hydrocephalus (NPH)
   b. Parkinson disease (PD)
   c. Progressive supranuclear palsy (PSP)
   d. Dementia with Lewy bodies (DLB)

Answer: c. Loss of vertical gaze that oculocephalic maneuvers overcome (see Fig. 18.11) points to PSP as the cause of the patient's parkinsonism, dementia, and apathy. The abnormal posture and loss of downward gaze, which led to the falling, also point to PSP. Apathy, which may masquerade as depression or severe dementia, is a frequent manifestation of frontal lobe dysfunction that, in turn, may result from multiple strokes, TBI, and numerous neurodegenerative illnesses. Dementia complicates PD, but usually only after at least 5 years of the illness' diagnosis. In another potential explanation, this patient's major findings – dementia and parkinsonism – overlap with those of dementia with Lewy bodies; however, his loss of vertical eye movements makes the PSP diagnosis inescapable.

241. A 30-year-old attorney, who delivered a healthy baby 3 months previously, sought a primary care physician's opinion regarding her lack of energy and failure to restart her menstrual cycle. Because he also elicited a history of unprovoked crying and

other symptoms of depression, he referred her to a psychiatrist. Although the psychiatrist suspected postpartum depression, she wanted to exclude an underlying medical condition. Which consultation should be solicited?
a. Endocrine
b. Nutrition
c. Psychopharmacology
d. None of the above

Answer: a. Postpartum lack of energy and failure to resume the menstrual cycle, even without the mood disorder, may indicate pituitary insufficiency. Unlike the dramatic cases of pituitary hemorrhage during a difficult delivery (Sheehan's syndrome), insidiously developing cases following an apparently uncomplicated delivery are more common. Physicians should include mild pituitary insufficiency or simply hypothyroidism, as well as panhypopituitarism, in the differential diagnosis of postpartum depression.

242. If an EEG shows K complexes, in which state of consciousness is the patient?
a. Coma
b. Deep sleep
c. Light sleep
d. Dreaming
e. Alert
f. Pretending to be unresponsive
g. Sedated by medications or drugs

Answer: c. K complexes are indicative of normal N2 stage of NREM sleep.

243. Which *two* conditions produce areflexic quadriparesis?
a. Hypokalemia
b. REM activity
c. Hyponatremia
d. Cocaine

Answer: a, b. Cataplexy, REM sleep, and hypokalemia from diuretic use or any other cause all produce areflexic quadriparesis. Hyponatremia, when severe, causes stupor and seizures, but not areflexic quadriparesis.

244. Regarding mtDNA, which statement is *true*?
a. Ragged red fibers in muscles are virtually pathognomonic of an mtDNA abnormality.
b. An individual's mtDNA is inherited exclusively from the mother.
c. mtDNA is not carried in the chromosomes.
d. mtDNA abnormalities do not follow a Mendelian pattern.
e. mtDNA abnormalities often elevate lactate and pyruvate serum concentrations.
f. All of the above.

Answer: f.

245. Several hours after a romantic fish dinner in a Caribbean resort, Ken and Barbie developed diarrhea, abdominal cramps, nausea, vomiting, and

fever. They reported to the local physician that they were beset with painful sensations in their fingers and toes. They also found that immediately before the onset of the nausea and vomiting, cold objects, such as glasses filled with ice water, felt hot to the touch and their lips felt tingling and numbness. Which is the most likely cause of their illness?
a. Guillain–Barré illness
b. *Salmonella* poisoning
c. Ciguatoxin poisoning
d. Malaria

Answer: c. Ken and Barbie probably consumed a medium or large reef fish, such as barracuda, grouper, or red snapper, which had eaten smaller fish, which in turn had eaten plankton contaminated with a poison, ciguatoxin. Because this toxin is thermostable, it persists in contaminated fish despite cooking. Ciguatoxin poisoning, common among Caribbean diners, is the most common fish-related food-borne disease. It increases nerve and muscle cell permeability to sodium by opening voltage-gated sodium channels in nerves and muscles. Its primary symptoms, besides headache, nausea, vomiting, and diarrhea, are an acute painful neuropathy and a peculiar sensory disturbance, "heat–cold reversal" or "dry ice effect," in which victims feel a burning hot sensation when touching cold objects.

246. Which description of myotonic dystrophy is *false*?
a. Females as well as males are susceptible to the illness.
b. It is a dystrophinopathy.
c. In successive generations, the disease appears at a younger age because of anticipation.
d. In successive generations, the disease is more severe because of anticipation.

Answer: b. Myotonic dystrophy, which is inherited in an autosomal dominant pattern, results from an excessive trinucleotide repeat mutation. Thus, it causes symptoms at an earlier age and with greater severity (anticipation) in successive generations. Because the muscle membrane defect in myotonic dystrophy consists of abnormal ion permeability, neurologists categorize it as a channelopathy. In contrast, because Duchenne and Becker dystrophies consist of defects in the muscle membrane protein dystrophin, neurologists categorize those muscle diseases as dystrophinopathies.

247–251. Match the following poisons with their mechanism of action.

247. Nerve gases
248. Tetanus
249. Botulism
250. Cyanide
251. Carbon monoxide
a. Blocks the release of glycine and GABA – both inhibitory neurotransmitters
b. Poisons the respiratory energy pathway
c. Interferes with the oxygen-carrying capacity of hemoglobin

d. Inactivates AChE, thereby causing excessive ACh activity

e. Blocks the release of ACh from the presynaptic membrane of the neuromuscular junction

f. Blocks the release of ACh from the presynaptic membranes in the brainstem

Answers: 247–d, 248–a, 249–e, 250–b, 251–c.

252–257. Match the following lifestyles (252–257) with their consequences (a–e). If appropriate, use more than one letter for each number.

252. Steroid injections for bodybuilding
253. Deer hunting in Connecticut
254. Using tryptophan-containing products as a hypnotic
255. Alcoholism
256. Eating undercooked game
257. Excessive pyridoxine (vitamin B_6) consumption
   a. Myositis
   b. Eosinophilia-myalgia syndrome
   c. Upper and lower facial nerve paresis
   d. Hypertrophied muscles, excessive facial hair, amenorrhea
   e. Peripheral neuropathy

Answers:
   252–d.
   253–c, e. Tics in Connecticut are vectors for Lyme disease, which may cause facial paresis or a peripheral neuropathy.
   254–b. Contaminated tryptophan preparations have caused myalgia with eosinophilia.
   255–e. Alcoholism, probably through the associated nutritional deficiency, causes peripheral neuropathy.
   256–a. *Trichinella*, which may survive in undercooked venison, causes trichinosis. The infection causes myositis because the larvae invade muscles.
   257–e. Taking excessive pyridoxine (vitamin B_6) causes a peripheral neuropathy.

258. Friends of a 24-year-old man, who has a history of substance abuse, found him standing in the local high-school football field at midnight in the middle of winter dressed only in short pants. In the ER, he was mute with his eyes open and unresponsive to physicians' questions and requests. He drooled and only stared at his friends and physicians. His blood pressure was elevated and his pulse rapid. On examination, he had intermittent three-direction nystagmus. His muscle tone was so great that it made him rigid. Which one of the following substances is most likely to have caused his condition?
   a. Alcohol
   b. Cocaine
   c. Methamphetamine
   d. PCP

Answer: d. His abnormal behavior and mental status, sometimes termed "wide awake coma," in combination with the nystagmus and muscle rigidity, is characteristic of PCP intoxication. The muscle rigidity mimics the neuroleptic malignant syndrome, but the nystagmus readily distinguishes the two conditions. Although Wernicke–Korsakoff syndrome causes nystagmus, it does not cause either muscle rigidity or mutism.

259. A 25-year-old right-handed epilepsy patient underwent a commissurotomy for intractable seizures. The procedure was successful, but the patient describes not being able to express himself. Which is the most likely explanation?
   a. Aphasia is a complication of the procedure.
   b. Commissurotomy patients lose cognitive function.
   c. Emotions and information generated in the left hemisphere are not as readily verbalized as those generated in the right hemisphere.
   d. Emotions and information generated in the right hemisphere are not as readily verbalized as those generated in the left hemisphere.

Answer: d. Information, ideas, and feelings generated in the right hemisphere no longer cross through the corpus callosum to the left hemisphere-based language circuit. Thus, patients who have undergone a commissurotomy have impairment in verbalizing some information, ideas, and feelings.

260. Of the following illnesses, which *four* are most consistent with this genetic pedigree?

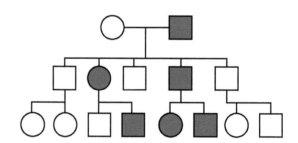

   a. Duchenne muscular dystrophy
   b. Myotonic dystrophy
   c. Phenylketonuria (PKU)
   d. Sickle cell disease
   e. Wilson disease
   f. Huntington disease
   g. Familial Alzheimer disease
   h. DYT1 dystonia

Answer: b, f, g, h. In the standard portrayal of genetic information, circles represent females and squares represent males. Shaded forms indicate affected individuals. In this and subsequent questions, paternity is assured, parents are unrelated by blood, and individuals who are not pictured are presumed to be free of the illness. This kindred illustrates an autosomal dominant disease that has affected both males and females. Myotonic dystrophy, Huntington disease, and early-onset torsion DYT1 dystonia are all autosomal illnesses, although they have different penetrance rates. Alzheimer disease is usually a sporadic illness, but about 10% of families, such as those carrying the presenillin gene, are affected through autosomal dominant inheritance. A recessive disorder, such as sickle cell disease or PKU, is unlikely because the female in generation 1 and two spouses in generation 2 (not represented) would need to be carriers.

261. The individual in this kindred developed a fatal genetic illness in childhood. Which *three* of the illnesses listed in the previous question are most likely to have been responsible?

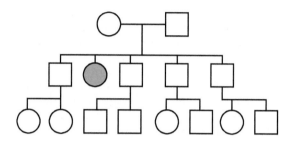

Answer: c, d, e. Her illness was autosomal recessive because neither parent had been affected. Because the victim was a girl, she probably did not have Duchenne muscular dystrophy or hemophilia, which are both X-linked recessive illnesses.

262. In this kindred, the woman in generation 2 is considering having another child. If she were to have another son, what is the probability that he would have the illness that affects his two older brothers?

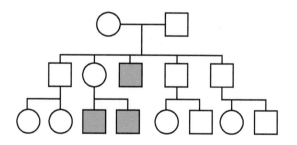

    a. 100%
    b. 75%
    c. 50%
    d. 25%
    e. 0%

Answer: c. Probably the illness is an X-linked disorder because the only affected family members are male and the woman with two affected sons has one normal and one abnormal gene, i.e., she is a heterozygote. Each of her sons has a 50% chance of inheriting the abnormal gene.

263. Of the illnesses listed in Question 260, which one is most likely to have affected the three individuals in Question 262?

Answer: a. Duchenne muscular dystrophy

264. In this kindred, five individuals are affected by a genetic illness that became fatal at the ages designated by the numerals. Of these illnesses, which one is most likely to be responsible?

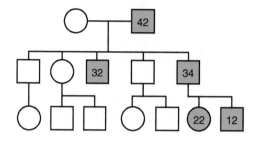

    a. Duchenne muscular dystrophy
    b. Myotonic dystrophy
    c. Hemophilia
    d. Sickle cell disease
    e. Wilson disease
    f. Huntington disease
    g. Alzheimer disease
    h. DYT1 dystonia

Answer: f. The illness is an autosomal dominant disorder that appeared and became fatal at a relatively young age. Although myotonic dystrophy and DYT1 dystonia become apparent in childhood and the young adult years, neither illness is usually fatal during that time. Familial Alzheimer disease becomes apparent before sporadically developing cases, but usually not until at least late middle age.

265. In Question 264, the disease becomes apparent at a younger age in successive generations. In which illnesses listed in Question 260 is that pattern characteristic?

Answer: b, f. Anticipation, the tendency of individuals in successive generations to show signs of a genetic illness at a younger age, is attributable to the instability of abnormal DNA. It is a characteristic of myotonic dystrophy, Huntington disease, and other illnesses associated with trinucleotide repeats.

266. A family is plagued by an illness that affects multiple members of both sexes for four generations (see pedigree below). The illness involves weakness but has variable other features. Symptoms appear between infancy and age 40 years with variable degrees of severity. Which inheritance pattern does the variable phenotype and this family tree indicate?
    a. Autosomal dominant
    b. Sex-linked dominant
    c. Autosomal recessive
    d. Sex-linked recessive
    e. None of the above

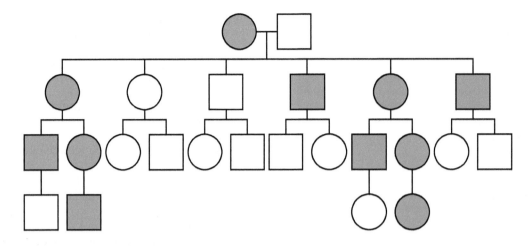

Answer: e. The family tree shows that, although both sexes develop the illness, only the mothers transmit it. A strictly maternal inheritance pattern indicates that mtDNA transmits the illness. Mitochondrial transmission is also fully consistent with the variable phenotype because mutations in mtDNA involve the threshold effect and organs being affected differently. The brain and muscles are particularly vulnerable because mitochondrial illness usually affects organs in proportion to their energy requirements.

267. Which of the following is a disconnection syndrome?
    a. Nonfluent aphasia
    b. Conduction aphasia
    c. Fluent aphasia
    d. Isolation aphasia

Answer: b. Disconnection syndromes generally refer to disorders that result from severed connections between primary neuropsychologic centers with the centers themselves remaining intact. Conduction aphasia results from separation of Wernicke's and Broca's areas.

268. Which *two* forms of communication are usually based, like speech and hearing, in the dominant hemisphere's perisylvian language arc?
    a. Reading
    b. Melody for most individuals
    c. American sign language in congenitally hearing-impaired individuals
    d. Cursing
    e. Prosody
    f. Body language

Answer: a, c.

269. Which is the common neurologic term for the zone of cerebral cortex between branches of the major cerebral arteries?
    a. Watershed area (border zone)
    b. Limbic system
    c. Cornea
    d. Arcuate fasciculus

Answer: a. Neurologists frequently speak of "watershed" areas when discussing regions of the cerebral cortex situated between the territories of major arteries. Only distal, thin branches of cerebral arteries perfuse these areas. This usage inverts the use of the term "watershed" which refers to the crest or ridge between or dividing two drainage systems. In other words, the neurologic term applies to supply of blood, but its origin derives from drainage of water.

270. Which condition is caused by hypoperfusion of the watershed area?
    a. Alexia without agraphia
    b. Fluent aphasia
    c. Hemiparesis
    d. Transcortical aphasia

Answer: d. The perisylvian language arc is well-perfused by relatively large branches of the middle cerebral artery. The more distal cortical regions, the watershed areas, have a tenuous blood supply from distal branches of the anterior, middle, and posterior cerebral arteries. With hypotension, the watershed areas often receive insufficient blood supply and develop ischemia; however, the language arc generally continues to receive an adequate supply. When the perisylvian language arc survives but the outlying cortex is damaged, language function is isolated. It will be devoid of cognitive input, and the patient will be able only to repeat.

271. Which cerebral artery perfuses the cerebral motor cortex for the contralateral leg?
    a. Anterior cerebral artery
    b. Middle cerebral artery
    c. Posterior cerebral artery

Answer: a.

272. A retired concert violinist sustained a stroke that produced left-sided sensory loss but little or no paresis. During the following days, his left hand began to make involuntary, small exploratory movements. The patient, initially unaware of the hand movements, alternately described the hand in derogatory terms, ignoring it, or claimed that it was his roommate's hand. Which condition best describes the situation?
    a. Hemiballismus
    b. Alien hand syndrome

c. Occupational dystonia
d. Aphasia
e. Anosognosia

Answer: b. The alien hand syndrome is the perceptual disorder that is often a component of the nondominant parietal lobe syndrome. Patients with this disorder typically believe the hand acts independently (an autonomous hand) or under the control of another person. They often employ various defense mechanisms.

273. Which of the following apraxias is most closely associated with dementia and incontinence?
 a. Ideational
 b. Gait
 c. Ideomotor
 d. Buccofacial

Answer: b. Patients with normal-pressure hydrocephalus have gait apraxia, urinary incontinence, and dementia. Of those symptoms, gait apraxia is the most characteristic and the one most readily responsive to insertion of a ventriculoperitoneal shunt.

274. As a teenager, a 40-year-old woman had episodic unilateral throbbing headaches several times a month. After she married and had two young children, she then experienced dull, pressure-like headaches several times a week in addition to the unilateral throbbing headaches. During the past 5 years, her headaches have become dull, symmetric, and nonthrobbing, and persist throughout every single day. She has come to rely on non-opioid prescription medications. When she has a flare-up of her headaches, which is about once a month, she visits an ER where physicians give her opioid injections. Further evaluation reveals no underlying neurologic or serious psychiatric disorder. How should physicians classify her continual headaches?
 a. Chronic daily headaches
 b. Tension headaches
 c. Status migrainosus
 d. Obsessive-compulsive disorder

Answer: a. This woman's headaches evolved from migraine to a mixture of tension-type and then into chronic daily headache (CDH). Use of excessive medications, particularly daily analgesics or vasoconstrictors, predisposes patients to CDH. Occasionally patients have been addicted to opioids, sedatives, or anxiolytics before or during CDH. In some patients depression leads to CDH, while in many others CDH leads to depression. Whichever the sequence, CDH and depression are frequently comorbid. CDH is a major management problem because patients request medication for their headaches, but the condition is medication-induced.

275. Patients often perceive migraine pain in or behind their eye (i.e., in the periorbital or retro-orbital location) even though the abnormality is in the meninges or extracranial vessels. Which is the best explanation for this pain pattern?

a. Intraocular pressure rises during migraines
b. Changes that occur in the ocular circulation produce pain
c. The trigeminal nerve innervates the meninges and the pain is referred
d. Nerve receptors for pain in the brain misperceive the location of pain
e. None of the above

Answer: c. The trigeminal nerve's first division (V_1) innervates the meninges, the eye, and its surrounding structures. In migraine and cluster headache, the eye and the periorbital or retro-orbital areas are structurally normal but seem painful because of referred pain. In contrast, the brain itself has no pain receptors. Thus, neurosurgeons can operate on the brain, once they have cut through skull and meninges, without using anesthesia.

276. In the ER, a farm worker who had a history of severe depression was confused and dysarthric. He had bradycardia, miosis, excessive salivation, sweating, and muscle weakness with fasciculations. Which of the following is the best treatment?
 a. Atropine
 b. Neostigmine
 c. Physostigmine
 d. None of the above

Answer: a. The physicians reasonably concluded that he attempted suicide with an organophosphate insecticide poison. The active ingredient of these poisons is an AChE inhibitor. He thus developed ACh (cholinergic) toxicity, which is characterized by miosis, bradycardia, and fasciculations. One readily available antidote for the CNS effects is atropine, an anticholinergic medication that crosses the blood–brain barrier. Physicians can also administer medications, such as pralidoxime (PAM), to reverse the cholinergic toxicity at the neuromuscular junction.

277. After a self-prepared meal, a novice plant lover develops excitation, restlessness, euphoria, dilated pupils, an uncomfortable dry mouth, and an intense thirst. Which of the following would be the best antidote?
 a. Atropine
 b. Neostigmine
 c. Physostigmine
 d. None of the above

Answer: c. This question is the counterpart of the preceding one. This patient has anticholinergic poisoning, readily diagnosed by his excitement, dry mouth, and dilated pupils. Physicians should counteract his excessive anticholinergic activity with an AChE inhibitor that crosses the blood–brain barrier and increases ACh concentrations. Atropine and physostigmine are essentially antagonists of each other.

278. Which *two* of the following statements are true regarding saccadic eye movements?
 a. Their speed is about 30°/s (degrees per second).
 b. Their speed is rapid and can reach 700°/s.
 c. They are governed by supranuclear centers.
 d. Abnormalities in saccades are present in the onset of Alzheimer disease.

Answer: b, c. Saccades are high-velocity conjugate gaze movements that originate in the cerebral conjugate gaze centers. For example, people use them to shift their visual attention from a book to someone entering the room, without looking at any object in between. Abnormal saccades are one of the first physical findings in Huntington disease. Physicians can also detect them in patients with schizophrenia.

279. A 30-year-old woman who has had migraines since adolescence presented to the ER with an unusually severe headache. Wanting to exclude a subarachnoid hemorrhage and meningitis, the physicians performed a lumbar puncture (LP) after obtaining a head CT. The CSF and CT were normal. The physicians concluded that she had only a severe migraine and treated her with a sumatriptan injection. For the next 2 weeks she complained of an incessant dull headache of a 4/10 severity when in bed that increased in severity to 9/10 when standing. Also when standing, she was lightheaded and nauseated. She was unable to eat, walk 20 feet, or go to work. She returned to the ER. A repeat head CT and routine blood tests were all normal. What would probably be the most effective treatment?
    a. Sumatriptan by injection
    b. A short course of opioids
    c. Metoclopramide
    d. Lumbar blood patch

Answer: d. When this patient came to the ER with an unusually severe headache, the physicians reasonably sought to exclude a subarachnoid hemorrhage and meningitis, regardless of her history of migraine. Unfortunately she developed a classic post-LP headache. It may also follow epidural anesthesia if the dura were accidently pierced. In both conditions, CSF presumably leaks and the reduced CSF volume lowers intracranial pressure. Insertion of the patient's own blood into the epidural space will stop the leak and almost immediately alleviate the symptoms. Physicians should avoid treating headaches with opioids. Metoclopramide is helpful in migraines because it suppresses the nausea and allows patients to sleep, which is often curative; however, like other dopamine-blockers, it may lead to dystonic reactions. Sumatriptan by injection is helpful for migraine when nausea and vomiting do not allow for oral medications; however, sumatriptan does not alleviate post-LP headaches.

280. Which condition does *not* cause unilateral miosis, ptosis, and anhidrosis?
    a. Pancoast tumors
    b. Cluster headache
    c. Migraine with aura
    d. Lateral medullary syndrome
    e. Midbrain infarction

Answer: c. Ptosis, miosis (small pupil), and anhidrosis (lack of sweating) comprise Horner's syndrome. Injury of the sympathetic pathway in the chest or neck is the most common cause. Thus, Pancoast tumors produce Horner's syndrome because they invade sympathetic ganglia in the chest. Carotid artery dissections produce it because they damage the sympathetic chain wrapped around the artery. Damage to the sympathetic tract in the upper and more frequently in the lower brainstem (the medulla) may also cause Horner's syndrome. Thus, it is common in lateral medullary strokes, but uncommon in midbrain strokes. In a common example, vigorous neck manipulation may lead to dissection of the vertebral artery, which causes posterior inferior cerebellar artery (PICA) occlusion and the lateral medullary infarction. The two most prominent elements of a Horner's syndrome – miosis and ptosis – are a classic finding in cluster headache.

281. To which *four* vision-impairing conditions are elderly individuals particularly susceptible?
    a. Cataracts
    b. Glaucoma
    c. Strabismus
    d. Amblyopia ex anopia
    e. Macular degeneration
    f. Temporal arteritis

Answer: a, b, e, f. Strabismus is congenital extraocular muscle weakness. If uncorrected, the affected eye will become blind from disuse, i.e., *amblyopia ex anopia*.

282. A neurologic examination of a 75-year-old man shows no abnormality of cognitive or physical function except for impairment of vibration sensation in his toes, absent ankle DTRs, and impaired tandem gait (walking with one foot in front of the other). Pain sensation is preserved. Plantar reflexes are flexor. Which is the most likely explanation for the findings?
    a. Combined system disease
    b. Diabetes
    c. MS
    d. None of the above

Answer: d. He merely has age-related peripheral nervous system changes, which include unsteady tandem gait, loss of DTRs, and impaired sense of vibration and temperature, with preserved pain sensation. Combined system disease and MS cause spasticity and Babinski signs (extensor plantar reflexes). Diabetic neuropathy, which usually develops only several years after the onset of the illness, causes loss of pain and temperature.

283. A 14-year-old boy with congenital cognitive delay has only second-grade academic and communications skills. He has a large forehead, large lobulated ears, and large testicles (macro-orchidism). He has repetitive, stereotyped movements of his face and fingers. His sister is reportedly physically normal, but is "slow" in school. His mother, who is 39 years old, is planning on remarrying a 49-year-old man. They expect to have another child. Which *two* of the following statements are *true*?

a. The boy probably has the fragile X mutation.

b. Because her son's condition is rare, the mother's next pregnancy has no greater risk than for other women of her age.

c. The sister probably is, as the mother claims, merely a mediocre student and does not need further evaluation.

d. Because she is 39 years old, close evaluation is indicated in future pregnancies.

Answer: a, d. The boy has moderate intellectual disability as part of the fragile X syndrome, which is the most frequent identifiable cause of inherited intellectual disability and accounts for about 10% of all cases of intellectual disability. A mutation on the X chromosome consisting of excessive trinucleotide repeats transmits fragile X syndrome. The woman must be concerned because she carries the fragile X mutation and could have another son with the disorder. She is also liable to conceive a child with trisomy 21 (Down syndrome) because she is almost 40 years old and her fiancée's advanced age increases the risk. In addition, because fragile X syndrome in girls appears in a modified form – mild intellectual disability – the boy's sister should undergo evaluation to determine if she carries the mutation.

284. A 17-year-old boy has a dozen light brown, flat "birthmarks," each larger than 3 cm by 1 cm, and axillary "freckles." He inquires about some nodules that have been developing on his arms and face. Which *two* statements concerning these new lesions are *true*?

a. They represent von Recklinghausen disease or neurofibromatosis (NF1).

b. They are closely associated with bilateral acoustic neuromas.

c. His siblings and parents ought to be examined because one of them is likely to have the same condition.

d. They are adenoma sebaceum (angiofibromas), which is the cutaneous manifestation of tuberous sclerosis.

Answer: a, c. He has neurofibromatosis type 1 (NF1), which is a common inherited neurocutaneous disturbance characterized by a triad of six or more *café-au-lait* spots and nodules (neurofibromas) on peripheral nerves that become apparent in adults. NF1 patients tend to develop meningiomas. Approximately 50% of patients acquire the disorder through inheritance. The others apparently acquire it by *de novo* mutation.

In contrast, neurofibromatosis type 2 (NF2), causes bilateral acoustic neuromas and sometimes several *café-au-lait* spots. NF1 and NF2 are transmitted on different autosomal chromosomes: NF1 is transmitted on chromosome 17 and NF2 on 22.

Tuberous sclerosis, an unrelated inherited neurocutaneous disorder, consists of a combination of nodules on the malar surface of the face and tubers in the brain. It causes seizures and mental deterioration. Depending on the mutation, chromosome 9 or 11 transmits tuberous sclerosis. Tuberous sclerosis and NF1 provide the clinician with an excellent opportunity to make a diagnosis by inspection.

285. A woman brought her 68-year-old husband to the ER after he called to say that he had become lost while visiting his customers in a neighboring town. Because he was agitated, a psychiatrist was asked to consult. She calmed him and then determined that his primary problem was memory impairment for recent events, including where he had traveled and the names of his customers. He retained basic, personal knowledge, such as his own name, telephone number, and social security number. He could not recall more than three of six digits, the name of the hospital, or even the name of the psychiatrist who had just introduced herself. She also established that he recognized his memory impairment. His physical neurologic examination, head CT, and routine blood tests were normal. By the end of several hours, the problem cleared. Which of the following conditions is the most likely diagnosis?

a. Transient global amnesia (TGA)

b. Focal seizure with altered awareness

c. Psychogenic amnesia

d. An anticholinergic medication

Answer: a. The salient feature of this hours-long episode of amnesia is the preservation of personal, deeply seated ("overlearned") information. He most likely experienced an episode of TGA. As in this case, TGA causes amnesia especially for recently acquired and newly presented information. In other words, TGA characteristically produces an anterograde amnesia, which contradicts the implication that the amnesia in TGA is global. Focal seizures with altered awareness and medication side effects are reasonable alternative explanations; however, those conditions usually cause clouding of consciousness and generalized memory impairment.

286. The parents of a 4-year-old girl, whom one physician previously diagnosed as autistic, noticed that she has begun to lose her clear voice and ability to converse. Moreover, she has developed a habit of incessantly playing with her hands. She seems to be washing them or clapping for hours at a time. The neurologist cannot keep her attention. He sees that the child's eyes are blue and her hair blond. Her head circumference is relatively small compared to her height and age. Which is the most likely disorder?

a. Down syndrome

b. Phenylketonuria (PKU)

c. Intellectual disability

d. Rett syndrome

Answer: d. The child probably has Rett syndrome, which causes intellectual disability, stereotypies, and regression or loss of language features. Although genetic testing will confirm the disorder, this condition is diagnosable on clinical grounds: young girls with acquired microcephaly who lose their verbal abilities and begin to perform repetitive, purposeless hand movements (stereotypies). The main features of Rett syndrome are often present, in retrospect, by age 2 years; however, physicians usually do not diagnose it until age 5 years. Almost all girls with Rett syndrome have a mutation in the gene for the methyl-CpG-binding protein 2 (MECP2) on the X chromosome. If she had had untreated PKU, which produces blue eyes and blond hair, she would likely have developed eczema, seizures, and severe intellectual disability.

287. Which one of the following structures is an intranuclear inclusion?
    a. Cowdry body
    b. Neurofibrillary tangle
    c. Pick body
    d. Lewy body
    e. Negri body

Answer: a. Cowdry bodies are intranuclear inclusions characteristic of SSPE. Negri bodies (which are found in rabies), neurofibrillary tangles, Pick bodies, and Lewy bodies are intracytoplasmic inclusions.

288. What is the usual effect of SSRI treatment on REM sleep?
    a. SSRIs increase REM sleep.
    b. SSRIs decrease REM sleep.
    c. SSRIs abolish REM sleep.
    d. SSRIs suppress behavior that interferes with REM sleep.

Answer: b. SSRIs usually enhance the restfulness and length of sleep, but they generally decrease REM sleep and increase its latency. Moreover, they may precipitate REM sleep behavior disorder and increase periodic movements. They occasionally cause insomnia.

289. A 77-year-old man described excessive and inappropriate sleepiness, but no naps, during most of his daytime hours for the previous 2 years. He takes no medications, does not use alcohol, and otherwise is in good health. During the night, his wife reports, he has violent movements of his whole body. She does not know if her husband's sleep is restful, but her own sleep is not. Which one of the following should be the next step?
    a. Delaying the sleep phase
    b. Additional blood tests
    c. Polysomnogram (PSG)
    d. EMG

Answer: c. Several conditions cause nocturnal movements in 77-year-old individuals: restless legs syndrome (RLS), sleep apnea, REM sleep disorder, and seizures. All these conditions interrupt the sleep of the bed partner as well as the patient, and cause excessive daytime sleepiness. Physicians should ideally send people with potentially injurious or even excessive movements during sleep for a PSG.

290. Which *four* effects can be attributed to benzodiazepines?

    a. Increase in total sleep time of 10%
    b. Increase in total sleep time of 33%
    c. Increase in total sleep time of 67% or more
    d. Reduced sleep fragmentation
    e. Increase in slow-wave NREM sleep
    f. Hip fractures from an increased tendency to fall
    g. Weight gain
    h. Lowered seizure threshold
    i. Anterograde amnesia

Answer: a, d, f, i.

291. From which structures do most subdural hematomas arise?
    a. Lacerated middle meningeal arteries
    b. Ripped bridging veins
    c. Lacerated great vein of Galen
    d. Aneurysms of the middle or anterior cerebral arteries

Answer: b. Venous bleeding, which is often so slow that it may be called "oozing," leads to subdural hematomas. Meningeal artery lacerations lead to epidural hematomas. Aneurysms lead to bleeding that is predominantly subarachnoid.

292. Which *three* of the following are closely associated with spastic cerebral palsy?
    a. Necrotic areas in the white matter around the ventricles (periventricular leukomalacia)
    b. Kernicterus
    c. Hyperactive DTRs and clonus
    d. Foreshortened, spastic limbs
    e. Thalidomide

Answer: a, c, d. Kernicterus, basal ganglia bilirubin staining, is associated with choreoathetotic cerebral palsy. Maternal thalidomide exposure causes congenital limb deformity (phocomelia).

293. Which one of the following is most closely associated with neonatal periventricular leukomalacia?
    a. Athetosis
    b. Spastic cerebral palsy, all varieties
    c. Spastic diplegia
    d. MS

Answer: c. Neonatal periventricular white matter necrosis leads to spastic diplegia. MS typically causes periventricular white matter changes, but not in neonates.

294. One hour after a grilled tuna fish dinner, a 29-year-old previously healthy physician develops profound nausea and vomiting. Colleagues find that she has beet-red skin and hypotension, but a temperature of only 100°F. In addition to general supportive measures, which one of the following is the best treatment?
    a. Antibiotics
    b. Antidiarrhea medication
    c. Antihistamines
    d. Antiparasitic medications

Answer: c. Even when eaten raw, tuna and most other deep-water fish are usually safe. However, if they are not refrigerated, bacteria in their gut and gills may proliferate and produce histidine. The histidine, which resists cooking, is transformed into histamine in the human intestine. As in this case, victims develop histamine poisoning. Thus, antihistamines are the best treatment. Antidiarrheal medications for fish poisons are ineffective and counteract the body's natural protective reaction to expel toxins.

295. Which one of the following is *false* regarding the Glasgow Coma Scale (GCS)?
    a. It measures three clinical parameters: eye opening, verbal response, and motor response.
    b. A high score indicates a greater depth of coma.
    c. GCS scores correlate with posttraumatic amnesia.
    d. GCS scores do not correlate with posttraumatic headaches.

Answer: b. GCS scores range from 3 to 15. Lower scores correlate with progressively less responsiveness, greater likelihood of death, and, with survival, longer posttraumatic amnesia. In contrast, GCS scores do not correlate with either posttraumatic headaches or whiplash injury.

296. Which one of the following statements is *false* regarding the relationship of alcohol to TBI?
    a. Alcohol is a frequent contributory factor in motor vehicle crashes that have resulted in TBI.
    b. Alcohol withdrawal may complicate recovery from posttraumatic coma.
    c. Alcohol use in patients surviving TBI increases the incidence of seizures.
    d. Alcohol is a good hypnotic and minor tranquilizer in survivors of TBI.
    e. Alcohol may precipitate violence in patients with posttraumatic dyscontrol.

Answer: d. Alcohol is neither a good hypnotic nor minor tranquilizer. Posttraumatic insomnia or anxiety requires medications, possibly antidepressants. In TBI patients, alcohol induces insomnia, irritability, and EDS. Excessive alcohol use, which occurs in many TBI patients, impairs memory and judgment. Physicians should assess TBI patients with prolonged anxiety and insomnia for surreptitious as well as overt alcohol abuse.

297. Physicians sometimes focus on head injuries when evaluating patients who have sustained multiple bodily injuries. However, the original trauma, extraction, transportation, or examination of the patient may have caused or exacerbated a cervical spine injury. Which of the following are complications of cervical spine injury?
    a. Respiratory failure
    b. Quadriplegia or paraplegia
    c. Herniated intervertebral disks
    d. Urinary retention
    e. Carotid artery dissection
    f. All of the above

Answer: f. Combined head and neck injuries occur in motor vehicle crashes in which the face or forehead strikes the windshield and the neck snaps backward (hyperextends). Facial and scalp lacerations, which bleed profusely, are dramatic and often overshadow cervical injuries. Forceful manipulation of the head and neck, especially with a cervical spine fracture, can wrench the cervical spinal cord. The same injury also occurs in accidents where divers strike their head in a shallow pool or on a diving board and hyperextend or compress their cervical spine.

298. Neuropathologists recognize several abnormalities that occur in the brain before Alzheimer disease patients fulfill clinical criteria for dementia. Which is the sequence of abnormalities?
    a. Development of cerebral atrophy, accumulation of tau, accumulation of amyloid
    b. Accumulation of amyloid, accumulation of tau, development of cerebral atrophy
    c. Accumulation of tau, accumulation of amyloid, development of cerebral atrophy
    d. Development of cerebral atrophy, accumulation of amyloid, accumulation of tau

Answer: b. Long before Alzheimer disease patients develop cognitive impairment, their brains show abnormal accumulations of amyloid and then tau. Cerebral atrophy begins with the appearance of mild cognitive impairment, but the atrophy is usually advanced by the time Alzheimer disease patients have deteriorated to the point of having dementia. For the DSM-5 "probable" diagnosis of Major Neurocognitive Disorder due to Alzheimer's Disease, the diagnostic criteria require evidence of either a genetic mutation causative of Alzheimer disease (based on family history or genetic testing) or gradual cognitive decline in at least two domains without extended plateaus in the absence of evidence of mixed etiology. There is no DSM-5 category corresponding to the concept of presymptomatic or preclinical Alzheimer disease.

299. Which *three* of the following tumors originate from glial cells?
    a. Astrocytomas
    b. Glioblastomas
    c. Oligodendrogliomas
    d. Lymphomas
    e. Meningiomas

Answer: a, b, c.

300. A 31-year-old right-handed waiter was diagnosed with focal epilepsy with impairment of consciousness (formerly "complex partial epilepsy," see Box 10.1) at the age of 16 years. His seizures frightened him away from working, traveling, or entering

romantic relationships. Only doses of AEDs that impair his cognition and mood suppress his seizures. EEG-TV monitoring documented a right-sided temporal lobe focus. MRI showed atrophy of the right hippocampus. Which of the following is probably the best therapy?

a. Partial right temporal lobectomy
b. A commissurotomy
c. Adding an antidepressant
d. None of the above

Answer: a. Surgery that removes a seizure focus has been a major medical advance that, in skilled hands, benefits about 75% of selected epilepsy patients. In surgical candidates, a Wada test or fMRI reliably predicts if the proposed surgery will lead to aphasia or permanent memory loss. A commissurotomy, which would block the spread to seizures through the corpus callosum, has limited usefulness and neurologists have mostly abandoned the procedure.

301. A 68-year-old woman loses her accuracy at her relatively complicated assembly-line job. Her family brings her for a psychiatric evaluation of depression and dementia. Soon after the interview begins, she becomes upset and attempts to put on her coat. She tries to put both hands through the left sleeve. She becomes confused and frustrated. Then she puts her coat on backward. Finally, she is perplexed as to how to extricate herself from it (see figure). Which condition is she displaying?

a. Dementia
b. Apraxia
c. Dressing apraxia
d. Left–right confusion
e. Neglect
f. Anosognosia
g. Inattention

Answer: c. Dressing apraxia, a dramatic manifestation of nondominant hemisphere injury, particularly of the parietal lobe, consists of inability to clothe oneself due to a combination of visual-spatial impairment, somatotop-agnosia, and motor apraxia. Like other apraxias, dressing apraxia is more than inattention, visual loss, weakness, or lack of sensation on one side of the body. Patients with dressing apraxia become stymied when attempting to put on a coat, shirt, or hospital robe. Unlike patients with anosognosia, those with dressing apraxia are aware of their problem and are frustrated.

Examiners wishing to demonstrate the phenomenon might ask patients to dress in a hospital robe with one sleeve turned inside out. Even when warned about the sleeve's being reversed, patients will usually be unable to dress. Not appreciating the problem or being unable to solve it, they tend to change the normal sleeve into an abnormal sleeve, reverse any of their corrections, put both arms through the same sleeve, or drastically misalign the two sides. In this patient's case, a glioblastoma in the parietal lobe caused her dressing apraxia.

302. Which statement regarding EEG changes following ECT is *false*?
a. Unilateral ECT induces bilateral β-activity.
b. Bilateral ECT induces bilateral theta and delta activity.
c. Greater post-ECT slowing is associated with greater antidepressant effect.
d. Greater post-ECT slowing is associated with greater amnesia.

Answer: a. Unilateral ECT is associated with unilateral EEG slowing (theta and delta activity) rather than fast (beta) activity.

303. After previously undergoing silicone breast implants, a 39-year-old dancer underwent placement of

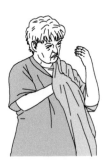
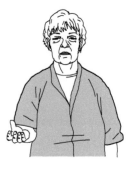
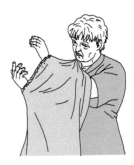
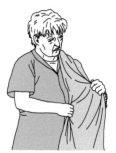
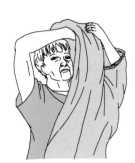
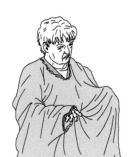

silicone implants into her buttocks. One week later her buttocks swelled beyond her expectations and then they became painful. Also, her ankles became weak. Which nerves have been injured?
a. Femoral
b. Sciatic
c. Fibular
d. Corticospinal

Answer: b. The silicone in her buttock implants probably leaked out and inflamed the sciatic nerves as well as the local tissue. The sciatic nerves in the buttocks are vulnerable to injury from pressure (as when individuals remain comatose while sitting on a toilet seat after a heroin overdose), buttock injections, stretching, blunt trauma, and penetrating wounds. Sciatic nerve injury leads to weakness of ankle dorsiflexion and plantarflexion, i.e., a "flail foot."

304. In which *two* of the following diseases is apoptosis the mechanism of cell death?
a. ALS
b. Head trauma
c. Huntington disease
d. Strokes

Answer: a, c. Apoptosis is programmed, energy-requiring cell death that does not elicit a cellular response from surrounding tissue. It occurs in some aspects of normal development, such as closure of the patent ductus arteriosus and involution of the thymus gland, as well as in many neurodegenerative disorders.

305. In which *two* of the following diseases is necrosis the mechanism of cell death?
a. ALS
b. TBI
c. Huntington disease
d. Strokes

Answer: b, d. Necrosis is death from catastrophic failure of structure or metabolism. Ischemic strokes and physical trauma are the most common causes. With the death of cells, a mononuclear infiltrate removes the cellular debris.

306. Which structure is immediately superior to the hypothalamus?
a. Thalamus
b. Subthalamic nucleus
c. Corpus callosum
d. Third ventricle

Answer: d. In other words, the hypothalamus is the floor of the third ventricle.

307. When a 60-year-old man being evaluated for dementia was asked to copy the sequence of figures on the top row, he produced the sequence on the bottom.

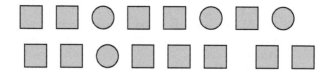

When he realized his error, he crumpled the paper, laughed uncontrollably, and then urinated in his pants. Which of the following conclusions can most reliably be drawn from his copying and behavior problems?

a. He has apraxia for figure copying, which indicates nondominant parietal lobe dysfunction.
b. He has dementia, but these problems are nonspecific.
c. These problems indicate subcortical dementia.
d. They indicate frontotemporal lobar degeneration.

Answer: d. The patient showed several signs of frontal lobe impairment. He showed perseveration when, after one appropriate change from copying squares to circles, he could not "switch sets" from squares to circles. He then demonstrated labile, impetuous, and uninhibited behavior (the laughing and urinating).

308. In which condition would evoked potential testing be *least* helpful?
a. Depression
b. Psychogenic blindness
c. MS
d. Optic neuritis
e. Deafness in uncooperative patients
f. Auditory capacity in autistic children

Answer: a. Brainstem auditory-evoked responses (BAERs), visual-evoked responses (VERs), and somatosensory-evoked potentials (SSEPs) can provide an objective measurement of the function, respectively, of the auditory, visual, and sensory systems. They provide no diagnostic help in depression or other psychiatric disease, except that normal VERs may indicate a psychogenic etiology in a seemingly blind patient. In MS patients, somatosensory-evoked potentials are often abnormal in patients with subclinical as well as overt spinal cord involvement, and visual-evoked responses are often abnormal in subclinical as well as overt optic nerve involvement. BAERs assess hearing in patients with auditory nerve damage and those who cannot cooperate because they are immature, cognitively impaired, or uncooperative.

309. Which *two* statements are true regarding the relationship of interictal violence to epilepsy?
a. Violent behavior is no more prevalent among patients with epilepsy with focal seizures with impairment of consciousness or awareness (formerly, complex partial seizures) than other varieties of epilepsy.
b. The consensus among neurologists is that epilepsy does not cause crime. Instead, epilepsy,

head trauma, and other brain injuries lead to conditions such as poor impulse control and lower socioeconomic status that predispose people to crime.

c. Interictal violence is associated with childhood-onset epilepsy.

d. Interictal violence can be reduced with benzodiazepines.

Answer: a, b.

310. In which *two* patients might a brain biopsy reveal Lewy bodies?

a. A 78-year-old person who had encephalitis as a young adult, with tremor, rigidity, and bradykinesia

b. A 70-year-old person who presents with 6 months of dementia, rigidity, and bradykinesia

c. A 40-year-old retired boxer with slurred speech, festinating gait, mild dementia, and resting tremor

d. A 30-year-old former intravenous drug abuser with tremor, rigidity, and bradykinesia

Answer: a, b. Lewy bodies are found in the substantia nigra in Parkinson disease, especially in the postencephalitic variety (Patient *a*). They are also found in dementia with Lewy bodies, which causes dementia and mild parkinsonism (Patient *b*). However, they are not found in chronic traumatic encephalopathy (Patient *c*) or MPTP-induced parkinsonism (Patient *d*).

311. Called to evaluate a 63-year-old man who demands to be released from the oncology service of a general hospital, a psychiatrist finds the patient to be relatively calm, oriented, and aware that he has "a melanoma that will be fatal in the near future." Physical examination and laboratory tests reveal no major abnormalities; however, the patient seems to fall to his left and be inattentive to friends and family who stand on his left side. Which of the following tests should the psychiatrist request before attempting to make a determination of the patient's competence?

a. Serum calcium determination

b. EEG

c. Mini-Mental Status Examination

d. MRI of the brain

Answer: d. Melanomas tend to spread widely via bloodborne dissemination. Although the patient seems to be making a rational decision, his left-sided inattention and motor difficulties indicate anosognosia. MRI would be the best test to detect metastases to the nondominant parietal lobe or elsewhere. Whether or not a lesion is present, the psychiatrist would have to assess his capacity.

312. A 67-year-old woman has just been admitted with an extensive right-sided cerebral infarction. Her physicians ask her to bisect a horizontal line. Which is the most likely result?

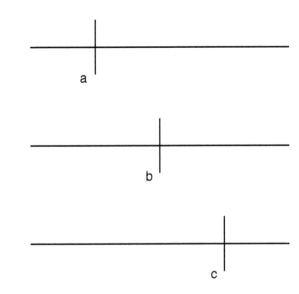

Answer: c. With or without a left homonymous hemianopia, she is likely be inattentive to her left visual field and her left arm and leg. Patients with hemi-inattention, which is a perceptual disorder, do not appreciate the left portion of the horizontal line and thus divide it off-center to the right.

313. Of the following, which is the single most frequent risk factor for falls in the elderly?

a. Transient ischemic attacks

b. Use of sedatives or hypnotics

c. Cardiac arrhythmias

d. Alzheimer disease

Answer: b.

314. A psychiatrist is asked to see a 25-year-old methadone maintenance patient hospitalized after his first seizure for agitated, belligerent behavior. MRI performed 3 days before the consultation revealed a single small, ring-enhancing lesion in the right frontal lobe. Physicians administered phenytoin and anti-toxoplasmosis medications. They also continued his methadone. Of the following, which is the most likely cause of his behavior?

a. Cerebral toxoplasmosis

b. AIDS dementia

c. Phenytoin-enhanced hepatic metabolism

d. Antitoxoplasmosis medications

Answer: c. Phenytoin induces hepatic enzymes that metabolize methadone and other medications. Thus, instituting phenytoin in methadone maintenance patients precipitates withdrawal. Individuals in methadone maintenance programs are often HIV-positive and many have AIDS. Some of them may have cerebral toxoplasmosis, but a single small lesion in the right, nondominant frontal lobe is unlikely to cause behavioral agitation.

315. Which are *two* characteristics of neurosyphilis in AIDS patients?
   a. Neurosyphilis testing often yields false-positive results.
   b. The diagnosis may be obscured by negative serologic tests.
   c. Treatment with penicillin may be deleterious.
   d. Neurosyphilis occurs rarely in AIDS patients.
   e. The usual doses of penicillin may be inadequate.

Answer: b, e.

316. Which *two* are the most powerful risk factors for HIV-associated dementia (HAD)?
   a. A CD4 count below 1000 cells/mL
   b. HIV load <75 copies/mL
   c. Anemia
   d. Depression
   e. Weight loss

Answer: c, e. Dementia usually does not complicate AIDS until immunodeficiency is pronounced, and anemia and systemic symptoms have developed. CD4 depletion, typically below 200 cells/mL, is a risk factor for AIDS dementia. On the other hand, patients on a HAART (highly active antiretroviral therapy) regimen may develop HAD and other complications even though they maintain a relatively normal CD4 count.

317. Although the value of the distinction has been questioned, many neurologists continue to divide dementia into cortical and subcortical varieties. Which of the following illnesses do neurologists consider examples of cortical dementia?
   a. HIV-associated dementia
   b. Alzheimer disease dementia
   c. Huntington disease dementia
   d. Normal-pressure hydrocephalus
   e. Parkinson disease dementia
   f. Frontotemporal lobar degeneration, including Pick disease
   g. Vascular disease

Answer: b, f. Neurologists typically offer Alzheimer disease dementia and frontotemporal lobar degeneration (including Pick disease) as examples of cortical dementia because aphasia, apraxia, and other higher cortical functions accompany the intellectual impairment, and patients have normal gait. In contrast, neurologists consider the dementia associated with HIV disease, Huntington disease, NPH, Parkinson disease, and vascular disease to be examples of subcortical dementia because, in these conditions, psychomotor retardation and gait abnormalities accompany the cognitive impairment. Nevertheless, the distinction is arbitrary and fallible because several of these illnesses have inconsistent or overlapping features. For example, the dementia in both HIV and Huntington diseases has cortical as well as subcortical features.

318. Which one of the following statements concerning hallucinations in Alzheimer disease is *false*?
   a. Hallucinations are almost always visual.
   b. They are associated with a rapid decline in cognitive function.
   c. They have little prognostic value.
   d. They are associated with clearly abnormal EEGs.

Answer: c. Hallucinations in Alzheimer disease indicate a poor prognosis.

319. If a man is 45 years old, in which decade of life is he?
   a. Third
   b. Fourth
   c. Fifth
   d. Sixth

Answer: c. The nomenclature is often a source of confusion. This man is in his fifth decade.

320. Which statement most closely describes the gate control theory of pain control?
   a. Descending pathways inhibit pain.
   b. Endogenous opioids suppress pain.
   c. Large-diameter, heavily myelinated fiber activity inhibits transmission of pain by small, sparsely myelinated fibers.
   d. Substance P and serotonin, carefully balanced, regulate pain transmission.

Answer: c.

321. Which one of the following statements is *true* regarding the periaqueductal gray matter?
   a. Stimulation of the periaqueductal gray matter produces analgesia by liberating endogenous opioids.
   b. Hemorrhage into the periaqueductal gray matter is associated with thiamine deficiency.
   c. The periaqueductal gray matter surrounds the aqueduct of Sylvius, which is the passage for CSF between the third and fourth ventricles.
   d. The periaqueductal gray matter is in the midbrain.
   e. All of the above.

Answer: e.

322. Which is not a characteristic of enkephalins?
   a. They are peptides
   b. They are neurotransmitters
   c. Naloxone inhibits enkephalins
   d. Serotonin inhibits enkephalins

Answer: d.

323. After a decade of progressively severe dementia, a former librarian died at the age of 49 years. At the onset of his illness, he showed rapid, varied, involuntary movements of each limb. Genetic

tests revealed a mutation in the short arm of chromosome 4. Postmortem examination of his brain would most likely stain for which protein?
a. Huntingtin
b. Dystrophin
c. Chorein
d. Frataxin

Answer: a. The brain of the patient, who died of Huntington disease, would show intraneuronal inclusions containing huntingtin. A deficiency or complete lack of dystrophin in the muscles characterizes Duchenne dystrophy. A deficiency or complete lack of serum chorein characterizes a rare neurodegenerative illness, neuroacanthocytosis. A deficiency or complete lack of serum frataxin, which has a role in mitochondrial iron metabolism, characterizes Friedreich ataxia.

324. During a summer vacation from college, where he excelled, a young man developed a pattern of sleeping 18 hours a day. His sleep was unrelated to night or daytime and was interrupted by his eating large amounts of food. His father attempted to wake him for work, but he was uncharacteristically surly and, on questioning, disoriented. When he arose for a few hours a day, he was apathetic and was found to be masturbating while gazing at a television. After refusing medical intervention for 2 weeks, the episode slowly cleared and he returned to his bright, cheerful, hard-working self. He remained entirely well – physically, mentally, and academically – for 8 months, when he lapsed into another episode of excessive sleeping, over-eating, and inappropriate sexual behavior. Before the full-blown symptoms emerged again, he reluctantly agreed to evaluation. His medical and neurological examinations were normal except for his somnolence. His routine laboratory tests, toxicology studies, CSF, MRI, and EEG were also normal. Which is the most likely diagnosis?
a. Kleine–Levin syndrome
b. Encephalitis
c. Tumor of the hypothalamus
d. Focal seizures with altered awareness
e. Klüver–Bucy syndrome
f. Drug abuse
g. Postconcussive syndrome
h. Depression

Answer: a. All of these conditions are tenable diagnoses on clinical grounds for the first episode of hypersomnia. If physicians had been able to perform the testing, they would have been able to exclude many of them. Once the second episode occurred and all the testing was unrevealing, Kleine–Levin syndrome (recurrent hypersomnia) emerges as the most likely diagnosis. This disorder, which is rare, usually affects males much more frequently than females and appears between the ages of 10 and 21 years. Kleine–Levin patients have attacks of hypersomnia lasting 1–4 weeks interrupted by hour-long periods of incomplete wakefulness during which they are dull, apathetic, withdrawn, amnesic, and confused. When awake, they eat voraciously and lose sexual inhibitions. Its main symptoms consist of the "3 *H*'s": hypersomnia, hypersexuality, and hyperphagia (morbid hunger).

325. What is the primary mechanism of action of NSAIDs?
a. They inhibit prostaglandin synthesis
b. They enhance serotonin activity
c. They enhance opioid activity
d. They cause opioid-like psychological side effects
e. All of the above

Answer: a.

326. Which fish has the highest concentration of mercury?
a. Herring
b. Bluefish
c. Sole
d. Tuna

Answer: d. As a general rule, the higher the fish lives in the food chain, the greater its mercury concentration. Tuna (especially its white meat), mackerel, Chilean sea bass, and swordfish carry the highest concentration of mercury. Another guideline is that mercury concentrations are greatest in river and lake fish and lowest in ocean fish.

327. A first-grade boy runs with his left thumb enclosed in his fisted hand. When asked to walk on the sides of his feet, the left thumb tends to flex toward the palm, as though he were starting to make a fist (see figure). Which *three* other stigmata of neurologic injury can be expected?
a. Hyperactive DTRs in the left arm
b. Intellectual disability
c. Clumsy movements with the left arm
d. Spasticity of the left arm
e. Hypoactive DTRs in the left arm
f. Athetosis

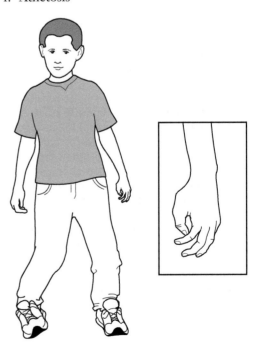

Answer: a, c, d. This boy's hand shows a "cortical thumb." In children and young adults, it often reflects congenital cerebral injury and is accompanied by hyperactive DTRs, spasticity, and clumsiness. In cases of unilateral involvement, the affected thumb, fingers, or entire arm may be smaller than their unaffected counterparts. In general, a cortical thumb in this age group, especially if accompanied by corticospinal tract signs, suggests "cerebral palsy." Adults may develop a cortical thumb after a cerebral infarction or TBI.

328. Match each enzyme (1–4) with the illness that results from its deficiency (a–d):
1. Hypoxanthine phosphoribosyl transferase (HPRT1)
2. Tyrosine hydroxylase
3. Phenylalanine hydroxylase
4. Arylsulfatase
   a. Phenylketonuria
   b. Lesch–Nyhan syndrome
   c. Metachromatic leukodystrophy
   d. Parkinson disease

Answers: 1–b, 2–d, 3–a, 4–c.

329. When a vagus nerve stimulator is implanted in an attempt to suppress seizures, where do the impulses first enter the CNS?
a. Temporal lobe
b. Diencephalon
c. Midbrain
d. Pons
e. Medulla

Answer: e. The vagus nerves' afferent fibers terminate in the solitary nucleus, which is located in the lateral portion of the medulla. Impulses are relayed from there to the more rostral portions of the brainstem and the cerebral cortex.

330. Match the speech pattern (a–c) with the disorder (1–3).
a. Strained and strangled
b. Hypophonic and monotonous
c. Scanning
   1. MS affecting the cerebellum
   2. Parkinson disease
   3. Spasmodic dysphonia

Answer: a–3, b–2, c–1.

331. Which finding is compatible with brain death?
a. Slow-wave activity on the EEG
b. Ocular movement artifact on the EEG
c. Presence of oculocephalic reflexes
d. Babinski signs and hyperactive Achilles reflexes

Answer: d. Spinal reflexes such as Babinski signs and hyperactive Achilles reflexes may persist despite brain death. EEG and clinical signs of brainstem activity, such as pupillary light and oculocephalic reflexes, indicate brainstem function and preclude a determination of brain death.

332. Why is succinylcholine used in conjunction with ECT?
a. It makes the brain more susceptible to the beneficial effects of ECT because it lowers the seizure threshold.
b. It paralyzes muscles by binding to the neuromuscular junction ACh receptors.
c. It reduces subsequent amnesia.
d. It is given to enhance ECT effect, but its usefulness has never been established.
e. It reduces oral secretions that the patient could aspirate.
f. It interferes with cerebral ACh and induces amnesia for the event.

Answer: b. Succinylcholine blocks the neuromuscular junction. It paralyzes muscles and prevents ECT-induced muscle contractions that can cause spine or limb fractures and other injuries. Succinylcholine does not cross the blood–brain barrier and thus does not affect the seizure threshold or memory pathways. Atropine reduces secretions.

333. A 32-year-old woman has developed slow and disordered thinking, word-finding difficulties, bilateral weakness and spasticity, and dysarthria and dysphagia. A noncontrast CT of the head and CSF analysis reveal no abnormalities, but an MRI shows numerous, large abnormal areas in the cerebral white matter. Which disorder can her physicians exclude at this point?
a. Toxoplasmosis
b. Adrenoleukodystrophy (ALD)
c. Toluene abuse
d. Progressive multifocal leukoencephalopathy (PML)
e. MS

Answer: b. Her neurologic signs – aphasia, pseudobulbar palsy, bilateral corticospinal tract signs, and possibly dementia – indicate diffuse cerebral injury that all the disorders cause. Except for toxoplasmosis, they are all demyelinating diseases. Physicians can exclude only ALD because it is an X-linked recessive disorder that develops only in males.

334. To which parts of the brain do the letters (A–E) in the figure refer? If appropriate, use more than one number for each letter.

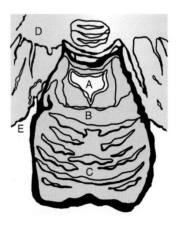

1. Lateral ventricle
2. Third ventricle
3. Aqueduct of Sylvius
4. Fourth ventricle
5. Midbrain
6. Pons
7. Medulla
8. Cerebellum
9. Cerebrum
10. Corticospinal tracts
11. Cerebellar tracts
12. Bulbar cranial nerves
13. Oculomotor cranial nerves
14. Cerebellopontine angle cranial nerves

Answer: The sketch shows the pons (B = 6), which is the bulky portion of the brainstem, and the inferior aspect of the cerebellum (D = 8). The fourth ventricle (A = 4) is located in the uppermost portion of the pons. Corticospinal and cerebellar tracts (C = 10 and 11) cross through the base of the pons. Cranial nerves 5, 7, and 8 emerge from the cerebellopontine angle (E = 14).

335. What is the mechanism of action of the hypnotic suvorexant (Belsomra)?
a. It stimulates melatonin receptors.
b. It antagonizes GABA$_A$ receptors.
c. It stimulates GABA$_A$ receptors.
d. It antagonizes orexin receptors.

Answer: d. Orexin, a naturally occurring neuropeptide synthesized in the lateral hypothalamus, promotes wakefulness. Suvorexant, a new hypnotic, antagonizes orexin receptors and thereby promotes sleep. Benzodiazepines and benzodiazepine agonists stimulate GABA$_A$ receptors.

336. A pediatric neurologist examines an 18-month-old boy who has developed seizures. His grandmother is worried that he has been losing developmental milestones since his first birthday. He is obviously retarded in mental and physical development, and he fails to track large, colorful objects. His head circumference is 50 cm. He is irritable and listless. His limbs are weak and spastic. Fundoscopic examination reveals a red spot near each macula. Which of the following enzymes is most likely to be deficient?
a. Hexosaminidase A
b. Sphingomyelinase
c. Arylsulfatase
d. Hypoxanthine phosphoribosyl transferase (HPRT1)

Answer: a. In view of the onset of intellectual disability, seizures, irritability, probable blindness, macrocephaly, and, especially the cherry red spot on the retinae, the child probably has Tay–Sachs disease. That illness, an autosomal recessive disorder almost entirely restricted to Ashkenazi Jews, results from a deficiency of hexosaminidase A. A deficiency of sphingomyelinase causes Niemann–Pick disease; a deficiency of

arylsulfatase, metachromatic leukodystrophy; and a deficiency of HPRT1, Lesch–Nyhan syndrome.

337. Which visual field cut is associated with alexia without agraphia? (Remember: the conventional display of visual fields appears from the patient's viewpoint, i.e., "right is right," and darkened or hatched areas are regions that the patient cannot see. Also, the left eye generally appears on the left, and right eye on the right.)

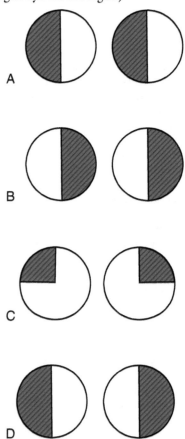

Answer: b. A right homonymous hemianopia is virtually a prerequisite for alexia without agraphia.

338. Which pattern on sequential mental status testing indicates Alzheimer disease?
a. A precipitous decline over 6 months
b. A decline over 6 months and then a plateau for 3 years
c. A steady borderline score in a well-educated individual
d. An uneven decline interrupted by several plateaus lasting 12 to 18 months

Answer: d. An uneven decline, including plateaus, is common in Alzheimer disease, but a precipitous decline suggests a "rapidly progressive dementia," such as CJD or a paraneoplastic syndrome. A plateau of more than 2 years is unusual for Alzheimer disease. A single borderline score in well-educated individuals is a common diagnostic dilemma. Such individuals might not have been very intelligent in the first place; they could have developed other problems, such as alcoholism; or they might have depression rather than dementia.

339. Match the view (a–c) with its common description (1–3).
   a. Axial
   b. Coronal
   c. Sagittal
      1. Front-to-back or head-on
      2. Top-down view
      3. Side view

Answer: a–2, b–1, c–3.

340. During the Vietnam War, numerous soldiers were exposed to Agent Orange. Which of the following neurologic problems have been found in rigorous scientific studies to be attributable to Agent Orange exposure?
   a. Brain tumors
   b. Peripheral neuropathy
   c. Cognitive impairment
   d. Neuropsychologic deficits
   e. None of the above

Answer: e. No reliable evidence has found a causal relationship between Agent Orange exposure and these problems.

341. During his recovery from a stroke, a 65-year-old retired high-school science teacher became sullen, despondent, and unnecessarily discouraged. He began to skip physical and occupational therapy sessions, regressed in his motor skills, and developed insomnia. His children reported that he was having needless, continual worries about his finances and their health. A reevaluation by the medical staff found no new neurologic injury, general medical disturbance, or medication that might be causing his feelings and concerns. Which is the most likely diagnosis?
   a. Poststroke depression
   b. Poststroke depression with comorbid anxiety
   c. Neurocognitive disorder due to vascular disease
   d. None of the above

Answer: b. The patient has developed poststroke depression with comorbid anxiety. Although most of its symptoms usually resolve within the first year after the stroke, poststroke depression leads to cognitive impairment, failure to participate in rehabilitation, and increased mortality. Most stroke patients with anxiety have comorbid depression.

342. Which *three* of the following medications elevate the serum prolactin concentration?
   a. Thorazine
   b. Bromocriptine
   c. Haloperidol
   d. Clozapine
   e. Pergolide
   f. Levodopa
   g. Risperidone

Answer: a, c, g. Dopamine and dopamine agonists inhibit the release of prolactin by acting on the tubero-infundibular tract. In contrast, dopamine-blocking neuroleptics trigger prolactin release and produce elevated serum prolactin concentrations. The prolactin level is also elevated for about 20 minutes after most generalized and focal seizures with altered awareness. Bromocriptine and other dopamine agonists can shrink prolactinomas, a common pituitary adenoma, and obviate surgery.

343. Which two of the following nuclei constitute the corpus striatum?
   a. Caudate
   b. Putamen
   c. Globus pallidus
   d. Subthalamic nucleus
   e. Substantia nigra

Answer: a, b.

344. In hepatolenticular degeneration, to which *two* structures does "lenticular" refer?
   a. Caudate
   b. Putamen
   c. Globus pallidus
   d. Subthalamic nucleus
   e. Substantia nigra

Answer: b, c. Resembling a pie-shaped or lens-shaped structure, the putamen and globus pallidus form the lenticular nuclei (see Fig. 18.1A). In hepatolenticular degeneration (Wilson disease), copper deposits damage these basal ganglia, the liver, and other organs. Deposits in the cornea form the characteristic Kayser–Fleischer rings.

345. Which *three* of the following findings suggest a deliberate head injury in an infant?
   a. Retinal hemorrhages
   b. Discrepancy between history and injuries
   c. An Arnold–Chiari malformation
   d. CT or MRI showing subdural hemorrhages of varying ages
   e. Absence of the corpus callosum
   f. Subconjunctival hemorrhages

Answer: a, b, d. Blood of varying ages in the face, retinae, subdural spaces, and brain of an infant indicates non-accidental head trauma, i.e., child abuse. Absence of the corpus callosum and Arnold–Chiari defects are congenital malformations. Retinal hemorrhages strongly suggest but do not prove trauma. Subconjunctival hemorrhages usually result from minimal trauma, minor illnesses, viral infection, and bleeding disorders.

346. With which phenomenon does the day's lowest body temperature coincide?
   a. Intense REM sleep
   b. Intense slow-wave sleep
   c. Sleep onset
   d. Noon
   e. 4:00 PM

Answer: a. In the early morning, when REM activity is most likely to be present, the body temperature reaches its low point (nadir).

347. A family brings their 72-year-old patriarch for an evaluation of dementia which has developed along with mild rigidity and bradykinesia during the past several months. He has been troubled primarily by visual hallucinations. Which is the probable pathology?
    a. Plaques and tangles in the hippocampus
    b. Lewy bodies in the cerebral cortex
    c. Lewy bodies in the substantia nigra
    d. Atrophy of the head of the caudate

Answer: b. Because this man presents with parkinsonism and dementia within 1 year (the "1 year rule") and visual hallucinations, he is unlikely to have Parkinson disease. Visual hallucinations are characteristic of dementia with Lewy bodies. Histologically, Lewy bodies in the cerebral cortex characterize this disorder. Lewy bodies in the substantia nigra characterize Parkinson disease, which does not cause dementia at its onset. Alzheimer disease causes plaques and tangles in the cerebral cortex and especially the hippocampus, but it does not present with either pyramidal or extrapyramidal signs. Atrophy of the head of the caudate nuclei characterizes Huntington disease.

348. Which receptors do dopamine agonists primarily stimulate when neurologists prescribe them to treat Parkinson disease?
    a. D1
    b. D2
    c. Both
    d. Neither

Answer: b. All commercially available dopamine agonists stimulate D2 receptors to alleviate the symptoms of Parkinson disease. In addition, dopamine agonists may either stimulate or inhibit D1.

349. The DSM-5 diagnostic criteria for most illnesses require that the patient show impaired performance, distress, or decreased social, occupational, or behavioral functioning. Which of the following illnesses has no such requirement?
    a. Tic disorders
    b. Conversion disorder
    c. Insomnia disorder
    d. Major neurocognitive impairment

Answer: a. The DSM-5 diagnostic criteria for Tic Disorders do not include impaired performance, distress, or decreased functioning. Indeed, individuals with tics and many with Tourette Disorder lead happy and productive lives. In contrast, the diagnostic criteria of Conversion Disorder require "clinically significant distress or impairment in social, occupational, or other important areas of functioning or warrants medical evaluation." Those for Insomnia Disorder require "clinically significant distress or impairment" in similar areas. Those for

Major Neurocognitive Disorder require that the deficits "interfere with independence in everyday activities."

350. A 50-year-old architect's hand forms a painful cramp several minutes after he begins to draw sketches. Early in his career, similar cramps developed but only after many hours of work. Which condition is responsible for forcing his hand into this position?

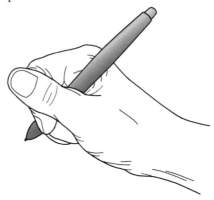

    a. Psychogenic disturbance
    b. Age-related disturbance
    c. Motor neuron disease
    d. Focal dystonia
    e. Exercised-induced cramp

Answer: d. He has developed writer's cramp, which neurologists label an occupational or task-specific focal dystonia. After several decades of work, musicians, writers, and architects may develop this disorder, which is a variety of focal dystonia. Other body parts used repetitively can also develop it. For example, professional wind instrument players may develop dystonia of their lip muscles. In all these conditions, botulinum toxin injections into the affected muscles may temporarily ameliorate the dystonia.

351. A 60-year-old man involuntary contractions of all his facial muscles. The contractions, which begin around the eyes, are bilateral and symmetric. They last for several seconds and prevent him from driving. He remains conscious during the contractions. His jaw, tongue, and ocular muscles are unaffected. Which type of illness is the most likely cause?

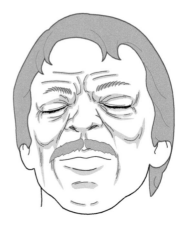

a. Seizure disorder
b. Iatrogenic illness
c. Meige syndrome
d. Psychogenic condition

Answer: c. Meige syndrome is more extensive than blepharospasm because it involves the lower as well as the upper face muscles. Unlike writer's cramp, it occurs spontaneously and is not occupational or task-specific. Most individuals with Meige syndrome have no history of psychiatric illness or exposure to neuroleptics. When the oral-buccal-lingual form of tardive dyskinesia involves facial muscles, it almost always involves the tongue and jaw muscles. Like other focal dystonias, cranial dystonia responds to botulinum injections. However, neurologists do not routinely inject the tongue because if the tongue is weakened it may fall back and occlude the airway. Also, if the injections were to cause bleeding, tongue swelling likewise may occlude the airway.

352. Which *five* illnesses result from trinucleotide repeats?
    a. Huntington disease
    b. Spinocerebellar atrophy
    c. Wilson disease
    d. DYT1 dystonia
    e. Fragile X syndrome
    f. Duchenne muscular dystrophy
    g. Myotonic dystrophy
    h. Friedreich ataxia

Answer: a, b, e, g, h.

353. In which *three* ways does juvenile Huntington disease differ from the common adult variety of the illness?
    a. Unlike the DNA in the adult variety, the DNA in juvenile Huntington disease typically has more than 60 trinucleotide repeats.
    b. The juvenile variety has a greater tendency toward anticipation in successive generations.
    c. The juvenile variety usually is inherited from the father.
    d. The juvenile variety tends to cause rigidity rather than chorea.
    e. The juvenile variety affects girls more often than boys.

Answer: a, c, d.

354. Having survived a cardiac arrest 6 months earlier, a 65-year-old retired judge has his eyes open during the daytime hours. He does not establish eye contact or respond to his health-care workers. He cannot name objects, repeat phrases, or follow requests. He lies in bed without any voluntary movement except that he uses a spoon to feed himself. Occasionally he responds to his wife's questions, such as "Is my name Mary?" or "Are we in a school building?" only with a smile or blink. Any verbal answers are partial and incorrect. Of the following would be the most accurate description of his level of consciousness?

a. Aphasia
b. Locked-in state
c. Minimally conscious state
d. Persistent vegetative state

Answer: c. By definition, patients in the minimally conscious state display certain behaviors on a reproducible and sustained basis. They follow one or more simple requests, gesture or say "yes" and "no" (regardless of accuracy), and may speak intelligible utterances. They appropriately, not reflexively, smile, cry, and use their hands to reach or manipulate objects. Although his answers are inaccurate, this patient expresses himself through gestures. In addition, he feeds himself. Postanoxic encephalopathy would be an acceptable alternative diagnosis.

355. A 33-year-old man with AIDS has sought medical attention because of gait impairment, confusion, and word-finding difficulties that have forced him to retire from work and turn over all his financial affairs to his partner. His MRI is shown below. Which process is causing his symptoms?

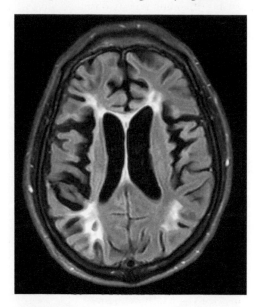

a. HIV encephalitis
b. MS
c. Toxoplasmosis
d. PML
e. Lymphoma

Answer: d. The patient has Major Neurocognitive Disorder due to HIV infection with PML as well as dementia. His MRI shows several hyperintense lesions in the white matter and marked cerebral atrophy. Unlike most intracerebral lesions, PML lesions are not surrounded by edema and do not exert mass effect (see Fig. 15.11). HIV encephalitis does not cause discrete lesions. Although MS attacks white matter, the plaques are typically periventricular (see Fig. 15.6). Toxoplasmosis, another complication of HIV infection, causes multiple circular lesions that have mass effect and usually occur in the basal ganglia (see Fig. 20.11). Cerebral lymphomas in AIDS patients are usually single large mass lesions.

356. During a 3-week vacation a 60-year-old man, who had been in excellent health, developed apathy, inattention, and a flattened affect. His MRI is shown below. Which is the most likely diagnosis?

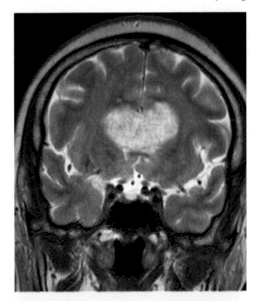

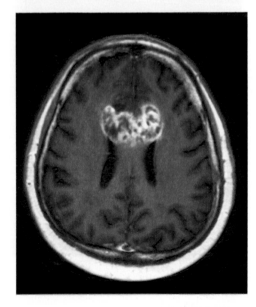

a. A frontal lobe glioblastoma
b. MS
c. Lymphoma
d. PML

Answer: a. The MRI shows a single, large hyperintense lesion extending into both frontal lobes through the corpus callosum in a "butterfly" pattern. The rapid course, clinical features, and MRI indicate that he is harboring a bilateral frontal lobe glioblastoma, which is a relatively common tumor in this age group. His age, absence of preceding episodes, and lack of risk factors argue against MS, lymphoma, and PML. Metastatic carcinoma is unlikely because metastases are usually multiple mass lesions surrounded by edema and do not spread across the corpus callosum. This case exemplifies that

frontal lobe glioblastomas frequently cause rapid onset of dementia or marked personality change in individuals aged 50 to 65 years.

357. Which of the following is a relay nucleus on the hearing pathway?
a. Lateral geniculate body
b. Medial geniculate body
c. Medial lemniscus
d. Substantia gelatinosa

Answer: b. The medial geniculate body is the relay nucleus in the hearing pathway just as the lateral geniculate body is the relay station for visual impulses. The medial lemniscus conveys position and vibration sensations ascending from the spinal cord, and the substantia gelatinosa relays pain sensation from the spinal dorsal nucleus to the lateral spinothalamic tract.

358. An examination by an audiologist determines that a 74-year-old man has bilateral impairment of speech discrimination, particularly for consonants. He has bilateral hearing loss particularly affecting high frequencies. Which is the most likely explanation?
a. He has NF2.
b. He has developed Alzheimer disease dementia.
c. Acoustic neuromas have developed bilaterally.
d. Age-related changes have developed.

Answer: d. He probably has normal age-related hearing loss (presbycusis). The development of bilateral acoustic neuromas is the signature of NF2. Alzheimer disease is associated with a loss of smell sensation (anosmia).

359. Which of the following is *not* a normal age-related change?
a. Small pupils
b. Loss of speech discrimination
c. Increased proportion of slow-wave sleep
d. Decreased vibration perception in the toes and ankles
e. Inability to perform tandem gait

Answer: c. Slow-wave sleep decreases with age. Elderly individuals can have all the other changes.

360. Which *three* of the following involuntary movements are typically preceded by an irresistible urge to move?
a. Periodic limb movements
b. RLS
c. Stereotypies
d. Akathisia
e. Chorea
f. Tics

Answer: b, d, f. Patients with certain movement disorders, including RLS, akathisia, and tics, typically have a preceding irresistible urge similar to a compulsion. Enacting the movements provides psychologic relief and reduces anxiety. Conversely, suppressing the movements leads to anxiety. In the case of tics, behavioral therapies may allow the patient to suppress the movements without causing undue anxiety.

361. Which *two* conditions typically produce brief, random, involuntary movements accompanied by motor impersistence that develop over several days in a 10-year-old child?
a. Tourette syndrome
b. Lyme disease
c. Mononucleosis
d. Sydenham chorea
e. Neuroleptic-induced dystonia
f. Withdrawal emergent dyskinesia

Answer: d, f. The child has suddenly developed chorea that – depending on the history – indicates either Sydenham chorea or withdrawal emergent dyskinesia. Tourette syndrome evolves over years and produces varied stereotyped movements (tics). Neuroleptic-induced dystonia produces sustained posturing, and extension of the head and neck (retrocollis) is particularly characteristic. Lyme disease and mononucleosis, which both occur in children, do not usually produce chorea.

362. Which one of the following children is most apt to have a mitochondria disorder?
a. A 10-year-old boy who develops dystonia of one foot that begins to spreads to his leg
b. An 8-year-old boy who has had a head toss for 2 years and then develops a cough for which there is no pulmonary explanation
c. A 6-year-old girl who develops polyuria and polydipsia
d. An 11-year-old autistic girl
e. A 9-year-old boy with mild intellectual disability
f. A 9-year-old boy who is short with mild intellectual disability, and has had repeated hospitalizations for lactic acidosis

Answer: f. Lactic acidosis indicates a mitochondrial disorder. The disorder characteristically becomes symptomatic on an intermittent basis.

363. Deficiency of which one of the following vitamins causes CNS demyelination?
a. Niacin (vitamin B_3)
b. Pyridoxine (vitamin B_6)
c. Cobalamin (vitamin B_{12})
d. Citric acid (vitamin C)

Answer: c. Vitamin B_{12} deficiency causes demyelination in the posterior tracts of the spinal cord, cerebrum, and other areas of the CNS. It also causes dementia and a peripheral neuropathy. Although neurologists often cite B_{12} deficiency as the quintessential cause of "reversible dementia," several studies have found that the dementia resists B_{12} repletion. Niacin deficiency causes pellagra with delirium and dementia. Pyridoxine deficiency causes a neuropathy and seizures. Citric acid deficiency causes scurvy.

364. This 65-year-old man has had weakness in all of his limbs, especially his right arm and leg, since age 4 years when he was hospitalized for 2 months and required a respirator for 2 weeks. He has remained confined to a wheelchair, but, with great effort and having considerable family financial resources, he was able to graduate from college, marry, and father three children. What does inspection of his limbs reveal?

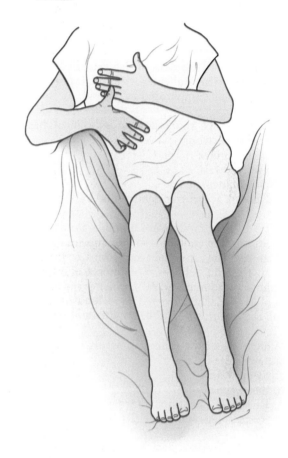

a. Dystonia
b. Spasticity
c. Smaller size and less muscle bulk on his right arm and leg
d. Pseudohypertrophy

Answer: c. This patient who undoubtedly survived poliomyelitis (polio) has the typical failure of development (growth arrest) of his weakened limbs. Note the guttering of the right hand's interosseous space, smaller circumference of the right calf, and the foreshortened right foot.

365. In regards to the patient in the previous question, which one of the following problems would probably be present?
a. Cognitive impairment
b. Severe erectile dysfunction
c. Diplopia from oculomotor motility
d. A raspy voice and dysphagia from bulbar palsy

Answer: d. Because poliovirus, an enterovirus, attacks lower motor neurons, survivors typically have a raspy voice and dysphagia from bulbar – not pseudobulbar – palsy. Also, despite quadriparesis, they retain cognitive, autonomic, sensory, sexual, and ocular function.

366. In addition to polio, which other virus produces acute lower motor neuron paresis?
   a. West Nile virus
   b. Measles
   c. HIV
   d. Dengue

Answer: a. West Nile virus, which is carried by birds, is similar to poliovirus and enterovirus 68. It produces an acute febrile illness complicated by paresis.

367. Which one of the following substances has an unpaired electron?
   a. Monoamines
   b. Free radicals
   c. Dopamine
   d. Choline acetyl transferase (ChAT)

Answer: b. Free radicals are unstable atoms or molecules because they contain a single, unpaired electron. They seize electrons from adjacent atoms or molecules. Loss of an electron oxidizes those atoms or molecules. Methylphenylpyridinium (MPP^+), which is the metabolic product of MPTP, when injected into laboratory animals, causes all the features of Parkinson disease.

368. Which one of the following occurs while patients are awake?
   a. Sleep walking
   b. Sleep apnea
   c. REM sleep behavior disorder
   d. Restless legs syndrome (RLS)

Answer: d. Restless legs movements occur while patients are trying to fall asleep but still awake. The movements prevent them from falling asleep. Once asleep, 80% of patients with RLS develop periodic leg movements.

369. A 19-year-old student has developed progressively severe intellectual impairment during the preceding year. Examination reveals a resting tremor, dysarthria, and rigidity. The cornea has a brown-green discoloration in its periphery. Liver function tests are abnormal. Which of the following is most likely to be found on further evaluation?
   a. Trinucleotide repeats
   b. Atrophy of the caudate nucleus
   c. Indications of drug abuse
   d. Decreased concentration of the serum protein that transports copper

Answer: d. He has Wilson disease. Tests would show that his serum contains a low concentration of ceruloplasmin, the primary copper-carrying protein. Trinucleotide repeats and atrophy of the caudate nucleus would indicate Huntington disease. Although not the explanation in this case, physicians should consider drug abuse in teenagers and young adults with progressive cognitive impairment.

370. A 66-year-old retired Air Force colonel who has had Parkinson disease for 12 years suddenly begins to invest his life's savings in stocks and spend inordinate time trading them. Many of the stocks are speculative. A psychiatrist finds that he has mild cognitive impairment and moderate tremor, rigidity, bradykinesia, and postural reflex impairment. What is the first best therapeutic strategy?
   a. Prescribe a mood-stabilizing medication
   b. Prescribe an anxiolytic antidepressant
   c. Send the patient to gamblers anonymous
   d. Reduce or remove dopamine agonist medication

Answer: d. The colonel has an impulse control disorder as a manifestation of Parkinson disease or its treatment. Although the expression of impulse control disorder depends on the patient's circumstances, most Parkinson disease patients with it excessively shop or gamble. Some seek inappropriate sexual activity. Buying stocks combines shopping and gambling. Using dopamine agonists such as ropinirole or pramipexole is a risk factor for impulse control disorder. Notably, impulse control disorder is neither mania nor bipolar disorder.

371. A 35-year-old woman reports weight loss, generalized weakness, darkening of her skin, amenorrhea, and depression. Her neurologic examination and head MRI are normal. However, her serum electrolytes show hyponatremia, hyperkalemia, and mild hypoglycemia. Which is the most likely cause of her symptoms?
   a. Adrenal failure
   b. Myasthenia gravis
   c. Diabetes
   d. Anorexia

Answer: a. Adrenal failure leads to hyponatremia, hyperkalemia, and hypoglycemia because of mineralocorticoid hormone deficiency. In adrenal failure, the pituitary secretes excess ACTH in an attempt to stimulate adrenal hormone production. It also secretes melanocyte-stimulating hormone, which darkens the skin. Secondary adrenal insufficiency due to pituitary insufficiency shares many of the same features as primary adrenal insufficiency; however, with ACTH deficiency, the skin does not darken.

372. Following cocaine use that led to small right parietal-occipital hemorrhages, a 28-year-old man said that he could not see out of his left eye. The examining physician found that his acuity was 20/25, and instead of having lost vision from the left eye, he had a left homonymous hemianopia. The patient then said that he could not distinguish similar items by sight but needed to "experience" them. For example, he was unable to identify a dog and cat unless he could pet and smell them. Also, he could not differentiate a pen and pencil unless

he wrote with each of them. Similarly, unless he spoke with family members, rather than just seeing them, he could not identify them. Nevertheless, he was able to name and state the use of all objects that he touched, repeat long and complicated phrases, and follow two- and three-step requests. Which is the best term for his disorder?
a. Cortical blindness
b. Aphasia
c. Hemi-inattention
d. Visual agnosia
e. A psychogenic disturbance
f. Delirium

Answer: d. Many individuals who develop a homonymous hemianopia believe that they have lost vision in one eye. This patient's disorder is visual agnosia, which is a perceptual problem. It prevents him from identifying objects that he sees. He also has prosopagnosia, a variety of visual agnosia, in which he cannot identify familiar faces. These conditions probably result from lesions that are just anterior to the occipital visual cortex and impair its communication with the parietal association areas. He does not have blindness because his visual acuity is 20/25; aphasia because he has normal language; hemi-inattention because he brings the objects into his consciousness through tactile routes; nor delirium because he remained alert and attentive during the testing.

373. A 35-year-old alcoholic man with mild chronic cirrhosis is brought to the ER because of agitation and belligerent behavior. Examination reveals disorientation, slurred speech, and asterixis. He has no nystagmus, extraocular paresis, pupillary abnormality, or lateralized signs. Laboratory data include the following: abnormal liver function tests, 26% hematocrit, and blood in the stool. Which condition is the most likely cause of his behavioral disturbances and confusion?
a. Wernicke encephalopathy
b. Alcohol-induced hypoglycemia

c. Hepatic encephalopathy
d. Subdural hematoma
e. Delirium tremens (DTs)

Answer: c. Hepatic encephalopathy from gastrointestinal bleeding is the most likely explanation. Laennec cirrhosis patients, for example, will develop hepatic encephalopathy when esophageal varices or gastric ulceration cause gastrointestinal bleeding, or even when they eat a high-protein meal. With both hemorrhage and a high-protein meal, protein breaks down in the intestine to form ammonia or other toxins. Asterixis and mental status changes often occur, as in this case, before liver function tests become abnormal. In this situation, physicians should avoid prescribing psychotropic medications that require hepatic metabolism.

374. All of the following conditions cause weakness. Which *three* of them result from impaired presynaptic ACh release?
a. Lambert–Eaton syndrome
b. Myasthenia gravis
c. Botulism
d. Tetanus
e. Insecticide poisoning
f. Botulinum treatment

Answer: a, c, f. In Lambert–Eaton syndrome, a paraneoplastic syndrome, antibodies block the influx of calcium ions into motor nerve terminals, thereby inhibiting the release of ACh packets. Similarly, botulism and botulinum toxin injections impair ACh release. In contrast, myasthenia gravis results from defective ACh postsynaptic receptors. Anticholinesterase insecticides cause paralyzing continual postsynaptic receptor stimulation. Tetanus results from loss of normal spinal cord inhibition because of impaired GABA activity.

375. After a several-day binge of using cocaine, a 33-year-old woman presents with hyperactivity of the hands and feet. She reports a "need" to move. She cannot

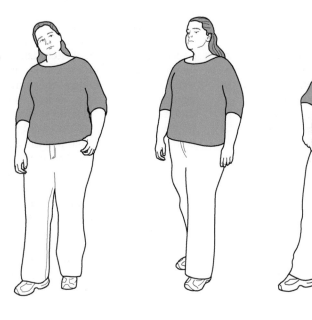

sit still or stand at attention. When walking, her gait is jerky. Of the following, which is the most likely cause of her movements?

a. Drug-induced psychosis
b. Akathisia
c. Sydenham chorea
d. Excessive dopamine activity
e. Alcohol withdrawal

Answer: d. Each of these conditions can cause chorea or similar hyperactive movements, particularly of the legs. Each may also incite an inner need to move. In this case, cocaine has increased dopamine activity to toxic levels, which has caused involuntary leg movements, i.e., "crack dancing." This condition usually subsides spontaneously over 1 to 3 days. If necessary, small doses of dopamine-blocking neuroleptics will suppress residual movements.

376. With which receptor does glutamate bind and lead to toxicity?

a. NMDA
b. Muscarinic ACh
c. Nicotinic ACh
d. Dopamine
e. Glutamate
f. None of the above

Answer: a. Glutamate–NMDA interactions are sometimes excitotoxic. In Huntington disease and possibly also in epilepsy and strokes, this mechanism may contribute to pathogenesis.

377. Which *four* of the following nuclei are pigmented?

a. Locus ceruleus
b. Oculomotor
c. Dorsal motor nucleus of X
d. Trigeminal motor
e. Substantia nigra
f. Nucleus basalis of Meynert
g. Red nucleus
h. Abducens

Answer: a, c, e, g. The red, the blue, and the black are pigmented: one red (red nucleus), one blue (locus ceruleus), and two black (substantia nigra and dorsal motor nucleus of the vagus nerve) nuclei are pigmented.

378. A janitor brings a 40-year-old tenant to the ER where he is initially belligerent and then stuporous. He is jaundiced, anemic, and has signs of a recent gastrointestinal hemorrhage. He has a history of chronic cirrhosis. A neurologic examination shows asterixis and bilateral Babinski signs but equal pupils and no hemiparesis. A CT of the head is normal. What would an EEG most likely reveal?

a. α-Activity
b. Electrocerebral silence
c. Triphasic waves
d. 3-Hz spike-and-wave activity

Answer: c. The patient has hepatic encephalopathy. In this disorder and other metabolic encephalopathies, the EEG shows disorganization and triphasic waves. In normal, alert, resting individuals who have their eyes closed, are free of anxiety and not concentrating, the EEG will show well-organized α-activity. In brain death, the EEG shows electrocerebral silence. The EEG hallmark of absence seizures is 3-Hz spike-and-wave discharges.

379. A 60-year-old man with Parkinson disease was under treatment with selegiline and carbidopa/levodopa. When depression developed, SSRI treatment was initiated. Two days later, he began to be agitated, confused, febrile (temperature 100°F), diaphoretic, rigid, and tremulous, and exhibited myoclonus. His CK was 120 U/L. Which syndrome has probably developed?

a. Dopamine intoxication
b. Neuroleptic malignant syndrome
c. Serotonin syndrome
d. None of the above

Answer: c. Following the administration of combinations of serotoninergic medications or a large dose of a single one, mental status changes, autonomic disturbances, myoclonus, and muscle breakdown indicate the serotonin syndrome. This iatrogenic disturbance has several features in common with the neuroleptic malignant syndrome (NMS), but its myoclonus, relatively low fever, and modest CK elevations help distinguish serotonin syndrome from NMS. Neurologic medications, including selegiline, (a MAO inhibitor selective for MAO-B at standard doses) sumatriptan (a serotonin agonist migraine medication), and antidepressants have precipitated the serotonin syndrome.

380. Which electrolyte disturbance characterizes the following conditions: laxative abuse, steroid abuse, and hydrochlorothiazide use?

a. Hyponatremia
b. Hypernatremia
c. Hypokalemia
d. Hyperkalemia

Answer: c. Each of these conditions leads to hypokalemia. Laxative abuse depletes potassium through excessive bowel movements. Steroids retain sodium at the expense of potassium. When hydrochlorothiazide promotes the renal clearance of sodium, compensatory mechanisms lead to a loss of potassium. Bulimia is associated with hypokalemia, but the effect is minor and often accompanied by mild hyponatremia.

381. A 76-year-old woman survived a nondominant cerebral hemisphere stroke but has residual left hemiparesis and sensory impairment. She sometimes finds that at night her left hand moves about and touches her leg or trunk (see figure). Sometimes she jolts upright after finding that the hand, which she believes is not hers, has been groping her. Similarly, during the daytime, she jokes that the

hand feels like her late husband's. Which is the most likely underlying problem?

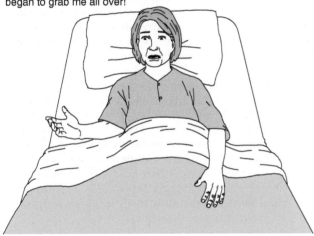

I was frightened, very frightened! In the middle of the night the hand began to grab me all over!

    a. Narcolepsy, with hallucinations
    b. Panic attacks
    c. Nocturnal epilepsy
    d. Alien hand syndrome
    e. A delusion

Answer: d. Patients with the alien hand syndrome, which typically follows a nondominant hemisphere stroke, have a sense of detachment from their own hand even though it retains rudimentary motor and sensory functions. Moreover, they typically believe that an external force governs it. The alien hand autonomously makes small semipurposeful movements, which explains the groping and would account for scratching, unbuttoning, and tugging.

382–389. In assigning a value to a biologic test for Alzheimer disease, what will be the effect of the following changes (382–389) on the test's sensitivity and specificity (a–i)?

382. Technical changes that increase false-negative results.

383. Technical changes that increase true-positive results.

384. Using the test on a population in which the disease is less prevalent.

385. Technical changes that increase false-positive results.

386. Technical changes that increase true-negative results.

387. Lowering the cut-off point of the test results so that both true- and false-positive results increase.

388. Changing the cut-off point of the test results so that both true- and false-negative results increase.

389. Testing for a disease in which individuals with and without the disease can be more readily identified.
    a. Sensitivity and specificity will both increase
    b. Sensitivity and specificity will both decrease
    c. Sensitivity and specificity will remain unchanged

    d. Sensitivity will increase and specificity will decrease
    e. Sensitivity will decrease and specificity will increase
    f. Sensitivity will increase
    g. Sensitivity will decrease
    h. Specificity will increase
    i. Specificity will decrease

Answers: 382–g, 383–f, 384–c, 385–i, 386–h, 387–d, 388–e, 389–a. Tests proposed for Alzheimer disease must be especially specific and sensitive because the clinical diagnosis is approximately 90% accurate. Sensitivity in testing for any disease is defined as the proportion of positive results that are true-positives. It equals true-positives/(true-positives + false-negatives). This formula is equivalent to true-positives/all positives. A highly sensitive test will detect almost all individuals with a disease; however, depending on its specificity, the test may also incorrectly identify individuals who do not actually have the disease.

Specificity in testing for any disease is defined as the proportion of valid negative results. It equals true-negatives/(true-negatives + false-positives). Specificity increases either when true-negatives increase or false-positives decrease, but it is not directly proportional to true positives. In other words, if a highly specific test is positive, the patient is very likely to have the illness; however, a negative result may not exclude it.

390. Which one of the following AEDs inhibits the hepatic cytochrome P-450 oxidases?
    a. Valproate (valproic acid/divalproex) (Depakote)
    b. Carbamazepine (Tegretol)
    c. Phenytoin (Dilantin)
    d. Gabapentin (Neurontin)
    e. Phenobarbital

Answer: a. Of the choices, valproate is the only one that inhibits the P-450 enzyme system. Carbamazepine, phenytoin, and phenobarbital all induce the enzyme system and thus reduce the effectiveness of oral contraceptives and other medications. Gabapentin, lamotrigine, and vigabatrin have little or no effect on the P-450 enzyme system.

391. Which of the following AEDs induces its own metabolism?
    a. Valproate (valproic acid/divalproex) (Depakote)
    b. Carbamazepine (Tegretol)
    c. Phenytoin (Dilantin)
    d. Gabapentin (Neurontin)
    e. Phenobarbital

Answer: b. Of the choices, only carbamazepine induces its own metabolism, i.e., "autoinduces" its metabolism. Thus, physicians must rapidly increase the dosage of carbamazepine at the start of treatment.

392. During her initial visit for a contact lens prescription, an ophthalmologist finds that a 17-year-old high-school student's left pupil is 6 mm and, even with bright light, constricts slowly and incompletely.

Her right pupil is 3 mm and constricts briskly and completely to bright light. Lenses correct her vision to 20/20 bilaterally. She has no diplopia, ptosis, headache, or other ophthalmologic symptom or sign; however, she has neither patellar nor Achilles' DTRs. Which test would most likely reveal the diagnosis?
a. Nerve conduction studies
b. CT or MRI of the head and orbits
c. Tensilon test
d. Instillation of dilute (0.1%) pilocarpine eye drops

Answer: d. Instillation of dilute pilocarpine eye drops will not affect the right (normal) pupil, but will constrict the dilated left pupil. Pupillary constriction when a dilute pilocarpine solution is applied indicates that its constrictor muscles have denervation supersensitivity (or hypersensitivity). The abnormality, which neurologists call an Adie's pupil, results from (parasympathetic) ciliary ganglion damage. For unknown reasons, loss of knee or ankle DTRs often accompanies an Adie's pupil. A Tensilon test, useful in detecting myasthenia gravis, would be superfluous because that illness does not affect the pupils and she has none of myasthenia's usual symptoms, such as diplopia, ptosis, dysarthria, and face weakness.

393. A 2-year-old boy with intellectual disability has dislocated ocular lenses, pectus excavatum, and increased height. An increased concentration of homocystine in his urine leads to a diagnosis of homocystinuria. Which of the following is the most common complication of the illness?
a. Dementia
b. Strokes
c. Autism
d. Epilepsy

Answer: b. Approximately 50% of individuals with homocystinuria suffer thromboembolic events, including strokes in one-third. Homocystinuria patients often have behavior disorders, obsessive-compulsive symptoms, and personality disturbances, but they do not show features of autism.

394. Deficiency of which enzyme causes homocystinuria?
a. Cystathionine β-synthase
b. Tyrosine hydroxylase
c. Hypoxanthine-guanine transferase (HGPRT)
d. Phenylalanine hydroxylase

Answer: a. Cystathionine β-synthase metabolizes homocysteine to cystathionine. Absence of this enzyme leads to an accumulation of plasma homocystine, total homocysteine, and urinary homocystine.

395. In homocystinuria patients, which *two* treatments will best lower the serum homocystine level?
a. A methionine-restricted diet
b. A homocysteine-free diet
c. Administration of folate and vitamins B_6 and B_{12}
d. L-DOPA

Answer: a, c. Restricting dietary methionine and administering folate and vitamins B_6 and B_{12} will reduce plasma homocysteine and total homocysteine levels. These vitamins will also reduce the incidence of intellectual disability and strokes in asymptomatic infants with homocystinuria. In the adult population, an elevated serum concentration of homocysteine is a risk factor for stroke. Contrary to expectations, although giving vitamin B_6 to otherwise normal adults with elevated serum homocystine concentration lowers the total homocysteine level, this treatment does not reduce the incidence of cerebral or myocardial infarction.

396. After playing in his backyard, a 4-year-old boy developed difficulty breathing because of excessive pulmonary secretions and general weakness. Physicians found that he had bradycardia and miosis. During the examination he vomited and had diarrhea. Which is the most likely category of toxin?
a. Sympathomimetic agent
b. Opioid
c. Anticholinesterase
d. SSRI

Answer: c. He has clear signs of cholinergic toxicity that stem predominantly from overstimulation of the parasympathetic muscarinic receptors. In addition to nerve gases, a wide variety of common substances contain an anticholinesterase (cholinesterase inhibitor). For example, insecticides (parathion, malathion), certain mushrooms, and an illegal but popular rice-shaped rat poison (*Tres Pasitos*) each contain potentially lethal concentrations of an anticholinesterase. By administering repeated doses of atropine, the physicians can correct the boy's breathing difficulty and bradycardia.

397. Having retired 5 years ago from her work as a government clerk, a 68-year-old widow comes to a psychiatrist because she feels tired, irritable, and inattentive. Her mood and her intellectual function are normal. However, she spontaneously awakes at 5 AM. Later in the morning she leaves to watch her grandchildren. She wants to take a nap in the afternoon, but she forces herself to remain awake. After she goes to bed at 9 PM, she falls asleep immediately. She is also frustrated because going to bed so early does not allow her to watch her favorite television shows or make telephone calls to her friends and other grandchildren. She uses no caffeine, alcohol, or medicines that would affect her sleep–wake cycle. Which would be the best treatment?
a. Sleep restriction
b. Amphetamines
c. Antidepressants
d. None of the above

Answer: d. This woman has normal age-related changes in her sleep–wake schedule consisting of a mild form of advanced sleep-phase syndrome and an almost irresistible afternoon sleepiness. Her sleep deprivation causes her to feel tired, irritable, and inattentive.

Somehow she must allow herself an afternoon nap – if only for the safety and well-being of her grandchildren. An afternoon nap will allow her to restore her energy, fall asleep later in the evening, and awake later in the morning.

Sleep restriction and other cognitive-behavioral therapies are helpful for sleep-onset insomnia. Amphetamines will intensify her irritability and not overcome her need to sleep in the afternoon or early evening.

398. Paramedics bring a young man to the ER after he swallowed almost an entire bottle of pills of an unknown medication. He is agitated, confused, combative, and unable to provide a coherent history or cooperate. His temperature is 104° and pulse 101. His skin is hot and dry. His pupils are large but reactive. He moves all his limbs, which have no tremor, rigidity, or increased tone. His bladder is distended and he has no bowel sounds. Which is the most likely category of medical intoxication?
   a. Opioid
   b. Serotonin reuptake inhibitor
   c. Anticholinesterase
   d. Anticholinergic

Answer: d. Anticholinergic medicines, such as scopolamine, cause agitated delirium, suppress parasympathetic activity, and allow excessive sympathetic activity. Lack of parasympathetic activity causes hot, dry skin and reduced bowel and bladder function, and unopposed sympathetic activity leads to tachycardia and mydriasis. Opioids cause small pupils and, with overdose, pulmonary edema. Anticholinesterases that do not cross the blood–brain barrier, such as pyridostigmine, do not alter mental status. Most that cross the blood–brain barrier, such as donepezil, can cause abdominal cramping and diarrhea from gastrointestinal hyperactivity.

399. Which of the following statements regarding prions is *false*?
   a. Inoculation may occur through non-neurologic as well as neurologic portals.
   b. The usually short incubation period lengthens with subsequent transmission.
   c. Individuals with a mutation on chromosome 20 are susceptible to prion infections.
   d. The infection strikes the brain predominantly or exclusively.

Answer: b. The incubation period is usually long, but it shortens with successive intraspecies and interspecies transmission. Prions enter the host through non-neurologic portals, such as when animals have eaten CNS tissue of infected animals. Prions also enter through as neurologic portals, as when infected CNS tissue is injected into the brain of a host animal. Individuals with a mutant PRNP gene, which is encoded on chromosome 20, are susceptible to CJD and variant CJD (vCJD). The brain remains the target organ, but the olfactory nerves and lymphatic tissue of the ileum also show signs of infection. Recent studies have also suggested that prions may be causative in several neurodegenerative illnesses.

400. A neurologist referred a 31-year-old woman to a psychiatrist because depression has complicated her migraines. She revealed to the psychiatrist that she also has had two miscarriages during the past year and a hospitalization for deep vein thromboses in one and then the other leg. A brain MRI and routine medical evaluation disclosed no underlying illness. Which one of the following tests would most likely indicate the diagnosis?
   a. VDRL
   b. Anticardiolipin antibodies
   c. HIV
   d. Thyroid function

Answer: b. Repeated miscarriages, migraines, and deep vein thromboses are major components of the antiphospholipid syndrome. Its other manifestations include myocardial infarctions and arterial and/or venous strokes. The presence of a serum lupus anticoagulant and anticardiolipin antibodies would confirm the diagnosis. On the other hand, these antibodies are not pathognomonic for the antiphospholipid syndrome. They are also detectable in older age, various inflammatory conditions, and systemic lupus erythematosus (SLE). While further testing is underway, physicians might administer antidepressants.

401. During evaluation of a 66-year-old man for the onset of dementia, the physician asked the patient to copy a sequence of four sets, each of three squares followed by a circle. After completing one set, the patient copied only the squares. When he was unable to complete the task, he shouted, cursed, and broke the pencil. An MRI showed generalized cerebral atrophy, especially in the frontal lobes. Of the following, which is the most likely underlying pathology?
   a. Plaques and tangles
   b. Spirochetes in gummas
   c. Intraneuronal argentophilic inclusions
   d. Intraneuronal eosinophilic intracytoplasmic inclusions

Answer: c. As in Question 307, this patient shows perseveration, easy frustration, emotional outburst, decrease in verbal output, and lack of inhibition. Although the underlying problem could reflect Neurocognitive Disorder due to Vascular Disease, these symptoms point to Neurocognitive Disorder due to Frontotemporal Lobar Degeneration. Intraneuronal argentophilic inclusions indicate Pick disease, which is a variety of Neurocognitive Disorder due to Frontotemporal Lobar Degeneration. Spirochetes in gummas characterize neurosyphilis. Intraneuronal eosinophilic intracytoplasmic inclusions are Lewy bodies, which indicate Neurocognitive Disorder due to Lewy Bodies.

402. The police bring a 17-year-old boy to the ER when, following a verbal fight with his parents, he seemed to develop quadriparesis and blindness. Nevertheless, his motor tone, DTRs, plantar reflexes, and cranial nerves are intact. His pupils are 4 mm,

round, and reactive to light. In addition, when a neurologist rotates a drum with vertical stripes in front of him, his eyes repetitively follow the stripes and then snap back. What is the implication of his ocular movements?
a. He has ingested PCP or related toxin.
b. He should be given thiamine.
c. His optokinetic nystagmus is intact.
d. He has sustained a traumatic injury to his occipital lobe.

Answer: c. His following the stripes on the drum shows that he has intact optokinetic nystagmus, which is an irresistible ocular motility reflex. The normal response indicates that his visual and ocular motility pathways are functioning normally. Its presence in someone who purports to be blind is strong evidence that the "visual loss" is psychogenic. Other tests may support a psychogenic diagnosis. A simple one is for the physician to smile, make ridiculous faces, or hold attractive pictures in front of a patient. Another one is for the physician to hold a mirror in front of the patient: if their vision is intact, people cannot resist following their image. An EEG will show occipital alpha rhythm in physiologically normal individuals when they are at rest, relaxed, and with their eyes closed; however, when they open their eyes and can see their surroundings, the alpha rhythm disappears. Thus, people with psychogenic blindness with their eyes closed will have alpha activity that vanishes when they open their eyes. Normal visual-evoked responses (VERs) also indicate an intact visual pathway.

403. A psychiatrist hospitalizes this 38-year-old woman for agitated depression with dangerous psychotic features. Despite treatment with antipsychotic and antidepressant medication, she remains agitated. She continually paces and, when sitting, has continual rhythmic adduction and abduction leg movements (see figure). Which is the *least* likely explanation for the leg movements?
a. Prolonged effect of an illicit drug, such as cocaine
b. Akathisia
c. Undertreatment of agitated depression
d. Chorea

Answer: d. Her movements present the dilemma of medication under-treatment failing to suppress symptoms versus over-treatment causing akathisia. Alternatively, cocaine or other stimulant use may cause mental and physical agitation. Chorea does not cause mental agitation or rhythmic movements.

404. Which statement is *true* concerning Angelman's syndrome?
a. Angelman's syndrome occurs exclusively in girls.
b. Children with Angelman's syndrome have imprinted behavior, as described by Konrad Lorenz.
c. Genomic imprinting largely determines the mutation's phenotype.
d. An Angelman's syndrome boy is likely to have a sister with Prader–Willi syndrome.

Answer: c. In Angelman's syndrome and its counterpart, Prader–Willi syndrome, the condition's phenotype often depends on which parent transmitted the mutation (genomic imprinting). Konrad Lorenz, who won the Nobel Prize in 1973, described a different phenomenon – behavioral imprinting – among social animals.

405. Which one of the following statements is *true* regarding adults with attention deficit hyperactivity disorder (ADHD)?
a. Although stimulants may be effective therapy in children with ADHD, they are usually ineffective in adults with ADHD.

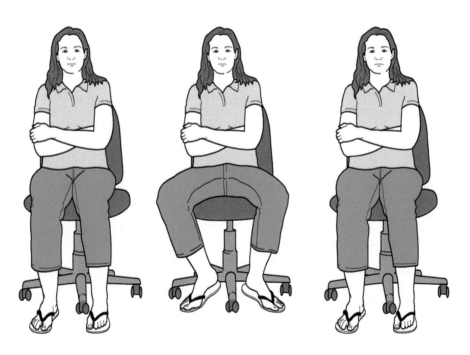

b. ADHD in children persists as they become adults.

c. Stimulants are contraindicated in ADHD patients with tic disorder.

d. ADHD adults are prone to develop antisocial personality disorder.

Answer: d. Stimulants are effective in adult as well as childhood ADHD. Only about 15% of children with ADHD grow into adults with ADHD. Stimulants are appropriately administered to patients with tic disorder who often have comorbid ADHD. However, phenobarbital and other sedatives are apt to precipitate paradoxical hyperactivity in both children and adults with ADHD. ADHD adults are prone to develop antisocial personality disorder, substance abuse, and other problems.

406. Which treatment might reduce involuntary hyperkinetic movements?
   a. Tetrabenazine
   b. Methyl-phenyl-tetrahydropyridine (MPTP)
   c. Magnetic stimulation
   d. Ropinirole

Answer: a. Tetrabenazine depletes presynaptic dopamine stores and thereby reduces chorea, tics, oral-buccal-lingual tardive dyskinesias, and other hyperkinetic movements. As a caveat, because tetrabenazine markedly reduces dopamine activity, it may lead to parkinsonism and depression. MPTP destroys neurons because it forms free radicals toxic to all neurons and causes parkinsonism. Magnetic stimulation has no proven role in treatment of these disorders. Ropinirole, a dopamine agonist, improves restless leg syndrome and increases mobility in Parkinson disease. Ropinirole and other dopamine agonists may cause dyskinesia, but they will not reduce involuntary hyperkinetic movements except for restless legs syndrome.

407. Match the sign (a–g) with its closest implication (1–6).
   a. Babinski
   b. Lhermitte
   c. Romberg
   d. Tinel
   e. Lasègue's
   f. Hoover
   g. Abductor
   1. Irritation of a lumbar nerve root
   2. Spinal cord posterior column impairment
   3. Corticospinal tract injury
   4. Cervical spinal cord irritation
   5. Psychogenic leg paresis
   6. Nerve entrapment

Answer: a–3, b–4 (typically elicited in MS), c–2 (tabes dorsalis and combined system degeneration), d–6 (carpal tunnel syndrome), e–1 (lumbar herniated disk), f–5, g–5.

408. In assessing an accomplished physician for neurocognitive disorder, which of the following is the *least* reliable indication of cognitive decline?

a. Results of a current neuropsychologic battery

b. Scores obtained on a current scholastic achievement test (SAT) compared to those in high school

c. Assessment of mathematical ability

d. Job performance

Answer: c. Mathematical ability is an isolated cognitive function that does not reflect overall cognition. Even in professionally successful, intellectual individuals, mathematical ability may not have been well developed during childhood. Moreover, with lack of use, mathematical skills atrophy. In contrast, vocabulary and reading skills are deeply ingrained.

409. Of the following, which medication produces the lowest relapse rate in chronic alcoholics?
   a. Naltrexone
   b. Disulfiram
   c. SSRIs
   d. Lithium

Answer: a.

410. On a neurologic examination, a 10-year-old boy with 6 months of behavioral and academic difficulties has clumsiness, Babinski signs, and inability to walk "in tandem" (one foot in front of the other [heel-to-toe walking]). The MRI shows extensive cerebral demyelination with surrounding inflammation. Testing also shows adrenal insufficiency. An older brother had the same symptoms and signs, but he succumbed to an adrenal crisis before it was diagnosed. Which one of the following statements is *false*?

a. The patient's urine will probably contain metachromatic granules.

b. Adrenal replacement therapy will correct any adrenal insufficiency but not the neurologic deterioration.

c. This condition can mimic MS; however, it typically occurs in boys, leads to death in approximately 5 years, and is characterized by adrenal failure.

d. This condition results from defective peroxisomes.

Answer: a. The boy and his brother have adrenoleukodystrophy (ALD), which is an X-linked leukodystrophy that first produces symptoms in childhood. ALD results from the accumulation of very long-chain fatty acids because of defective peroxisomes, which are intracellular organelles. As its name indicates, ALD leads to demyelination of the CNS. The first signs of ALD are typically behavioral, emotional, and cognitive difficulties. Soon afterward corticospinal tract and cerebellar signs develop and predominate. At the same time, the adrenal glands fail.

Metachromatic granules in the urine would indicate metachromatic leukodystrophy (MLD), which is another CNS demyelinating disease. It usually presents in childhood, but often not until the young adult years. Unlike

ALD, MLD is inherited in an autosomal recessive pattern and does not cause adrenal insufficiency.

411. In treating erectile dysfunction, what is the role of nitric oxide?
    a. It leads to vasoconstriction.
    b. It promotes the production of cGMP-phosphodiesterase.
    c. It promotes cGMP activity.
    d. It leads to amnesia.

Answer: c. Nitric oxide promotes cyclic guanosine monophosphate (cGMP) activity, which leads to vasodilation. The vasodilation leads to genital engorgement.

412. What is the mechanism of action of sildenafil (Viagra)?
    a. It increases cGMP activity.
    b. It enhances cGMP-phosphodiesterase.
    c. It promotes the production of cyclic guanylate cyclase monophosphate (cGMP).
    d. It provokes the release of nitric oxide (NO).

Answer: a. As presaged by the previous question, sildenafil (Viagra) increases cGMP activity by inhibiting its metabolic enzyme (cGMP-phosphodiesterase).

413. Emergency room physicians admit a 43-year-old school bus driver to the hospital because of acute severe painful incapacitating torticollis. He denied taking medicines or illicit drugs. Aside from continual forceful turning of his head and neck in one direction for a few minutes and then to the other direction for a few minutes, the neurologic examination revealed no abnormalities. An EEG and routine blood and urine tests, including ones for dopamine-blocking medicines and illicit substances, also disclosed no abnormalities. While awaiting an MRI, a medical student recognized the patient as having been admitted elsewhere 6 months before with a tremor that remained undiagnosed but finally disappeared after 5 days. Searching his old records, another student found that he had been admitted 2 years previously for a 1-week episode of apparent myoclonus. What is the MRI most likely to show?
    a. Diffuse demyelination
    b. Multiple areas of periventricular demyelination
    c. Bilateral frontal lobe lesions
    d. No abnormality

Answer: d. Psychogenic movement disorders occur less frequently than psychogenic seizures or most other conversion disorders, such as psychogenic hemiparesis or elective mutism. Neurologists suspect a psychogenic basis for a movement disorder if it has an acute onset, exhibits inconsistent or variable features, has accompanying non-movement deficits, such as paresis or blindness, and causes more functional disability than clear-cut cases. Neurologists also suspect psychogenic tremor if they can entrain it. Sometimes a movement's bizarre appearance suggests a psychogenic basis. Ingestion of dopamine-blocking medicines could have caused transient torticollis and tremor, but not myoclonus, and the history and tests on the blood and urine excluded this possibility. Diffuse demyelination characterizes certain storage diseases, such as metachromatic dystrophy, and abuse of volatile hydrocarbons, such as toluene. Multiple areas of periventricular demyelination characterize MS.

414. The ER staff requested a psychiatric consultation to assist in managing a 55-year-old woman. She had a history of anxiety disorder for which her psychiatrist prescribed benzodiazepines. She had presented to the ER with a 36-hour history that began with constipation and increasing abdominal pain; then dysarthria, dyspnea, and dysphagia; and finally diplopia and blurred vision. With the onset of the dyspnea, she developed fearfulness and mental and physical agitation. A neurologist found that she had bilateral ptosis, dilated and unreactive pupils, paresis of one medial rectus muscle and the contralateral lateral rectus, bilateral face and palate weakness, and hypophonia. Her gag and jaw jerk reflexes were absent. She had generalized mild weakness. Her temperature, pulse, and blood pressure were mildly elevated. How should the physicians proceed?
    a. Administer naloxone
    b. Give a benzodiazepine
    c. Intubate her
    d. Administer edrophonium

Answer: c. Because the immediate problem is potential airway occlusion manifest by her anxiety and agitation as well as dyspnea, physicians must intubate her to secure a patent airway. Afterwards they can treat her with benzodiazepines to allow her to tolerate an endotracheal tube, allay her anxiety, and enable her to cooperate in gathering additional history and cooperating with complete examination and testing. In situations where impaired breathing or substantial bleeding is the immediate issue, physicians must support vital signs before reaching a specific diagnosis. Giving benzodiazepines to a patient with delirium and dyspnea risks suppressing their respiratory drive. Moreover, the delirium may, in part, reflect hypoxia.

415. To which disorder should her physicians attribute her dysarthria, dysphagia, dyspnea, and probable vocal cord paralysis?
    a. Bulbar palsy
    b. Pseudobulbar palsy
    c. Myasthenia gravis
    d. Polymyositis

Answer: a. The paresis of the oculomotor, facial, and abducens nerves, and probably masseters and vocal cord muscles, with absence of her gag and jaw jerk reflexes indicates paresis of cranial nerves V through XI. Myasthenia gravis might have been responsible except that she has dilated unreactive pupils, fever, and constipation.

Polymyositis in adults strikes the proximal limb muscles and does not involve the pupillary sphincter muscles.

416. Of the following possible etiologies, which is the *least* likely?
   a. West Nile virus infection
   b. Guillain–Barré syndrome
   c. Botulism
   d. ALS

Answer: d. All of these illnesses may cause bulbar palsy and the symptoms that brought her to the ER. However, ALS develops over months and does not involve the pupils or gastrointestinal tract. This woman's illness is most likely botulism, which characteristically presents with constipation and then bulbar palsy accompanied by facial diplegia and large unreactive pupils.

417. A 26-year-old woman consults a neurologist because she has had 6 weeks of recurring headaches. She had no history of migraine or tension headache, trauma, infections, or risk factors for HIV disease. She is obese and has irregular menses, but she is not pregnant. She has florid papilledema and bilateral abducens nerve palsies. She is fully alert and able to ambulate. She has no ataxia. Of the following, which should be the next diagnostic step?
   a. Perform tests for AIDS
   b. Obtain a head CT or MRI
   c. Perform an LP, which will be therapeutic as well as diagnostic
   d. None of the above

Answer: b. This patient's age, obesity, menstrual irregularity, and absence of focal findings indicate that she has idiopathic intracranial hypertension (pseudotumor cerebri). Before performing an LP to confirm the diagnosis, she should undergo either a CT or MRI to exclude a mass lesion and hydrocephalus. In some cases of idiopathic intracranial hypertension, an obstructed intracranial venous sinus is responsible for the disorder.

418. What is the effect of dopamine's stimulating D2 receptors?
   a. The interaction increases adenylate cyclase activity.
   b. The interaction decreases adenylate cyclase activity.
   c. The interaction has no effect on adenylate cyclase activity.

Answer: b. Dopamine–D1 receptor interaction increases adenylate cyclase activity, but dopamine–D2 receptor interaction reduces adenylate cyclase activity.

419. A 6-year-old boy began to have inward turning of his feet most pronounced after he finishes school at 3 pm. One trick that he shows his parents is that when he walks backward, the foot assumes a normal position. At a mid-afternoon examination, the boy's pediatrician attributed the problem to a subtle, previously undiagnosed congenital cerebral injury ("cerebral palsy" or "CP"). Later that day, when a pediatric neurologist evaluated the boy, both legs had sustained, inward turning and his lower trunk was rotated (see figure). Even though the boy's DTRs were normal, the neurologist concurred with the diagnosis of CP. However, having second thoughts, the neurologist reexamined the boy the next morning and found no abnormalities in either movement or posture. Which test will most likely indicate the diagnosis?
   a. A psychiatric evaluation
   b. A therapeutic trial of levodopa
   c. Muscle biopsy
   d. Determine the serum ceruloplasmin concentration
   e. Genetic tests for the DYT1 mutation

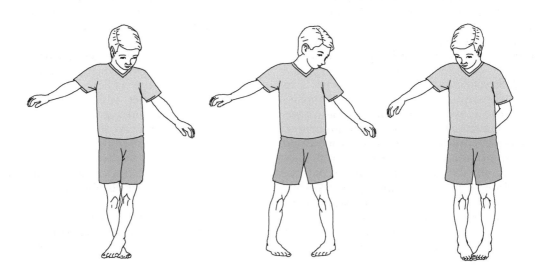

Answer: b. The boy has developed dystonia – involuntary twisting movements of his trunk and limbs. "Tricks" that temporarily abolish the movements – walking backward, skipping, dancing, or applying pressure to the involved limb – are fully consistent with that diagnosis. Moreover, the diurnal fluctuation of his dystonia strongly supports dopamine-responsive dystonia (DRD). Other causes of dystonia in childhood include early-onset torsion dystonia, which is found predominantly in Ashkenazi Jews and identified by the DYT1 gene test, and Wilson disease; however, neither of these illnesses produces a diurnal fluctuation. Intellectual disability but not dystonia characterizes phenylketonuria (PKU), which becomes apparent in infancy. Physicians have misdiagnosed DRD as either a congenital cerebral injury or a psychogenic movement disorder.

420. A 39-year-old housewife has reported to many physicians and other health-care providers that she has chronic fatigue, insomnia, and the need to sleep during most of the daytime. She also reports having fibromyalgia, chronic daily headaches, and irritable bowel syndrome. Routine examinations, blood tests, and neurologic evaluations have revealed no abnormalities. A PSG showed markedly reduced slow-wave and REM sleep but excessive spindles and β-activity. Which test should her physicians perform, whether or not she has already had one done?
a. Mononucleosis test
b. Lyme titer
c. Urine for toxicology
d. Epstein–Barr virus serology

Answer: c. The most important PSG finding is loss of slow-wave and REM sleep, as this explains her EDS. Using alcohol, hypnotics, opioids, and amphetamines would explain her excessive daytime sleepiness, other symptoms, and PSG abnormalities.

421. A junior faculty member who was denied tenure swallowed a strychnine-containing liquid. Violent muscle spasms convulsed her body. Her face was drawn tight and her back arched. After turning blue, she died. What was the mechanism of her death?
a. Poisoning of her mitochondria
b. Status epilepticus
c. Impaired release of presynaptic glycine and GABA
d. Blockade of postsynaptic glycine and GABA receptors

Answer: d. Strychnine's mechanism of action is to block postsynaptic receptors of the inhibitory neurotransmitters glycine and GABA. Uninhibited activity causes violent muscle contractions (spasms) that mimic seizures. Muscles spasms prevent breathing because they occlude the airway and prevent coordinated chest wall contractions and relaxations. By way of a comparison, tetanus impairs the release of presynaptic glycine and GABA, causing uninhibited persistent muscle contractions. Cyanide poisons mitochondria.

422. Which one of the following illnesses is *not* a polyglutamine disease?

a. Huntington disease
b. Duchenne muscular dystrophy
c. Fragile X
d. Myotonic dystrophy

Answer: b. Polyglutamine diseases include Huntington disease, fragile X, myotonic dystrophy, and many spinocerebellar ataxias. Neurologists refer to these illnesses, which are carried by excessive CAG trinucleotide repeats, as polyglutamine diseases because that mutation leads to excessive polyglutamine synthesis.

423. A young woman joined a new friend at a bar. After a few drinks, they went to a hookah lounge. While smoking tobacco through the hookah, she became euphoric and then developed a seizure. In the ER, she awoke and had no deficits. Blood and urine tests, including toxicology screen, disclosed no abnormalities. Which is the most likely scenario?
a. Someone laced the tobacco with marijuana.
b. Someone laced the tobacco with synthetic marijuana.
c. She had epilepsy and had not disclosed it to her new friend.
d. Someone added GHB to the tobacco.

Answer: b. The ER physicians had a difficult time deciding on a diagnosis. Unlike garden-variety marijuana, synthetic versions induce euphoria and they also cause seizures. Because of their chemical variability, synthetic marijuanas escape detection on standard urine toxicology screening. Synthetic marijuana users often add them to tobacco, actual marijuana, e-cigarettes, energy drinks, or illicit drugs. These drugs may cause delirium, psychotic reactions, and strokes as well as seizures. Simply smoking unadulterated tobacco does not precipitate seizures in individuals with epilepsy. Although smoking pure tobacco through a hookah appears to add an element of safety from a water filter, the smoke still contains the same dependence-inducing nicotine, cancer-causing agents, and toxic carbon monoxide as smoking tobacco. Gamma-hydroxybutyrate (GHB, or the "date-rape drug") causes a deep sleep followed by amnesia but not seizures.

424. Which one of the following statements regarding radioligands in PET is *true*?
a. These radioligands have a half-life that typically exceeds 7 days.
b. In PET, the radioligands release positrons, which interact with electrons. The reaction annihilates both particles. Their combined mass converts into two photons.
c. In PET, radioligands produce an anatomic image that has the same resolution as CT.
d. PET radioligands are specific enough to diagnose Alzheimer disease.

Answer: b. PET produces a gross anatomic image but a good picture of the brain's metabolism. Results are not sufficiently sensitive or specific for definitive diagnosis of Alzheimer disease.

425. A 33-year-old man with MS has paraparesis and a left-sided scotoma. On testing, he states that the neurologist's red tie appears maroon when he uses his left eye, but red when he uses his right eye. Which is the most likely explanation for his visual distortion?
   a. He has color blindness.
   b. The MS has affected his occipital cortex.
   c. He has a persistent ocular migraine.
   d. He has color desaturation.
   e. He has developed a psychogenic disturbance.

Answer: d. He has color desaturation, which is a common manifestation of optic neuritis. Optic neuritis is a frequently occurring manifestation of MS but also can result from other etiologies. Color blindness, especially the red–green variety, is a sex-linked genetic disorder, detectable from childhood. It affects both eyes. MS can affect the occipital lobe, but lesions there would cause hemianopia rather than color desaturation.

426. In which condition is a patient unable to perceive pain and suffering?
   a. Locked-in syndrome
   b. Persistent vegetative state
   c. Dementia
   d. Aphasia
   e. None of the above

Answer: b. Although patients in the locked-in syndrome or with dementia or aphasia may experience pain and suffering because they are conscious, those in the persistent vegetative state cannot consciously perceive pain or suffering. According to some reports, patients in the minimally conscious state are capable of perceiving pain. This distinction has medicolegal ramifications.

427. This is the MRI of a 23-year-old man who had noticed that he had been losing hearing ability in his left ear for 1 year. The MRI was performed following infusion of gadolinium. Where is the lesion located?

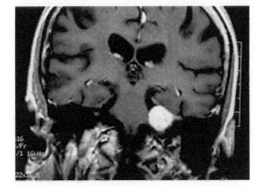

   a. Lateral to the pons
   b. In the pons
   c. In the temporal lobe
   d. None of the above

Answer: a. The round hyperintense lesion is located in the left cerebellopontine angle. It arises from the acoustic nerve, which can be seen as a bright streak above and medial to the lesion.

428. The man described in the previous question underwent gamma-knife surgery. The surgeon was able to remove most of the lesion and preserve facial strength and most of his hearing. What is the most likely histology of the lesion?
   a. Glioblastoma
   b. Medulloblastoma
   c. Acoustic neuroma
   d. Meningioma

Answer: c. Although a meningioma is possible, the lesion proved to be an acoustic neuroma. Glioblastomas and medulloblastomas are intra-axial.

429. In a postoperative evaluation, the surgeon discovered that the man in the previous two questions had three small *café-au-lait* spots. He remained asymptomatic for several years, but then the hearing in his right ear began to fail. A repeat MRI showed a lesion on the right side similar to the initial, left-sided one present on the initial MRI. Which is the most likely underlying diagnosis?
   a. Neurofibromatosis type 1 (NF1)
   b. Neurofibromatosis type 2 (NF2)
   c. Metastatic carcinoma
   d. A mitochondrial disorder

Answer: b. Bilateral acoustic neuromas indicate that he has neurofibromatosis type 2 (NF2), which is inherited on chromosome 22 in an autosomal dominant pattern. NF2 produces fewer neurofibromas or *café-au-lait* spots, than the more common variety of neurofibromatosis, NF1, which is carried on chromosome 17. Neurologists require six *café-au-lait* spots each larger than 5 mm in children and 1.5 cm in adults to diagnosis NF1. Genetic tests can establish the diagnosis of either variety.

430. Which statement is *true* regarding meningomyelocele?
   a. Meningomyelocele is a minor congenital defect.
   b. Although MRI can make an early and accurate diagnosis of meningomyelocele, ultrasound testing cannot detect it.
   c. Folic acid (folate) diet supplements have reduced the incidence of meningomyelocele.
   d. The neural tube normally forms during the second trimester of pregnancy.

Answer: c. The neural tube forms during the first trimester of gestation. During this period, if the lower (caudal) end of the neural tube fails to close, the failure will cause spina bifida, a meningocele, or a meningomyelocele – in increasing order of severity of neural tube defects. If the upper (rostral) end fails to close, the failure will cause an encephalocele or the more severe anencephaly. Prescribing prenatal vitamins with folic acid and supplementing breakfast cereals with folic acid have lowered the incidence of neural tube defects. Nevertheless, it remains unsafe for pregnant women to take medicines associated with the defect. MRI and ultrasound may each detect a meningomyelocele, but most physicians prefer an ultrasound examination. Elevated levels of maternal serum alpha-fetoprotein suggest the presence of a meningomyelocele. Studies have not shown an increased incidence of meningomyelocele with all mood stabilizers taken during pregnancy. The ones that remain closely linked are valproate and, to a lesser extent, carbamazepine. Studies have also linked toxins and mutations to the defect.

431. An 85-year-old retired millionaire is brought to the hospital by his lifelong butler. The patient, who had a 10-year history of Parkinson disease complicated by dementia, had experienced a seizure. His psychiatrist has been prescribing haloperidol at bedtime because of nocturnal hallucinations, delusions, screaming, and a tendency to wander; however, neither haloperidol nor any other antipsychotic controlled his thought disorder or abnormal behavior. A CT showed a small acute and a large chronic subdural hematoma. After neurosurgeons drained the subdural hematomas, the patient returned to his usual state. One month later, the patient was readmitted with a fracture-dislocation of shoulder and the following month with another subdural hematoma. What is the most likely cause of the repeated hospitalizations?
a. Parkinson disease
b. Other forms of trauma
c. Adverse reactions to medications
d. Age-related deterioration

Answer: b. The first admission probably resulted from a combination of acute traumatic bleeding superimposed on a chronic subdural hematoma. The second admission may have been due to a fall or deliberate trauma. Undoubtedly, Parkinson disease and age-related neurologic and orthopedic changes are risk factors for falls. However, physicians should remain vigilant for abuse in elderly patients who repeatedly sustain trauma.

432. A 73-year-old woman was admitted to the hospital immediately after the sudden onset of left-sided hemiparesis. Diagnosing an acute stroke, neurologists administered tPA. During the next 3 days, she became agitated and belligerent. She accused the staff of keeping her in the hospital even though nothing was wrong with her. What is the most likely cause of her feeling that "nothing is wrong"?
a. The tPA has caused a delirium.
b. A new stroke developed on the third day of hospitalization.
c. Anosognosia has emerged.
d. She has developed dementia.

Answer: c. The thrombolytic agent tPA has some potentially serious side effects, such as intracerebral bleeding, but delirium is not one of them. Patients with anosognosia often do not appreciate their situation and treatment. In fact, patients with acute strokes complicated by anosognosia might refuse tPA.

433. As part of a re-evaluation of the patient in the preceding question, this CT was obtained on the fifth hospital day. What does it reveal?

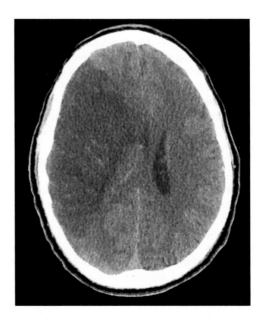

a. A right middle cerebral artery stroke
b. A right cerebral tumor
c. A left middle cerebral artery stroke
d. Occlusion of the right internal carotid artery
e. Occlusion of the left internal carotid artery

Answer: a. In keeping with the convention, this CT displays the patient's right side on the left. The CT shows the territory of the right middle cerebral artery to be dark (hypodense) due to occlusion of that artery and consequent infarction of the brain tissue it irrigates. (The tPA failed to dissolve the clot, and a stroke ensued.)

434. One sunny spring afternoon, several middle-school girls, who were all cheerleaders, complain of dizziness and begin to have incessant jerking movements of their arms. Soon all the girl cheerleaders and then almost all the 50 girls in the grade have the same symptom and movements. The press and worried families appear. The school principal rushes in a toxicologist and neurologist to diagnose the problem. Which is the neurologist's most likely diagnosis?
a. Substance abuse
b. NMDA receptor encephalitis
c. Sydenham chorea
d. Mass hysteria

Answer: d. Mini-epidemics among adolescents have consisted of rapid, widespread common symptoms, such as dizziness, fainting, sickness, and dyspnea. Falling to the floor, seizure-like episodes, and chorea-like jerking may follow. Usually the symptoms and signs primarily or exclusively affect girls, often begin with the most popular individuals, and spread explosively within their cliques and then the larger group. For the affected student, the diagnosis would be Conversion Disorder, acute episode, with a psychological stressor. Chorea, whether from Sydenham chorea, chorea gravidarum, oral contraceptive use, or lupus, can develop in adolescent girls. Only Sydenham chorea occurs in mini-epidemics, but its onset is gradual and spread is limited.

435. Which is the best initial strategy for dealing with the adolescents in the preceding question?
a. Convene group meetings of the "victims."
b. Meet with family units.
c. Allow the press to interview each victim.
d. Separate "victims" from each other, their family, and the press.

Answer: d. To stop the spread of the problem and reduce the symptoms, authorities should ideally isolate and evaluate each student. Some of the students may have a neurologic or psychiatric illness.

436. Which electrolyte disturbance characterizes the following conditions: primary adrenal failure, psychogenic polydipsia, SIADH, and use of diuretics, carbamazepine (Tegretol), and oxcarbazepine (Trileptal)?
a. Hyponatremia
b. Hypernatremia
c. Hypokalemia
d. Hyperkalemia

Answer: a. Each of these conditions leads to hyponatremia but through different mechanisms. Primary adrenal failure (Addison disease) leads to a deficiency of mineralocorticoid hormone. Psychogenic polydipsia and SIADH cause dilutional hyponatremia. Diuretics (especially hydrochlorothiazide), carbamazepine, and oxcarbazepine impair renal retention of sodium. In addition, diabetic ketoacidosis leads to hyponatremia because of the loss of all electrolytes from the polyuria and the dilutional effect of hyperglycemia.

437. Which of the following statements correctly describes the actions of serotonin in migraine treatment?
a. Sumatriptan acts as a 5-$HT_{1B/1D}$ agonist.
b. Sumatriptan–5-$HT_{1B/1D}$ receptor interactions produce vasodilation.
c. Sumatriptan acts as a 5-$HT_{1B/1D}$ antagonist.

Answer: a. Sumatriptan acts as a 5-$HT_{1B/1D}$ agonist and alleviates migraine's autonomic nervous system disturbances as well as its headache.

438. Which is the phenotype of untreated infants with congenital absence of phenylalanine hydroxylase?
a. Intellectual disability, deafness, and epilepsy
b. Episodes of encephalopathy and lactic acidosis
c. Self-mutilation, intellectual disability, hyperuricemia, dystonia, and spasticity
d. Intellectual disability, eczema, and fair complexion
e. Rigidity, dystonia, and gait impairment that occur in the late afternoon

Answer: d. Infants with congenital absence of phenylalanine hydroxylase have phenylketonuria (PKU). The phenylalanine hydroxylase deficiency causes intellectual disability, eczema, and lack of pigment in the hair and eyes. If the disease remains undiagnosed or untreated, epilepsy develops. Intellectual disability, deafness, and epilepsy are the cardinal features of congenital rubella infection. Episodic encephalopathy and lactic acidosis suggest a mitochondrial DNA disorder. The combination of intellectual disability, self-mutilation, hyperuricemia, dystonia, and spasticity in a boy indicates Lesch–Nyhan syndrome. Rigidity, dystonia, and gait impairment that occur in the late afternoon indicate dopamine-responsive dystonia.

439. On which chromosome is the gene that codes for amyloid precursor protein (APP)?
a. 4
b. 17
c. 21
d. X

Answer: c. A credible theory suggests that Alzheimer disease develops in almost all trisomy 21 individuals, if they live long enough, because they have three APP-carrying chromosomes.

440. A 60-year-old woman reports having had several episodes, each lasting several hours, of incapacitating "dizziness." The symptom develops suddenly and is associated with nausea, but not tinnitus or hearing loss. The physician determines that the dizziness is actually vertigo and that it is present only when her head changes position. During the examination, when she lies supine with her head and neck hyperextended and rotated 45° to the right, she develops vertigo and nystagmus. The rest of her neurologic examination, audiometry, and an MRI scan of her brain are normal. Which is the best treatment?
a. Neurosurgery for an acoustic neuroma
b. Canalith repositioning maneuvers
c. ASA for basilar artery TIAs
d. An SSRI for panic attacks

Answer: b. The nystagmus elicited by the Dix–Hallpike maneuver indicates that she has benign positional vertigo, which probably results from debris (otoliths) in a semicircular canal. Canal repositioning is a therapeutic maneuver that consists of the physician's hyperextending and then rotating the patient's head, which hopefully moves otoliths from the semicircular canal to the utricle.

441. Which of the following antidepressants is most likely to cause priapism?
a. Fluvoxamine
b. Fluoxetine
c. Bupropion
d. Trazodone
e. Paroxetine

Answer: d.

442. Physicians hospitalized a 45-year-old inveterate smoker of two to four packs of cigarettes each day for cardiac monitoring. After being unable to smoke for 2 days, he became agitated, loud, and then disoriented. Which would best relieve his nicotine craving?

a. Benzodiazepine
b. Ethanol
c. Varenicline
d. Haloperidol

Answer: c. Nicotine withdrawal is a major problem in hospitals where smoking is forbidden in almost all areas. It routinely causes anxiety and may induce delirium and even violent behavior. This case shows that delirium can manifest as a hyperalert rather than a somnolent state. Unlike alcohol withdrawal, nicotine withdrawal does not lead to hallucinations or seizures. Varenicline (Chantix), a nicotinic ACh receptor agonist, would probably alleviate his nicotine withdrawal symptoms and allow his medical care to proceed. Alternatively, bupropion, a nicotine antagonist, may help.

443. The physicians gave the patient in the previous question nicotine medications, but they failed to quell his delirium. Then they arranged for him to smoke, but that strategy also did not reduce his delirium and it failed to stop his disruptive behavior. After applying psychologic measures and seeing them fail, which group of medicines would be most helpful?
    a. Benzodiazepine
    b. Antipsychotic
    c. Opioid
    d. Benzodiazepine receptor agonist

Answer: b. Benzodiazepines and opioids carry the potential adverse effect of respiratory depression. In this situation, small doses of antipsychotics are probably the most likely to help without undue potential adverse effects. Of course, physicians should search for causes of delirium other than nicotine withdrawal, including alcohol withdrawal, hypoxia, paraneoplastic syndromes and medicines that induce abnormal behavior, such as levetiracetam (Keppra).

444–446. A wife sent her 63-year-old husband for psychiatric consultation because of inappropriate behavior. The psychiatrist, finding that the patient had headaches, cognitive impairment, and a mild left-hemiparesis, requested an MRI.

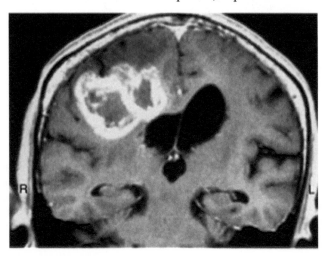

444. Which view has been displayed?
    a. Axial
    b. Sagittal
    c. Coronal

Answer: c.

445. Where is the lesion?
    a. Right frontal-parietal lobe
    b. Left frontal-parietal lobe
    c. Right temporal lobe
    d. Left temporal lobe
    e. Right occipital lobe
    f. Left occipital lobe

Answer: a. The lesion is in the right cerebral hemisphere. (Note again that images are conventionally presented with the right side of the brain on the left side of the page.) The lesion is superior and lateral to the lateral ventricle and well above the Sylvian fissure.

446. Based on this MRI, which of the following is the most likely etiology?
    a. Hemorrhagic stroke
    b. Thrombotic stroke
    c. Meningioma
    d. Glioblastoma
    e. MS
    f. PML

Answer: d. The lesion is most likely a glioblastoma because it is a ring-like, lobulated mass arising in the white matter. It compresses the adjacent lateral ventricle and shifts midline structures. MS plaques and PML, which also arise in the white matter, do not create mass effect. Strokes usually conform to the distribution of cerebral arteries and usually have a wedge shape.

447. A psychiatrist is called to evaluate a 13-year-old girl who, after receiving successful treatment for status epilepticus, remains withdrawn, depressed, and amnestic for all events that occurred during the several weeks before the episodes. She had no history of seizures or drug abuse; however, she had had multiple recent admissions for abdominal pain and headaches. The EEG was normal, but a head CT showed a linear, nondepressed skull fracture. Her phenytoin level was in the therapeutic range. Her routine blood tests and toxicology screens were all unremarkable. Which would be the best course of action for the psychiatrist?
    a. Use a tricyclic antidepressant
    b. Use an SSRI
    c. Change her AED
    d. Stop all AEDs
    e. None of the above

Answer: e. Certainly in view the skull fracture, the psychiatrist should suspect child abuse or nonaccidental head injury. Multiple admissions for different undiagnosed pain syndromes are another clue. A history of sexual or physical abuse is common but far from universal in children with psychogenic nonepileptic seizures (PNES), which neurologists previously named pseudoseizures.

448. During the course of an annual check-up, a 50-year-old car salesman mentioned to his physician that during the last 6 months he must have two glasses of Scotch to help him sleep at night. Otherwise, he remains awake and paces around his bedroom. He also reported mild anxiety and a 15-lb. weight loss despite increased appetite. The physician found no physical abnormality on an examination and referred the patient to a psychiatrist at a substance abuse program. The psychiatrist, finding no major psychiatric abnormality, advised the patient to stop drinking alcohol. The patient rapidly stopped all alcohol, but 6 weeks later he returned complaining of insomnia. What is the next step?
a. Treat the patient for substance/medication-induced sleep disorder.
b. Treat the patient for bipolar disorder.
c. Send the patient for cognitive behavior therapy (CBT).
d. Send the patient back to the primary care physician for further evaluation.

Answer: d. Although the initial diagnosis may reasonably have been Substance-Induced Sleep Disorder, his insomnia should have improved by 4 weeks once he stopped his alcohol consumption. Thus, the diagnosis of Substance-Induced Sleep Disorder is untenable. Yet, before diagnosing Insomnia Disorder and either prescribing a hypnotic or referring the patient for CBT, the primary care physician should exclude systemic medical conditions. Further testing showed that this patient had hyperthyroidism.

449. An aunt brought her 5-month-old nephew, who has recently come to the United States from a developing country, to the ER because his right arm and left leg became weak during the previous day. In the ER, the child was lethargic, in general pain, and febrile. His neck was rigid. The entire right arm had flaccid paresis and absent deep tendon reflexes (DTRs). He had no rash, organomegaly, or abnormalities on chest examination. A lumbar puncture (LP) disclosed CSF with 100 lymphocytes/mm³, glucose of 35 mg/dL, and protein of 80 mg/dL. Which of the following conditions is the most likely diagnosis?
a. Trauma
b. Brachial plexus inflammation (plexitis) following a vaccination
c. Werdnig–Hoffman disease
d. Poliomyelitis

Answer: d. Although poliomyelitis has been almost entirely eradicated, small epidemics still plague citizens of Middle Eastern and African countries. As in this case, poliovirus infection causes flaccid, areflexic weakness in an asymmetric pattern, fever and nuchal rigidity, and a lymphocytic pleocytosis in the CSF. Werdnig–Hoffman

disease is a genetic autosomal recessive lower motor neuron disease that appears in infancy. Accidental or deliberate ("nonaccidental") trauma in infants and children causes limb pain and immobility. Postvaccinial plexitis rarely occurs but it causes fever, pain, and flaccid limb weakness without nuchal rigidity or CSF abnormalities. Reports have implicated West Nile virus and enterovirus 68 infections as causes of flaccid paresis.

450. A 60-year-old man who was recently placed in a nursing home requested a psychiatric consultation because he began to experience episodes of visual hallucinations. A typical hallucination consisted of multiple glowing lamps in the left visual field that were reproductions of a table lamp located in the right side of his room. The hallucinations' most remarkable aspect, he explained, was that the visions occurred entirely in his left visual field, which had been rendered blind by a stroke the previous year. The stroke had also caused left-sided sensory loss and mild hemiparesis. Another aspect of the hallucinations was that they consisted of single or multiple replications of objects that he had recently seen in his intact right visual field. The episodes lasted for several minutes and occurred once or twice daily. During them, he remained fully alert but mesmerized. At most other times, he was despondent, discouraged about his health, and unable to sleep restfully. Of the following, which investigation is most likely to be diagnostic?

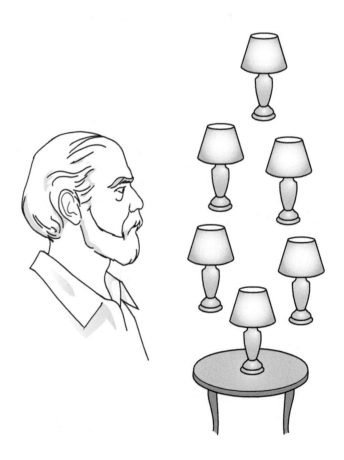

a. Visual-evoked potentials
b. Beck depression inventory
c. EEG
d. Slit-lamp examination
e. Cerebral angiogram

Answer: c. The patient is experiencing palinopsia. This disorder, which is also called visual perseveration, consists of recurrent images within an area of visual loss. These visual hallucinations typically occur in a left homonymous hemianopia. They are usually duplications of individuals or objects in the intact right visual field. Although palinopsia has reportedly resulted from depression, hallucinogens, other toxins, and metabolic aberrations, most cases result from a lesion in the right occipital lobe such as stroke, neoplasm, or trauma. If palinopsia is due to seizures arising from right occipital cortex, EEG should be confirmatory. When strokes lead to depression, the lesion is usually situated in the frontal lobes or subcortical structures, but generally not in the occipital lobes. This syndrome should be differentiated from the visual release phenomenon of Charles Bonnet syndrome, in which the patients may see nondescript shapes or complex visual hallucinations in areas of prior vision loss (see Chapter 12).

451. Which mode of inheritance does this genotype suggest (see figure below)?
a. Autosomal dominant
b. Autosomal recessive
c. Sex-linked dominant
d. Sex-linked recessive
e. None of the above

Answer: e. The inheritance, which is strictly maternal, indicates a mitochondrial DNA mutation syndrome, such as mitochondrial encephalomyelopathy, lactic acidosis, and stroke-like episodes (MELAS) or myoclonic epilepsy and ragged-red fibers (MERRF).

452. Which of the following disorders does *not* result from a calcium channel defect?
a. Myasthenia gravis
b. Lambert–Eaton syndrome
c. Malignant hyperthermia
d. Familial hemiplegic migraine

Answer: a. All the others result from a calcium channel defect.

453. Which *three* of the following neurocognitive disorders are classified as tauopathies?
a. Alzheimer disease
b. Frontotemporal dementia
c. Dementia with Lewy bodies
d. Parkinson disease
e. Progressive supranuclear palsy (PSP)

Answer: a, b, e. Neurologists classify Alzheimer disease, frontotemporal lobar degeneration, and PSP as tauopathies. They classify dementia with Lewy bodies and Parkinson diseases as synucleinopathies.

454. Which one of the following AEDs is *least* likely to lead to osteoporosis?
a. Valproate
b. Phenytoin
c. Carbamazepine

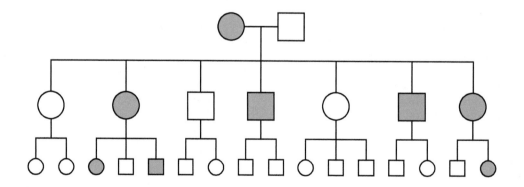

d. Phenobarbital

e. Lamotrigine

Answer: e. Most older AEDs accelerate demineralization and leave epilepsy patients, especially women and those receiving little sunlight, vulnerable to osteoporosis.

455. Of the following AEDs, which one does *not* induce cytochrome P-450 enzymes?

a. Valproate

b. Phenytoin

c. Carbamazepine

d. Phenobarbital

Answer: a. Unlike the other older AEDs, valproate does not induce cytochrome P-450 enzymes, but it still accelerates bone loss.

456. A 41-year-old schoolteacher began to smoke crack cocaine on weekends. After several years of this substance use, which slowly increased after he retired, he began to have periods lasting for 1 to 2 hours of wrapping and unwrapping small objects in tissue paper or placing a dozen playing cards in various patterns. During these periods, his friends could only briefly interrupt him and engage in short coherent conversations, but he was uninterested in them and had an expressionless face. When asked about these activities, the former teacher claimed that, although he "loved" the cocaine, he was compelled to perform the activities and performing them gave him no pleasure except to reduce an urge or need. Which is the best term to describe his behavior?

a. Intoxication

b. Focal seizure activity

c. Dementia

d. Punding

Answer: d. He is punding, which is performing mindless, repetitive, purposeless, and unrewarding activities. Punding, which is similar to stereotypies or obsessive-compulsive activity, includes incessantly arranging clothing in a drawer, building and taking apart paper constructions, and repeatedly aligning pens and pencils into diagrams, as well as this teacher's activities. Parkinson disease patients as well as individuals who use amphetamines or cocaine engage in punding. Excessive dopamine activity is its most likely cause.

457. Which condition is associated with hypernatremia?

a. Diabetic ketoacidosis

b. Use of oxcarbazepine

c. Diabetes insipidus

d. Addison disease

e. SIADH

f. Polydipsia

Answer: c. Nephrogenic and neurogenic diabetes insipidus both cause hypernatremia and serum hyperosmolality. Nephrogenic diabetes insipidus results from the kidneys being unresponsive to ADH. Neurogenic diabetes insipidus results from decreased synthesis of ADH due to dysfunction of the hypothalamic–pituitary axis. The other conditions all cause hyponatremia. Carbamazepine and oxcarbazepine enhance ADH activity or act like ADH in the kidney. SIADH and compulsive water drinking dilute serum sodium and cause hypoosmolality as well as hyponatremia.

458. During a vacation, immediately after having sex with his wife, a healthy 70-year-old man could not find his cigarettes for a postcoital smoke, and he was unable to recall the next day's itinerary for the European city, the hotel's name, or their new travel companions. His wife brought him to the local hospital's ER where his vital signs, general physical examination, and physical neurologic examination were normal; however, he was distraught, befuddled, and unable to recall the name of the physician examining him, more than two of six digits, or any of three objects after 3 minutes. Nevertheless, he was physically comfortable, fully alert and attentive, and able to state – without hesitancy – his home address, his wife's cell phone number, and his social security number. After 3 hours his memory, orientation, and other cognitive functions returned to normal. What is the most likely diagnosis?

a. Side effect of a phosphodiesterase inhibitor

b. Focal seizure with impaired consciousness or awareness

c. Transient global amnesia (TGA)

d. Dissociative amnesia

Answer: c. This man had an episode of TGA that consisted of a several-hour period of almost entirely anterograde amnesia. During that time, he retained personal, well-learned information. Physically stressful activities, sexual intercourse, swimming, and exposure to cold most often serve as precipitants of TGA. Episodes rarely recur. Postulated mechanisms have included TIAs, cerebral venous insufficiency, and focal seizures. In contrast to TGA, the DSM-5 diagnostic criteria for Dissociative Amnesia require loss of important autobiographical information, usually of a traumatic or stressful event, or generalized amnesia for identity and life history, and that the amnesia cause distress or functional impairment. Dissociative Identity Disorder's criteria essentially require two or more personality states as well as amnesia for autobiographical information or traumatic events, and distress or functional impairment. Because he was fully alert and attentive, he could not have been having a focal seizure with impaired consciousness or awareness. Sildenafil (Viagra) and other phosphodiesterase inhibitors often cause headache, dizziness, and nasal congestion, and they may cause amnesia.

459. A 19-year-old Marine recruit suddenly developed a temperature of 103°F and then stupor. In the ER, medics find that he has nuchal rigidity. Which *three* therapies and diagnostic tests should the medical staff perform as soon as possible?

a. Intravenous fluids and electrolytes

b. Oral AEDs

c. Thiamine

d. LP

e. Antibiotic

Answer: a, d, e. Small epidemics of bacterial meningitis frequently erupt in groups of children or young adults brought together in kindergartens, colleges, and military barracks from different geographic locations. Acute bacterial meningitis is fatal unless treated promptly with intravenous antibiotics. Physicians often institute antibacterial therapy even before establishing a diagnosis because the disease's progression is often explosive. In this patient, fever, stupor, and nuchal rigidity indicate meningitis. Examination of the spinal fluid by the LP can confirm the diagnosis of bacterial meningitis, as well as rule out alternative possibilities, such as subarachnoid hemorrhage. Over the past decade, vaccinations have greatly reduced the incidence of bacterial meningitis. Nevertheless, it remains a potential cause of life-threatening illness in military and educational institutions.

460. Since his teenage years, a 30-year-old man has shown aggressive behavior and other antisocial activities. His EEG shows an isolated, phase-reversed spike focus intermittently over the left frontal lobe. Which statement is most likely?
    a. In retrospect, focal seizures with impaired consciousness or awareness have been the cause of the behavioral disturbances.
    b. The EEG has absolutely no bearing on the case.
    c. The EEG of individuals with antisocial personality almost always shows specific EEG abnormalities.
    d. Both the EEG and the behavior may reflect cerebral damage.

Answer: d. Although the EEG indicates an area with epileptic potential in the left frontal lobe, the patient does not display stereotyped behavior. Depending on the circumstances, further testing may be appropriate. Individuals with antisocial personality disorder have a higher frequency of EEG abnormalities than the general population, but the abnormalities are minor, nonspecific, and inconsistent from person to person.

461. A 30-year-old journalist who had just returned from reporting abroad awoke with decreased vision in her left eye. She also had pain in and around that eye when she looked from side to side. An ophthalmologist found that she had a central scotoma and visual acuity of 20/300 in her left eye. The globe and the fundi, including the optic disks, were normal. The pupils were both 5 mm in room light and, when the ophthalmologist aimed a flashlight at her right eye, both pupils constricted to 2 mm; however, when the ophthalmologist swung the light to the left eye, both pupils dilated back to 5 mm. What is the explanation for this abnormal pupillary reaction to light?
    a. Posterior communicating artery aneurysm
    b. Efferent pupillary defect
    c. Acute glaucoma
    d. Afferent pupillary defect

Answer: d. Instead of remaining constricted, both pupils dilated when the ophthalmologist swung the flashlight from the normal to the affected eye in the "swinging flashlight test." This response signifies decreased light input (decreased afferent stimulation) into the light reflex pathway (see Fig. 4.2). In this patient's case, inflammation of the left optic nerve – optic neuritis – impaired the direct and consensual light reflex when light was shone into the left eye. Neurologists sometimes call the afferent pupillary defect a "Marcus Gunn pupil." Because it is a sign of optic neuritis, the Marcus Gunn pupil is often a harbinger of MS. An expanding or ruptured posterior communicating artery aneurysm may cause ocular pain, but it usually causes a generalized headache. More importantly, it usually causes a third cranial nerve palsy with a fixed, dilated pupil, i.e., the pupil has no direct or consensual response to light. In acute glaucoma, the lens is "cloudy," the sclera injected, and the pupil fixed to light. An ophthalmologist should measure the intraocular pressure in cases of sudden, painful visual loss.

462. Which one of the following patients is most likely to have a seizure?
    a. A 65-year-old man with left Bell's palsy
    b. A 70-year-old woman with a right third cranial nerve palsy and left hemiparesis
    c. A 55-year-old woman with rapidly progressive paresis and sensory loss in her left arm and more so her left leg, which has hyperactive DTRs and a Babinski sign
    d. A 40-year-old man who, after an upper respiratory tract infection, develops ascending flaccid, areflexic weakness of both legs

Answer: c. This patient has a lesion involving the right cerebral cortex that could cause seizures. She may have a glioblastoma, abscess, or parasagittal (parafalcine) meningioma. Lesions located outside of the cerebral cortex – such as the left seventh cranial nerve (a), right midbrain (b), or peripheral nerves, including the Guillain–Barré syndrome (d) – are unlikely to cause seizures.

463. Which *four* conditions are inherited in an autosomal recessive pattern?
    a. Duchenne muscular dystrophy
    b. Hemophilia
    c. Sickle cell disease
    d. Phenylketonuria
    e. Homocystinuria
    f. Red–green color blindness
    g. Wilson disease

Answer: c, d, e, g. Duchenne dystrophy, hemophilia, and red–green color blindness are X-linked.

464. After a prolonged but eventually successful resuscitation from a cardiac arrest, a 70-year-old man has apathy and psychomotor retardation. He says only a few simple words. However, he repeats many long, complex phrases, and he accompanies singers on the radio. He can move all his limbs, but he is too weak to walk. What is the nature of this patient's language impairment?
    a. Nonfluent aphasia
    b. Fluent aphasia

c. Frontal lobe dysfunction

d. Transcortical (isolation) aphasia

Answer: d. Anoxic destruction of the cerebral cortex surrounding the perisylvian language arc – Broca's area, the arcuate fasciculus, and Wernicke's area – isolates it from the remaining cerebral cortex and produces transcortical (isolation) aphasia. Anoxia, as occurs with cardiac arrest and carbon monoxide poisoning, is the most common cause of this variety of aphasia. Although patients are able to repeat words, phrases, and songs because the language arc itself remains intact, they are unable to utilize other cognitive functions because anoxia has damaged the rest of the cerebral cortex.

465. Below are six sketches of spinal cords portrayed with normal myelin stained black, demyelinated areas white (unstained), and central gray areas *crosshatched*. Match the sketches (a–f) with the descriptions of the clinical associations (1–6).

1. During the previous 4 years, a 45-year-old man has had progressively severe intellectual and personality impairment. He has loss of vibration and position sensation, absent reflexes in the legs, and a floppy-foot gait. His pupils are miotic. They constrict to closely regarded objects but not to light.

2. A 65-year-old man who underwent a complete gastrectomy 4 years ago now has dementia, hyperactive DTRs, bilateral Babinski signs, and loss of vibration.

3. During the previous 4 months, a 70-year-old woman has developed weakness of her left leg, right arm, and neck muscles. She has atrophy of limb muscles. The physician sees fasciculations in her tongue and atrophy of several muscles. Despite her disability, she has normal cognitive function.

4. A 35-year-old man has optic neuritis, internuclear ophthalmoplegia, and gait impairment from ataxia and spasticity.

5. A 40-year-old woman and her sister have pes cavus, intention tremor on finger-to-nose testing, and loss of position and vibration sensation.

6. A 47-year-old man who has confusion, nystagmus, and bilateral abducens nerve palsy.

Answers:

4–a: The spinal cord shows multiple areas (plaques) of demyelination (sclerosis). The patient has signs of optic nerve, brainstem, and spinal cord dysfunction. Both the clinical and pathologic information indicate MS.

3–b: The spinal cord shows demyelination of the lateral corticospinal tracts and loss of the anterior horns, which contain the motor neurons. This is the typical picture of ALS, the most common form of motor neuron disease, in which both the upper and lower motor neuron systems degenerate but cognitive function remains intact.

5–c: The spinocerebellar, posterior column, and corticospinal tracts have undergone demyelination. Their loss would cause intention tremor, position and vibration sense loss, and a foot deformity (pes cavus). This clinical and pathologic pattern indicates a spinocerebellar ataxia.

1–d: The spinal cord shows demyelination of the posterior columns. Loss of these tracts impairs position sensation and forces patients to walk with a high, uncertain, and awkward pattern (a steppage gait). This patient also has Argyll–Robertson pupils. This is a case of neurosyphilis of the brain and spinal cord (tabes dorsalis).

2–e: The spinal cord shows demyelination of the posterior columns and the lateral corticospinal tracts. This pattern, combined system degeneration, is associated with vitamin B_{12} deficiency from pernicious anemia or surgical removal of the stomach because both conditions remove intrinsic factor. In addition, B_{12} deficiency is associated with prolonged exposure to nitrous oxide because it oxidizes the cobalt in B_{12} (cobalamin) to an inactive form. Combined system degeneration causes dementia, paraparesis, hyperactive DTRs, and position and vibration sense loss. These findings are similar to those of tabes dorsalis with dementia; however, while combined-system degeneration causes hyperactive DTRs and Babinski signs, tabes dorsalis causes hypoactive DTRs and Argyll–Robertson pupils but neither spasticity nor Babinski signs.

6–f: The spinal cord remains normal despite Wernicke's encephalopathy.

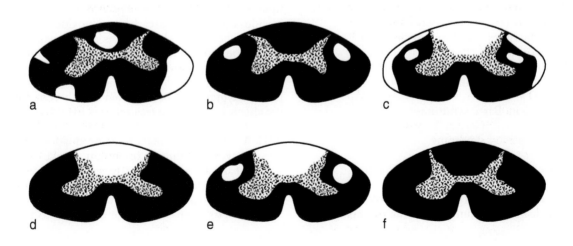

a   b   c

d   e   f

466. Which of the following is *not* a complication of lithium toxicity?
a. Cerebellar damage
b. SIADH
c. Hypothyroidism
d. Tremor

Answer: b. SIADH and its concomitant hyponatremia are not manifestations of lithium toxicity. In fact, lithium toxicity inhibits antidiuretic hormone and the lack of antidiuretic hormone activity causes a renal concentration defect (diabetes insipidus) that leads to hypernatremia. Lithium toxicity may also cause irreversible cerebellar damage.

467. A 50-year-old worker in a poorly ventilated battery factory developed excitability, memory loss, insomnia, and then delirium. On neurologic examination, he had poor handwriting, tremor on finger-to-nose and heel-to-shin testing, and gait ataxia. His gums each had developed a black horizontal line. Which was the most likely toxin?
a. Toluene
b. Arsenic
c. Mercury
d. Lead

Answer: c. In addition to his cognitive and personality changes, this man has cerebellar dysfunction. That combination is attributable to several conditions, including alcoholism and mercury intoxication. Mercury intoxication produces a black "gum line." Inhalation of mercury vapors in industrial settings is the most common cause of mercury intoxication. The FDA has determined the mercury level emanating from dental fillings is safe. Excessive exposure to toluene, ethanol, and, in adults, lead may cause a peripheral neuropathy and cerebellar dysfunction.

468. Despite some false-positive and false-negative results, neurologists associate several CSF abnormalities with certain neurologic illness. Match the CSF abnormalities (a–g) to the diseases (1–6) that they indicate.
a. Oligoclonal bands
b. 14-3-3 protein
c. Increased levels of tau
d. Myelin basic protein
e. Antimeasles antibodies
f. Albumino-cytologic disassociation
g. Anti-glutamic acid decarboxylase (GAD) antibodies
   1. Alzheimer disease
   2. Multiple sclerosis
   3. CJD
   4. Guillain–Barré syndrome
   5. SSPE
   6. Stiff-person syndrome

Answers: a–2, b–3, c–1, d–2, e–5, f–4, g–6.

469. One evening the emergency health service workers bring a disheveled gaunt man to the psychiatry ER.

Lice infest his hair. A thick, burn-like rash covers his hands and circles his neck. He has loose, watery bowel movements. His level of consciousness fluctuates between inattention and lethargy. When responsive, he cannot state the month, year, or place. He has poor anterograde and retrograde memory, judgment, and language ability. Eye movements are full and without nystagmus. He has no paresis or ataxia. His reflexes are hypoactive. Which is the most specific immediate treatment?
a. Thiamine
b. Referral to alcoholics anonymous
c. Pyridoxine
d. Niacin

Answer: d. His dermatitis, diarrhea, and delirium (the "3D's") indicate that he has pellagra ("rough skin," from the Italian, *pelle*, skin and *agro*, rough). A necklace-like rash is characteristic. Pellagra, which was endemic in rural southeastern United States in the early 1900s, results from absence of niacin in the diet. This nutritional deficiency illness was common in this region because the natives subsisted on maize, which lacks niacin (vitamin B3) and its precursor, tryptophan. Use of isoniazid can also cause pellagra. With nutritional deprivation, Wernicke–Korsakoff disease may be comorbid with pellagra. The treatment of pellagra is niacin. Physicians usually add thiamine and nutrients to the medical regimen.

470. The family of a 30-year-old woman with a history of focal seizures refractory to AEDs and surgery found her in a car with its engine running in a closed garage. In the ER, she is stuporous, but has round, equal, and reactive pupils. Her extraocular movements are intact. Staff members note that her skin color is pink or cherry-red. Which of the following laboratory abnormalities is most likely to be present?
a. Toxic concentrations of blood alcohol
b. Elevated concentration of carboxyhemoglobin in her blood
c. Toxic concentrations of an AED
d. Toxic concentrations of an opioid

Answer: b. Depression and suicide are comorbid with epilepsy, especially when it is refractory or requires multiple AEDs. In this case, the patient undoubtedly made a suicide attempt using carbon monoxide. Although the pink or cherry-red skin color is almost pathognomonic for carbon monoxide poisoning, this coloration occurs in less than 10% of cases of carbon monoxide poisoning and it also follows cyanide poisoning. Carbon monoxide displaces oxygen from hemoglobin and thereby causes carboxyhemoglobin. The treatment is hyperbaric oxygen.

471. A 70-year-old man remains quadriplegic 1 year after sustaining a brainstem stroke. He cannot speak or use his arms to gesture or write. He is dependent on a tracheostomy and ventilator, a gastrotomy tube, and intravenous fluids and antibiotics. His sleep–wake cycle conforms to the nursing home's schedule. Although a naïve observer would probably judge him to be devastated, the patient establishes eye contact with visitors and can blink once for "yes" and twice for "no." His brother, who is his sole living relative and health-care proxy, has established detailed communication with the patient using a system of eye movements and eyelid blinks. One day, the brother announces that the patient, who has had full knowledge of his condition and prognosis, has now decided to terminate his life by having the artificial ventilation withdrawn. The nursing home staff disagrees, stating that the patient is incompetent and cannot make medical decisions. A psychiatry consultation is brought in to determine if the patient possesses decisional capacity. What will the psychiatrist probably determine?

a. The patient lacks decisional capacity because the stroke impaired his cognitive ability. The health-care proxy should make medical decisions on his behalf.
b. The patient is naturally depressed by the total loss of function and therefore lacks decisional capacity. The health-care proxy should make medical decisions on his behalf.
c. Despite the devastation, the patient comprehends his situation and the consequences of his plans, and therefore retains his autonomy and decisional capacity.
d. The patient's decisional capacity cannot be determined.

Answer: c. The patient is in the locked-in state. Characteristically, he can communicate with eye movements and eyelid blinks. Assuming that the psychiatry consultant confirms the brother's ability to communicate and elicits the same information from the patient as the brother did, the psychiatrist will confirm that the patient retains his autonomy and possesses decisional capacity. Most cases of locked-in syndrome result from an occlusion of the basilar artery causing a brainstem stroke. Other causes are brainstem trauma, amyotrophic lateral sclerosis (ALS), and, usually temporarily, Guillain–Barré syndrome.

472. A bariatric surgeon referred a 30-year-old woman for psychiatric evaluation because of persistent vomiting and personality change 8 weeks after gastric bypass for obesity. The psychiatrist found that the patient had apathy, poor memory, and gait ataxia. Which is the most likely explanation of these findings?
a. Dumping syndrome
b. Wernicke encephalopathy
c. Intermittent intestinal obstruction
d. Persistent bulimia

Answer: b. Intestinal obstruction, malabsorption problems, and persistent eating disorders may complicate gastric bypass and other bariatric surgical procedures. As in this case, Wernicke encephalopathy may complicate such surgery. Wernicke encephalopathy tends to occur 4

to 12 weeks postoperatively, especially in young women with vomiting. Unless the patient takes nutrients and can absorb them, vitamin B deficiency and malabsorption syndromes may also complicate the patient's course.

473. Which aspect of ECT treatment of depression is the most powerful risk factor for subsequent amnesia?
a. Nondominant electrode placement
b. Use of alternating current
c. Subthreshold energy for seizures
d. Treatment of middle-aged rather than elderly patients

Answer: b. Use of alternating or sine wave current rather than brief pulses of direct current is the most powerful risk factor for subsequent amnesia. Bilateral and dominant hemisphere electrode placement is not only associated with persistent amnesia but also other neuropsychiatric complications. The crucial therapeutic step in ECT is its producing seizures. Subthreshold energy produces fewer side effects, but also little benefit. Elderly individuals are especially vulnerable because they are more likely than younger ones to have underlying mild cognitive impairment.

474. This 32-year-old schoolteacher came to the ER reporting that, for the previous 2 hours, he has had the worst headache of his life. The pain is centered in and around his right eye. His vital signs are normal. Despite the right eye's pain and tearing, his visual acuity is 20/20 OU. His eyes have full range of movement and he reports no diplopia. His neck muscles are supple and he has no paresis, ataxia, or abnormality in his reflexes (see figure). Which is the most likely diagnosis?

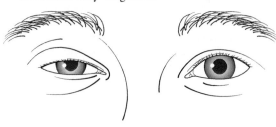

a. Herniation
b. Subarachnoid hemorrhage from a right posterior communicating aneurysm
c. Cluster headache
d. Glaucoma

Answer: c. The sketch shows that he has developed a right-sided Horner's syndrome (miosis and ptosis) with compensatory elevation of the eyebrow. He has most likely developed the first in a series of cluster headaches in view of its unilateral, orbital area pain and Horner's syndrome with no other physical abnormalities. Future attacks will also probably be located in the right periorbital region. Nevertheless, because he has described this headache as the worst in his life, physicians should exclude a subarachnoid hemorrhage. Those due to a ruptured right posterior communicating aneurysm might cause paresis of the ipsilateral third cranial nerve, which would result in ocular deviation and ptosis as well as a dilated, unreactive pupil – the opposite of this case. Moreover, the lack of nuchal rigidity speaks against his having sustained a subarachnoid hemorrhage. Herniation is unlikely in a fully alert patient. Glaucoma is unlikely given his normal visual acuity and lack of conjunctival injection.

475. A 60-year-old woman, a successful novelist, had been institutionalized for a decade for psychosis and suicide attempts. She had been maintained on conventional antipsychotic medications. She maintained her antipsychotic and other drug regimen until she was transferred for emergency major abdominal surgery, which was performed without complications. Several days postoperatively, she began to make grimaces, lip smacking, tongue protrusion, and jerky limb movements. She also had respiratory tics in which she would seem to gasp for air. When the movements began, they were only bothersome, but after several days they interfered with her eating, speaking, sitting in a chair, and occasionally breathing. They even interfered with her undergoing mental status evaluation and imaging studies. Which would be the best strategy?
    a. Administer general anesthesia to obtain a CT or MRI
    b. Obtain an EEG
    c. Empirically treat her with dopamine-blocking antipsychotic drugs
    d. None of the above

Answer: c. She has developed withdrawal-emergent dyskinesia, which is a variety of tardive dyskinesia. Her presurgical antipsychotic regimen had probably suppressed latent or subtle oral-buccal-lingual dyskinesia. Being unable to take her antipsychotic medications led to the appearance (emergence) of involuntary movements (dyskinesias). Restoring her medicine will suppress the movements and allow her to eat, breath, and speak.

476. A disheveled, cachectic homeless man staggered into the ER and said that he was "blind drunk" after drinking his friend's "booze." The physicians found that the man was lethargic, disoriented, confused, and obstreperous. They determined that his vision was less than 20/200. His pupils were equal and reacted slowly to light. He had no papilledema. He had no nystagmus but he was so ataxic and weak that he could not walk 6 feet. His breathing rate was 40/minute and his blood pressure was 80/40. Blood tests showed a pronounced anion gap and metabolic acidosis. As the physicians were administering injections of thiamine, niacin, and glucose, the friend arrived and showed the staff that the "booze" was a mixture of cheap red wine and Sterno. Which is the most likely intoxicant?
    a. Methanol
    b. Ethanol
    c. Isopropyl alcohol
    d. Ethylene glycol

Answer: a. Alcoholics occasionally adulterate their wines and hard liquors with nonethanol alcohols from commercial and home products, including lacquer, antifreeze, engine coolant, or, as in this case, methanol-based Sterno. Methanol intoxication, like ethanol intoxication, causes depressed sensorium, confusion, and ataxia. In contrast to ethanol intoxication, methanol intoxication characteristically causes blurred, hazy, or snow-filled vision, sluggish pupil reaction to light, and a potentially fatal pronounced anion gap with metabolic acidosis.

477. In regards to the previous question, as his physicians put supportive measures into place, they consider several specific treatments to reverse the poisoning. Which one of the following is *inappropriate*?
    a. Bicarbonate
    b. Ethanol
    c. Fomepizole
    d. Hemodialysis
    e. Peritoneal dialysis

Answer: e. Although large quantities may be necessary, physicians administer bicarbonate to reverse the acidosis and reduce the anion gap. In addition, they must combat the body's naturally occurring alcohol dehydrogenase, which converts methanol to its toxic metabolites, formaldehyde and formic acid. Giving ethanol diverts alcohol dehydrogenase from metabolizing methanol and thereby slows the production of its toxic metabolites. Giving fomepizole also slows the production of the metabolites because fomepizole is a competitive inhibitor of alcohol dehydrogenase. (Administering fomepizole is more effective than giving ethanol.) Hemodialysis will clear the methanol and its metabolites. Surprisingly, peritoneal dialysis is relatively ineffective.

478. If treatment saves the man's life in the previous question, which deficits will likely persist?
    a. Peripheral neuropathy
    b. Blindness and parkinsonism
    c. Facial diplegia and deafness
    d. None of the above

Answer: b. Methanol poisoning typically results in optic atrophy and necrosis of the putamen, which lead to blindness and parkinsonism.

479. A woman found her 5-year-old grandson unconscious in her daughter's apartment, next to a bottle of rubbing alcohol. In the ER, he was confused and unable to follow requests. He had no signs of abuse. His breath smelled of acetone. His pupils were equal and normally reactive to light. Extraocular movements were full and he had no nystagmus. He was generally weak and had hypoactive DTRs. In addition to the supportive measures, which treatment should the physicians institute?
    a. Bicarbonate
    b. Ethanol
    c. Fomepizole
    d. Hemodialysis

Answer: d. The boy probably ingested isopropanol (isopropyl alcohol). Unlike methanol intoxication, isopropanol intoxication causes ketosis without acidosis accompanied by only nonspecific and inconsistent neurologic signs. Alcohol dehydrogenase metabolizes isopropyl alcohol to acetone, which is responsible for the ketosis and the smell of his breath. Because isopropyl alcohol ingestion does not cause acidosis, administering bicarbonate will not help. Similarly, ethanol and fomepizole will provide small benefit. The most effective treatment would be hemodialysis. In many states, the staff must report childhood poisoning cases.

480. Family members of a 45-year-old car mechanic found him unresponsive next to a suicide note and a canister of antifreeze. In the ER, he was stuporous, but when roused, he seemed grossly disoriented and hallucinating. He was hypotensive, tachypneic, and hypothermic. His pupils were 4 mm and reactive. Extraocular movements were full and he had no nystagmus. Blood tests showed renal failure and metabolic acidosis with a pronounced anion gap. Urine sediment contained abundant crystals. Wood's light shone on the urine produced fluorescence. Which is the most likely toxin?

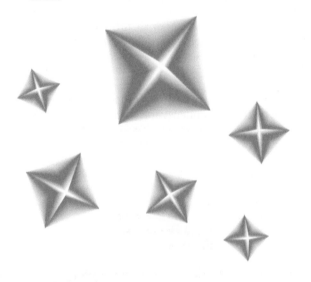

a. Methanol
b. Ethanol
c. Isopropyl alcohol
d. Ethylene glycol

Answer: d. Antifreeze often contains methanol, but its major toxic ingredient is ethylene glycol. Ethylene glycol forms calcium oxalate crystals in the urine (shown above). Antifreeze additives that reveal leaks in a car's radiator fluid cause urine to fluoresce when exposed to a Wood's light. In other words, it is not the ethylene glycol itself that fluoresces. Like methanol, ethylene glycol is a toxic alcohol that produces an anion gap with metabolic acidosis. The treatment of ethylene glycol poisoning is the same as treatment of methanol poisoning: bicarbonate, inhibition of alcohol dehydrogenase with ethanol or fomepizole, and hemodialysis.

481. Which are neurologic sequelae of ethylene glycol poisoning?
a. Ataxia, peripheral neuropathy, and amnesia
b. Facial diplegia, deafness, and changes in personality and cognition
c. Blindness and parkinsonism
d. Dry and hot skin, dilated and unreactive pupils, blurred vision, tachycardia, and delirium

Answer: b. Ethylene glycol poisoning causes inflammation at the base of the brain that most often damages the seventh and eight cranial nerves. It also causes permanent cerebral damage that results in cognitive and personality changes. Chronic, common ethanol use (alcoholism) with concomitant nutritional deficiency causes Wernicke–Korsakoff syndrome. Methanol poisoning causes blindness and parkinsonism. Plants containing belladonna, such as jimson weed or nightshade, which is a powerful anticholinergic, cause dry and hot skin, dilated and unreactive pupils, blurred vision, tachycardia, and delirium. That combination of signs has given rise to the adage describing anticholinergic poisoning, "Hot as a hare, red as a beet, dry as a bone, blind as a bat, and mad as a hatter." If belladonna victims develop hallucinations, physicians should not administer antipsychotic agents with anticholinergic side effects, such as phenothiazine.

482. Of the following, which is the most frequently occurring problem in advanced dementia?
a. Seizures
b. Pain
c. Eating disorders
d. Stroke

Answer: c. Refusal to eat, inability to manipulate utensils or food, pseudobulbar and bulbar palsy, infections and other dental problems, and pocketing or "cheeking" food – which may occur alone or in various combinations – frequently prevent the severely demented patient from receiving adequate nutrition. If physicians cannot identify a readily correctable problem, such as a dental abscess, they may recommend a feeding tube or intravenous feeding, which are usually futile, or hand feeding. Pain, decubiti, aspiration pneumonia, sepsis, episodes of delirium, and even seizures also complicate end-stage dementia.

483. Which of the following defines heteroplasmy?
a. The admixture of normal and mutant mtDNA in a single cell
b. The uneven distribution of mutant mtDNA among various organs
c. The susceptibility of different organs to mutations in mtDNA
d. The inheritability of mtDNA mutations exclusively from the mother

Answer: a. The admixture of mitochondria containing mutant and normal mtDNA in a single cell defines heteroplasmy. It is a consequence of random mitotic segregation of mitochondria, i.e., uneven distribution of mitochondria in daughter cells. Organs with great energy requirements, such as the brain, heart, and skeletal muscles, are especially susceptible to mtDNA mutations. Neurologists say that these organs have a low "threshold" or that they show a "threshold effect." The loss of sperm mitochondria during fertilization explains the maternal inheritance of mtDNA disorders.

484. A 59-year-old retired counter-terrorism agent developed short- and long-term memory impairment. Otherwise his cognitive abilities, affect, and behavior were normal, and he had no physical neurologic deficit. His EEG shows bitemporal spikes and a head MRI shows high signal intensity in his medial temporal lobes. A general medical evaluation found small-cell carcinoma of the lung. Which serologic test is most likely to be positive?
a. Arsenic
b. Thallium
c. Radium
d. Anti-Hu antibodies

Answer: d. His illness consists exclusively of memory impairment, i.e., isolated amnesia. The EEG and MRI abnormalities confirm that the primary problem originates in the temporal lobes. Commonly cited causes of isolated amnesia are Wernicke–Korsakoff syndrome, TBI with temporal lobe contusions, frontotemporal lobar degeneration, strokes of the posterior cerebral arteries, herpes simplex encephalitis, ECT, and, as in this case, limbic encephalitis as a paraneoplastic syndrome. Serum anti-Hu or similar antibodies are frequently detectable in this disorder. Physicians should consider paraneoplastic syndromes as potential causes of dementia that develops rapidly (within 6 months to 2 years) and dementia developing in relatively young individuals (younger than 60 years) as well as in isolated amnesia. Arsenic, thallium, and radium poisonings do not cause amnesia or other specific neuropsychologic deficits. Also, they do not preferentially strike the temporal lobes.

485. The family of a 75-year-old retired physician solicits a psychiatric consultation because she has begun to experience visual hallucinations that sometimes agitate and confuse her. They began after ocular surgery several months before the visit that left her blind. During the periods of hallucinations, which consist of different but familiar scenes and people, she remains fully alert, lucid, and aware that they are not "real." She is cognizant of her blindness and makes allowances for it. She has no cognitive impairment. Which is the most likely explanation for the patient's hallucinations?
a. Anton's syndrome
b. Charles Bonnet syndrome
c. Focal seizures with altered awareness
d. Focal seizures originating in the occipital lobe
e. Major Neurocognitive Disorder due to Lewy body disease

Answer: b. In keeping with a general rule that sensory deprivation leads to spontaneous cerebral activity, blindness leads to visual hallucinations. This patient has the classic neuropsychiatric disorder, Charles Bonnet syndrome, which consists of visual hallucinations following the onset of blindness. The blindness may have resulted from either ocular or occipital cortex injury. In this syndrome, visual hallucinations may occur only in the "blind field" of patients with homonymous hemianopia as well as in the entire field of vision of individuals who are completely blind. Anton syndrome, another neuropsychiatric disorder, usually consists of patients denying their blindness, confabulating, and acting as though their sight were normal. In this question, the patient's hallucinations are not seizures because they differ from episode to episode and her level of consciousness remains intact. They are also not a manifestation of Major Neurocognitive Disorder due to Lewy body disease because she has neither dementia nor parkinsonism.

486. In the patient described in the previous question, reassurance and other nonpharmacologic methods failed to suppress the hallucinations. Which medication or category of medication should the psychiatrist prescribe?
a. Antiepileptic drug
b. Modafinil
c. Antipsychotic
d. Benzodiazepine

Answer: c. Small doses of an antipsychotic will usually suppress these hallucinations. The other medications will not help, except to sedate her or render her oblivious to the hallucinations.

487. The school psychologist refers this 9-year-old boy, who has had epilepsy for several years, for a psychiatric examination. He has begun to regress in his interpersonal skills, language use, and academic performance. Moreover, he has begun a rocking movement while sitting in class (see figure). Which is the most likely diagnosis?

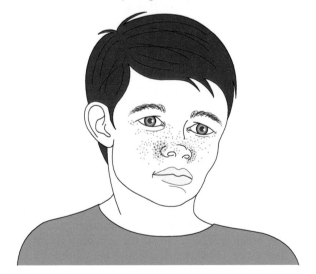

a. Autistic spectrum disorder
b. Intellectual disability
c. Tuberous sclerosis
d. Antiepileptic drug toxicity

Answer: c. Although antiepileptic drugs may impair his cognitive abilities and interpersonal skills, the combination of facial adenomas, epilepsy, and autistic symptoms indicate that he has tuberous sclerosis. CT and MRI of his head would probably show subependymal giant-cell astrocytomas (SEGAs). Genetic testing may confirm the diagnosis. In a major medical advance, studies have shown that inhibitors of the *mammalian target of rapamycin (mTOR)*, such as everolimus and sirolimus, shrink subependymal giant-cell astrocytomas. Topically applied, they also shrink facial adenomas. Fragile X, Angelman, and Rett syndromes, as well as tuberous sclerosis, produce symptoms of autistic spectrum disorder.

488. A 60-year-old retired police officer who has had Parkinson disease for 12 years developed hallucinations, paranoid ideation, and physical agitation. In conjunction with a psychiatrist, the neurologist reduced his Parkinson medication regimen. Although the change greatly reduced the psychosis, it left him rigid and immobile. During the day, he had numerous periods of being "on," when he could freely walk, eat, and shower. However, more frequently he had periods of being "off," which confined him to bed or his wheelchair. Which therapy should the neurologist suggest?
    a. The addition of an antipsychotic
    b. The addition of an antidepressant
    c. Administer a course of ECT
    d. Refer for deep-brain stimulation (DBS)

Answer: d. DBS has been a major advance in treatment of Parkinson disease, dystonia, and essential tremor. DBS in Parkinson disease enhances "on" periods and allows a reduction of the dopaminergic medications, which decreases iatrogenic psychosis and dyskinesias. If depression had been the main problem and was unresponsive to conventional antidepressants, ECT would improve the patient's mood and at least temporarily reverse his rigidity and bradykinesia.

489. The wife of a 65-year-old retired screen actor brings him for a consultation because he has developed cognitive impairment and occasional daytime visual hallucinations. The most troublesome symptom is that during sleep he swings his arms as though he were boxing. He has fallen from bed and fractured his wrist. He has also struck the wife. If she wakes him during these episodes, he explains that he has been dreaming that he is defending both of them from attack. Neurologic examination reveals that he has a flat affect, moderate cognitive impairment, rigidity, and bradykinesia. To address the primary symptom the psychiatrist orders a PSG. What would it most likely show?
    a. Epileptic discharges
    b. Excess β activity
    c. REM with atonia
    d. REM without atonia

Answer: d. Parkinsonism accompanying the onset of visual hallucination and dementia with sleep disturbances suggests a diagnosis of Major Neurocognitive Disorder due to Lewy Body Disease. The physical activity accompanying dreams (dream enactment) indicates REM sleep behavior disorder. The PSG correlate of REM sleep behavior disorder is persistence of muscle tone during REM sleep, i.e., REM without atonia. Not only is REM sleep behavior disorder a common comorbidity of Major Neurocognitive Disorder due to Lewy Body Disease, REM sleep behavior disorder frequently precedes all other manifestations of it. Of note, this patient's illness is not Parkinson disease dementia, because in that condition, physical changes must be present for 1 year before the onset of cognitive impairment.

490. In the preceding case, which is the most likely neuropathology?
    a. Beta-amyloid (Aβ) deposits
    b. Accumulation of α-synuclein
    c. Abnormalities in tau
    d. Multiple small cerebral infarctions

Answer: b. Accumulation of α-synuclein characterizes Lewy body disease and Parkinson disease, i.e., the synucleinopathies. Aβ deposits accumulate as plaques in Alzheimer disease. Tau accumulates in frontotemporal lobar degeneration, in progressive supranuclear palsy, and, to a limited extent, in Alzheimer disease. Multiple small cerebral infarcts reflect vascular disease.

491. The daughters of a 62-year-old professor of literature bring their father for consultation. During the previous 6 months, they report, he has rapidly lost his cognitive ability. At the onset of the decline, obvious only in retrospect, he had been morose and paranoid. On examination, he has impairment in all cognitive domains and psychomotor retardation. He has no lateralized signs, ocular motility abnormality, or involuntary movements. His gait is slow and uncertain. His MRI shows only appropriate age-related atrophy. His EEG shows theta activity. Routine blood tests show no significant abnormality. Which is the most likely category of illness?
    a. Alzheimer-like illness
    b. Delirium
    c. Depression (pseudodementia)
    d. Rapid-onset dementia

Answer: d. Frequent causes of rapidly evolving dementia, assuming that the patient has no overt underlying medical illness and that imaging studies exclude a mass lesion, include frontotemporal lobar degeneration, Lewy body disease, CJD, paraneoplastic syndromes, HIV infection, and normal-pressure hydrocephalus. All of these conditions cause psychomotor retardation and gait impairment, as well as dementia, because they predominantly affect subcortical structures and the frontal lobe. This dementia's rapid onset is inconsistent with Alzheimer disease. He does not have delirium because he has remained lucid and has no autonomic dysfunction. His gait abnormality and slowed EEG weigh heavily against depression.

492. A 55-year-old airline pilot who has had an HIV infection for 8 years presents with 2 weeks of progressively severe left hemiparesis. He denies having a headache and neurologists find no signs of increased intracranial pressure or meningeal irritation. His MRI, shown below, reveals an abnormality in his right cerebral hemisphere. His CD4 count is 180 cell/mm³. Which test is most likely to be positive?

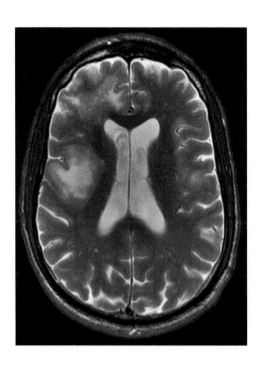

a. CSF PCR analysis for JC virus antigen
b. Serum toxoplasmosis titer
c. CSF analysis for antimeasles antibody
d. CSF analysis for 14-3-3 protein

Answer: a. He probably has PML, in which case a CSF PCR analysis for JC virus antigen will be positive. The MRI shows a prominent white matter hyperintense lesion in his right posterior subcortical frontal lobe. In addition he has a similar lesion in his right frontal pole and a suggestion of one in his left posterior subcortical frontal lobe. All the lesions follow the "U-shaped" white matter tracts and exert no mass effect. In most cases of PML, PCR testing of the CSF will detect JC virus antigen. However, if he were following a HAART regimen, testing his CSF may yield a false-negative result. AIDS patients with relatively normal CD4 counts develop PML and other complications of the disease if they do not rigidly adhere to the HAART regimen or if some of its components do not cross the blood–brain barrier. Toxoplasmosis, which is a relatively frequent complication, is less likely in this case because the lesion has no mass effect and is situated in the cerebral hemisphere rather than the basal ganglia, the more usual location for toxoplasmosis. CSF antimeasles antibodies would indicate SSPE. Finding the 14-3-3 protein in the CSF would support CJD, but the test has a significant level of false-positive results.

493. Which neurotransmitter does the pair of pigmented nuclei synthesize (see figure)?
a. ACh
b. Dopamine
c. Norepinephrine
d. Serotonin

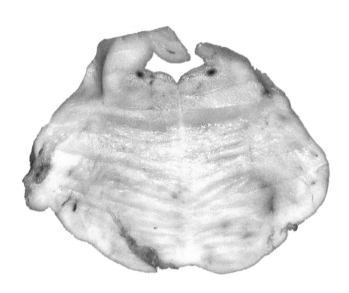

Answer: c. The pigmented nuclei, which are situated inferior and lateral to the 4th ventricle, are the loci cerulei. These nuclei synthesize norepinephrine. In Parkinson disease, the loci cerulei lose their pigmentation and ability to synthesize norepinephrine (see Fig. 21.2 for another view of the pons, 4th ventricle, and overlying cerebellum).

494–496. A neurologist was asked to evaluate a 30-year-old man who had just begun to work as a messenger but was unable to deliver packages to the correct address. Moreover, he would frequently drop the packages. The problem was immediately obvious. He could not remember directions or read the city map and he was clumsy. Somehow he knew that he did not speak until 24 months or walk until 30 months. He had had school difficulty as far back as the 8th grade and was unable to complete vocational high school. An examination showed that he had a head circumference of 61 cm. He had psychomotor retardation and a short attention span. His gait was broad-based and he was unable to perform tandem gait, i.e., walk heel-to-toe. This is his MRI.

494. Into which category should the neurologist place the diagnosis?
a. Neurodegenerative disease
b. Static encephalopathy
c. Developmental coordination disorder
d. Neuronal storage disease

Answer: b. The steady, life-long cognitive and physical disabilities allow the neurologist to place the disorder into the category of static encephalopathy, which some physicians still call "mental retardation with cerebral palsy" or intellectual disability. Developmental coordination disorder is not applicable because the DSM-5 excludes cases where neurologic conditions impair movement. Neuronal storage diseases, such as Niemann–Pick or Tay–Sachs diseases, cause macrocephaly, as in this case, but they typically have a fatal outcome in infancy or early childhood.

495. In this abnormal MRI, which shows hydrocephalus, to which numbers (1–7) do the structures (a–i) refer?
a. Lateral ventricles
b. Third ventricle
c. Fourth ventricle
d. Corpus callosum
e. Midbrain
f. Pons
g. Medulla
h. Cerebellum
i. Posterior fossa

Answers:
1–i. The posterior fossa usually contains the cerebellum, pons, and medulla. In this axial view MRI, a gaping hole, a cyst, occupies the area where the cerebellum usually sits. The sagittal view reveals a small pons and medulla.
2–a. The posterior fossa cyst is accompanied by hydrocephalus. The axial view MRI shows dilated temporal horns of the lateral ventricles. The hydrocephalus has led to macrocephaly.
3–e. The midbrain, the uppermost part of the brainstem.
4–i. The sagittal MRI shows the large posterior fossa cyst and absence of cerebellar tissue.
5–b. The third ventricle is also dilated, reflecting hydrocephalus.
6–d. The expanded third ventricle has compressed the corpus callosum.
7–g. The pons, another posterior fossa structure, is present but compressed by the cyst.

496. Which condition is causing this patient's symptoms and signs?
a. Meningomyelocele
b. Anencephaly
c. Dandy–Walker syndrome
d. Aqueductal stenosis

Answer: c. Dandy–Walker syndrome is a congenital malformation that consists of absence of the cerebellum and adjacent structures, which are replaced by a cyst, hydrocephalus, and macrocephaly. It causes clumsiness, gait impairment, and cognitive impairment; however,

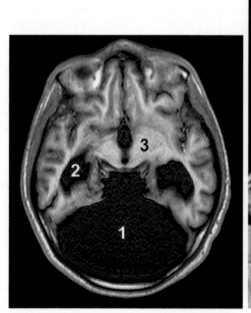

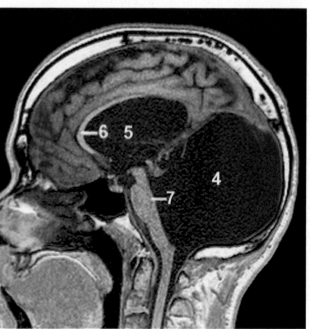

patients are able to ambulate and have grossly coordinated activities. Ultrasound examinations will detect the posterior fossa cyst in a fetus. Some neurologists consider the disorder a neural tube defect. Genetic studies have linked several different mutations to the syndrome.

497–499. A trainer sent a 58-year-old semi-retired left-handed major league baseball pitcher for a neurology consultation because at winter batting practice he has become especially slow in practice pitching and he has tripped and fallen when walking up the mound. The trainer has seen that at "Old-Timer Baseball Shows," the pitcher covers his left hand with his gloved right hand to cover a tremor and he has stopped signing baseballs because his signature has become so small and shaky that it is illegible and therefore worthless.

497. Of the following, which is the neurologist most likely to find?
   a. Cognitive impairment
   b. Tremor and rigidity equally severe in the elbows and wrists symmetrically
   c. Brown-green rings at the periphery of each cornea
   d. Tremor and rigidity at the left but not right elbow and wrist
   e. Impairment of downward gaze
   f. Use of dopamine-blocking medicines

Answer: d. The patient has left-sided rigidity, bradykinesia, and tremor – a triad that indicates idiopathic Parkinson disease. He probably also has micrographia and left leg rigidity and bradykinesia. Cognitive impairment complicates Parkinson disease but usually only after the motor impairments have been present for 5 years. In contrast, cognitive impairment presents simultaneously or within 1 year of the motor impairment in most other conditions that cause parkinsonism, such as dementia with Lewy bodies, progressive supranuclear palsy (PSP), Wilson disease, and sometimes drug-induced parkinsonism. Although relatively young, his age is compatible with the onset of Parkinson disease but incompatible with the onset of Wilson disease, which would have been further indicated by Kayser–Fleischer corneal rings. Drug- or medication-induced parkinsonism almost always causes bilateral signs. Impairment of downward gaze, which is usually accompanied by impairment of upward gaze and a tendency to fall, would have indicated PSP; however, the presence of tremor and the unilateral findings, as well as the absence of ophthalmoparesis, make PSP an unlikely diagnosis.

498. The neurologist diagnoses the pitcher with Parkinson disease. He considers several methods to confirm his diagnosis. Which of the following tests will be most informative?
   a. Diffusion-weighted imaging (DWI)
   b. Diffusion tensor imaging (DTI)
   c. Dopamine transporter scan (DaTscan)
   d. MRI

Answer: c. A DaTscan, using single-positron emission computed tomography (SPECT), can determine the level and location of dopamine transporter activity. If this patient has left-sided Parkinson disease signs, the test will show abnormally low DaT activity in his right-sided putamen. The rationale of the test is that dopamine transporters, which return dopamine from the synaptic cleft back into the presynaptic dopamine neurons' nerve ending, are depleted in Parkinson and other diseases associated with loss of presynaptic basal ganglia neurons. DaTscans show decreased dopamine transporter activity in the basal ganglia in Parkinson disease, PSP, and dementia with Lewy bodies, but normal dopamine transporter activity in essential tremor, neuroleptic drug-induced parkinsonism, and psychogenic tremor. Diffusion-weighted imaging (DWI) is an MRI sequence that reveals changes due to acute injury from strokes. Diffusion tensor imaging (DTI) shows white matter tracts. Neither MRI nor CT shows characteristic changes in Parkinson disease.

499. The insurance company refuses to authorize any confirmatory test. Which strategy would be the most helpful?
   a. Start a therapeutic trial of carbidopa/levodopa
   b. Start a therapeutic trial of a dopamine agonist
   c. Begin an MAOIs
   d. Begin amantadine

Answer: a. Most neurologists would offer this patient a therapeutic trial of carbidopa/levodopa. If he responds, the patient has had a successful treatment as well as a diagnosis. If the patient fails to respond, the neurologist must reconsider the diagnosis. Administering a dopamine agonist may, in the long run, reduce the incidence of dyskinesias, but its effectiveness is less assured and failure to respond is a less reliable guide to etiology. Other agents, such as an MAOI and amantadine, are helpful as adjunctive therapy, but neither is a good initial therapy.

500. Which statement is *false* regarding diffusion tensor imaging (DTI)?
   a. DTI relies on detection of anisotropy.
   b. DTI can perform tractography.
   c. DTI readily detects gray matter abnormalities and is therefore helpful in the diagnosis of Alzheimer disease.
   d. DTI readily detects white matter abnormalities and is therefore helpful in the diagnosis of TBI, corticospinal tract diseases and injuries, and CNS demyelinating illnesses.

Answer: c. In fact, DTI has little or no ability to detect gray matter disorders. Relying on detecting diffusion of water (anisotropy) within neurons, DTI can identify myelinated CNS tracts (perform tractography), sheared neurons in closed head injury, and degeneration of the corticospinal tract from strokes and ALS.

501. EMS workers bring a stuporous middle-aged, apparently healthy, and well-dressed man to the ER

with the history from his companions that he suddenly lost urinary continence and had convulsive movements of all his limbs. On examination, he only moaned in pain, but breathed easily and moved all his limbs. His pupils were 6 mm and reactive. Flecks of white powder coated his nostrils. His blood pressure was 210/140 and his pulse was 100. A head CT showed a small cerebral hemorrhage. Which would be the most appropriate initial management?
a. Perform an EEG
b. Lower his blood pressure to prevent extension of the hemorrhage and reduce the likelihood of another
c. Administer naloxone to reverse the opioid intoxication
d. Administer meperidine for pain

Answer: b. Classic teaching is that the first seizure in an adult most often results from a brain tumor and slightly less often from a stroke. Today, among middle-aged individuals, use of cocaine, another stimulant, or synthetic marijuana is probably more often the cause of a first seizure. In contrast, intoxication with heroin or benzodiazepines does not cause seizures. The flecks of white powder in this man's nostrils indicated that he used cocaine, which caused the cerebral hemorrhage, seizure, and hypertension. Giving meperidine to an individual with cocaine intoxication may cause fatal hypertension.

502. Why does gadolinium infusion during MRI produce hyperintensity in acute MS lesions?
a. Acute lesions disrupt the blood–brain barrier
b. MS lesions create artifacts
c. The abnormal lymphocytes absorb the gadolinium
d. Altered metabolism in acute lesions attracts the gadolinium

Answer: a. Gadolinium enhances the signal from neoplastic, infectious, and inflammatory as well as acute demyelinating lesions because these conditions disrupt the blood–brain barrier. In MS, MRI with gadolinium helps distinguish acute from long-standing, inactive lesions. Seeing new lesions allows neurologists to determine the disease activity and response to immunomodulatory drugs.

503. Asked to evaluate a 60-year-old woman admitted to the Medicine Service, a neurology consultant finds her to have shaking of the limbs on both sides of the body, but she is able to answer simple questions and follow requests. Which of the following is the *least* likely cause of her movements?
a. Psychogenic movement disorder
b. Hyperthyroidism
c. Rigors
d. Essential tremor
e. Generalized tonic-clonic seizure

Answer: e. If the patient were truly having a generalized seizure, she would be unable to talk or follow requests.

504. An 11-year-old girl who had "strep throat" a month earlier presents with hyperactivity, poor attention, and rapid movements randomly flowing from one body part to another. An antistreptolysin O (ALSO) titer is elevated. What is the most important next investigation?
a. MRI of the brain
b. Lumbar puncture
c. Trial of oral levodopa
d. Genetic testing
e. Urine toxicology screen
f. Echocardiogram

Answer: f. She has Sydenham chorea, which is one of the major Jones criteria for rheumatic heart disease. Carditis is present in up to 80% of patients with Sydenham chorea and must be excluded. Early diagnosis of rheumatic fever may be life-saving.

505. A 56-year-old woman has action tremor of both arms. There is no family history of tremor and her examination is otherwise normal. Which of her medications is most likely to induce tremor?
a. Topiramate
b. Sertraline
c. Simvastatin
d. Gabapentin
e. Atenolol

Answer: b. Tremor occurs in as many as 11% of patients treated with sertraline. Topiramate, gabapentin, and atenolol can be useful in the treatment of essential tremor. Simvastatin can cause myopathy but not tremor.

506. A 67-year-old inpatient with worsening renal failure has irregular jerking movements of his arms and legs. Which of his medications is likely to be responsible?
a. Gabapentin
b. Valproic acid
c. Levetiracetam
d. Clonazepam
e. Atorvastatin

Answer: a. Gabapentin and pregabalin can cause myoclonus, especially in the setting of end-stage renal disease. Valproic acid, levetiracetam, and clonazepam are useful in treating post-anoxic myoclonus.

507. A 29-year-old man has sustained twisting of his neck, trunk, and limbs throughout the day (see figure). The movements, which remit during sleep, began at age 8 with inward turning of his right ankle with walking and spread over subsequent years. Which of the following therapies would be *least* likely to stop the abnormal movement?

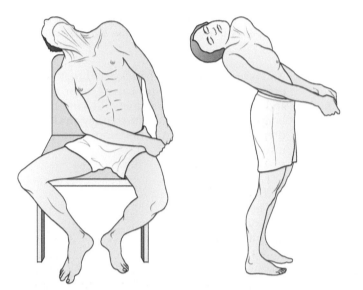

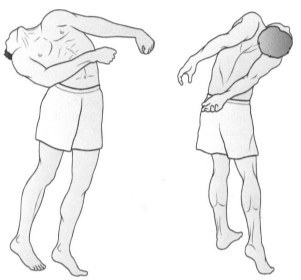

a. Diazepam
b. Trihexyphenidyl
c. Baclofen
d. Carbamazepine
e. DBS

Answer: d. This patient has generalized dystonia, and the history is suggestive of DYT1 dystonia. Benzodiazepines, anticholinergic agents, and baclofen can help with symptoms, and DBS can be very effective. There is no role for carbamazepine.

508. A 59-year-old man has noted slowing of his gait for the past 8 months. Examination shows that when asked to rapidly raise his arms above his head, the left arm moves upward slowly and incompletely (see figure). Which of the following is *least* likely to be true?

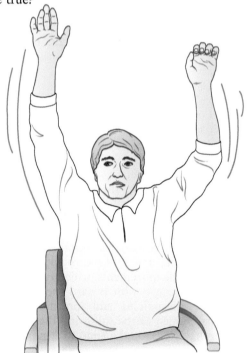

a. A SPECT scan with iodine-123 (DaTscan) will show reduced uptake in the right basal ganglia.
b. He has Parkinson disease.
c. He has corticobasal degeneration.
d. MRI of the brain will be normal.
e. He has neuroleptic-induced parkinsonism.

Answer: e. Both Parkinson disease and corticobasal degeneration are associated with asymmetric rigidity and bradykinesia. In both conditions MRI should be normal, but DaTscan should show decreased dopamine transporter density in the contralateral striatum. Drug-induced parkinsonism produces symmetric parkinsonism.

509. Several students brought a middle-aged high-school teacher who lived alone and had no known family or close friends to the ER after they discovered him in a classroom on Monday morning. He apparently had remained in the room all weekend. The ER staff noted that his eyes were open and he showed no sign of pain. His vital signs, pupils' size and reactivity, and extraocular movements were normal. However, he was unresponsive to verbal or tactile stimulation, he had no spontaneous movements, and he made no effort to communicate. When the staff raised his limbs, they remained elevated and in fixed positions for 15 to 30 min. When the staff elevated his arms in pretzel-like positions, they remained contorted and raised for longer times than any of the staff were able to mimic. After 3 hours, he began to repeat the examiners' questions and requests, but he had no spontaneous speech or conversation. Routine blood tests, a head MRI, toxicology, EEG, and other testing revealed no abnormalities. A slip of paper in his wallet listed a psychiatrist as his primary physician, but the ER staff could not reach him. After concluding that there was no neurologic or internal medical explanation for the patient's behavior, the ER staff requested that the hospital psychiatrist see the patient. Which term best describes the patient's presentation?

a. Catatonia
b. Delirium
c. Cataplexy
d. Stiff person syndrome

Answer: a. The patient has catalepsy (maintaining postures against gravity), waxy flexibility, and echolalia. Psychiatrists would also say that he was in a stupor because he had no psychomotor activity and was not relating to his environment. Thus, this patient fulfills the DSM-5 diagnostic criteria for Catatonia. In contrast, neurologists expect patients in stupor to have a markedly impaired level of consciousness. They also expect that catatonic patients show no spontaneous movements that the DSM-5 includes as manifestations of Catatonia, such as mannerisms, stereotypies, echolalia, and echopraxia. He does not have delirium because he has no fluctuating level of consciousness. Cataplexy is loss of motor tone that accompanies narcolepsy. Stiff person syndrome, a slowly developing disorder, is often a paraneoplastic syndrome. It causes stiffness but not changes in mental status, waxy flexibility, or behavioral disturbances.

510. In regard to the previous question, which of the following conditions most often underlies the presentation?
a. Thought disorders
b. Mood disorders
c. Dissociative disorders
d. Obsessive disorders

Answer: b. Bipolar and depressive disorders most frequently underlie catatonia. Of course, schizophrenia and other mental disorders also may underlie catatonia. In addition, other conditions – dystonic reactions to antipsychotics, neuroleptic malignant syndrome, PCP intoxication, and delirium – may also cause muscle rigidity and inability to speak. Finally, tetanus, meningitis, and various toxins may cause similar features.

511. After further testing and speaking with his psychiatrist, the ER psychiatrist and other staff conclude that the patient in the previous question has Catatonia associated with Major Depressive Disorder. Which would be the best immediate treatment?
a. ECT
b. An SSRI
c. A benzodiazepine
d. An antipsychotic

Answer: c. Although his illness may eventually require the other agents, the immediate treatment is a benzodiazepine.

512. After receiving treatment with an antipsychotic medicine, a 44-year-old woman developed urinary retention. She had had the same complication for 1 week with a similar medicine 1 year before. A urologic evaluation at that time found no urinary outlet obstruction. Which strategy would most likely relieve her urinary retention?
a. Prescribe a cholinergic medicine
b. Prescribe an anticholinergic medicine
c. Prescribe a sympathomimetic medicine
d. Prescribe a β-blocker

Answer: a. Many antipsychotics and other medicines cause central and peripheral anticholinergic effects, such as urinary retention. As long as the patient has no mechanical blockage of urinary outflow or neurologic illness causing the retention, the medicines most likely to relieve the problem are ones that stimulate the cholinergic system, such as bethanechol (Urecholine). Ones that stimulate the sympathetic system would exacerbate the problem. β-Blockers would not help.

INDEX

Page numbers followed by "*f*" indicate figures, "*t*" indicate tables, and "*b*" indicate boxes.